ESSENTIAL PATHOLOGY

ESSENTIAL PATHOLOGY

Edited by

Emanuel Rubin, MD

Gonzalo E. Aponte Professor and Chairman
Department of Pathology
Jefferson Medical College
Thomas Jefferson University
Philadelphia, Pennsylvania

John L. Farber, MD

Professor of Pathology
Jefferson Medical College
Thomas Jefferson University
Philadelphia, Pennsylvania

With 39 contributors

Illustrations by
Dimitri Karetnikov

J. B. Lippincott Company
Philadelphia

Grand Rapids   New York   St. Louis   San Francisco
London   Sydney   Tokyo

Acquisitions Editor: Lisa McAllister
Developmental Editor: Richard Winters
Project Editor: Marian A. Bellus
Indexer: Julia Schwager
Cover Designer: Miriam Recio
Art Director: Susan Hess Blaker
Production Manager: Carol A. Florence
Production Coordinator: Pamela Milcos
Compositor: TAPSCO
Printer/Binder: R. R. Donnelley & Sons Co.

6 5 4 3 2 1

Library of Congress Cataloging in Publication Data

Essential pathology/edited by Emanuel Rubin, John L. Farber; with
    39 contributors; illustrations by Dimitri Karetnikov.
        p.   cm.
        Based on: Pathology/edited by Emanuel Rubin, John L.
    Farber. c 1988.
        ISBN 0-397-51003-9
        1. Pathology.   I. Rubin, Emanuel, 1982–   II. Farber,
    John L.   III. Pathology.
        [DNLM: 1. Pathology—handbooks.   QZ 39 E78]
    RB25.E77   1990
    616.07—dc20
    DNLM/DLC
    for Library of Congress   89-12195
                                                          CIP

To our parents:
    Jacob and Sophie Rubin,
    Lionel and Freda Farber

and our wives:
    Linda Anne and Susan

CONTRIBUTORS

Vernon Armbrustmacher
Col USAF, MC
Deputy Director
Armed Forces Institute of
    Pathology
Washington, DC

Károly Balogh, MD
Associate Professor
Department of Pathology
Harvard Medical School
Pathologist
New England Deaconess Hospital
Boston, Massachusetts

Sue A. Bartow, MD
Associate Professor
Department of Pathology
University of New Mexico School
    of Medicine
Albuquerque, New Mexico

Earl P. Benditt, MD
Professor Emeritus
Department of Pathology
University of Washington School
    of Medicine
Distinguished Physician
Veterans' Administration Medical
    Center
Seattle, Washington

Hugh Bonner, MD
Adjunct Associate Professor of
    Pathology and Pathology in
    Medicine
University of Pennsylvania School
    of Medicine
Philadelphia, Pennsylvania
Pathologist
Chester County Hospital
West Chester, Pennsylvania

Thomas W. Bouldin, MD
Associate Professor of Pathology
    and Ophthalmology
University of North Carolina
    School of Medicine
Associate Attending Physician
The North Carolina Memorial
    Hospital
Chapel Hill, North Carolina

Stephen W. Chensue, MD, PhD
Assistant Professor of Pathology
University of Michigan Medical
    School
Staff Pathologist
Veterans' Administration Medical
    Center
Ann Arbor, Michigan

Wallace H. Clark, Jr., MD
Professor of Dermatology and
    Pathology
Hospital of the University of
    Pennsylvania School of Medicine
Philadelphia, Pennsylvania

Daniel H. Connor, MD, CM
Visiting Professor
Georgetown University School of
    Medicine
Washington, DC

John E. Craighead, MD
Professor and Chairman
Department of Pathology
University of Vermont College of
    Medicine
Director of Laboratories
Medical Center Hospital of
    Vermont
Burlington, Vermont

Ivan Damjanov, MD, PhD
Professor of Pathology
Jefferson Medical College
Thomas Jefferson University
Philadelphia, Pennsylvania

Maire Duggan, MD, MRC, Path FRCP(C)
Associate Professor of Pathology
University of Calgary
Staff Pathologist
Foothills Hospital
Calgary, Alberta, Canada

Joseph C. Fantone, MD
Associate Professor
Department of Pathology
University of Michigan Medical School
Ann Arbor, Michigan

John L. Farber, MD
Professor of Pathology
Jefferson Medical College
Thomas Jefferson University
Philadelphia, Pennsylvania

Cecilia M. Fenoglio-Preiser, MD
Professor of Pathology
University of New Mexico School of Medicine
Chief of Laboratory Services
Veterans' Administration Medical Center
Albuquerque, New Mexico

Dean W. Gibson, PhD
Special Assistant to the Director
National Museum of Health and Medicine
Armed Forces Institute of Pathology
Washington, DC

Victor E. Gould, MD
Otho S. A. Sprague Professor of Pathology
Rush Medical College
Senior Attending Pathologist
Rush-Presbyterian-St. Luke's Medical Center
Chicago, Illinois

Donald B. Hackel, MD
Professor of Pathology
Duke University Medical Center
Associate Pathologist
Duke Hospital
Durham, North Carolina

Robert B. Jennings, MD
James B. Duke Professor
Department of Pathology
Duke University Medical Center
Durham, North Carolina

Kent J. Johnson, MD
Professor of Pathology
University of Michigan Medical School
Ann Arbor, Michigan

Robert Kisilevsky, MD, PhD, FRCP(C)
Professor and Head
Department of Pathology
Queen's University
Pathologist-in-Chief
Kingston General Hospital
Kingston, Ontario, Canada

Gordon K. Klintworth, MD, PhD
Professor of Pathology
Joseph A. C. Wadsworth Research Professor of Ophthalmology
Duke University Medical Center
Durham, North Carolina

Steven L. Kunkel, PhD
Associate Professor of Pathology
The University of Michigan Medical School
Ann Arbor, Michigan

Robert J. Kurman, MD
Richard W. Te Linde Professor of Gynecologic Pathology
Johns Hopkins School of Medicine
Baltimore, Maryland

Antonio Martinez-Hernandez, MD
Professor of Pathology
Jefferson Medical College
Director of Autopsy Service
Thomas Jefferson University Hospital
Philadelphia, Pennsylvania

Wolfgang J. Mergner, MD, PhD
Professor of Pathology
University of Maryland School of Medicine
Director
Anatomic Pathology
University of Maryland Medical Systems
Baltimore, Maryland

Robert O. Petersen, MD, PhD
Senior Staff Pathologist
Fox Chase Cancer Center
Philadelphia, Pennsylvania

Stanley J. Robboy, MD
Professor of Pathology
New Jersey Medical School
University of Medicine and Dentistry of New Jersey
Newark, New Jersey

Emanuel Rubin, MD
Gonzalo E. Aponte Professor and Chairman
Department of Pathology
Jefferson Medical College
Thomas Jefferson University
Attending Physician-in-Chief (Pathology)
Thomas Jefferson University Hospital
Philadelphia, Pennsylvania

Dante G. Scarpelli, MD, PhD
Professor and Chairman
Department of Pathology
Northwestern University Medical School
Chief Pathologist
Northwestern Memorial Hospital
Chicago, Illinois

Alan L. Schiller, MD
Irene Heinz Given and John LaPorte Given Professor and Chairman
Department of Pathology
Mount Sinai Medical Center
New York, New York
Consulting Pathologist
Massachusetts General Hospital
Boston, Massachusetts

Stephen M. Schwartz, MD, PhD
Professor of Pathology and
    Director of the Cardiovascular
    Pathology Training Program
Department of Pathology
University of Washington School
    of Medicine
Seattle, Washington

Sheldon C. Sommers, MD
Clinical Professor of Pathology
Columbia University College of
    Physicians and Surgeons
Consultant in Pathology
Lenox Hill Hospital
New York, New York

Benjamin H. Spargo, MD
Professor of Pathology
University of Chicago
Director of Renal Pathology
University of Chicago Medical
    Center
Chicago, Illinois

James R. Taylor, MD
Clinical Assistant Professor
University of Oklahoma
Tulsa Medical College
Pathologist
St. Francis Hospital
Tulsa, Oklahoma

**William M. Thurlbeck, MB,
    FRCP(C)**
Professor of Pathology
University of British Columbia
Pathologist
British Columbia Children's
    Hospital
Consultant in Pathology
University Hospital
Vancouver, British Columbia,
    Canada

Benjamin F. Trump, MD
Professor and Chairman
Department of Pathology
University of Maryland School of
    Medicine
Baltimore, Maryland

F. Stephen Vogel, MD
Professor of Pathology
Duke University Medical Center
Durham, North Carolina

Peter A. Ward, MD
Professor and Chairman
Department of Pathology
University of Michigan Medical
    School
University of Michigan Hospitals
Ann Arbor, Michigan

PREFACE

The widespread acceptance of our recently published textbook, *Pathology,* and the novel didactic and graphic principles embodied in it, have led to requests for a companion volume that can serve as a concise and selective reference and review for students of pathology. We have, therefore, prepared *Essential Pathology* to meet this need. This text is based upon the larger one, and represents a summary of contemporary general and systemic pathology. To accomplish this end, we have omitted most of the discussions of normal anatomy and physiology, as well as the descriptions of less frequently encountered diseases. In addition, many sections dealing with the clinical and experimental support for the statements in the text have been shortened. Thus, *Essential Pathology* presents the reader with all the key concepts of the evolution and expression of disease and assigns priorities based upon the clinical importance and heuristic relevance of individual disorders.

As we emphasized in the preface to the original comprehensive volume, because graphic images take advantage of pattern recognition, one of the most fundamental characteristics of the human brain, they are powerful tools for communicating abstract and complex material. We have, therefore, retained the majority of the graphics, which students have already come to rely upon as a crucial aid in the learning of both pathogenesis and descriptive pathology. These color drawings provide a direct route to the important principles —a "road map" to the essential concepts of pathology.

In the preparation of *Essential Pathology,* as well as *Pathology* itself, we were mindful of the unparalleled advances in biology that have occurred over the past half century. The towering achievements in the study of ultrastructure, biochemistry, immunology, and molecular genetics have had a profound effect on current thinking about the pathogenesis of disease. At the same time, we remained dedicated to Virchow's original concept that ". . . the cell is really the ultimate morphological element in which there is any manifestation of life, and . . . we must not transfer the seat of real action to any point beyond the cell." The marriage of classical morphological descriptions of disease and contemporary concepts summarized in this book serves to join traditional pathology with the modern revolution in biology.

Emanuel Rubin
John L. Farber

CONTENTS

ESSENTIAL
PATHOLOGY

1

CELL INJURY

EMANUEL RUBIN AND JOHN L. FARBER

CELLULAR PATTERNS OF RESPONSE TO STRESS

Pathology is the study of cell injury and the expression of a pre-existing capacity to adapt to such injury, on the part of injured or intact cells.

All cells have efficient mechanisms to deal with shifts in environmental conditions. Thus, ion channels open or close, harmful chemicals are detoxified, metabolic stores such as fat or glycogen are mobilized, and catabolic processes lead to the segregation of internal particulate materials. It is when environmental changes exceed the capacity of the cell to maintain normal homeostasis that we recognize acute cell injury. If the stress is removed in time, or if the cell is able to withstand the assault, cell injury is reversible, and complete structural and functional integrity is restored. The cell can also be exposed to persistent, sublethal stress, in which case it has time to adapt to reversible injury. On the other hand, if the stress is severe, irreversible injury leads to death of the cell. The precise moment when reversible gives way to irreversible injury, the "point of no return," cannot at present be identified. **The morphologic pattern of cell death occasioned by disparate exogenous environmental stresses is coagulative necrosis.** This type of necrosis is common to almost all forms of cell death and precedes the other forms described below.

REVERSIBLE CELL INJURY

HYDROPIC SWELLING

Acute cell injury may result from such disparate causes as chemical and biological toxins, viruses or bacterial infections, ischemia, excessive heat or cold, and so on. Regardless of the cause, reversibly injured cells are often enlarged. The greater volume reflects an increased water content and is known as **hydropic swelling, a condition characterized by a large, pale, cytoplasm and a normally located nucleus** (Fig. 1-1). The number of organelles is unchanged, although they appear dispersed in a larger volume. Hydropic swelling results from impairment of cellular volume regulation, a process which controls ionic concentrations in the cytoplasm.

ULTRASTRUCTURAL CHANGES

Changes in the ultrastructure of intracellular organelles occur in reversibly injured cells.

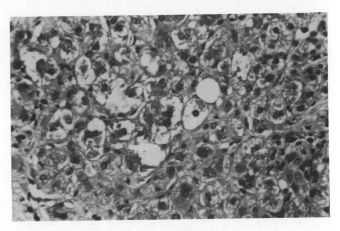

Figure 1-1. Hydropic swelling of liver cells in alcoholic liver injury. The hepatocytes in the center show central nuclei and cytoplasm distended (ballooned) by excess fluid.

Endoplasmic Reticulum With swelling of the cell the cisternae of the endoplasmic reticulum become dilated, presumably because of shifts in ions and water (Fig. 1-2). Independently, membrane-bound polysomes may undergo disaggregation and detach from the surface of the rough endoplasmic reticulum (Fig. 1-3).

Mitochondria In some forms of injury, particularly ischemia, mitochondria swell (Fig. 1-4). Amorphous densities rich in phospholipid may appear, but these effects are fully reversible upon recovery.

Plasma Membrane Blebs of the plasma membrane—that is, focal extrusion of the cytoplasm—are occasionally noted. These can be pinched off and released, while the cell remains viable.

Nucleolus In the nucleus, reversible injury is reflected principally in changes in the nucleolus, characterized by separation of fibrillar and granular components, or a diminution in the latter, leaving naked fibrillar cores.

It is important to recognize that after withdrawal of an acute stress that has led to reversible cell injury, by definition, the cell returns to its normal state.

MORPHOLOGIC REACTIONS TO PERSISTENT STRESS

Permanent organ injury is usually associated with the **death of individual cells.** By contrast, the cellular response to **persistent, sublethal injury,** whether chemical or physical, reflects **adaptation of the cell** to a hostile environment. Thus **at the cellular level** it is more appropriate to speak of **chronic adaptation** than

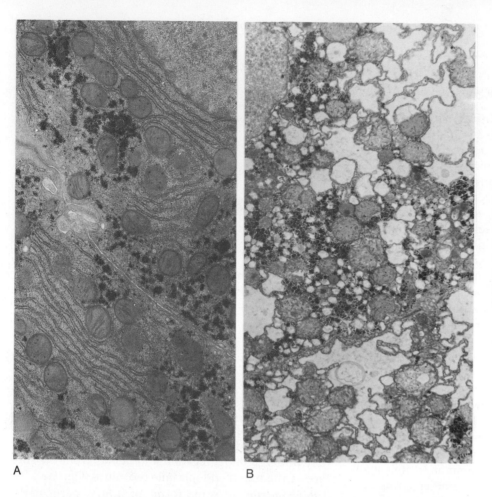

A   B

Figure 1-2. Ultrastructure of hydropic swelling of a liver cell. (*A*) Two apposed normal hepatocytes with tightly organized, parallel arrays of rough endoplasmic reticulum. (*B*) Swollen hepatocyte in which the cisternae of the endoplasmic reticulum are dilated by excess fluid.

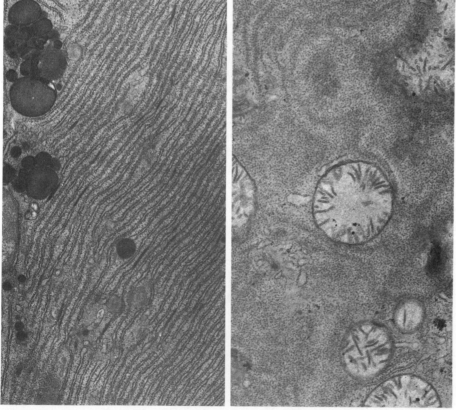

A   B

Figure 1-3. Disaggregation of membrane-bound polyribosomes in acute, reversible liver injury. (*A*) Normal hepatocyte, in which the profiles of endoplasmic reticulum are studded with ribosomes. (*B*) An injured hepatocyte, showing detachment of ribosomes from the membranes of the endoplasmic reticulum and the accumulation of free ribosomes in the cytoplasm.

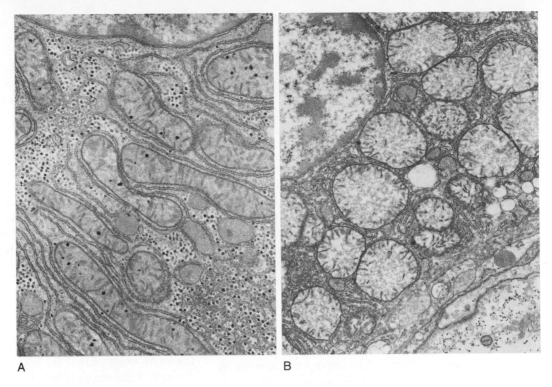

A   B

Figure 1-4. Mitochondrial swelling in acute ischemic cell injury. (*A*) Normal mitochondria are elongated and display prominent cristae, which traverse the mitochondrial matrix. (*B*) Mitochondria from an ischemic cell are swollen and round, and exhibit a decreased matrix density. The cristae are less prominent than in the normal organelle.

of **chronic injury** (Fig. 1-5). The major adaptive responses are **atrophy, hypertrophy, metaplasia, dysplasia, and intracellular storage.**

ATROPHY

Atrophy is a decrease in the size and function of a cell. It is often seen in areas of vascular insufficiency or chronic inflammation and may result from disuse in skeletal muscle. Atrophy may be thought of as an adaptive response to stress in which the cell shrinks in volume and shuts down its differentiated functions, thus reducing its need for energy to a minimum. Upon restoration of normal conditions, atrophic cells are fully capable of resuming their differentiated functions.

REDUCED FUNCTIONAL DEMAND

The most common form of atrophy follows reduced functional demand. For example, after immobilization of a limb in a cast as treatment for a bone fracture, or after prolonged bed rest, muscle cells atrophy, and muscular strength is reduced. With resumption of normal activity, normal size and function are restored.

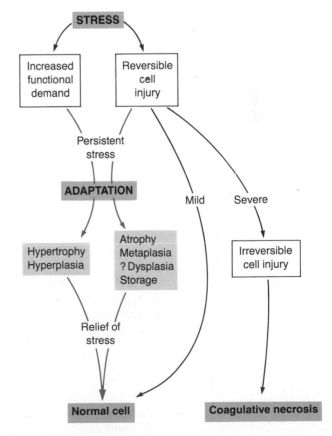

Figure 1-5. Reaction of cells to stress.

INADEQUATE SUPPLY OF OXYGEN OR NUTRIENTS

Interference with blood supply to tissues is known as ischemia. Total ischemia, with cessation of oxygen perfusion of tissues, results in cell death. Partial ischemia occurs after incomplete occlusion of a blood vessel or in areas of inadequate collateral circulation following complete vascular occlusion. This results in a chronically reduced oxygen supply, a condition often compatible with cell viability. Under such circumstances, cell atrophy is common. It is frequently seen around the inadequately perfused margins of ischemic necrosis (infarcts) in the heart, brain and kidneys following vascular occlusion in these organs. Starvation or inadequate nutrition associated with chronic disease leads to cell atrophy, particularly in skeletal muscle.

INTERRUPTION OF TROPHIC SIGNALS

The demands placed upon the cell by the actions of hormones or, in the case of skeletal muscle, by synaptic transmission, can be eliminated by removing the source of the signal. This can be accomplished through, for example, ablation of an endocrine gland or by denervation. If the anterior pituitary is surgically resected, the loss of thyroid-stimulating hormone (TSH), adrenocorticotropic hormone (ACTH), and follicle-stimulating hormone (FSH) results in atrophy of the thyroid, adrenal cortex, and ovaries, respectively. Atrophy secondary to endocrine insufficiency is not restricted to pathological conditions—witness the atrophy of the endometrium caused by the decreased estrogen levels following menopause. Neurological conditions resulting in denervation of muscle, and thus in loss of the neuromuscular transmission necessary for muscle tone, cause atrophy of the affected muscles. The wasting caused by poliomyelitis or traumatic paraplegia falls into this category.

PERSISTENT CELL INJURY

Persistent cell injury is most commonly caused by chronic inflammation associated with prolonged viral or bacterial infections. Cells in areas of chronic inflammation are often atrophic. Persistent toxic injury, as exemplified by the action of cigarette smoke on the bronchial mucosa, can also cause atrophy. Even physical injury, such as prolonged pressure in inappropriate locations, produces atrophy.

AGING

One of the hallmarks of aging, particularly in non-replicating cells such as those of the brain and heart, is cell atrophy. The size of all the parenchymal organs of the body decreases with age. The size of the brain is invariably decreased, while in the very old the size of the heart may be so diminished that the term "senile atrophy" has been used.

HYPERTROPHY

Hypertrophy is an increase in size of a cell accompanied by an augmented functional capacity. Physiological hypertrophy occurs during maturation under the influence of a **variety of hormones.** Sex hormones at puberty lead to hypertrophy of the juvenile sex organs and organs associated with secondary sex characteristics. The lactating woman, under the influence of prolactin and estrogen, exhibits hypertrophy (and hyperplasia) of breast tissue.

Hypertrophy caused by an **increased functional demand** is exemplified by increased muscle size and strength following repeated exercise. In an analogous fashion, one places an **exogenous** metabolic demand on the liver cell by administering drugs that must be detoxified by the mixed-function oxidase system. The liver cell responds with hypertrophy.

Increased demand occurs under pathological conditions as well. The heart may be called upon to increase its contractile force because of mechanical interference with the aortic outflow or because of systemic hypertension (Fig. 1-6). The myocardial cells enlarge, and the heart may double in weight. Increased demand also results from the loss of functional mass. If one kidney is surgically removed or rendered inoperative because of vascular occlusion, the contralateral kidney hypertrophies to accommodate the increased demand.

HYPERPLASIA

An organ may augment function by increasing **the number of cells,** a process known as **hyperplasia.** Hypertrophy and hyperplasia are not mutually exclusive, and are often seen concurrently. **Hormonal signals** can induce a physiologic hyperplastic effect. For example, the normal increase in estrogen levels at puberty and during the early phase of the menstrual cycle leads to an increased number of both endometrial and uterine stromal cells. Hormones produced by tumors can also lead to hyperplasia. For example, secretion of erythropoietin by cancer of the kidney leads to an increase in the number of red blood cell precursors in the bone marrow.

Hyperplasia, like hypertrophy, may also follow **increased physiologic demand.** Residence at high alti-

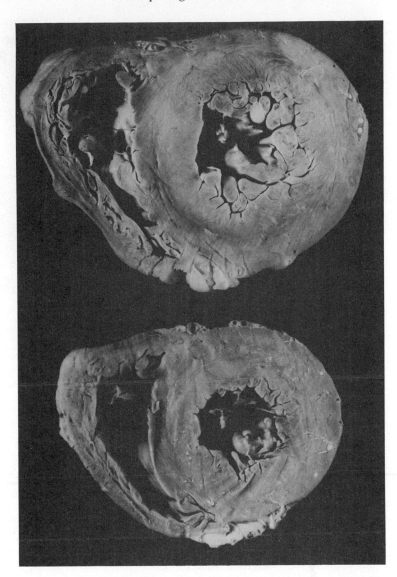

Figure 1-6. Myocardial hypertrophy. Cross section of the heart of a patient with longstanding hypertension (*top*), contrasted with a normal heart (*bottom*). The hypertensive left ventricle is uniformly thickened because of muscular hypertrophy.

tude, where the oxygen content of the air is relatively low, leads to compensatory hyperplasia of red blood cell precursors in the bone marrow and an increased number of circulating red blood cells (secondary polycythemia). Similarly, chronic blood loss, as in abnormal uterine bleeding, causes hyperplasia of erythrocytic elements. The immune system's response to many antigens—a vital mechanism for protection from foreign invaders—constitutes another example of demand-induced hyperplasia.

Persistent cell injury may lead to hyperplasia. For instance, pressure from ill-fitting shoes causes hyperplasia of the skin of the foot, so-called corns or calluses. Chronic inflammation of the bladder (chronic cystitis) commonly causes hyperplasia of the bladder epithelium.

METAPLASIA

Metaplasia is the replacement of one differentiated cell type by another, the most common sequence being the replacement of a glandular epithelium by a squamous one. It is almost invariably a response to persistent injury and can be thought of as an adaptive mechanism. Prolonged exposure of the bronchi to tobacco smoke leads to squamous metaplasia of the bronchial epithelium. A comparable response, associated

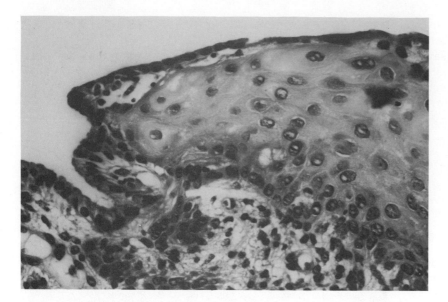

Figure 1-7. Squamous metaplasia. A section of endocervix shows the normal columnar epithelium on the left and metaplastic squamous epithelium on the right.

with chronic infection, is seen in the endocervix (Fig. 1-7).

Metaplasia may also consist of replacement of one glandular epithelium by another. In chronic gastritis, a disorder of the stomach characterized by chronic inflammation, atrophic gastric glands are replaced by cells resembling those of the small intestine.

Neoplastic transformation may occur in metaplastic epithelium; cancers of the lung, cervix, stomach, and bladder have their origin in such areas.

Metaplasia is fully reversible. If the stimulus is removed—for example, when one stops smoking—the metaplastic epithelium returns to normal.

DYSPLASIA

Dysplasia means that the monotonous appearance of an epithelium is disturbed by variations in the size and shape of the cells; by enlargement, irregularity, and hyperchromatism of the nuclei; and by disorderly arrangement of the cells within the epithelium. Dysplasia occurs most commonly in hyperplastic squamous epithelium, as seen in epidermal actinic keratosis (caused by sunlight), and in areas of squamous metaplasia, such as in the bronchus or the cervix. It is not, however, exclusive to squamous epithelium. Ulcerative colitis, an inflammatory disease of the large intestine, often is complicated by dysplastic changes in the mucosal cells.

Dysplasia shares many cytologic features with cancer and is usually considered a preneoplastic lesion.

INTRACELLULAR STORAGE

The normal storage functions of specialized cells are exaggerated under a variety of circumstances encountered in human disease. This can lead to the excess intracellular accumulation and storage of a number of substances, such as lipids, pigments, and dusts. For instance, when the delivery of free fatty acids to the liver is increased, as in diabetes, or when the intrahepatic metabolism of lipids is disturbed, as in alcoholism, triglycerides accumulate in the liver cell. Fatty liver is recognized morphologically by the presence of lipid globules in the cytoplasm.

Hemosiderin is a partially denatured form of ferritin that easily aggregates and is recognized microscopically as yellow-brown granules in the cytoplasm. Increasing the body's total iron content results in a progressive accumulation of hemosiderin, a condition labelled "hemosiderosis". In this condition, iron is present not only in the organs in which it is normally found, but also throughout the body, in such places as the skin, pancreas, heart, kidneys and endocrine organs. There are a number of situations in which the increase in total body iron is extreme; we then speak of **hemochromatosis,** a disorder in which iron deposition is so severe that it damages vital organs—the heart, liver and pancreas.

The storage of other metals also presents dangers. In Wilson's disease, a hereditary disorder of copper metabolism, storage of excess copper in the liver and brain leads to severe chronic disease of those organs.

IRREVERSIBLE CELL INJURY

If the acute stress to which a cell must react is too great, the resulting changes in structure and function lead to the death of the cell. Among the more common causes of cell death are viruses, reduction in blood supply (ischemia), and physical agents such as ionizing radiation, extreme temperatures, or toxic chemicals. Cell death is invariably accompanied by a number of morphological changes recognizable by the naked eye and by light microscopy, and labelled **coagulative necrosis** (Figs. 1-8 and 1-9).

When stained with the usual combination of hematoxylin and eosin, the cytoplasm of such a necrotic cell is more eosinophilic, because of an increased affinity of the cytoplasmic proteins for eosin. The nucleus becomes smaller and stains deeply basophilic as chroma-

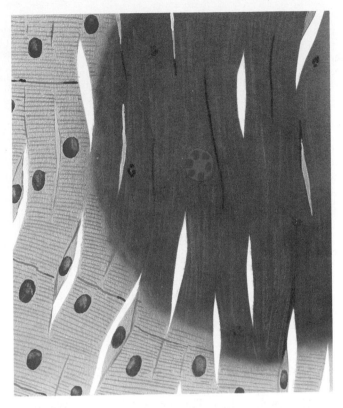

Figure 1-9. Acute myocardial infarction. Obstruction of a coronary artery leads to coagulative necrosis of the myocardium in the ischemic area. The deeply eosinophilic necrotic cells have lost their nuclei and cross striations.

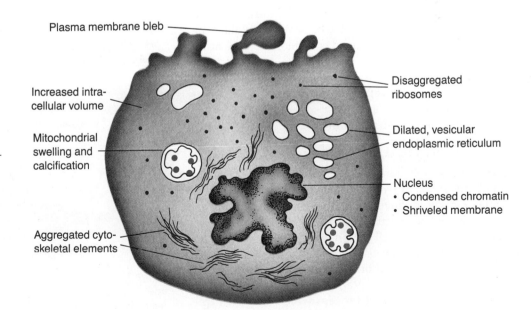

Figure 1-8. Ultrastructural features of coagulative necrosis.

Plasma membrane bleb

Increased intra-cellular volume

Mitochondrial swelling and calcification

Aggregated cyto-skeletal elements

Disaggregated ribosomes

Dilated, vesicular endoplasmic reticulum

Nucleus
• Condensed chromatin
• Shriveled membrane

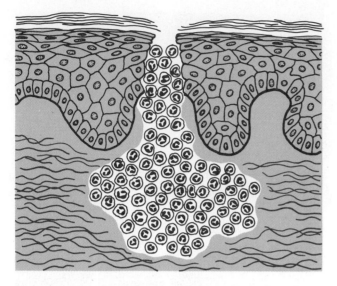

Figure 1-10. Liquefactive necrosis in the epidermis and dermis in an abscess of the skin. The abscess cavity is filled with polymorphonuclear leukocytes.

tin clumping occurs. This process is called **pyknosis.** The pyknotic nucleus may break up into many smaller fragments scattered about the cytoplasm, an appearance termed **karyorrhexis.** Alternatively, the pyknotic nucleus may be extruded from the cell, or it may manifest progressive loss of chromatin staining. We then use the term **karyolysis.**

There are two circumstances in which the rate of dissolution of the necrotic cells is considerably faster than the rate of repair. The polymorphonuclear leukocytes of the acute inflammatory reaction are endowed with potent hydrolases capable of completely digesting dead cells. A sharply localized collection of these acute inflammatory cells, generally in response to a bacterial infection, produces the rapid death and dissolution of tissue, so-called **liquefactive necrosis.** The result is often an **abscess** (Fig. 1-10).

Fat necrosis specifically affects adipose tissue, and most commonly results from pancreatitis or trauma (Fig. 1-11). The process is begun when digestive enzymes, normally found only in the pancreatic duct and small intestine, are released from injured pancreatic acinar cells and ducts into the extracellular spaces. Upon extracellular activation these enzymes digest the pancreas itself, as well as the surrounding tissues, including adipose cells. Phospholipases and proteases attack the plasma membrane of the fat cells, releasing their stored triglycerides. Pancreatic lipase then hydrolyzes the triglycerides, a process which produces free fatty acids. The fatty acids are precipitated as calcium soaps, which accumulate microscopically as amorphous, basophilic deposits at the periphery of the irregular islands of necrotic adipocytes. On gross examination, fat necrosis appears as an irregular, chalky white area embedded in otherwise normal adipose tissue. In the case of traumatic fat necrosis, we presume that triglycerides and lipases are released from the injured adipocytes.

Caseous necrosis is characteristic of tuberculosis (Fig. 1-12). The lesions of tuberculosis are the tuberculous granulomas or tubercles. In the center of such a granuloma, the necrotic cells do not retain their cellular outlines. The dead cells persist indefinitely as amorphous, coarsely granular, eosinophilic debris. Grossly, this debris appears greyish-white and is soft and friable. It resembles clumpy cheese, hence the name *caseous* necrosis.

Finally, there is an alteration of blood vessels known as **fibrinoid necrosis** (Fig. 1-13). In this case, the proximity of the blood allows insudation and accumulation of plasma proteins that cause the injured vessels to stain intensely eosinophilic.

THE PATHOGENESIS OF COAGULATIVE NECROSIS

The morphologic changes constituting the coagulative necrosis of cells are not specific for a particular insult. The morphologic manifestation of cell death—coagulative necrosis—is the same regardless of whether the cells have been killed by a virus, by ionizing radiation, or by interruption in blood supply.

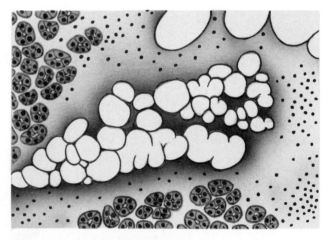

Figure 1-11. Fat necrosis in acute pancreatitis. The release and activation of lipolytic pancreatic enzymes results in the necrosis of surrounding adipose tissue. The hydrolysis of the triglycerides releases free fatty acids, which precipitate as calcium soaps in the necrotic debris.

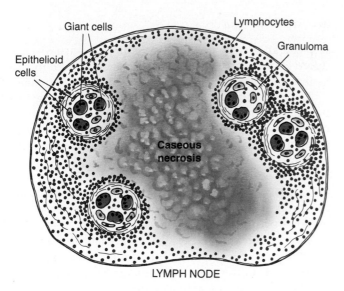

Figure 1-12. Caseous necrosis in a tuberculous lymph node, showing the typical amorphous, granular, eosinophilic, necrotic center surrounded by granulomatous inflammation.

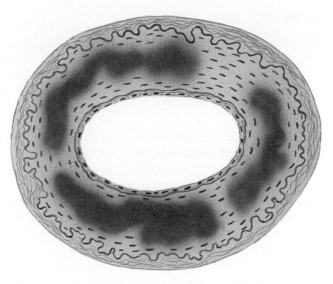

Figure 1-13. Fibrinoid necrosis in a medium-sized artery. The muscular media contains sharply demarcated, homogeneous, deeply eosinophilic areas of necrosis.

With cell death, the gradients between the internal and external environments are dissipated. The largest gradient in all living cells is that of calcium.

Coagulative necrosis is, therefore, accompanied by the accumulation of calcium ions in the dead cells (Fig. 1-14). The influx and accumulation of calcium ions, and the resultant morphological changes of coagulative necrosis, can account for the common morphology of cell death. The sequence of events leading to coagulative necrosis may then be described as (1) irreversible injury; (2) loss of the plasma membrane's ability to maintain a gradient of calcium ions; (3) the influx and accumulation of calcium ions in the cell, and (4) the morphologic appearance of coagulative necrosis.

Alternatively, cell injury may lead to potentially reversible plasma membrane damage. As a result of this damage, however, the large gradient of calcium ions can no longer be maintained. Excess calcium ions then may accumulate in the injured cells and **cause** coagulative necrosis.

In summary, the disruption of the permeability barrier of the plasma membrane seems to be a critical event in lethal cell injury. Loss of the plasma membrane's barrier function results in an equilibration of the concentration gradients that characterize living cells.

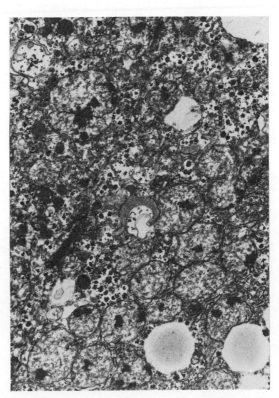

Figure 1-14. Calcium deposits in mitochondria with ischemic necrosis.

ISCHEMIC CELL INJURY

The interruption of blood flow—ischemia—is probably the most important cause of coagulative necrosis in human disease. The complications of atherosclerosis, for example, are generally the result of ischemic cell injury in the brain, heart, small intestine, kidneys and lower extremities.

The effects of ischemic injury are all reversible if the duration of ischemia is short. For example, changes in myocardial contractility, membrane potential, metabolism, and ultrastructure are short-lived if the circulation is rapidly restored. However, when ischemia persists the affected cells become irreversibly injured—that is, the cells continue to deteriorate and become necrotic, despite reperfusion with arterial blood.

A definitive understanding of the mechanism underlying membrane damage in irreversible ischemic injury remains elusive. There are potential candidates for this mechanism.

Activated Oxygen

A popular theory postulates a role for partially reduced—and thereby activated—oxygen species in the genesis of membrane damage in irreversible ischemia.

Toxic oxygen species are generated not during the period of ischemia itself but rather upon restoration of blood flow, or reperfusion—hence the term **reperfusion injury.** A hypothetical scheme holds that ischemia results in an overproduction of toxic oxygen species on restoration of the oxygen supply. On return of the oxygen supply, the abundant purines derived from the catabolism of ATP allow oxygen species to be overproduced.

Another form of cell injury is characterized by the development of lethal cell injury during a longer period of ischemia. In this case, cell damage is not dependent on the formation of activated oxygen species. When cells are reperfused after periods of ischemia that produce this type of injury, there is an explosive accumu-

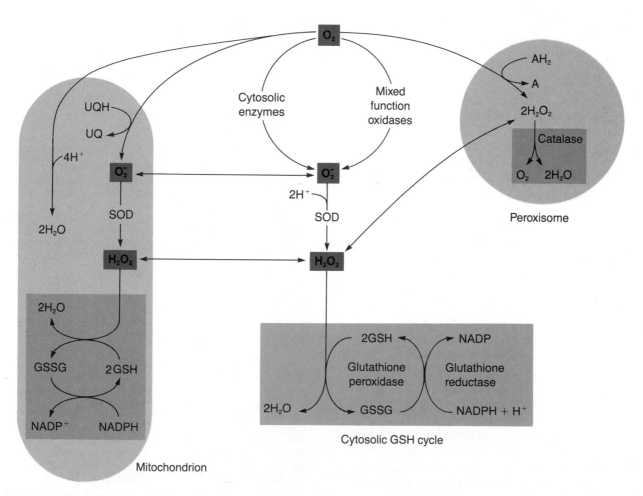

Figure 1-15. Cellular metabolism of oxygen and the accompanying antioxidant defense mechanisms.

lation of sodium and calcium ions in the cells. This accumulation is a result of plasma membrane damage that developed during the period of ischemia—not during reperfusion.

A number of mechanisms have been postulated to cause ischemic membrane damage, although none are proved:

1. Accelerated degradation of membrane phospholipids has been demonstrated in experimental ischemia.
2. Ischemia results in blebs of the plasma membrane, which seem to originate in damage to the cytoskeleton.
3. Cellular anoxia leads to the dissipation of the mitochondrial membrane potential, thereby causing mitochondrial calcium to be released into the cytoplasm. An increase in cytosolic free calcium may activate membrane-associated phospholipases, thus causing membrane injury.
4. There are three partially reduced species that are intermediate between O_2 and H_2O, representing transfers of varying numbers of electrons. They are O_2^-, superoxide (one electron); H_2O_2, hydro-gen peroxide (two electrons); and OH·, the hydroxyl radical (three electrons). These partially reduced oxygen species are derived from enzymatic and nonenzymatic reactions (Fig. 1-15).

Partially reduced oxygen species have been identified as the likely cause of cell injury in an increasing number of diseases (Fig. 1-16). We referred earlier to reperfusion injury in ischemia. The inflammatory process, whether acute or chronic, can cause considerable tissue destruction. Partially reduced oxygen species produced by phagocytic cells are important mediators of cell injury in such circumstances. Damage to cells resulting from oxygen radicals formed by inflammatory cells has been implicated in diseases of the joints and of many organs, including the kidney, lungs, and heart. The toxicity of many chemicals may reflect the formation of toxic oxygen species. The killing of cells by ionizing radiation is most likely the result of the direct formation of hydroxyl radicals from the radiolysis of water.

Cells also may be injured when oxygen is present at concentrations greater than normal. In the past, this occurred largely in those therapeutic circumstances in which oxygen was given to patients at concentrations greater than the normal 20% of inspired air. The lungs of adults and the eyes of premature newborns were the major targets of such oxygen toxicity.

Hydroxyl Radicals and Lipid Peroxidation

The hydroxyl radical (OH·) is an extremely reactive species, and there are several mechanisms by which it might damage membranes. The best known relates to OH· as an initiator of lipid peroxidation (Fig. 1-17). The hydroxyl radical removes a hydrogen atom from the unsaturated fatty acids of membrane phospholipids, a process that forms a free lipid radical. The lipid radical, in turn, reacts with molecular oxygen and forms a lipid peroxide radical. Like the hydroxyl radical, this peroxide radical can function as an initiator, removing another hydrogen atom from a second unsaturated fatty acid. A lipid peroxide and a new lipid radical result, and a chain reaction is initiated.

Antioxidants, such as vitamin E, prevent the injury that usually follows exposure of cells to partially reduced oxygen species. This protection is attributed to the inhibition of lipid peroxidation by antioxidants.

Hydroxyl radicals may also damage membranes by interacting with proteins. They may cause cross-linking of membrane proteins through the formation of disulfide (S—S) bonds. The SH groups of membrane proteins can also be modified by the formation of mixed disulfides in a reaction with GSH, a process dependent on the hydroxyl radical.

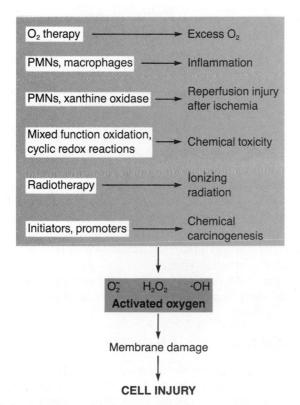

Figure 1-16. The role of activated oxygen species in human disease.

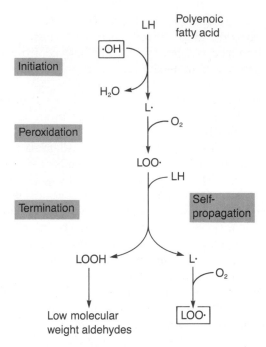

Figure 1-17. Lipid peroxidation initiated by the hydroxyl radical.

The discussion of activated oxygen species can be extended to include the mechanism by which ionizing radiation injures cells. The adjective "ionizing" in reference to electromagnetic radiation connotes an ability to effect the radiolysis of water, thus directly forming hydroxyl radicals. These **radicals can also interact with DNA.** An important functional consequence of such damage is the inhibition of DNA replication. For a nonproliferating cell, such as a hepatocyte or a neuron, the inability to replicate DNA is of little consequence. For a proliferating cell, however, the inability to replicate DNA represents a catastrophic loss of function. Experimental data suggest that once a proliferating cell is prevented from replicating, a mechanism is set in motion that leads to its demise.

HOW VIRUSES KILL CELLS

Viruses kill cells in two distinct ways. The infection of a cell by a **directly cytopathic virus** leads to lethal injury without the participation of the host immune system. **Indirectly cytopathic viruses** on the other hand, require the participation of the immune system.

The polio virus is typical of the group of viruses that is **directly cytopathic.** It consists of a single strand of RNA surrounded by a protein capsule. After binding to specific receptors on the surface of the target cell, the virus is internalized by endocytosis. The endosome

fuses with a cellular lysosome to form a phagolysosome, after which the protein capsule is removed by proteolysis. The viral genome is released into the cytosol and is recognized by the protein synthetic apparatus as just another messenger RNA molecule. As a result the viral genome is translated by the host cell into capsular proteins and a specific RNA polymerase. The polymerase, in turn, leads to replication of the viral genome. Virally coded proteins insert into the host cell plasma membrane and form a pore, or channel, that disrupts the permeability barrier, allowing equilibration of ionic gradients. Potassium ions leave, and sodium and calcium ions enter. The cell is dead.

The hepatitis B virus is an example of an **indirectly cytopathic** virus. This agent consists of a double-stranded DNA genome enclosed in a protein capsule. Like the polio virus, the hepatitis B virus binds to specific receptors on the target cell surface, is internalized, and the capsule removed by acidic proteases after the phagosome fuses with a lysosome. Unlike the polio virus, however, the viral DNA genome cannot be directly translated by the protein synthetic machinery. It must first be transcribed into viral messenger RNA before it can be translated into viral proteins. The transcription of the viral DNA genome is accomplished in the nucleus by the host cell DNA-dependent RNA polymerase. The resulting viral RNAs are transported to the cytoplasm, where they are translated into proteins. The viral proteins include a DNA polymerase that replicates the viral genome and the capsular proteins. Progeny viruses are assembled and released from the host cell without lethal cell injury. Yet all is not well. It is thought that the process of viral assembly or release exposes viral proteins on the external surface of the plasma membrane. These proteins are recognized as non-self, or foreign, antigens. A cellular and humoral immune response develops in reaction to the viral proteins on the surface of the infected host cells. **It is this immune response that seems to be responsible for the lethal injury of the virus-infected cell.** T cells recognizing the viral antigens release a protein that interacts with the target cell plasma membrane. Disruption of membrane's functional integrity and cell death proceed in a manner similar to that seen with the directly cytopathic viruses.

Figure 1-18 summarizes the mechanisms of cell killing by directly and indirectly cytopathic viruses.

HOW CHEMICALS KILL CELLS

There are innumerable chemicals that can damage almost any cell in the body. Toxic chemicals are divided into two general classes: those that interact directly

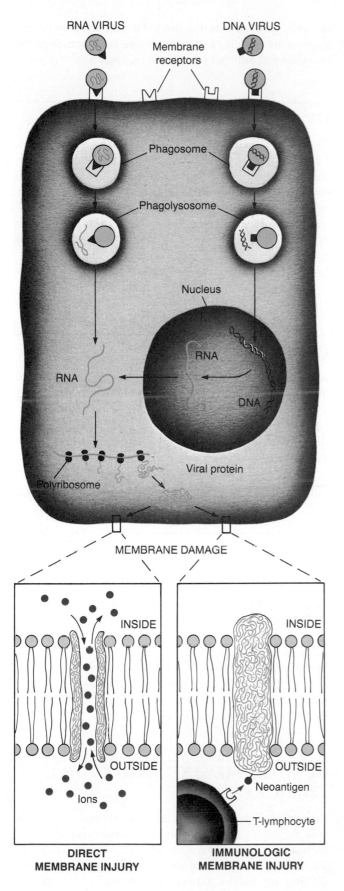

RNA VIRUS

DNA VIRUS

Membrane receptors

Phagosome

Phagolysosome

Nucleus

RNA

RNA

DNA

RNA

Viral protein

Polyribosome

MEMBRANE DAMAGE

INSIDE

INSIDE

OUTSIDE

OUTSIDE

Ions

Neoantigen

T-lymphocyte

DIRECT MEMBRANE INJURY

IMMUNOLOGIC MEMBRANE INJURY

with cellular constituents without requiring metabolic activation, and those that are themselves not toxic but are metabolized to yield an ultimate toxin which interacts with the target cell. This target cell need not be the same cell that metabolizes the toxin.

Toxic Liver Necrosis

Carbon tetrachloride, acetaminophen, and bromobenzene are well-studied hepatotoxins. Each is metabolized by the mixed function oxidase system of the endoplasmic reticulum, and each causes liver cell necrosis.

ACETAMINOPHEN AND BROMOBENZENE It has been suggested that the hepatotoxicity of the two model hepatotoxins, bromobenzene and the analgesic, acetaminophen, might reflect covalent binding of electrophilic metabolites to critical cellular macromolecules. Bromobenzene is metabolized to a reactive, electrophilic epoxide, which can react with glutathione (GSH). If glutathione is depleted, the epoxide is free to react with cellular macromolecules. Acetaminophen is also metabolized to an electrophilic intermediate, which can react with both GSH and cellular macromolecules. However, recent studies of the mechanisms by which bromobenzene and acetaminophen kill liver cells have suggested an alternative to the covalent binding of electrophilic metabolites. It has been possible to dissociate covalent binding from cell killing, and it is possible that liver necrosis is actually related to the toxicity of activated oxygen species.

To summarize, the metabolism of hepatotoxic chemicals by mixed function oxidation leads to irreversible cell injury through mechanisms that may be unrelated, at least in part, to the covalent binding of their reactive metabolites. What is emerging is a common theme of membrane damage as a result of the peroxidation of the constituent phospholipids. Lipid peroxidation is initiated by a metabolite of the original compound (CCl_4) or by activated oxygen species formed during the metabolism of the toxin (as with acetaminophen), the latter augmented by weakened anti-oxidant defenses.

Figure 1-18. Mechanisms of cell killing by directly and indirectly cytopathic viruses. Membrane damage is the final common pathway by which both types of viruses produce cell death. The directly cytopathic viruses create a transmembrane channel by inserting their proteins into the plasmalemma, disrupting its function as a permeability barrier. The indirectly cytopathic viruses also insert into the plasma membrane and create a target for cytotoxic T-lymphocytes.

Chemicals That Are Not Metabolized

Directly cytotoxic chemicals do not have to be metabolized in order to injure the target cell. Such compounds are inherently reactive and combine directly with cellular constituents. The class of directly cytotoxic chemicals includes many of the cancer chemotherapeutic agents and toxic heavy metals, such as mercury, lead, and iron. Because of the inherent reactivity of directly cytotoxic chemicals, many of the constituents of the target cell are damaged. This plethora of alterations has made it difficult to single out the critical interaction that leads to irreversible cell injury. We suspect that directly cytotoxic chemicals either interact directly with the plasma membrane or produce plasma membrane injury as a consequence of their interaction with other cellular constituents, such as glutathione.

Figure 1-19 reviews the various mechanisms we have discussed by which cellular membranes may be damaged in human disease. The functional consequence of these changes is usually coagulative necrosis.

CALCIFICATION

Dystrophic calcification refers to the macroscopic deposition of calcium salts in injured tissues. This type of calcification represents an extracellular deposition of calcium from the circulation or interstitial fluid. Dystrophic calcification apparently requires the persistence of necrotic tissue; it is often visible to the naked eye, and ranges from gritty, sandlike grains to firm, rock-hard material. Dystrophic calcification may occur in crucial locations, such as the mitral or aortic valves after rheumatic fever. In such instances, calcification leads to impaired blood flow because it produces inflexible valve leaflets and narrowed valve orifices (mitral and aortic stenosis). Dystrophic calcification in atherosclerotic coronary arteries contributes to narrowing of those vessels.

Metastatic calcification reflects deranged calcium metabolism, a change associated with an increased serum calcium concentration (hypercalcemia). In general, almost any disorder that increases the serum calcium level can lead to calcification in such inappropriate locations as the alveolar septa of the lung, renal tubules, and blood vessels. Calcification is seen in varied disorders, including chronic renal failure, vitamin D intoxication, and hyperparathyroidism. In contrast to dystrophic calcification, the metastatic variety does not require pre-existing cell injury.

Another form of pathologic calcification is represented by the formation of stones containing calcium carbonate in sites such as the gall bladder, renal pelvis, bladder, and pancreatic duct. Under certain circumstances the mineral salts precipitate from solution and crystallize about foci of organic material.

HYALINE

The word hyaline refers to any material that exhibits a reddish, homogeneous appearance when routinely stained with hematoxylin and eosin. The various lesions called hyaline actually have nothing in common. Alcoholic hyaline is composed of cytoskeletal filaments; the hyaline found in arterioles of the kidney is derived from basement membranes; and hyaline membranes consist of plasma proteins deposited in alveoli. The term is anachronistic and of questionable value, except as a handy morphologic descriptor.

CELLULAR AGING

Aging must be distinguished from mortality, on the one hand, and from disease on the other. Death is an accidental event; an aged individual who does not succumb to the most common cause of death, will die from the second, third, or fourth most common cause. While the increased vulnerability to disease among the elderly is an interesting problem, disease itself is entirely distinct from aging.

LIFE SPAN

The maximum human life span has remained constant at about 110 years. What would happen if diseases associated with old age, such as coronary artery disease and cancer, were eliminated? Such triumphs might lead to an **ideal survival curve,** but only a modest increase in average life expectancy. A long period of good health and low mortality would inevitably be followed by a precipitously increased mortality, owing to aging itself; the life span would, for practical purposes, remain on the lower side of 100.

FUNCTIONAL AND STRUCTURAL CHANGES

Beginning in the fourth decade of life there is a progressive decline in many physiologic functions (Fig. 1-20), including such easily measurable parameters as muscular strength, cardiac reserve, nerve conduction time, pulmonary vital capacity, glomerular filtration, and

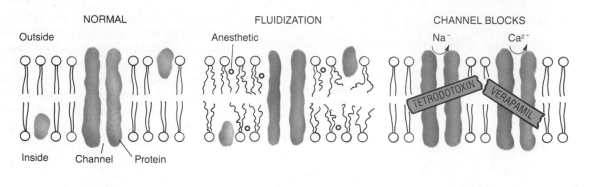

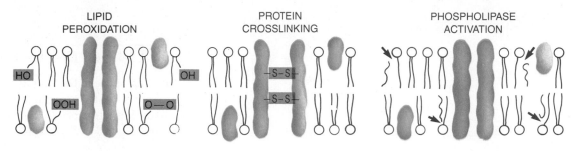

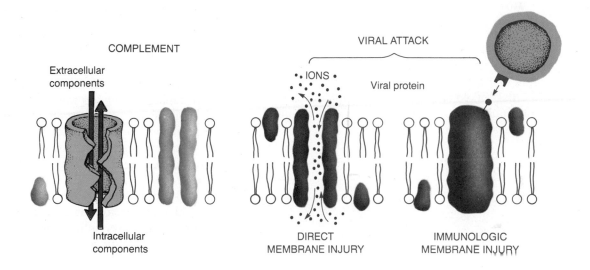

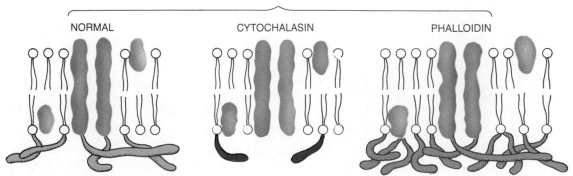

Figure 1-19. Mechanisms of membrane damage in disease.

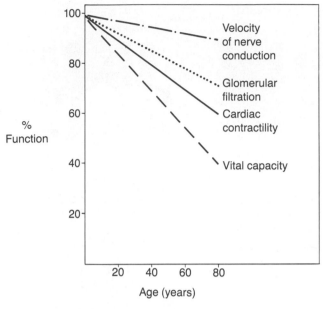

Figure 1-20. Decrease in human physiological capacities as a function of age.

The salient characteristic of aging is not so much a decrease in basal functional capacity as it is a reduced ability to adapt to environmental stress. Although the resting pulse is unchanged, the maximal increase with exercise is reduced with age, and the time required for the return to a normal heart rate is prolonged. Similarly, the aged show an impaired adaptive response to ingested carbohydrates. Although the fasting blood sugar level in old age is normal compared to that of the young, it rises higher after a carbohydrate meal and declines more slowly.

THE CELLULAR BASIS OF AGING

Current theories propose that aging results either from **extrinsic** events that progressively damage cells or from **intrinsic** characteristics of the cell, such as genetic programming.

vascular elasticity. These functional deteriorations are accompanied by structural changes (Fig. 1-21). Lean body mass decreases, and the proportion of fat rises. Constituents of the connective tissue matrix are progressively cross-linked. Lipofuscin ("wear and tear") pigment accumulates in the cytoplasm of organs such as the brain, heart and liver.

RANDOM EVENT (STOCHASTIC) THEORIES

The **somatic mutation theory** is based on the notion that background radiation produces random genetic damage in all cells. When enough genetic loci are altered, critical functions are impaired and the cell dies. The theory relies heavily on the observations that irradiation of experimental animals shortens life span. There is, however, no direct evidence linking the accelerated aging produced by radiation to normal aging. If the theory were true, one might expect a difference in aging between those living at high altitude, where background radiation is more intense, and those at sea level. No such difference has been reported. There are also experimental observations that are not consistent with a theory of somatic mutation.

The **error theory of aging,** also based on random or stochastic events, holds that erroneous copies of protein molecules associated with the chromosomes may lead to genetic abnormalities, which in turn, result in persistently abnormal protein synthesis. An eventual "error catastrophe" destroys the cell. The error theory is conceptually elegant but devoid of adequate supporting data.

DEVELOPMENTAL-GENETIC THEORIES

The distinctive life spans of different species and the invariable senescence of certain cells and organs during embryogenesis suggest that aging is controlled by some intrinsic program, probably linked to the genetic apparatus. **Neuroendocrine** theories emphasize the role of

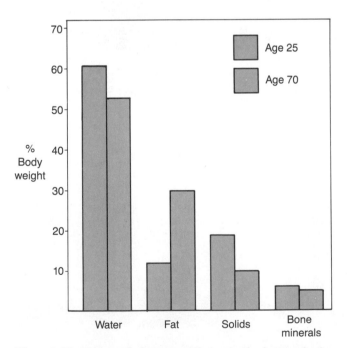

Figure 1-21. Structural changes with age in the human body.

the hypothalamic-pituitary system as the master time-keeper of the body. An age-related loss of functions in the cells of this system leads to hormonal deficits, and thus to decreased systemic function.

In an attempt to bridge the differences between stochastic theories and the perceived genetic basis of the maximum life span, the **theory of intrinsic mutagenesis** holds that the regulation of the fidelity of genetic replication is different for each species. As a consequence, the genetic error rate is different for each species; thus, the life span varies. Although there is some evidence for a rough correlation between the levels of DNA repair mechanisms with species life spans, there are exceptions, and the theory remains controversial.

The functional capacity of the immune system—for example, T cell function—declines with age. Moreover, its fidelity appears to be impaired, as indicated by an age-related increase in autoimmune phenomena. These observations have led to an **immunologic theory of aging.** The immune theory suffers from a lack of universality because it does not explain aging in simple animals lacking a well-developed immune system.

LIPID PEROXIDATION

Aging is accompanied by the deposition of lipofuscin pigment, principally in nonreplicating cells of organs such as the brain, heart and liver. This brown pigment is located in lysosomes and contains products of the peroxidation of unsaturated fatty acids. Although no functional derangements are directly attributed to the accumulation of lipofuscin, it has been proposed that the presence of this pigment reflects continuing lipid peroxidation of cellular membranes, as a result of inadequate defenses against the stress of activated oxygen. Presumably, an overload of rancid lipids results in persistent cell injury and, consequently, to aging. This theory is based to some extent on several observations: that the generation of activated oxygen species is directly related to body size; the metabolic rate is inversely related to body size (the larger the animal, the lower the metabolic rate); and that larger animals usually have longer life spans than smaller ones. As with most theories of aging, the evidence for lipid peroxidation is entirely circumstantial.

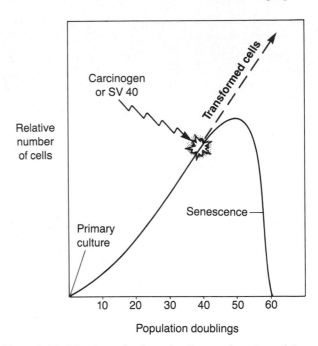

Figure 1-22. Number of cultured cells as a function of the number of population doublings. Note that after about 50 population doublings the cells no longer divide and the culture dies out. However, if the cells are transformed with a virus or a chemical, cellular senescence is not seen, and the cells continue to divide indefinitely.

AGING AS A GENETIC PROGRAM

Every species has an appointed life span which, within limits, is immutable. Given an adequate environment, life span may be genetically determined.

Major support for the concept of a genetically programmed life span comes from studies of replicating cells in tissue culture. Unlike cancer cells, normal cells in tissue culture do not exhibit an unrestrained capacity to replicate. Cultured human fibroblasts undergo about 50 population doublings, after which they no longer divide, and the culture dies out (Fig. 1-22). If the cells are transformed into cancer cells, by exposure to the SV 40 virus or a chemical carcinogen, they continue to replicate; in a sense, they become immortal. A rough correlation between the of population doublings in fibroblasts life span has been reported in several species.

2

INFLAMMATION

JOSEPH C. FANTONE AND PETER A. WARD

Inflammation is a reaction of the microcirculation characterized by movement of fluid and white blood cells from the blood into extravascular tissues. This is frequently an expression of the host's attempt to localize and eliminate metabolically altered cells, foreign particles, microorganisms, or antigens.

Under normal conditions the inflammatory response eliminates the pathogenic insult and removes injured tissue components. This process accomplishes either regeneration of the normal tissue architecture and return of physiologic function or the formation of scar tissue to replace what cannot be repaired. Further extension of injury or the effects of the inflammatory response itself may lead to loss of function of the organ or tissue. Under certain conditions the ability to clear injured tissue and foreign agents is impaired, or the regulatory mechanisms of the inflammatory response are altered. In these circumstances inflammation is harmful to the host and leads to excessive tissue destruction and injury. In other instances, an immune response to residual microbial products or to altered tissue components also triggers a persistent inflammatory reaction.

Initiation of the inflammatory response following tissue injury occurs within the microvasculature at the level of the *capillary and post capillary venule.* Following injury to a tissue, changes occur in the structure of the vascular wall, leading to a loss of endothelial cell integrity, leakage of fluid and plasma components from the intravascular compartment, and emigration of both red and white blood cells from the intraluminal space into the extravascular tissue.

Specific inflammatory mediators produced at the sites of injury (Fig. 2-1) regulate the response of the vasculature to injury. Among these mediators are vasoactive molecules that act directly on the vasculature to increase vascular permeability. In addition, chemotactic factors are generated that recruit white blood cells from the vascular compartment into the injured tissue. Once present in tissues, recruited white blood

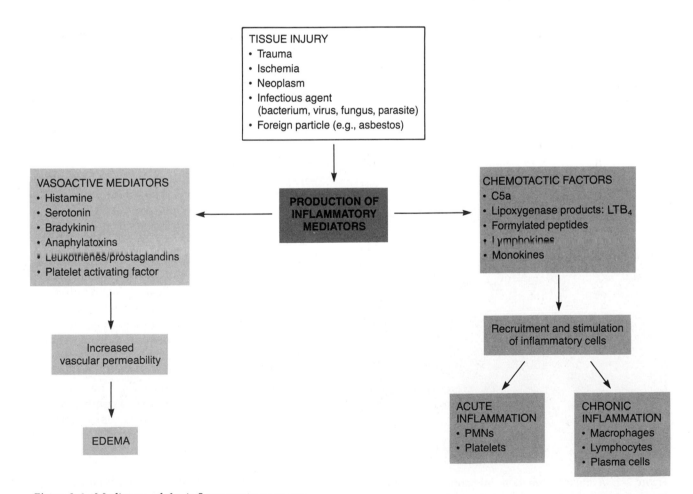

Figure 2-1. Mediators of the inflammatory response.

cells secrete additional inflammatory mediators that either enhance or inhibit the inflammatory response.

Historically, inflammation has been referred to as either **acute or chronic inflammation,** depending on the persistence of the injury, its clinical symptomatology, and the nature of the inflammatory response. **The hallmarks of acute inflammation include accumulation of fluid and plasma components in the affected tissue, intravascular stimulation of platelets, and the presence of polymorphonuclear leukocytes** (Fig. 2-2). **By contrast, the characteristic cell components of chronic inflammation are macrophages, lymphocytes, and plasma cells** (Fig. 2-3).

Activation of the inflammatory response results in one of three distinct outcomes. Under ideal conditions the source of the tissue injury is eliminated, the inflammatory response resolves, and normal tissue architecture and physiologic function are restored. In some cases, however, the nature of the acute inflammatory reaction is such that the area is walled off by the collection of inflammatory cells, a process that results in destruction of the tissue by products of the polymorphonuclear leukocytes (also known as neutrophils). This is the mechanism by which an **abscess** is formed. Alternatively, if the tissue is irreversibly injured despite elimination of the initial pathologic insult, the affected tissue's normal architecture is often replaced by scar. The third possibility is that the inflammatory cells may fail to eliminate the pathologic insult, in which case the inflammatory reaction persists. The areas of chronic inflammation often expand, leading to fibrosis and scar formation.

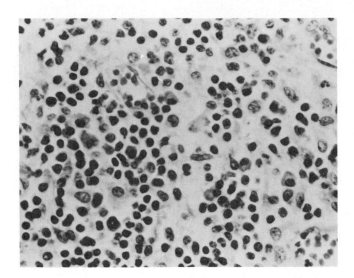

Figure 2-3. Chronic inflammation. Macrophages, lymphocytes, and plasma cells predominate.

VASCULAR PERMEABILITY

Alterations in the anatomy and function of the microvasculature are among the earliest responses to tissue injury (Fig. 2-4). An early vascular response to mild injury of the skin involves a transient vasoconstriction of arterioles at the site of injury. This **vasoconstriction** is mediated by both neurogenic and chemical mediator systems, and usually resolves within seconds to minutes. **Vasodilatation** of precapillary arterioles follows, with an increase in blood flow to the tissue. **This vasodilatation is caused by the release of specific mediators and is responsible, in part, for the redness and warmth at sites of tissue injury.**

In conjunction with the vasodilatation and increased blood flow, alterations in the permeability of the endothelial cell barrier result in increased leakage of fluid from the intravascular compartment into extravascular spaces. If not effectively cleared by lymphatics, fluid accumulates in the extravascular space. A net increase in extravascular fluid is called **edema;** its clinical manifestation is swelling. The loss of fluid from the intravascular compartment as blood passes through the capillary venules leads to local stasis and plugging of dilated small vessels with red blood cells. These changes are reversible following mild injury. Within several minutes to several hours the extravascular fluid is cleared through lymphatics, the endothelial injury is reversed, and the normal structure of the microcirculation is reestablished.

Injury to the vasculature is a dynamic event and frequently involves sequential physiologic and patho-

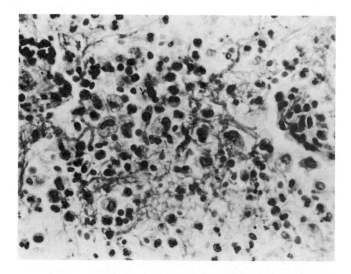

Figure 2-2. Acute inflammation. Interstitial edema and numerous polymorphonuclear leukocytes are present.

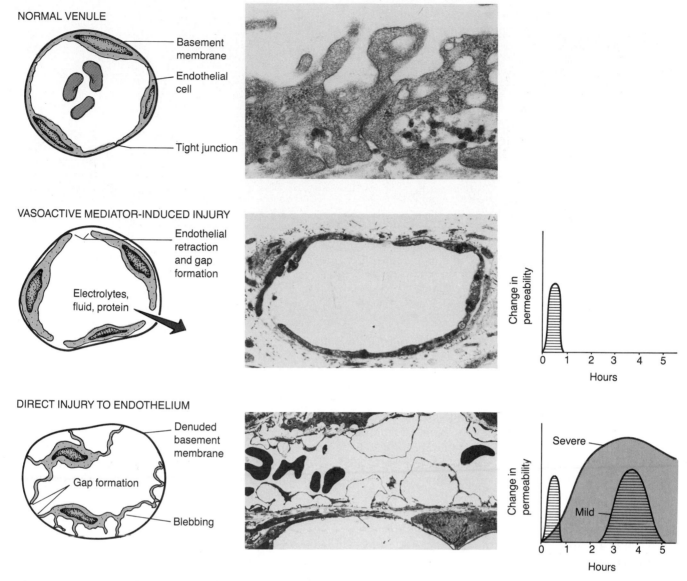

Figure 2-4. Response of the microvasculature to injury. The wall of the normal venule is sealed by tight junctions between adjacent endothelial cells. During mild injury, the endothelial cells separate and permit the passage of the fluid constituents of the blood. With severe direct injury, the endothelial cells form blebs and separate from the underlying basement membrane. Areas of denuded basement membrane allow a prolonged escape of fluid elements from the microvasculature.

logic changes. **Vasoactive mediators,** originating from both plasma and cellular sources, are generated at sites of tissue injury by a variety of mechanisms (Fig. 2-5). These mediators bind to specific receptors on vascular endothelial and smooth muscle cells.

Binding of vasoactive mediators to endothelial cells results in a complex series of biochemical events causing endothelial cell contraction and gap formation. This break in the endothelial barrier leads to an extravasa-

tion (leakage) of intravascular fluids into the extravascular space. **The postcapillary venule is the primary site at which the vasoactive mediators induce endothelial changes.** Endothelial retraction and gap formation is a reversible process. By contrast, direct injury to the endothelium, such as that caused by burns or caustic chemicals, may result in irreversible damage. In such cases the endothelium is separated from the basement membrane, an effect that leads to cell bleb-

SOURCE   MEDIATOR

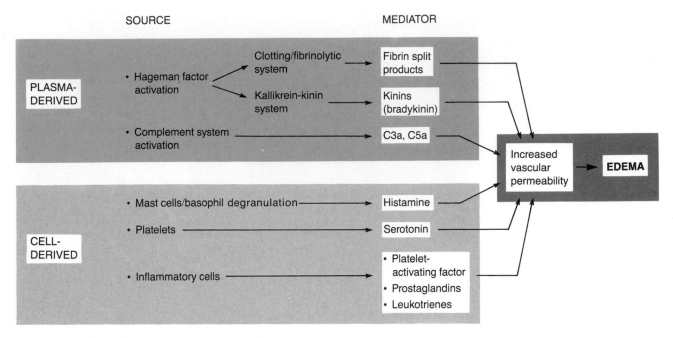

Figure 2-5. Vasoactive mediators of increased vascular permeability.

bing, that is, the appearance of blisters or bubbles between the endothelium and the basement membrane, and areas of denuded basement membrane. Mild, direct injury to the endothelium may result in a biphasic response: an early change in permeability occurs 15 to 30 minutes after the injury, followed by a second increase in vascular permeability after 3 to 5 hours. When damage is severe the exudation of intravascular fluid into the extravascular compartment increases progressively, reaching a peak between 3 to 4 hours after injury.

Accumulation of fluid within the extravascular compartment and interstitial tissues is referred to as **edema;** excess fluid in the cavities of the body is labeled an **effusion.** Edema fluid with a low protein content (specific gravity of <1.010) is called a **transudate.** Edema fluid with a high protein concentration (specific gravity >1.010) is termed an **exudate;** it is frequently characterized by a high lipid content and cellular debris. Exudates are observed early in acute inflammatory reactions and are produced by mild injuries, such as sunburn or traumatic blisters. When exudates or effusions occur in tissues in the absence of a prominent cellular response, they are termed **serous.** A serous fluid usually has a yellow, strawlike color. When red blood cells are present the fluid has a red tinge and is referred to as **serosanguineous.** Under conditions that activate the coagulation system, large amounts of fibrin may be deposited in tissues, a process that results in a **fibrinous** exudate. An inflammatory exudate or effu-

sion that contains prominent cellular components is described as **purulent. Purulent exudates and effusions are frequently identified with pathologic conditions such as pyogenic bacterial infections, in which the predominant cell type is the polymorphonuclear leukocyte.**

SOURCES OF VASOACTIVE MEDIATORS

The primary sources of vasoactive mediators are cells and plasma. Important cellular sources of vasoactive mediators are circulating platelets, tissue mast cells, and basophils.

Platelets play a primary role in normal homeostasis and in the initiation and regulation of clot formation. When platelets come in contact with fibrillar collagen (following vascular injury that exposes the interstitial matrix proteins) or thrombin (following activation of the coagulation system), platelet adherence, aggregation, and degranulation may occur. Degranulation is associated with the release of **serotonin (5-hydroxytryptamine) and histamine,** mediators that directly induce changes in vascular permeability. In addition, the arachidonic acid metabolite **thromboxane A_2** is produced. Thromboxane A_2 not only plays a key role in the second wave of platelet aggregation, but also possesses smooth muscle constrictive properties.

Mast cells and basophils are additional cellular sources of vasoactive mediators. Histamine is released from electron-dense cytoplasmic granules into extracellular tissues when IgE-sensitized cells are stimulated with antigen or the anaphylatoxins C3a and C5a (derived from the third and fifth components of the complement system). Degranulation of mast cells and basophils may also be induced by physical agonists, such as cold and trauma. When injected into skin, both histamine and serotonin induce reversible endothelial cell contraction, gap formation, and edema. Histamine's action on the vasculature is a result of its binding to specific H_1 receptors in the vascular wall. This effect can be inhibited pharmacologically by H_1-receptor antagonists.

Stimulation of mast cells and basophils also leads to the release of products of arachidonic acid metabolism, including the so-called **slow-reacting substances of anaphylaxis (SRS-As). The SRS-As consist of leukotriene C_4 (LTC$_4$), leukotriene D_4 (LTD$_4$), and leukotriene E_4 (LTE$_4$).** These lipoxygenase products of arachidonic acid metabolism induce smooth muscle contraction and increase vascular permeability in the skin. They produce their effects by binding to specific receptors on cell membranes and are important in delayed changes in vascular permeability at sites of inflammation.

Stimulation of mast cells and leukocytes results in the generation of another class of vasoactive mediators having the structure of an acetylated lysophospholipid, and called platelet activating factor (PAF). PAF induces platelet aggregation and degranulation at sites of tissue injury and enhances the release of serotonin and histamine, thereby causing changes in vascular permeability. In addition, it enhances arachidonic acid metabolism in neutrophils, an effect associated with increased motility, superoxide production, and degranulation of the polymorphonuclear leukocyte. PAF also has direct effects on the microvasculature, causing vasodilatation and enhancing vascular permeability at sites of tissue injury.

Additional sources of vasoactive mediators are generated within plasma. Plasmin generated by activated Hageman factor (clotting factor XII) induces fibrinolysis (Fig. 2-6). **The products of fibrin degradation augment vascular permeability in both the skin and the lung. In addition, plasmin cleaves components of the complement system in an action that generates bio-**

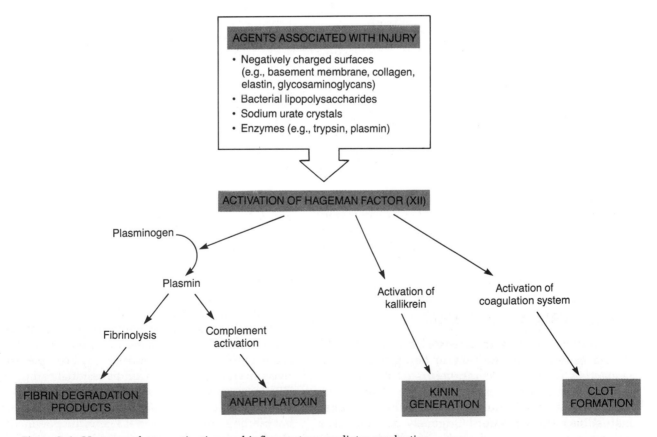

Figure 2-6. Hageman factor activation and inflammatory mediator production.

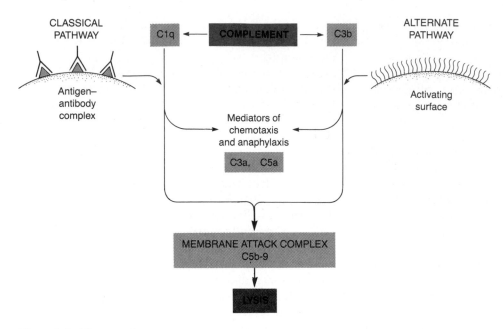

Figure 2-7. The complement system.

logically active products, including the anaphylatoxins C3a and C5a. C3a and C5a increase vascular permeability in the skin both directly and indirectly
(e.g., by a mast cell-dependent mechanism).

Plasma kallikrein generated by activated Hageman factor cleaves high-molecular-weight kinino-
gen, thus generating several vasoactive low-molecular-weight peptides, collectively referred to as
kinins. The best characterized of these vasoactive
kinins is bradykinin.

The permeability changes induced by the vasoactive
mediators are enhanced by the local production of vasodilative substances. In particular, the vasodilative
prostaglandins (PGI_2, PGE_2, and PGD_2) increase edema
formation when injected locally at sites of tissue injury.
One proposed mechanism for the anti-inflammatory
effects of aspirin, indomethacin, and other nonsteroidal anti-inflammatory drugs is their inhibition of prostaglandin production.

COMPLEMENT SYSTEM

The complement system consists of a group of 20
plasma proteins. In addition to being a source of
vasoactive mediators, components of the complement system are an integral part of the immune system and play an important role in host defense
against bacterial infection. Originally described as a
biologic effect of serum responsible for the lysis of an-

tibody-coated cells, it is now known that this activity is
present in an inactive form in plasma. These proteins
are sequentially activated by two independent pathways, termed "classical" and "alternative" (Fig. 2-7).

CLASSICAL PATHWAY

Activators of the classical pathway (Table 2-1) include
antigen-antibody immune complexes and products of
bacteria and viruses. The activation of the classical
pathway inolves recognition of the inflammatory agent
by the first component of complement, C1. C1 consists
of three separate proteins. C1q, C1r, and C1s. Two
additional components of the complement system, C4
and C2, serve as the substrate for the enzymatically
active C1s. The action of C1s on C4 and C2 is responsible for the release of the first soluble anaphylatoxin,
C4a, and the generation of the complex C4b2a. This
complex, in turn has proteolytic activity for the C3 molecule, generating a second soluble anaphylatoxin molecule, C3a, and a residual product of C3 cleavage, C3b.
The resulting multimolecular complex formed with
C4b2a binds C5 and initiates hydrolysis of the C5 molecule, a process that generates a third complement-de-
rived anaphylatoxin, C5a, and a residual component of
C5 cleavage, C5b. The C5b molecule serves as a nucleus on target cell surface membranes for the sequential binding of C6, C7, and C8, and the polymerization
of C9 molecules. This cascade leads to the formation of

Table 2-1 Activators of the Complement System

CLASSICAL	ALTERNATIVE
Immune complexes (IgM, IgG)	Zymosan (yeast cell wall)
Aggregated antibody	Cobra venom factor (CVF)
Proteases	Endotoxin (lipopolysaccha-
	rides)
Urate crystals	Polysaccharides
Polyanions (polynucleotides)	X-ray contrast media
	Dialysis membranes
	Parasites, fungi, and viruses

a macromolecular complex termed the **membrane attack complex.**

Morphologically, the injury by the membrane attack complex appears as a cylindrical hole in the cell membrane. As a consequence of its highly lipophilic nature, the membrane attack complex alters the phospholipid bilayer and membrane functions, which may ultimately result in the loss of cell membrane integrity, followed by cell lysis.

ALTERNATIVE PATHWAY

Activation of the alternative pathway of the complement system is initiated through derivative products of infectious organisms and through foreign materials (see Table 2-1) via a cascadelike interaction of specific plasma proteins. In the alternative pathway, unlike the classical pathway, C1, C4, and C2 are not involved. Activation of the alternative pathway occurs through the binding of C3 with two plasma proteins, factor B and factor D. This results in the formation of an enzymatically active derivative of factor B. The larger fragment, termed Bb, catalyzes the conversion of C3 to C3b and C3a. When C3b is bound to Bb, a C3 convertase is generated, thus greatly amplifying subsequent conversion of C3 and generating additional C3b and C3a. In addition, C5 convertase is formed, which in turn generates C5b (soluble C5a), and the membrane attack complex is subsequently assembled. **Thus, whether the alternative or the classical complement pathway is activated, the end result is the same: formation of a membrane attack complex capable of inducing cell lysis and generation of the biologically active anaphylatoxins C3a and C5a.**

ANAPHYLATOXINS

The anaphylatoxins C3a, C4a, and C5a are important products of complement activation via the classical pathway. Each of these molecules has been shown to have potent effects on smooth muscle and the vasculature, including enhancement of smooth muscle contraction and increasing vascular permeability (Fig. 2-8). Both C3a and C5a also induce mast cell and basophil degranulation, and the consequent release of histamine further potentiates the increase in vascular permeability. In addition to their effects on vascular smooth

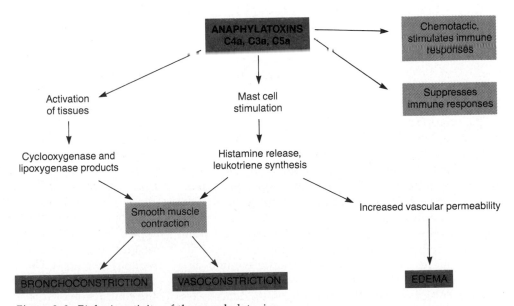

Figure 2-8. Biologic activity of the anaphylatoxins.

muscle, the anaphylatoxins stimulate contraction of bronchial smooth muscle and cause airway narrowing. This effect is produced in two ways. The first is dependent on arachidonic acid metabolism in the lung; the second is mediated by the release of mast cell products.

C5a is also a potent chemotactic factor for neutrophils, monocytes, eosinophils, and basophils and induces low levels of neutrophil degranulation and superoxide anion production.

REGULATION OF THE COMPLEMENT SYSTEM

Activation of the complement system is regulated by three mechanisms. One mechanism involves the spontaneous decay of the individual enzymatically active complexes C4b2a, C3bBb, or cleavage products C3b and C4b. A second regulatory mechanism involves the proteolytic inactivation of specific components by inhibitors present in plasma, including factor I (an inhibitor of C3b and C4b) and serum carboxypeptidase N (SCPN). A third mechanism of regulation of the complement system relates to the binding of active components by specific proteins in the plasma, including C1 esterase inhibitor (C1INA).

The complement system plays an important role in many forms of immunologic tissue injury (see Chapter 4). In addition, it is an important host defense mechanism against bacterial infection. Once the complement system is activated, bacteriolysis may follow, either by means of the assembled membrane attack complex or by enhanced bacterial clearance following opsonization. Bacterial **opsonization** is the process by which a specific molecule (e.g., IgG or C3b) binds to the surface of the bacterium. The process enhances phagocytosis by enabling receptors on the phagocytic cell membrane (e.g., the Fc or the C3b receptor) to recognize and bind to the opsonized bacterium. Viruses, parasites, and transformed cells also activate the complement system by similar mechanisms, resulting in their inactivation or death.

The importance of an intact and appropriately regulated complement system as a component of host defense is exemplified in individuals who have deficiencies of either specific complement components or regulatory proteins. **Deficiencies of complement components may be either acquired or congenital.** The most common congenital defect is a C2 deficiency, which is inherited as an autosomal codominant trait. Acquired deficiencies of early complement components may occur in patients with certain autoimmune diseases, especially those associated with circulating immune complexes. Patients with congenital deficiencies in the early components of the complement system have recurrent symptoms resembling those of systemic lupus erythematosus. Patients with deficiencies of the middle (C3, C5) and terminal (C6, C7, or C8) complement components are particularly susceptible to pyogenic bacterial and neisserial infections, respectively. Congenital defects have been reported in regulatory proteins of the complement system, including deficiencies of C1INA and SCPN.

PHOSPHOLIPID METABOLISM AND ARACHIDONIC ACID METABOLITES

Among the mediators generated by inflammatory cells and injured tissues, certain derivatives of phospholipids and fatty acids are important. Depending on the specific inflammatory cell and the nature of the stimulus, activated cells generate arachidonic acid from membrane phospholipids (Fig. 2-9). Once generated, arachidonic acid, a polyunsaturated (20:4) fatty acid, is metabolized via two pathways: cyclooxygenation, with the subsequent production of prostaglandins and thromboxanes; and lipoxygenation, to form monohydroxyeicosatetranoic and dihydroxyeicosatetranoic acids (HETEs and diHETEs) and leukotrienes. The production of specific arachidonic metabolites is highly dependent on the characterization of the inflammatory cell and stimulus.

The primary cyclooxygenase metabolite in platelets is thromboxane A_2; endothelial cells secrete principally PGI_2. Macrophages, depending on their state of activation, produce any or all of the derivative products, PGG_2, PGH_2, PGI_2, $PGF_{2\alpha}$, PGE_2, PGD_2, and thromboxane A_2.

PGI_2 **and** PGE_2, **due to their vasodilatory effects, enhance vascular permeability at sites of inflammation;** **thromboxane** A_2 **is a potent vasoconstrictor and plays an important role in the mediation of the "second wave" of platelet aggregation** (Table 2–2). PGI_2 and PGE_2 bind to specific receptors on inflammatory cells, activating adenylate cyclase and increasing intracellular cyclic adenosine monophosphate (cAMP) levels, and thereby inhibit their functional responses to other inflammatory stimuli.

In the neutrophil and in certain macrophage populations, an important lipoxygenase product is leukotriene B_4, a compound with potent chemotactic activity for neutrophils, monocytes, and macrophages. In other cell types, especially mast cells, basophils, and macrophages, leukotrienes C_4, D_4, and E_4 are formed. These leukotrienes are collectively known as **slow-reacting substances of anaphylaxis (SRS-As).** They stimulate the contraction of smooth muscle and enhance vascular permeability. The generation of leukotriene B_4 at sites of tissue injury plays an important role in the recruit-

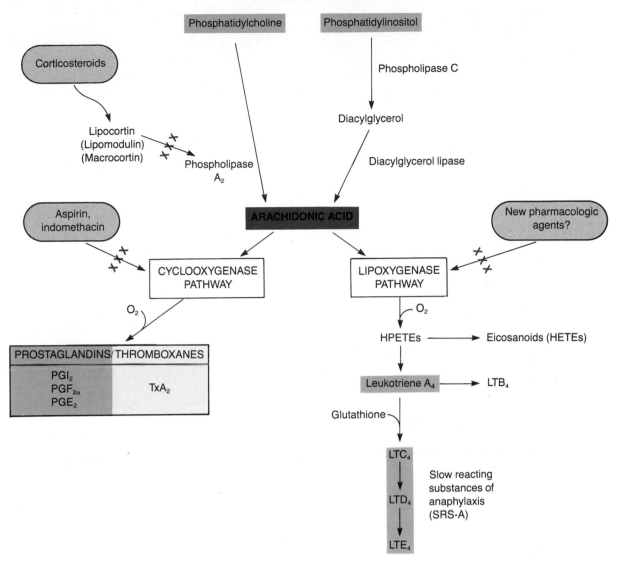

MEMBRANE PHOSPHOLIPIDS

Figure 2-9. Arachidonic acid metabolism.

ment of polymorphonuclear leukocytes, while the production of leukotrienes C_4, D_4, and E_4 is responsible for the development of much of the clinical symptomatology associated with allergic-type reactions.

The importance of arachidonic acid metabolites in mediating many of the effects of the inflammatory response is demonstrated by the ability of inhibitors of the involved enzymes to attenuate both the pathologic changes and clinical symptomatology. Corticosteroids are widely used to inhibit the tissue destruction associated with many inflammatory diseases, including allergic responses, rheumatoid arthritis, and systemic lupus erythematosus. Corticosteroids induce the synthesis of lipocortin, an inhibitor of phospholipase A_2, and block the release of arachidonic acid in inflammatory cells.

Table 2-2   Biologic Activity of Arachidonic Acid Metabolites

METABOLITE	BIOLOGIC ACTIVITY
PGE_2, PGD_2	Induce vasodilatation, bronchodilation Inhibit inflammatory cell function
PGI_2	Induces vasodilatation, bronchodilation Inhibits inflammatory cell function
$PGF_{2\alpha}$	Induces vasodilatation, bronchoconstriction
TxA_2	Induces vasoconstriction, bronchoconstriction Enhances inflammatory cell functions (esp. platelets)
LTB_4	Chemotactic for phagocytic cells Stimulates phagocytic cell adherence Enhances microvascular permeability
LTC_4, LTD_4, LTE_4	Induce smooth-muscle contraction Constrict pulmonary airways Increase microvascular permeability

A second class of anti-inflammatory agents that is widely used in the treatment of inflammatory diseases is the nonsteroidal anti-inflammatory drugs. These compounds—including aspirin, indomethacin, ibuprofen, and piroxicam—inhibit cyclooxygenase, and thus the synthesis of prostaglandins and thromboxanes. A third class of compounds that block specific lipoxygenase activities in inflammatory cells is currently being developed.

CELLULAR RECRUITMENT

The second phase of the acute inflammatory response involves the accumulation of leukocytes—especially polymorphonuclear leukocytes (PMNs)—at sites of tissue injury (Fig. 2-10). During the first 24 hours (and sometimes even in the first few hours) after initiation of injury, many polymorphonuclear leuko-

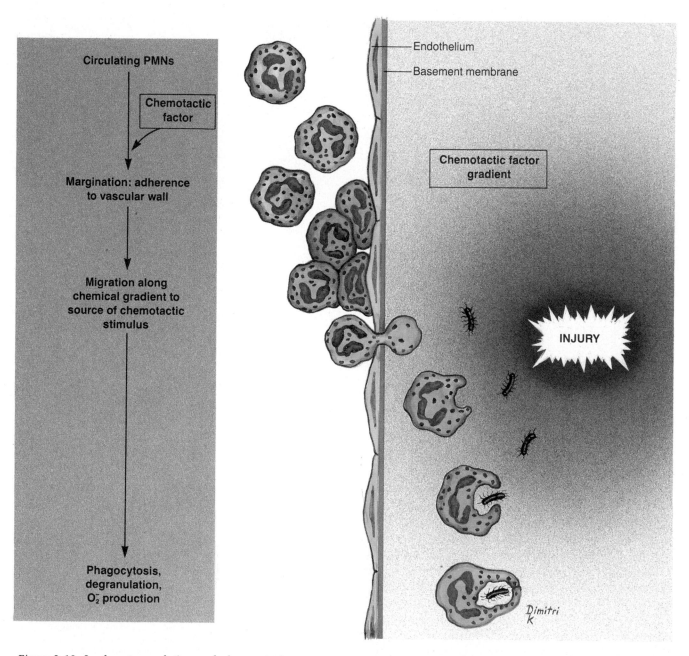

Circulating PMNs

Chemotactic factor

Margination: adherence to vascular wall

Migration along chemical gradient to source of chemotactic stimulus

Phagocytosis, degranulation, O_2^- production

Endothelium

Basement membrane

Chemotactic factor gradient

INJURY

Dimitri K

Figure 2-10. Leukocyte exudation and phagocytosis.

cytes accumulate. This accumulation at inflammatory sites is initiated by locally generated soluble chemical mediators. These mediators, collectively referred to as **chemotactic factors,** are generated in high concentration at sites of tissue injury, with a progressively decreasing gradient away from the injured tissue.

The physiologic responses of circulating leukocytes exposed to chemotactic factors include margination of the cells along the vascular wall, adherence of the leukocytes to the endothelium or vascular basement membrane, emigration through the vascular wall, and unidirectional migration toward increasing concentrations of the chemotactic agent **(chemotaxis).** The most important chemotactic factors for polymorphonuclear leukocytes are C5a derived from complement, low-molecular-weight N-formylated peptides (such as N-formyl-methionyl-leucylphenylalanine) derived from bacteria and mitochondria, and specific products of lipid metabolism, including leukotriene B_4.

Chemotactic factors for other cell types, including monocytes, lymphocytes, basophils, and eosinophils, are also produced at sites of tissue injury. Low-molecular-weight secretory products of lymphocytes (referred to as lymphokines) are chemotactic, as are secretions of monocytes and tissue macrophages (monokines). Proteases from neutrophils and macrophages also cleave C5 to generate C5a or C5a-related peptides.

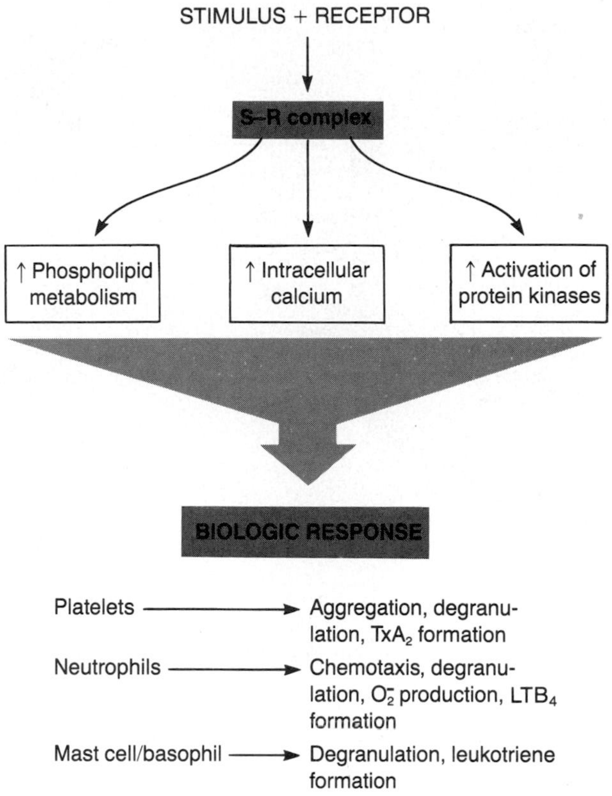

Figure 2-11. Mechanisms of inflammatory cell activation.

INFLAMMATORY CELL ACTIVATION

Polymorphonuclear leukocytes, mast cells, mononuclear phagocytic cells, and platelets are important cellular components of the inflammatory reaction. Once stimulated, these cells release inflammatory mediators that cause tissue injury.

The polymorphonuclear leukocyte is activated in response to phagocytic stimuli or by binding of chemotactic mediators or antibody-antigen complex to specific receptors on its cell membrane. Neutrophil receptors react with the Fc portion of IgG and IgM molecules; with complement system components C5a, C3b, and C3bi; with arachidonic acid metabolites (e.g., leukotriene B_4); and with formylated low-molecular-weight chemotactic peptides.

Mast cells, platelets, and mononuclear phagocytic cells are also activated in a receptor-specific manner. **The process by which diverse stimuli lead to the functional responses of inflammatory cells (e.g., degranulation or aggregation) is referred to as "stimulus-response coupling."** Common pathways associated with inflammatory cell activation are stimulus-induced increases in phospholipid metabolism of cell membranes, raised intracellular calcium levels, and augmented protein kinase activity within the cell (Fig. 2-11).

MODULATION OF INFLAMMATORY CELL FUNCTION

The pharmacologic modulation of inflammatory cell activation is exemplified by the inhibitory effects of E-series prostaglandins and PGI_2 on the functional responses of mast cells, neutrophils, macrophages, and platelets. Prostaglandins of the E series and PGI_2 inhibit inflammatory cell function by activating adenylate cyclase and increasing intracellular cAMP levels. Treatment of inflammatory cells with an inhibitor of cyclic nucleotide phosphodiesterase, such as theophylline, increases levels of cAMP within the cells and enhances inhibition by adenylate cyclase agonists of cell functional responses.

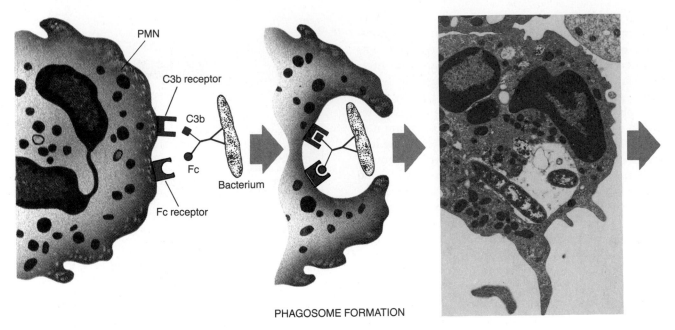

PHAGOSOME FORMATION

Figure 2-12. Mechanisms of polymorphonuclear leukocyte bacterial phagocytosis and cell killing.

Adenylate cyclase agonists and phosphodiesterase inhibitors also affect target tissues of inflammatory mediators. For instance, an increased cAMP level in bronchiolar smooth muscle causes relaxation and blocks the effects of mediators that promote bronchoconstriction. This is the basis for using phosphodiesterase inhibitors in the pharmacologic modulation of mast cell degranulation and the arrest of clinical symptoms associated with certain allergic reactions.

MECHANISMS OF INJURY PRODUCED BY POLYMORPHONUCLEAR LEUKOCYTES

The process of engulfment and internalization of foreign agents or injured cell material is termed phagocytosis, and cells that possess this function are referred to as phagocytic cells. Among these cells are polymorphonuclear leukocytes, monocytes, and tissue macrophages (including Kupffer cells).

The process of phagocytosis of a bacterium or foreign material may be enhanced by the opsonization of that particle by antibody or the fixation of C3b on its surface (Fig. 2-12). As described above, phagocytic cells pos-

sess specific receptors for C3b, C3bi, and the Fc fragment of immunoglobulin molecules. The engulfment of a foreign agent by the cell membrane results in the formation of a phagolysosome, which then fuses with a lysosome to form a phagosome. The release of lysosomal contents into the phagolysosome exposes the engulfed particle to the degradative properties of lysosomal hydrolases, which are activated by acidification within the phagolysosome.

Three distinct granules in the cytoplasm of polymorphonuclear leukocytes are designated primary, secondary, and tertiary granules. Each granule displays a unique spectrum of enzymes that are capable of degrading components of the extracellular matrix and possess bactericidal activity. **Primary granules** contain potent acid hydrolases capable of digesting mucopolysaccharides (glycosaminoglycans). The granules also contain elastase and cathepsin G, which are serine proteases capable of digesting structural proteins of tissues, including elastin and collagen. Other enzymes in the primary granule with known bactericidal activity are lysozyme and phospholipase A_2, which degrade bacterial cell walls and membranes, respectively. Myeloperoxidase, an enzyme also present in these granules, enhances cytotoxicity by metabolizing hydrogen peroxide in the presence of halide ions (e.g., Cl^- or I^-) to form hypohalous acid (see below). **Secondary gran-**

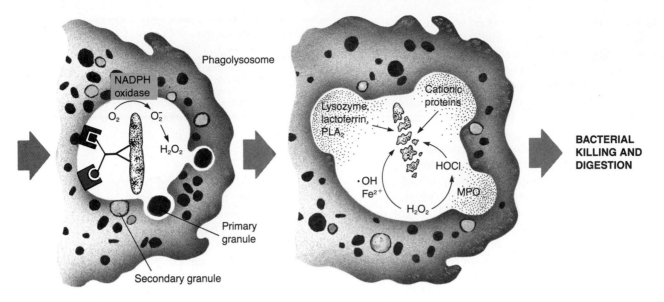

DEGRANULATION AND NADPH OXIDASE ACTIVATION

ules contain phospholipase A_2, lysozyme, the cationic protein lactoferrin, a vitamin B_{12}-binding protein, and a collagenase against type IV collagen. **Tertiary granules,** also referred to as C particles, contain acid hydrolases and gelatinase, the latter an enzyme that digests basement membrane and denatured collagen. Similar granules are present in monocytes and macrophages. Monocytes possess myeloperoxidase, but tissue macrophages do not. Both monocytes and macrophages contain varying amounts of acid hydrolase activity, collagenase, and gelatinase. However, there is a paucity of elastase and cathepsin G in both cell types. An additional neutral protease, plasminogen activator, is also secreted by both neutrophils and mononuclear phagocytic cells. Plasmin, the product of the cleavage of plasminogen by plasminogen activator, attacks several substrates, including fibrin, complement, and fibronectin. Therefore, both neutrophils and mononuclear phagocytic cells have the ability to degrade fibrin at sites of tissue injury and activate the complement system.

The biologic activities of proteases, such as elastase and cathepsin G, are regulated by inhibitors in plasma and tissue fluids. α_1-Antiprotease is synthesized by hepatocytes and is the primary inhibitor of neutrophil elastase. The importance of this protein's inhibitory activity is evident in patients with a genetic deficiency of

α_1-antiprotease; such patients develop pulmonary emphysema, presumably as a result of the lack of elastase inhibitory activity. A second antiprotease in plasma is α_2-macroglobulin, a protein that also inhibits elastase and cathespin G activities. Additionally, both α_1-antiprotease and α_2-macroglobulin inhibit plasmin, trypsin, and chymotrypsin activities. Thus, circulating serum inhibitors not only block protease activity derived from phagocytic cells, but also inhibit protease activity generated within the plasma and tissues.

In addition to releasing granular enzymes into the phagolysosome, phagocytosis activates an NADPH oxidase in the cell membrane (see Fig. 2-12). The ac-

Table 2-3   Reactions Involving Reactive Oxygen Metabolites Produced by Phagocytic Cells

Reduction of Molecular Oxygen	
$O_2 + e^- \rightarrow O_2^-$	Superoxide anion
Dismutation of O_2^-	
$O_2^- + O_2^- + 2H^+ \rightarrow O_2 + H_2O_2$	Hydrogen peroxide
Haber-Weiss Reaction	
$H_2O_2 + O_2^- \rightarrow OH^- + \cdot OH$	Hydroxyl radical
Fenton Reaction (iron-catalyzed)	
$H_2O_2 + Fe^{2+} \rightarrow Fe^{3+} + OH^- + \cdot OH$	Hydroxyl radical
Myeloperoxidase Reaction	
$H_2O_2 + Cl^- + H^+ \rightleftharpoons H_2O + HOCl$	Hypochlorous acid

tivation of this enzyme is associated with an increase in oxygen consumption and activation of the hexose-monophosphate shunt. Together these cell responses are referred to as the **"respiratory burst."** NADPH oxidase reduces molecular oxygen to the superoxide anion, O_2^-. Almost all the oxygen consumed following initiation of the respiratory burst can be accounted for by the generation of O_2^-.

Superoxide anion is reduced to hydrogen peroxide via a dismutation reaction at the cell surface and within phagolysosomes. As discussed above, hydrogen peroxide can react with myeloperoxidase in the presence of a halide to form hypohalous acid (Table 2-3). The most prominent halogen present in biologic systems is chlorine, and hypochlorous acid is produced following neutrophil stimulation. This acid is a more potent oxidant and bactericidal agent than hydrogen peroxide. As noted in Chapter 1, further reduction of H_2O_2 occurs via a Haber-Weiss reaction that forms the highly reactive hydroxyl radical $\cdot OH$. At physiologic pH this reaction occurs slowly. However, reduction of hydrogen peroxide is facilitated by reduced transition metals, such as ferrous iron. The mechanisms by which reactive oxygen metabolites may initiate cell and tissue injury include initiation of lipid peroxidation, DNA scission and cross linking, sulfhydryl group oxidation in proteins, and depolymerization of glycosaminoglycans (e.g., hyaluronic acid).

Reactive oxygen metabolites and lysosomal enzymes are synergistic in producing tissue injury. Proteins and glycosaminoglycans exposed to oxidants are rendered more susceptible to degradation by proteases and acid hydrolases, respectively. For example, oxidants in cigarette smoke and from activated phagocytic cells react with a methionine residue on α_1-antiprotease to render it inactive. This inactivation of α_1-antiprotease enhances elastase activity at sites of tissue injury.

Monocytes, macrophages, and eosinophils also may produce superoxide anion and hydrogen peroxide, depending on their state of activation and the stimulus to which they are exposed. The production of reactive oxygen metabolites by these cells has been implicated in their bactericidal and fungicidal activity, as well as in their ability to kill certain parasites.

The importance of oxygen-dependent mechanisms in phagocytic cell function is exemplified in patients who suffer from a defect in NADPH oxidase. Chronic granulomatous disease of childhood is characterized by an inherited defect in NADPH oxidase or in its expression, and by a failure to produce superoxide anion and H_2O_2 during phagocytosis. Patients with this disorder are susceptible to recurrent infections, especially by gram-positive cocci (Tables 2-4, 2-5).

Depending on the nature of the tissue injury and the size of the phagocytized particle, varying amounts of lysosomal enzymes are released into the extracellular milieu. Prolonged activation of NADPH oxidase may result in the release of hydrogen peroxide and superoxide anion into the adjacent tissues. Under these conditions the activation of phagocytic cells is harmful to the host, since it leads to tissue damage. Such mechanisms of tissue injury play an important role in the pathogenesis of several diseases, including pulmonary emphysema, rheumatoid arthritis and other immune complex diseases, and the adult respiratory distress syndrome.

Table 2-5 Causes of Acquired Defects in Phagocytic Cell Locomotion

Overwhelming infections
Severe trauma or burn
Diabetes mellitus
Chronic debilitating disease

Table 2-4 Congenital Defects in Phagocytic Cell Function

DEFECT	AFFECTED GROUP	CLINICAL EFFECT
Defect in NADPH oxidase: deficient O_2^-, H_2O_2 production	Those with chronic granulomatous disease of childhood (CGD). CGD has several forms; it is most commonly inherited as X-linked recessive	Increased risk of infection with pyogenic bacteria and fungi
Myeloperoxidase deficiency	Heterogeneous group of patients	Increased risk of *Candida* infections
Defect in adherence proteins: MO-1, GP 150,95	Heterogeneous group of patients	Increased risk of recurrent bacterial infections
Lysosomal granule defect	Those with Chédiak-Higashi syndrome, a rare disorder with large cytoplasmic inclusions	Defective bacterial killing and cell locomotion

CELL ADHERENCE AND TISSUE INJURY

The adherence of inflammatory cells to the endothelium or vascular basement membrane is critical for recruitment of these circulating cells to sites of tissue injury. Under normal conditions inflammatory cell membranes and vascular basement membrane possess mutually repulsive negative charges. The number of anionic sites (and hence, negative charges) on the surface of endothelial cells and basement membrane decreases after injury, resulting in a concomitant decrease in the repulsion between the circulating inflammatory cells and the vascular wall. Other components of plasma, vascular wall, and phagocytic cell membranes participate in modulating cell adherence reactions. Fibronectin, a glycoprotein present in plasma, basement membranes, and, to a lesser degree, phagocytic cell membranes, is important in modulating the attachment of phagocytic cells to vascular walls. Following injury to the vascular wall or tissues, increased amounts of fibronectin are deposited at the injury site. Fibronectin also is a potent opsonin that enhances phagocytosis of bacteria and phagocytic cell adherence.

Membrane glycoproteins that promote adherence are among the factors that enhance phagocytic cell attachment to vascular walls and phagocytic particles. The adherence glycoproteins of human leukocytes are a family of molecules designated MO-1, LFA-1 (leukocyte function antigen-1), and p150,95. Activation of phagocytic cells by chemotactic stimuli increases the expression of these adherence molecules on the cell surface. Persons deficient in MO-1, or GP 150,95 are susceptible to recurrent bacterial infection. Thus, the expression of these glycoproteins on phagocytic cell surfaces plays an important role in the localization of cells within the vasculature at sites of tissue injury and in the host defense against bacterial infection.

The adherence of phagocytic cells to their targets is associated with an increased cytotoxicity and degradation of substrates. The ability of a phagocytic cell to recognize its target and to adhere to it serves to "focus" the functional responses of the cell along the adherent surface. When stimulated phagocytic cells adhere to basement membranes, the production of reactive oxygen metabolites is greatest along the adherent surface. The fact that this is also the site of greatest lysosomal degranulation indicates a close approximation of the generation and release of these potentially injurious agents. In addition, close approximation of the phagocytic cell to its target serves to exclude macromolecular inhibitors, such as α-1-antiprotease, from the cell-substrate interface. **In summary, phagocytic cell adherence, secretion of reactive oxygen metabolites, and the release of lysosomal enzymes, function in a synergistic manner to enhance cytotoxicity and tissue degradation.**

CHRONIC INFLAMMATION

Following acute injury of tissue, polymorphonuclear leukocytes are replaced over several days by lymphocytes, mononuclear phagocytic cells, and plasma cells. This "subacute inflammatory response" represents the early stages of resolution leading to the formation of granulation tissue. **Granulation tissue is characterized by the proliferation of endothelial cells and fibroblasts into the area of injury** (Fig. 2-13). Proliferation of endothelial cells leads to the formation of small capillaries and restoration of the vascular supply. The fibroblast restores the connective tissue matrix in the injured tissue by increased synthesis of glycosaminoglycans and collagen types I and III. Proliferation of endothelial cells and fibroblasts is regulated by specific mediators secreted by activated macrophages and T-lymphocytes. Plasma and platelet-derived factors also regulate endothelial and fibroblast growth. These factors cause an increased proliferation of cells and, in the case of fibroblasts, increased connective tissue synthesis and deposition.

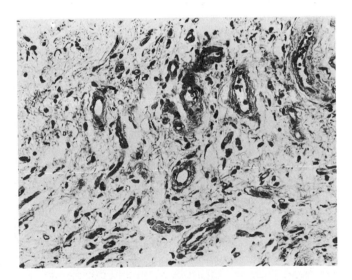

Figure 2-13. Granulation tissue. Chronic inflammatory cells, fibroblasts, loose connective tissue, and abundant blood vessels are evident.

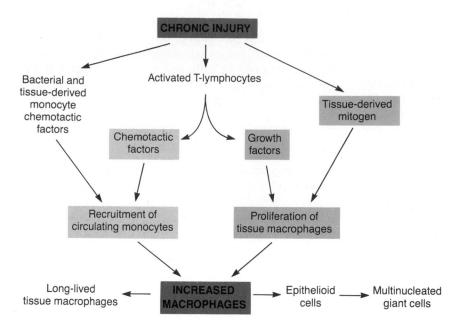

Figure 2-14. The accumulation of macrophages in chronic inflammation.

Under conditions in which the inflammatory response is unable to eliminate the injurious agent or restore injured tissue to its normal physiologic state, there may be progression to a state of chronic inflammation. The primary cellular components of the chronic inflammatory response are macrophages, plasma cells, lymphocytes, and, in certain conditions, eosinophils. Chronic inflammation is mediated by both immunologic and nonimmunologic mechanisms and is frequently observed in conjunction with granulation tissue. The macrophage is the pivotal cell in regulating these reactions because it functions as a source of both inflammatory and immunologic mediators. The accumulation of **macrophages** occurs primarily as a consequence of recruitment of circulating monocytes by chemotactic stimuli and their differentiation in tissues (Fig. 2-14). In addition to generating inflammatory mediators, macrophages regulate lymphocyte responses to antigen and secrete mediators that modulate the proliferation and function of fibroblasts and endothelial cells.

Plasma cells and **lymphocytes** are also prominent features of chronic inflammatory reactions. While **eosinophils** are occasionally a conspicuous component of the chronic inflammatory response, their precise role is not clear. They are particularly evident during allergic-type reactions and parasitic infections. Eosinophils share many functional features with the neutrophil. Their rhomboid, crystalloid granules are rich in acid

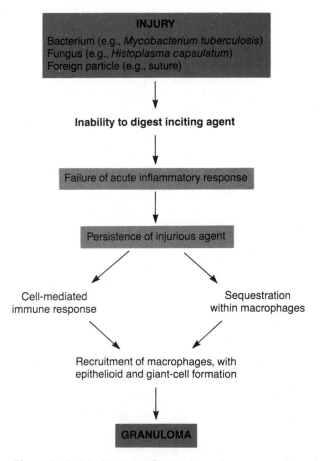

Figure 2-15. Mechanism of granuloma formation.

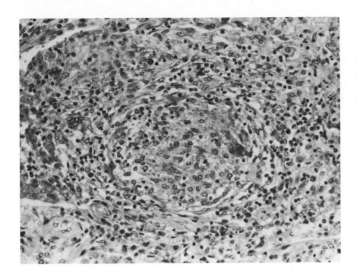

Figure 2-16. Granulomatous inflammation. A granuloma displays epithelioid cells in the center, surrounded by a rim of lymphoid cells. Several multinucleated giant cells are present.

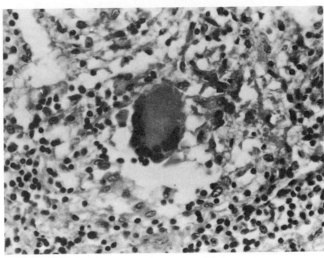

Figure 2-17. Langhans' giant cell. A number of nuclei are arranged on the periphery of an abundant cytoplasm.

phosphatase and have a specific peroxidase activity. The granules also contain a unique eosinophil basic protein that is toxic to certain parasites and normal host cells. **Polymorphonuclear leukocytes,** although characteristic of acute inflammation, may also be observed at sites of chronic inflammation. **Acute and chronic inflammation represent ends of a dynamic continuum, in which the morphologic features of the inflammatory response frequently overlap.**

GRANULOMATOUS INFLAMMATION

As we have seen, phagocytosis followed by digestion is the mechanism by which neutrophils inactivate and remove agents that incite an acute inflammatory response. However, there are circumstances in which the substances that provoke the acute inflammatory reaction are not digestible by the reacting neutrophils, namely **granulomatous inflammation** (Fig. 2-15).

Granulomatous inflammation is typical of the tissue response elicited by fungal infections, tuberculosis, leprosy, schistosomiasis, and the presence of foreign material (e.g., suture or talc). The principal cells involved in granuloma formation are macrophages and lymphocytes. Macrophages are much longer-lived than neu-

trophils. They are not killed by the pathogenic agent that incites the inflammatory reaction, and they can store it in their cytoplasm for indefinite periods. Such intracellular sequestration of the noxious agent prevents it from continuing to provoke an acute inflammatory reaction. Upon phagocytizing and retaining substances that they cannot digest, the macrophages lose their motility and remain in place. A characteristic change in their structure follows that transforms them into so-called **epithelioid cells. Nodular collections of epithelioid cells form the granulomas that are the morphologic hallmark of granulomatous inflammation.**

Granulomas are usually small (usually <2 mm), and the collections of epithelioid cells are frequently surrounded by a rim of lymphocytes (Fig. 2-16). Unlike circulating monocytes, epithelioid cells have abundant cytoplasm and numerous lysosomal granules. An additional feature of granulomas is the presence of multinucleated giant cells. These cells are large, contain numerous (up to 40 to 50) nuclei, and are formed from the cytoplasmic fusion of macrophages. When the nuclei are arranged around the periphery of the cell in a horseshoe-shaped pattern, the cell is termed **Langhans' giant cell** (Fig. 2-17). Frequently one can identify a foreign pathogenic agent (e.g., silica or a *Histoplasma* spore) or other indigestible material within the cytoplasm of a multinucleated giant cell. These cells are referred to as **foreign body giant cells**

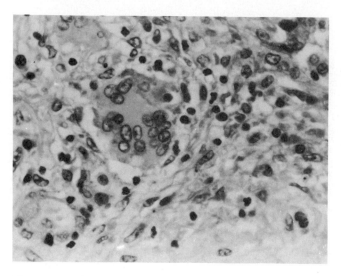

Figure 2-18. Foreign body giant cell. The numerous nuclei are randomly arranged in the cytoplasm.

(Fig. 2-18). Giant cells are functionally inactive, especially when compared to macrophages. In association with the granuloma, one may also see all the other cell types characteristic of chronic inflammation.

Cell-mediated immune responses to the inciting agent may occur and, in turn, modify the basic granulomatous reaction by recruiting and activating more macrophages and lymphocytes. The contribution of the immune system to the evolution of chronic granulomatous inflammation varies with the immunogenicity of the inciting agent. Figure 2-15 summarizes the mechanisms in the generation of granulomatous inflammation.

SYSTEMIC MANIFESTATIONS OF INFLAMMATION

One of the important manifestations of localized inflammatory injury is the subsequent reaction in lymphatics and lymph nodes that drain the tissue. Inflammatory mediators generated at sites of injury, as well as necrotic debris, drain into the lymphatic system and flow to the regional lymph nodes. Under conditions of severe injury there is secondary inflammation of the lymphatic channels (lymphangitis) and the lymph nodes (lymphadenitis). Clinically, the inflamed lymphatic channels in the skin manifest as red streaks, and the lymph nodes themselves are enlarged and

painful. Lymph nodes can exhibit hyperplasia of the lymphoid follicles (follicular hyperplasia) and proliferation of mononuclear phagocytic cells in the sinuses (sinus histiocytosis).

A clinical hallmark of inflammation is **fever.** Pyrogens are released into the circulation from exogenous sources, such as bacteria, or are produced endogenously. The primary endogenous pyrogen is interleukin-1, a protein secreted primarily by macrophages, which regulates lymphocyte activation during immune responses. Interleukin-1 acts on the thermoregulatory centers within the hypothalamus to initiate the fever response. Interleukin-1 stimulates arachidonic acid metabolism within the hypothalamus, thus leading to prostaglandin synthesis. Inhibitors of cyclooxygenase (e.g., aspirin) block the fever response by inhibiting interleukin-1-stimulated PGE_2 synthesis in the hypothalamus.

An additional systemic effect of local inflammation is an increase in the numbers of circulating white blood cells **(leukocytosis).** Leukocytosis is commonly manifested as a two- to threefold increase in the number of white blood cells and reflects principally an increase in circulating polymorphonuclear leukocytes (neutrophilia). In addition, an increase in the number of immature polymorphonuclear leukocytes ("band" forms) is also seen in the peripheral blood. The mechanism for increasing circulating white blood cells involves the release of specific mediators that promote an accelerated release of polymorphonuclear leukocytes from the bone marrow and an increased proliferation of bone marrow precursors. One of the best characterized of the mediators responsible for the increased cell proliferation is a group of compounds referred to as **colony stimulating factors.** These factors are produced by macrophages and T-lymphocytes and stimulate mitotic activity in myeloid precursors in the bone marrow. The circulating levels of the myeloid precursors of leukocytes often may become extremely high, reaching levels of 40,000 to 100,000 cells per mm^3. This extreme elevation in the circulating white blood cell count has been referred to as a **"leukemoid reaction"** and must be differentiated from leukemia. Neutrophilia is most frequently seen in association with bacterial infections and with infarction of tissues. In contrast, viral infections, including infectious mononucleosis, are characterized by an absolute increase in the number of circulating lymphocytes **(lymphocytosis).** During parasitic infections and certain allergic reactions, one may observe an increase in the number of eosinophils in the peripheral blood without an increase in the absolute white blood cell count **(eosinophilia).** Eosinophils, which normally constitute 1% to 3% of peripheral white blood cells, can reach a level of 10% to 15% or more in eosinophilia.

Under conditions of chronic inflammation, particularly in patients who are nutritionally deprived or who suffer from chronic debilitating disease such as disseminated cancer, an absolute decrease in circulating white blood cell counts may be observed **(leukopenia).** The mechanisms responsible for the suppression of leukopoiesis are not well understood. They presumably represent an imbalance in the production of mediators that regulate myeloid and lymphoid precursors in the bone marrow.

3

REPAIR, REGENERATION, AND FIBROSIS

ANTONIO MARTINEZ-HERNANDEZ

THE EXTRACELLULAR MATRIX

The extracellular matrix is a stable complex of macromolecules that underlies epithelia and surrounds connective tissue cells. It has a crucial role in wound healing through its chemotactic, opsonic, and attachment properties. The strength of the wound and the properties of the scar ultimately depend on the deposition of an adequate extracellular matrix.

The extracellular matrix has five major components: collagens, basement membranes, elastic fibers, fibronectin, and proteoglycans.

COLLAGENS

The collagens are a closely related family of proteins having common properties. They contain triple helical domains with a repeating amino acid sequence (Gly-X-Y triplets) and are rich in the two hydroxylated amino acids, hydroxyproline and hydroxylysine. A glycine in every third position imparts a right handed helicity to the collagenous chain. The collagen molecule is formed by three polypeptide chains that intertwine in a left-handed supercoil to form a triple helical rope. The individual polypeptide chains are designated by the Greek letter α, and an Arabic numeral after the α characterizes the constituent chains of the trimer. For example,

type I collagen consists of two $\alpha 1$ chains and one $\alpha 2$ chain. The different trimers are designated by Roman numerals and represent the collagen types. The chains of different collagens are distinguished by placing the Roman numeral of the corresponding type in parentheses after the Arabic numeral—for example, $\alpha 1(I)$ and $\alpha 1(III)$. The composition and distribution of 10 collagen types are summarized in Table 3-1.

COLLAGEN BIOSYNTHESIS

The steps in the synthesis, secretion, and assembly into definitive extracellular structures of collagen are a complicated sequence. The individual polypeptide chains are synthesized on membrane-bound ribosomes. Like other export proteins, these pre-procollagen chains contain signal sequences at the amino-terminal end that are cleaved shortly after translation. The resulting procollagen chains display extension peptides (propeptides) at both ends of the molecule. The pro-α chains therefore have three major domains: the α-chain, the amino-terminal peptide, and the carboxy-terminal peptide. In the cisternae of the rough endoplasmic reticulum, three pro-α chains interact to form a procollagen molecule. Hydroxylation of proline and lysine residues, glycosylation, chain association, disulfide bonding, and triple helix formation take place before secretion. **Hydroxylation requires vitamin C, a need that explains the inadequate wound healing characteristic of vitamin C deficiency (scurvy).** Ex-

---

Table 3-1   Genetically Distinct Vertebrate Collagen Types

TYPE	CHAINS	MACROMOLECULAR ASSOCIATION	AGGREGATE FORM	LOCALIZATION
I	$\alpha 1(I)$, $\alpha 2(I)$			Most abundant collagen: Ubiquitous—skin, bone, etc.
II	$\alpha 1(II)$			Major cartilage collagen: Cartilage, vitreous humor
III	$\alpha 1(III)$			Abundant in pliable tissues: Blood vessels, uterus, skin, etc.
IV	$\alpha 1(IV)$, $\alpha 2(IV)$			All basement membranes
V	$\alpha 1(V)$, $\alpha 2(V)$, $\alpha 3(V)$	???		Minor component of most interstitial tissues
VI	$\alpha 1(VI)$, $\alpha 2(VI)$			Abundant in most interstitial tissues
VII	$\alpha 1(VII)$			? Anchoring fibrils
VIII	$\alpha 1(VIII)$	???		Produced by some endothelia
IX	$\alpha 1(IX)$, $\alpha 2(IX)$, $\alpha 3(IX)$	???		Cartilage
X	$\alpha 1(X)$	???		Mineralizing cartilage

tracellular processing of collagen types I, II, III, and V is needed before the definitive structures can be assembled. The extension peptides are cleaved by aminoproteases and carboxyproteases. These enzymes act independently; partially processed collagen forms have been identified. Inappropriate action of the aminoprotease leads to retention of the N-terminal propeptide and defective fiber formation, as in the case of the hereditary disease Ehler-Danlos type VII. After removal of the extension propeptides, collagen molecules interact and aggregate to form collagen fibers. However, the full tensile strength of collagen fibers is not achieved until a series of intramolecular and intermolecular bonds form. Some of these bonds result from the action of specific enzymes, such as lysyl oxidase. This enzyme is a metalloenzyme that requires copper as cofactor. Chelation of copper by nitriles, a toxic disorder called lathyrism, or inherited diseases of copper metabolism result in reduced lysyl oxidase activity and poorly cross-linked collagen fibers that lack tensile strength.

COLLAGEN CATABOLISM

Collagen has a slow turnover (months) in adult tissues. Native collagen is resistant to most nonspecific proteases. **Collagenases** are enzymes that digest native triple-helical collagen. In general, the same collagenase cleaves collagen types I, II, and III, although the rates of cleavage are different with each type. Type IV and V collagens are not degraded by the same collagenases that cleave types I, II, and III, but are degraded by another family of collagenases.

Fibroblasts are the main source of collagenases, although other cells, including macrophages, epithelial cells, and endothelial cells, also produce them. Several collagenase inhibitors are present in plasma, including α_2-macroglobulin, α_1-antitrypsin, and β_1-globulin. Fibronectin, a plasma and tissue protein, has a specific binding site for collagen. The point at which it binds to the collagen molecule is adjacent to the collagenase-susceptible bond. It is likely that fibronectin bound to collagen fibers protects them from the action of collagenases.

MORPHOLOGY AND FUNCTIONS

Collagen molecules self-assemble nonenzymatically to form **collagen fibrils,** the smallest collagen structures recognizable by conventional electron microscopy. Fibrils appear as thin (4-nm diameter) filaments consisting of four or five quarter-staggered collagen molecules. Several fibrils are aligned in parallel to form **collagen fibers.** The characteristic cross-banding of fibers at 67-nm periods reflects the staggered array of the collagen molecules. Groups of collagen fibers ori-

ented along the same axis are called **collagen bundles.** Several collagen types may participate in bundle formation: type I fibers form the backbone and types III, V, and VI are attached to it. Collagen bundles have various sizes and orientations, depending on the organ and function. For example, tendons consist of dense, parallel bundles composed almost exclusively of type I collagen. By contrast, the cornea is formed by orthogonal layers (lamellae) of type I collagen, with some filaments of collagen types V and VI. Collagen fibers are beyond the resolving power of the light microscope, and only large bundles can be identified. The reticulin stain (a silver impregnation) demonstrates the fine reticular connective-tissue network of many organs. In recent years there have been attempts to equate the components reacting with this stain with specific connective tissue components, such as collagen type III or fibronectin. The reality is that the reticulin stain demonstrates various glycoproteins, including fibronectin and several collagen types; therefore, reticulin cannot be identified with a single molecular species.

The best-known function of the collagens is physical support. Type I collagen predominates in organs in which tensile strength is needed, such as tendon and bone, whereas type III is found in organs with some plasticity, such as blood vessels, uterus, gastrointestinal tract, and adventitial dermis. Nevertheless, collagens should not be regarded as merely passive, inert scaffolds. They bind to cell surfaces and modulate morphogenesis, chemotaxis, platelet adhesion and aggregation, cell attachment, and cell phenotype.

BASEMENT MEMBRANES

Basement membranes are delicate structures, found at the interface between cells and stroma, that contain type IV collagen and laminin. By light microscopy they appear as pale, amorphous structures that react with histochemical stains for carbohydrate groups (e.g., periodic acid-Schiff [PAS]). By electron microscopy most basement membranes have two layers with distinct electron densities. The layer of lower electron density, the lamina rara or lucida, is adjacent to the cell membrane, whereas the layer of higher electron density, the lamina densa, is adjacent to the stroma. In most tissues both laminae are of equal thickness, 40 to 60 nm. Some basement membranes—for example, lens capsule and Descemet's membrane—have only a lamina densa. The mature glomerular basement membrane, on the other hand, is trilaminar, with a central lamina densa of double thickness between two outer 40-nm lamina rarae. This trilaminar appearance results from the fusion of the developmentally distinct endothelial and epithelial basement membranes. Segments of the alveolar basement membrane in the lung are also trilaminar.

Basement membranes are found in every organ. **All epithelia, whether epidermal, endocrine, genitourinary, respiratory, or gastrointestinal, are separated from the stroma by continuous basement membranes.** The liver is an exception, since hepatocytes lack a basement membrane. The central nervous system has only vascular basement membranes. In the peripheral nervous system, Schwann cells are surrounded by a basement membrane. **All endothelial cells are separated from the underlying stroma by a basement membrane, except for the sinusoidal endothelium of the bone marrow, spleen, lymph nodes, and liver.** Adipocytes and cardiac, skeletal, and smooth muscle cells are individually surrounded by a basement membrane. All other cells of mesodermal origin—that is, fibroblasts, histiocytes, synovial cells, and lymphoid and other blood cells—lack a basement membrane. Basement membranes are complex structures that result from the interaction of several macromolecules: type IV collagen, laminin, entactin, and heparan sulfate proteoglycan (Table 3-2).

They have significant tensile strength and provide physical support to structures resting on or enclosed by them. They also function as a site for cell attachment. Many cells have a membrane protein that specifically binds to laminin. Basement membranes also serve as filters. This function is more obvious in capillaries and has been extensively studied in the renal glomerulus. Initially it was assumed that basement membranes filtered molecules on the basis of their size and shape. It is now thought that the high anionic charge of the basement membrane plays the crucial role in filtration.

ELASTIC FIBERS

Tissues such as the uterus, blood vessels, skin, and lung require elasticity in addition to tensile strength for their function. **Whereas tensile strength is provided by members of the collagen family, the ability to recoil after transient stretching is provided by elastic fibers.** By electron microscopy elastic fibers have two distinct components, a central amorphous core and a peripheral rim of microfibrils. Elastic fibers vary in size from large sheets visible by light microscopy (elastic lamellae of large arteries) to delicate fibers demonstrable only by electron microscopy.

The central core of elastic fibers consists of **elastin,** a 70,000-dalton glycoprotein. Like collagen, elastin is rich in glycine and proline, but unlike collagen, it contains practically no hydroxylated amino acids. Elastin molecules are cross-linked to form an extensive network. Unlike most other proteins, elastin does not form definitive folds, but oscillates between different states to form **random coils.** It is this cross-linked, random-coiled structure of elastin that determines the capacity of the network to stretch and recoil. The interwoven and inelastic collagen fibers limit elasticity and maintain tissue integrity. The exact composition and function of the elastic fibers' peripheral microfibrils is unknown.

Table 3-2 Basement Membrane Components

COMPONENT	CONSTITUENT CHAINS	MOLECULAR COMPOSITION	SUPRAMOLECULAR AGGREGATE	FUNCTION
Type IV collagen	$\alpha1$(IV), $\alpha2$(IV)	Three α chains		Network Structural
Laminin	A, B_1, B_2	One A and two B chains		Cell attachment
Entactin	Single polypeptide chain	Single polypeptide chain		? Unknown
Heparan sulfate proteoglycan	Polypeptide chain, glycosaminoglycan side chains	Protein core, glycosaminoglycan side chains		Electrostatic charge

FIBRONECTIN

In addition to collagens and elastin, the extracellular matrix contains several other glycoproteins, of which **fibronectin** is the best characterized. Fibronectin exists in two major forms, plasma and tissue fibronectin.

Fibronectins have two nearly identical polypeptide chains held together by disulfide bridges. Each polypeptide chain has a molecular weight of about 200,000 daltons. All forms of fibronectin are derived from a single gene. **Specific binding sites in specialized domains of the fibronectin molecule allow it to bind avidly to collagens, proteoglycans, glycosaminoglycans, fibrinogen, fibrin, cell surfaces, bacteria, and DNA.** The varied binding properties of fibronectin (*nectere = to bind*) allow it to connect cells with other components of the extracellular matrix, thus integrating the tissue into a functional unit. Through the action of transglutaminase (factor XIII of the clotting cascade) fibronectin is covalently cross-linked with itself, fibrinogen, fibrin, or collagen. This cross-linking is probably of great importance in the early phases of wound healing.

Like other plasma proteins, plasma fibronectin is synthesized and secreted by hepatocytes. Most mesenchymal cells, including fibroblasts and endothelial cells, secrete tissue fibronectin. Fibronectin is ubiquitous in the extracellular matrix, where it is found as delicate filaments, as small aggregates, attached to collagen fibers, and on cell surfaces. Tissue fibronectin is one of the first structural macromolecules to be deposited during embryonic development. It forms a "primitive" matrix that allows the initial organization to be replaced by the definitive, organ-specific matrix. This role of tissue fibronectin as the initial, "undifferentiated" matrix is recapitulated in the early phases of wound healing.

PROTEOGLYCANS

Molecules formed by long, unbranched polysaccharide chains are major constituents of the extracellular matrix. These carbohydrate polymers, formerly termed the "**mucopolysaccharides**," are referred to as **glycosaminoglycans** because one of the sugar residues in the repeating disaccharide unit is always an amino sugar. With the exception of hyaluronic acid, glycosaminoglycans are covalently bound to a protein core, in which form they are termed **proteoglycans.** Up to 95% of the dry weight of proteoglycans consists of carbohydrate. Glycosaminoglycans are negatively charged, extended molecules that occupy large volumes. They are also highly hydrophilic, and form hydrated gels even at low concentrations. Proteoglycans are widely distributed in all extracellular matrices, and they are also found in cell surfaces and in most biologic fluids.

Proteoglycan and glycosaminoglycan distribution is tissue-specific. Cartilage contains abundant chondroitin 4-sulfate, keratan sulfate, and hyaluronic acid but no heparan sulfate or dermatan sulfate. Basement membranes contain heparan sulfate whereas the dermis contains hyaluronic acid, chondroitin sulfate, and dermatan sulfate. Proteoglycan hydrated gels help maintain tissue turgor. Their high charge density also allows them to act as selective filters. Heparan sulfate seems to provide most of the charge selectivity of basement membranes. In tissues, proteoglycans are often bound to collagen fibers, elastic fibers, and fibronectin. Through these interactions, they may participate in the organization of the extracellular matrix. In cartilage, where they are particularly abundant, proteoglycans modulate and regulate the size of type II collagen fibers. As organizers of the extracellular matrix, proteoglycans are deposited in the early phases of wound healing before collagen deposition becomes prominent.

THE REPAIR REACTION

Following the initial influx of hematogenous inflammatory cells into a wound site, additional cells—fibroblasts—move into the injured area. Inactive fibroblasts, seen by light microscopy as oval cells with an indistinct cytoplasm and an elongated, homogenous nucleus, comprise at least three functionally distinct mesenchymal cell types, all of which are important in the repair response. These cells are stem cells of connective tissues, cells with Fc receptors and phagocytic capacities (histiocytes), and cells specialized in the synthesis of extracellular matrix components (fibrocytes). In addition, endothelial cells, macrophages, platelets, and the parenchymal cells of the injured organ itself participate in the repair reaction.

LABILE CELLS

When more than 1.5% of the cells of a normal adult tissue are in mitosis, the tissue is said to be composed of **labile cells.** Not all of the cells in labile tissues are continuously dividing. Rather, these tissues have special cells, called **stem cells,** that are programmed to divide continuously. The basal cells of the epidermis and of the gastrointestinal crypts are such stem cells. In the case of some stem cells, the progeny differentiates into only one type of cell. For instance, the daughter cells of a basal epidermal cell mature only into keratinized cells that will eventually desquamate. This type of

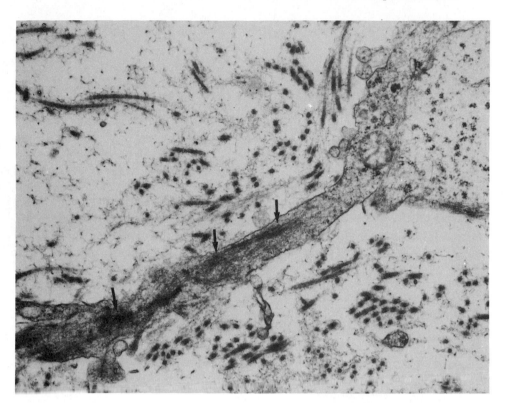

Figure 3-1. Myofibroblast viewed by electron microscopy. Myofibroblasts have an important role in the repair reaction. These cells, with features intermediate between those of smooth muscle cells and fibroblasts, are characterized by the presence of discrete bundles of myofilaments in the cytoplasm (*arrows*).

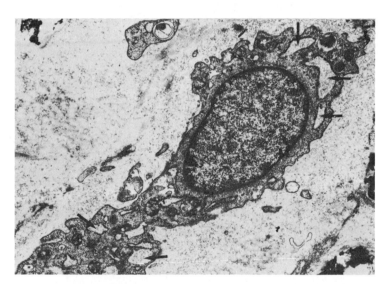

Figure 3-2. Fibroblast viewed by electron microscopy. This elongated cell, with multiple, delicate cell processes and an oval nucleus, is an active fibroblast. During the repair reaction fibroblasts secrete extracellular matrix components. This activity is manifested by the distended rough endoplasmic reticulum cisternae (*arrows*). The loose extracellular matrix characteristic of this early stage of the repair process contains mostly proteoglycans, type III collagen, and fibronectin. Only a few type I collagen fibers are present.

stem cell is **unipotent.** Other stem cells give rise to more than one cell type. Hemocytoblasts of the bone marrow yield red blood cells, neutrophils, eosinophils, basophils, monocytes, lymphocytes, and megakaryocytes. This type of stem cell is **pluripotent. Tissues composed of labile cells regenerate after injury, provided that enough stem cells remain.**

STABLE CELLS

When fewer than 1.5% of the cells in a normal adult tissue are in mitosis, the tissue is said to be composed of **stable** cells. Stable tissues—for example, endocrine glands, endothelium, and liver—do not have stem

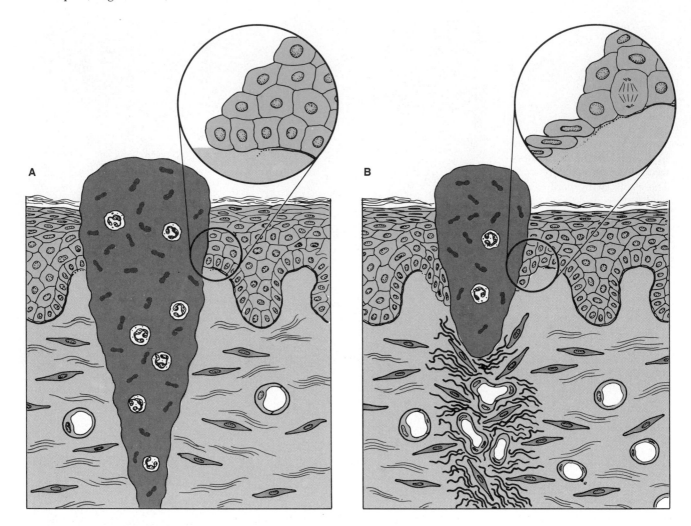

Figure 3-3. Skin healing. (*A*) In any wound, the initial gap is filled by blood that upon clotting (formation of fibrin polymers) provides the initial stability to the wound. Plasma fibronectin, present in the clot, can be cross-linked with extracellular matrix components and fibrin to bridge the clot and tissues. (*B*) As a consequence of the wound, the epidermal cells at its edges lose contact with other epithelial cells and with their basement membrane. This loss of contact probably acts as a signal triggering migration of the cells. Concurrently, basal epidermal cells adjacent to the migrating cells undergo division. The result of this coordinated migration and cell division is the gradual covering of the epidermal defect. The breakdown products from the injured cells, fibronectin, and lysosomal enzymes from blood cells act as chemoattractants, resulting in an influx of macrophages, myofibroblasts, and fibroblasts. Simultaneously, endothelial cells proliferate and neovascularization begins. The phagocytic cells attracted to the wound remove part of the clot, while fibroblasts and myofibroblasts begin to deposit a new extracellular matrix.

cells. Rather, the cells of these stable tissues divide mostly under the proper stimulus. **It is the potential to replicate and not the actual number of mitoses that determines the organ's ability to regenerate.** The liver, a stable tissue with less than one mitosis for every 15,000 cells, regenerates after a loss of 75% of its mass.

PERMANENT CELLS

A tissue in which no cells are in mitosis is composed of **permanent** cells. Neurons, cardiac myocytes, and cells of the lens are permanent cells. **If lost, permanent cells cannot be replaced.**

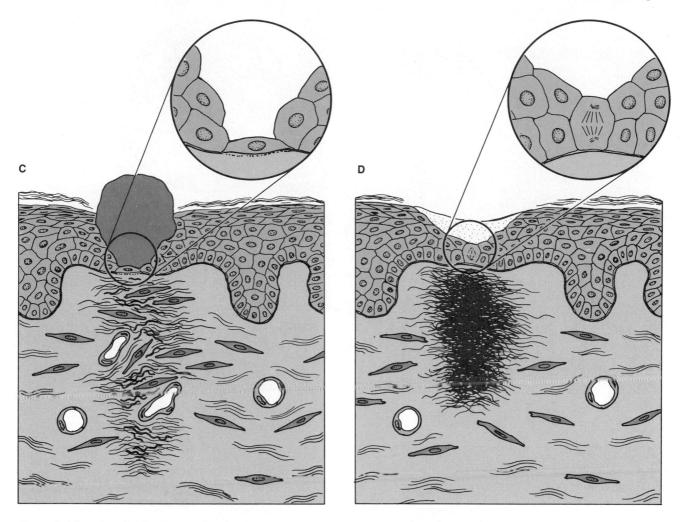

Figure 3-3 (continued). (C) The concentric migration of epidermal cells, sustained by the mitotic activity of the trailing cells, fills the wound gap and displaces the remnants of the original clot (scab) toward the surface. Contact with other epidermal cells is the signal that stops migration. The trailing cells not only divide, but also secrete basement membrane components. In this manner the continuity of the epidermal basement membrane is restored. In a similar fashion, the concerted activity of fibroblasts, myofibroblasts, macrophages, and endothelial cells fill the dermal gap. At this point, the number of macrophages and myofibroblasts declines. Those capillaries that failed to establish a definitive flow pattern begin to be obliterated and accumulation of the definitive extracellular matrix is initiated. (D) The gap created by the wound has been repaired. The mitotic activity of the epidermal cells will restore the epidermal thickness. Most capillaries of the initial granulation tissue have been reabsorbed, and the dermal gap has been filled with a dense, almost avascular, hypocellular extracellular matrix, composed predominantly of type I collagen.

WOUND HEALING

Healing is the replacement of dead by living tissue. The initial inflammatory phase of the healing process leads to the formation of an exudate rich in fibrin and fibronectin. The dead cells and all other debris resulting from the injury are removed by a process termed **demolition,** achieved by the phagocytic cells of the inflammatory response. Following the inflammatory phase, three mechanisms—**contraction, repair,** and **regeneration**—complete the healing process. In most instances, all three mechanisms are operative; thus, in a

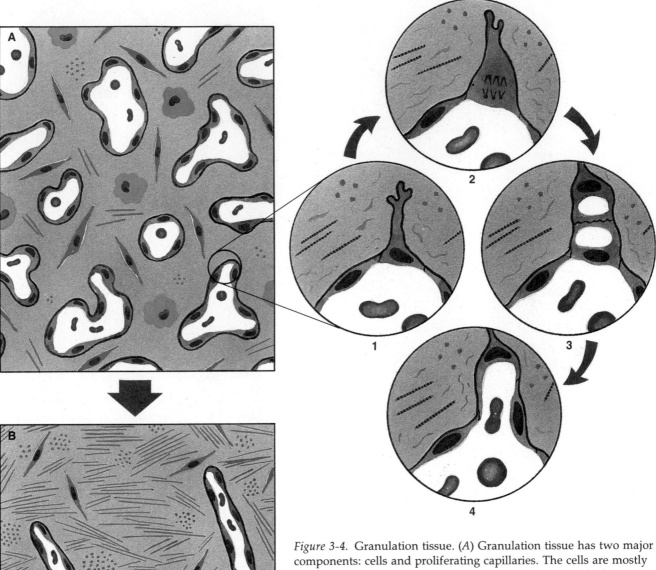

Figure 3-4. Granulation tissue. (*A*) Granulation tissue has two major components: cells and proliferating capillaries. The cells are mostly fibroblasts, myofibroblasts, and macrophages. The macrophages are derived from monocytes and histiocytes. The fibroblasts and myofibroblasts derive from mesenchymal stem cells, and the capillaries arise from adjacent vessels by division of the lining endothelial cells (*detail*) in a process termed *angiogenesis.* Endothelial cells put out cell extensions, called *pseudopodia,* that grow toward the wound site. Cytoplasmic growth enlarges the pseudopodium and eventually the cell divides. Vacuoles formed in the daughter cells eventually fuse to create a new lumen. The entire process continues until the sprout encounters another capillary, with which it will connect. At its peak, granulation tissue is the most richly vascularized tissue in the body. (*B*) Once repair has been achieved, most of the newly formed capillaries are obliterated and then reabsorbed, leaving a pale avascular scar.

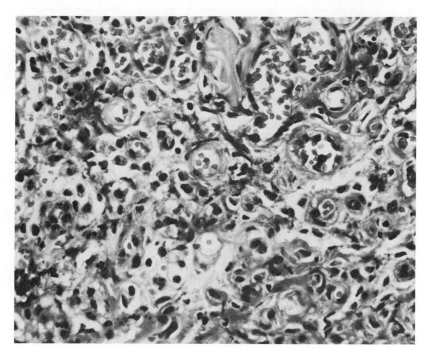

Figure 3-4 (continued). (C) At this stage, granulation tissue consists mostly of thin-walled vessels embedded in a loose connective tissue matrix containing mesenchymal cells and occasional inflammatory cells.

skin wound, part of the defect is closed by wound contraction, part by granulation tissue, and part by epithelial cells.

CONTRACTION

Contraction is the mechanical reduction in the size of the wound defect as a result of the action of myofibroblasts. Under some circumstances contraction reduces the size of the original defect by as much as 70%. **Thus, faster healing results, since only one-third to one-half of the original defect has to be replaced.** If contraction is prevented, large, unsightly scars result. On the other hand, excessive contraction may lead to **contractures.**

Myofibroblasts appear in the wound area 2 or 3 days after injury, and migrate into the wound. Their active contraction decreases the size of the defect. Myofibroblasts have features intermediate between those of a fibroblast and a smooth muscle cell (Fig. 3-1). Their nuclei are irregular and indented, and the cytoplasm contains actin and myosin bundles and occasional dense bodies resembling those of smooth muscle cells. The rough endoplasmic reticulum and the Golgi complex are prominent. Myofibroblasts have cell junctions and occasionally are surrounded by a basement membrane.

REPAIR

Repair is the replacement of dead tissue by granulation tissue that eventually matures to scar tissue (Figs. 3-2 and 3-3). In wounds in which only the lining epithelium is affected, we speak of **erosions.** These lesions heal exclusively by regeneration; that is, proliferation of the surrounding epithelial cells covers the defect. In wounds where the injury extends to the connective tissue, the dermis in the skin, or the submucosa in the gastrointestinal tract, mesenchymal or stem cells are activated and proliferate, giving rise to **active fibroblasts.** These cells synthesize and secrete extracellular matrix components, including fibronectin, proteoglycans, and collagen types I and III.

A striking vascular proliferation starts 48 to 72 hours after injury and lasts for several days. Endothelial cells near the injury divide and form solid sprouts extending from the preexisting vessels (Fig. 3-4). Frequently, these sprouting capillaries protrude from the surface of the wound as minute red granules; hence the term **granulation tissue.**

Early wound healing by granulation tissue is characterized by inflammatory cells, some debris, and a copious accumulation of fibroblasts and capillaries. Fibroblasts actively secrete extracellular matrix components: hyaluronic acid initially and sulfated pro-

(Text continues on p. 52)

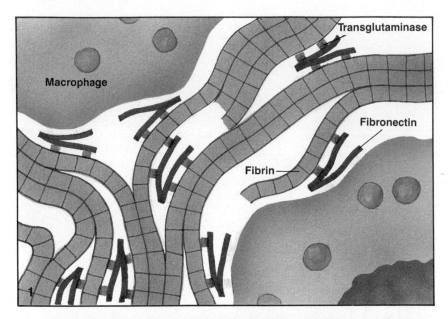

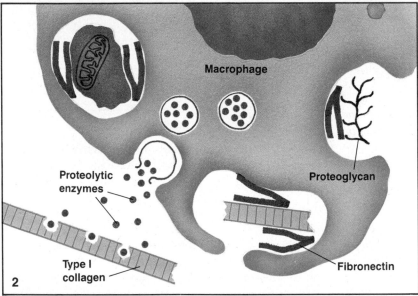

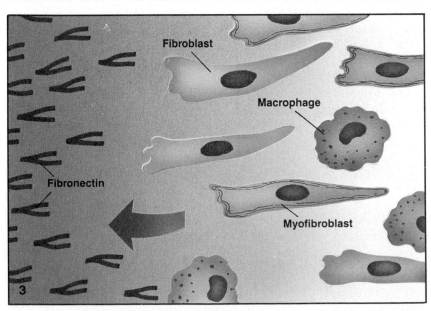

Figure 3-5. Summary of the healing process: The initial phase of the repair reaction, which typically begins with hemorrhage into the tissues. (*1*) A fibrin clot forms and fills the gap created by the wound. Fibronectin in the extravasated plasma can be cross-linked to fibrin, collagen, and other extracellular matrix components by the action of transglutaminases. This cross-linking provides a provisional mechanical stabilization of the wound. (*2*) Macrophages recruited to the wound area process cell remnants and damaged extracellular matrix. Fibronectin binding to cell membranes, collagens, proteoglycans, DNA, and bacteria facilitates phagocytosis (opsonization) of these elements; collagenases and other proteases secreted by leukocytes and macrophages contribute to the removal of debris. (*3*) Fibronectin, cell debris, and bacterial products are chemoattractants for a variety of cells that are recruited to the wound site.

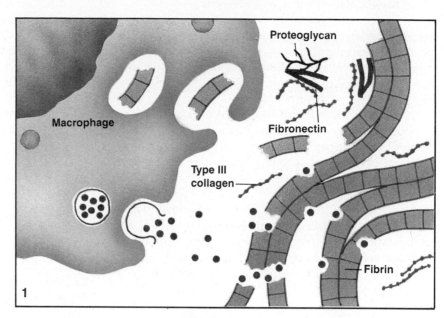

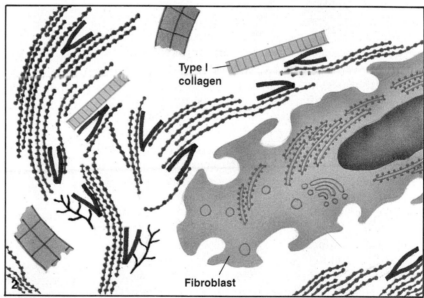

Figure 3-5 (continued). Intermediate phase of the repair reaction. (*1*) As a new extracellular matrix is deposited at the wound site, the initial fibrin clot is lysed by a combination of extracellular proteolytic enzymes and phagocytosis. (*2*) Concurrent with fibrin removal there is deposition of a temporary matrix formed by proteoglycans, glycoproteins, and type III collagen. (*3*) Final phase of the repair reaction. Eventually the temporary matrix is removed by a combination of extra- and intracellular digestion, and the definitive matrix, rich in type I collagen, is deposited.

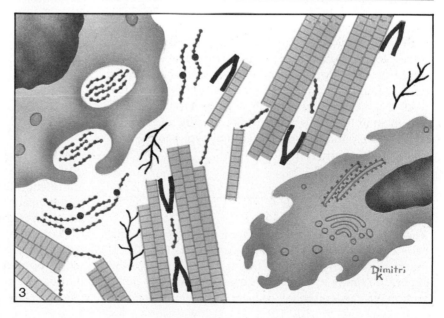

teoglycans later. Since proteoglycans are very hydrophilic, their accumulation contributes to the edematous appearance of wounds. Simultaneously with the synthesis and secretion of proteoglycans, fibronectin is produced.

In synthesis of collagen by fibroblasts begins within 24 hours of the injury although its deposition in the tissues is not apparent until 4 days. Initially, type III collagen predominates, but by day 7 to 8, type I is prominent, and it eventually becomes the major collagen of mature scar tissue.

After the initial stages of wound healing, tensile strength is established, capillaries are resorbed, and mobilization of the tissue begins. It is therefore necessary for collagen fibers and bundles to be reoriented according to new lines of stress. This reorientation is achieved by removal of the initially deposited collagen fibers and deposition of new ones. Despite an increased collagenase activity in the wound, collagen accumulates at a steady rate, usually reaching a maximum 2 to 3 months after the injury. **The tensile strength of the wound continues to increase many months after the collagen content has reached a maximum, a physical change that is clearly related to an increase in collagen cross-linking.** As the collagen content of the wound increases, many of the newly formed vessels disappear. This vascular involution, or **devascularization,** which takes place in a few weeks, dramatically transforms a richly vacularized tissue into a pale, avascular scar. Maturation of a scar, or **organization,** involves a devascularization, a decrease in the rate of collagen degradation, and the formation of stable intramolecular and intermolecular collagen cross-links.

We can summarize the process of wound healing (Fig. 3-5) as follows: the initial event at the site of injury is hemorrhage and clotting. The fibrin clot in stabilized by the cross-linking of fibronectin to fibrin by transglutaminases. Fibronectin, in turn, is chemotactic for macrophages and fibroblasts. The fibroblasts attracted to the area, perhaps stimulated by macrophage factors, secrete extracellular matrix components. The newly secreted proteoglycans and type III collagen specifically bind to fibronectin and provide tensile strength to the wound while the fibrin mesh is being lysed. Eventually, most of the proteoglycans, fibronectin, and type III collagen are removed and replaced by type I collagen to form a permanent scar.

REGENERATION

Regeneration is the replacement of lost tissue and cells by new tissues and cells. As long as there is no injury to underlying connective tissue, damage to the superficial lining epithelium is easily repaired by poliferation of the epithelial cells at the wound margin.

These cells detach from the underlying basement membrane and migrate into the denuded area without cell division. Division occurs in cells that are slightly behind the advancing edge. When the wound surface is completely covered, the cells attach themselves to the basement membrane. Differentiation proceeds and the normal thickness of the epithelium is restored.

A number of growth factors including **brain-, epidermal-, macrophage-, nerve-, and platelet-derived growth factors,** have been implicated in regeneration. Insulin, glucagen, and thyroid hormones, and even the extracellular matrix components fibronectin and laminin, also play a role.

HEALING BY PRIMARY AND SECONDARY INTENTION

It is traditional to make a distinction between the healing of the opposed edges of a cleanly incised wound—**healing by primary intention**—and the separated edges of a gouged wound—**healing by secondary intention.** Although the end results—minimal and prominent scarring, respectively—are clearly different, the basic mechanism is the same for both. The differences are quantitive, not qualitative (Fig. 3-6).

HEALING OF WOUNDS WITH APPOSED EDGES

In well-approximated wounds, within 48 hours a continuous layer of epithelial cells covers the wound. By the third or fourth day, granulation tissue (myofibroblasts, fibroblasts, and budding capillaries) invades the wound and collagen deposition begins. For the first month, tensile strength closely parallels the collagen content of the wound. The epithelial cells on the surface divide and differentiate, thus restoring a multilayered epithelium. As devascularization takes place in the granulation tissue, the scar decreases in **size** and changes from red to white. **Healing by primary intention is the desired result in surgical incisions.**

HEALING OF WOUNDS WITH SEPARATED EDGES

When there is extensive tissue loss, or simply a failure to approximate the wound edges, the defect is filled by granulation tissue. The main difference, therefore, between healing by primary and healing by secondary intention is the large defect that has to be replaced in the latter. **The difference is in the type of wound, not in the healing process.** Whereas healing of a wound with opposed edges is fast and leaves a small, often inapparent scar, healing of wounds with separated edges is slow and can result in large, deforming scars.

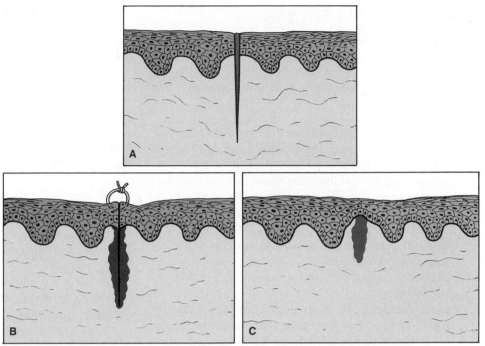

HEALING BY PRIMARY INTENTION (WOUNDS WITH APPOSED EDGES)

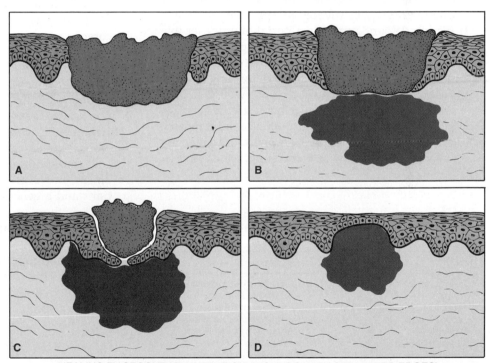

HEALING BY SECONDARY INTENTION (WOUNDS WITH SEPARATED EDGES)

Figure 3-6. Healing by primary intention: A wound with closely apposed edges and minimal tissue loss requires only minimal cell proliferation and neovascularization to heal. The result is a small scar. Healing by secondary intention: A gouged wound, in which the edges are far apart and in which there is substantial tissue loss, requires extensive cell proliferation, neovascularization, and scar formation to heal. Although the actual repair process is similar to that of healing by primary intention, healing by secondary intention results in a large scar that is functionally and cosmetically unsatisfactory.

FACTORS INFLUENCING WOUND HEALING

LOCAL FACTORS

A variety of local agents are known to influence wound healing (Table 3-3):

Type, size, and location of the wound. A clean, aseptic wound produced by the surgeon's scalpel heals faster than a wound produced by blunt trauma, which exhibits abundant necrosis and irregular edges. Small wounds of the latter type heal faster than large ones, and wounds in richly vascularized areas (e.g., the face) heal faster than those in poorly vascularized areas (e.g., the foot). Adhesion to bony surfaces, as in wounds over the tibia, prevents contraction and adequate apposition of the edges.

Vascular supply. Wounds with poor blood supply heal slowly. For example, the healing of leg wounds in patients with varicose veins is prolonged. Ischemia due to pressure produces bed sores and then prevents their healing. Ischemia due to arterial obstruction also prevents healing.

Infection. Wounds provide a portal of entry for microorganisms. Infection delays or prevents healing, promotes exuberant granulation tissue (proud flesh), and may result in large, deforming scars.

Movement. Early motion subjects the wound to persistent trauma. Exercise also increases the circulating levels of glucocorticoids, which inhibit repair.

Ionizing radiation. Irradiation leaves vascular lesions that interfere with blood supply and result in slow healing. Irradiation of the wound blocks cell proliferation, inhibits contraction, and retards granulation tissue formation.

Ultraviolet light. Exposure of wounds to ultraviolet light accelerates the rate of healing.

SYSTEMIC FACTORS

The following systemic factors influence wound healing (see Table 3-3).

Circulatory status. Cardiovascular status, because it determines the blood supply to the injured area, is important in wound healing. Poor healing attributed to old age is often due largely to impaired circulation.

Infection. Systemic infections delay wound healing.

Metabolic status. Poorly controlled **diabetes mellitus** prevents wound healing. Wounds in diabetics often become infected, and, in turn, an infection makes the control of diabetes difficult. The result is severe retardation or actual failure of healing. **Malnutrition** impedes wound healing. Methionine is needed for proper healing. Zinc, a cofactor of several enzymes, promotes faster healing in experimental animals. Vitamin C is required for collagen synthesis and secretion; **vitamin C deficiency (scurvy)** results in grossly deficient wound healing, with a lack of vascular proliferation and collagen deposition.

Hormones. Cortisone and other steroids impair wound healing, an effect attributed to inhibition of collagen synthesis. These hormones have many effects, however, including anti-inflammatory actions and a general depression of protein synthesis. It is therefore difficult to attribute their action on wound healing to any specific mechanism. Thyroid hormones, androgens, estrogens, and growth hormone have some influence on wound healing. This influence, however, may be due more to their effect on general metabolic status than to a specific effect on the healing process.

Table 3-3   Factors Influencing Wound Healing

LOCAL	SYSTEMIC
Type, size, and location of wound	Circulatory status (age)
Adequacy of blood supply	Metabolic status
Presence of infection	Presence of infection, diabetes, or neoplasia
Movement	Adequacy of levels of
Exposure to ionizing radiation	Vitamin C
Exposure to ultraviolet light	Amino acids (methionine)
Temperature deviation	Zinc
	Hormones
	Corticoids
	ACTH
	Iodothyronines
	Estrogens
	Growth hormone
	Temperature elevation

COMPLICATIONS OF WOUND HEALING

Abnormalities in any of the three basic healing processes—repair, contraction, and regeneration—result

---
Table 3-4 Complications of Wound Healing

Deficient Scar Formation
　　Dehiscence
　　Incisional hernias
　　Ulceration
　　　Vascular
　　　Neuropathic

Excessive Scar Formation
　　Hypertrophic scars and keloids

Excessive Contraction
　　Contracture of cicatrization

Excessive Regeneration

Miscellaneous
　　Painful scars
　　Pigmentary changes
　　Implantation

---

in the complications of wound healing summarized in Table 3-4.

DEFICIENT SCAR FORMATION

Inadequate formation of granulation tissue or inability to form a suitable extracellular matrix leads to deficient scar formation.

Wound Dehiscence and Incisional Hernias

Dehiscence, the bursting open of a wound, is of most concern after a laparotomy. Dehiscent abdomen, which occurs in 0.5% to 5% of all abdominal operations, carries a mortality of 30%. Increased mechanical stress on the wound from vomiting, coughing, or ileus is a factor in over 90% of the cases. Systemic factors include poor metabolic status, such as vitamin C deficiency, hypoproteinemia, and neoplasia. If insufficient extracellular matrix is deposited or there is inadequate cross-linking of the matrix, weak scars result. Incisional hernia is the late consequence of a weak abdominal scar.

Ulceration

Wounds ulcerate because of inadequate blood supply and vascularization. For example, leg wounds in persons with varicose veins or severe atherosclerosis typically ulcerate. Nonhealing wounds develop in areas devoid of sensation. Such **trophic or neuropathic ulcers** are occasionally seen in patients with spinal involvement from tertiary syphilis (tabes dorsalis) and in leprosy.

EXCESSIVE SCAR FORMATION

An excessive deposition of extracellular matrix at the wound site results in **hypertrophic scars** and **keloids.** Histologically there are abundant, broad, and irregular collagen bundles, with more capillaries and fibroblasts than expected for a scar of the same age. The rate of collagen synthesis, the ratio of type III to type I collagen, and the number of reducible cross-links remain high, a situation that indicates a "maturation arrest," or block, in the healing process.

EXCESSIVE CONTRACTION

A decrease in wound size depends on the presence of myofibroblasts, development of cell-cell contacts, and sustained cell contraction. An exaggeration of these processes is termed **contracture** and results in severe deformity of the wound and surrounding tissues. Interestingly, the regions that normally show minimal wound contraction (such as the palms of the hands, the soles of the feet, and the anterior aspect of the thorax) are the ones prone to contractures. Contracture is particularly dramatic in the healing of skin burns, especially second- and third-degree burns. A contracture can be severe enough to block joints and close natural openings. Contracture also has serious consequences in the gastrointestinal tract, where an excessive proliferation of myofibroblasts leads to constrictive rings. Esophageal stricture following the ingestion of a caustic chemical is an example.

HEALING IN SPECIFIC TISSUES

LIVER

Liver injury results in complete parenchymal regeneration, scar formation, or a combination of both. The outcome depends on the location, extent, and chronicity of the insult.

Recovery after focal necrosis is by regeneration. The normal architecture is restored and no fibrosis occurs, because the extracellular matrix framework is not affected. After massive hepatic necrosis, in patients who survive, the remaining hepatocytes regenerate. However, because the extracellular matrix framework is destroyed, regeneration forms irregular hepatocyte nodules that are separated by broad scars. Repeated hepatic injury that destroys the extracellular matrix framework elicits a mixture of regeneration and fibrosis; the result is **cirrhosis.**

KIDNEY

The kidney has a limited regenerative capacity. If the injury is not extensive and the extracellular matrix framework is not destroyed, tubular epithelium regenerates. In most clinically relevant lesions, however, there is some destruction of the extracellular matrix framework. Regeneration is incomplete, and repair with scar formation is the usual outcome. The regenerative capacity of renal tissue is maximal in cortical tubules, minimal in medullary tubules, and nonexistent in glomeruli.

CORTICAL TUBULES

The outcome of injury to renal tubules depends on whether or not the tubular basement membrane is ruptured. If the injury does not produce discontinuities in the tubular basement membrane, the surviving tubular cells in the vicinity of the wound flatten, acquire a squamoid appearance, and migrate into the necrotic area along the basement membrane. Mitoses are frequent, and occasional clusters of epithelial cells project into the lumen. Within a week, the flattened cells are more cuboidal, and differentiated cytoplasmic elements appear. Tubular morphology and function are normal by 3 to 4 weeks.

When the tubular basement membrane is ruptured, we speak of **tubulorrhexis.** The sequence of events resembles that for tubular damage in which the basement membrane is intact, except that interstitial changes are more prominent. There is fibroblast proliferation, increased extracellular matrix deposition, and collapse of the tubular lumen. The final result is regeneration of some tubules and fibrosis of others, usually with a loss of functional nephrons.

MEDULLARY TUBULES

If the lesion is not fatal, the necrotic tissue sloughs into the urine. The surviving stump heals, and extensive fibrosis produces intrarenal obstruction. Although there is some epithelial proliferation, there is no significant regeneration.

GLOMERULI

Unlike tubules, glomeruli do not regenerate. Injuries that produce necrosis of glomerular endothelial or epithelial cells, whether focal, segmental, or diffuse, heal by scarring (glomerulosclerosis). Mesangial cells seem to have some capacity for regeneration.

LUNG

ALVEOLAR INJURY WITH INTACT BASEMENT MEMBRANES

Alveolar injury occurs in many pneumonitides and with acute exposures to toxic fumes. Following injury, there is a variable degree of alveolar cell necrosis. The alveoli are flooded with an inflammatory exudate particularly rich in plasma proteins. **As long as the alveolar basement membrane remains intact, healing is by regeneration, and the alveolar exudate is cleared by neutrophils and macrophages.** If these fail to lyse the alveolar exudate, it is organized by granulation tissue, and intra-alveolar fibrosis results. The alveolar type II pneumocytes are the alveolar reserve cells. After injury they migrate to denuded areas and undergo mitosis to generate cells with features intermediate between those of type I and type II pneumocytes. As they establish contact with other epithelial cells, mitosis stops and the cells differentiate into type I pneumocytes.

ALVEOLAR INJURY WITH RUPTURED BASEMENT MEMBRANES

Extensive damage to the alveolar basement membrane usually elicits a repair reaction that results in scarring and fibrosis. Mesenchymal cells from the alveolar septa proliferate and differentiate into fibroblasts and myofibroblasts. The myofibroblasts and fibroblasts migrate into the alveolar space, where they secrete extracellular matrix components—mainly type I collagen and proteoglycans. Scarring is the end result.

HEART

Myocardial cells have no regenerative capacity. Therefore, irreversible injuries to the heart heal only by repair, with formation of granulation tissue and scarring.

NERVOUS SYSTEM

Mature neurons are permanent post-mitotic cells and cannot divide. Following trauma, neuronal connections can be reestablished only by regrowth and reorganization of the cell processes of surviving neurons. Whereas the peripheral nervous system has the capacity for axonal regeneration, the central nervous system lacks it.

CENTRAL NERVOUS SYSTEM

Axonal regeneration seems to require contact with extracellular fluid containing plasma proteins. Any damage to the brain or spinal cord is followed by capillary growth and **astrocytic** and **microglial proliferation. Gliosis** in the central nervous system is the equivalent of scar formation elsewhere; once established, it remains permanently. Axonal regeneration does occur in the hypothalamic–hypophyseal region, where glial and capillary barriers do not interfere with axonal regeneration.

PERIPHERAL NERVOUS SYSTEM

Neurons in the peripheral nervous system can regenerate their axons, and under ideal circumstances section of a peripheral nerve eventuates in complete functional recovery. However, if the cut ends are not in perfect alignment, granulation tissue grows between them, resulting in a traumatic neuroma. The regenerative capacity of the peripheral nervous system can be ascribed to the late restoration of the blood–nerve barrier (2 to 3 months) and to the presence of Schwann cells with basement membranes.

4

IMMUNOPATHOLOGY

KENT J. JOHNSON, STEPHEN W. CHENSUE, STEVEN L. KUNKEL, AND PETER A. WARD

CELLULAR COMPONENTS OF THE IMMUNE RESPONSE

The immune system comprises an exquisitely complex network of cellular and humoral elements that promote defense against a vast spectrum of microbial agents, ranging from viruses to multicellular parasites. Many of the cellular and humoral components of this system have been described in Chapter 2. Here, we extend the discussion of the cells that orchestrate immune responses and describe the immunopathologic manifestations of exaggerated or dysfunctional immune responses.

LYMPHOCYTES

Lymphocytes, because they have the capacity to recognize and react with specific foreign molecules, are primary directors of antigen-specific immune responses. In the traditional model of lymphocyte development all followed one of two major pathways of development (Fig. 4-1). They originate from primitive yolk sac stem cell precursors that, depending on subsequent migration and molecular signals, become either T cells or B cells. However, a third class of lymphocytes lacking the defining characteristics of T and B cells has also been recognized. The ontogeny of these "null" cells is unclear. The natural killer cells, which are described later, belong in this category. T- and B-lymphocytes are defined on the basis of several functional and phenotypic characteristics acquired during their ontogeny.

T CELLS

Figure 4-2 summarizes T cell ontogeny in the thymus. The stem cell precursors interact with thymic epithelium, which provides the molecular signals that cause sequential expression of genes conferring the specific functional and phenotypic characteristics of T cells. A spectrum of functionally related T cell membrane antigens has been defined with monoclonal antibody reagents, thus enabling the maturational stage of the T cell to be identified. **T cells at different stages of maturation are characterized by the surface markers they express.** T cells acquire a different complement of markers as they migrate from cortex to medulla and finally to peripheral blood and lymphatics.

In the medulla, the T4 and T8 antigens define two separate cell populations, which display helper and suppressor/cytotoxic functions, respectively. **In the blood and peripheral lymphoid organs, T4+ cells comprise 65% and T8+ cells 35% of all T cells.**

T cells recognize specific antigens—usually proteins or haptens bound to proteins—and respond as directed by endogenous maturational factors and exogenous molecular signals. Experimental studies suggest that T4+ and T8+ cells are, in fact, subsets of T cells that have varied effector or regulatory functions. **Effector functions include secretion of proinflammatory mediators and cytotoxic responses to cells containing foreign or altered membrane antigens. Regulatory functions include augmentation or suppression of immune responses, usually by secretion of specific helper or suppressor molecules.** One such helper molecule is **interleukin-2 (IL-2),** which promotes the growth of activated T cells. **In general, T4+ cells perform helper functions and secrete proinflammatory lymphokines. By contrast, T8+ cells generally perform suppressor and cytotoxic functions.** Clearly, however, there is overlap, since T8+ cells secrete lymphokines and T4+ cells induce suppressor activity. A summary of some of the important T cell lymphokines and their effects is provided in Table 4-1.

An interesting aspect of T cell antigen recognition is the requirement for antigens to be presented in the context of self-histocompatibility membrane proteins. In other words, T cells have a membrane receptor complex that, for a maximal immune response, must interact not only with foreign but also with self-histocompatibility molecular structures. The relevant histocompatibility antigens are derived from genes in the **major histocompatibility complex** (MHC). This region codes for class I and class II membrane proteins, a subject that will be discussed in greater detail below.

B CELLS

B cells are defined as lymphocytes that bear membrane immunoglobulin and under appropriate conditions differentiate into antibody-secreting cells. B cell maturation is illustrated in Figure 4-1.

Pre-B cells contain cytoplasmic heavy-chain μ immunoglobulins but no light-chain or surface immunoglobulins. Immature B cells are recognized by the appearance of surface monomeric IgM. With subsequent maturation involving gene rearrangements, B cells acquire surface IgD.

The next stage of B cell development involves further gene rearrangements, a process that results in **isotype switching.** In other words, in the absence of antigenic stimulation, a proportion of the B cell clones proceed to express other heavy-chain isotypes: IgG (γ_1, γ_2, γ_3), IgA (α_1 or α_2), or IgE (ϵ). In the presence of antigen, T

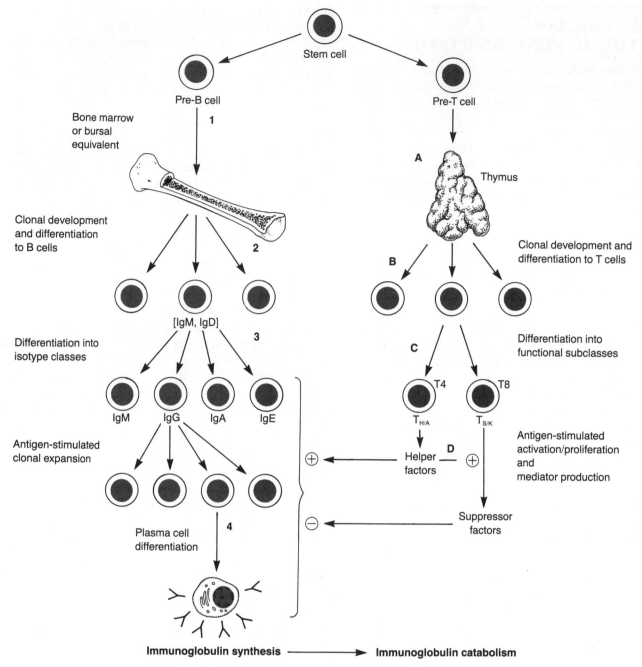

Figure 4-1. Major maturational stages of lymphocytes.

cells produce differentiation factors that either stimulate B cell isotype switching or induce the proliferation of particular committed isotype populations.

Mature B cells are primarily in a resting state, awaiting activation by foreign antigen. Activation involves cross-linking of membrane immunoglobulin receptors by antigens presented on accessory cells. This initial stimulus leads to proliferation and clonal expansion, which can be amplified by macrophage-and T cell-derived factors, such as interleukin-1 (IL-1) and B cell growth factor. If no further signal is provided, the proliferating B cells return to the resting state and enter the **memory cell** pool.

The final stage of B cell differentiation into antibody-synthesizing plasma cells generally requires exposure to additional T cell products—for instance, B

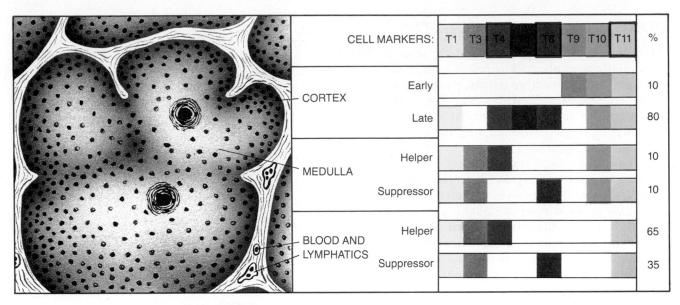

Figure 4-2. Membrane marker changes during thymic T cell maturation.

cell differentiation factors. This is the case for responses to most protein antigens. However, some polyvalent agents directly induce B cell proliferation and antibody synthesis, bypassing the requirements for B cell growth and differentiation factors. Such agents are called polyclonal B cell activators because they do not interact with antigen-binding sites and hence are not antigen-specific. Examples of these antigens are bacterial products (lipopolysaccharide, protein A) and certain viruses (Epstein-Barr virus, cytomegalovirus).

It is noteworthy that the spectrum of immunoglobulins produced during immune responses changes with age. Neonates tend to produce predominantly IgM; in contrast, older children and adults show rapid shifts toward IgG synthesis following antigenic challenge. Thus, B cell responses continue to be modified during early childhood.

In addition to antibodies, B cells also produce lymphokines that modulate immune responses.

NATURAL KILLER CELLS

One population of lymphocytes has the capacity to recognize directly and kill various tumor and virus-infected cells in vitro. These large lymphocytes with cytoplasmic granules cannot be precisely classified as T, B, or myelomonocytic cells. Thus, they represent a subset of so-called **null** cells and are termed **natural killer (NK) cells.** These cells may have several receptors for various target cell membrane structures.

Natural killer cells are affected by several molecular mediators. For example, interleukin-2 supports their growth, and interferons promote their killing activity. By contrast, prostaglandin E_2 is highly suppressive of NK cell activity.

NK cells also seem to have Fc receptors and thus kill target cells by an antibody-dependent mechanism. This null cell function was previously attributed to a population of K (killer) cells.

Table 4-1   T Cell Products and Their Biologic Activity

LYMPHOKINE	TARGET CELL AND ACTION
B cell growth factor (BCGF)	Stimulates proliferation and differentiation of B cells
B cell differentiation factor (BCDF)	Causes differentiation of terminal plasma cells
Colony stimulating factor (CSF)	Stimulates differentiation of monocytes from bone marrow stem cells
Fibroblast activating factor (FAF)	Promotes proliferation of fibroblasts
Gamma-interferon (γIF)	Activates macrophages and promotes cytotoxic functions
Interleukin-2 (IL-2)	Stimulates proliferation of activated T cells
Interleukin-3 (IL-3)	Stimulates differentiation of bone marrow stem cells
Leukocyte inhibition factor (LIF)	Inhibits random migration of neutrophils
Lymphotoxin (LT)	Kills target tumor or virus-infected cells
Migration inhibition factor (MIF)	Inhibits random migration of macrophages

MONONUCLEAR PHAGOCYTES

"Mononuclear phagocyte" is a general term applied to populations of phagocytic cells found in virtually all organs and connective tissues. Among these cells are macrophages, monocytes, Kupffer cells of the liver, and the so-called histiocytes. These cells are identified by their nonsegmented nuclei, relatively abundant cytoplasm, and phagocytic function. In the lung, liver, and spleen, large numbers of macrophages populate sinuses and capillaries to form an effective filtering system that removes effete cells and foreign particulate material from the blood. This system was formerly known as **the reticuloendothelial system** but is also termed the **mononuclear phagocytic system.** In addition to this housekeeping role, macrophages play a critical role in the induction of immune responses, as well as in the maintenance and resolution of inflammatory reactions.

Macrophages are important accessory cells by virtue of their expression of class II histocompatibility antigens. They actively ingest and process antigens for presentation to T cells in conjunction with class II antigens. The subsequent T cell responses are further amplified by macrophage-derived monokines. One of the best-characterized of these is interleukin-1 (previously known as T cell growth factor), which promotes the expression of interleukin-2 receptor by T cells, thereby augmenting interleukin-2-driven T cell proliferation. **Interleukin-1 also has a broad spectrum of effects on other tissues and, in general, prepares the body to combat infection—for example, it induces fever and promotes catabolic metabolism.**

Macrophages are dominant participants in subacute and chronic inflammatory reactions. During inflammation, increased numbers of monocytes are recruited from the bone marrow. Under chemotactic influences they migrate to sites of inflammation and mature into macrophages. Both recruited and local tissue macrophages participate and proliferate at these foci. Table 4-2 summarizes some of the many secretory products of macrophages that can play a role at sites of inflammation. Among these are proteins, lipids, nucleotides, and reactive oxygen metabolites. Functionally, these molecules are digestive, opsonic, cytotoxic, growth promoting, or growth inhibiting. Thus, macrophages are ideal cells both to effect and to direct inflammatory events, locally and systemically.

The functional activity of macrophages and the spectrum of molecules they produce are regulated by external factors, such as T cell-derived lymphokines. Macrophages exposed to such factors become "activated"; that is, they acquire a greater capacity to release oxygen metabolites and kill tumor cells and intracellular microbes.

Table 4-2   *Major Macrophage Products*

Proteins

Enzymes:
  Neutral proteinases (e.g., plasminogen
    activator, elastase, collagenases)
  Lysozyme
  Arginase
  Lipoprotein lipase
  Angiotensin-converting enzyme
  Acid hydrolases
Plasma proteins:
  Coagulation proteins
  Complement components
  α_2-Macroglobulin
  Fibronectin
Monokines:
  Interleukin-1
  Tumor necrosis factor
  Interferon alpha
  Angiogenesis factor

Reactive Oxygen Species

Superoxide anion
Hydrogen peroxide
Oxygen radicals

Bioactive Lipids

Prostaglandin E_2
Prostacyclin I_2
Thromboxane B_2
Leukotriene B_4, C_4, D_4, E_4
Hydroxyeicosatetraenoic acids

Nucleotides

Thymidine, uracil
cAMP
Uric acid

MAJOR HISTOCOMPATIBILITY COMPLEX (MHC)

The major histocompatibility complex (MHC) antigens or **human leukocyte antigens (HLA)** are proteins that are highly polymorphic within the human population. They are **the main target antigens during rejection of transplanted organs.** Such antigens allow for self-recognition during cell-cell interactions, especially in immune responses.

The HLA gene complex is located on the short arm of chromosome 6 (Fig. 4-3). Three major classes of molecules, designated I, II, and III, are coded for.

The class I antigens, the first MHC antigens to be defined using the sera of multiparous women, are coded for by genes in the A, B, and C regions. The alleles that occupy these three class I loci are expressed codominantly. Thus, tissues bear antigens for both parents. **Class I antigens are recognized by cytotoxic T cells during graft rejection or during killing of virus-infected cells.**

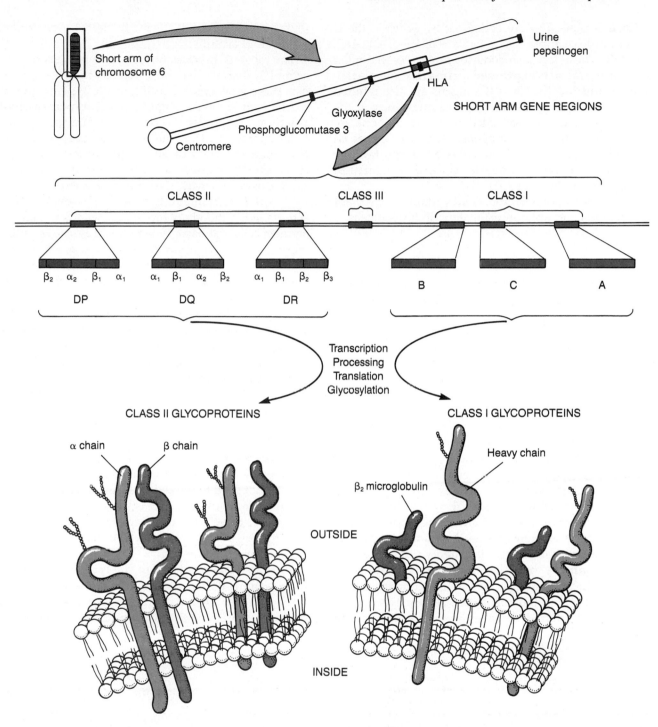

Figure 4-3. The genes of the human major histocompatibility complex (MHC) and their protein products.

Class II molecules are coded for by genes in the D region; at least three major loci are defined: DP, DQ, and DR. These loci also code for molecules of similar structure and **are expressed primarily on macrophages and B cells.** Class II antigens are also referred to as Ia antigens because they are analogous to the mouse MHC genes associated with the immune response. As with class I antigens, alleles are expressed codominantly. **Class II molecules are important for interactions between immune cells, particularly in antigen presentation to T cells.**

The class III antigens represent certain complement components and are not histocompatibility antigens.

IMMUNOLOGICALLY MEDIATED TISSUE INJURY

Although the immune response is a protective mechanism, it is apparent that immune responses often lead to tissue damage. Many inflammatory diseases are based on immune mechanisms. A wide variety of foreign substances (dust, pollen, bacteria, viruses, etc.) are capable of acting as antigens and provoking a protective immune response. In certain situations the protective effects of the immune response give way to deleterious events that may produce temporary discomfort or substantial injury to the host. For example, in the process of phagocytizing and destroying bacteria, phagocytic cells (neutrophils and macrophages) often cause injury to the surrounding tissue. **An immune response that results in tissue injury is broadly referred to as a "hypersensitivity" reaction and is associated with a group of diseases categorized as immune or immunologically mediated disorders.** Immune-or hypersensitivity-mediated diseases are common; among

them are asthma, hay fever, hepatitis, glomerulonephritis, and arthritis.

The most useful classification of hypersensitivity reactions is that of Gell and Coombs (Table 4-3), which lists these reactions according to the type of immune mechanism involved. **Types I to III hypersensitivity reactions all require the formation of a specific antibody against an exogenous or endogenous antigen. However, the class of antibody formed varies, and the antibody class is a critical determinant in the mechanism by which tissue injury occurs.**

In **type I, or immediate-type, hypersensitivity reactions,** IgE antibody is formed and binds to receptors on mast cells and basophils. In the presence of antigen reactive with the IgE, products are released from these cells—a sequence that results in the development of the characteristic symptoms of diseases such as asthma or anaphylaxis.

In **type II hypersensitivity reactions,** IgG or IgM antibody is formed against an antigen, usually on a cell surface or (less commonly) on a component of extracellular matrix, such as basement membrane. This antigen–antibody coupling causes complement activation, which in turn is responsible for causing lysis (cytotoxicity) of the cell or damage to the extracellular matrix.

In **type III hypersensitivity reactions,** the antibody responsible for tissue injury is also IgM or IgG, but here the mechanism of tissue injury differs. The antigen is usually not fixed to the cell surface, but circulates in the vascular compartment and is eventually deposited in tissues. In those sites complement activation leads to recruitment of leukocytes, which are responsible for the subsequent tissue injury.

Type IV (cell-mediated or delayed-hypersensitivity) reactions do not require the formation of an antibody. Rather, there is antigenic activation of T-lymphocytes, usually with the help of macrophages. The

Table 4-3   Classification of Hypersensitivity Reactions

TYPE	IMMUNOLOGIC MECHANISM	EXAMPLES
Type I (anaphylactic type): Immediate hypersensitivity	IgE antibody mediated—mast cell activation and degranulation	Hay fever, asthma, anaphylaxis
Type II (cytotoxic type): Cytotoxic antibodies	Cytotoxic (IgG, IgM) antibodies formed against cell surface antigens. Complement is usually involved.	Autoimmune hemolytic anemias, antibody-dependent cellular cytotoxicity (ADCC), Goodpasture's disease
Type III (immune complex type): Immune complex disease	Antibodies (IgG, IgM, IgA) formed against exogenous or endogenous antigens. Complement and leukocytes (neutrophils, macrophages) are often involved.	Autoimmune diseases (SLE, rheumatoid arthritis), most types of glomerulonephritis
Type IV (cell-mediated type): Delayed type hypersensitivity	Mononuclear cells (T lymphocytes, macrophages) with interleukin and lymphokine production	Granulomatous diseases (tuberculosis, sarcoidosis)

products of either activated lymphocytes or macrophages lead to subsequent tissue injury.

TYPE I HYPERSENSITIVITY: IMMEDIATE TYPE OR ANAPHYLAXIS

Immediate-type hypersensitivity or anaphylaxis is manifested by a localized or generalized reaction that occurs immediately (within minutes) after exposure to an antigen to which the individual has previously become sensitized. The reactions depend on the site of antigen exposure. For example, when the reactions involve the skin, the characteristic local reaction is swelling and edema **(hives).** Another common example of the localized manifestations of immediate hypersensitivity is hay fever, which involves the upper respiratory tract and conjunctiva, causing sneezing and conjunctivitis. In its generalized, most severe form, the immediate hypersensitivity reaction is associated with bronchial constriction, airway obstruction, and circulatory collapse, as seen in the **anaphylactic syndrome.** Fortunately, severe anaphylaxis reactions are rare, even though immediate-type hypersensitivity reactions, particularly of the localized variety, are common (millions of people every year have allergic rhinitis).

The mechanism involved in all immediate hypersensitivity reactions is related to the formation of IgE antibody. **IgE antibodies are formed by a T cell-dependent mechanism and bind avidly to Fc receptors on mast cells and basophils.** This avid and specific binding accounts for the term "cytotropic" antibody. An individual, once exposed to a specific allergen that has resulted in formation of IgE, is "sensitized," in the sense that subsequent responses to the allergen induce the immediate hypersensitivity reaction. It should also be stressed that IgE bound to receptors on mast cells and basophils persists for long periods of time (weeks), a feature unique to IgE. **The reaction of antigen with IgE coupled to the surface receptor activates mast cells and basophils, an event that releases the potent inflammatory mediators that are responsible for the development of the hypersensitivity reactions.** As shown in Figure 4-4, the antigen (allergen) binds to IgE antibody via its Fab sites. A binding or bridging of the antigen to more than one IgE antibody molecule, attached to receptors on mast cells and basophils, activates the cells. Cells can also be activated by agents other than antibodies. As shown in Figure 4-4, the complement anaphylatoxin peptides, C3a and C5a, directly stimulate mast cells by a different receptor-mediated process to cause release of granule constituents

or the rapid synthesis and release of other mediators. Other compounds, including mellitin (from bee venom) and drugs (morphine, for example), also directly activate mast cells and cause release of granule constituents.

No matter how the mast cell activation sequence is initiated, calcium influx into the cell cytoplasm is required, with the subsequent secretion of two main groups of products: preformed and inflammatory mediators. Potent preformed mediators are rapidly released from granules. Because they are preformed and stored in granules, these mediators exert immediate biologic effects following their release. Of the granule constituents listed in Figure 4-5, histamine is perhaps the most important. **Histamine causes rapid contraction of airway smooth muscles as well as an increase in vascular permeability. These effects account for the classic early manifestations of immediate hypersensitivity: bronchospasm, vascular congestion, and edema.** Other preformed products released from mast cell granules are heparin, proteolytic enzymes, and at least two chemotactic factors: a neutrophil chemotactic factor and an eosinophil chemotactic factor, the latter being responsible for the accumulation of eosinophils so characteristic of immediate hypersensitivity.

When the mast cell is activated, the synthesis of potent inflammatory mediators is also initiated. Foremost among these mediators are the various products of the arachidonic acid pathway that are formed following the activation of phospholipase, as discussed in Chapter 2. Another inflammatory mediator synthesized by the mast cell is platelet activating factor (PAF), a lipid derived from phospholipids (see Chapter 2).

In summary, the type I (immediate) hypersensitivity reaction is characterized by a specific cytotropic antibody that binds to receptors on basophils and mast cells and reacts with a specific antigen. This results in the activation of mast cells and basophils and the release of preformed (granule) products as well as the synthesis of mediators that cause the classic manifestations of immediate hypersensitivity.

TYPE II HYPERSENSITIVITY: CYTOTOXIC TYPE

Type II hypersensitivity reactions are also caused by an antigen–antibody reaction but, as the name implies, the antibodies formed are often cytotoxic and are directed against antigens on cell surfaces or in connective tissues. IgG and IgM are the classes of antibody usually involved in these reactions. The most

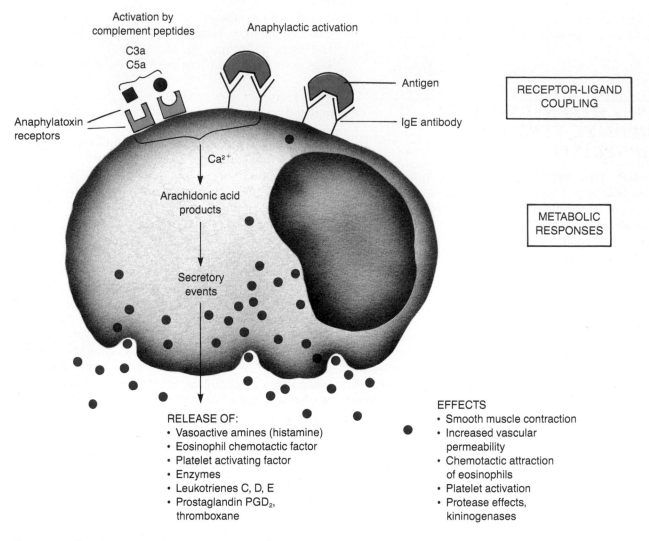

Activation by
complement peptides

Anaphylactic activation

C3a
C5a

Antigen

RECEPTOR-LIGAND
COUPLING

Anaphylatoxin
receptors

IgE antibody

Ca²⁺

Arachidonic acid
products

METABOLIC
RESPONSES

Secretory
events

RELEASE OF:
• Vasoactive amines (histamine)
• Eosinophil chemotactic factor
• Platelet activating factor
• Enzymes
• Leukotrienes C, D, E
• Prostaglandin PGD₂,
  thromboxane

EFFECTS
• Smooth muscle contraction
• Increased vascular
  permeability
• Chemotactic attraction
  of eosinophils
• Platelet activation
• Protease effects,
  kininogenases

Figure 4-4. Type I hypersensitivity. Activation of the mast cell and the potent inflammatory mediators released or synthesized by the cell.

important characteristic of these antibodies is their ability to activate the complement system via Fc receptors. There are several antibody-dependent mechanisms of cytotoxicity.

The classical model of antibody-mediated cytotoxicity of red blood cells is illustrated in Figure 4-5. IgM or IgG antibody binds to an antigen on the surface of the erythrocyte membrane. As discussed in Chapter 2, this antibody binding induces activation of the complement system via the classical pathway through interaction with C1q. Once activated, complement leads to the destruction of the target cell by two distinct mechanisms. Complement products directly lyse the target cells, as shown in Figure 4-5, by the formation of a complex of C5b–9 complement components. This complex is referred to as the "membrane attack com-

plex" because of its ability to form "holes" or ionic channels in the cell membrane, thus inducing lysis of the cell. This type of cell lysis in human diseases is exemplified in certain types of autoimmune hemolytic anemias caused by the formation of cold reactive antibodies against erythrocyte blood group antigens. In transfusion reactions, in which hemolysis occurs as a result of a major blood group incompatibility, there is a potent activation of complement and red blood cell destruction because the isoantibodies (anti A and anti B) of humans are of the IgM class.

Complement also indirectly enhances the destruction of a target cell by opsonization. As shown in Figure 4-6, this involves complement interaction on the target cell surface, with the formation of C3b. Many phagocytic cells, including neutrophils and macrophages,

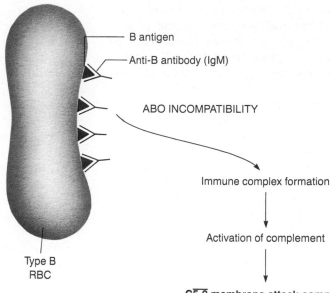

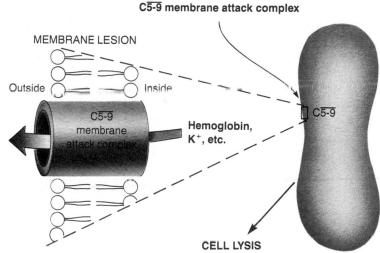

Figure 4-5. Type II hypersensitivity. Antibody- and complement-mediated red cell lysis due to complement activation and the formation of the C5–9 membrane attack complex (MAC).

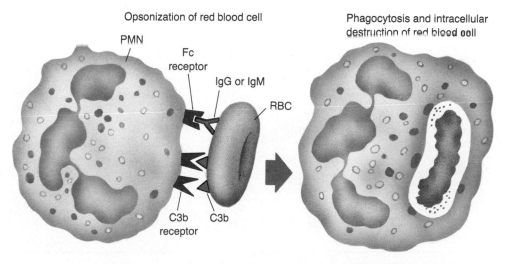

Figure 4-6. Type II hypersensitivity. Antibody- and complement-dependent opsonization.

contain receptors for C3b on the cell membrane. Thus, **C3b bridges the target cell and the effector (phagocytic) cell, enhancing phagocytosis and intracellular destruction of the complement-coated cell.** Certain types of autoimmune hemolytic anemias and some drug reactions are mediated by this type of complement-associated opsonization.

In the two examples of type II hypersensitivity (cytotoxicity) already discussed, complement activation is required for the destruction of the target cell. There is another type of antibody-mediated cytotoxicity that does not require participation of the complement system. **This type of cytotoxicity is referred to as antibody-dependent, cell-mediated cytotoxicity (ADCC) and involves the destruction of antibody-coated cells by leukocytes that attack the antibody-coated target cells via Fc receptors.** Effector cells involved in these types of reactions are phagocytic cells, as well as a type of lymphocyte referred to as a null or K cell. The mechanism by which the target cell is destroyed in these reactions is not clear. It appears that these effector cells synthesize homologues of terminal complement proteins, and these homologues may be related to the cytotoxic events. Antibody-dependent, cell-mediated cytotoxicity may be involved in the pathogenesis of some autoimmune diseases, such as autoimmune thyroiditis.

In some type II reactions, antibody binding to a specific target cell receptor does not lead to death of the cell, but rather to physiologic changes in the target cells. As shown in Figure 4-7, the autoimmune diseases thyroiditis (Grave's disease) and myasthenia gravis feature autoantibodies against cell receptors for hormones such as TSH and acetylcholine, respectively. In thyroiditis the autoantibody against the receptor (referred to as "long-acting thyroid stimulator") mimics the effect of TSH, thereby stimulating thyroid acinar cells. By contrast, in myasthenia gravis the autoantibody competes for the acetylcholine receptor in the neuromuscular end plate and inhibits synaptic transmission. Autoantibodies have also been described for receptors for insulin, prolactin, and growth hormone.

Finally, some type II hypersensitivity reactions occur as a result of the formation of antibody against a connective tissue component. Classic examples are Goodpasture's syndrome and the bullous skin diseases pemphigus and pemphigoid. In these diseases there is evidence of a circulating antibody against a fixed connective tissue antigen. The antibody binds to the antigen in the tissues and evokes a local inflammatory response. In the case of Goodpasture's disease (Fig. 4-8), an autoantibody binds to an antigen, or antigens, in pulmonary and glomerular basement membranes.

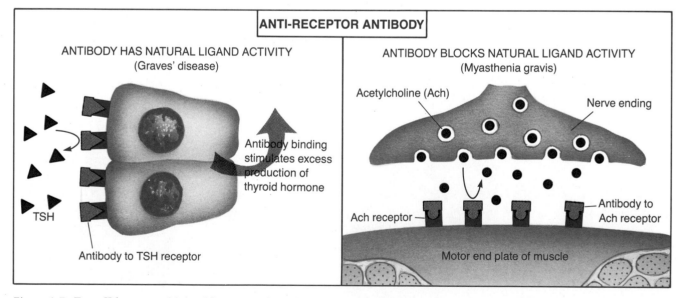

Figure 4-7. Type II hypersensitivity. Noncytotoxic antireceptor antibody in Graves' disease and myasthenia gravis.

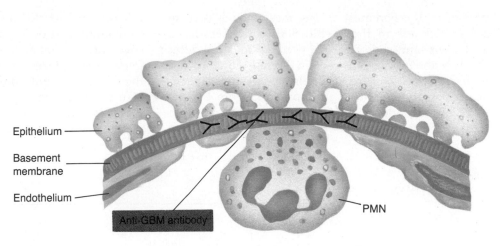

Figure 4-8. Type II hypersensitivity. Antibody against glomerular basement membrane antigens in Goodpasture's disease.

Complement activation occurs locally, and injury develops because of recruitment of neutrophils into the site, although direct complement damage to the basement membrane via formation of the membrane attack complex may also be involved.

In summary, type II hypersensitivity reactions are generally directly or indirectly cytotoxic and involve the formation of antibodies against antigens on cell surfaces or in connective tissues. Complement is required for many of these cytotoxic events. Lysis is mediated directly by complement or indirectly by opsonization or the chemotactic attraction of phagocytic cells. Complement-independent reactions, such as antibody-dependent, cell-mediated cytotoxicity also fall into this category. Many human diseases, including the autoimmune hemolytic anemias, Goodpasture's syndrome, pemphigus and pemphigoid, Graves' disease, and myasthenia gravis are mediated by type II hypersensitivity reactions.

TYPE III HYPERSENSITIVITY: IMMUNE COMPLEX DISEASES

Type III hypersensitivity reactions involve tissue injury mediated by immune complexes. IgM, IgG, or IgA is formed against a circulating antigen or one derived from tissues. Primarily on the basis of the physiochemical characteristics of the immune complexes, such as size, charge, and so on, antigen–antibody complexes formed in the circulation are deposited in tissues, including the renal glomerulus, skin capillary venules, choroid plexus, lung, and synovium. Once deposited in tissues, immune complexes call forth an inflammatory response by activating complement, thereby leading to chemotactic recruitment of neutrophils or macrophages to the site. These cells are then activated and release their tissue-damaging substances, such as proteases and oxygen radicals.

Immune complexes have been implicated in the pathogenesis of many human diseases. The most compelling case is one in which the demonstration of immune complexes in the injured tissue correlates with the development of the injury. A convincing example of this is the lesions of periarteritis nodosa, in which medium-size arteries contain immune complexes of IgG and the hepatitis virus antigen (HB$_s$Ag) in the vessel wall. In many diseases immune complexes are detected in plasma without concomitant evidence of tissue injury. The physiochemical properties of circulating complexes differ from those of complexes deposited in tissues, the presence of which is correlated with tissue injury. The diseases that seem to be most clearly attributable to immune complexes are autoimmune diseases of connective tissue, such as systemic lupus erythematosus and rheumatoid arthritis, some types of vasculitis, and most varieties of glomerulonephritis.

Several experimental models of immune complex injury allow a precise definition of the mediation of this type of injury. Foremost among these models is acute serum sickness in the rabbit. Serum sickness is an acute, self-limited disease that occurs 6 to 8 days after the injection of a foreign protein (bovine albumin) and is characterized by fever, arthralgias, vasculitis, and an acute glomerulonephritis. As shown in Figure 4-9, the levels of exogenously injected antigen in the circulation remain constant until about day 6, at which time they fall rapidly. At the same time, immune complexes (containing IgM or IgG and the antigen) appear in the circulation. Simultaneously, some of these circulating immune complexes begin to deposit in tissues such as the renal glomeruli and blood vessels. As shown in Figure 4-9, tissue deposition of these immune complexes is enhanced by their interaction with the complement system, a process that renders the complexes

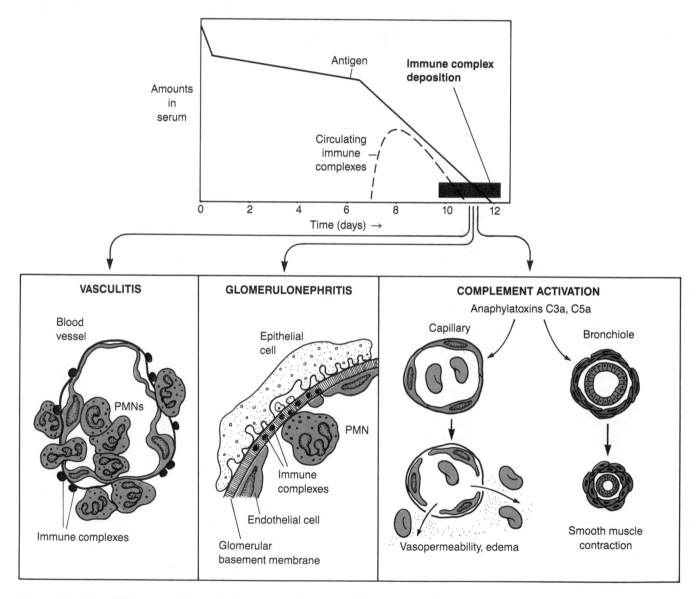

Figure 4-9. Type III hypersensitivity. In the serum sickness model of immune complex tissue injury, antibody forms against a circulating antigen and immune complexes form in the circulation. These complexes deposit in tissues such as blood vessels and glomeruli and, augmented by complement activation, induce tissue injury.

more soluble. The interaction with complement also generates C3a and C5a, which increase vascular permeability.

Once immune complexes are deposited in tissues, they induce an inflammatory response. The mediation of this response revolves around the local activation of the complement system by the complexes and the resulting formation of C5a, which functions as a chemoattractant for the accumulation of neutrophils. Once neutrophils arrive they are activated, usually through contact with and ingestion of immune complexes. In the process they release many inflammatory mediators, such as proteases, oxygen radicals, and arachidonic acid products, which collectively produce tissue injury. The serum-sickness-induced injury, such as that seen in the renal glomerulus, mimics the histologic appearance of many types of human glomerulonephritis.

An example of a localized injury induced by immune complexes is an experimental vasculitis model, the Arthus reaction (Fig. 4-10). This reaction is classically induced in the dermal blood vessels by the local injection of an antigen to which the animal has been previously sensitized (i.e., against which it has circulating antibody). The circulating antibody and locally injected antigen diffuse toward each other and form immune complex deposits in the walls of small blood vessels. The ensuing vascular injury is mediated by complement activation, followed by recruitment and stimulation of neutrophils, which release their tissue-damaging factors. Because the injury is caused by recruited neutrophils and their products, several (2 to 6) hours are required for evidence of tissue injury, in marked contrast to type I hypersensitivity reactions. Histologically, the affected vessels show large numbers of neutrophils and evidence of damage to the vessel, with edema and hemorrhage into the surrounding tissue (see Fig. 4-10). In addition, the presence of fibrin creates the classic appearance of an immune-complex-induced vasculitis referred to as **fibrinoid necrosis**. This experimental model of localized vasculitis is the prototype for many types of vasculitis seen in man— for example, the various types of cutaneous vasculitides seen in drug reactions.

In summary, type III hypersensitivity reactions represent the classic example of immune complex-mediated injury, in which antigen–antibody complexes, which are usually not organ-specific, are formed in the circulation and directly in the tissues. Once deposited in the tissues, these complexes induce an inflammatory response by activating the complement system, consequently attracting neutrophils and macrophages. Activation of these cells by **the immune complexes, with the release of potent inflammatory mediators, is directly responsible for the injury. Many human diseases, including autoimmune diseases such as systemic lupus erythematosus, as well as most types of glomerulonephritis, appear to be mediated by type III hypersensitivity reactions.**

TYPE IV HYPERSENSITIVITY: CELL-MEDIATED IMMUNITY

Cell-mediated hypersensitivity is defined as an antigen-elicited cellular immune reaction that results in tissue damage and does not require the participation of antibodies. Cellular immune reactions often occur together with superimposed antibody reactions, which makes it difficult to define them under natural circumstances. Studies with several experimental models suggest that the type of tissue response largely depends on the nature of the inciting agent.

DELAYED-TYPE HYPERSENSITIVITY

Classically, delayed-type hypersensitivity is defined as a tissue reaction, primarily involving lymphocytes and mononuclear phagocytes, that occurs in response to the subcutaneous injection of a soluble protein antigen and reaches greatest intensity 24 to 48 hours after injection. A naturally occurring example of this reaction is the contact sensitivity response to poison ivy. Although the chemical ligands in poison ivy are not proteins, they bind covalently to cell membrane proteins and are therefore recognized by antigen-specific lymphocytes.

Figure 4-11 summarizes the main stages of the delayed-type hypersensitivity reaction. In the initial phase, foreign protein antigens or chemical ligands interact with accessory cells bearing class II, HLA-D molecules. Soluble protein antigens are actively processed by macrophages and then presented in conjunction with HLA-D molecules. Small reactive chemical ligands interact directly with membrane proteins and thereby alter their structure. The foreign antigens are then recognized by antigen-specific T cells. The latter are called T effector or delayed hypersensitivity cells, and usually have the T4 phenotype. These cells become activated and begin the synthesis of a spectrum of lymphokines (see Table 4-1). The lymphokines recruit and activate lymphocytes, monocytes, fibrocytes,

(Text continues on p. 74)

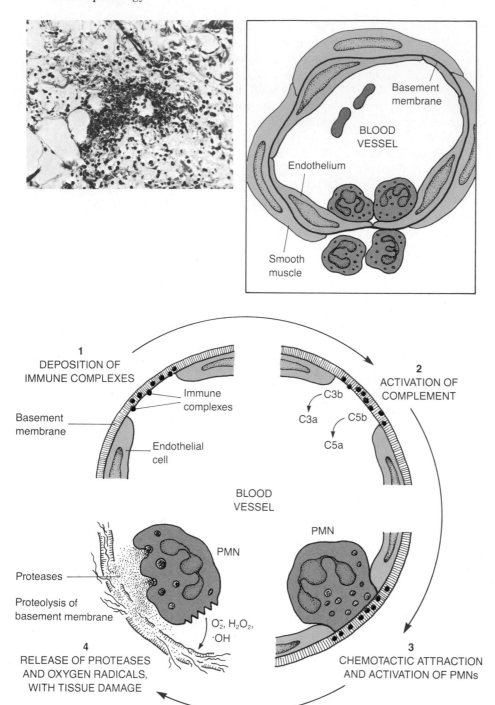

Figure 4-10. Type III hypersensitivity. Localized immune-complex-induced vasculitis in the Arthus reaction is depicted. The formation of immune complexes in the vessel wall leads to localized complement activation and the recruitment of neutrophils as shown in the photomicrograph. The neutrophils induce injury to the vessel wall with edema, hemorrhage, and fibrin deposition.

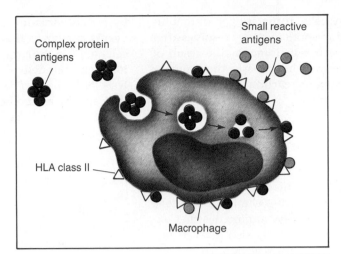

**ANTIGEN PROCESSING
AND PRESENTATION**

- Complex protein antigens are ingested by macrophages, processed, and then presented on the surface in association with class II HLA molecules
- Small reactive antigens may bind directly to class II molecules

Figure 4-11. Delayed-type hypersensitivity reaction.

(*Panel 1*) Complex antigens are phagocytosed and "processed" by macrophages, then presented in the membrane complexes with class II (Ia) antigens. Chemically reactive ligands then may bind directly to macrophage membrane proteins.

(*Panel 2*) Antigen-specific T cells recognize the membrane protein-antigen complexes and receive growth promoting signals (monokines), such as interleukin-1, from macrophages. T cells then become activated and begin synthesis and secretion of molecular mediators (lymphokines).

(*Panel 3*) The generated lymphokines, as well as monokines, recruit additional inflammatory cells, predominantly mononuclear cells.

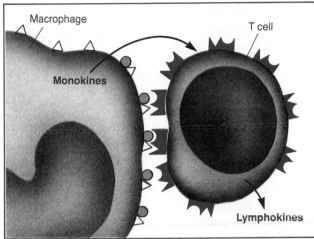

**ANTIGEN RECOGNITION
AND T CELL ACTIVATION**

- Antigen-specific T cells recognize antigen plus class II molecules
- T cells are stimulated to synthesize and release lymphokines; macrophage-derived monokines promote this activation

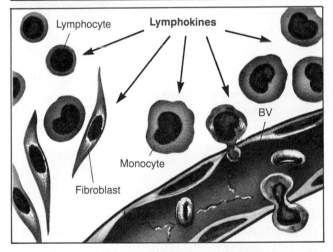

**AMPLIFICATION AND
RECRUITMENT**

- Lymphokines produce numerous effects, including recruitment of additional inflammatory cells and activation of macrophages and fibroblasts and other inflammatory cells. If the antigenic stimulus is eliminated, the reaction spontaneously resolves after 48 hours, with only a scar remaining, as the result of fibroblast activity. If the stimulus persists, the response evolves into a granulomatous reaction in an attempt to sequester the inciting agent.

T CELL–MEDIATED CYTOTOXICITY

Another mechanism by which T cells injure tissue is the direct cytolysis of target cells. This immune mechanism is important for the destruction and elimination of cells infected by viruses and, possibly, tumor cells that express neoantigens. Cytotoxic T cells also play an important role in graft or transplant rejection.

Figure 4-12 summarizes the events in T cell-mediated cytotoxicity. In contrast to the delayed hypersensitivity reaction, the cytotoxic or killer T cell must interact with both the target and the class I major histocompatibility complex (MHC) antigens, HLA-A, B, or C. In the case of virus-infected and tumor cells, self-MHC antigens are recognized in addition to the viral antigens or tumor neoantigens. In graft rejection, foreign MHC antigens are potent activators of killer cells. T-killer cells bear the T8 phenotype marker. Once activated by the antigenic stimulus, the proliferation of these cells is promoted by helper or amplifier cells. This amplification is mediated by soluble growth factors such as interleukin-1. An expanded population of antigen-specific killer cells is thus generated for attacking target cells. The actual killing event requires energy-dependent binding of the killer to the target cell. The killer cell next delivers a molecular signal that disrupts the membrane permeability of the target, causing an influx of sodium, calcium, and water, and ultimate lysis. Once the cytotoxic signal is delivered, the subsequent lytic events are energy-independent and irreversible.

NATURAL KILLER CELL–MEDIATED CYTOTOXICITY

The defining characteristics of natural killer (NK) cells have been described, but the extent to which such cells participate in tissue-damaging immune reactions is unclear. Mounting evidence indicates that they have both important effector and immunoregulatory functions.

Figure 4-13 summarizes the events of target-cell killing by NK cells. Unlike T-killer cells, NK cells recognize a variety of target cells. Thus, they bear receptors that recognize either several different antigenic structures or similar antigens on different target cells. The target antigens are membrane glycoproteins that are expressed by certain virus-infected or tumor cells. In a series of events similar to that described for killer T cells, NK cells bind to the target cell via their membrane receptors and then deliver a molecular signal that results in lysis. NK cells also have membrane Fc receptors. Thus, they acquire antibodies that allow for binding and killing of target cells by an antibody-directed mechanism —that is, antibody-dependent cell-mediated cytotoxicity.

In summary, the type IV hypersensitivity reaction, unlike the other types of hypersensitivity reactions, is not an antibody-mediated response. Rather, antigens are processed by macrophages and presented to antigen-specific T-lymphocytes. These lymphocytes become activated and release a variety of mediators termed lymphokines, which recruit and activate lymphocytes, macrophages, and fibroblasts. The resulting injury is caused by the T-lymphocytes themselves, the macrophages, or both. The granulomatous inflammation of diseases such as sarcoidosis or tuberculosis is an important example of type IV granulomatous reactions in human disease.

IMMUNE REACTIONS TO TRANSPLANTED ORGANS AND TISSUES

The introduction of organ transplantation has initiated intense investigation into the immune mechanisms that cause rejection. **These efforts have revealed the role of histocompatibility antigens as the critical immunogenic molecules that stimulate rejection episodes.**

HOST VERSUS GRAFT

The histopathologic features of graft rejection are well demonstrated in rejected renal allografts. Three major types of rejection, based on the time of onset of the rejection episode and corresponding histologic features, have been described. These three types—hyperacute, acute, and chronic rejection—are illustrated in Figure 4-14.

Hyperacute rejection of the kidney occurs within the first days after transplantation and is manifested clinically as a sudden cessation of urine output accompanied by fever and pain in the area of the graft site. This reaction necessitates prompt surgical removal of the kidney. **The histologic features of hyperacute rejection within the transplanted kidney are vascular congestion, fibrin-platelet thrombi within capillar-**

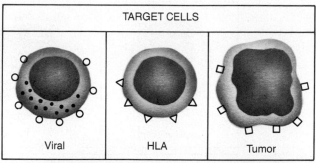

TARGET CELLS

Viral   HLA   Tumor

TARGET ANTIGENS
- Virally-coded membrane antigen
- Foreign or modified histocompatibility antigen
- Tumor-specific membrane antigens

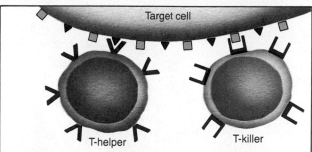

Target cell

T-helper   T-killer

RECOGNITION OF ANTIGEN BY T CELLS
- T-helper cells recognize antigen plus class II molecules
- T-cytotoxic/killer cells recognize antigen plus class I molecules

Figure 4-12. T cell-mediated cytotoxicity.

(*Panel 1*) Potential target cells of T cells include virally infected cells, histoincompatible cells (e.g., transplanted organ), and tumor cells expressing neoantigens.

(*Panel 2*) T cells recognize foreign antigens and class I histocompatibility antigens.

(*Panel 3*) T cells become activated and begin to proliferate. T-helper cells release lymphokines that amplify proliferation.

(*Panel 4*) T-killer cell binds to target cell and delivers a signal, resulting in disruption of the sodium-potassium pump. The target cell is then lysed.

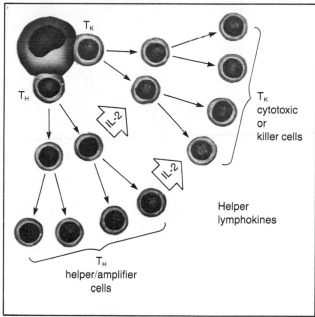

T_K

T_H

IL-2

IL-2

T_K cytotoxic or killer cells

Helper lymphokines

T_H helper/amplifier cells

ACTIVATION AND AMPLIFICATION
- T-helper cells activate and proliferate, releasing helper molecules (e.g., IL-2)
- T-cytotoxic/killer cells proliferate in response to helper molecules

T_K

T_K binding to target cell

T_K

Ca^{2+}
Na^+

K^+

Membrane leakage

T_K

Target lysis

TARGET CELL KILLING
- T-cytotoxic/killer cells bind to target cell
- Killing signals released and target cell loses membrane integrity
- Target cell undergoes lysis

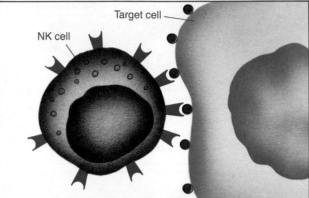

Figure 4-13. Natural killer cell-mediated cytotoxicity.
(*Panel 1*) Potential targets of natural killer cells include virally infected cells and tumor cells.
(*Panel 2*) Recognition of antigen. Natural killer cells bear receptors for a variety of membrane glycoproteins, allowing for cell–cell binding.
(*Panel 3*) Following binding, the NK cell delivers the killer signal. The target cell sodium-potassium pump is disrupted, and the target cell is lysed.

TARGET CELLS
- Virally-infected cells
- Tumor cells

RECOGNITION
- The natural killer (NK) cell binds to target via undefined receptor (possibly involving transferrin receptor)

TARGET CELL KILLING
- NK cell releases signals that commit target to lysis
- Target membrane integrity is lost, NK cell is detached
- Target undergoes lysis

Virally infected

Tumor

Target cell

NK cell

NK-target cell interaction

K⁺

Na⁺
Ca²⁺

Membrane leakage

Target cell lysis

ies, neutrophilic vasculitis with fibrinoid necrosis, prominent interstitial edema, and neutrophilic infiltrates. This rapid form of rejection is mediated by preformed antibodies and complement activation products, including chemotactic and other inflammatory mediators. Fortunately, this form of rejection is not common if appropriate antibody screening is per-

formed, using recipient lymphocytes as the target cell for the antibody assay.

Acute rejection characteristically occurs in the first few weeks or months after transplantation. Clinically, there is a sudden onset of azotemia and oliguria, which may be associated with fever and graft tenderness. A needle biopsy is often performed to differentiate be-

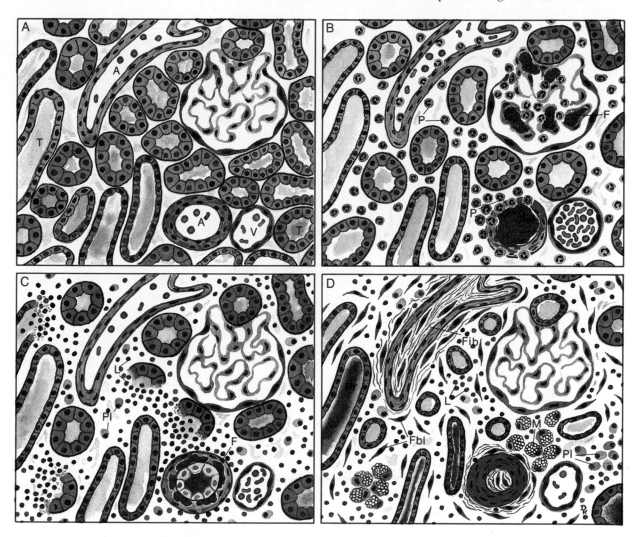

Figure 4-14. Histologic features of major forms of renal transplant rejection. (*A*) Normal kidney. (*B*) Hyperacute rejection occurs in minutes to hours and is characterized by interstitial edema, infiltrates of polymorphonuclear leukocytes, intravascular fibrin-platelet thrombi, and fibrinoid necrosis of arterioles. (*C*) Acute cellular rejection occurs in the first weeks to months and is characterized by interstitial edema, infiltrates of mononuclear cells, tubular damage, and vasculitis associated with thrombosis and fibrinoid necrosis. (*D*) Chronic rejection occurs months to years after transplantation and is characterized by arterial and arteriolar sclerosis, tubular atrophy, interstitial fibrosis, and glomerular capillary wall thickening. *P*, polymorphonuclear leukocyte; *F*, fibrin; *T*, tubule; *A*, artery; *V*, vein; *Fbl*, fibroblast; *Pl*, plasma cell; *L*, lymphocyte; *M*, macrophage; *Fib*, fibrous tissue.

tween a rejection episode and acute tubular necrosis or toxicity from immunosuppressive agents. **The microscopic findings of acute graft rejection include interstitial infiltrates of lymphocytes and macrophages, with associated edema. In addition, there is lymphocytic tubulitis and tubular necrosis. The most severe form also shows vascular damage, manifested as an arteritis, with thrombosis and fibrinoid necrosis.** Vascular involvement is an ominous sign because it usually means the rejection episode will be refractory to therapy. Acute cellular rejection likely involves both cell-mediated and humoral mechanisms of tissue damage. If detected in its early stages, acute rejection can be reversed with immunosuppressive therapy.

Chronic rejection occurs several months to years after transplantation. Clinically, the patient develops progressive azotemia, oliguria, hypertension, and weight gain. If indeed there is chronic rejection, a biopsy specimen will show the characteristic histologic picture. **The dominant features of chronic rejection are arterial and arteriolar intimal thickening, causing stenosis or obstruction. This is associated with thick glomerular capillary walls, tubular atrophy, and interstitial fibrosis.** The interstitium often has scattered mononuclear infiltrates and tubules containing proteinaceous casts. Chronic rejection may be the end result of repeated episodes of cellular rejection, either clinical or subclinical in presentation. This advanced state of damage is not responsive to therapy.

It should be noted that the histologic features described above may overlap and vary in degree, such that a distinct picture may not be apparent on renal biopsy. Moreover, immunosuppressive drugs, such as cyclosporin, have complicated the histologic diagnosis by modifying immune responses as well as by exerting direct toxic effects on renal tubular cells.

GRAFT VERSUS HOST

In recent years, bone marrow transplantation to bone marrow-depleted or immunodeficient patients has resulted in the complication of **graft-versus-host (GVH) disease.** Immunocompetent lymphocytes in the grafted marrow attempt to reject the host tissues. GVH disease also occurs when severely immunodeficient patients are transfused with blood products containing HLA-incompatible lymphocytes.

Clinically, GVH disease manifests as skin rash, diarrhea, abdominal cramps, anemia, and liver dysfunction. Histologically, the skin and gut show mononuclear cell infiltrates and epithelial cell necrosis. The liver displays periportal inflammation, damaged bile ducts, and liver cell injury. A chronic form of GVH disease is characterized by dermal sclerosis, sicca syndrome (dry eyes and dry mouth secondary to chronic inflammation of the lacrimal and salivary glands), and immunodeficiency. Treatment of GVH disease usually involves immunosuppressive therapy.

ASSESSMENT OF IMMUNE STATUS

Immunodeficiency is usually suspected in an infant or adult with chronic, recurrent, or unusual infections. The specific type of immunodeficiency is suggested by the kinds of infections developed and other clinical features. However, diagnosis and confirmation usually require laboratory studies. A number of laboratory methods are used to assess the various components of immunity—that is, antibody-mediated immunity (B cells), cell-mediated immunity (T cells), phagocytosis, and complement.

Immunoglobulin levels are crudely measured by **serum protein electrophoresis.** In this technique, serum proteins are separated electrophoretically, stained, and then quantitated by densitometry. Figure 4-15A shows the characteristic patterns of both a normal and a hypogammaglobulinemic individual, and their corresponding densitometric tracings. The immunoglobulins comprise the gammaglobulin fraction, which migrates cathodically and is significantly reduced in hypogammaglobulinemic patients.

Immunoglobulins (Ig) are more precisely measured by quantitation of individual Ig subclasses. Various methods are used (radial immunodiffusion, nephelometry, radioimmunoassay), but all employ antibodies directed against the different heavy-chain isotypes. Quantitation allows the detection of selective deficiencies of Ig subclasses and provides a measure of total available Ig. A number of conditions have been described in which there is a specific deficiency of IgA, IgM, or IgG.

Serologic methods for evaluating antibody-dependent immunity measure levels of circulating antibodies to specific antigens to which a person has been introduced through vaccination or environmental exposure (tetanus, diphtheria, typhoid, rubella, and major blood groups). These methods uncover subtle deficiencies that may be present even when levels of immunoglobulin are normal.

Cell-mediated immunity is also evaluated by a number of techniques. Since most blood lymphocytes are T cells, the total lymphocyte count is a crude indication of cell-mediated immunity. Functional screening of delayed hypersensitivity is done through intradermal injection of antigens to which most of the population should be sensitive (*Candida albicans*, tetanus toxoid, streptokinase, streptodornase). A normal response is notable swelling, redness, and induration (>5 mm) at the skin injection site.

More sophisticated methods assess T-lymphocyte function in vitro. Figure 4-15B diagrams a commonly employed assay in which lymphoid cells are isolated from a blood sample and then incubated with a polyclonal T cell mitogen (phytohemagglutinin), a common microbial antigen (*Candida*, streptokinase, etc.), or histoincompatible cells. Normal T cells proliferate in response to such stimuli. A poor or absent response suggests a qualitative, quantitative, or regulatory lymphocyte defect.

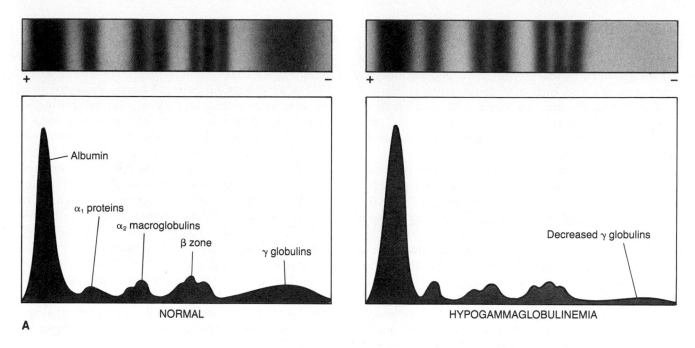

NORMAL

HYPOGAMMAGLOBULINEMIA

A

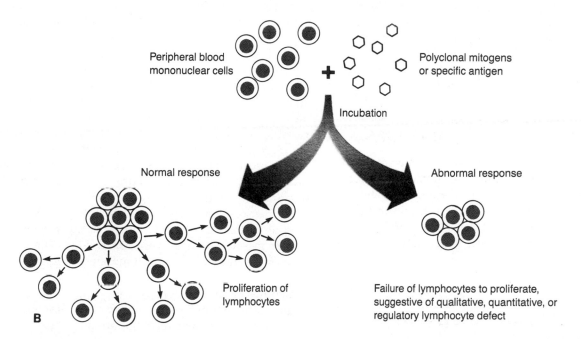

B

Figure 4-15. (*A*) Normal and hypogammaglobulinemic serum protein electrophoresis (SPEP). The SPEP provides a relatively rapid means to evaluate the major protein components of serum. (*B*) T cell mitogenic or blastogenic response assay. This assay tests the capacity of peripheral blood T cells to respond to mitogenic or antigenic stimuli.

Both antibody-mediated and cell-mediated immunity are evaluated by quantitation of peripheral blood T- and B-lymphocyte populations. For example, T cells are measured by their ability to bind sheep erythrocytes spontaneously and form rosettes in vitro. B cells are easily identified with fluorochrome-labeled rabbit or goat antibodies directed against human immunoglobulins. These antibodies bind to B cells, which are identified by fluorescence microscopy.

Recently, the development of laser technology and monoclonal antibodies with specificities for lymphocyte subpopulations has enabled more detailed analyses of lymphoid cells by the method of **flow cytometry.** The principles of this method are outlined in Figure 4-16. Briefly, lymphocyte preparations are stained with a fluorochrome-labeled monoclonal antibody specific for the target population—for instance, T4, T8, and so on. The cells are then passed individually through a narrow beam of laser light of appropriate wavelength. Diffracted light is analyzed by a forward light scatter detector. Various blood cell types, lymphocytes, neutrophils, monocytes, and so on, are recognized by their characteristic forward light scatter pattern. A second detector positioned at 90° to the incident beam monitors cells for fluorescent intensity. The information from both detectors is subjected to computer analysis.

IMMUNODEFICIENCY DISEASES

Immunodeficiency disorders are classified into antibody (B cell), cellular (T cell), and combined T and B cell deficiencies. In many cases functional defects are localized to particular points in the ontogeny of the immune system. The defects are congenital or acquired and their precise etiologies are often unclear.

DEFICIENCIES OF ANTIBODY (B CELL) IMMUNITY

Congenital (Bruton's) X-linked infantile hypogammaglobulinemia is generally observed in male infants at 5 to 6 months of age, the time when maternal antibody levels begin to decline. The infant usually presents with recurrent pyogenic infections, severe hypogammaglobulinemia, and an absence of mature peripheral blood B cells. Pre-B cells, however, can be detected. Thus, there is a defect early in the maturation of B cells, at the point at which pre-B cells receive the maturation signal from the bursal equivalent (see Fig. 4-1, step 2). A flow cytometry profile of a patient with

Bruton's agammaglobulinemia is shown in Figure 4-17. Note that the levels of mature B cells are severely decreased, whereas pre-B cells are still detectable by the HLA-D/DR marker.

Another congenital form of hypogammaglobulinemia is known as **transient hypogammaglobulinemia of infancy.** The condition is characterized by prolonged hypogammaglobulinemia after maternal antibodies have reached a nadir. Some affected infants develop recurrent infections and require therapy, but all eventually produce immunoglobulins. Such infants have mature B cells that are temporarily unable to produce antibodies. The defect is thought to be at the level of the helper T cell signal.

An interesting congenital immunodeficiency exhibits low levels of IgG and IgA, but normal to elevated levels of IgM. The defect appears to be at the level of the "switch" to other heavy-chain isotopes (see Fig. 4-2, step 3); in this condition, B cells, although capable of producing IgM, secrete inadequate levels of other isotypes.

Common variable immunodeficiency is a severe hypogammaglobulinemia (IgG) that is manifested years to decades after birth. The mean age of onset is 31 years. Patients present with recurrent, severe pyogenic infections, especially pneumonia, as well as diarrhea, often due to *Giardia lamblia.* Different maturational and regulatory defects of the immune system result in the same clinical presentation, recognized as common variable immunodeficiency. Thus, this disorder probably represents several diseases rather than one.

The most common immunodeficiency syndrome, selective IgA deficiency, occurs in one of every 700 persons. Individuals with IgA deficiency are asymptomatic or present with severe respiratory or gastrointestinal infections. There is also a strong predilection for allergies and collagen vascular diseases. These individuals generally have normal numbers of IgA-bearing B cells. Therefore, their defect seems to be an inability to synthesize and secrete IgA (see Fig. 4-2, step 4). Similar selective deficiencies have been described for the IgG subclasses and IgM, but are quite rare.

DEFICIENCIES OF CELL-MEDIATED (T CELL) IMMUNITY

DiGeorge syndrome is one of the severest forms of deficient T cell immunity. The disease usually presents in an infant with congenital heart defects and severe hypocalcemia (due to hypoparathyroidism) and is recognized shortly after birth. Infants who survive the neonatal period are subject to recurrent or chronic viral, bacterial, fungal, and protozoal infections. **The condi-**

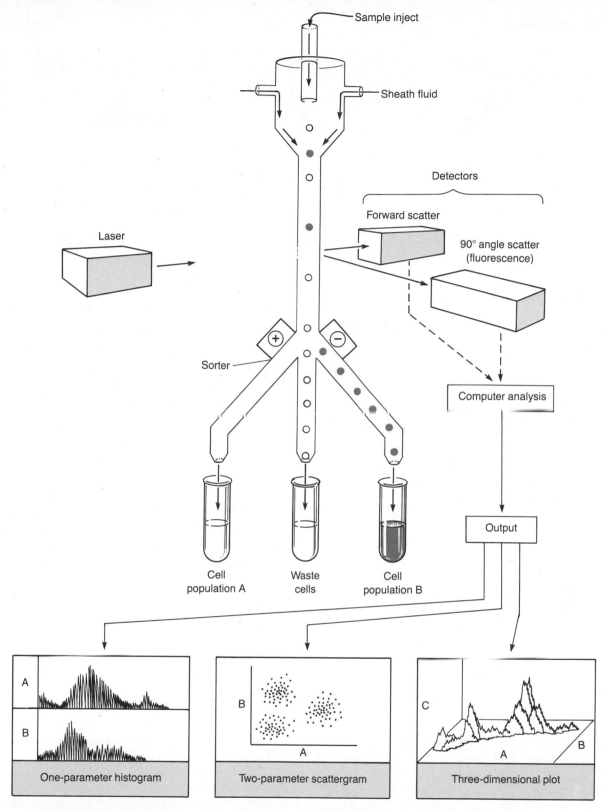

Figure 4-16. Schematic of flow cytometric analysis of cell populations. Cells treated with population-specific antibodies labeled with fluorochromes are passed individually through an incident beam of laser light. The diffracted and fluorescent light is monitored by forward scatter and 90° angle fluorescent light detectors. The monitored light is subjected to computer analysis. Cells with specific markers can be sorted and collected using electroplates.

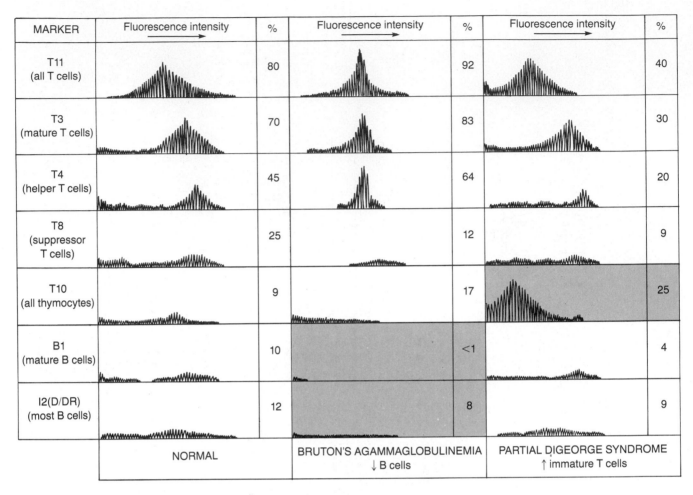

MARKER	Fluorescence intensity →	%	Fluorescence intensity →	%	Fluorescence intensity →	%
T11 (all T cells)		80		92		40
T3 (mature T cells)		70		83		30
T4 (helper T cells)		45		64		20
T8 (suppressor T cells)		25		12		9
T10 (all thymocytes)		9		17		25
B1 (mature B cells)		10		<1		4
I2(D/DR) (most B cells)		12		8		9
	NORMAL		BRUTON'S AGAMMAGLOBULINEMIA ↓ B cells		PARTIAL DIGEORGE SYNDROME ↑ immature T cells	

Figure 4-17. Flow cytometric profiles in immunodeficiency states. Bruton's agammaglobulinemia: marked reduction in the number of circulating mature B cells (B1 marker); some immature B cells present (D/DR marker). Partial DiGeorge's syndrome: marked decrease in the number of mature T cells (T3, T4, T8 markers); increased numbers of immature T cells present (T11 marker). Acquired immunodeficiency syndrome (AIDS): decreased numbers of helper T cells (T4 marker); normal or decreased numbers of suppressor T cells (T8 marker). B cell leukemia: increased B cells; decreased T cells.

tion is caused by defective embryologic development of the third and fourth pharyngeal pouches, which become the thymus and parathyroid glands. In the absence of a thymus, T cell maturation is interrupted at the pre-T cell stage (see Fig. 4-1, stage A). The disease can be corrected by transplanting thymic tissue.

Some patients have a **partial DiGeorge syndrome,** in which a small remnant of thymus is present. With time, these individuals recover T cell function without treatment. Figure 4-18 shows a flow cytometric profile of such a patient. Before thymic function has fully recovered, a large proportion of peripheral T cells still express the T10 marker, having not quite reached maturity.

Chronic mucocutaneous candidiasis, another congenital defect in T cell function, is characterized by susceptibility to candidal infections. The condition is associated with an endocrinopathy (hypoparathyroidism, Addison's disease, diabetes mellitus). Although most T cell functions are intact, there is a defective response to *Candida* antigens. The precise cause of the defect is unknown, but it could occur at any of several points during T cell development. Among the possibilities are failure to develop T cell clones that are specific

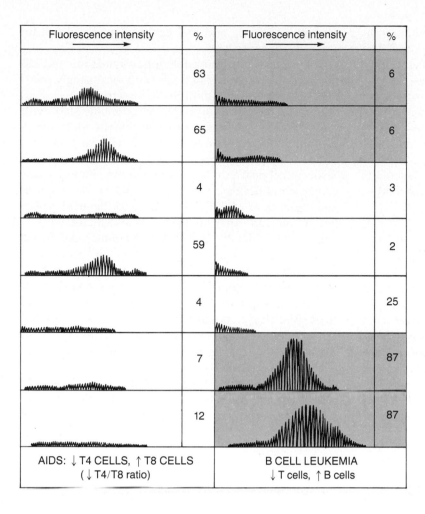

Fluorescence intensity	%	Fluorescence intensity	%
	63		6
	65		6
	4		3
	59		2
	4		25
	7		87
	12		87
AIDS: ↓ T4 CELLS, ↑ T8 CELLS (↓ T4/T8 ratio)		B CELL LEUKEMIA ↓ T cells, ↑ B cells	

for *Candida* antigens (see Fig. 4-1, stage B) and failure to proliferate and produce inflammatory mediators in response to *Candida* antigens (see Fig. 4-1, stage D).

COMBINED T AND B CELL DEFICIENCIES

Severe combined immunodeficiency disease is characterized by recurrent viral, bacterial, fungal, and protozoal infections with onset at about 6 months of age. The disease occurs in X-linked and autosomal recessive (Swiss type) forms. Both forms are associated with a virtually complete absence of T cells and severe hypogammaglobulinemia. Many of these infants have severely reduced lymphoid tissue and an immature thymus that lacks lymphocytes. In some patients, the undefined defect or defects manifest very early in the developing immune system. Specifically, lymphocytes fail to develop beyond the pre-B and pre-T cell level (see Fig. 4-1, stages 1 and A). In other patients, mature lymphocytes are present but fail to function, possibly because of a lack of helper cell activity.

In about half of patients with the autosomal recessive form of combined immunodeficiency, production of adenosine deaminase is defective. This enzyme takes part in the catabolism of purine nucleotides, specifically converting adenosine to inosine or deoxyadenosine to deoxyinosine. If it is defective or absent, deoxyadenosine and deoxy-ATP accumulate. Deoxy-ATP then inhibits ribonucleotide reductase, causing depletion of deoxyribonucleoside triphosphates and defective lymphocyte function. The clinical manifestations of adenosine deaminase deficiency range from mild to severe dysfunctions of T and B cells.

ACQUIRED IMMUNODEFICIENCY

Immunodeficiency states can be secondary to a large number of conditions, including infections (viral, bacterial, and fungal), malnutrition, autoimmune diseases (systemic lupus erythematosus, rheumatoid arthritis), nephrotic syndrome, uremia, sarcoidosis, cancer (lymphoid and nonlymphoid), and treatment with immunosuppressive agents (radiation, steroids, chemotherapy, cyclosporin A, etc.). The widespread use of immunosuppressive agents is today the main cause of immunodeficiency and the resulting increased risk for opportunistic infection.

The **acquired immunodeficiency syndrome (AIDS)** has become recognized as a fatal and increasingly prevalent disease. AIDS exhibits a spectrum of clinical manifestations, including an asymptomatic state with only laboratory evidence of immunodeficiency; a prodromal state manifested by fever, weight loss, and lymphadenopathy; and the classic picture of opportunistic infections and Kaposi's sarcoma. Kaposi's sarcoma, a multicentric vascular neoplasm, develops in about one-third of AIDS patients, and the incidence of lymphoma and other neoplasms is also increased.

Epidemiologically, in the United States AIDS has been largely restricted to homosexual men, intravenous drug abusers, hemophiliacs and other recipients of blood products, and Haitians. In Africa heterosexual transmission appears to be common. Table 4-4 summarizes the current classification of AIDS, issued by the Centers for Disease Control in 1986. Figure 4-18 summarizes a few of the common conditions associated with the classic form of AIDS.

Immunologically, AIDS patients show defects in both T cell and B cell function: delayed-type hypersensitivity is impaired, T cell cytotoxicity is reduced, and

Table 4-4   Classification of HIV Infections

GROUP	TYPE	DESCRIPTION
Group I	Acute infection	Mononucleosis-like syndrome with associated seroconversion for HIV antibody
Group II	Asymptomatic infection	No signs or symptoms of HIV. There may or may not be laboratory evidence of disease.
Group III	Persistent generalized lymphadenopathy	Lymphadenopathy ($\geq$1 cm) at two or more extrainguinal sites persisting for more than 3 months in the absence of a condition other than HIV infection to explain the findings. There may or may not be laboratory evidence of disease.
Group IV	Other disease	*Subgroup A.* Constitutional disease, fever (>1 month), weight loss (>10% of baseline), or diarrhea (>1 month), in the absence of a condition other than HIV infection to explain the findings.

Subgroup B. Neurologic disease such as dementia, myelopathy, or peripheral neuropathy in the absence of a condition other than HIV infection to explain the findings.

Subgroup C. Diagnosis of an infectious disease associated with HIV infection or at least moderately indicative of a defect in cell-mediated immunity.

    Category C-1. Disease due to at least one of the following:

Pneumocystis carinii	Cytomegalovirus
Toxoplasma	Cryptosporidia
Stronglyoides (extraintestinal)	Isosporidia
Cryptococcus	*Candida* (esophageal, pulmonary or bronchial)
Atypical mycobacteria (*avium* complex or *kansasii*)	*Candida* (chronic mucocutaneous)
	Histoplasma
Progressive multifocal leukoencephalopathy	Herpes simplex (disseminated)

    Category C-2. Disease due to one of the following:

Oral hairy leukoplakia	Multidermatomal herpes zoster
Nocardia	*Salmonella* bacteremia (recurrent)
Tuberculosis	
Oral candidiasis	

Subgroup D. Secondary cancers known to be associated with HIV infection; Kaposi's sarcoma, non-Hodgkin's lymphoma, or primary lymphoma of the brain

Subgroup E. Clinical conditions not defined above that may be due to HIV infection or indicative of defective cell-mediated immunity. Also included are patients with signs and symptoms that may be due to HIV or other clinical illness.

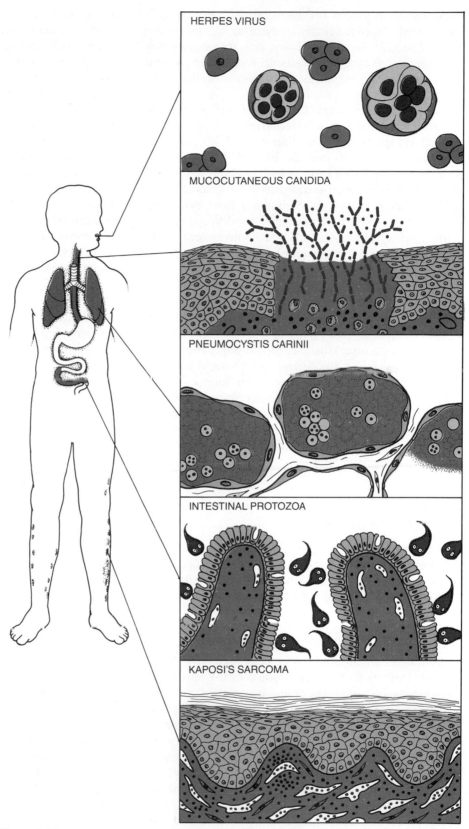

Figure 4-18. Diseases and opportunistic infections of AIDS.

responses to mitogens and histocompatibility antigens are stunted. There is usually an increase in total plasma gammaglobulin level, but this is due to a nonspecific polyclonal activation of B cells. In fact, AIDS patients fail to mount specific antibody responses to immunizing antigens.

The major laboratory features of AIDS are lymphopenia and the loss of circulating T4 (helper/amplifier) lymphocytes. The numbers of T8 (suppressor/cytotoxic) cells can be elevated, normal, or decreased. The **T4:T8 ratio,** which is about 2:1 in normal individuals, can be completely inverted (0.5) in AIDS patients. Figure 4-17 shows a flow cytometric profile of an AIDS patient. Other conditions, such as acute viral infections, can also cause inversions of the T4:T8 ratio, but these are not usually associated with a net loss of T4 cells.

The etiologic agent of AIDS is now known to be a retrovirus "human immunodeficiency virus" (HIV). This RNA virus is one of a family of human T cell viruses that cause leukemias and lymphomas. HIV specifically infects and kills the T4 subpopulation of T-lymphocytes (Fig. 4-19). However, it should be noted that HIV has also been recovered from monocytes and macrophages. The broad immunosuppressive action of the disease reflects the importance of T4 cells in amplifying immune responses. The only practical serologic test detects serum antibodies against HIV.

AUTOIMMUNITY

Autoimmunity implies that an immune response has been generated against self-antigens (autoantigens). Central to the concept of autoimmunity is the breakdown in the ability of the immune system to differentiate between self- and nonself-antigens. The **regulated** production of autoantibodies is a normal event. However, when the normal regulatory mechanisms are in some way deranged, the uncontrolled production of autoantibodies, or the appearance of abnormal cell-cell recognition, produces disease. The mere presence of autoantibodies is not sufficient for a designation of autoimmune disease. It is necessary to demonstrate a cause and effect relationship in which the autoimmune reaction (whether cellular or humoral) is directly related to the disease process. At present only a few diseases, such as lupus erythematosus and thyroiditis, fit this criterion.

An abnormal autoimmune response to self-antigens implies that there is a loss of immune tolerance. The term "tolerance" traditionally denotes a condition in which there is no measurable immune response to specific (usually self-) antigens. Experimental studies suggest that normal tolerance to self-antigens is an active process requiring contact between self-components and immune cells. In the fetus, tolerance is readily established to antigens that in the adult cause vigorous immune responses. Induction of tolerance to an antigen is partly related to the dose of antigen to which cells of the intact organism are exposed. In contrast to the classical theory of Burnet, who postulated that tolerance is caused by "clonal deletion" of antigen-reactive T cells, there is extensive evidence that induction of tolerance is an active immune response that can be produced in a variety of ways. **Tolerance is best looked on as a diversion of the immune system to an active state of nonreactivity: that is, the immune response is blocked by inhibitory products.** Both T and B cells are rendered tolerant—T-helper cells after exposure to low doses of the antigen and B cells after large doses.

In the following sections we will briefly describe those systemic diseases for which there is good evidence of an autoimmune etiology.

SYSTEMIC LUPUS ERYTHEMATOSUS

Systemic lupus erythematosus (SLE) is a chronic multisystem, inflammatory disease that may involve almost any organ but characteristically affects the kidneys, joints, serosal membranes, and skin (Table 4-5). It is the prototype of a systemic autoimmune disease in which autoantibodies are formed against a variety of self-antigens, including plasma proteins (complement components and clotting factors), cell surface antigens (lymphocytes, neutrophils, platelets, erythrocytes), and intracellular cytoplasmic and nuclear components (microfilaments, microtubules, lysosomes, ribosomes, DNA, RNA, histone).

The most important autoantibodies are those against nuclear antigens—in particular, antibody to double-stranded DNA and to the SM antigen, a soluble nuclear antigen. A high titer of these two autoantibodies (called antinuclear antibodies) is pathognomonic of SLE. These antinuclear antibodies are usually not directly cytotoxic by themselves. Antigen–antibody complexes form in the circulation and deposit in tissues, creating the characteristic injury of vasculitis, synovitis, and glomerulonephritis. It is for this reason that SLE is considered the prototype of type III hypersensitivity reactions.

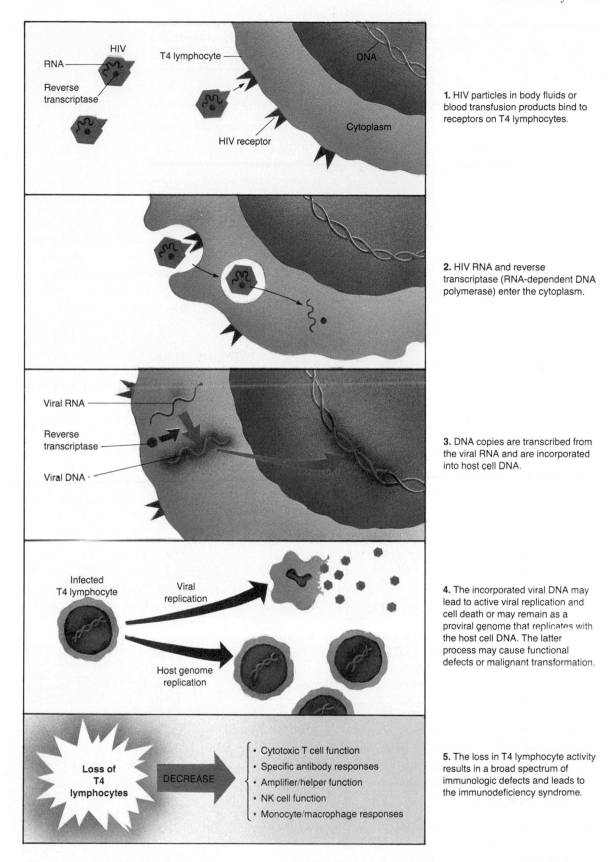

Figure 4-19. Pathogenesis of AIDS.

1. HIV particles in body fluids or blood transfusion products bind to receptors on T4 lymphocytes.

2. HIV RNA and reverse transcriptase (RNA-dependent DNA polymerase) enter the cytoplasm.

3. DNA copies are transcribed from the viral RNA and are incorporated into host cell DNA.

4. The incorporated viral DNA may lead to active viral replication and cell death or may remain as a proviral genome that replicates with the host cell DNA. The latter process may cause functional defects or malignant transformation.

5. The loss in T4 lymphocyte activity results in a broad spectrum of immunologic defects and leads to the immunodeficiency syndrome.

Table 4-5   Primary Organ System Involvement in Systemic Lupus Erythematosus

ORGAN SYSTEM	PERCENTAGE	CHARACTERISTIC PATHOLOGY
Joints	90	Nonerosive synovitis with neutrophils and mononuclear cells
Kidney	75	Immune complex glomerulonephritis, interstitial nephritis
Serosal membranes	35	Pluritis, pericarditis peritonitis secondary to immune complex deposition
Heart	45–50	Pericarditis, myocarditis, endocarditis

ETIOLOGY

The etiology of SLE is unknown. The characteristic feature of the disease—the presence of numerous autoantibodies, particularly antinuclear antibodies—suggests that there is a breakdown in the normal immune surveillance mechanisms, a defect that leads to a loss of the normal self-tolerance mechanisms.

There is a clear female predisposition for SLE, women accounting for 90% of cases between ages 12 and 40. For unknown reasons, this female-to-male predominance is true for all autoimmune diseases. Sex hormones may in part be the explanation.

There also appears to be some genetic predisposition to lupus, and a higher incidence is described in families and monozygotic twins. The incidence of lupus (and the other autoimmune diseases) is higher among those exhibiting certain HLA and DR antigens of the major histocompatibility complex (MHC)—in the case of lupus, DR2 and DR3. **Many genetic factors seem to predispose to SLE, including defects in both immunoregulation and immune effector mechanisms.**

IMMUNOLOGIC ABNORMALITIES

As noted earlier, **autoantibody production to nuclear antigens is characteristic of SLE.** This autoantibody production is linked to B cell hyperreactivity, the major effector mechanism of this disease. B cell hyperreactivity is genetically determined (DR locus) and, being polyclonal, is independent of T cells. B cells from patients with lupus show greatly increased spontaneous proliferation and antibody formation, and the antibodies formed are not exclusively against self-antigens.

PATHOGENESIS

The evidence for the hypothesis that SLE is caused by a type III hypersensitivity reaction is as follows: During the active disease stages of lupus it is often possible to measure the levels of circulating immune complexes that contain nuclear antigens. Secondly, in lupus-induced tissue injury—for example, vasculitis or glomerulonephritis—immune complexes are identified in injured tissues by immunofluorescence. Finally, immune complexes extracted from the tissues contain nuclear antigens. Thus, there is good evidence that the bulk of the injury seen in lupus is due to immune complexes formed against self, particularly against DNA. Type II hypersensitivity reactions may also have a role in lupus, since cytotoxic antibodies against leukocytes, erythrocytes, and platelets have been described.

Because circulating immune complexes deposit in almost all tissues, virtually every organ in the body can be involved. Skin involvement is common and is manifested by an erythematous rash in sun-exposed sites, a "butterfly" malar rash being the most characteristic. Microscopically, the skin exhibits a perivascular lymphoid infiltrate and liquefactive degeneration of the basal cells. The organs with the most serious involvement by SLE are shown in Figure 4-20 and Table 4-5.

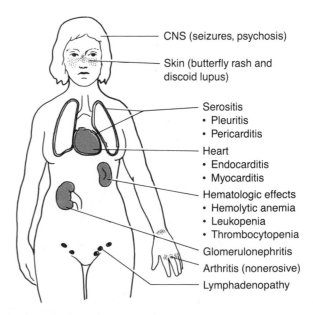

Figure 4-20. Complications of systemic lupus erythematosus.

Joint involvement is the most common manifestation of SLE; over 90% of patients have polyarthralgias. Although an inflammatory synovitis occurs, unlike rheumatoid arthritis there is usually no injury to the joint itself.

While the deposition of preformed circulating immune complexes in tissues may be responsible for the bulk of the tissue injury in SLE and other immune complex diseases, in situ formation of immune complexes in the tissues also appears to be important.

Renal involvement, in particular glomerulonephritis, is very common and as **many as 75% of patients with SLE have evidence of renal disease at autopsy.** The mildest form of renal involvement is **mesangial lupus nephritis.** In this disorder immune complexes and complement deposit almost exclusively in the mesangial regions of the glomeruli, but there are only slight increases in mesangial cells and mesangial matrix (Fig. 4-21). These patients have only mild renal dysfunction, characterized by mild proteinuria and hematuria. The prognosis is excellent.

The next category is **focal proliferative lupus nephritis.** Some glomeruli, but not all (focal), show increased cellularity (Fig. 4-22) characterized both by a proliferation of resident glomerular endothelial and mesangial cells and by infiltrating neutrophils and monocytes. Necrosis and fibrin deposition are also often present. Immunofluorescence studies and electron microscopy demonstrate deposition of immunoglobulin and complement, primarily in the mesangial regions of the glomeruli. The prognosis of patients with

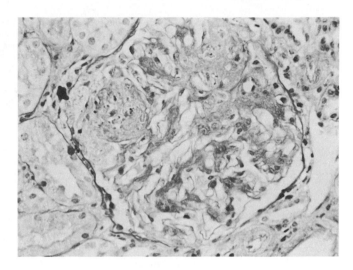

Figure 4-22. Focal proliferative lupus nephritis. Note the segmental necrosis in the glomerulus.

this form of lupus nephritis is mixed. Some remain with only mild disease, whereas others progress to renal failure.

The third type, **diffuse proliferative lupus nephritis,** is the most serious. It occurs in as many as 50% of lupus patients with renal involvement and is associated with conspicuous increases in glomerular cellularity, fibrin deposition, and necrosis (Fig. 4-23). Epithelial crescents are also commonly seen. By immunofluorescence and electron microscopy widespread

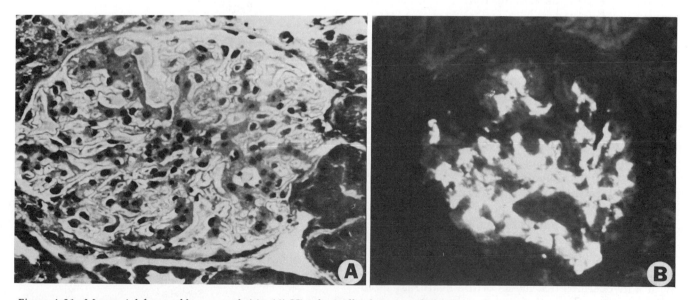

Figure 4-21. Mesangial form of lupus nephritis. (*A*) Histologically there is a slight increase in mesangial matrix and cellularity. (*B*) Immunofluorescence studies reveal immunoglobulin and complement deposition in the mesangium.

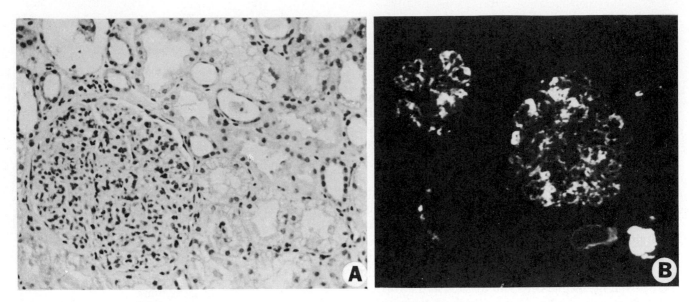

Figure 4-23. Diffuse proliferative lupus nephritis. (*A*) Marked diffuse cellularity increase in the glomerulus. (*B*) Immunofluorescence showing intense immunoglobulin and complement deposition in mesangial and capillary wall locations.

deposition of immune complexes is seen throughout the glomeruli, primarily in the mesangium and underneath the glomerular basement membrane (subendothelial). Many patients with this form of lupus nephritis progress to renal failure.

The final type of lupus nephritis is **membranous lupus nephritis,** which is associated with massive proteinuria. Membranous lupus nephritis resembles other forms of membranous glomerulonephritis. There is no hypercellularity, but instead diffusely thickened glomerular capillary loops caused by the deposition of immunoglobulin and complement on the epithelial surface of the glomerular basement membrane (subepithelial). This pattern of lupus involvement is usually not associated with renal failure.

Involvement of serous membranes is common in SLE. More than a third of patients have a pleuritis and a pleural effusion. Pericarditis and peritonitis occur less frequently.

Cardiac involvement is also common in SLE, but congestive heart failure is rare and is usually associated with a myocarditis. All layers of the heart may be involved, with pericarditis being the most common finding. Endocarditis is usually not clinically significant and is characterized by small vegetations along the lines of

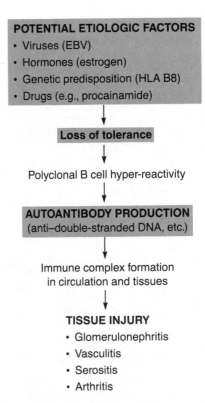

Figure 4-24. Pathogenesis of systemic lupus erythematosus.

closure of the valve leaflets. These small nonbacterial vegetations constitute **Libman–Sacks endocarditis,** and they should be differentiated from the larger, bulkier vegetations of bacterial endocarditis.

Involvement of the central nervous system is a life-threatening complication of lupus. Its nature is not well understood, but vasculitis, hemorrhage and infarction of the brain may be seen.

In summary, the primary abnormality in systemic lupus erythematosus is polyclonal B cell hyperactivity, which is associated with a loss of normal self-tolerance and autoantibody formation to a variety of self-antigens, the most important of which is against DNA (Fig. 4-24). The reason for this B cell hyperactivity is not clear, but it is not associated with consistent T cell abnormalities. The systemic injury seen in lupus is caused by the deposition of these autoantibodies in tissues, which triggers acute inflammation.

SJÖGREN'S DISEASE

Sjögren's disease is an autoimmune disorder characterized by keratoconjunctivitis sicca (dry eyes) and xerostomia (dry mouth) in the absence of other connective tissue diseases. The main target in Sjögren's disease is the major and minor salivary glands, but other organs are frequently involved, including the thyroid gland, the lung, and the kidney.

Primary Sjögren's disease is the second most common connective tissue disorder, after lupus. Like most autoimmune diseases, it occurs primarily in women (30–65 years). There are strong associations between primary Sjögren's disease and certain HLA types, notably HLA-DW3, DR3, DW2, and MT2, a B cell alloantigen. Familial clustering occurs, and in these families there is also a high incidence of other autoimmune diseases.

IMMUNOLOGIC ABNORMALITIES

Production of autoantibodies, particularly antinuclear antibodies, occurs in patients with Sjögren's disease. These autoantibodies may be directed against DNA, histones, or nonhistone proteins in the nucleus. **Autoantibodies to the soluble nuclear nonhistone proteins characterize primary Sjögren's disease, particularly the antigens SS-A and SS-B; however, autoantibodies to DNA or histones are rare. The presence of these antibodies suggests secondary Sjögren's disease due to lupus.** Rheumatoid factor is also commonly present in saliva, tears, and the circulation.

PATHOGENESIS

The etiology of Sjögren's disease is unknown, and the autoantibody production appears to be caused by a polyclonal B cell proliferation. This proliferation is possibly triggered by the Epstein-Barr virus or cytomegalovirus.

PATHOLOGY

Sjögren's disease is characterized by an intense lymphocytic infiltrate of the major and minor salivary glands (Fig. 4-25). Minor salivary glands are the usual biopsy sites, and focal lymphocytic infiltrates are initially observed in a periductal location. The lymphoid infiltrates destroy acini and ducts, and the latter often become dilated and filled with cellular debris. The infiltrates in the glands are predominantly T cells.

Involvement of extraglandular sites is common in Sjögren's disease. Pulmonary involvement occurs in most patients, and bronchial glands atrophy following lymphoid infiltration. This causes thick tenacious secretions, focal atelectasis, recurrent infections, and bronchiectasis.

The disease also affects the gastrointestinal tract, and many patients have difficulty in swallowing (dysphagia). The submucosal glands of the esophagus are infiltrated by lymphocytes. In addition, atrophic gastritis occurs secondary to lymphoid infiltrates of the gastric mucosa. Liver involvement is present in 5% to 10% of patients and is associated with cholangitis and nodular lymphoid infiltrates.

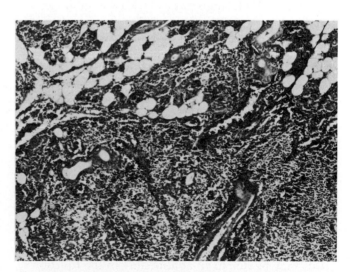

Figure 4-25. Sjögren's disease involving a major salivary gland. Focal intense lymphoid infiltrates are destroying the gland acini but sparing the ducts.

PROGRESSIVE SYSTEMIC SCLEROSIS (SCLERODERMA)

Progressive systemic sclerosis, or scleroderma, is an autoimmune disease of connective tissue characterized by excessive collagen deposition in the skin and in internal organs.

The disease occurs primarily in women, but familial incidence is not a feature. There is also no association between HLA haplotypes and scleroderma. Nevertheless, almost all (96%) of patients with scleroderma have chromosomal abnormalities, such as chromatid breaks, translocations, and deletions. These abnormalities appear to be acquired rather than transmitted and are associated with a "serum breaking factor." The significance of these chromosomal abnormalities is unclear.

IMMUNOLOGIC ABNORMALITIES

Patients with scleroderma exhibit abnormalities of the humoral and cellular immune systems. The number of circulating B-lymphocytes is normal, but there is evidence of hyperactivity, as manifested by hypergammaglobulinemia and cryoglobulinemia. Antinuclear antibodies are commonly present, but are usually in a lower titer than in lupus. However, **some types of antinuclear antibodies—for example, nucleolar autoantibody—are highly specific for scleroderma. Even more specific for scleroderma are antibodies to ScL-70, a nonhistone nuclear protein, and anticentromere antibodies.** Anticentromere antibodies are present in the milder CREST variant of scleroderma, a form that is characterized by calcinosis (C), Raynaud's phenomenon (R), esophageal dysfunction (E), sclerodactyly (S), and telangiectasia (T). Rheumatoid factor is commonly present, and autoantibodies are occasionally directed against other tissues, such as smooth muscle, the thyroid gland, and salivary glands. Antibodies against types I and IV collagen have been described, and may be relevant to the pathogenesis of this disease.

Cellular immune derangements in progressive systemic sclerosis include a decrease in the number of circulating T cells, a decrease in T-helper cells, and an increase in T-suppressor cells.

PATHOGENESIS

Progressive systemic sclerosis is characterized by excessive collagen deposition in many tissues. This fibrosis may be due to an abnormality in the function of fibroblasts. Fibroblasts from patients with this disorder show spontaneously increased collagen synthesis in tissue culture.

PATHOLOGY

The skin in scleroderma displays early edema and then induration, the latter characterized by the following:

- A striking increase in collagen fibers in the reticular dermis
- Thinning of the epidermis with loss of rete pegs
- Atrophy of dermal appendages
- Hyalinization and obliteration of arterioles
- Variable mononuclear infiltrates, consisting primarily of T cells

The induration stage may progress to atrophy or revert to normal.

The most significant systemic involvement occurs in the kidneys, lungs, and heart. The kidneys, which are involved in more than half of the patients with scleroderma, show marked vascular changes, often with focal hemorrhage and cortical infarcts. Among the most severely affected vessels are the interlobular arteries and afferent arterioles. Early fibromuscular thickening of the subintima causes luminal narrowing, which is followed by fibrosis (Fig. 4-26). "Fibrinoid" necrosis is commonly seen in afferent arterioles. The glomerular alterations are nonspecific, and focal changes range from necrosis extending from the afferent arterioles to fibrosis. There is diffuse deposition of immunoglobulin, complement, and fibrin in affected vessels early in the disease, probably because of increased vascular permeability.

In the **lungs** the primary abnormality is diffuse interstitial fibrosis. The lungs may progress to endstage fibrosis, eventuating in a "honeycomb" lung.

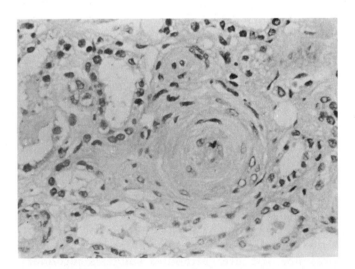

Figure 4-26. Scleroderma with characteristic renal vascular involvement. The interlobular artery shows a marked intimal thickening with virtual obliteration of the lumen.

Primary myocardial necrosis is seen with progressive systemic sclerosis, but does not reflect obstruction of the coronary arteries and ischemic necrosis. It is, rather, a primary event. In a quarter of patients the myocardial fibrosis is extensive, involving 10% or more of the myocardium.

Finally, progressive systemic sclerosis can involve any portion of the **gastrointestinal tract.** Esophageal dysfunction is typically the most significant gastrointestinal complication. Atrophy of the smooth muscle and fibrous replacement are seen in the lower esophagus.

POLYMYOSITIS/DERMATOMYOSITIS

Polymyositis/dermatomyositis is a multisystem autoimmune disease primarily involving skin and muscle. It occurs in both children and adults, and there is an increased frequency of HLA-B8 and DR3 in the childhood form of the disease. Women are affected twice as frequently as men.

IMMUNOLOGIC ABNORMALITIES

Defects in both cellular and humoral mechanisms occur in these patients. Various autoantibodies against muscle are commonly present, and almost all patients (90%) have antibodies against myosin. Antibodies to myoglobin are also common. Various antinuclear and anti-DNA autoantibodies are found, including antibodies to ribonucleoprotein (RNP).

PATHOGENESIS

In polymyositis/dermatomyositis, as in all of the systemic autoimmune diseases, the causative agent is not known. Both humoral and cell-mediated immune mechanisms have been suggested to play a role.

PATHOLOGY

The diagnosis of polymyositis rests not only on the histologic appearance of the involved muscles but also on the location of the involved muscles, on electromyographic alterations, and on elevated activities of muscle enzymes in the blood, including the MM isoenzyme of creatine phosphokinase (CPK) and aldolase. The disease typically involves proximal muscle groups of the upper and lower extremities, and is symmetrical. Skin involvement may or may not be present. Histologically, the skeletal muscle shows evidence of necrosis, regeneration, and a mononuclear inflammatory infiltrate. In chronic cases dense fibrous tissue replaces muscle fibers.

Skin involvement occurs in about 40% of patients and is manifested by an erythematous rash on the face resembling that seen in SLE. However, the rash is also present elsewhere; if it involves the eyelids (heliotropic rash), it is considered specific for dermatomyositis. The skin changes, as in SLE, involve a perivascular lymphoid infiltrate and liquefactive degeneration of the basal epithelial cells. Immunofluorescence studies of skin are helpful to differentiate these two entities. In SLE, granular immunoglobulin and complement deposition at the dermal–epidermal junction, which occurs in uninvolved and involved skin, is virtually pathognomonic. By contrast, dermatomyositis is not associated with the deposition of immune components at the dermal–epidermal junction. Other organ systems are involved, including joints, kidneys, lungs, and gastrointestinal tract. In the childhood form of the disease, a vasculitis may also be present. Many patients with polymyositis/dermatomyositis, particularly adult men, are also at increased risk for developing cancers. Renal involvement was initially thought to be rare, but newer reports suggest that a small percentage of patients (5% to 10%) do have immune complex renal disease. Dermatomyositis usually responds to treatment with adrenocortical steroids, and the prognosis is generally considered good. Some patients, however, develop classic scleroderma, and others have significant pulmonary and brain involvement.

MIXED CONNECTIVE TISSUE DISEASE

Mixed connective tissue disease (MCTD) combines features of SLE (skin rash, Raynaud's phenomenon, arthritis, arthralgias), scleroderma (swollen hands, esophageal hypomotility, pulmonary interstitial disease), and polymyositis (inflammatory myositis). Some patients also develop symptoms suggestive of rheumatoid arthritis. Patients with this disease have been reported to respond well to corticosteroid therapy, although newer studies have challenged this assertion.

Between 80% and 90% of patients are female, and most are adults (mean age 37 years).

Patients with MCTD often have hypergammaglobulinemia and a positive rheumatoid factor. Antinuclear antibodies are present, but, unlike in SLE, are usually not against double-stranded DNA. The most distinctive antinuclear antibody is directed against an extractable nuclear antigen.

The etiology and pathogenesis of this malady are unknown. Whether MCTD represents a distinct entity or just an "overlap" of symptoms from patients with other types of collagen vascular diseases remains an open question.

5

NEOPLASIA

EMANUEL RUBIN AND JOHN L. FARBER

Cancer is an uncontrolled proliferation of cells that express varying degrees of fidelity to their precursors. The structural resemblance of the cancer cell to its putative cell of origin enables specific diagnoses as to the source and potential behavior of the neoplasm. Although the causes of most cancers are not identified and the mechanisms of carcinogenesis remain obscure, considerable data on the biologic attributes of neoplasia are available. A wide variety of human and experimental data suggests that the neoplastic process entails not only cellular proliferation but also a modification of the differentiation of the involved cell types. Thus, in a sense cancer may be viewed as a burlesque of normal development.

A neoplasm is an abnormal mass of cells that exhibits uncontrolled proliferation and that persists after cessation of the stimulus that produced it. In general, neoplasms are irreversible, and their growth is, for the most part, autonomous. Several observations are important at this point: First, neoplasms are derived from cells that normally maintain a proliferative capacity. Thus, mature neurons and cardiac myocytes do not give rise to tumors. Second, a tumor may express varying degrees of differentiation, from relatively mature structures that mimic normal tissues to a collection of cells so primitive that the cell of origin cannot be identified. Third, the stimulus responsible for the uncontrolled proliferation may not be identifiable; in fact, it is not known for most human neoplasms.

BENIGN VERSUS MALIGNANT TUMORS

Benign tumors remain as localized overgrowths in the area in which they arise. By definition, benign tumors do not penetrate (invade) adjacent tissue borders, nor do they spread (metastasize) to distant sites. As a rule, benign tumors are more differentiated than malignant ones—that is, they more closely resemble their tissue of origin. By contrast, malignant tumors, or cancers, have the added property of invading contiguous tissues and metastasizing to distant sites, where subpopulations of malignant cells take up residence, grow anew, and again invade.

In common usage the terms "benign" and "malignant" refer to the overall biologic behavior of a tumor rather than to its morphologic characteristics. As a general rule, malignant tumors kill and benign ones do not. However, so-called benign tumors in critical locations can be deadly. For example, a benign intracranial tumor of the meninges (meningioma) can kill by exerting pressure on the brain. A minute benign tumor of the ependymal cells of the third ventricle (ependymoma) can block the circulation of cerebrospinal fluid, and the resulting hydrocephalus is lethal. A benign mesenchymal tumor of the left atrium (myxoma) may kill suddenly by blocking the orifice of the mitral valve. In certain locations the erosion or necrosis of a benign tumor of smooth muscle can lead to serious hemorrhage—witness the peptic ulceration of a gastric leiomyoma. On rare occasions a functioning, benign endocrine adenoma can be life-threatening, as in the case of the sudden hypoglycemia associated with an insulinoma of the pancreas or the hypertensive crisis produced by a pheochromocytoma of the adrenal medulla. Conversely, certain types of malignant tumors are so indolent that many are curable by surgical resection. In this category are a considerable proportion of cancers of the breast and some malignant tumors of connective tissue, such as fibrosarcoma.

CLASSIFICATION OF NEOPLASMS

The primary descriptor of any tumor, benign or malignant, is its cell or tissue of origin. The classification of benign tumors is the basis for the names of their malignant variants. Benign tumors are identified by the suffix "oma," which is preceded by reference to the cell or tissue of origin. For instance, a benign tumor that resembles chondrocytes is termed a "chondroma" (Fig. 5-1). If the tumor resembles the precursor of the chondrocyte, it is labeled a "chondroblastoma". When a chondroma is located entirely within the bone, it is designated an "enchondroma". Tumors of epithelial origin are given a variety of names based on what is thought to be their outstanding characteristic. Thus, a benign tumor of the squamous epithelium may be called simply an "epithelioma" or, when branched and exophytic, may be termed a "papilloma". Benign tumors arising from glandular epithelium, such as in the colon or the endocrine glands, are termed "adenomas". Accordingly, we refer to a thyroid adenoma (Fig. 5-2) or an islet cell adenoma. In some instances the predominating feature is the gross appearance, in which case we speak, for example, of an "adenomatous polyp" of the colon or the endometrium. Benign tumors that arise from germ cells and contain derivatives of different germ layers are labeled "teratomas". These occur principally in the gonads and occasionally in the mediastinum and may contain a variety of structures, such as skin, neurons and glial cells, thyroid, intestinal epithelium, and cartilage. Localized, disordered differentiation during embryonic development results in a "hamartoma", a disorganized caricature of

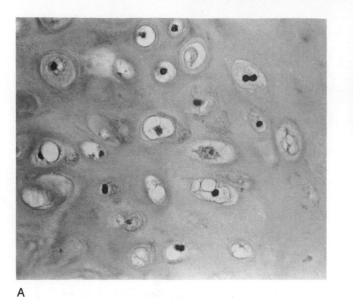 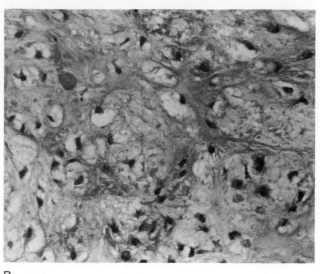

A   B

Figure 5-1. Benign chondroma. (*A*) Normal hyaline cartilage. (*B*) A benign chondroma closely resembles normal cartilage.

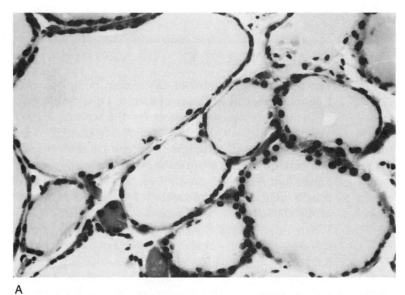

A

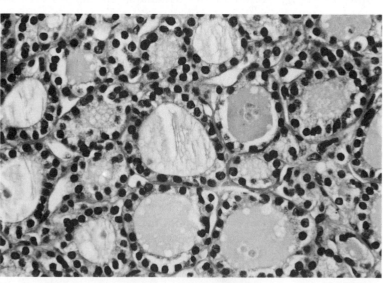

B

Figure 5-2. Benign thyroid adenoma. (*A*) Normal thyroid. (*B*) The follicles of a thyroid adenoma are similar to those of the normal thyroid tissue. Both types of follicles (shown here at the same magnification) are lined by regular epithelial cells and contain colloid.

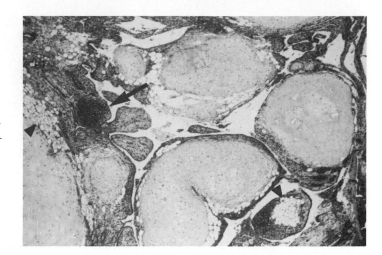

Figure 5-3. Hamartoma of the lung. The tumor contains islands of cartilage and clefts lined by a cuboidal epithelium. A lymphoid follicle (*arrow*) and foci of fat cells (*arrowheads*) are evident.

normal tissue components (Fig. 5-3). Such tumors, which are not strictly neoplasms, contain varying combinations of cartilage, ducts or bronchi, connective tissue, blood vessels, and lymphoid tissue. Certain benign growths, recognized clinically as tumors, are not truly neoplastic but rather represent overgrowth of normal tissue elements. Examples are vocal cord polyps, skin tags, and hyperplastic polyps of the colon.

In general, the malignant counterparts of benign tumors carry the same name, except that the suffix **carcinoma** is applied to epithelial cancers and **sarcoma** to those of mesenchymal origin. For instance, a malignant tumor of the stomach is a "gastric adenocarcinoma" or "adenocarcinoma of the stomach." "Squamous cell carcinoma" is an invasive tumor of the skin (Fig. 5-4) or the metaplastic squamous epithelium of the bronchus or endocervix, and "transitional cell carcinoma" is a malignant neoplasm of the bladder. By contrast, we speak of "chondrosarcoma" (Fig. 5-5) or "fibrosarcoma." Sometimes the name of the tumor suggests the tissue type of origin, as in "osteogenic sarcoma" or "bronchogenic carcinoma." Some tumors display neoplastic elements of different cell types but are not germ cell tumors. For example, fibroadenoma of the breast, composed of epithelial and stromal elements, is benign, whereas, as the name implies, "adenosquamous carcinoma" of the uterus or the lung is malignant. A rare malignant tumor that contains intermingled carcinomatous and sarcomatous elements is known as "carcinosarcoma."

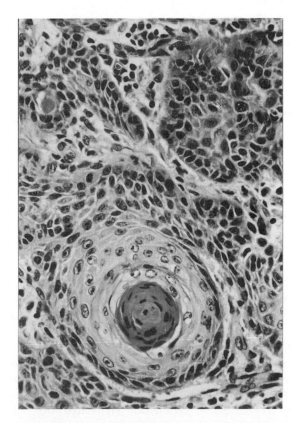

Figure 5-4. Squamous cell carcinoma of the skin. The tumor is composed of islands of neoplastic squamous cells. In the lower portion of the field, well-differentiated keratinized tumor cells have degenerated to form a concentric mass of keratin and pyknotic nuclei, termed an epithelial "pearl."

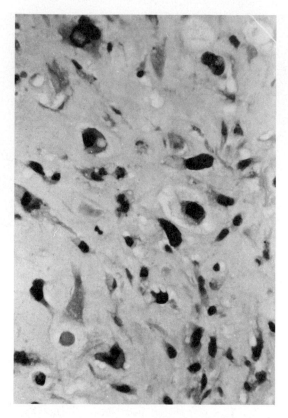

Figure 5-5. Chondrosarcoma of bone. The tumor is composed of malignant chondrocytes, which have bizarre shapes and irregular, hyperchromatic nuclei, embedded in a cartilaginous matrix. Compare with Figure 5-1.

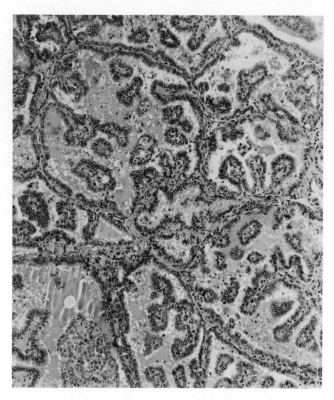

Figure 5-6. Papillary adenocarcinoma of the thyroid. The tumor exhibits numerous fronds, lined by malignant thyroid epithelium, which project into distended colloid-containing follicles.

The persistence of certain historical terms adds a note of confusion. "Hepatoma" of the liver, "melanoma" of the skin, "seminoma" of the testis, and the lymphoproliferative tumor, "lymphoma," are all highly malignant. On the other hand, basal cell carcinoma is labeled by many as "basal cell epithelioma" to emphasize its localized nature. **Tumors of the hematopoietic system** are a special case in which the relationship to the blood is indicated by the **suffix "emia."** Thus "leukemia" refers to a malignant proliferation of white blood cells.

Secondary descriptors (again, with some inconsistencies) refer to a tumor's morphologic and functional characteristics. For example, the term "papillary" refers to a frondlike structure (Fig. 5-6) "Medullary" signifies a soft, cellular tumor with little connective stroma, while "scirrhous" or "desmoplastic" implies a dense fibrous stoma (Fig. 5-7). "Colloid" carcinomas secrete abundant mucus in which float islands of tumor cells. "Comedocarcinoma" is an intraductal neoplasm in which necrotic material can be expressed from the ducts. Certain visible secretions of the tumor cells lend their characteristics to the classification—for example, production of mucin or serous fluid. A further designation describes the gross appearance of a cystic mass. From all these considerations we derive such common terms as "papillary serous cystadenocarcinoma" of the ovary, "comedocarcinoma" of the breast, "adenoid cystic carcinoma" of the salivary glands, "polypoid adenocarcinoma" of the stomach, and "medullary carcinoma" of the thyroid. Finally, tumors in which the histogenesis is poorly understood are often given an eponym—as in, for example, Hodgkin's disease, Ewing's sarcoma of bone, or Brenner tumor of the ovary.

HISTOLOGIC DIAGNOSIS OF MALIGNANCY

The criteria used to assess the biologic nature of any tumor are based not on scientific principles, but rather on a historical correlation of histologic and cytologic

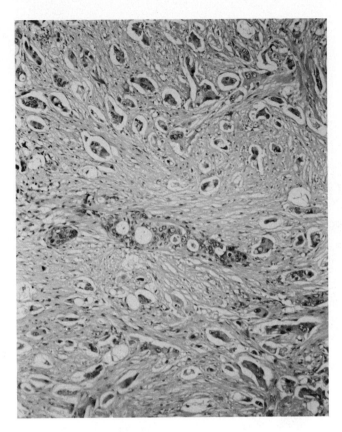

Figure 5-7. Scirrhous adenocarcinoma of the breast. Nests of cancer cells are embedded in a dense fibrous stroma.

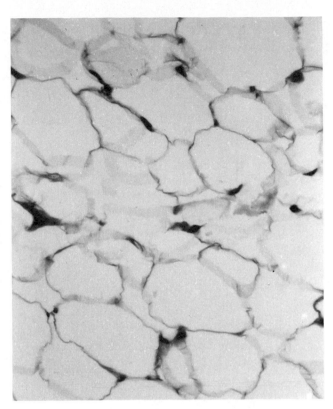

Figure 5-8. Lipoma. This nodular tumor of adipocytes is grossly and microscopically indistinguishable from normal fat.

patterns with clinical outcomes. Established criteria are recognized for various organ and tumor types but must be used with caution in specific cases. For instance, while the reactive proliferation of connective cells termed "nodular fasciitis" has a more alarming histologic appearance than many fibrosarcomas, it is benign, and misdiagnosis can lead to unnecessary surgery. Conversely, many well-differentiated endocrine adenocarcinomas are histologically indistinguishable from benign adenomas.

Benign tumors in general resemble their parent tissues, both histologically and cytologically. For example, lipomas, despite their often lobulated gross appearance, seem to be composed of normal adipocytes (Fig. 5-8). Fibromas are composed of mature fibroblasts and a collagenous stroma. Chondromas exhibit chondrocytes dispersed in a cartilaginous matrix. Thyroid adenomas form acini and produce thyroglobulin. The gross structure of a benign tumor may depart from the normal and assume papillary or polypoid configurations, as in papillomas of the bladder and skin and adenomatous polyps of the colon. However, **the lining epithelium of a benign tumor resembles that of the normal tissue.** Although many benign tumors are circumscribed by a connective tissue capsule, many equally benign neoplasms are not encapsulated. In the latter category are such benign tumors as papillomas and polyps of the visceral organs, hepatic adenomas, many endocrine adenomas, and hemangiomas. **It bears repetition that the definition of a benign tumor resides above all in an inability to invade adjacent tissue and to metastasize.**

Malignant tumors depart from the parent tissue morphologically and functionally, although an accurate diagnosis of their origin depends not only on the location but also on a histologic and cytologic resemblance to a normal tissue. The lack of differentiated features in a cancer cell is referred to as **anaplasia** or **cellular atypia,** and in general the degree of anaplasia correlates with the aggressiveness of the tumor. Cytologic evidence of anaplasia includes variation in the size and shape of cells and cell nuclei ("pleomorphism"), enlarged and hyperchromatic nuclei with coarsely clumped chromatin and prominent nucleoli, atypical

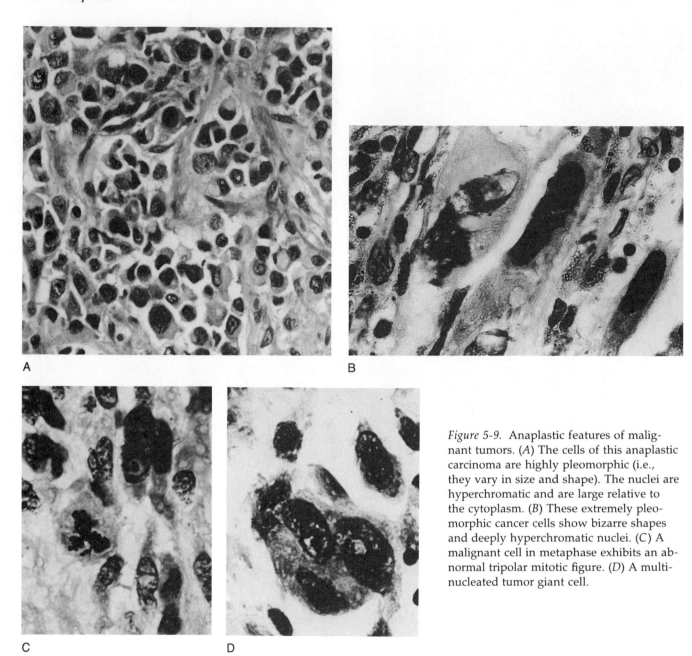

A

B

C

D

Figure 5-9. Anaplastic features of malignant tumors. (*A*) The cells of this anaplastic carcinoma are highly pleomorphic (i.e., they vary in size and shape). The nuclei are hyperchromatic and are large relative to the cytoplasm. (*B*) These extremely pleomorphic cancer cells show bizarre shapes and deeply hyperchromatic nuclei. (*C*) A malignant cell in metaphase exhibits an abnormal tripolar mitotic figure. (*D*) A multinucleated tumor giant cell.

mitoses, and bizarre cells, including tumor giant cells (Fig. 5-9). Abundant mitoses are characteristic of many malignant tumors, but are not a necessary criterion. However, in some cases—for example, leiomyosarcomas—the diagnosis of malignancy is based on the finding of even a few mitoses. Malignancy is proved by the demonstration of invasion, particularly of blood vessels and lymphatics. In some circumstances, such as squamous carcinoma of the cervix or carcinoma arising in an adenomatous polyp, the diagnosis of malignant transformation is made on the basis of local invasion. It is intuitively obvious that the presence of metastases identifies a tumor as malignant, but occasionally it reveals the true nature of a tumor previously considered benign. In metastatic disease that was not preceded by a clinically diagnosed primary tumor, the site of origin is often not readily apparent from the morphologic characteristics of the tumor. In such cases electron microscopic examination and the demonstration of a specific tumor marker may establish the correct diagnosis.

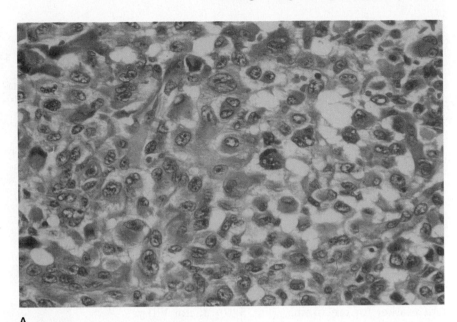

A

Figure 5-10. Tumor markers in the identification of undifferentiated neoplasms. (*A*) A metastatic undifferentiated malignant melanoma stained with hematoxylin and eosin does not exhibit melanin pigment by light microscopy. (*B*) An immunoperoxidase stain of the same tumor shows numerous cells positive for S-100 protein, a commonly used marker for cells of melanocytic origin.

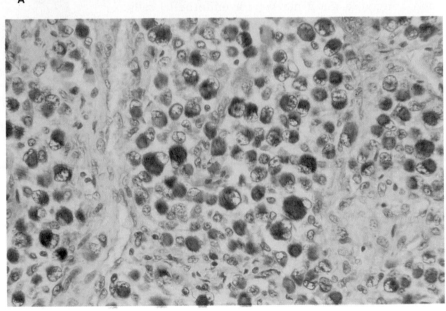

B

TUMOR MARKERS

Metastatic tumors may be so undifferentiated microscopically as to preclude even the distinction between an epithelial and a mesenchymal origin. Tumor markers rely on the preservation of characteristics of the progenitor cell or the synthesis of specialized proteins by the neoplastic cell to make this distinction. For example, they can be used to determine the presence of neuroendocrine features in apparently undifferentiated small cell carcinomas. One of the markers used in this determination is **neuron specific enolase** (NSE), a glycolytic enzyme of normal neurons and neuroendocrine cells that is also produced by their transformed counterparts.

Intermediate filaments serve as immunomarkers. These filaments tend to be cell type-specific, and that relative specificity is retained after neoplastic transformation. Thus, antibodies to intermediate filaments allow a reliable discrimination among poorly differentiated epithelial, mesenchymal, and neural neoplasms.

Intermediate filaments fall within five distinct classes:

Cytokeratins, a multigene family of proteins comprising at least 19 distinct polypeptides, are characteristic of epithelial cells and carcinomas.

Vimentin is found in mesenchymal cells and sarcomas.

Desmin is found in smooth muscle and striated muscle cells and neoplasms.

Glial filament protein, also known as glial fibrillary acidic protein (GFAP), is typical of glial cells and gliomas.

Neurofilament proteins are apparent in neurons and paraganglia cells and in neurogenic neoplasms.

Other diagnostically significant, though not pathognomonic, tumor markers are S-100 protein, an excellent marker for melanomas (Fig. 5-10); factor VIII-related antigen, a good marker for endothelial cells; alpha-fetoprotein, which exists in hepatocellular carcinomas and yolk sac carcinomas; thyroglobulin, which may help in identifying thyroid carcinomas; prostatic acid phosphatase and prostate-specific antigen, which are useful for the differentiation between prostatic carcinomas and carcinomas of other sites; and human chorionic gonadotropin, which marks trophoblastic tumors. Carcinoembryonic antigen (CEA), although neither site-nor tumor-specific, is nevertheless a useful marker for gastrointestinal and related cancers.

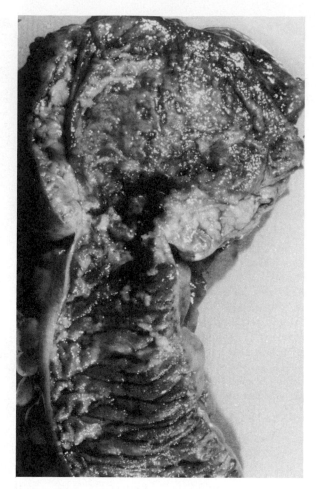

Figure 5-11. Adenocarcinoma of the colon with intestinal obstruction. The lumen of the colon at the site of the cancer is narrowed. The colon proximal to the obstruction is dilated.

INVASION AND METASTASIS

The two properties that are unique to cancer cells are the capacity to invade locally and the capacity to metastasize to distant sites. It is these properties that are responsible for the vast majority of deaths from cancer; the primary tumor itself is generally amenable to surgical extirpation.

PATTERNS OF SPREAD

DIRECT EXTENSION

Malignant tumors characteristically grow within the tissue of origin, where they enlarge and infiltrate normal structures. They may also extend directly beyond the confines of that organ to involve adjacent tissues. In some cases the growth of the cancer may be so extensive that replacement of the normal tissue results in functional insufficiency of the organ. Such a situation is not uncommon in primary cancer of the liver.

Tumors of the brain, such as astrocytomas, infiltrate the brain until they compromise vital regions. The direct extension of malignant tumors within an organ may also be life-threatening because of their location. A common example is the intestinal obstruction produced by cancer of the colon (Fig. 5-11).

The invasive growth pattern of malignant tumors often leads to their direct extension outside the tissue of origin, in which case the tumor may secondarily impair the function of an adjacent organ. Squamous carcinoma of the cervix often grows beyond the genital tract to produce vesicovaginal fistulas and obstruction of the ureters. Neglected cases of breast cancer are often complicated by extensive ulceration of the skin. Even small tumors can produce severe consequences when they invade vital structures. A small cancer of the lung can cause a bronchopleural fistula when it penetrates the bronchus, or exsanguinating hemorrhage when it erodes a blood vessel. The agonizing pain of pancreatic carcinoma results from direct extension of the tumor to the celiac nerve plexus. Tumor cells that reach serous cavities—for example, those of the peritoneum or pleura—spread easily by direct extension or can be carried by the fluid to new locations on the serous membranes. The most common example is the seeding of the peritoneal cavity by certain types of ovarian cancer (Fig. 5-12). Although malignant brain tumors do not customarily metastasize extracranially, cells that reach the cerebrospinal fluid may be transported to other sites within the central nervous system.

METASTATIC SPREAD

The invasive properties of malignant tumors bring them into contact with blood and lymphatic vessels. **In the same way that they can invade parenchymal tissue, neoplastic cells also can penetrate vascular and lymphatic channels. For metastases to appear, after the invasion of lymphatics or blood vessels the neoplastic cells must be released from the primary tumor, be transported through the circulation, lodge in the microcirculation of an organ, penetrate the vessel in the reverse direction, and grow autono-**

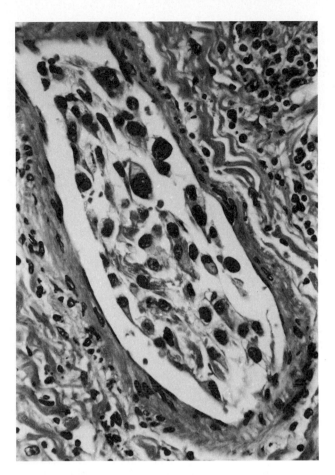

Figure 5-13. Hematogenous spread of cancer. Malignant cells fill a small pulmonary artery.

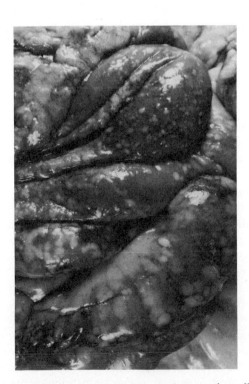

Figure 5-12. Peritoneal carcinomatosis. Loops of small intestine show peritoneal seeding by metastatic carcinoma, which appears as small whitish plaques on the serosal surface.

mously in this new location. In general, metastases resemble the primary tumor histologically, although they are occasionally so anaplastic that their cell of origin is obscure.

Hematogenous Metastases

Cancer cells commonly invade capillaries and venules, whereas the thicker-walled arterioles and arteries are relatively resistant. Before they can form viable metastases, circulating tumor cells must lodge in the vascular bed of the metastatic site (Fig. 5-13). Here they presumably attach to the walls of blood vessels, either to endothelial cells or to naked basement membranes, although the mechanisms remain a matter of speculation. This sequence of events explains why the liver and the lung are so frequently the sites of metastases. Because abdominal tumors seed the portal system, they lead to hepatic metastases, while other tumors penetrate systemic veins that eventually drain into the vena cava and hence to the lungs. In this respect it should be noted that some tumor cells released into the venous system survive passage through the microcirculation and are thereby transported to more distant organs. For instance, tumor cells may traverse the liver and produce pulmonary metastases, and neoplastic cells may also survive passage through the pulmonary microcirculation to reach the brain and other organs via arterial dissemination. Neoplastic cells arrested in the microcirculation are thought to penetrate the vessel walls at the site of metastasis by the same mechanisms with which the primary tumor invades.

Lymphatic Metastases

A historical dogma of metastatic spread held that epithelial tumors (carcinomas) preferentially metastasize through lymphatic channels whereas mesenchymal neoplasms (sarcomas) are distributed hematogenously. This distinction is no longer considered valid, because of clinical observations of metastatic patterns and the demonstration of numerous connections between the lymphatic and vascular systems. Tumors arising in tissues that have a rich lymphatic network—for instance, the breast—often metastasize by this route, although the particular properties of specific neoplasms may play a role in the route of spread.

Basement membranes envelop only the large lymphatic channels; they are lacking in the lymphatic capillaries. Thus, there is reason to believe that invasive tumor cells may penetrate lymphatic channels more readily than blood vessels. Once in the lymphatic vessels, the cells are carried to the regional draining lymph nodes, where they initially lodge in the marginal sinus and then extend throughout the node. Lymph nodes bearing metastatic deposits may be enlarged to many times their normal size, often exceeding the diameter of the primary lesion. The cut surface of the lymph node usually resembles that of the primary tumor in color and consistency and may also exhibit the necrosis and hemorrhage commonly seen in primary cancers (Fig. 5-14).

The regional lymphatic pattern of metastatic spread is most prominently exemplified by cancer of the breast. In breast cancer the initial metastases are almost always lymphatic, and these regional lymphatic metastases have considerable prognostic significance. Cancers that arise in the lateral aspect of the breast characteristically spread to the lymph nodes of the axilla, whereas those arising in the medial portion drain to the internal mammary lymph nodes in the thorax.

Lymphatic metastases are occasionally found in lymph nodes distant from the site of the primary tumor; these are termed **"skip" metastases.** For example, abdominal cancers may initially be signaled by the

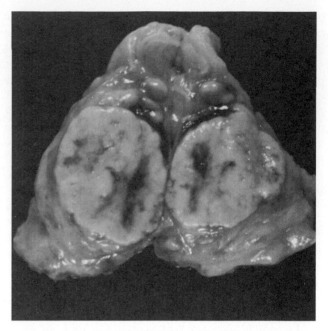

Figure 5-14. Metastatic carcinoma in a lymph node. The bisected node, embedded in fat tissue, is enlarged and indurated by metastatic carcinoma of the colon. Necrosis and hemorrhage are seen as dark, irregular areas.

appearance of an enlarged supraclavicular node, the so-called sentinel node.

BIOLOGY OF INVASION AND METASTASIS

It is intuitively clear that for invasion to occur, tumor cells must escape the confines of the basement membrane of their tissue of origin, traverse the extracellular matrix of the surrounding normal tissues, and penetrate the basement membranes of blood vessels. Invasive cancers, unlike their benign counterparts, do not generally produce basement membranes.

The penetration of the basement membrane of the host tissue and the invasion of the surrounding extracellular environment is thought to involve three steps (Fig. 5-15): (1) binding of the tumor cell to a matrix component; (2) enzymatic lysis of this structure, and (3) movement through the resulting defect. The initial binding may involve such tissue matrix components as fibronectin, laminin, proteoglycans, and collagen, which may be lysed by certain proteases and collagenases found in tumor cells. An attractive hypothesis holds that binding occurs by way of specific laminin receptors on the tumor cell membrane. It is postulated that the enhanced attachment of tumor cells to con-

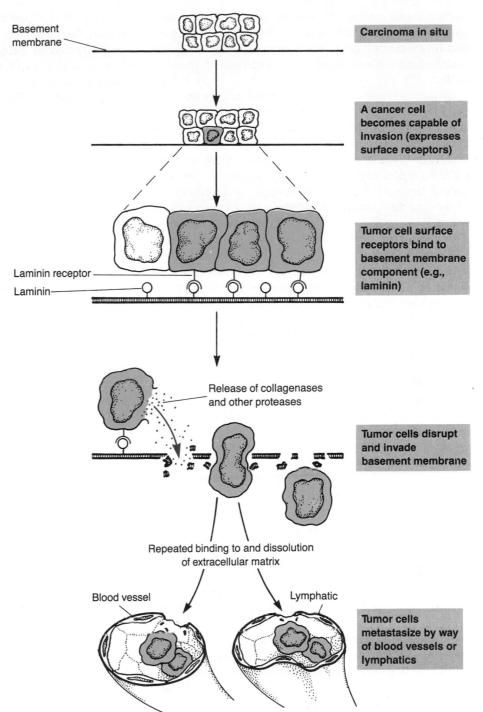

Basement membrane

Carcinoma in situ

A cancer cell becomes capable of invasion (expresses surface receptors)

Laminin receptor

Laminin

Tumor cell surface receptors bind to basement membrane component (e.g., laminin)

Release of collagenases and other proteases

Tumor cells disrupt and invade basement membrane

Repeated binding to and dissolution of extracellular matrix

Blood vessel

Lymphatic

Tumor cells metastasize by way of blood vessels or lymphatics

Figure 5-15. Mechanisms of tumor invasion. The mechanism by which a malignant tumor initially penetrates a confining basement membrane and then invades the surrounding extracellular environment is thought to involve three steps. The tumor must first acquire the ability to bind to a component of the basement membrane. This is depicted as the acquisition of receptors that bind to laminin, one component of the basement membrane. As a consequence of the binding to laminin, collagenases and other proteases are released from the tumor cells, and the basement membrane is lysed. The cancer cell then moves through the defect in the basement membrane into the extracellular environment. By repeatedly binding to and lysing components of the extracellular matrix, the invading tumor penetrates farther into the extracellular environment. The invasion of blood vessels and lymphatics occurs by essentially the same mechanisms.

nective tissue matrix components permits collagenases and other proteases to lyse the basement membrane and other connective tissue elements, after which the ameboid movement of the tumor exploits the resulting fault.

Although it appears that malignant tumors have the capacity to destroy connective tissue, they also frequently stimulate fibrosis, a process termed "desmoplasia." In some tumors the desmoplastic response, rather than the accumulation of tumor cells, accounts for the clinical appearance of the cancer. In this category is the hard lump of infiltrating carcinoma of the breast and the "leather bottle stomach" of gastric carcinoma.

The anatomy of the vascular system and the vascularity of specific organs unquestionably influence the pattern of metastatic spread, but it is also true that certain tumors seem to prefer some organs over others, presumably because of interactions between tumor cells and the host organ. It is noteworthy that despite their size and abundant blood flow, neither the spleen nor skeletal muscle are common sites of metastases.

Cancer is generally monoclonal—that is, the tumor is derived from the transformation of a single cell. This circumstance might lead to the expectation that the progeny of the originally transformed cell are all alike. This assumption is not true. **Tumors are composed of heterogeneous cell populations.** This fact has important implications for the metastatic potential of tumors. A tumor must surmount a variety of hurdles before becoming established as a metastasis. When neoplastic cells are injected into an animal, as few as one in a thousand survives to establish a metastasis. Mechanical factors and host defenses undoubtedly play an important role in this reduction, but the question remains whether the survivors are selected randomly or are endowed with specific properties not inherent in the other elements of the primary neoplastic population.

It has long been known that by transplanting successive generations of metastatic cells from one animal to another it is possible to produce cells that have a far greater metastatic potential than the original tumor cells. In vitro, certain properties of neoplastic cells correlate with metastatic potential, including resistance to immunologic attack, the ability to invade other tissues, the capacity to digest type IV collagen, and detachment from a monolayer culture. Cells selected for such properties in vitro show enhanced metastatic potential in vivo.

An important demonstration of tumor heterogeneity has come from experiments in which a variety of epithelial and mesenchymal tumors were cloned in vitro and each clone was individually injected into a host animal. If the tumor cells were originally homogeneous, then a comparable number of metastases would be expected in each animal. In fact, however, the clones, which had not been treated or selected in any manner, displayed widely varying metastatic activity. **This heterogeneity of the primary tumor suggests that the survival of malignant cells in the form of metastases is not due to a random process, but rather is a manifestation of the selective growth of subpopulations of cells that are endowed with the properties necessary for survival and growth in potentially inhospitable places.** This concept of tumor heterogeneity extends beyond metastatic potential to include the expression of hormone receptors and, of great importance, sensitivity to chemotherapeutic agents.

GRADING AND STAGING OF CANCERS

In an attempt to predict the clinical behavior of a malignant tumor and to establish criteria for therapy, many cancers are classified according to a cytologic and histologic grading scheme or by staging protocols that describe the extent of spread. **Cytologic/histologic grading, which is necessarily subjective and at best semiquantitative, is based on the degree of anaplasia and on the number of proliferating cells.** The degree of anaplasia is determined from the shape and regularity of the cells, and the presence of distinct differentiated features, such as functioning glandlike structures in adenocarcinomas or epithelial pearls in squamous carcinomas. Evidence of rapid or abnormal growth is provided by large numbers of mitoses, the presence of atypical mitoses, nuclear pleomorphism, and tumor giant cells. Most grading schemes classify tumors into three or four grades of increasing degrees of malignancy (Fig. 5-16). The general correlation between the cytologic grade and the biologic behavior of a neoplasm is not invariable: There are many examples of tumors of low cytologic grades with substantial malignant properties.

The choice of surgical approach or the selection of treatment modalities is influenced more by the stage of a cancer than by its cytologic grade. Moreover, most statistical data related to cancer survival are based on the stage rather than the cytologic grade of the tumor. Clinical staging according to the extent of spread of the tumor is independent of cytologic grading. **The significant criteria used for staging vary with different organs. Commonly used criteria include tumor size; the extent of local growth, whether within or without the organ; the presence of lymph**

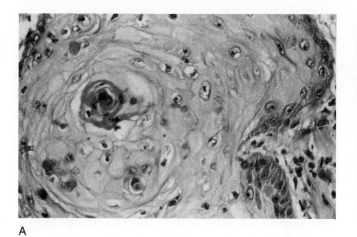

A

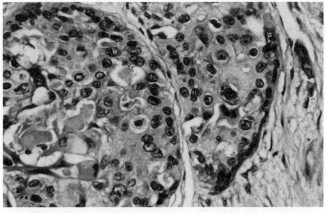

B

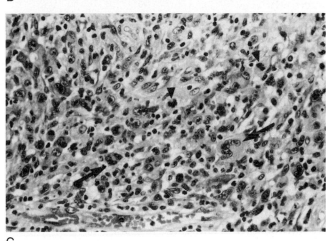

C

Figure 5-16. Cytologic grading of squamous cell carcinoma of the lung. (*A*) Well-differentiated (grade 1) squamous cell carcinoma. The tumor cells bear a strong resemblance to normal squamous cells and are synthesizing keratin, as evidenced by the epithelial pearl. (*B*) Moderately differentiated (grade 2) squamous cell carcinoma. The tumor cells are more pleomorphic and are less similar to squamous cells than those in A. Individual cells still produce keratin. (*C*) Poorly differentiated (grade 3) squamous cell carcinoma. The malignant cells are no longer identifiable as of squamous origin. Tumor giant cells (*arrows*) and atypical mitoses (*arrowhead*) are present.

node metastases; and the presence of distant metastases. These criteria have been codified in the international **TNM cancer staging system,** in which *T* refers to the size of the primary tumor, *N* to the number and distribution of lymph node metastases, and *M* to the presence and extent of distant metastases.

In some cases the distinction between benign and malignant tumors is based solely on size, as in the case of renal carcinoma. On the basis of clinical experience, tumors below 2 cm in diameter are considered benign adenomas, whereas those of larger size are labeled carcinomas. The choice of surgical therapy is often influenced by size alone. For example, a primary breast cancer smaller than 2 cm in diameter can be treated with local excision and radiation therapy, whereas larger masses necessitate mastectomy. Local extension, too, can be used to estimate prognosis, as in the Dukes classification of colorectal cancer. Penetration of the tumor into the muscularis and serosa is associated with a poorer prognosis than that of a more superficial tumor. Clearly, the presence of lymph node metastases

mandates more aggressive treatment than their absence, whereas the presence of distant metastases is generally a contraindication to surgical intervention other than for palliation.

BIOCHEMISTRY OF THE CANCER CELL

Despite more than a half-century of intensive investigation of the biochemical basis of neoplasia, no alterations unique to cancer cells or crucial to carcinogenesis have emerged. Among the earliest studies the most prominent were those of Warburg, who proposed that the biochemical basis of neoplasia was the dependence of tumor cells on anaerobic glycolysis rather than aerobic respiration. According to Warburg's theory the neoplastic stimulus is an irreversible injury to respiration, followed by a compensatory increase in fermentation and the production of a neoplastic cell. However, although it is true that most cancers do display high glycolytic rates, many display normal rates. An increase in glycolysis seems, therefore, to be a characteristic of only some tumors and to be an effect rather than a cause of neoplastic transformation. Later investigations found an association between neoplasia and numerous enzyme deficits, lowered protein levels, the appearance of unusual isozymes, and the production of fetal proteins. However, detailed studies of tumors with varying degrees of differentiation have clearly shown that this phenotypic heterogeneity of cancer cells simply reflects the variable degree of differentiation. **The search for a common qualitative biochemical defect to explain neoplasia has to date been unsuccessful.**

GROWTH OF CANCERS

CELL CYCLE KINETICS

The fact that **tumor cells do not necessarily proliferate at a faster rate than their normal counterparts** is now well established. This suggests that tumor growth depends on other factors, such as the proportion of cycling cells (growth fraction) and the rate of cell death. In normal proliferating tissues, such as the intestine and the bone marrow, an exquisite balance between cell renewal and cell death is strictly maintained. By contrast, **the major determinant of tumor growth is clearly the fact that more cells are produced than die in a given time.**

The growth of a tumor may be expressed in terms of the **doubling time**—that is, the time taken for the number of cells in the mass to double. Importantly, it has been shown in experimental and human tumors that the doubling time is not necessarily correlated with the growth fraction. Since the duration of mitosis in cancer cells is often prolonged, the number of mitoses in a histologic section can be misleading as an indicator of overall growth. For example, a doubling in mitotic time will result in twice as many visible mitoses without any real increase in the rate of growth. In most cases the theoretical tumor doubling time, calculated from the growth fraction and the cell cycle time, bears little relation to the actual clinical situation. For example, if a tumor weighing 1 g (often the smallest size clinically detectable) produces about two new cells per 1000 cells in each mitotic cycle the theoretical net increase would be a staggering 10^6 cells per hour, a figure totally at variance with the experience with most solid tumors. **Because of this difference between the theoretical and observed growth of tumors, it has been estimated that in human skin tumors as many as 97% of proliferated cells die spontaneously.** The causes of tumor cell death are not precisely defined, but probably include such factors as inherent genetic programs (programmed cell death); inadequate blood supply with consequent ischemia; a paucity of nutrients; and vulnerability to specific and nonspecific host defenses.

GROWTH FACTORS AND NEOPLASIA

The recent discovery of polypeptide growth factors (PGFs) has led to an enormous research effort aimed at defining their roles in the regulation of normal growth and the preservation of viability of many cell types. PGFs have been implicated in the regulation of embryogenesis, growth and development, selective cell survival, hematopoiesis, tissue repair, immune responses, atherosclerosis, and neoplastic growth. The molecular structures of a number of PGFs—for example epidermal growth factor (EGF), interleukin-2 (T-cell growth factor), nerve growth factor (NGF), and platelet-derived growth factor (PDGF)—have been determined. Numerous other growth factors have been partially characterized, while a number of naturally occurring substances, such as insulin, prolactin, thrombin, and transferrin, have been identified as growth regulators.

For a substance to qualify as a PGF, its production, transportation, and interaction with target cells must occur in a fashion consistent with a normal or regulated physiologic process. PGFs have the following characteristics: (1) most of the structure consists of polypeptide material, (2) binding at the cell surface initiates the cellular response, (3) the response is initiated exclusively by the formation of a specific PGF-receptor complex, (4) a specific hypertrophic or hyperplastic response is produced by the PGF-receptor complex, and (5) the PGF-receptor complex is internalized by receptor-mediated endocytosis.

A direct link between PGFs and events involved in the initiation or expression of the neoplastic state remains to be proved, but several important facts suggest that a relationship indeed exists:

- In some instances PGFs related to EGF and derived from both normal and neoplastic cells have the capacity to transform normal cells in vitro.
- PGDF is virtually identical to a major sequence found in the product of a viral oncogene. A viral oncogene is a genetic locus of an RNA-transforming virus (retrovirus) whose activity is responsible for the initiation and maintenance of neoplastic

transformation. The oncogenes of retroviruses are, in turn, close copies of cellular genes, known as proto-oncogenes or cellular oncogenes. In this context it is intriguing that PDGF is also involved in the normal proliferative responses of wound healing and repair—processes that have classically been thought to have certain analogies with neoplasia.

- The receptors for PDGF, EGF, and insulin possess tyrosine-specific kinase (phosphorylating) activity. The product of the Rous sarcoma viral oncogene displays similar activity.
- EGF enhances the synthesis of a viral gene product (poly(A^+)RNA, known as VL 30) that has been linked to the growth response of normal and transformed cells.
- Certain chemicals (phorbol esters) that promote the development of skin tumors in vivo can regulate the affinity and number of EGF receptors.
- A PGF coded for by an oncogene can, in turn, induce the expression of a second oncogene, an observation that is consistent with the multistep nature of carcinogenesis.
- Small molecules, such as retinoids, that under certain circumstances prevent the development of cancer modulate the expression of oncogenes or PGFs.

CAUSES OF CANCER

The morphologic appearance and biologic behavior of established cancers are well known. The underlying mechanisms of carcinogenesis, however, and the molecular description of the neoplastic state remain mysterious. Although we know of many agents that can cause cancer in man and experimental animals, we are ignorant of the proportion of human cancers that may be attributed to them. In some instances, it is clear that the majority of the cancers relate to a specific agent. For instance, most cancers of the lung are unquestionably examples of chemical carcinogenesis by tobacco smoke. On the other hand, although both high-dose radiation and an aromatic hydrocarbon, benzene, are known to cause leukemia, we do not know whether radiation- or chemical-induced leukemias comprise more than a small proportion of all granulocytic leukemias. Notwithstanding correlations with age, hormonal status, diet, genetic factors, and environmental agents, the etiology of many of the most common cancers, such as those of the breast, colon, and prostate, remains obscure. Despite the enormous gaps in our knowledge, an appreciation of carcinogenesis associated with chemicals, viruses, and physical agents is important, because

the mechanisms of these processes may also underlie the induction of the majority of cancers, which are of unknown etiology.

CHEMICAL CARCINOGENESIS

The entire field of chemical carcinogenesis originated some two centuries ago in descriptions of an occupational disease. This was not the first recognition of an occupation-related cancer (a peculiar predisposition of nuns to breast cancer was appreciated even earlier), but to the English physician Sir Percival Pott goes the credit for relating cancer of the scrotum in chimney sweeps to a specific chemical exposure, namely soot. Almost a century elapsed between these observations and the realization that other products of the combustion of organic materials are responsible for a man-made epidemic of cancer: cancer of the lung in cigarette smokers.

The experimental production of cancer by chemicals dates to 1915, when Japanese investigators produced skin cancers in rabbits with coal tar. Since that time, many more organic and inorganic materials have been proved to be carcinogens, including many compounds that are relatively inert in terms of chemical reactivity. This paradox was explained in the early 1960s, when it was shown that **most, although not all, chemical carcinogens require metabolic activation before they can react with cell constituents.** On the basis of those observations and the close correlation between mutagenicity and carcinogenicity, an in vitro test for screening potential chemical carcinogens—the Ames test—was developed a decade later. The experimental study of the actions of carcinogenic chemicals also led to the realization that **cancer is the result of a multistep process.** Initially, it was found that a single application of a carcinogen to the skin of a mouse is not, by itself, sufficient to produce cancer (Fig. 5-17). However, when a proliferative stimulus is then applied locally, in the form of a second, noncarcinogenic, irritating chemical —for example, a phorbol ester—tumors appear. The first effect is irreversible but not detectable by current methods, and is termed **initiation.** The action of the second, noncarcinogenic chemical is called **promotion.** This concept of a two-stage carcinogenic process has been expanded to a multistep process by numerous further experiments, principally centered on the liver.

CHEMICAL CARCINOGENS AND THEIR METABOLISM

Chemicals cause cancer either directly or, more often, after metabolic activation. The direct-acting carcino-

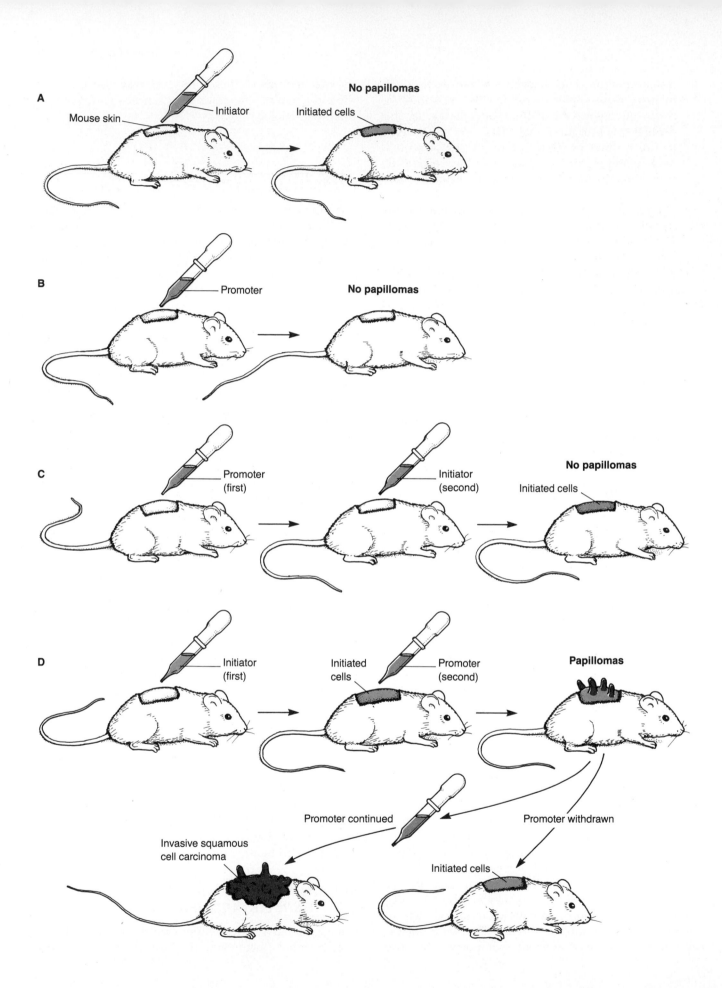

A

Mouse skin — Initiator

No papillomas

Initiated cells

B

Promoter

No papillomas

C

Promoter
(first)

Initiator
(second)

No papillomas

Initiated cells

D

Initiator
(first)

Initiated
cells

Promoter
(second)

Papillomas

Promoter continued

Promoter withdrawn

Invasive squamous
cell carcinoma

Initiated cells

gens are inherently sufficiently reactive to bind covalently to cellular macromolecules. In addition to a number of organic compounds, such as nitrogen mustard, bis(chloromethyl)ether, and benzyl chloride, certain metals are included in this category. The great majority of organic carcinogens, however, require conversion to an ultimate, more reactive compound. This conversion is enzymatic and, for the most part, is effected by the cellular systems involved in drug metabolism and detoxification. Many cells in the body, particularly liver cells, possess enzyme systems that are capable of converting procarcinogens to their active forms. Each carcinogen has its own spectrum of target tissues, often limited to a single organ. The basis for organ specificity in chemical carcinogenesis is not well understood, but there is experimental evidence to suggest that other factors are required for initiation in certain tissues, such as the suspected role of cystitis in bladder cancer.

The **polycyclic aromatic hydrocarbons,** originally derived from coal tar, are among the most extensively studied carcinogens. In this class are such model compounds as benzo(a)pyrene, 3-methylcholanthrene, and dibenzanthracene. These compounds have a broad range of target organs and generally produce cancers at the site of application. The specific type of cancer produced varies with the route of administration and includes tumors of the skin, soft tissues, and breast. Since polycyclic hydrocarbons have been identified in cigarette smoke, it has been suggested that they may be involved in the production of carcinoma of the lung.

Polycyclic hydrocarbons are metabolized by cytochrome P_{450}-dependent mixed function oxidases to electrophilic epoxides, which in turn react with proteins and nucleic acids. The formation of the epoxide depends on the presence of an unsaturated carbon–carbon bond. For example, **vinyl chloride,** the simple two-carbon molecule from which the widely used plastic polyvinyl chloride is synthesized, is metabolized to an epoxide, which is why it has carcinogenic properties. Workers exposed to the vinyl chloride monomer in the ambient atmosphere later developed angiosarcomas of the liver.

In contrast to the polycyclic hydrocarbons, which are for the most part formed either by the combustion of organic material or synthetically, a heterocyclic hydrocarbon, **aflatoxin B_1, is a natural product of the fungus** *Aspergillus flavus.* Like the polycyclic aromatic hydrocarbons, aflatoxin B_1 is metabolized to an epoxide, which is either detoxified or binds covalently to DNA (Fig. 5-18).

Aromatic amines and **azo dyes,** in contrast to the polycyclic aromatic hydrocarbons, are not ordinarily carcinogenic at the point of application but commonly produce bladder and liver tumors, respectively, when fed to experimental animals. Both aromatic amines and azo dyes are primarily metabolized in the liver. The activation reaction undergone by aromatic amines is N-hydroxylation to form the hydroxylamino derivatives, which are then detoxified by conjugation with glucuronic acid. In the bladder, hydrolysis of the glucuronide releases the reactive hydroxylamine. **Occupational exposure to aromatic amines in the form of aniline dyes has resulted in bladder cancer.**

Carcinogenic **nitrosamines** are a subject of considerable study because it is suspected that they may play a role in human gastrointestinal neoplasms and possibly other cancers. The simplest nitrosamine, dimethylnitrosamine, produces kidney and liver tumors in rodents. Nitrosamines are also potent carcinogens in primates, although unambiguous evidence of cancer induction in humans is lacking. Nitrosamines are activated by hydroxylation, followed by formation of a reactive alkyl carbonium ion. A carbonium ion is also formed in the liver by the metabolism of carcinogenic **pyrrolizidine alkaloids,** which are important constituents of medicinal bush and herbal teas in undeveloped countries.

A number of metals or metal compounds can induce cancer, but the mechanisms by which they do so are unknown. Most metal-induced cancers occur in an

---

Figure 5-17. The concept of initiation and promotion. (A) The single application of an initiator to the skin of a mouse produces initiated cells, but no papillomas form. (B) Likewise, the application of a promotor alone to the skin produces no papillomas. (C) If the promoter is applied to the skin before the application of the initiator, no papillomas form, although initiated cells are present. (D) When the skin is first exposed to the initiator, the subsequent application of the promoter results in papillomas. If the promoter is withdrawn, the papillomas regress, leaving initiated cells in their place. When the promoter is applied to mouse skin bearing papillomas, invasive squamous cell carcinomas are produced.

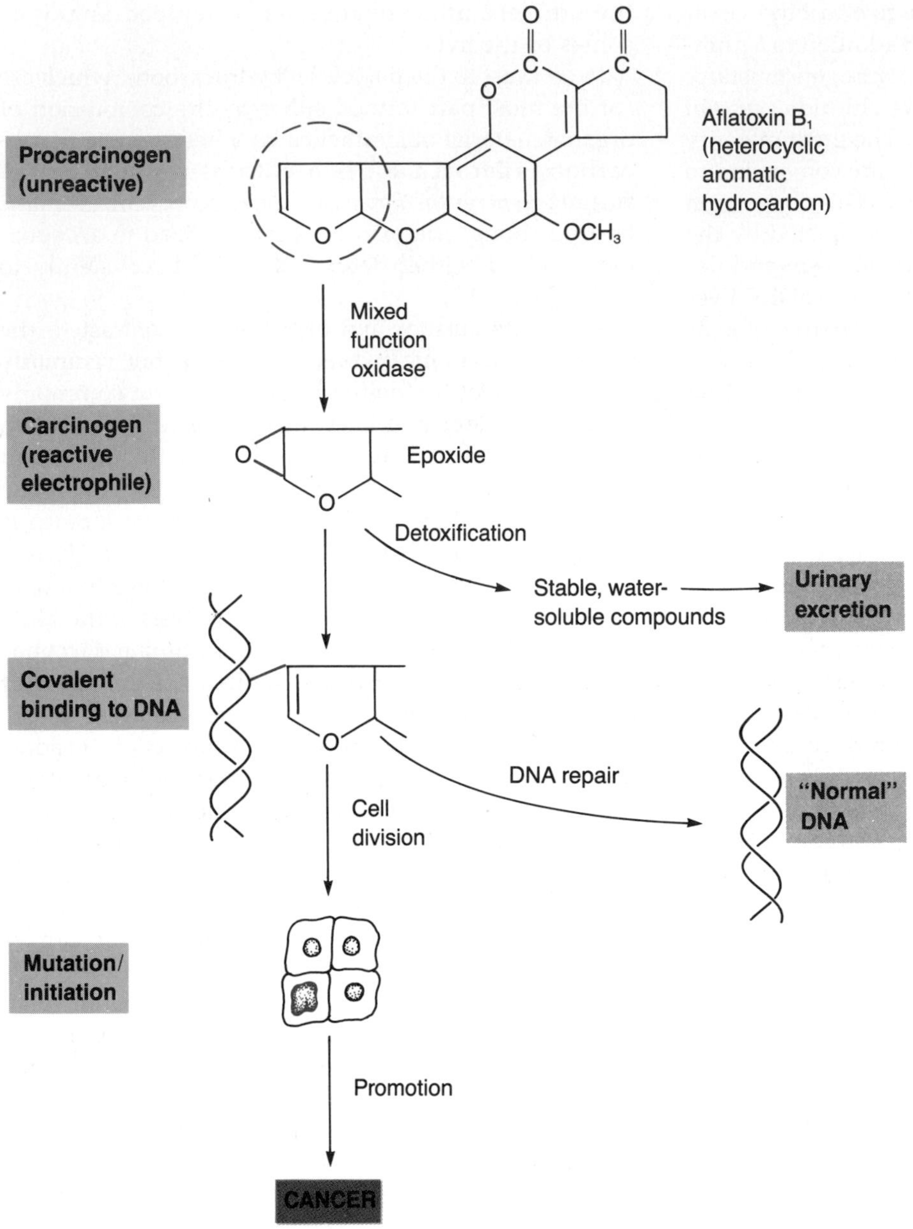

Procarcinogen (unreactive)

Aflatoxin B₁ (heterocyclic aromatic hydrocarbon)

Mixed function oxidase

Carcinogen (reactive electrophile)

Epoxide

Detoxification

Stable, water-soluble compounds → **Urinary excretion**

Covalent binding to DNA

DNA repair → **"Normal" DNA**

Cell division

Mutation/ initiation

Promotion

CANCER

Figure 5-18. Metabolic activation of aflatoxin B_1. The unreactive procarcinogen aflatoxin B_1 is metabolized by the mixed function oxidase of the hepatic endoplasmic reticulum to yield an epoxide. This electrophilic metabolite can be detoxified by conjugation with GSH and excreted in the urine. Alternatively, the epoxide of aflatoxin B_1 can covalently bind to liver cell macromolecules, and in particular can bind to DNA. The resulting DNA damage can be repaired, a process that restores the integrity of the DNA. If the hepatocyte divides before DNA repair is complete, initiated liver cells result. With the appropriate regimen, these initiated hepatocytes can be promoted to a hepatocellular carcinoma.

occupational setting, and the subject is, therefore, discussed in more detail in Chapter 8, which deals with environmental pathology.

FACTORS INFLUENCING CHEMICAL CARCINOGENESIS

Chemical carcinogenesis in experimental animals is influenced by a variety of factors, including species and strain, age and sex of the animal, hormonal status, diet, and the presence or absence of inducers of drug-meta-bolizing systems and tumor promoters. A similar role for such factors in humans has been postulated on the basis of epidemiologic studies. In the context of chemical carcinogenesis, it is appropriate to focus on the effects of modifiers of the metabolism of carcinogens.

The activity of the **mixed function oxidases** is genetically determined, and a correlation has been observed between the levels of these enzymes in various strains of mice and their sensitivity to chemical carcinogens.

The effects of **sex and hormonal status** are important determinants of susceptibility to chemical carcinogens but are highly variable and in many instances not readily predictable. In most experimental species, male animals are more susceptible to the aromatic amine liver carcinogens than are females. By contrast, female mice are more sensitive to the carcinogenic effects of aminoazotoluene and diethylnitrosamine.

The **composition of the diet** can affect the level of drug-metabolizing enzymes. A low-protein diet, which reduces the hepatic activity of mixed function oxidases, is associated with a decreased sensitivity to hepatocarcinogens. Much attention has recently been focused on an alleged association between fat in the diet and the incidence of breast and colon cancers. It has been clearly shown experimentally that a diet high in fat increases susceptibility to chemically produced breast cancer. Dietary fiber has also been suggested as an influence on the occurrence of colorectal cancer. In this case a plausible explanation lies in the effect of fiber on increasing the motility of the gut and thereby hastening the elimination of potentially harmful chemicals in the fecal stream. However, despite the recommendations of health officials and the claims of manufacturers of certain foods, there is no clinical or epidemiologic evidence that the introduction of more fiber into the Western diet reduces the risk of colorectal cancer.

CHEMICAL CARCINOGENS AS MUTAGENS

The search for rapid, reproducible, and reliable screening assays for potential carcinogenic activity has centered on the relationship between carcinogenicity and mutagenicity. **A mutagen is an agent that can permanently alter the genetic constitution of a cell.** The most widely used screening test, **the Ames test,** utilizes the appearance of mutants in a culture of bacteria of the *Salmonella* species. About 90% of known carcinogens are mutagenic, as shown by this test. Moreover, most, but not all, mutagens are carcinogenic. (This close correlation between carcinogenicity and mutagenicity presumably reflects the fact that both damage DNA.) Thus, while not infallible, the in vitro mutagenicity assay has proved to be a valuable tool in screening for the carcinogenic potential of chemicals.

CHEMICAL CARCINOGENESIS AS A MULTISTEP PROCESS

We have previously mentioned that experimentally chemical carcinogenesis is a multistep process, the details of which have been best defined in the rodent liver. The carcinogenic process in the liver from the administration of the carcinogen to the appearance of a hepatocellular carcinoma has been dissected into at least seven steps (Fig. 5-19):

1. **Biochemical lesion.** Most hepatocarcinogens react with DNA as the initial event. If this damage is not repaired, such an interaction may result in mutations, chromosomal translocations, inactivation of regulatory genes, or more subtle changes.

2. **Fixation of the biochemical lesion by cell proliferation.** Most chemical carcinogens do not produce tumors in the normal adult liver even though they damage DNA. If initiation is to occur there must be cell proliferation before DNA repair is completed. Such proliferation can be induced by partial hepatectomy; by toxic necrosis, produced by either the carcinogen itself or another nonspecific agent; or by the physiologic growth of the newborn animal.

3. **Microscopic foci of altered cells.** During the process of promotion, initiated cells grow to form microscopic foci of phenotypically altered cells.

4. **Hepatocyte nodules.** Nodules are defined as macroscopically visible focal proliferations of altered hepatocytes that compress the surrounding liver. They may measure up to 1 cm in diameter in the rat liver. On removal of the promoting stimulus, the vast majority of nodules (95% to 98%) eventually remodel to the appearance of normal liver as their cells return to a more differentiated state. However, the preneoplastic process is evidenced by the persistence of a small minority of nodules (2% to 5%). These persistent nodules exhibit autonomous cell proliferation and are the precursors of the eventual hepatocellular carcinoma.

5. **Cell proliferation and cell death in the persistent nodules.** The persistent nodules at first display synchronous cell proliferation, which may be ten times faster than that of the surrounding normal liver. This growth is almost always balanced by an accelerated cell death, and the nodules, therefore, enlarge only slowly.

6. **Defective control of the cell cycle.** Eventually, a small subset of hepatocytes in the persistent nodules acquire a new property: namely, the capacity to continue cycling indefinitely, without the usual arrest after one or two cell divisions. For the first time these cells will form nodules, and eventually hepatocellular carcinomas, on transplantation to the spleen.

7. **Progression to hepatocellular carcinoma.** This step probably consists of a number of separate and distinct events, but the nature of these is obscure. It is clear that progression to cancer is subject to delay by dietary and hormonal influences. By 9 to 12 months after initiation, unequivocal hepatocellular carcinomas are seen.

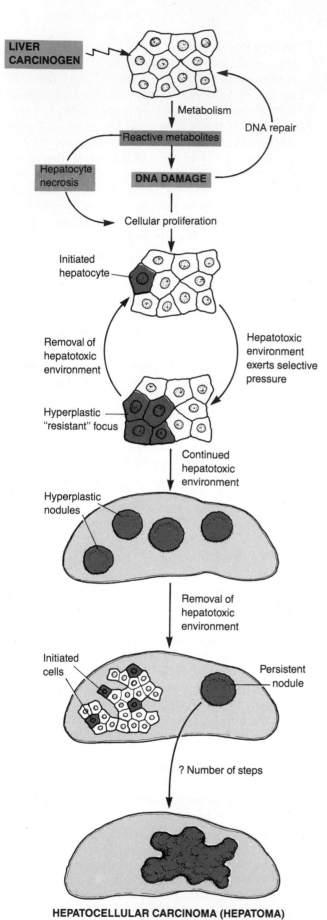

LIVER CARCINOGEN

Metabolism

Reactive metabolites

DNA repair

Hepatocyte necrosis

DNA DAMAGE

Cellular proliferation

Initiated hepatocyte

Removal of hepatotoxic environment

Hepatotoxic environment exerts selective pressure

Hyperplastic "resistant" focus

Continued hepatotoxic environment

Hyperplastic nodules

Removal of hepatotoxic environment

Initiated cells

Persistent nodule

? Number of steps

HEPATOCELLULAR CARCINOMA (HEPATOMA)

Figure 5-19. Hepatocarcinogenesis in the rat.

From these observations, one can abstract four hypothetical stages of chemical carcinogenesis. The first stage, **initiation,** is followed by a stage of **promotion,** which is characterized by an excess of cell proliferation over cell death. During this second stage the altered cells do not exhibit autonomous growth, but remain dependent on the continued presence of the promoting stimulus. In the third stage, growth is autonomous, and **progression** to cancer is independent of the carcinogen or the promoter. When the cells acquire the capacity to invade and metastasize, the tumor is labeled **"cancer."**

PHYSICAL CARCINOGENESIS

There are significant implications for public health stemming from the diagnostic and therapeutic use of x-rays and radioisotopes in medicine, and widespread concern about the safety of nuclear reactors and the dangers of atomic war. Radiation carcinogenesis is discussed in Chapter 8, which is concerned with environmental pathology. The physical agents of carcinogenesis discussed here are ultraviolet light, asbestos, and foreign bodies.

ULTRAVIOLET RADIATION

Appreciation of the carcinogenic effect of ultraviolet (UV) radiation in humans is based principally on clinical and epidemiologic observations. **Cancers attributed to sun exposure—namely basal cell carcinoma, squamous carcinoma, and melanoma—occur predominantly in whites;** the skin of the darker races is presumably protected by the increased concentration of melanin pigment, which absorbs UV radiation. In fair-skinned people the areas exposed to the sun are most prone to develop skin cancer. Moreover, there is a direct correlation between total exposure to sunlight and incidence of skin cancer.

It now appears that the most important biochemical effect of UV radiation is the formation of **pyrimidine dimers in DNA,** although other photoproducts may also play a role. Pyrimidine dimers may form between thymine and thymine, between thymine and cytosine, or between cytosine pairs alone.

The importance of DNA repair in protecting against the harmful effects of UV radiation is exemplified by the autosomal recessive disease **xeroderma pigmentosum.** In this rare disease a sensitivity to sunlight is accompanied by a high incidence of skin cancers, including basal cell carcinoma, squamous cell carcinoma, and melanoma. Both the neoplastic and non-neoplastic disorders of the skin in this disease are attributed to an impairment in the excision of UV-damaged DNA.

ASBESTOS

The characteristic tumor associated with asbestos exposure is malignant mesothelioma of the pleural and peritoneal cavities. This cancer, which is exceedingly rare in the general population, has been reported to occur in 2% to 3% (in some studies even more) of heavily exposed workers. The latent period—that is, the interval between exposure and the appearance of a tumor—is usually about 20 years, but may be twice that figure. Fibrotic pleural lesions are often found in those exposed to asbestos but are not related to the development of malignant mesothelioma.

The pathogenesis of asbestos-associated mesotheliomas is obscure. In rats the dimensions of the fiber, rather than its chemical composition, were reported to be crucial. Long, thin fibers deposited in the pleural space produced tumors, while short, thick fibers did not. This finding is compatible with the clinical observation that the long, thin crocidolite fibers are associated with a considerably greater risk of mesothelioma than the shorter and thicker amosite fibers of the flexible chrysotile fibers. However, the distinction between these fibers in the causation of human disease should not be taken as absolute, particularly since mixtures of these fibers are characteristically found in human lungs.

An association between cancer of the lung and asbestos exposure is clearly established in smokers. A small increase in the prevalence of lung cancer has been found in nonsmokers exposed to asbestos, but the data base of the studies was small, and the subject would benefit from further investigation. An increased incidence of cancer of the larynx has also been reported among asbestos workers who smoke. Claims that exposure to asbestos increases the risk of gastrointestinal cancer have not withstood statistical analysis of the collected data.

Pulmonary asbestosis and asbestosis-associated neoplasms are discussed in Chapter 12, which deals with diseases of the lungs.

FOREIGN BODY CARCINOGENESIS

A number of different sarcomas have been induced in rodents by the implantation of inert materials, such as plastic and metal films, various fibers (including fiberglass), plastic sponges, glass spheres, and dextran polymers. The chemical nature of these implants does not seem to be the critical feature, since disks made of pure carbon also produce sarcomas. Rather, the size, smoothness, and durability of the implanted surface are important. This form of cancer is highly species-specific. For example, rats and mice are highly susceptible to foreign-body carcinogenesis but guinea pigs are resistant. Humans are certainly highly resistant, as evidenced by the lack of cancers following the implantation of prostheses constructed of plastics and metals.

VIRAL CARCINOGENESIS

The role of viruses in the spontaneous appearance and experimental induction of cancer in animals is thoroughly established. The strongest associations between viruses and cancer in humans are the RNA retrovirus HTLV I and T cell leukemia/lymphoma; the human papillomavirus (DNA) and squamous carcinoma of the cervix; and the hepatitis B virus (DNA) and primary hepatocellular carcinoma.

DNA VIRUSES

Papillomaviruses

A viral etiology of human cancers has yet to be proved conclusively, but the evidence that human papillomaviruses (HPV) can induce cancer in man is highly suggestive. In humans, as in animals, HPV causes benign lesions of squamous epithelium, including warts, laryngeal papillomas, and condylomata accuminata (genital warts) of the vulva, penis, and perianal region. Occasionally condylomata accuminata and laryngeal papillomas undergo malignant transformation to squamous cell carcinoma. It is noteworthy that malignant transformations of benign squamous lesions in animals and humans exemplify the multistep nature of cancer development, proceeding through dysplasia and carcinoma in situ to frank invasion. It is of great interest that **HPV has now been associated with the development of cervical intraepithelial neoplasia and invasive squamous carcinoma.**

Polyomaviruses

Polyomavirus produces tumors in a wide variety of organs in newborn mice or hamsters. **SV-40,** another important virus of this group, produces tumors only in the baby hamster, including lymphocytic leukemia,

lymphoma, and osteogenic sarcoma. Two widespread human viruses, BK and JC viruses, are closely related to SV-40 and are responsible for a fatal demyelinating disease, **progressive multifocal leukoencephalopathy (PML).**

Transformation by polyomaviruses has been a widely studied model for in vitro viral tumorigenesis (Fig. 5-20). Cells are transformed if they do not permit replication of the virus or if they are infected with inactivated viral particles. This observation is explained by the fact that before transformation can occur, viral DNA must be integrated into the DNA of the host cell. In such a location the viral genome is not replicated independently of the host genome, as it is in a productive, lytic infection. Rather, the viral genome is expressed as a cellular gene. Only that portion of the viral genome that encodes for tumor antigens is expressed. These proteins initiate and maintain the transformed state, but their specific functions are unknown.

Herpesviruses

Many herpesviruses produce lymphomas in animals or transform cells in vitro. In humans the Epstein-Barr virus (EBV) has been strongly associated with certain cancers.

EBV is so widely disseminated that 80% of adults in the world have antibodies to it. This virus infects B lymphocytes in humans and other primates, a situation similar to the tropism of other herpesviruses of nonhuman primates. Of all cells only B lymphocytes possess receptors for EBV, which transforms these cells into lymphoblasts with an indefinite lifespan. In a small proportion of primary infections with EBV, this lymphoblastoid transformation is manifested as **infectious mononucleosis.** However, in Africa, principally in children, and in sporadic cases elsewhere, EBV has been closely associated with **Burkitt's lymphoma,** a B-cell neoplasm in which the neoplastic lymphocytes contain EBV in DNA and manifest EBV-related antigens. A similar correlation, though perhaps not as persuasive, is reported with **nasopharyngeal carcinoma.** It remains to be proved whether the association of EBV with these tumors is causal.

Figure 5-20. The cellular consequences of infection with a DNA tumor virus. Cells are either killed or transformed, depending on whether or not the viral DNA is integrated into the host genome. Viral replication directed by unintegrated viral DNA results in cell death. By contrast, integration of the viral genome into the host DNA results in the cellular expression of viral antigens, presumably associated with the process of transformation.

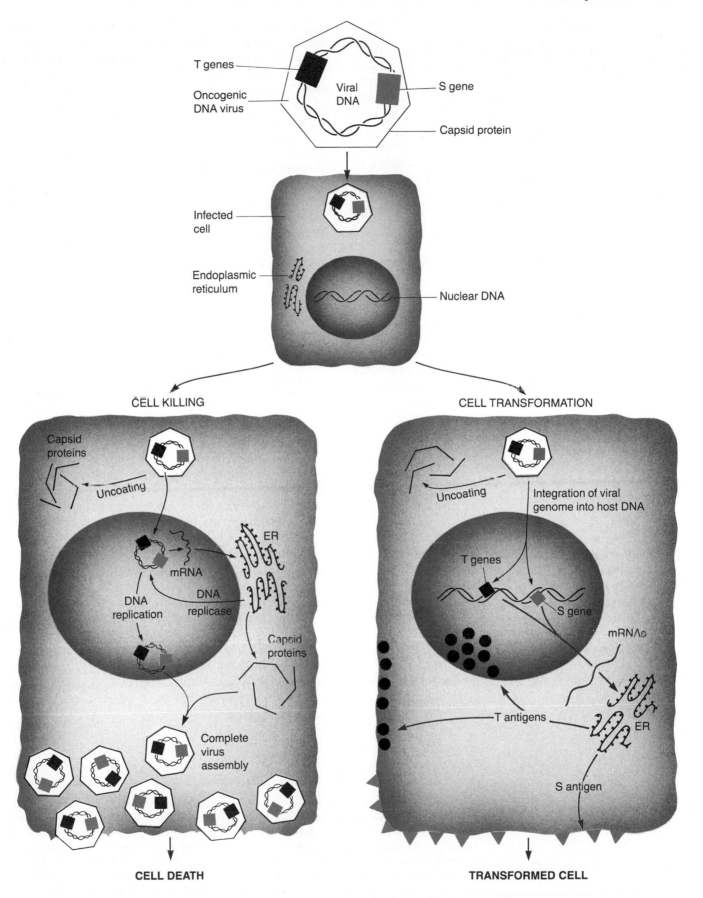

Hepatitis B virus (HBV)

Hepatitis B virus, a partially double-stranded DNA virus, infects only humans, although separate, closely related viruses infect woodchucks, ground squirrels, and domestic ducks. Epidemiologic studies have clearly established an association between chronic infection with HBV and the development of primary hepatocellular carcinoma. Animals chronically infected with related hepatitis viruses also exhibit a high incidence of primary hepatocellular carcinoma. The demonstration that the HBV genome is integrated into host liver cell DNA suggests that this virus should now be considered a putative oncogenic virus.

RNA VIRUSES (RETROVIRUSES) AND THE GENETIC BASIS OF CANCER

While DNA viruses have been closely associated with the development of a number of epithelial, mesenchymal, and hematopoietic cancers, the RNA viruses to date have been implicated in only one human cancer, the rare T cell leukemia/lymphoma seen in Japan and the Caribbean region. Despite this apparently slight clinical impact, experimental studies of these viruses have added considerably to our understanding of the molecular biology of cancer.

Research on retroviruses has pointed to the existence of cellular genes, termed **proto-oncogenes,** which, in another form—namely, as **oncogenes**—may play a central role in neoplasia.

Retroviral Oncogenes

Infection by a retrovirus introduces new genetic material into the host cell. The viral RNA is transcribed into DNA by reverse transcriptase, and this DNA is then integrated into the host's chromosomal DNA. In this position there are two general mechanisms by which the viral DNA can influence the transformation of the cell (Fig. 5-21). In one, cellular genes undergo abnormal regulation by the viral genome. This process has been named **insertional mutagenesis.** In the second, genetic recombination causes cellular genes to be implanted within the viral genome, in which case the cellular gene may become a viral oncogene. The process by which retroviral oncogenes are formed from such cellular proto-oncogenes is termed **transduction.** To date, close to two dozen retroviral oncogenes have been recognized, each of which encodes a protein whose biochemical action is amenable to study. In almost half of these viral oncogenes, corresponding cellular proto-oncogenes have been implicated in carcinogenesis. Despite the large number of viral and cellular oncogenes identified, only four biochemical mechanisms by which they may act have been recognized. These are protein phosphorylation of tyrosine or serine and threonine; metabolic regulation by proteins that bind GTP, in a manner resembling the normal B or N proteins; control of gene expression by influence on the biogenesis of mRNA; and participation in the replication of DNA. Many of these biochemical mechanisms relate, in turn, to the actions of polypeptide growth factors (Fig. 5-22).

The question arises: What are the properties of the transduced oncogenes of retroviruses—presumably formed from apparently innocuous cellular genes—that cause them to be tumorigenic? The answer is twofold. In the first place, the expression of the transduced oncogenes is stimulated by signals from the viral genome in a manner not coordinated with the ordinary metabolism of the cell. Second, during the recombinations that lead from a proto-oncogene to a viral oncogene, the transduced genes often undergo mutations, such as point mutations, deletions, and genetic substitutions. Such mutations have been shown in some cases to increase the activities of the gene products, particularly tyrosine kinases. In other words, **transformation may induce sustained high levels of otherwise normal biochemical activities.**

It is not necessary for a retrovirus to possess an oncogene in order for it to cause cancer. In some virally induced tumors, a cellular proto-oncogene—for example, *c-myc* or *c-ras*—is activated by the insertion of retroviral sequences adjacent to it, a process that results in the ungoverned expression of the previously regulated or silent gene. The integrated viral DNA may function as a powerful promotor itself or it may activate a host promotor.

Figure 5-21. Mechanisms of tumorigenesis by RNA retroviruses. Acute transforming RNA viruses contain a viral oncogene formed by transduction of a cellular proto-oncogene. Infection of a cell by such a virus results in the integration and expression of the viral oncogene, presumably leading to neoplastic transformation. By contrast, long-latency RNA-transforming viruses do not contain a viral oncogene, but rather a promoter gene. The integration of this promoter gene deregulates the expression of a cellular proto-oncogene (a process called insertional mutagenesis), again presumably leading to neoplastic transformation.

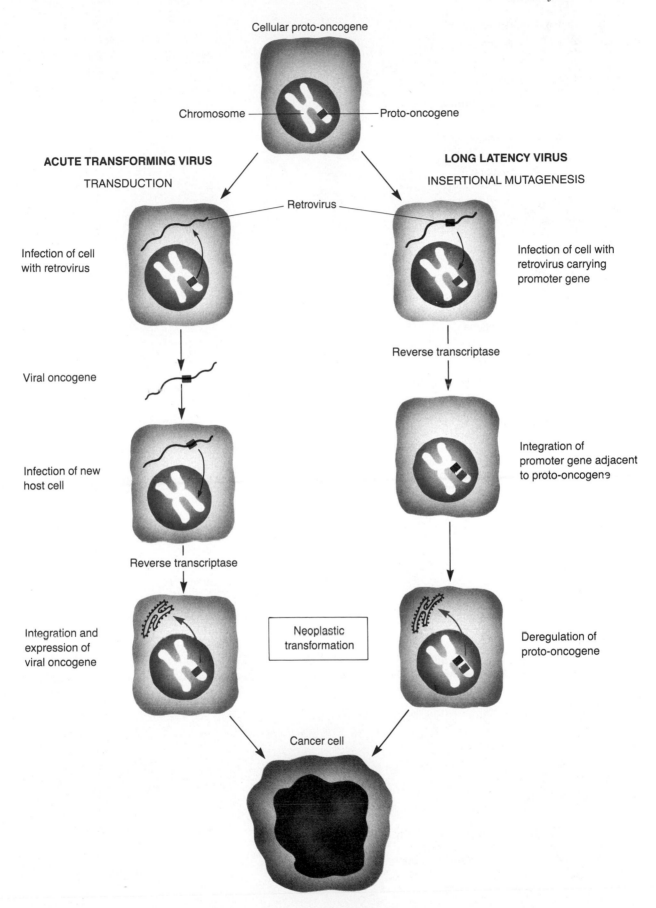

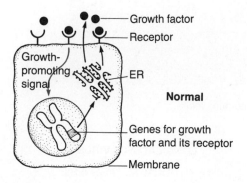

Growth factor
Receptor
Growth-
promoting
signal
ER
Normal
Genes for growth
factor and its receptor
Membrane

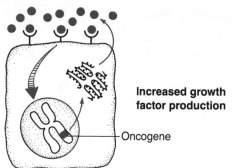

**Increased growth
factor production**

Oncogene

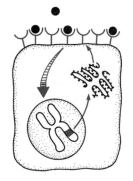

**Increased number
of receptors**

Figure 5-22. Possible interactions between oncogenes and growth factors. Oncogenes may code directly for growth factors, alter the number or affinity of growth factor receptors, or change the sensitivity of the cell to growth factors.

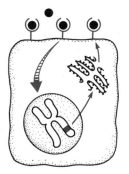

**Increased affinity
of receptors**

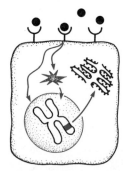

**Increased sensitivity
of cell (cytoplasm
or nucleus) to signal**

CHROMOSOMAL ALTERATIONS AND CANCER

It is now well recognized that specific alterations in particular chromosomes are associated with certain types of tumors or with neoplasia in general. The study of these nonrandom karyotypic changes, particularly the **reciprocal chromosome translocations** in Burkitt's lymphoma and chronic myelogenous leukemia, has shed further light on the potential role of cellular proto-oncogenes in neoplasia. Most cases of Burkitt's lymphoma exhibit a reciprocal translocation involving chromosomes 8 and 14. The human *c-myc* gene on chromosome 8 has been mapped to the break point on that chromosome in Burkitt's lymphoma, and the immunoglobulin genes on chromosome 14 have also been traced to the break point. The translocation of the *c-myc* gene to the region adjacent to the immunoglobulin genes on chromosome 14 presumably leads to the deregulation of the expression of the *c-myc* oncogene (Fig. 5-23). The *c-myc* gene product is a nuclear protein whose normal function is believed to involve the growth regulation of lymphocytes and other cells. Thus, theoretically, deregulation of this gene in Burkitt's lymphoma could provide an unremitting growth stimulus to the cell.

The first and still the best-known example of an acquired chromosomal anomaly in a human cancer is the **Philadelphia chromosome, found in most cases of chronic myelogenous leukemia.** The anomaly has now been identified as a translocation of the *c-abl* cellular proto-oncogene from its site on chromosome 9 to a critical region of chromosome 22. Unlike the situation in Burkitt's lymphoma, in which the *c-myc* gene product is unchanged in structure, the translocation producing the Philadelphia chromosome leads to a tran-

script that codes for an abnormal protein that has a much greater tyrosine kinase activity than the normal *c-abl* gene product. In other words, **the translocation produces a mutation that affects the biochemical function (a qualitative change) rather than the level of expression (a quantitative change) of a gene product.**

Reciprocal translocations are not the only form of chromosomal alterations that may be involved in carcinogenesis. Other nonrandom karyotypic abnormalities are trisomies, which represent the gain of a whole chromosome, and monosomies, which reflect a loss. For instance, trisomy 8 is common in acute leukemia and trisomy 12 in chronic B-cell leukemia. Extra copies of chromosome 7 have been noted in many melanomas and are consistently associated with the expression on the tumor cells of the receptor for epidermal growth factor. **A nonrandom loss of a whole chromosome or chromosomal segment is common in many leukemias.**

Gene deletion has been most extensively studied in children who harbor a hereditary predisposition to develop retinoblastoma, an otherwise rare ocular neoplasm. The disease is inherited as an autosomal recessive trait. These children typically show deletion of a segment of both copies of chromosome 13. Although the missing gene product has not been identified, some suspect it to be an inhibitor of a normal process, possibly involving growth regulation.

Another type of genetic aberration that has been associated with changes in the function of oncogenes is gene dosage, represented by the term **gene amplification.** This may take the form of many chromosomal copies of either the same gene or labile alternative forms. In some instances these changes have been shown to involve cellular or proto-oncogenes. Interestingly, it has been shown in cases of neuroblastoma that

Figure 5-23. Chromosomal translocation in Burkitt's lymphoma. During interphase, the cellular *myc* gene (*c-myc*) on chromosome 8 is translocated to chromosome 14 adjacent to the gene coding for the constant region of an immunoglobulin heavy chain (C$_H$). A reciprocal translocation of the gene coding for the variable region of the heavy chain (V$_H$) from chromosome 14 to chromosome 8 occurs. During metaphase the altered chromosomes are duplicated, a process that results in both chromatids of each chromosome bearing the translocated genes. The expression of *c-myc* is enhanced by its new association with the actively transcribed immunoglobulin genes.

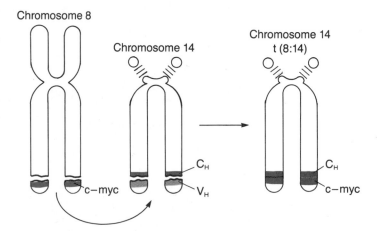

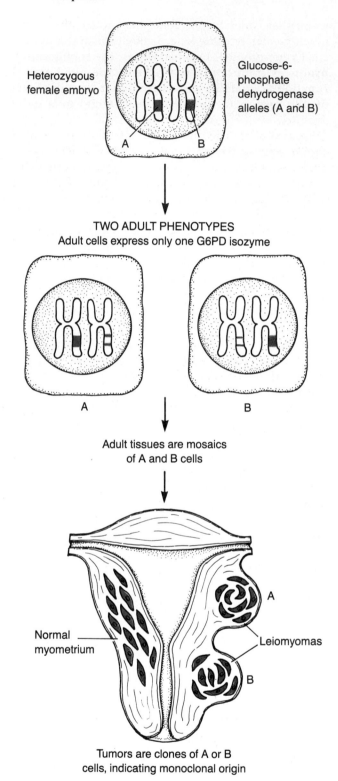

Heterozygous female embryo

Glucose-6-phosphate dehydrogenase alleles (A and B)

A   B

TWO ADULT PHENOTYPES
Adult cells express only one G6PD isozyme

A   B

Adult tissues are mosaics
of A and B cells

Normal myometrium

Leiomyomas

A

B

Tumors are clones of A or B
cells, indicating monoclonal origin

Figure 5-24. Monoclonal origin of human tumors.

multiple copies of the *c-myc* gene are associated with the more aggressive stages of the tumor. Furthermore, amplification of a gene in the *erb* oncogene family to more than double the normal activity was a significant predictor of overall survival and time to relapse in patients with carcinoma of the breast.

CLONAL ORIGIN OF CANCER

Studies of human and experimental tumors have provided strong evidence that most cancers arise from a single transformed cell. This theory has been most thoroughly examined in connection with proliferative disorders of the hematopoietic system. The most common piece of clinical evidence in its favor is the production of a single immunoglobulin unique to that patient by the neoplastic plasma cells of multiple myeloma. Indeed, such a "monoclonal spike" in the serum electrophoresis in a patient with suspected myeloma is regarded as conclusive evidence of the disease.

One of the most important observations in regard to the monoclonal origin of cancer was derived from the study of glucose-6-phosphate dehydrogenase in women who were heterozygous for its two isozymes, *A* and *B* (Fig. 5-24). These isozymes are encoded in genes located on the X chromosome, but only one of these genes is expressed in any given cell. Thus, whereas the genotypes of all cells are the same, their phenotypes vary with regard to the expression of isozyme *A* or *B*. An examination of benign uterine smooth muscle tumors (leiomyomas or "fibroids") revealed that all the cells in an individual tumor expressed only *A* or *B*, indicating that those cells were all derived from a single progenitor cell.

CANCER AS ALTERED DIFFERENTIATION

In many tumors **most of the neoplastic cells are outside the cell cycle and, thus, do not contribute to the malignancy of the tumor.** For example, as previously noted, fewer than 3% of the cells in a squamous carcinoma maintain the malignant potential of the tumor, and most differentiate and die spontaneously. **When such terminally differentiated tumor cells are transplanted into appropriate hosts, they do not grow, whereas their undifferentiated counterparts from** the same tumor form typical squamous carcinomas. Such observations raise the interesting possibility that the initial step in the development of some cancers is a **failure of the stem cell to differentiate normally.**

Evidence to support the concept of cancer as a failure of differentiation has come from the study of experimental, malignant germ cell tumors (teratocarcinomas). A single embryonal carcinoma cell, the stem cell of a teratocarcinoma, when transplanted into a mouse, gives rise to a tumor that contains cells derived from all three germ layers. Clearly, the progeny of the original transplanted tumor cell differentiate into more mature cells, which express recognizable phenotypes of more fully differentiated tissues. When these differentiated tissues of the teratocarcinoma are separated from the malignant embryonal cells and transplanted into compatible hosts, they not only survive, but function with no detriment to the host. These cells are clearly benign, and the dogma that "once a cancer cell, always a cancer cell" does not hold in this case.

In normal hematopoietic maturation, differentiation is tightly coupled to proliferation—that is, terminally differentiated cells are continually lost, to be replaced by newly proliferated and differentiated cells. By contrast, **certain leukemias and lymphomas may not be truly proliferative disorders, but rather reflect an uncoupling of differentiation from proliferation, with the resulting accumulation of cells that have not attained terminal differentiation.** According to this theory, leukemia and lymphoma may represent the stabilization of a phenotype that is also expressed, though only transiently, in developing normal cells.

TUMOR IMMUNOLOGY

It is clear from animal experiments that immune defenses against malignant tumors exist and may be important in humans. To invoke a role for an immune defense against cancer, it is necessary to postulate that tumor cells express antigens that are different from normal cells and that are recognized as foreign by the host. Such a condition has been indirectly demonstrated in experiments with inbred mice (Fig. 5-25). When cells from a chemically or virally induced tumor are transplanted into a syngeneic mouse, the cells form a tumor. When cells from this tumor are passed into a second mouse, they again form a tumor. On the other hand, if the first transplanted tumor is removed before it metastasizes (i.e., the mouse is cured of its tumor),

re-injection of the tumor cells back into the cured mouse will not produce a tumor. **The transplanted tumor is rejected because of immunity acquired as a result of the first tumor transplant.** Moreover, irradiated tumor cells or preparations of tumor cell membranes, when injected experimentally, augment resistance to tumor growth.

MECHANISMS OF IMMUNOLOGIC CYTOTOXICITY

The specific rejection of transplanted tumors is mediated by T cells, as evidenced by the demonstration that lymphocytes from tumor-bearing hosts can transfer tumor immunity when injected into normal animals. Moreover, the transferred immunity is eliminated by the administration of antibodies directed against T cell antigens. The mechanisms of T-cell mediated immunologic cell killing are discussed in Chapter 4.

Another set of lymphocytes, the **natural killer (NK) cells,** have tumoricidal activity that is not dependent on prior sensitization. NK cells are identical with the large granular lymphocytes. Although tumors vary in their sensitivity to NK cells, these lymphocytes are generally more effective in killing tumor cells than untransformed cells. A different population of naturally occurring lymphocytes, **natural cytotoxic (NC) cells,** exerts a tumoricidal effect on some target cells that are resistant to NK cells. These lymphoid cells are clearly different from NK cells in their response to stimulation by interleukin-2 and in their resistance to corticosteroids. Proliferation of a third group of cells, the **lymphokine-activated killer (LAK) cells,** is also stimulated by interleukin-2, an effect that has been reported to hold some promise for cancer treatment. **Macrophages are capable of killing tumor cells nonspecifically.** Of the many lymphokines that stimulate macrophages, the most potent appears to be gamma interferon.

Although tumor-associated antigens are capable of eliciting a humoral antibody response, these immunoglobulins by themselves are not capable of killing tumor cells. However, as discussed in Chapter 4, such antibodies can participate in antibody-dependent cell-mediated cytotoxicity and complement-dependent cell killing.

The mechanisms underlying immunologic cytotoxicity are summarized in Figure 5-26.

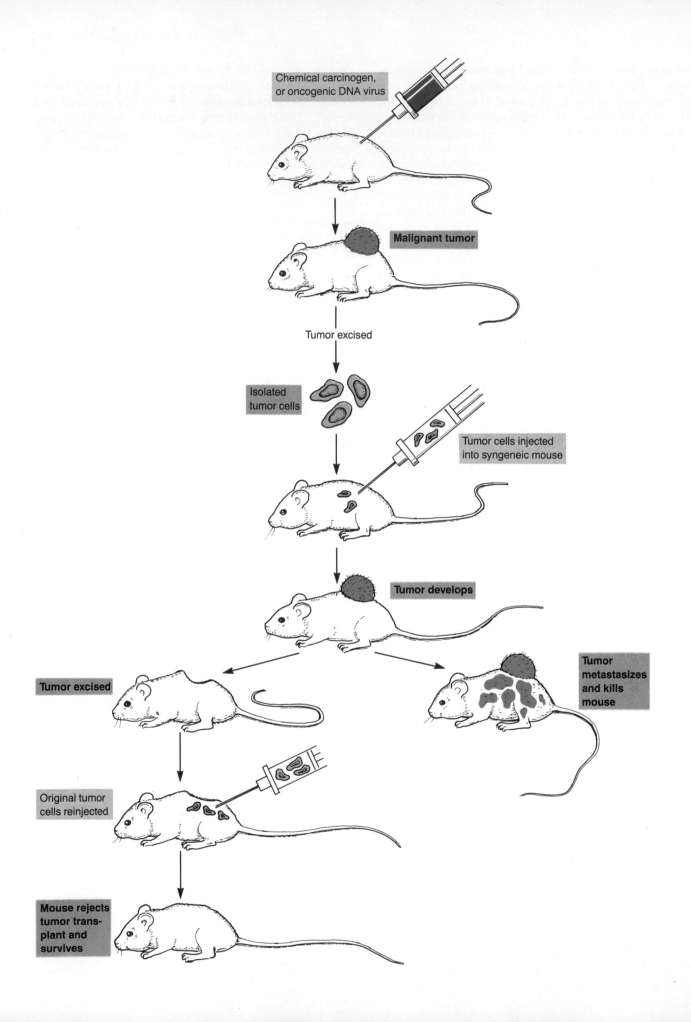

Chemical carcinogen, or oncogenic DNA virus

Malignant tumor

Tumor excised

Isolated tumor cells

Tumor cells injected into syngeneic mouse

Tumor develops

Tumor excised

Tumor metastasizes and kills mouse

Original tumor cells reinjected

Mouse rejects tumor transplant and survives

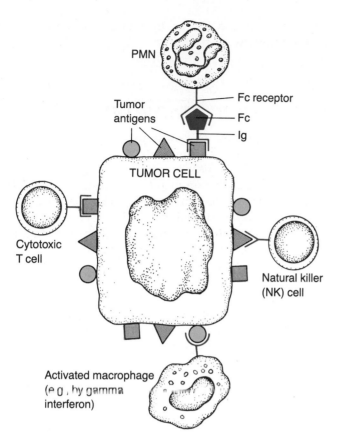

Figure 5-26. Mechanisms of immunologic tumor cytotoxicity.

IMMUNE SURVEILLANCE

Considering the enormous number of chemical, viral, and physical agents that have been identified as potential carcinogens, it seems remarkable that the incidence of cancer is not far greater than current statistics indicate. Although it may be argued that exposure to these factors is random and that cancer develops only in those who are particularly susceptible, an equally attractive hypothesis holds that incipient neoplasms appear in the population at large with considerable frequency but are immediately recognized and eliminated. Shortly after the promulgation of the clonal selection theory of immune reactivity, it was postulated that cell-mediated immune responses recognize and expunge mutant clones with neoplastic potential.

This theory of **immune surveillance** has been supported by a number of experimental and clinical observations. The strongest evidence for immune surveillance by T cells comes from the observation that there is an increase in tumor induction by oncogenic DNA viruses in T-cell-deficient mice. (This increase is evident both in naturally deficient mice and in mice made deficient by thymectomy or treatment with thymus-specific antibodies.) About 10% of patients with a genetic T-cell deficiency develop cancer, principally of the lymphoproliferative variety. The occurrence of cancers in immunosuppressed patients with AIDS also supports the immune surveillance concept. Immunosuppression to prevent transplant rejection has also been followed by a higher incidence of certain cancers.

It has been pointed out that the evidence for immune surveillance—that is, for a common mechanism for the elimination of all incipient neoplasms—is indirect, and wanting in many respects. Although a strong case can indeed be made in the case of highly antigenic oncogenic DNA-viruses, the theory appears weak with respect to other mechanisms of carcinogenesis. Nude mice, which are genetically deficient in T cells, do not exhibit an increased incidence of spontaneous tumors and are not more susceptible to tumor induction by RNA viruses or carcinogenic chemicals.

REMOTE EFFECTS OF CANCER ON THE HOST

The symptoms of cancer are, for the most part, referable to the local effects of either the primary tumor or its metastases. However, in a minority of patients, cancer produces remote effects that are not attributable to tumor invasion or to metastasis, and that are collectively termed **paraneoplastic syndromes.**

ANOREXIA AND WEIGHT LOSS

A paraneoplastic syndrome of anorexia, weight loss, and cachexia is very common in patients with cancer, often appearing before its malignant cause becomes apparent. Although cancer patients often have a decreased caloric intake because of anorexia and abnor-

Figure 5-25. Immunogenicity of tumors. Cancer cells injected into a syngeneic mouse form tumors, which metastasize and kill the animal. Excision of the tumor before it has metastasized allows the rejection of a second tumor implant, presumably as a consequence of immunity acquired from exposure to the original tumor.

malities of taste, restricted food intake does not explain the profound wasting so common among them; in fact, the mechanisms responsible are poorly understood. Of note is the recent discovery that **tumor necrosis factor,** a macrophage-derived substance that mediates tumor cell necrosis, is identical with **cachectin,** a similarly derived factor, which has profound catabolic effects at the cellular level.

ENDOCRINE SYNDROMES

Malignant tumors may produce a number of peptide hormones whose secretion is not under normal regulatory control.

CUSHING'S SYNDROME

Ectopic secretion of adrenocorticotropic hormone (ACTH) by a tumor leads to features of Cushing's syndrome, including hypokalemia, hyperglycemia, hypertension, and muscle weakness. The other prominent features of this syndrome, such as obesity, buffalo hump, and a moon facies, are less common. ACTH production is most commonly seen with cancers of the lung, particularly small cell (oat cell) carcinoma. It also complicates carcinoid tumors, thymomas, and neuroendocrine tumors, such as pheochromocytomas, neuroblastomas, and medullary carcinomas of the thyroid.

HYPERCALCEMIA

Hypercalcemia, a paraneoplastic complication that afflicts 10% of all cancer patients, is usually caused by metastatic disease of bone. However, in about one-tenth of cases it occurs in the absence of bony metastases. In the latter situation, the tumor may produce parathormone, prostaglandins, osteoclast activating factor, and possibly other osteolytic agents. Hypercalcemia from bony involvement is most common with cancer of the breast and multiple myeloma; in the absence of metastases lung cancer is the usual culprit.

HYPOGLYCEMIA

The best-understood cause of hypoglycemia associated with tumors is excessive insulin production by islet cell tumors of the pancreas. Other tumors, especially large mesotheliomas and fibrosarcomas, and primary hepatocellular carcinoma, are associated with hypoglycemia. The cause of hypoglycemia in nonendocrine tumors is not established, but the most likely candidate is production of somatomedins, a family of peptides normally produced by the liver under regulation by growth hormone.

NEUROLOGIC SYNDROMES

A small proportion of cancer patients suffer from a variety of neurologic complaints without any demonstrable cause. Such disorders are thought to reflect remote effects of cancer on the nervous system. Cerebral complications may present as dementia, subacute cerebellar degeneration, or limbic encephalitis. In the spinal cord, a subacute motor neuropathy characterized by slowly developing lower motor neuron weakness without sensory changes is so strongly associated with cancer that an intensive search for an occult neoplasm, often a lymphoma, should be made in patients who present with these symptoms. In addition, a form of amyotrophic lateral sclerosis is well described among cancer patients, and conversely, many patients with this disease are found to have cancer. A rapidly ascending motor and sensory paralysis to the thoracic level, with severe destruction of gray and white matter, has been described.

The peripheral nerves are also the site of paraneoplastic effects. A sensorimotor peripheral neuropathy, characterized by distal weakness and wasting and sensory loss, is common in cancer patients, and when not associated with an overt neoplasm suggests the possibility of an occult tumor.

Paraneoplastic effects are also seen in the muscle and neuromuscular junction. Patients with dermatomyositis or polymyositis have an incidence of cancer five to seven times higher than the general population. The association is most striking in affected men over the age of 50 years, in whom more than 70% have a cancer. In most cases the muscle disorder and cancer present within a year of each other. The association of myasthenia gravis with thymoma is well recognized, although a wide variety of other tumors have on occasion been linked to this disorder of the neuromuscular junction.

HEMATOLOGIC SYNDROMES

The most common hematologic complications of neoplastic disease result either from direct infiltration of the marrow or from treatment. However, hematologic paraneoplastic syndromes, which antedate the modern era of chemotherapy and radiotherapy, are well described. Cancer-associated erythrocytosis is a complication of some tumors, particularly renal cell carcinoma, primary hepatocellular carcinoma, and cerebellar hemangioblastoma. Interestingly, benign kidney disease, such as cystic disease or hydronephrosis, and uterine myomas can lead to erythrocytosis. Elevated erythropoietin levels are found in the tumor and in the serum in about half of the patients with erythrocytosis.

One of the most common findings in patients with cancer is anemia, but the mechanism for this disorder is not clear. The anemia is usually normocytic and normochromic, although iron deficiency anemia is common in cancers that bleed into the gastrointestinal tract, such as colorectal cancers.

Between 30% and 40% of cancer patients exhibit a thrombocytosis, with platelet counts above 400,000/μl. The platelet count usually returns to normal with successful treatment of the malignant disease.

THE HYPERCOAGULABLE STATE

The association between cancer and **thrombophlebitis** was noted more than a century ago. Since then other abnormalities resulting from a hypercoagulable state —for example **disseminated intravascular coagulation** and **nonbacterial thrombotic endocarditis**— have been recognized. The cancers most commonly associated with thrombophlebitis are carcinoma of the lung, pancreas, and gastrointestinal tract, but tumors of the breast, ovary, prostate, and other organs may also lead to this complication. The cause of this hypercoagulable state is debated.

CUTANEOUS SYNDROMES

Pigmented lesions and keratoses are well-recognized paraneoplastic effects. **Acanthosis nigricans,** a cutaneous disorder marked by hyperkeratosis and pigmentation of the axilla, neck, flexures, and anogenital region is of particular interest. **More than half of patients with acanthosis nigricans have cancer.** Development of the disease may precede, accompany, or follow the detection of the cancer. Over 90% of the cases occur in association with gastrointestinal carcinomas, tumors of the stomach accounting for one-half to two-thirds. Regression of the skin lesions after removal of the cancer has been recorded in a few cases. In rare instances the sudden development or rapid increase in the size of **seborrheic keratoses** heralds the presence of a malignant tumor. Certain lymphomas and Hodgkin's disease are complicated by an **exfoliative dermatitis** without any cutaneous involvement by tumor.

AMYLOIDOSIS

About 15% of cases of **amyloidosis** occur in association with cancers, particularly with multiple myeloma and renal cell carcinoma, but also with other solid tumors and lymphomas. The presence of amyloidosis implies a poor prognosis; in myeloma patients with the disorder the median survival is 14 months or less.

HEREDITY AND CANCER

Hereditary tumors can be arbitrarily divided into three categories: malignant tumors inherited as such—for example, retinoblastoma, Wilms' tumor, and many endocrine tumors; benign inherited tumors that remain benign or have a malignant potential, as in familial polyposis of the colon; and inherited syndromes associated with a high risk of malignant tumors, such as Bloom syndrome and ataxia-telangiectasia. Most of these are discussed in detail in the chapters dealing with specific organs, and selected examples are given in Table 5-1. In most cases the underlying genetic defect responsible for the tumor development is totally unknown, but in a few cases there are hints as to the underlying abnormality. Patients with Bloom syndrome, ataxia-telangiectasia, and Fanconi's anemia display defects in DNA repair. Adenomatous polyps are the precursor of most colorectal adenocarcinomas, and it is not surprising that familial polyposis of the colon is associated with a high incidence of intestinal cancer. Similarly, von Recklinghausen's disease (neurofibromatosis) is complicated by malignant schwannomas and neurogenic sarcomas, and hereditary multiple trichoepitheliomas convert to basal and squamous cell carcinomas.

EPIDEMIOLOGY OF CANCER

INCIDENCE OF CANCER IN THE UNITED STATES

Cancer accounts for one-fifth of the total mortality in the United States, and is the second leading cause of death after cardiovascular diseases and stroke. For most cancers death rates in the United States have largely remained flat over the last 50 years, with some notable exceptions (Fig. 5-27). The death rate from cancer of the lung among men has risen dramatically from 1930, when it was an uncommon tumor, to the present, when it is by far the most common cause of

(Text continues on p. 130)

Table 5-1   Inherited Neoplastic Syndromes

DISEASE	ASSOCIATED NEOPLASMS	INHERITANCE*
Chromosomal Instability Syndromes		
Bloom syndrome	Leukemia, gastrointestinal cancer	R
Fanconi's anemia	Leukemia, squamous cell carcinoma, hepatoma	R
Werner syndrome	Sarcomas	R
Hereditary Skin Diseases		
Nevi	Malignant melanoma	D
Giant hairy nevi	Malignant melanoma	D
Xeroderma pigmentosum	Skin cancers	R
Multiple trichoepitheliomas	Basal and squamous cell carcinomas	D
Epidermodysplasia verruciformis	Basal cell carcinoma, Bowen's disease, squamous carcinoma	R
Familial atypical nevi	Malignant melanoma	D
Nevoid basal carcinoma syndrome	Basal cell carcinoma, medulloblastoma, ovarian carcinoma	D
Tylosis	Esophageal cancer	D
Endocrine System		
Multiple endocrine neoplasia syndromes	Adenomas of endocrine glands	D
Nervous System		
Retinoblastoma	Retinoblastoma	D
Neuroblastoma	Neuroblastoma	R
Phacomatoses		
Neurofibromatosis (von Recklinghausen's disease)	Fibrosarcoma, schwannoma, meningioma, optic glioma	D
Tuberous sclerosis	Glial tumors, rhabdomyoma of heart, angiomyolipoma of kidney	D
von Hippel-Lindau syndrome	Cerebellar hemangioblastoma, retinal angioma, other hemangiomas	D and R
Sturge-Weber syndrome	Multiple angiomas	D
Gastrointestinal System		
Familial polyposis coli	Intestinal polyps and carcinomas	D
Gardener's syndrome	Intestinal polyps and cancers, osteomas, fibromas	D
Peutz-Jeghers syndrome	Intestinal polyps and cancers	D
Vascular Syndromes		
Osler-Weber-Rendu syndrome	Angiomas	D
Multiple angiolipomas	Angiolipomas	D
Ataxia-telangiectasia	Lymphoma, leukemia, gastric cancer, brain tumors	R
Urogenital System		
Gonadal dysgenesis	Gonadoblastoma, dysgerminoma	R
Wilms' tumor		R and D
Immunologic Syndromes		
Agammaglobulinemia (Swiss type)	Lymphoma, leukemia	R
X-linked agammaglobulinemia	Lymphoma, leukemia	XR
DiGeorge syndrome	Squamous carcinoma of upper respiratory tract	D
Wiskott-Aldrich syndrome	Lymphoma	XR
Severe combined immunodeficiency	Lymphoma, leukemia, sarcoma	XR
Family Cancer Syndrome	Carcinomas of colon, breast, endometrium, lung	D

* D, autosomal dominant; R, autosomal recessive; XR, X-linked recessive

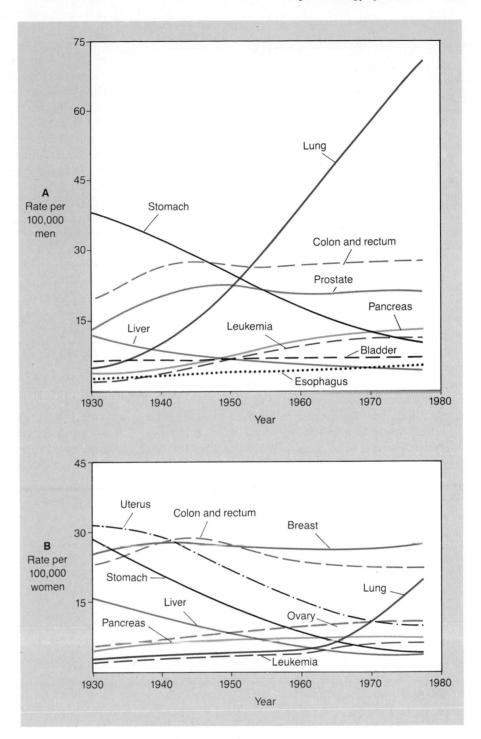

Figure 5-27. Cancer death rates in the United States over the last 50 years. (*A*) In men a striking increase in the incidence of cancer of the lung is attributable to smoking, whereas the sharp decline in stomach cancer is unexplained. (*B*) Increased smoking among women has led to a corresponding increase in cancer of the lung. The unexplained decrease in cancer of the stomach has been paralleled by a similar reduction in cancer of the uterus.

Table 5-2   Most Common Tumor Types in Men and Women

MEN		WOMEN	
TYPE	%	TYPE	%
Lung	20	Breast	27
Prostate	20	Colon and rectum	16
Colon and rectum	14	Lung	11
Urinary	10	Uterus	10
Leukemia and lymphoma	8	Leukemia and Lymphoma	7
Oral	4	Ovary	4
Skin	3	Urinary	4
Pancreas	3	Pancreas	3
All others	18	Skin	3
		Oral	2
		All others	13

death from cancer in men. As discussed in Chapter 8, the entire epidemic of lung cancer deaths is attributable to smoking. Among women, smoking did not become fashionable until World War II. Considering the time lag needed between starting to smoke and the development of cancer of the lung, it is not surprising that the increased death rate from cancer of the lung in women did not become significant until after 1965. By 1983 the death rate from lung cancer in women exceeded that for breast cancer in nine states, and it is now, as in men, the most common fatal cancer. By contrast, for reasons difficult to fathom, cancer of the stomach, which in

1930 was by far the most common cancer in men and was only slightly less common than breast cancer in women, has shown a remarkable and sustained decline in frequency. Similarly, there has been an unexplained decline in the death rate from cancer of the uterus, although better screening, diagnostic, and therapeutic methods may account for some of this reduction. The ranking of the incidence of tumors in men and women in the United States is shown in Table 5-2.

Individual cancers have their own age-related profiles, but for most, increased age is associated with an increased incidence. The most striking example of the dependency on age is carcinoma of the prostate, in which the incidence increases 30-fold between age 50 and 85 years. Certain neoplastic diseases, such as acute lymphoblastic leukemia in children and testicular cancer in young adults, show different age-related peaks of incidence (Fig. 5-28).

STUDIES OF MIGRANT POPULATIONS

Although planned experiments on the etiology of human cancer are hardly feasible, certain populations have unwittingly performed such experiments by migrating from one environment to another. Initially at least, the genetic characteristics of such people re-

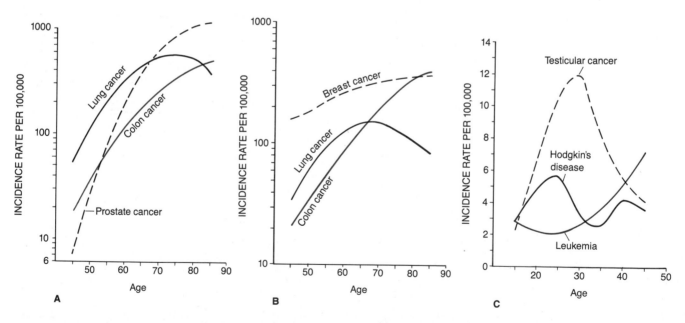

Figure 5-28. Incidence of specific cancers as a function of age. (*A*) Men. (*B*) Women. (*C*) Testicular cancer in men and Hodgkin's disease and leukemia in both sexes. The incidence of these cancers in *C* peaks at younger ages than do those in *A* and *B*.

mained the same, but the new environment differed in climate, diet, infectious agents, occupations, and so on. Consequently, **epidemiologic studies of migrant populations have provided many intriguing clues to the factors that may influence the pathogenesis of cancer.** The United States, which has been the destination of one of the greatest population movements of all time, is the source of most of the important data in this field.

CANCER OF THE STOMACH

A study of Japanese residents of Hawaii found that migrants from Japanese regions with the highest risk of stomach cancer continued to exhibit an excess risk in Hawaii. By contrast, their offspring who were born in Hawaii had the same incidence of this cancer as American whites. Although a diet including large quantities of foods such as pickled vegetables and salted fish has been postulated to account for the higher incidence in Japan and the lower incidence in Hawaii, no firm evidence has been adduced to support this contention. More recently it has been shown in Japan that the population in regions at high risk for stomach cancer also display a high prevalence of chronic atrophic gastritis with intestinal metaplasia, lesions that are considered precursors of gastric cancer. Interestingly, when individuals from these regions move to low-risk areas, they carry the high prevalence of intestinal metaplasia with them. Thus, the environmental factors associated with stomach cancer may not be directly carcinogenic but rather may be related to atrophic gastritis and intestinal metaplasia.

COLORECTAL, BREAST, ENDOMETRIAL, OVARIAN, AND PROSTATIC CANCER

Migrant studies of the incidence of colorectal cancer show opposite trends to those of stomach cancer. Migrants from low-risk areas in Europe and Japan exhibit an increased risk of colorectal cancer in the United States. Moreover, their offspring continue at higher risk and reach the incidence levels of the general American population. This rule for colorectal cancer also holds for cancers of the breast, endometrium, ovary, and prostate.

BURKITT'S LYMPHOMA

Emigrants to lowland areas from highland regions in Central Africa, where Burkitt's lymphoma is rare, develop tumors at an older age than do those born in endemic areas. This presumably reflects a later age of exposure to the Epstein-Barr virus or a more potent stimulation of the antigenic response by malaria. Moreover, the incidence of Burkitt's lymphoma is higher among emigrants to high-risk areas than among the same group who stay in the low-risk areas, and, indeed, higher than among adults who were born in the high-risk area. It is probable that many adults in the high-risk areas who have escaped Burkitt's lymphoma in their youth are immune to the disease.

6

DEVELOPMENTAL AND GENETIC DISEASES

IVAN DAMJANOV

Disorders that can be traced to prenatal stages of human development form a heterogeneous group that is best considered as a broad spectrum. At one end of the spectrum are diseases caused by adverse exogenous influences. At the other end are disorders that are genetically determined and are not related to environmental factors. Between these two extremes are numerous pathologic conditions that are genetically predetermined but have a pathogenesis that depends largely on the interaction between the developing organism, the maternal body, and other external influences.

For didactic purposes it is customary to classify the origins of developmental and genetic disorders as **errors of morphogenesis, cytogenetic (chromosomal) abnormalities, single-gene defects, or multifactorial (polygenic) inheritance.** For the sake of completeness, we also include fetopathies due to **adverse transplacental influences** during intrauterine life, **fetal deformities and injuries** caused by mechanical intrauterine and intrapartal trauma, and **diseases of infancy and childhood.** Worldwide, at least 1 in 50 newborn infants has a major congenital anomaly, about 1 in 100 has a single-gene abnormality, and about 1 in 200 has a major chromosomal abnormality. In more than two-thirds of all birth defects diagnosed clinically, the cause is not determined. In a minority of cases the defect can be related to uterine factors (<1%), maternal factors, such as metabolic imbalance (1% to 2%), maternal infections during pregnancy (2% to 3%), or other adverse environmental influences, such as exposure to drugs, chemicals, or radiation (1% to 3%). Genetic diseases account for the remaining 15% to 20% of disorders. In 3% to 5% of children born with a congenital anomaly, cytogenetic analysis reveals an abnormal karyotype (i.e., a structural or numerical chromosomal abnormality).

Although chromosomal abnormalities account for only a small fraction of birth defects in newborn infants, cytogenetic analysis of fetuses spontaneously aborted in early pregnancy indicates that approximately two-thirds show chromosomal abnormalities. The incidence of specific numerical chromosomal abnormalities in the abortuses is several times higher than in term infants, indicating that **most inborn chromosomal defects are lethal.** The conceptus with a chromosomal defect typically dies in early pregnancy; only a small number of children with cytogenetic abnormalities are born alive.

PRINCIPLES OF TERATOLOGY

The discipline concerned with the study of developmental anomalies is called **teratology** (Greek *teraton*, "monster"). Chemical, physical, and biological agents that cause developmental anomalies are known as **teratogens.** There are very few agents of proven teratogenicity in humans, but many drugs and chemicals are teratogenic in animals and should, therefore, be considered as potentially teratogenic for humans.

A morphologic defect or abnormality of an organ, part of an organ, or anatomical region that results from perturbed or abnormal morphogenesis is called a **malformation.** Exposure to a known teratogen may, but does not invariably, result in a malformation. These and similar observations have led to the formulation of the following five general principles of teratology.

Susceptibility varies with the individual. The genotypes of the conceptus and the mother are the primary determinants of susceptibility to teratogens. Some strains of inbred mice are susceptible to particular exogenous stimuli to which other strains are resistant. This principle is the one most likely operative in humans. A good example is the fetal alcohol syndrome, which affects only some children born to alcoholic mothers, whereas others do not bear the stigmata of this disorder.

Susceptibility is specific for each developmental stage. Most agents are teratogenic only during critical stages of development. For example, maternal rubella infection causes abnormalities in the fetus only during the first 3 months of pregnancy.

Pharmacologic or biologic mechanisms are specific for each teratogen. The teratogenicity of each chemical depends, to a large extent, on the mechanisms of its action. Teratogenic drugs inhibit the activity of crucial enzymes or receptors, interfere with the formation of the mitotic spindle, or block energy sources, and thus inhibit metabolic steps critical for normal morphogenesis. Many drugs and viruses affect specific tissues ("neurotropism," "cardiotropism") and thus damage some developing organs more than others.

Response is related to dose. Teratogens act in a dose-dependent manner, a higher dose being more toxic than a smaller one. Theoretically this means that for each teratogen one can determine a "safe" dose, which should have no consequences. In practice, however, because of the multiple determinants of teratogenesis, all established teratogens should be avoided during human pregnancy; an absolutely safe dose cannot be predicted for each individual.

The outcome of teratogenic influences is death, growth retardation, malformation, or functional impairment. The outcome depends on the interaction between the teratogenic influences, the maternal organism, and the fetal placental unit.

The list of proven human teratogens includes most cytotoxic drugs, alcohol, some antiepileptic drugs, heavy metals, and thalidomide, among others. On the other side of the spectrum are the drugs and chemicals that have been declared as safe for use during pregnancy, primarily on the basis of a negative outcome of teratogenic studies in laboratory animals. However, there is species specificity for every drug, and the fact that a drug is not teratogenic for mice and rabbits is not necessarily evidence that it is innocuous for humans.

ERRORS OF MORPHOGENESIS

Abnormally activated or structurally abnormal genes in the zygote and early embryonic cells result in early death. Malformations resulting from nonlethal injuries during preimplantation stages of embryogenesis are rare, since few embryos survive injury at early stages of development. Injury during the first 8 to 10 days after fertilization usually results in an incomplete separation of blastomeres, an effect that leads to the formation of **double monsters.** Symmetrical double monsters represent incompletely separated twins ("Siamese twins") joined at various anatomical sites, such as the head (craniopagus), thorax (thoracopagus) or rump (ischiopagus). Asymmetrical double monsters have one well-developed and one rudimentary or hypoplastic twin.

Disorganized or disrupted morphogenesis may have minor or major consequences at the level of cells and tissues, organs or organ systems, and anatomical regions. Representative examples given here reflect the disturbance of some specific morphogenetic processes.

Agenesis is the complete absence of an organ primordium. It may manifest as complete absence of an organ, as in unilateral or bilateral agenesis of kidneys; as the absence of part of an organ, as in agenesis of the corpus callosum of the brain; or as the absence of tissue or cells within an organ, as in the absence of testicular germ cells in congenital infertility ("Sertoli cell only" syndrome).

Aplasia is absence of the organ coupled with persistence of the organ anlage or a rudiment that never developed completely. Thus, aplasia of the lung refers to a condition in which the main bronchus ends blindly in nondescript tissue composed of rudimentary ducts and connective tissue.

Hypoplasia refers to reduced size due to the incomplete development of all or part of an organ. Examples are microphthalmia (small eyes), micrognathia (small jaw), and microcephaly (small brain and head).

Dysraphic anomalies are defects caused by failure to fuse. Spina bifida is an anomaly in which the spinal canal has not closed completely and the overlaying bone and skin have not fused, thus leaving a midline defect.

Involution failures are defects due to the persistence of embryonic or fetal structures that should involute at certain stages of development. A persistent thyroglossal duct is the result of incomplete involution of the tract that connects the base of the tongue with the developing thyroid.

Division failures are defects caused by incomplete cleavage, when that process depends on the involution and programmed death of cells. Fingers and toes are formed at the distal end of the limb bud through programmed death of cells between the primordia that contain the cartilage. If these cells do not die in a predetermined manner, the fingers will be conjoined or incompletely separated ("syndactyly").

Atresia refers to defects caused by incomplete formation of a lumen. Many hollow organs originate as strands and cords of cells, the centers of which are programmed to die, thus forming a central cavity or lumen. Atresia of the esophagus is characterized by partial occlusion of the lumen, which was not fully established in embryogenesis.

Dysplasia is a defect caused by abnormal organization of cells into tissues, a situation that results in abnormal histogenesis. ("Dysplasia" has a different meaning here from that used in characterizing the precancerous lesion, epithelial dysplasia [see Chapter 1]. Tuberous sclerosis is a striking example of dysplasia, being characterized by abnormal development of the brain, which contains aggregates of normally developed cells arranged into grossly visible "tubers."

Ectopia or heterotopia is an anomaly in which an organ is outside its normal anatomical site. Thus, ectopic heart is located outside the thorax. Heterotopic parathyroid glands can be located within the thymus in the anterior mediastinum. **Dystopia** denotes the retention of an organ in a site at which it is usually located during development. For example, the kidneys are initially located in the pelvis, and move thereafter into a more cranial lumbar position. Dystopic kidneys are those that remain in the pelvis. Dystopic testes are retained in the inguinal canal, not having completed their descent into the scrotum.

Multiple anomalies that are pathogenetically related form a **developmental syndrome.** The term "syndrome" implies a single cause for anomalies in anatomically distant organs that have been damaged by the same polytopic effect during a critical developmental period. Many of the developmental syndromes are related to chromosomal abnormalities or single-gene defects. The nonrandom occurrence of multiple anomalies not due to the polytopic field defect (sequence or syndrome) is called **developmental association or syntropy.** This term refers to multiple anomalies that are associated statistically but do not necessarily share the same pathogenetic mechanisms.

After the third month of pregnancy, exposure of the human fetus to teratogenic influences rarely results in major errors of morphogenesis. However, subcellular, histologic, and, especially, functional consequences are still found in children exposed to exogenous teratogens during the fetal stages of development —that is, the second and third trimesters of pregnancy.

Most anatomical defects caused by adverse influences in the fetal stage of pregnancy fall into the category of **deformations,** defined as abnormalities of form, shape, or position of a part of the body caused by mechanical forces. These forces may be external—for instance, amniotic bands in the uterus—or intrinsic, as in fetal hypomobility due to a central nervous system injury. Thus, a deformity known as equinovarus foot can be due to the compression of the extremities by the uterine wall in oligohydramnios or to spinal cord abnormalities that lead to defective innervation and movement of the foot.

CLINICALLY IMPORTANT MALFORMATIONS

ANENCEPHALY AND SPINA BIFIDA

Anencephaly is a dysraphic defect of neural tube closure. Anencephalic fetuses lack the calvarium and the soft tissues of the cranium. The defective closure may involve only the calvarium and the brain (acrania) or may extend into the spinal cord and vertebral column (craniorachischisis). **Spina bifida,** the incomplete closure of the spinal cord canal and vertebral column, is usually localized to the lumbar region and represents the mildest dysraphic anomaly of the central nervous system.

Anencephaly is a typical multifactorial birth defect. The disorder affects female fetuses twice as often as male ones, and it occurs with higher incidence in certain families. It has been calculated that there is a 5% chance of recurrence in the same marriage; if two offspring are affected the risk rises to 20% to 25% for each subsequent pregnancy. Thus, genetic factors also play a role.

Children born with anencephaly are shortlived; most, in fact, are stillborn. Spina bifida, with or without myelomeningocele, is compatible with life, and the degree of neurologic impairment depends on the extent of the lesion.

THALIDOMIDE-INDUCED MALFORMATIONS

Limb-reduction deformities, involving from one to all four extremities, are rare congenital defects of unknown origin. In the 1960s a sudden increase in the incidence of limb-reduction deformities in Germany and England was epidemiologically linked to maternal intake of a sedative, thalidomide, during the early stages of pregnancy. This drug is teratogenic between the 28th and 50th day of pregnancy. Many of the children born to mothers exposed to thalidomide presented with skeletal deformities and pleomorphic defects in other organs, most commonly the ears **(microtia and anotia)** and the heart. Typically, the arms of the affected children were short and malformed and resembled the flippers of the seal **(phocomelia).** Sometimes limbs were completely missing **(amelia).**

FETAL ALCOHOL SYNDROME

Although the association between alcohol intake and malformations has only recently been recognized, **ethyl alcohol is today one of the best known human teratogens.** Alcohol consumption during pregnancy increases the rate of miscarriages and stillbirths. Perinatal mortality is also augmented. The syndrome is both dose-dependent and under the influence of genetic factors. Approximately 30% to 50% of all children born to chronic alcoholic women who consume more than 125 grams of ethanol per day are born with the fetal alcohol syndrome, but even as little as 28 to 36 grams of pure ethanol (about 3 ounces of 86-proof whiskey) per day may adversely affect the conceptus.

Most children suffering from the fetal alcohol syndrome exhibit growth retardation, microcephaly, and mild-to-moderate mental retardation. Typical facial features include short palpebral fissures, epicanthal folds, ptosis, a short nose, a hypoplastic philtrum, and a thinned vermilion border of the upper lip. Commonly, the children have a short, upturned nose and a hypoplastic maxilla. Other malformations involve the extremities, kidneys, and heart.

TORCH COMPLEX

Neonatologists dealing with infants who were damaged in utero or perinatally by infectious agents noticed that the same complex of symptoms is produced by different microorganisms. **Toxoplasma, rubella, cytomegalovirus, and herpes simplex virus** were found to be the most frequent causes of this syndrome, and their initials were used to form the acronym **TORCH.** In this term the only unaccounted letter, namely ''O'', stands for all **Others.** The term was coined to alert pediatricians to the fact that the infections in fetus and newborn by TORCH agents are usually indistinguishable from each other, and that testing for one of the four major TORCH agents should include testing for the other three and for some possible ''others'' as well (Fig. 6-1).

All microorganisms of the TORCH complex cross the placenta and infect the conceptus, even before the placenta is functional. Toxoplasma is usually transmitted from a recently infected mother who experienced her primary infection while pregnant. Chronic infection is not unduly hazardous for the fetus, although women with chronic toxoplasmosis have a high rate of spontaneous abortions. This suggests that the full-blown syndrome is not seen in the offspring because the infected embryo is aborted early in pregnancy. Cytomegalovi-

Table 6-1   Pathologic Findings in the Fetus and Newborn Infected with TORCH Agents

General	Prematurity, intrauterine retardation
Central Nervous System	Encephalitis Microcephaly Hydrocephaly Intracranial calcifications Psychomotor retardation
Ear	Inner ear damage with hearing loss
Eye	Chorioretinitis (TCH) Pigmented retina (R) Keratoconjunctivitis (H) Cataracts (RH) Glaucoma (R) Visual impairment (TRCH)
Liver	Hepatomegaly Liver calcifications (R) Jaundice
Hematopoietic System	Hemolytic and other anemias Thrombocytopenia Splenomegaly
Skin and Mucosae	Vesicular or ulcerative lesions (H) Petechiae and ecchymoses
Cardiopulmonary System	Pneumonitis Myocarditis Congenital heart disease
Skeleton	Various bone lesions

T, toxoplasma; R, rubella; C, cytomegalovirus; H, herpes virus

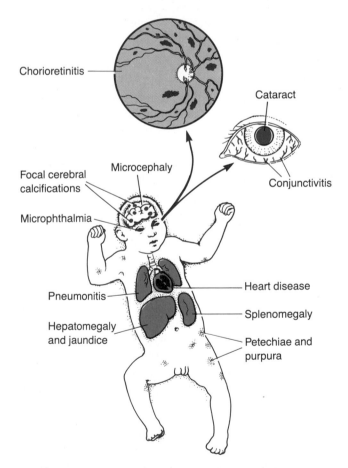

Figure 6-1. TORCH complex. Children infected in utero with toxoplasma, rubella, cytomegalovirus, or herpes simplex virus show remarkably similar symptoms.

rus and herpes simplex virus infections are transmitted to the fetus from chronic carrier mothers; activation of the virus presumably facilitates its transmission to the infant. Herpes-related blisters in the vagina or the vulva are a major source of perinatal herpes infection. Cytomegalovirus infection of the genitalia is usually inapparent, but as many as 20% of asymptomatic women have the virus in the cells of the cervix and vagina.

Rubella virus harms the fetus only during acute infection, and only if the acute infection occurs during the first 20 weeks of pregnancy. Infection within the first 10 weeks is more dangerous than infection during the period from 10 to 20 weeks of gestation. Transplacental transmission of the virus to the fetus rarely occurs after the 20th week of pregnancy; infections in late pregnancy usually do not produce malformations. Active immunity to the rubella virus, due to a previous infection or active immunization, usually provides protection.

Clinical and pathologic findings in the symptomatic fetus and newborn infected with TORCH agents vary, and only a minority present with a multisystemic disease and the full-blown syndrome (Table 6-1).

Congenital rubella is a prototype of the entire syndrome. In the classic form the syndrome includes ocular defects, cardiac defects, and sensorineural deafness. Most infants also have thrombocytopenia, hepatosplenomegaly, and lesions of the central nervous system. Toxoplasmosis is usually dominated by chorioretinitis and calcifications in the brain. Hepatosplenomegaly, thrombocytopenia, and brain lesions characterize congenital cytomegalovirus infection. Herpes simplex infection presents with brain or hepatosplenic involvement, and the diagnosis is facilitated by the presence of mucocutaneous vesicles.

TORCH complex infections are major causes of morbidity among newborn children in the United States.

The most serious pathologic changes in TORCH-infected children are found in the brain. Acute encephalitis is associated with foci of necrosis, which are initially surrounded by inflammatory cells. In later stages the lesions become calcified and are visible radiologically, most prominently in congenital toxoplasmosis. Microcephaly and hydrocephalus are frequently evident on gross examination.

Ocular symptoms are prominent in the TORCH complex. Rubella embryopathy, found in more than 70% of all affected children, typically presents with unilateral or bilateral **cataracts** and **microphthalmos.** Other ocular abnormalities include **glaucoma, chorioretinitis,** and **coloboma** of the retina. Chorioretinitis is also very common in congenital toxoplasmosis and cytomegalovirus infection. **Keratoconjunctivitis** is the most common ocular lesion in children afflicted with herpes simplex. **Cardiac defects** occur in many children with the TORCH complex, but are most typical of congenital rubella. The commonest lesions are patent ductus arteriosus and various septal defects.

CONGENITAL SYPHILIS

Infection with *Treponema pallidum* is transmitted to fetuses in utero by mothers who acquire syphilis during pregnancy. There is a possibility that the fetus will be infected if the mother became infected in the 2 years preceding the pregnancy and was not treated adequately, but the actual risk cannot be accurately assessed.

Children born with congenital syphilis are initially normal or show symptoms clinically indistinguishable from the TORCH complex. Many are asymptomatic, only to develop the typical stigmata of tardive syphilis several years later. Skin lesions include **macules, papules,** and **vesicular and annular skin eruptions.** Palmar and plantar sloughing of the epithelium, and circumoral and circumanal **rhagades,** with oozing, may be the only signs of intrauterine infection. Involvement of the nasopharynx presents as a serosanguineous nasal discharge **(sniffles).** Anemia, hepatosplenomegaly, jaundice, and signs of mild meningeal irritation are common. Osteochondritis involves the long bones, and occasionally the small bones of the extremities. Pneumonitis **(pneumonia alba)** is found only in severe congenital syphilis. All of these lesions contain spirochetes. The tissues are infiltrated with lymphocytes and plasma cells, and show inflammatory changes of small arteries and arterioles and fully developed gummas. Late symptoms of congenital syphilis become apparent many years after birth. Most of them reflect slowly evolving tissue destruction and repair of subclinical lesions, and are also due to the immune response of the body.

Prominent among the symptoms of tardive syphilis is the **Hutchinson's triad,** considered for many years to be the hallmark of the disease. It includes interstitial **keratitis,** sensorineural **deafness,** and **deformed teeth.** Dental lesions typically involve permanent teeth. Notched edges of the anterior teeth, which are usually narrower at the apical than the basal side, produces a typical change known as **Hutchinson's teeth.** Deformed molars, known as **mulberry molars,** are another sign of deranged dentition and impaired enamel formation. Other symptoms of tardive syphilis are predominantly found in the skeleton; they include **saddle deformity** of the nose, perforation of the hard palate, and **saber deformity** of the shin. Perforation of the palate and saddle deformity of the nose are caused by the destruction of the facial bones by gummas. Disturbed ossification and chronic periostitis lead to the "sabre deformity" of the shin, which can be traced to anterior bowing of the tibia and thinning of cortical bone in one area in conjunction with excessive formation of subperiosteal bone in other parts. Symptoms of brain involvement are protean.

CHROMOSOMAL ABNORMALITIES

NORMAL CHROMOSOMES

Cytogenetic analysis can be performed on any spontaneously dividing cell. However, in most instances the analysis is performed on circulating lymphocytes. Mitotic cells are treated with colchicine to arrest them in metaphase, after which they are spread on glass slides to disperse the chromosomes. The chromosomes are stained with standard hematologic stains and by more sophisticated techniques that enable more precise identification of chromosomes on the basis of distinct bands. Using hematologic stains such as Giemsa, the chromosomes are classified according to their **length** and the positioning of the constriction, or **centromere.** The centromere is the point at which the two identical double helices of the chromosomal DNA, called sister **chromatids,** attach to each other. The location of the centromere is used to classify the chromosomes as **metacentric, submetacentric,** or **acrocentric.** In metacentric chromosomes (numbers 1, 3, 19, and 20) the centromere is exactly in the middle. In submetacentric chromosomes the centromere divides the chromosomes into a short arm (p—from French *petit*), and a long arm (q—next letter in the alphabet). Acrocentric chromosomes (numbers 13, 14, 15, 21, 22, and Y) have very short arms or stalks and satellites attached to an eccentrically located centromere.

STRUCTURAL ABNORMALITIES

Structurally abnormal chromosomes arise during cell division (Fig. 6-2). In dividing somatic cells, these abnormalities usually either are of no consequence or lead to lethal traits that cause extinction of the abnormal cell clone. It has become evident that some structural chromosomal abnormalities are pathogenetically related to some forms of cancer. However, most of these **somatic cell mutations** are limited to a few cell lines and have little effect on fetal development. **Much more important from the embryologic point of view are the structural chromosomal abnormalities that originate during gametogenesis, because these are transmitted to all somatic cells and result in hereditary transmissible traits.**

During meiosis homologous chromosomes pair to form bivalents. Their chromatids are broken, and crossing of portions of chromatids normally occurs. Exchange of fragmented chromatids during the first meiotic division also occurs between nonhomologous chromosomes, a process that results in **translocation.** In **reciprocal translocation** acentric segments of chromatid from one chromosome are exchanged for a similar segment from a heterologous chromosome.

Robertsonian translocations, or centric fusion, involve the centromere and can be recognized in routine chromosomal preparations. In such cases two acrocentric chromosomes, broken near the centromere, exchange two arms and form a new, large, metacentric chromosome and a small fragment. This fragment is devoid of a centromere and is usually lost during subsequent divisions. If there is no loss of genetic material, this translocation is called **balanced.** Individuals with such abnormalities are usually normal, but may suffer from infertility.

The overall risk for the development of cancer because of translocations in germ cells is only now being assessed. Nevertheless, it is already evident that certain forms of translocation in somatic cell lineages are associated with an increased risk of tumor formation. The best examples are the translocations between chromosomes 8 and 14 and between 22 and 9 in malignant lymphomas and leukemias. The Robertsonian translocation of chromosome 21 plays a role in hereditary Down's syndrome.

Meiotic disturbances, or single breaks of chromatids in somatic cells, induced by physical, chemical, and biological agents cause formation of acentric fragments that are not incorporated into any of the 46 chromosomes and may be lost in subsequent cell divisions. This loss of genetic material is called **deletion** and involves either the terminal or the intercalary (middle) portion of a chromosome. Deletion is pathogenetically related to several cancers in man, including some hereditary forms of cancer. For example, **retinoblastomas** are associated with the deletion of the long arm of chromosome 13. **Wilms' tumor aniridia syndrome** is associated with deletion of the short arm of chromosome 11.

The break of a chromosome at two points, followed by **inversion** of the intermediate segment and reunion, results in the formation of chromosomes with a rearranged distribution of genes in the restructured chromatid. Inversions are called **pericentric** or **paracentric,** depending on whether the rotation occurs around the centromere or only on the acentric portion of the arm.

Ring chromosomes are formed by a break involving both telomeric ends of a chromosome, followed by deletion of the broken acentric fragment and end-to-end fusion of the remaining portion.

Isochromosomes are formed by the faulty division of the centromere. Normally, centromere division occurs in a plane parallel to the long axis of the chromosome, leading to the formation of two identical hemichromosomes. If the centromere divides transversely to the long axis, pairs of isochromosomes are formed, one corresponding to the short arms attached to the upper portion of the centromere and the other to the long arms attached to the lower segment. The most important clinical condition involving isochromosomes is **Turner's syndrome.**

NUMERICAL ABERRATIONS

Every mammalian species has a characteristic number of chromosomes corresponding to two **haploid** sets of homologous chromosomes. In man each haploid set includes 23 chromosomes; the **diploid** number is,

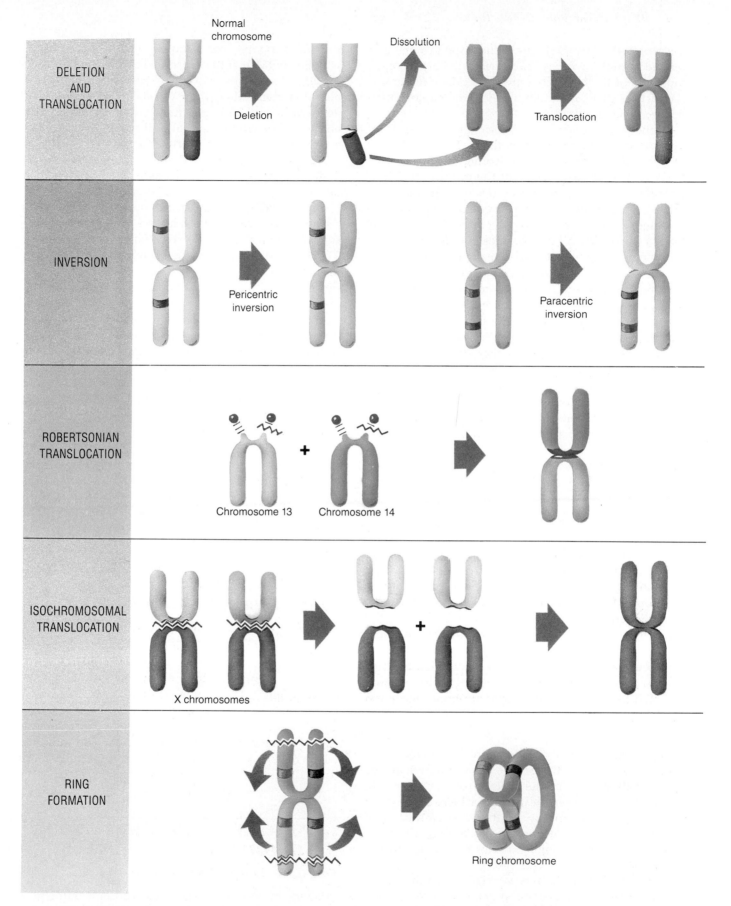

Figure 6-2. Structural abnormalities of human chromosomes. Such abnormalities evolve during either mitosis or meiosis.

therefore, 46. Any multiple of the haploid number is termed **euploid,** whereas karyotypes that are not exact multiples of the haploid number are called **aneuploid.** Karyotypes that contain multiples of the haploid number are labeled **polyploid.**

Numerical chromosomal abnormalities arise primarily from **nondisjunction. Nondisjunction is a failure of paired chromosomes or chromatids to separate and move to opposite poles of the mitotic spindle at anaphase.** Nondisjunction occurs during mitosis or meiosis. It leads to aneuploidy if only one pair of chromosomes is involved and to polyploidy if the entire set fails to divide and all the chromosomes are segregated in a single daughter cell. In somatic cells aneuploidy due to nondisjunction results in one daughter cell exhibiting **trisomy** and the other **monosomy** for the affected chromosome pair (2n + 1 or 2n − 1). Aneuploid germ cells have two copies of the same chromosome or lack the affected chromosome entirely (n + 1 or n − 1).

The causes of chromosomal aberrations are obscure. Putative exogenous factors, such as radiation, viruses, and chemicals, affect the mitotic spindle or DNA synthesis and produce mitotic and meiotic disturbances in experimental animals. However, the role of these factors in the production of human chromosomal abnormalities remains conjectural.

There are only two phenomena known to be of importance in aberrations of human development:

Disturbances of meiotic division are more common in individuals with structurally abnormal chromosomes. This is probably related to the fact that structurally abnormal chromosomes do not pair or segregate as readily as normal chromosomes, and therefore nondisjunction occurs more frequently.

Children born to older women show chromosomal aberrations more frequently than those born to younger mothers. Maternal age obviously plays an important role, but there is no precise explanation for the higher incidence of nondisjunction in older women.

Abnormal ova or spermatozoa resulting from nondisjunction transmit the genetic defect through all cell lineages derived from the division of the zygote. In most instances the genetic imbalance has a lethal effect on the developing conceptus and leads to early death of the embryo or spontaneous abortion in the early stages of pregnancy. Most major chromosomal abnormalities are, thus, incompatible with life.

Autosomal aneuploidies associated with the loss of genetic material (monosomies) generally do not even reach the terminal stages of pregnancy. **Monosomy** of sex chromosomes, on the other hand, is compatible with life, but only if the conserved chromosome is an X. Female fetuses with only one X chromosome (45,X) are also less viable than their normal counterparts and about 90% are lost in pregnancy. The karyotype 45,Y absolutely precludes normal embryonic development and invariably results in early abortion.

Autosomal trisomies—that is, aneuploidies with an additional chromosome—are associated with several developmental abnormalities. Many fetuses with trisomy are viable throughout the pregnancy, and some are even liveborn. Liveborn infants with autosomal trisomy die soon after birth, except for those with trisomy 21. These infants express the stigmata of **Down's syndrome,** and can survive for years. Sex chromosome trisomies may result in abnormal development but are not lethal.

Mitotic nondisjunction may involve embryonic cells during early stages of development and result in chromosomal aberrations. These are transmitted selectively through some cell lineages but not through others. The condition in which the body contains two or more karyotypically different cell lines is called **mosaicism.** Like all chromosomal abnormalities related to nondisjunction, mosaicism may involve autosomes or sex chromosomes. Autosomal mosaicism is rare, most likely because this condition is usually lethal. On the other hand mosaicism involving sex chromosomes is common and is found in patients with gonadal dysgenesis who present with Turner's or Klinefelter's syndromes.

NOMENCLATURE OF CHROMOSOMAL ABERRATIONS

According to an international convention, 47,XX +21 denotes trisomy 21 in a female with Down's syndrome. The first number, indicating the total number of chromosomes, is followed by the symbols for the two sex chromosomes. The plus sign denotes an additional chromosome 21. The designation 46,XX del (5) (qter p 13): denotes deletion of the terminal portion of the long arm of chromosome 5. The colon at the end indicates where the break occurred and that the segment distal to band 13 of the chromosome 5 has been deleted.

CLINICALLY IMPORTANT SYNDROMES

TRISOMY 21 (DOWN'S SYNDROME)

Trisomy 21 is one of the most common clinically recognized chromosomal disorders and also the sin-

gle most common cause of mental retardation. Life expectancy is also reduced: 30% die within the first year of life, 50% succumb before the age of 5 years and only 8% survive beyond 40 years.

Most patients with Down's syndrome (92% to 95%) have trisomy 21. **The extra chromosome in classical trisomy is the result of nondisjunction during meiosis in one of the parents. The incidence of trisomy 21 correlates strongly with maternal age.** The risk of giving birth to abnormal children rises with age, which suggests that **nondisjunction during oogenesis is the underlying cause of this chromosomal anomaly,** at least in older mothers. The risk of giving birth to a trisomic child is constant at about 0.9 per 1000 liveborns for women in their mid- to late thirties. The risk then dramatically increases, to reach an incidence of 1 in 30 pregnancies at age 44 years. In the small percentage of patients with Down's syndrome that is not due to trisomy 21, the trisomy found in one of the somatic cell lines is due to **mitotic nondisjunction in early stages of embryogenesis.**

The infant with Down's syndrome is hypotonic and displays typical craniofacial features (Fig. 6-3). These include a flat facial profile, a low-bridged nose, reduced interpupillary distance, oblique palpebral fissures, and epicanthal folds on the eyes, imparting an Oriental appearance. The iris may be speckled (Brushfield spots). The mouth is often open and the tongue is enlarged, protruding, coarsely furrowed, and without a central fissure. The hands are broad and short and exhibit a transverse simian crease. The middle phalanx of the fifth finger is hypoplastic, a feature resulting in clinodactyly (inward curvature). The feet and toes show equivalent abnormalities. Other skeletal defects include those of the rib cage, pelvis, and long bones, which are shorter than average. Congenital heart defects are common. Malformations of other organ systems occur at an increased rate but are not standard features of this syndrome. **Mental retardation is usually severe, and the intelligence quotient (IQ) is, in most instances, lower than 50.**

Down's syndrome is associated with an increased incidence of acute lymphoblastic and myeloblastic leukemia. Neuropathologic changes indistinguishable from those in Alzheimer's disease occur in adults who survive into their 40s and 50s.

SEX CHROMOSOME TRISOMIES

Trisomies of sex chromosomes (Fig. 6-4) are considerably more common than those involving autosomes.

Individuals born with an extra Y chromosome (47,XYY) are phenotypically male, and although very tall, do not exhibit any symptoms. Multiplicity of X chromosomes over the normal XX or XY complement is often accompanied by mental retardation, which

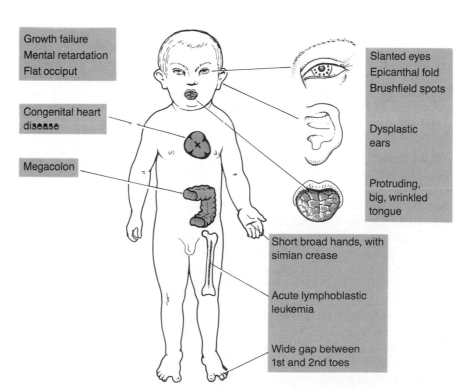

Growth failure
Mental retardation
Flat occiput

Congenital heart disease

Megacolon

Slanted eyes
Epicanthal fold
Brushfield spots

Dysplastic ears

Protruding, big, wrinkled tongue

Short broad hands, with simian crease

Acute lymphoblastic leukemia

Wide gap between 1st and 2nd toes

Figure 6-3. Clinical features of Down's syndrome.

Gametes	SPERM	X		Y		XY		0	
	OVUM								
X		XX Normal ♀	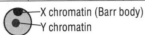	XY Normal ♂		XXY Klinefelter ♂		XO Turner ♀	
XX		XXX Triple X ♀		XXY Klinefelter ♂		XXXY Klinefelter ♂		XXO Normal ♀	
XXX		XXXX 48, XXXX ♀		XXXY Klinefelter ♂		XXXXY 49, XXXXY ♂		XXXO Triple X ♀	
0		OX Turner ♀		OY LETHAL		OXY LETHAL		OO LETHAL	

X chromatin (Barr body)
Y chromatin

Figure 6-4. Pathogenesis of sex chromosome aberrations. Non-disjunction in either the male or female gamete is the principal cause of these numerical chromosomal abnormalities.

roughly correlates with the number of extra X chromosomes. This is especially true in males, who also show some degree of feminization. Females with three X chromosomes are usually normal, whereas those with four or five are mentally retarded. The reasons for the adverse effects of extra X chromosomes are not obvious, since all the X chromosomes but one are inactivated and attached to the nuclear membrane as heteropyknotic chromatin, or **Barr body.**

Klinefelter's syndrome, or testicular dysgenesis, is the most important sex chromosome trisomy (Fig. 6-5). The syndrome is related to the presence of one or more X chromosomes in excess of the normal male XY complement. Approximately 80% of those affected have a 47,XXY karyotype. The remainder are mosaics or have more than two X chromosomes. The additional chromosome affects the development of the gonads and of intelligence. Abnormalities of sexual development and intelligence are usually not apparent until later in childhood. The testicles are small, and at puberty the body does not assume the typical male characteristics and proportions. Individuals with Klinefelter's syndrome are tall, with long arms and legs, and have a small penis. Feminization is typified by a female pattern of pubic hair, gynecomastia, and a high-pitched voice. All these changes are related to hypogonadism and inadequate Leydig cells. Low levels of testosterone in serum and urine are associated with elevated serum levels of follicle-stimulating hormone (FSH), indicating that the pituitary is normal but that the testicular hormone-producing cells do not respond to the stimulus. Testicular biopsy reveals prominent interstitial fibrosis replacing normal Leydig cells and surrounding atrophic

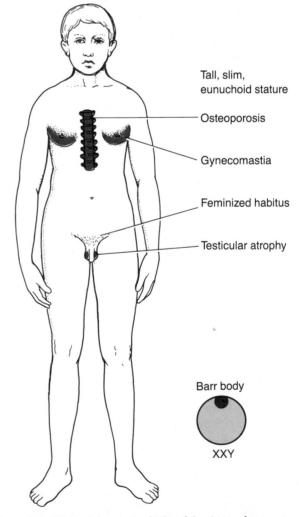

Tall, slim, eunuchoid stature

Osteoporosis

Gynecomastia

Feminized habitus

Testicular atrophy

Barr body

XXY

Figure 6-5. Clinical features of Klinefelter's syndrome.

tubules. A low sperm count or aspermatogenesis is reflected in infertility.

MONOSOMY X

The X chromosome is essential for the viability of the fetus, and those missing both X chromosomes or having the 45,Y karyotype die in utero. Almost all fetuses with the 45,X karyotype are spontaneously aborted.

Infants born with the 45,X karyotype display the clinical features of **Turner's syndrome** (Fig. 6-6). In 80% of these cases, the single X chromosome is of maternal origin, indicating that the **missing X was most commonly lost in paternal meiosis.** Approximately half of patients with Turner's syndrome have classic monosomy X, whereas the others have variant forms —namely, mosaicism and abnormal X chromosomes. **Structurally abnormal chromosomes are often of paternal origin, and this anomaly may be causally related to advanced age of the father.** The constant and typical features of the syndrome are the streak gonads and growth retardation.

In most children with Turner's syndrome, primordial follicles completely disappear from the ovaries by the time of puberty. Such gonads, devoid of oocytes, transform into fibrous streaks, but the fallopian tubes, uterus, and vagina develop normally. Menarche does not occur, and sterility is the rule.

Other somatic features of Turner's syndrome are highly variable, depending on the nature of the chromosomal defect. Common features are a short, broad neck with low hairline, web neck (**"pterygium coli"**),

shield chest with widely spaced nipples, cubitus valgus, short metatarsal and metacarpal bones, numerous pigmented nevi, lymphedema of hands and feet, hypoplasia of nails, miscellaneous renal malformations, coarctation of the aorta, ventricular septal defect, and craniofacial peculiarities, such as epicanthal folds, abnormal teeth, and a high arched palate. In most instances intelligence is normal.

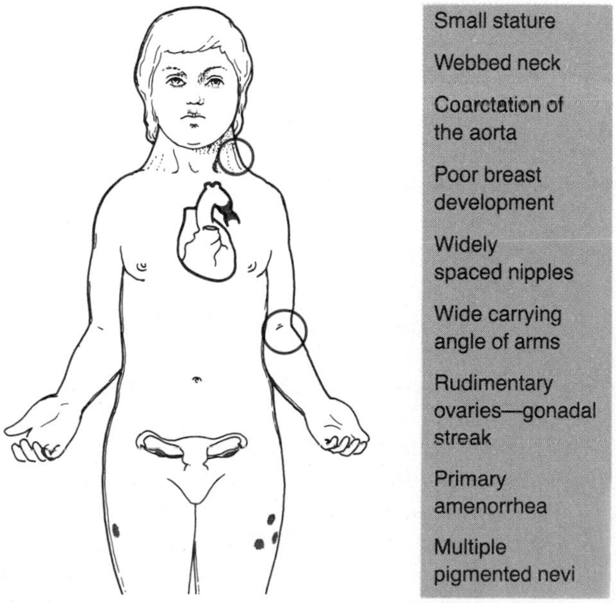

SINGLE-GENE ABNORMALITIES

Single genes that **encode identifiable traits, segregate sharply within families, and transmit according to the classic laws of inheritance outlined by Gregor Mendel are called "mendelian."** Each mendelian trait is specified by two variants of the same gene, called **"alleles,"** which are located on the same locus of two homologous chromosomes. Genes are classified as **autosomal** if located on autosomes and as **sex-linked** if located on the X and Y chromosomes. Genes that are expressed only when they present in identical form on both chromosomes (i.e., when the individual is homozygous for that pair of genes) are called **recessive.** Genes that require only one copy—that is, genes that are expressed in homozygous and heterozygous form —are called **dominant.** A variant of dominance in which both alleles in a heterozygous gene pair are fully expressed is called **codominance**—an example is provided by the AB blood group genes. Mendelian traits are classified as autosomal dominant or recessive and sex-linked dominant or recessive. Sex-linked dominant traits are rare and of little practical significance.

THE BIOCHEMICAL BASIS OF SINGLE-GENE ABNORMALITIES

Mendelian traits can be identified only by a study of pedigree and transmission patterns through generations; they cannot be recognized by chromosomal analysis.

A series of genes codes for a series of enzymes of a specific metabolic pathway, which catalyzes the conversion of substrate A through several intermediate metabolites (B and C) to the final product, D.

$$A \rightarrow B \rightarrow C \rightarrow D$$

A		D
initial substrate	intermediary metabolites	end product

A single-gene defect can have several possible consequences:

Small stature
Webbed neck
Coarctation of the aorta
Poor breast development
Widely spaced nipples
Wide carrying angle of arms
Rudimentary ovaries—gonadal streak
Primary amenorrhea
Multiple pigmented nevi

Figure 6-6. Clinical features of Turner's syndrome.

- **Failure to complete a metabolic pathway.** In this situation the end product is not formed because an enzyme that is essential for the completion of a metabolic sequence is missing.

$$A \rightarrow B \rightarrow C \rightarrow (D)$$

An example is albinism due to tryosinase deficiency. Tyrosinase catalyzes the formation of dihydroxyphenylalanine (DOPA), an intermediary metabolite in the metabolic pathway leading to the synthesis of melanin from tyrosine. In the absence of this enzyme, melanin is not formed, and the affected individual is devoid of pigment (albino) in all organs that normally contain it, primarily the eyes and skin.

- **Accumulation of unmetabolized substrate.** In these circumstances the enzyme that converts the initial substrate into the first intermediary metabolite is missing. Absence of the enzyme results in an excessive accumulation of the initial substrate.

$$A(\uparrow) \overset{x}{\underset{x}{\longrightarrow}} x\ B(\downarrow)C(\downarrow)D(\downarrow)$$

A typical example of this sequence of events is glycogenosis caused by a deficiency of glucose-6-phosphatase. Defective mobilization of glycogen leads to low blood glucose levels, which in turn produce other metabolic disturbances in a number of organs.

- **Storage of an intermediary metabolite.** In this situation an intermediary metabolite, which is readily processed into the final product and is normally present only in minute amounts, accumulates in large quantities. The subsequent intermediary metabolites and the end product are reduced in amount.

$$A \rightarrow B(\uparrow)C(\downarrow)D(\downarrow)$$

Lysosomal storage diseases are typical examples of this metabolic derangement. An enzyme deficiency causes intermediary metabolites to accumulate in the lysosomes in various conditions, such as Tay-Sachs disease, Niemann-Pick disease, and other gangliosidoses, mucopolysaccharidoses, and lipid storage diseases.

- **Activation of an alternate metabolic pathway.** In this sequence of events, an enzyme deficiency leads to the accumulation of intermediary metabolites, which are then channeled into an alternate pathway. Metabolites normally formed in minute amounts are produced excessively and accumulate in the body.

$$A \rightarrow B \rightarrow C(\downarrow)D(\downarrow)$$
$$\rightarrow XYZ$$

This type of genetic disorder is exemplified by phenylalanine hydroxylase deficiency, the major cause of phenylketonuria. The deficiency of this enzyme, which catalyzes the conversion of phenylalanine to tyrosine, results in both the accumulation of toxic phenylketones and a deficiency in the normal end products of tyrosine metabolism, a pathway essential for the functioning of many cell systems.

- **Formation of abnormal end product.** In this situation an altered genetic code perturbs the synthesis of a structural protein that will form the normal equivalent.

$$A \rightarrow B \rightarrow C \rightarrow d$$

In sickle cell anemia, one such defect, the sequencing of amino acids is normal, except that valine is substituted for glutamine at the sixth position of the beta chain of hemoglobin.

AUTOSOMAL DOMINANT DISORDERS

The salient features of autosomal dominant traits are the following:

- The gene is located on an autosome.
- The gene produces its effects in both the homozygous and heterozygous states.
- The trait transmitted by the gene appears in every generation, unless it has a low penetrance or its expression has been modified by additional mutations.
- Unaffected members of the family do not transmit the trait to their offspring.
- Affected individuals are usually heterozygous for the trait and transmit it to only one half of their offspring.
- Males and females are equally affected.

Figure 6-7 illustrates the pattern of inheritance of autosomal dominant traits. **More than a thousand human diseases are inherited as autosomal dominant traits, but most of them are rare.** Examples of such diseases are systemic disorders of connective tissue (the Marfan syndrome), skeletal abnormalities

AUTOSOMAL DOMINANT

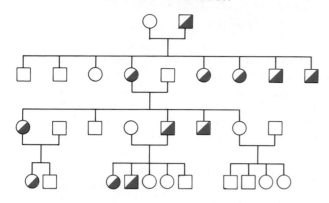

■, ◑ Heterozygote with disease

Figure 6-7. Autosomal dominant inheritance. Only symptomatic individuals transmit the trait to the next generation, and heterozygotes are symptomatic. Both males and females are affected.

(achondroplastic dwarfism), developmental disturbances of the kidneys (polycystic kidneys), maladies of the brain (tuberous sclerosis, Huntington's chorea), hemoglobinopathies (sickle cell anemia, thalassemia), impaired metabolism of cholesterol (familial hypercholesterolemia), and even familial tumors, such as polyposis coli and neurofibromatosis.

CLINICALLY IMPORTANT AUTOSOMAL DOMINANT DISORDERS

THE MARFAN SYNDROME

The hallmarks of the Marfan syndrome are structural abnormalities of the skeletal system, the cardiovascular system, and the eye. The skeletal derangements are characterized by dolichomorphism (Greek *dolichos* means long).

The patients are usually (but not invariably) tall, and the lower body segment (pubis-to-sole) is longer than the upper body. A slender habitus, which reflects a paucity of subcutaneous fat, is complemented by long, thin extremities and fingers, the latter accounting for the term "arachnodactyly" (spider fingers) (Fig. 6-8).

Disorders of the ribs are conspicuous and produce pectus excavatum (concave sternum) and pectus carinatum (pigeon breast). The tendons, ligaments, and joint capsules are weak, a condition that leads to hyperextensibility of the joints (double-jointedness), dislocations, hernias, and kyphoscoliosis, the last often severe.

The most important cardiovascular defect resides in the aorta, in which the principal lesion is a faulty media. Weakness of the media leads to variable dilatation of the ascending aorta and to a high incidence of dissecting aneurysms. Dilatation of the aortic ring results in aortic regurgitation, which may be so severe as to produce angina pectoris and congestive heart failure. The mitral valve may exhibit redundant valve leaflets and chordae tendineae—changes that result in the so-called floppy valve syndrome.

Microscopic examination of the aorta reveals a conspicuous fragmentation and loss of elastic fibers, accompanied by an increase in metachromatic mucopolysaccharides (glycosaminoglycans). Focally, the defect in the elastic tissue results in discrete pools of amorphous metachromatic material. Cardiovascular disorders particularly dissecting aortic aneurysm, are the most common causes of death in the Marfan syndrome.

The ocular changes reflect the generalized weakness in the structure of collagen and include subluxation (dislocation) of the lens, cataracts (opacification of the lens), and retinal detachments.

The molecular defect in the Marfan syndrome has not been unequivocally identified.

NEUROFIBROMATOSIS (VON RECKLINGHAUSEN'S DISEASE)

Neurofibromatosis is one of the most common autosomal disorders. It has been estimated that in the United States there are three million people with some features of this syndrome. At least 50% of cases represent new mutations. In the classic form, neurofibromatosis presents with a triad consisting of **multiple nerve**

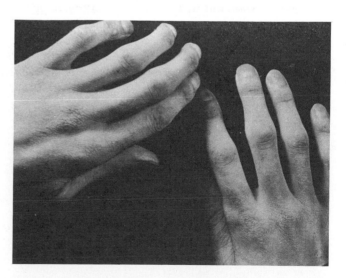

Figure 6-8. Arachnodactyly of Marfan's syndrome.

tumors (neurofibromas and neurilemmomas), **pigmented skin macules** called "café au lait spots", and **pigmented nodules of the iris** (Lisch nodules).

Abnormalities of other organ systems are common. About one-third of patients have skeletal lesions, such as scoliosis of the spine, multiple intraosseous and subperiosteal cysts, and various degenerative changes of the joints. Affected individuals are at high risk for developing various tumors—most commonly pheochromocytoma, meningioma, Wilms' tumor, and medullary carcinoma of the thyroid.

ACHONDROPLASTIC DWARFISM

Achrondroplastic dwarfs have short limbs and a large head, with a bulging forehead and a deeply indented bridge of the nose. The abnormal gene affects the proliferation of cartilage cells and causes impaired epiphyseal bone growth (see Chapter 26). The condition is more severe in homozygotes, who usually die in early infancy.

FAMILIAL HYPERCHOLESTEROLEMIA

Familial hypercholesterolemia is one of the most common autosomal dominant disorders and affects at least one in 500 adults in the United States. The genetic defect involves the low density lipoprotein (LDL) receptor on the cell surface, which is crucial for the regulation of the level of LDL and cholesterol in plasma and of cholesterol metabolism in the cells. In familial hypercholesterolemia a deficiency of LDL receptors prevents entry of LDL-cholesterol into the cell, and endogenous cholesterol synthesis is, therefore, not regulated. Overproduction and maldistribution of cholesterol at the cellular level and in various compartments of the body leads to severe complications, primarily affecting the cardiovascular system. In heterozygotes suffering from familial hypercholesterolemia, the number of cell surface receptors for LDL is reduced to a variable extent; in homozygotes they may be lacking entirely. Cholesterol–LDL complexes are still removed from the blood, but only through a less efficient, receptor-independent mechanism. Heterozygotes have a twofold to three-fold elevation of plasma cholesterol, whereas in homozygotes the cholesterol levels are five to six times higher than normal. **Patients with hypercholesterolemia develop atherosclerosis at an accelerated rate and suffer at an early age from myocardial infarction, cerebrovascular accidents, and occlusive peripheral vascular disease.**

AUTOSOMAL RECESSIVE DISORDERS

Essentially all clinically identified inborn errors of metabolism and storage diseases, and many of the hereditary traits that have only marginal significance for the practice of medicine, exhibit an autosomal recessive pattern of inheritance. The characteristics of this pattern are as follows:

- The gene is located on an autosome.
- The effects of the gene are obvious only in the homozygous state.
- Both parents are usually heterozygous for the trait and are clinically unaffected.
- Symptoms appear in one-quarter of the offspring.
- One-half of all siblings are heterozygous for the trait and are thus asymptomatic.
- Males and females are equally affected.

Figure 6-9 illustrates the pattern of autosomal recessive inheritance. The pathogenesis of these disorders follows the principle of "one gene, one enzyme." The deficient enzyme has been identified in many conditions, among them lysosomal storage diseases (glycogenoses, lipidoses, mucopolysaccharidoses), deficiencies of synthetic enzymes (agammaglobulinemia, albinism), transport enzymes (cystinuria), and many others.

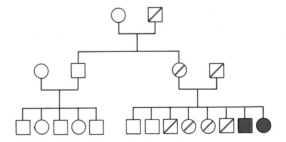

AUTOSOMAL RECESSIVE

■, ● Homozygote with disease
▨, ⊘ Heterozygote without disease (silent carrier)

Figure 6-9. Autosomal recessive inheritance. Symptoms of the disease appear only in homozygotes, male or female. Heterozygotes are asymptomatic carriers.

CLINICALLY IMPORTANT AUTOSOMAL RECESSIVE DISEASES

CYSTIC FIBROSIS

Cystic fibrosis is the most common clinically important autosomal recessive disorder in white children, having an incidence of 1 in 2500 newborns. More than 95% of cases have been recorded in whites. The disease is found only exceptionally in blacks and almost never in Orientals. Since the condition is autosomal recessive, the afflicted children are obviously homozygous for the trait. Recombinant DNA technology has enabled the identification in fetal tissue of restriction fragment length polymorphisms (RFLPs) within the human *mer* gene that predict inheritance of cystic fibrosis.

Cystic fibrosis is a systemic disease that affects essentially all exocrine glands of the body and results in abnormal sweat electrolyte content and hyperviscous secretions in the pancreas, biliary tract, and bronchial tree. The original name, "cystic fibrosis of the pancreas," denotes foremost the typical changes in that organ. The ducts are cystically dilated, and fibrosis replaces pancreatic acini destroyed by stagnant pancreatic enzymes. Viscous mucus, which accounts for the synonymous term **"mucoviscidosis,"** causes comparable changes in salivary and other mucus-secreting glands, and in organs containing mucus-secreting cells, such as the bronchi, biliary tree, epididymis, and intestine (Fig. 6-10). The basic defect in cystic fibrosis is not known. Electrolyte disturbances are detectable in the sweat of affected individuals and serve as a test for early diagnosis. **The sodium and chloride content of sweat is two to three times normal, and levels of 60 mEq/liter are diagnostic.** This basic test for the diagnosis of cystic fibrosis has an accuracy of over 95%.

Clinically the condition presents even in utero. Viscous contents of the gut **(meconium)** cause obstruction. This blockage results in ileus or peritonitis due to the extravasation of intestinal contents **(meconium peritonitis).** In infancy and early childhood, nutritional deficiency is the major clinical problem. Because the pancreatic ducts are obstructed, digestive enzymes do not reach the intestine. Consequently, the patient shows the typical symptoms of malabsorption, such as lipid intolerance, bulky fatty stools **(steatorrhea),** and deficiencies of the fat-soluble vitamins (A,D,K). Obstruction of the biliary tree is another contributory cause of malabsorption. Children who survive infancy show stunted growth and suffer predominantly from bronchopulmonary infections, which account for most of the morbidity. Even with modern antibiotic therapy, the average life expectancy for girls is 12 years and for boys 16 years.

Pathologic changes in the pancreas and the salivary glands are found in practically all instances. Excretory ducts are dilated and plugged with inspissated mucus. Acini are atrophic and are replaced by fibrous tissue. About one-third of patients show some degree of endocrine pancreatic insufficiency. Bile ducts are also obstructed, and 2% to 3% of older patients show signs of **secondary biliary cirrhosis.** Mucous obstruction of the bronchopulmonary spaces, combined with superimposed infections, leads to **recurrent bronchitis, bronchiectasis, and bronchopneumonia.** Chronic infection

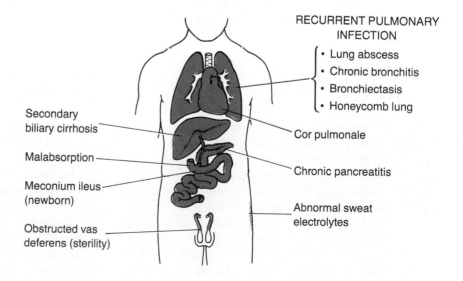

Figure 6-10. Clinical features of cystic fibrosis.

and obstruction of the air passages promote recurrent and persistent pneumonia and pulmonary fibrosis. The resulting pulmonary hypertension causes chronic cor pulmonale and right ventricular hypertrophy.

STORAGE DISEASES

Deficiencies of enzymes involved in complex metabolic pathways lead to the accumulation of the unmetabolized initial substrate or one of the intermediary metabolites. Conditions characterized by excessive accumulation of unmetabolized substrates or intermediary metabolites are called **storage diseases.** Since the lysosomes are a major site of intracellular catabolism and are the primary cytoplasmic organelle involved in the storage of the accumulated material, these disorders are also known as **lysosomal diseases.** In these diseases the deficient enzyme is usually a lysosomal hydrolase. Storage diseases are conventionally classified according to the stored material and are labeled **glycogenoses, lipidoses, mucopolysaccharidoses,** and **mucolipidoses.**

Glycogenoses

Glycogenoses are inborn errors of glycogen catabolism, at least eight distinct enzyme deficiencies having been identified. These disorders have been classified according to numerical and eponymic designations, but a nomenclature based on the enzyme deficiency is preferable (Fig. 6-11).

Glycogenoses may be divided into those presenting with hepatomegaly and those presenting primarily as muscle disease. Deficiencies of lysosomal glucosidase and the debrancher enzyme cause severe metabolic disturbances and are associated with a high mortality in infancy. Other glycogenoses are associated with mild clinical symptoms.

Sphingolipidoses

The sphingolipidoses are the most important group of disorders involving disturbances of lipid metabolism (Fig. 6-12). Sphingolipidoses are inborn errors of metabolism that are characterized by deficiencies of lysosomal enzymes responsible for cleaving various moieties from cerebrosides and gangliosides in the catabolic pathway that ends in sphingosine and fatty acids. Cerebrosides, gangliosides, and various degradation products accumulate in lysosomes, which contain whorls of concentrically layered membranes. The specific enzyme deficiency is determined biochemically in cultured cells from a skin biopsy, blood, or amniotic fluid.

Tay-Sachs disease, an autosomal recessive disorder, primarily afflicts Ashkenazi Jews. Approximately 1 in 30 Ashkenazi Jews is a carrier of the defective gene. Tay-Sachs disease has mental deterioration and blindness as the major clinical findings. Initially, affected newborns appear normal, but in early infancy the disease evolves rapidly, and most children succumb by the age of 3 years. The basic defect is a deficiency of hexosaminidase A, with a compensatory increase in hexosaminidase B. **GM_2 ganglioside accumulates in the lysosomes of all organs, but the neurons and retinal cells are affected most dramatically.** Owing to the pallor of the lipid-laden retinal cells, the normal red color of the choroid of the macula appears more prominent and is labeled the **cherry-red spot.** The lipid-laden neurons appear enlarged and vacuolated in histologic sections. Electron microscopy reveals lipid accumulation in lysosomes, which appear filled with whorls of lipid-rich membranes ("myelin figures" (Fig. 6-13). Heterozygous carriers are detected with appropriate biochemical tests, and the affected fetus can be identified by amniocentesis or chorionic villus sampling.

Gaucher's disease reflects a deficiency of glucocerebrosidase, the lysosomal enzyme that cleaves glucose from the ceramide backbone. This enzyme degrades glycolipids formed continuously from the turnover of lipid-rich cell membranes. For example, it is involved in the degradation of glycolipids liberated from the membranes of senescent red blood cells taken up by the reticuloendothelial cells in the liver and spleen. Since the brain contains more lipid than most other tissues, and since the reticuloendothelial cells of the spleen and liver are the major degradation sites for the senescent erythrocytes, it is understandable that deficiency of glucocerebrosidase primarily affects those organs.

There are three forms of Gaucher's disease. In the most common form—type I or **adult Gaucher's disease,** found primarily in Ashkenazi Jews—the disease presents with hepatosplenomegaly, but without any neurologic symptoms. The adult form does not produce any serious symptoms and does not shorten the life span. In the type II form, also called **infantile Gaucher's disease,** both the brain and the reticuloendothelial system are involved. The disease, which shows no predilection for Jews, begins in early infancy, and death occurs early. The third form of the disorder is termed **juvenile Gaucher's disease.** There is no ethnic predominance, and the clinical presentation is intermediate between the adult and infantile forms. Patients with type I disease have reduced levels of glucocerebrosidase, patients suffering from type II disease have no measurable enzyme activity, and type III patients are in between. Although all three forms of

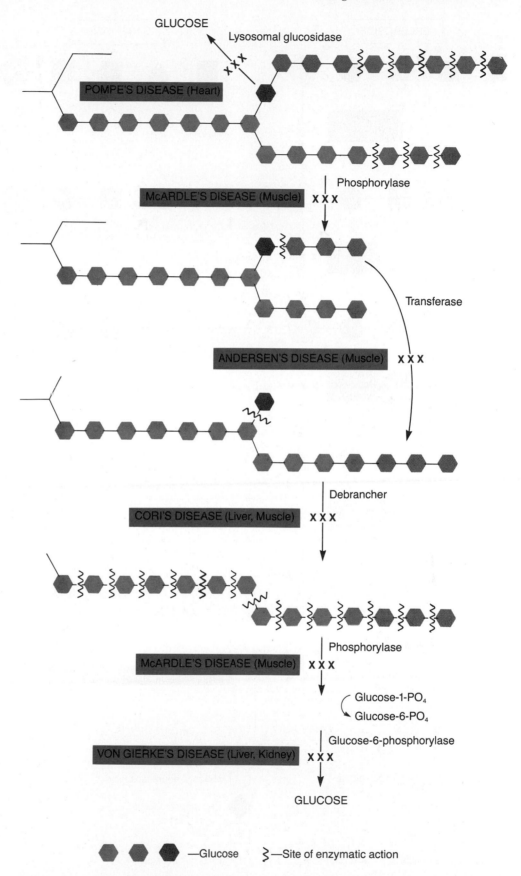

Figure 6-11. Schematic outline of the catabolism of glycogen and the enzymes that are missing in various glycogenoses.

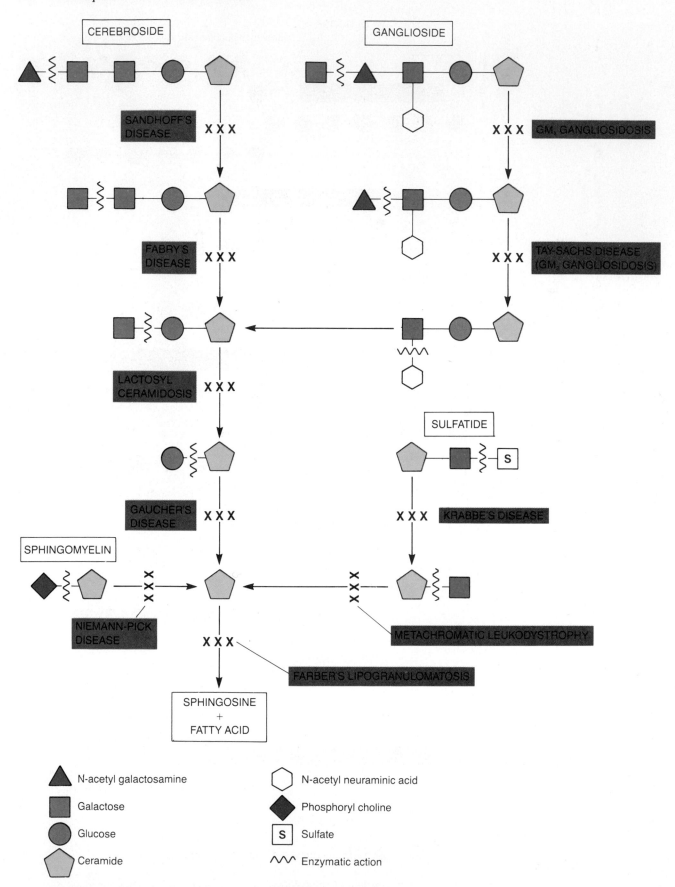

Figure 6-12. Disturbances of lipid metabolism in various sphingolipidoses.

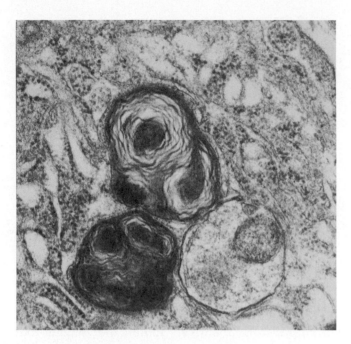

Figure 6-13. Tay-Sachs disease. The cytoplasm of the nerve cell contains lysosomes filled with whorled membranes.

Gaucher's disease involve the same enzyme, the differences in enzyme activity indicate that the disorders may be caused by different mutations.

Mucopolysaccharidoses

Mucopolysaccharides (glycosaminoglycans) are high-molecular-weight polymers composed of hexosamines and hexuronic acid. Complexed with protein to form proteoglycans, they are integral components of the extracellular matrix. Connective tissue cells synthesize the mucopolysaccharides and are also involved in their degradation.

Mucopolysaccharidoses are inborn errors of metabolism involving the lysosomal enzymes engaged in the degradation of mucopolysaccharides (Fig. 6-14). Fibroblasts and other connective tissue cells that produce mucopolysaccharides excrete most of the synthesized material. However, a small fraction remains in the cytoplasm and is degraded by lysosomal enzymes, such as alpha-L-iduronidase or beta-glucosaminidase. A lack of one of these enzymes results in the **accumulation of mucopolysaccharides in the lysosomes,** primarily in connective tissue cells but also in other cells, most notably neurons. Although there are several dis-

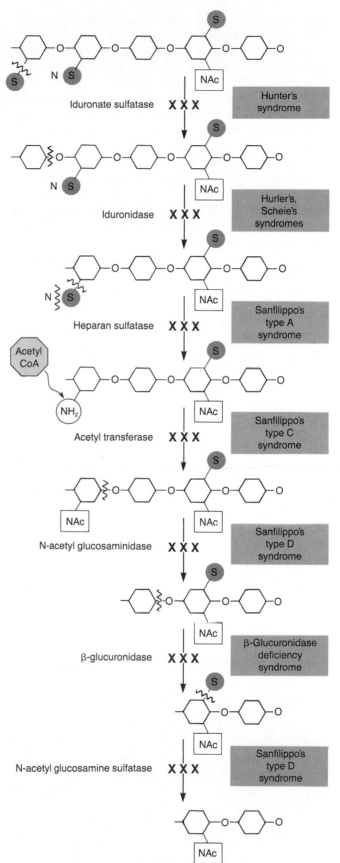

Figure 6-14. Metabolic disturbances in various mucopolysaccharidoses.

tinct clinical entities having different underlying enzyme deficiencies, in all cases the storage material consists of one or more of the four mucopolysaccharides: heparan sulfate, dermatan sulfate, keratan sulfate, and chondroitin sulfate.

The clinical presentation of each disease has its own peculiarities, but most mucopolysaccharidoses also have certain common features, including skeletal deformities, aortic and cardiac valvular lesions, and corneal clouding. Mental retardation is invariably present in all mucopolysaccharidoses. Many of the patients are dwarfs and show coarse facial features and hepatosplenomegaly, a picture resembling the gargoyle figures from Gothic cathedrals. Hence, the term "gargoylism" applied to patients with the prototype of this group of disorders, namely **Hurler's syndrome.** Most patients with mucopolysaccharidoses have a shortened life span. Cardiovascular changes, due to deposits of mucopolysaccharides in the coronary arteries and valves and the aorta are major causes of morbidity and mortality. Except for Hunter's syndrome, which is X-linked recessive, all are autosomal recessive traits. Excessive amounts of mucopolysaccharides in the blood,

urine, and amniotic fluid serve as the basis for diagnosis. This is confirmed by analyzing the cells (skin or amniotic fluid) for specific enzyme deficiencies.

INBORN ERRORS OF AMINO ACID METABOLISM

Many enzyme deficiencies involve the metabolism of amino acids. Some present serious clinical problems, whereas others are of lesser importance. (Fig. 6-15).

Phenylketonuria

In phenylketonuria **a deficiency of phenylalanine hydroxylase** prevents the conversion of phenylalanine into tyrosine, and all the dietary phenylalanine is shunted into the formation of phenylketones. Early in childhood, neurologic dysfunction, typified by hyperirritability, tremor, and hypertonicity, gives rise to slowly progressive mental deterioration. The phenylketones also competitively inhibit the enzyme that mediates the conversion of tyrosine to melanin. The children are, therefore, fair-haired and have hypopigmented skin. Elevated levels of serum phenylalanine

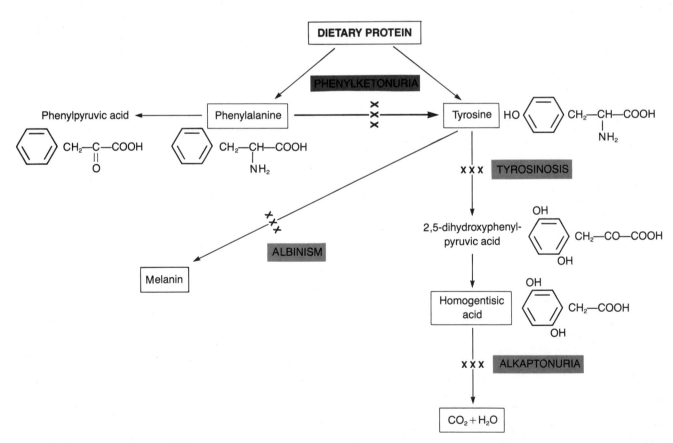

Figure 6-15. Disturbances of phenylalanine and tyrosine metabolism causing albinism, tyrosinosis, and alkaptonuria.

and urinary phenylketones can be detected biochemically in newborn infants, but not prenatally.

If an affected child is placed on a phenylalanine-deficient diet early in life, mental retardation can be prevented. A phenylalanine-deficient diet is of no help after 1 year of age.

Albinism

Albinism is a common inborn error of metabolism that is related to several defects in the synthesis of melanin. Melanin synthesis starts with the initial conversion of tyrosine to 3,4-dihydroxyphenylalanine (DOPA), which is then converted to melanin. Both steps are catalyzed by tyrosinase, and a deficiency of this enzyme results in deficient melanin synthesis, or albinism. The skin and eyes of those affected are devoid of pigment. It should be noted that tyrosine deficiency accounts for only some forms of albinism.

SEX-LINKED DISORDERS

The term "sex-linked inheritance' primarily denotes conditions that are recessive and caused by genes located on the X chromosome. Recessive mutations involving genes on the X chromosome are not expressed in females, because the homologous X chromosome contains the dominant allele. If the same recessive gene is present in the male, however, there is no hindrance to its expression, since the Y chromosome does not have a homologous allele. X-linked recessive genes may be expressed in females, but only in individuals homozygous for the trait.

The pattern of X-linked recessive inheritance is illustrated in Figure 6-16. The principles of this form of inheritance are as follows:

- The gene is located on the X chromosome.

- The recessive traits are fully expressed in heterozygous males and rarely in homozygous females.
- Partial expression may occur in heterozygous females, a phenomenon that reflects the random inactivation of one X chromosome.
- A trait is usually transmitted by asymptomatic females.
- Each son of a heterozygous female carrier has a 1 in 2 chance of being affected.
- Unaffected males do not transmit the gene.
- Affected males do not transmit the trait to their sons, but only to daughters. These daughters then become asymptomatic carriers. Rarely, if they inherit the second recessive allele from a carrier mother, daughters homozygous for the trait may present with symptoms.

There are close to 100 identified genes on the X chromosomes. Important clinical conditions inherited as X-linked recessive traits include hemophilia A and B, red–green color blindness, Duchenne's muscular dystrophy, glucose-6-phosphate dehydrogenase deficiency, diabetes insipidus, and some congenital immunodeficiency syndromes, such as Bruton's agammaglobulinemia, the Wiskott-Aldrich syndrome, and the Lesch-Nyhan syndrome.

CLINICALLY IMPORTANT SEX-LINKED DISORDERS

HEMOPHILIA

Hemophilia is an inborn bleeding disorder that occurs in two forms, known as hemophilia A (classic hemophilia) and hemophilia B (Christmas disease). Factor VIII:C is missing in hemophilia A, and factor IX in hemophilia B. Since the gene for factor VIII:C is very

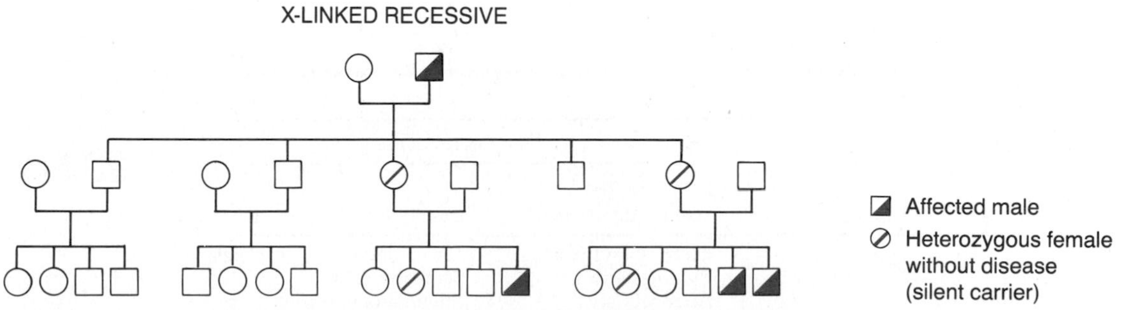

X-LINKED RECESSIVE

■ Affected male
⊘ Heterozygous female without disease (silent carrier)

Figure 6-16. X-linked recessive inheritance. Only males are affected; females are asymptomatic carriers. Asymptomatic males of the kindred do not transmit the trait.

large and occupies about 0.1% of the entire X chromosome, it is understandable that point mutations or deletions occur more often in this region than in the smaller region that codes for factor IX. Accordingly, hemophilia A occurs six times more often (1:5000 males) than hemophilia B (1:30,000 males).

MUSCULAR DYSTROPHY

Duchenne's muscular dystrophy is the most important of the three clinically distinct forms of muscle disease transmitted as X-linked recessive traits. The disease is rare, affecting one to four males per 100,000.

Symptoms appear in early childhood, and by school age most patients are incapacitated. The muscle wasting first involves the pelvic and femoral muscles, but the disease progressively spreads to the extremities and finally paralyzes the truncal muscles. Most affected individuals are confined to a wheelchair by puberty and do not survive beyond 20 years. All of them also have reduced intelligence. Histologically, the dystrophic muscles show degeneration and necrosis, and compensatory hypertrophy of the remaining fibers.

MULTIFACTORIAL INHERITANCE

Most human traits are inherited neither as dominant nor as recessive mendelian characteristics, but in a more complex manner known as **multifactorial inheritance.** This type of inheritance is determined by a combination of many genetic and nongenetic factors, each of which exerts a minor, but nonetheless distinct, effect.

Most of the quantifiable traits—for example, height or intelligence—have a distribution in the general population that corresponds to the gaussian (bell-shaped) curve. These traits are examples of **continuous multifactorial** characteristics that exhibit a range of values, with a continuous gradation between two extremes. Arterial hypertension and diabetes mellitus type 2 are diseases that belong to this category.

The so-called **discontinuous multifactorial traits,** less common but pathogenetically more important, account for a considerable number of **congenital malformations and common adult diseases** (Table 6-2). The following characteristics of multifactorial inheritance are useful in distinguishing between multifactorial and single-gene traits:

- The expression of symptoms is proportional to the number of mutant genes. The chances of expressing the same number of mutant genes are highest in identical twins, who express the trait concordantly about one-third of the time.
- Environmental factors influence the expression of the trait. Thus, concordance of the expression is seen in fewer than half of monozygotic twin pairs.
- Relatives of those affected have an increased risk of disease.
- The probability of the trait's being expressed in later offspring is influenced by whether or not it was expressed in earlier offspring. If one or more children are born with a multifactorial defect, the overall chances for recurrence rise from between 2% and 7%, and in some cases up to 9%. This contrasts with mendelian traits, in which the probability of occurrence is independent of the number of affected siblings.
- The more severe the defect the higher are the chances that it will be transmitted to offspring or recur in subsequent pregnancies. Individuals with more severe defects have presumably more mutant or inactive genes, and their offspring thus have a greater chance of inheriting some of the abnormal genes than offspring of less affected persons.

CLINICALLY IMPORTANT DISORDERS

CLEFT LIP AND CLEFT PALATE

At about the 35th day of pregnancy, the frontal prominence fuses with the maxillary process to form the

Table 6-2   Multifactorial Traits

CONTINUOUS		DISCONTINUOUS	
TRAITS	DISEASES	CONGENITAL MALFORMATIONS	DISEASES
Height	Hypertension	Cleft lip and palate	Manic-depressive psychosis
Intelligence	Diabetes	Pyloric stenosis	Schizophrenia
Blood pressure		Anencephaly	Rheumatoid arthritis
Skin color		Congenital heart	
Metabolic		disease	
parameters			

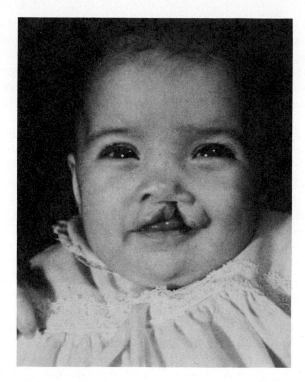

Figure 6-17. Cleft palate.

upper lip. **Many chromosomal processes of upper lip formation are easily disturbed, thereby leading to malformations.** Any disturbance of morphogenesis of the facial structures may interfere with the proper fusion of the fetal rudiments and lead to cleft lip, with or without cleft palate (Fig. 6-17). Sixty percent of affected individuals are male. The clinical consequences vary from a minor cosmetic defect to a serious anatomic anomaly that impairs normal speech and feeding.

Cleft lip and cleft palate are an excellent paradigm to illustrate the principles of multifactorial inheritance. If one child is born with cleft lip, the chances are 4% that the second child will also exhibit the defect. If the first two children have the defect, the risk increases to 9% for the third child. The severity of the defect also influences the risk.

PRENATAL DIAGNOSIS OF GENETIC DISORDERS

Amniocentesis and chorionic villus biopsy are the most important diagnostic methods for the diagnosis of developmental and genetic disorders. Both procedures are safe, reliable, and easily performed. The indications for chorionic villus biopsy or amniocentesis in pregnant women are as follows:

- **Age 35 years old and over.** The risk of having a child with Down's syndrome is about 1 in 300 for a 40-year-old woman, compared to 1 in 1200 at age 25.
- **Previous chromosomal abnormality.** The risk of recurrence of Down's syndrome in a succeeding child of a woman who has already borne an infant with trisomy 21 (Down's syndrome) is about 1%.
- **Translocation carrier.** Estimates of risks to the offspring of translocation carriers vary from 3% to 15% for D/G translocation carriers to 100% for 21/21 translocation carriers.
- **History of familial inborn errors of metabolism.** Recessive inborn errors of metabolism have a risk of 25% for each child.
- **Identified heterozygotes.** Carrier detection programs, such as the Tay-Sachs Disease Prevention Program, detect couples in which both spouses are carriers of the same recessive gene. Each pregnancy to such couples has a 25% risk of an affected child.
- **Family history of X-linked disorders.** Fetal sex determination, using amniotic cells, should be offered to women known to be carriers for X-linked disorders.
- **Occurrence of neural tube anomalies in a previous pregnancy.** The recurrence risk for a neural tube disorder, when a couple has had such a child, is 15%.

DISEASES OF INFANCY AND CHILDHOOD

DISORDERS RELATED TO MATURITY OF THE NEONATE

The term **prematurity,** indiscriminately applied to all neonates weighing less than 2500 g or born before term, is clinically useful. **The maturity of the neonate is the sum of the maturity of its organs, which may be precisely evaluated and expressed in functional terms.**

In contrast to birth at term, deliveries before the 38th week are called **preterm,** and those after the 42nd week **post-term.** Term babies who weigh less than 2500 g are called **small for gestational age** (SGA), while other newborns are labeled **appropriate for gestational age** (AGA) and **large for gestational age** (LGA) infants. Preterm babies may also be SGA, and a combination of these two factors doubles the risk of neonatal death and adversely affects life expectancy.

The causes of intrauterine growth retardation that result in an SGA birth belong to several classes: fetal factors, maternal factors, and defined environmental influences. In one-third of SGA infants the cause of intrauterine growth retardation cannot be determined. **Placental insufficiency,** an imprecise term, has been invoked to explain some idiopathic cases.

When intrauterine growth retardation exists in the presence of an adequate nutritional supply and in the absence of adverse environmental or maternal metabolic conditions, it is usually due to fetal abnormalities. These include various genetic metabolic disorders, chromosomal anomalies, and developmental malformations. **Identifiable exogenous causes include infections, smoking, alcohol, and drug abuse.** Inadequate maternal nutrition may be a significant contributory factor, but no clearcut relationship between SGA and nutritional factors has been established. Maternal diabetes and renal and cardiac disease all predispose to intrauterine growth retardation. SGA babies usually reach normal size by late infancy or early childhood. Identifiable fetal abnormalities, low gestational age, and serious postnatal complications adversely affect the neural development of SGA babies, which is the most serious consequence of this condition.

The **maturity of the lungs** is of paramount importance for normal postnatal life. Fetal alveoli are only partially expanded and are filled with amniotic fluid.

At the time of birth the amniotic fluid pours out of the lungs and air expands most of the respiratory spaces. Sluggish respiratory movements do not suffice to evacuate the amniotic fluid from the lungs, and those neonates who die at this point have incompletely expanded lungs. On histologic examination the alveolar ducts, bronchioles, and larger bronchi contain squames, lanugo hair, and protein-rich amniotic fluid. Some alveoli contain the same material, whereas most of the others appear collapsed; that is, they display **atelectasis.** This residual amniotic fluid is often called **amniotic fluid aspiration,** although this "aspiration" reflects only the inability of the fetus to expel all the fluid from the lungs.

Before the 35th week of pregnancy the immature fetal lungs secrete surfactant that differs from adult surfactant in several respects: (1) it contains a higher proportion of sphingomyelin; (2) instead of the surface-active dipalmitic lecithin, it contains alpha palmitic, beta myristic lecithin; and (3) it does not contain phosphatidylglycerol. Fetal pulmonary surfactant is released into the amniotic fluid, which can be sampled in pregnancy to determine fetal lung maturity. Most often, a lecithin:sphingomyelin ratio above 2:1 indicates that the fetus will survive without developing the respiratory distress syndrome. The appearance of

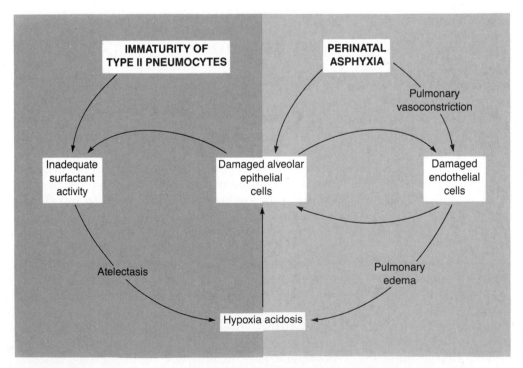

Figure 6-18. Pathogenesis of the idiopathic respiratory distress syndrome of the neonate. Immaturity of the lungs and perinatal asphyxia are the major pathogenetic factors.

phosphatidylglycerol is the best available biochemical proof of fetal lung maturity. This compound is not present in fetal lungs before the 35th week and is, therefore, of little practical significance before that time.

The most obvious evidence of hepatic immaturity is the inability of the liver to conjugate and excrete bilirubin—a failure that leads to jaundice. Jaundice **(icterus neonatorum),** due in part to the rapid destruction of fetal erythrocytes and in part to a deficiency of glucuronyl transferase, appears often in neonates. It is more pronounced in premature babies and usually lasts longer in these infants than in those born at term.

RESPIRATORY DISTRESS SYNDROME OF THE NEWBORN

The respiratory distress syndrome is one of the major clinical problems affecting premature babies. It is related to or caused by immaturity of the lung and inadequate release or storage of surfactant by type II pneumocytes.

A basic defect causing the idiopathic respiratory distress syndrome in preterm babies is the immaturity of the lungs, particularly type II pneumocytes (Fig. 6-18). Fetal surfactant is less efficient than adult surfactant in lowering the alveolar surface tension and keeping the alveoli open. Because lung compliance is low, the critical negative pressure needed to allow influx of air into the lungs cannot be attained. The collapse of alveoli (atelectasis) not adequately coated with surfactant reduces the pulmonary surface, allowing exchange of gases only through the walls of alveolar ducts and terminal bronchioles—structures that are not suitable for that purpose. Anoxia and hypercapnia cause acidosis, leading to peripheral vasodilatation and pulmonary vasoconstriction. This situation, in turn, leads to the reestablishment of a partial fetal circulatory pattern. Right-to-left shunting of unoxygenated blood through the ductus arteriosus and foramen ovale further contributes to hypoperfusion of the lungs, jeopardizing the respiratory oxygen supply even more. Hypoxia adversely affects pulmonary cells, and necrosis of endothelial, alveolar, and bronchial cells takes place. Vascular disruption causes transudation of plasma into the alveolar spaces and layering of fibrin ("hyaline membranes") along the surface of alveolar ducts and respiratory bronchioles partially denuded of their normal cell lining. This in turn further impedes the passage of oxygen from the alveolar spaces across the respiratory surface into the pulmonary vasculature. Moreover, extravasation of blood into the respiratory passages, combined with the collapse of the alveoli, further contributes to the consolidation of the lungs. In terminal stages air is found only in bronchi and dilated bronchioles, and the rest of the lung is consolidated and airless.

On histologic examination the lungs have a characteristic appearance. The alveoli are collapsed and the alveolar ducts and respiratory bronchioles are dilated. Within these spaces cellular debris, proteinaceous edema fluid, and some red blood cells accumulate. The lining of the dilated alveolar ducts is covered with fibrin-rich hyaline membranes. The walls of the collapsed alveoli are thick, the capillaries are congested, and the lymphatics are filled with proteinaceous material (Fig. 6-19).

The outcome of the idiopathic respiratory distress syndrome of the neonate depends on the severity of the disease, the gestational age of the infant at birth, and the presence of complications or aggravating conditions. The overall mortality is still about 30%, and in infants born before 30 weeks of pregnancy it is over 50%. Aggravating factors, such as maternal diabetes, anoxia during delivery, or extensive blood loss, also adversely influence the outcome. Rapid development of profound respiratory insufficiency unresponsive to standard treatment is a bad omen and is associated with high mortality. Mild cases can be salvaged with oxygen alone, whereas more serious distress requires intensive care to correct acidosis, sustain the failing circulation, and assist the respiration.

Major complications of the idiopathic respiratory distress syndrome of the neonate are **intraventricular cerebral hemorrhage,** persistence of the **patent ductus**

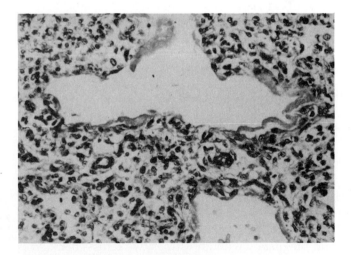

Figure 6-19. The lung in idiopathic respiratory distress syndrome of the neonate. The alveoli are atelectatic, and the dilated alveolar ducts are lined with fibrin-rich hyaline membranes.

arteriosus, and **necrotizing enterocolitis.** These complications are consequences of anoxia, hypercapnia, and acidosis.

ERYTHROBLASTOSIS FETALIS AND NEONATAL HEMOLYTIC ANEMIA

Erythroblastosis fetalis is defined as hemolytic disease in the fetus or newborn caused by transplacental passage of maternal antibodies directed against paternally inherited antigens on fetal red blood cells. **Such maternal–fetal blood group incompatibility may result in hemolytic anemia in the fetus.**

The **Rh blood group system** consists of a group of some 25 components, of which only the alleles cde/CDE are strong antigens. In practice, Rh serotyping is limited to the strongest of these three antigens, namely d/D—D denoting Rh-positive, and d Rh-negative individuals. Rh-negative persons comprise approximately 15% of the Euro-American white population, and 5% of Afro-American blacks. Japanese, Chinese, and North American Indian populations contain essentially no Rh-negative individuals.

In contrast to the naturally occurring antibodies against the major ABO blood group antigens, antibodies to Rh antigens are found only in Rh-negative people who are immunized with Rh-positive blood. Typical antibodies to ABO are of the IgM class, and only some persons of type O have natural IgG anti-A or anti-B. Whereas the initial immunization with Rh-positive cells produces a surge of IgM antibodies, the second exposure leads to the production of IgG antibodies. This is of particular importance in pregnancy, since **only IgG crosses the placenta.**

A characteristic sequence leading to Rh-related erythroblastosis fetalis starts with immunization of an Rh-negative mother with blood of an Rh-positive infant, who has inherited the D antigen from an Rh-positive father (Fig. 6-20). Immunization usually occurs at the time of delivery, owing to the passage of fetal blood into maternal uterine veins. Immunization can also occur during the late stages of pregnancy because of **transplacental transfusions,** but since only minute amounts of fetal blood cross the placenta, this is rarely the case. This initial exposure to Rh-positive blood leads to IgM antibody formation, which is of little clinical significance. A surge of IgG antibodies after the second exposure to Rh-positive blood—usually a second pregnancy with an Rh-positive fetus—hemolyzes the fetal red blood cells.

An Rh-positive fetus in an isoimmunized Rh-negative mother develops normally through the first two trimesters. As the transplacental transport of immunoglobulins becomes more efficient in the third trimester, and as the paternal antigens become fully expressed on fetal red blood cells, immune hemolysis increases. Fetal injury presents in three clinical forms of graded severity. The most severe is **hydrops fetalis.** Less severe is **icterus gravis,** and the mildest form is **congenital anemia of the newborn.** Because of the destruction of red blood cells, generalized anoxia develops, affecting most prominently the heart, liver, and brain. Hypoxic liver cells produce less serum proteins, an effect that decreases the oncotic pressure of the plasma. Together with the inefficient pumping of blood by the anoxic heart, this leads to generalized edema, or hydrops fetalis.

Hemolyzed red blood cells release hemoglobin, which is degraded to bilirubin. **In the fetus or neonate, an oversupply of bilirubin, combined with functional immaturity of the liver and anoxia of liver cells, leads to jaundice.** Unconjugated bilirubin is normally bound to albumin in the serum. Since dysfunction of the liver cells leads to hypoalbuminemia, much of the bilirubin is not complexed to albumin and crosses the blood–brain barrier, to be deposited in the brain substance. Unconjugated bilirubin is toxic to the brain and causes edema and yellowish discoloration, most prominently in the basal ganglia. Jaundice of basal nuclei is known by the German term **kernicterus** (*kern* = nucleus).

With appropriate medical care erythroblastosis fetalis can be almost completely prevented. **Rh immunoprophylaxis is based on the administration of anti-D immunoglobulin to all Rh-negative women within 72 hours after delivery of an Rh-positive infant.** This treatment interdicts isoimmunization of 98% of all Rh-negative women and efficiently prevents erythroblastosis fetalis.

Because of the efficient immunoprophylaxis of erythroblastosis fetalis due to Rh incompatibility, hemolytic disease of the newborn caused by **ABO and other minor blood group antigens** has achieved relative prominence. Fortunately, hemolysis of fetal red blood cells in these cases is usually much milder than with Rh incompatibility. One might expect a considerable number of pregnancies to exhibit maternal–fetal incompatibility of the ABO system, but only 10% of these children show mild hemolysis, and only 1 in 200 presents with symptoms that require treatment. Usually the hemolytic disease occurs in group O mothers carrying an A, B, or AB fetus. Infants with the A$_1$ blood group antigen, which is usually strongly expressed on fetal red blood cells, are at highest risk. Some blood group O mothers have peculiar natural IgG antibodies to AB antigens. Since these antibodies are not elicited by previous sensitization in pregnancy, the first infant may also be affected.

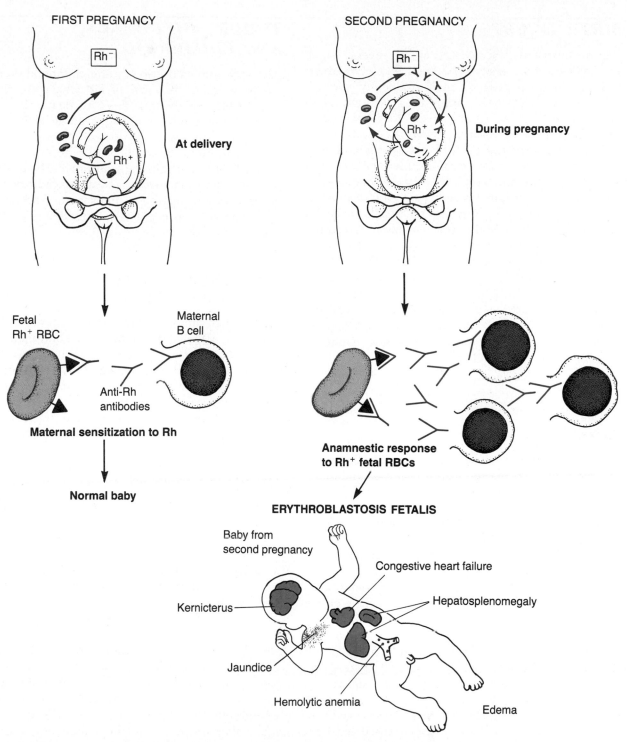

Figure 6-20. Pathogenesis of erythroblastosis fetalis due to maternal-fetal Rh incompatibility. Immunization of the Rh-negative mother with Rh-positive erythrocytes in the first pregnancy leads to the formation of anti-Rh antibodies of the IgG type. These antibodies cross the placenta and damage the Rh-positive fetus in subsequent pregnancies.

BIRTH INJURY

Natural birth lasts, in most instances, several hours, and injuries occur easily. The **head, skeleton, liver, and peripheral nerves** are most frequently affected. Compression of the head during the passage through the birth canal or delivery by forceps may cause a tear in the falx cerebri, tentorium cerebelli, or dural sinuses, with massive **subdural or epidural hematomas.** The fragile brain tissue is also easily bruised, especially in premature infants and term infants large for gestational age. Massive intracranial hemorrhage causes an acute onset of neurologic symptoms and results in death. Birth injury of the brain can also have disturbing chronic consequences, including **cerebral palsy.** Bones are easily **fractured** during birth, but many of these fractures are partial and heal easily, and they are generally subclinical. Birth trauma may affect nerves and result in subsequent paralysis. **Facial nerve injury** and **tearing of the brachial plexus** are the most common forms of injury, again reflecting the most common, head-first form of natural birth.

SUDDEN INFANT DEATH SYNDROME (SIDS)

The sudden infant death syndrome (SIDS), also known as "crib death," is a term given to "sudden and unexpected death of an infant who was either well or almost well prior to death, and whose death remains unexplained after the performance of an adequate autopsy." SIDS is one of the major causes of infant mortality, an estimated 10,000 cases occurring annually in the United States.

Typically, SIDS occurs in 2- to 4-month old infants, most of whom seem perfectly healthy or have only a minor respiratory illness. The infants usually die unexpectedly during the night. There are no satisfactory explanations for the occurrence of sudden death, and there are no reliable means to identify children at risk. Autopsy usually reveals minor signs of anoxia, but the findings are nonspecific and cannot be interpreted unequivocally. There are children who experienced prolonged apnea but were saved and resuscitated by a watching parent. Such cases, which are considered to represent "near misses," suggest that some infants in this age group have labile cardiorespiratory centers that inadequately control cardiovascular function. However, it is uncertain whether central disturbances of respiration or heart function indeed represent the basic defect in all affected infants, or whether the condition has more than one cause and pathogenetic pathway.

TUMORS OF INFANCY AND CHILDHOOD

Although tumors of infancy and childhood do not account for more than 2% of all neoplasms, they are responsible for about 10% of all deaths in this age group. Some tumors are diagnosed at birth or in the immediate neonatal period and have obviously evolved in utero. In addition to these **developmental tumors,** others originate in **abnormally developed organs, organ primordia, and displaced organ rests,** an observation suggesting that somatic and neoplastic development represent two diametrically opposite aspects of ontogenesis.

BENIGN TUMORS AND TUMOR-LIKE CONDITIONS

Most benign tumors encountered in infancy and childhood are actually developmental abnormalities and cannot be clearly separated from hamartomas and choristomas. Traditionally, **nevocellular nevi** in the skin are considered to be hamartomas, whereas **hemangiomas** are considered tumors. Some inflamed hemangiomas cannot be distinguished from **pyogenic granuloma,** which is an inflammatory lesion.

MALIGNANT TUMORS

The spectrum of malignant tumors of infancy and childhood differs from that in adults. Furthermore, each period of prepubertal life is characterized by the predominance of different forms of cancer. In infants and children under 5 years of age, the most prominent tumors are **embryomas** or **blastomas**—so classified because they consist of cells that resemble embryonic or partially differentiated cells forming the primordium or the blastema of the organs and tissues. These include the eight most common tumors of infancy and early childhood: **lymphoblastic leukemia, neuroblastoma, nephroblastoma** (Wilms' tumor), **hepatoblastoma, retinoblastoma, rhabdomyosarcoma, teratoma,** and **ependymoma.** In the 5- to 9-year age group, acute leukemia is the most common malignancy; at later ages soft tissue and bone tumors comprise the largest group.

These age-dependent changes in the prevalence of various tumors reflect, at least in part, their etiology and time of onset. For example, **nephroblastomas** are most common in infants and young children because these tumors develop from disorganized renal blastema. Renal blastema is formed in the first trimester, and the origin of nephroblastoma is related to the early stages of intrauterine development corresponding to the differentiation of the kidney anlage. Similarly, the **hereditary retinoblastomas,** which regularly show chromosomal abnormalities, originate in genetically abnormal fetal eyes and are recognized in many cases even at birth.

Some tumors are apparently initiated in utero but become evident only later in life. An example is the **clear cell adenocarcinoma** of the vagina in offspring of mothers who received **diethylstilbestrol** (DES) in pregnancy. These tumors developed at puberty and even later, years after the mother's exposure to DES. By contrast, **Burkitt's lymphoma,** a tumor that occurs in older children, is thought to be related to an acquired infection with the **Epstein-Barr virus.** Since the Epstein-Barr virus induces tumors after a latent period and the infection rarely occurs in infants, these tumors are rare at an early age. **Bone tumors** have a peripubertal peak that correlates with the complex changes in the epiphyseal growth plate that occur in that life period. **Hepatoblastoma** is composed of cells that resemble fetal liver cells, and its peak incidence is in infancy. **Hepatocellular carcinoma,** on the other hand, occurs in older children and does not differ from similar tumors originating in the liver of adults.

Many neonatal and childhood tumors are part of **developmental complexes.** An example is the complex of **Wilms' tumor** (nephroblastoma), aniridia, genitourinary malformations, and mental retardation. Hemihypertrophy of the body is associated with several tumors, most notably nephroblastoma, hepatoblastoma, and adrenal carcinoma. The hereditary and chromosomal bases of some forms of neoplasia in infancy and childhood have already been mentioned.

7

HEMODYNAMIC DISORDERS

WOLFGANG J. MERGNER AND BENJAMIN F. TRUMP

DISORDERS OF PERFUSION

HEMORRHAGE

Hemorrhage (bleeding) is a discharge of blood from the vascular compartment to the exterior of the body or into nonvascular body spaces. The most common and obvious cause is trauma. A blood vessel may be ruptured in ways other than laceration. For instance, severe atherosclerosis may so weaken the wall of the abdominal aorta that it balloons to form an aneurysm, which then bleeds into the retroperitoneal space. By the same token, an aneurysm may complicate a congenitally weak cerebral artery (berry aneurysm) and lead to cerebral (subarachnoid) hemorrhage.

Hemorrhage also results from damage at the level of the capillaries—for instance, the rupture of capillaries by blunt trauma. Increased venous pressure also causes extravasation of blood from capillaries in the lung. Vitamin C deficiency is associated with capillary fragility and bleeding, due to a defect in the supporting structures. It is important to recognize that the capillary barrier by itself is not sufficient to contain the blood within the intravascular space. The minor trauma imposed on small vessels and capillaries by normal movement requires an intact coagulation system to prevent hemorrhage. Thus, a severe decrease in the number of platelets (thrombocytopenia) or a deficiency of a coagulation factor (e.g., factor VIII in hemophilia) is associated with spontaneous hemorrhages unrelated to any apparent trauma.

A person may exsanguinate into an internal cavity, as in the case of gastrointestinal hemorrhage from a peptic ulcer (arterial hemorrhage) or esophageal varices (venous hemorrhage). In such cases large amounts of fresh blood fill the entire gastrointestinal tract. When a large amount of blood accumulates in soft tissue, we speak of a **hematoma.** Such a collection of blood can be merely painful, as in a muscle bruise, or fatal, if located in the brain.

Diffuse superficial hemorrhages in the skin are termed **purpura** or **ecchymoses.** Following a bruise or in association with a coagulation defect, an initially purple discoloration of the skin turns green and then yellow before resolving, a sequence that reflects the progressive oxidation of bilirubin released from the hemoglobin of degraded red blood cells. A good example of an ecchymosis is a "black eye."

A minute punctate hemorrhage, usually in the skin or conjunctiva, is labeled a **petechia.** This lesion represents the rupture of a capillary or arteriole and is seen in conjunction with coagulopathies or vasculitis, the latter classically associated with bacterial endocarditis.

HYPEREMIA

Hyperemia, defined simply as an excess amount of blood in an organ, may be caused either by an increased supply of blood from the arterial system (active hyperemia) or by an impediment to the exit of blood through venous pathways (passive hyperemia or congestion).

ACTIVE HYPEREMIA

An augmented supply of blood to an organ is usually a physiologic response to an increased functional demand, as in the case of the heart and skeletal muscle during exercise. Hyperemia of the skin in febrile states serves to dissipate heat. The increased blood supply is brought about by arteriolar dilatation and recruitment of inactive or latent capillaries. The most striking active hyperemia occurs in association with inflammation. Vasoactive materials released by inflammatory cells cause dilatation of blood vessels; in the skin this results in the classic "tumor, rubor, and calor" of inflammation. Since inflammation can also damage endothelial cells and increase capillary permeability, the hyperemia of inflammation is often accompanied by edema (i.e. the accumulation of a transudate in the extravascular tissue) and the local extravasation of red blood cells.

PASSIVE HYPEREMIA (CONGESTION)

Any obstruction to the return of blood results in a generalized increase in venous pressure, slower blood flow, and a consequent increase in the volume of blood in many organs, including the liver, spleen, and kidneys. In **acute passive congestion** affected organs increase in size and assume a bluish color because of the presence of large amounts of deoxygenated blood.

The Lung

Chronic failure of the left ventricle constitutes an impediment to the exit of blood from the lungs and leads to **chronic passive congestion** of the lungs. As a result, the pressure in the alveolar capillaries is increased, and these vessels become engorged with blood. The increased pressure in the alveolar capillaries has four major consequences:

- **Microhemorrhages** release red blood cells into the alveolar spaces, where they are phagocytosed and degraded by alveolar macrophages. The released iron, in the form of hemosiderin, remains in the macrophages, which are then termed "heart failure cells."

- **The increased hydrostatic pressure forces fluid from the blood into the alveolar spaces, resulting in pulmonary edema,** a dangerous condition that interferes with gas exchange in the lung.
- **The increased pressure, together with other poorly understood factors, stimulates fibrosis** in the interstitial spaces of the lung. The presence of fibrosis and iron is viewed grossly as a firm, brown lung ("brown induration").
- **The increased capillary pressure is transmitted to the pulmonary arterial system, a condition labeled pulmonary hypertension.** This disorder leads to right-sided heart failure and consequent generalized venous congestion.

The Liver

The liver, with the hepatic veins emptying into the vena cava immediately inferior to the heart, is particularly vulnerable to chronic passive congestion. The central veins of the hepatic lobule become dilated. The increased venous pressure is transferred to the sinusoids, where it leads to dilatation of the sinusoids with blood and pressure atrophy of the centrilobular hepatocytes. Grossly, the cut surface of the liver exhibits dark foci of centrilobular congestion surrounded by paler zones of unaffected peripheral portions of the lobules. The result is a curious reticulated appearance, resembling a cross section of a nutmeg, and is appropriately termed "nutmeg liver" (Fig. 7-1). Prolonged venous congestion of the liver eventually leads to thickening of the central veins and centrilobular fibrosis. Only in the most extreme cases of venous congestion (e.g., constrictive pericarditis or tricuspid stenosis) is the fibrosis sufficiently generalized and severe to justify the label "cardiac cirrhosis."

The Spleen

Increased pressure in the liver, whether from cardiac failure or from an intrahepatic obstruction to the flow of blood (e.g., cirrhosis), results in higher splenic vein pressure and congestion of the spleen. The organ becomes enlarged and tense, and the cut section oozes dark blood. In longstanding congestion diffuse fibrosis of the spleen is seen, together with iron-containing, fibrotic, and calcified foci of old hemorrhage (Gamna-Gandy bodies).

Edema and Ascites

Venous congestion impedes the flow of blood in the capillaries, thus increasing hydrostatic pressure and promoting edema formation. The accumulation of edema fluid in heart failure is particularly noticeable in dependent tissues: the legs and feet in ambulatory patients and the back in bedridden individuals. Ascites, the accumulation of fluid in the peritoneal space, reflects (among other factors) the lack of tissue rigor, a condition in which there is no countervailing external pressure to oppose hydrostatic pressure.

ALTERED REGIONAL PERFUSION

VASCULAR STENOSIS

Vascular stenosis, a lesion that causes reduced blood flow, is most commonly a result of atherosclerotic lesions—for example, in the extramural coronary arteries. Factors recognized as affecting flow in stenotic lesions are the entrance of a blood stream into a stenotic lesion, frictional loss of energy in the stenotic segment, and turbulence at the exit.

VASCULAR SPASM

Vascular spasm in the coronary circulation can produce ischemic attacks (Printzmetal's angina). Candidates for substances that can produce spasm are thromboxanes, platelet aggregates, catecholamines, histamine, and serotonin.

TOTAL OCCLUSION OF ARTERIAL CIRCULATION

When an artery is suddenly occluded, ischemia occurs in the vascular bed it supplies. The subsequent area of ischemic necrosis (infarct), however, may not extend over the whole area served by the occluded vessel. The principal determinants of the size of this area are the extent to which perfusion has been reduced and the perfusion through the collateral circulation. The flow through collaterals is determined by the size and diameter of the collateral vascular bed and by the pressure gradient between the perfused and occluded vascular bed.

PATHOLOGY OF REDUCED PERFUSION

Total occlusion of an artery produces an area of coagulative necrosis called an infarct. Partial occlusion—that is, stenosis—occasionally causes necrosis, but more commonly leads to a variety of degenerative cell changes. These changes include vacuolization of cells, atrophy, loss of muscle cell myofibrils, and interstitial fibrosis. Infarction of vital organs such as the heart, brain, and intestine may be life-threatening.

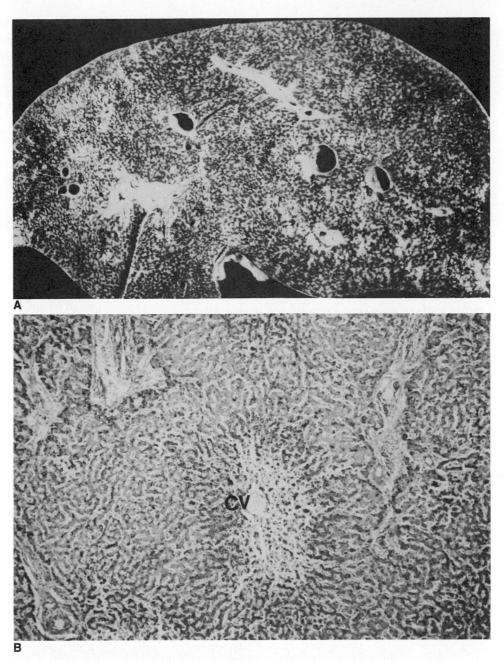

Figure 7-1. Passive congestion of the liver. (*A*) A gross photograph shows the pattern of chronic passive congestion, in which lighter-appearing tissue segments form an interlacing pattern with dark-staining centrilobular blood spaces. (*B*) In histologic sections of liver tissue from patients with chronic passive congestion, the central vein (*CV*) and central sinusoids appear distended. Adjacent liver cells may become atrophic because of hypoxia or compression. Chronic passive congestion of the liver may cause central hemorrhagic necrosis, the distinguishing features of which are marked centrilobular sinusoidal dilatation and necrosis of adjacent hepatocytes.

INFARCT MORPHOLOGY

A fresh infarct is pale because of the loss of red blood cells, an appearance reflected in the terms "white" or "pale" infarct (Fig. 7-2). Infarcts can also be hemorrhagic and therefore red, particularly in the lung and the intestine. The border of an infarct is often hemorrhagic. With time, the tissue surrounding an infarct forms granulation tissue rich in sprouting capillaries. As an infarct ages it undergoes fibrosis, reduces in size, and ultimately shrinks below the surface of the organ. Figure 7-3 details the organs most commonly affected by infarction.

Myocardial Infarcts

Myocardial infarcts are **transmural** or **subendocardial.** A transmural infarct results from complete occlusion of a major extramural coronary artery. A myocardial infarct is initially pale, but hemorrhage occurs after reflow into an injured vascular bed. Subendocardial infarction reflects ischemia caused by partially occluding stenotic lesions when the requirement for oxygen outstrips the supply.

Pulmonary Infarcts

Only about 10% of pulmonary emboli elicit clinical evidence of pulmonary infarction, usually after occlusion of a middle-sized pulmonary artery. **Infarction occurs if the circulation from the bronchial arteries inadequately compensates for the loss of supply from the pulmonary arteries.** Infarcts of the lung are pyramidal in shape with the base toward the pleural surface. Hemorrhage into the alveolar spaces of the necrotic lining tissue occurs within 48 hours.

Cerebral Infarcts

Infarction of the brain may be the result of local ischemia or of a generalized reduction in blood flow. A generalized reduction in blood flow resulting from systemic hypotension, as in shock, produces infarction in the border zones between the distributions of the major cerebral arteries. If prolonged, severe hypotension can cause widespread brain necrosis. The occlusion of a single vessel in the brain—for example, after an embolus has lodged—causes ischemia and necrosis in a well defined area. This type of cerebral infarct may be pale (nonhemorrhagic) or red (hemorrhagic), the latter being common with embolic occlusions. Infarcts in the areas supplied by small penetrating arteries are referred to as "lacunar infarcts." The occlusion of a large artery produces a wide area of necrosis that may ultimately resolve as a large fluid-filled cavity in the brain (Fig. 7-4).

Intestinal Infarcts

Severe ischemia leads to hemorrhagic necrosis of the intestinal submucosa and muscularis. Small mucosal infarcts heal in a few days, but more severe injury leads to ulceration. These ulcers can eventually re-epithelialize. If the ulcers are large they are repaired by scar tissue, a process that may lead to strictures. Severe

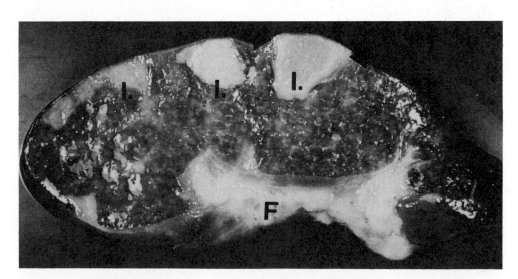

Figure 7-2. Spleen infarction. The gross photograph shows three wedge-shaped, pale infarcts of the spleen (*1*) bulging above the contour of the spleen and lifting the capsule. The pale region at the bottom (*F*) is hilar adipose tissue. Splenic infarcts are often encountered during autopsies and are often due to emboli that arise in the heart.

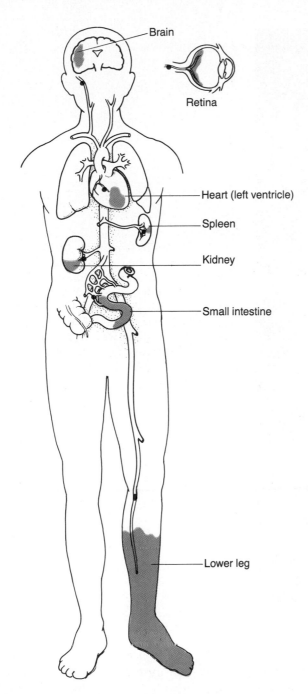

Figure 7-3. Common sites of systemic infarction from arterial emboli.

transmural necrosis may be associated with massive bleeding or perforation, complications that often result in irreversible shock, sepsis, and death.

Renal Infarcts

Renal infarcts are pyramidal in shape, with the base toward the capsule. These pale infarcts acquire a hemorrhagic border.

DISORDERS OF WATER AND ELECTROLYTES

EFFECTS AND CAUSES OF EDEMA

Mild degrees of **edema,** an excess of interstitial fluid, are not detectable clinically. More severe derangements, however, appear as pitting edema over the extremities, as pleural or abdominal effusions, or as edema over soft connective tissue, such as that of the orbit. Edema can be caused by an imbalance between the perfusion pressure and the osmotic pressure. **Edema can be generalized or localized. Local edema** may be caused by local deep venous obstruction, by a thrombus, or by obstruction of lymphatic drainage by a tumor. The mechanisms of edema formation are summarized in Table 7-1 and in Figure 7-5.

GENERALIZED EDEMA AND SALT METABOLISM

The kidney controls sodium homeostasis, thereby maintaining the intravascular volume and blood pressure. Normally a reduction in perfusion pressure is sensed by baroreceptors in the kidney, which respond by activating the renin–angiotensin–aldosterone regulatory mechanism for sodium conservation. **Paradoxically, in certain disease states—for example, congestive heart failure, ascites, and the nephrotic syndrome—a counter-regulation augments, rather than decreases, sodium retention. This effect contributes to the formation of edema. Although the conditions responsible for systemic edema differ, they share a deranged regulatory mechanism for sodium homeostasis.**

CONGESTIVE HEART FAILURE

Congestive heart failure results from impaired cardiac emptying, which leads to a rise in ventricular end-diastolic pressure. Increased end-diastolic pressure is transmitted to the venous system as increased venous pressure. High venous pressure promotes exudation of fluid by several mechanisms: decreased reabsorption, altered neurogenic precapillary resistance, hepatic congestion (which impairs renin clearance by the liver), and altered lymphatic drainage.

The clinical manifestations of congestive heart failure reflect either inadequate cardiac output or increased venous pressure. The major effects are, therefore, divided into "forward failure" and "backward failure," respectively. Failure to deliver blood as a re-

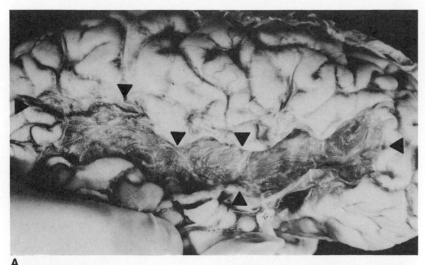

A

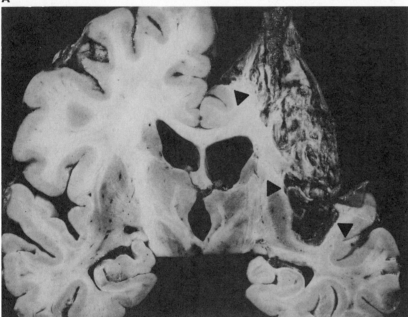

B

Figure 7-4. Cerebral infarction. (*A*) An old cystic infarction of the brain (*arrows*) is seen in the distribution of the middle cerebral artery. Cerebral infarctions are frequently pale and nonhemorrhagic. As seen here, healing of a cerebral infarct may lead to the development of large cystic spaces. (*B*) A coronal cross section through the frontal lobe reveals a focal area of infarction. Note the destruction of the cortex.

Table 7-1   Mechanisms of Edema Formation

Hydrostatic pressure	Increase in capillary transmural pressure caused by:
	Severe arteriolar dilatation
	Increased venous pressure due to venous obstruction, left or right ventricular failure, or hypervolemia
	Increased gravitational pressure (postural)
Oncotic pressure	Decreased oncotic transmural pressure due to:
	Plasma protein depletion
	Plasma protein dilution
Increased capillary permeability	Defective removal of interstitial fluid due to lymphatic obstruction

sult of insufficient cardiac output eventually can result in cardiogenic shock, manifested clinically as impaired perfusion. Mental confusion, oliguria, and acidosis ensue. Backward failure results in increased hydrostatic pressure in the venous system. In left ventricular failure this leads to pulmonary edema, whereas in right ventricular failure, peripheral edema is seen.

In congestive heart failure the heart is enlarged and the chambers are dilated. Visible edema is more severe in the dependent body regions: the legs in upright patients and the back in bedridden ones. The condition is called "pitting edema," because when the skin is depressed it does not immediately rebound, leaving a "pit."

EDEMA IN CIRRHOSIS OF THE LIVER

Cirrhosis obstructs the liver's portal flow and leads to **portal hypertension,** a condition that increases the hydrostatic pressure in the splanchnic circulation. Cirrhosis also augments **vasodilatation** and opens arteriovenous bypasses. This situation is compounded by a **decreased synthesis of albumin** as a result of hepatic dysfunction. In combination these changes are sensed as a decrease in the effective blood volume and stimulate the **renin–angiotensin–aldosterone** mechanism. Elevated levels of these hormones are complicated by impairment of renin inactivation in the liver. A vicious cycle thus leads to chronic sodium retention. Furthermore, the increased **transudation of lymph from the liver capsule** adds to the accumulation of fluid in the peritoneal space.

NEPHROTIC SYNDROME

The nephrotic syndrome is caused by a massive loss of protein in the urine that exceeds the rate at which albumin is replaced by the liver. The resulting decline in the concentration of plasma proteins reduces the colloid–osmotic pressure in the venous circulation and diminishes the ability of the vascular system to reabsorb water from the extracellular space; both effects promote the formation of edema. These events also decrease the blood volume, thereby stimulating the renin–angiotensin–aldosterone mechanism, leading to a further increase in sodium retention.

The edema in the nephrotic syndrome shows a direct correlation with the plasma albumin concentration. The edema is generalized, but appears preferentially in soft connective tissues, the eyes, eyelids, and subcutaneous tissue. Ascites and pleural effusions also occur

EDEMA IN SPECIAL ORGANS
CEREBRAL EDEMA

Edema of the brain is extremely dangerous because the confined space of the cranium allows little expansion. The resulting increased intracranial pressure compromises the blood supply and integrity of the brain.

At autopsy, a diffusely edematous brain is soft and heavy. The gyri are flattened and the sulci narrowed. Severe cerebral edema leads to herniation of the cerebral tonsils.

PULMONARY EDEMA

Pulmonary edema refers to increased fluid in the interstitium of the lung or in the alveolar spaces. Pulmonary edema leads to decreased gas exchange in the lung, causing hypoxia and hypercapnia.

The lung is a loose tissue without much connective tissue support and, therefore, requires mechanisms to prevent the development of edema. Among these mechanisms are:

- Low hydrostatic pressure in the lung capillaries due to low right ventricular pressure
- Effective draining of the interstitial space of the lung by lymphatics, which are under a slightly negative pressure and can accommodate up to 10 times the normal lymph flow
- Tight cellular junctions between endothelial cells, which control capillary permeability
- Surfactant protection of the alveolar surface against the exudation of fluid into the alveoli

If these protective mechanisms are perturbed, pulmonary alveolar edema results. Prolonged interstitial edema is also a strong stimulus for interstitial fibrosis in the lung. Clinical conditions that induce the formation of edema are **hemodynamic diseases** (including left heart failure, mitral valve stenosis or insufficiency, pulmonary veno-occlusive disease, and the physiologic effects of high altitude) or **changes in capillary permeability** (produced by irritant gases, aspiration of acidic material, near drowning, shock lung, fat embolism, viral infections, and uremia).

Pulmonary fluid accumulation may go unnoticed initially, but eventually dyspnea and coughing become prominent. If the edema is severe, large amounts of frothy sputum, often pink, are expectorated. Hypoxemia is manifested as cyanosis.

Pulmonary function is restricted in severe congestion and in interstitial pulmonary edema because the accumulation of fluid in the interstitial space causes reduced compliance—that is, a stiffening of the lung tissue. Thus, increased respiratory work is required to maintain ventilation. Since the alveolar walls are thickened, there is a greater barrier to the exchange of oxygen and carbon dioxide. As a result of capillary damage, which frequently accompanies vascular congestion, proteins and electrolytes drain into the interstitial space. Fluid accumulation in pulmonary alveoli (i.e., alveolar edema) further restricts the surface for pulmonary gas exchange.

In conditions of severe endothelial damage, a protein-rich fluid leaks into the alveoli. Sections of the lung reveal severely congested alveolar capillaries and

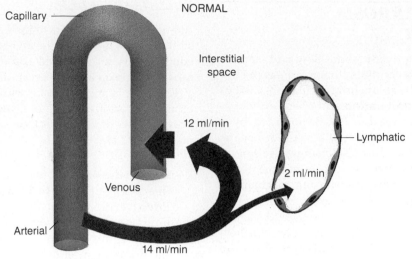

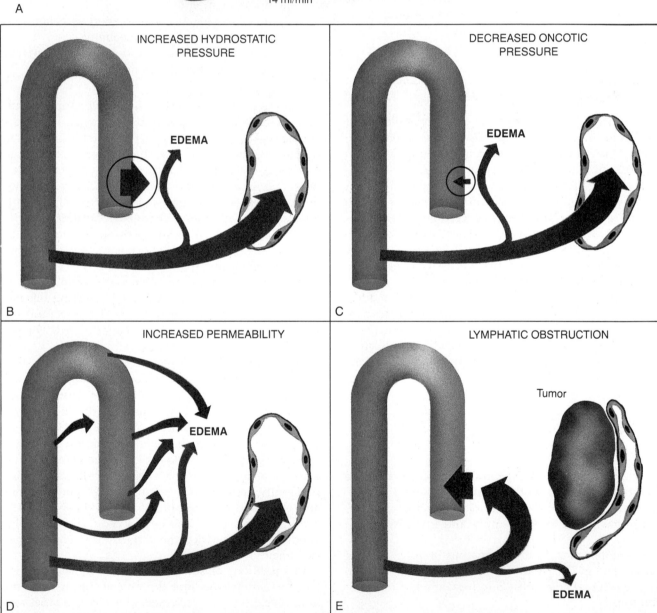

alveoli filled with a homogeneous, pink-staining fluid permeated by air bubbles. Cell debris, fibrin, and proteins may form films of proteinaceous material, called "hyaline membranes."

FLUID ACCUMULATION IN BODY CAVITIES

The body cavities, such as the pericardium and the pleural and peritoneal spaces, are extensions of the interstitial space. Fluid accumulates in them as an expression of generalized edema.

PLEURAL SPACE

Fluid in the pleural space, also called **pleural effusion,** is a straw-colored transudate of low specific gravity that contains few cells (mainly exfoliated mesothelial cells). Fluid commonly accumulates as an expression of a generalized tendency to form edema in diseases such as the nephrotic syndrome, cirrhosis, and congestive heart failure. It may also accumulate in response to an inflammatory process or a tumor in the lung or on the pleural surface.

PERICARDIUM

Fluid in the pericardium may accumulate slowly or quickly. A rapid accumulation is poorly tolerated. Because the distensibility of the pericardium is limited, pericardial pressure rises rapidly. This effect—termed tamponade—interferes with cardiac function. If the fluid accumulates slowly, the pericardium expands without an increase in pericardial pressure. Although the upper tolerable limit may be 90 to 120 ml of fluid when a pericardial effusion forms quickly, a liter or more of fluid may be tolerated when the process is gradual.

PERITONEUM

Peritoneal effusion, also called **ascites,** causes distension of the abdomen. The main causes of ascites are cirrhosis, abdominal tumors, pancreatitis, cardiac failure, the nephrotic syndrome, and hepatic venous obstruction. The pathogenesis of ascites in cirrhosis was discussed earlier. Complications of ascites derive from increased abdominal pressure and include anorexia and vomiting, dyspnea, ventral hernia, and leakage of fluid into the pleural space.

EMBOLISM

Embolism is the passage through the venous or arterial circulations of any material capable of lodging in a blood vessel and thereby obstructing the lumen. The usual embolus is a thromboembolus—that is, a blood clot formed in one location that detaches from the vessel wall and travels to a distant site.

PULMONARY THROMBOEMBOLISM

The majority of emboli arise from the deep veins of the lower extremities; most of the fatal ones originate in the ileofemoral veins (Fig. 7-6). Only half of patients with pulmonary thromboembolism have signs of thrombophlebitis. Some thromboemboli arise from the pelvic venous plexus and others from the right

Figure 7-5. The capillary system and mechanisms of edema formation. (*A*) **Normal:** The differential between the hydrostatic and oncotic pressure at the arterial end of the capillary system is responsible for the filtration into the interstitial space of approximately 14 ml of fluid per minute. This fluid is reabsorbed at the venous end at the rate of 12 ml/min. It is also drained through the lymphatic capillaries at a rate of 2 ml/min. Proteins are removed by the lymphatics from the interstitial space. (*B*) **Hydrostatic edema:** If the hydrostatic pressure at the venous end of the capillary system is elevated, reabsorption is decreased. As long as the lymphatics are able to drain the surplus fluid, no edema results. If their capacity is exceeded, however, edema fluid accumulates. (*C*) **Oncotic edema:** Edema fluid also accumulates if reabsorption is diminished by a decrease in the oncotic pressure of the vascular bed, owing to a loss of albumin. (*D*) **Inflammatory and traumatic edema:** Edema, either local or systemic, results if the vascular bed becomes leaky following injury to the endothelium. (*E*) **Lymphedema:** Lymphatic obstruction causes the accumulation of interstitial fluid because of insufficient reabsorption and deficient removal of proteins, the latter increasing the oncotic pressure of the fluid in the interstitial space.

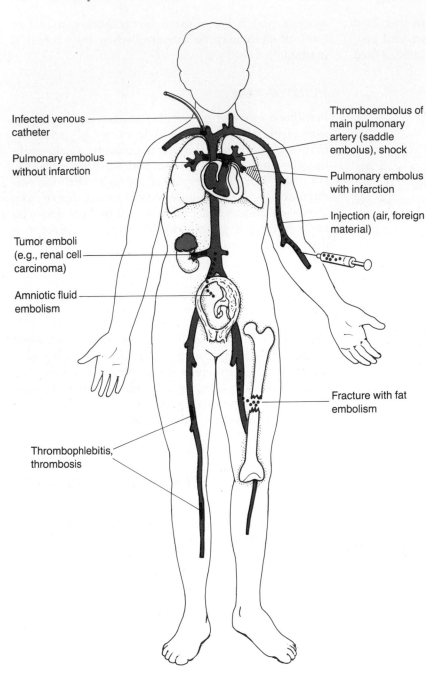

Infected venous catheter

Pulmonary embolus without infarction

Tumor emboli (e.g., renal cell carcinoma)

Amniotic fluid embolism

Thrombophlebitis, thrombosis

Thromboembolus of main pulmonary artery (saddle embolus), shock

Pulmonary embolus with infarction

Injection (air, foreign material)

Fracture with fat embolism

Figure 7-6. Sources of venous emboli.

heart. The upper extremities are a rare source of thromboemboli. Conditions that favor the development of pulmonary thromboembolism are:

- Stasis (heart failure, chronic venous insufficiency)
- Injury (trauma, surgery, parturition)
- Oral contraceptive use
- Immobilization (orthopedic, paralysis, bed rest)
- Sickle cell disease

CLINICAL FEATURES

Pulmonary thromboembolism with infarction clinically resembles pneumonia. Patients experience cough, stabbing pleuritic pain, shortness of breath, and occasionally hemoptysis. Pleural effusion is common and often bloody. Pathologically, pyramidal segments of hemorrhagic infarction are seen at the periphery of the lung.

Pulmonary thromboembolism may also occur without infarction. Under these circumstances the patient may suffer from dyspnea, cough, chest pain, and hypotension, with attacks of shortness of breath. Embolism produces pulmonary hypertension by mechanical blockage of the arterial bed. Reflex vasoconstriction and bronchial constriction due to release of vasoactive substances may contribute to a reduction in the size of the functional pulmonary vascular bed.

Massive pulmonary emboli cause sudden obstruction of blood flow through one or both of the major pulmonary arteries. The patient often goes into shock immediately—presumably because of certain neurologic reflexes—and may die within minutes. This catastrophe is characteristically precipitated when a patient who has been recuperating from surgery gets out of bed for the first time. Venous thrombi in the legs, formed because of stasis, are dislodged and travel to the lungs, resulting in **sudden death.**

FATE OF PULMONARY THROMBOEMBOLI

Small pulmonary emboli may completely resolve, depending on the embolic load, the adequacy of the pulmonary vascular reserve, the state of the bronchial collateral circulation, and the activity of the thrombolytic process. Thromboemboli may become organized and leave strings of fibrous tissue in the lumen of pulmonary arteries.

EMBOLI IN PERIPHERAL ARTERIES

The heart is the most common source of systemic emboli (Fig. 7-7), which usually arise from mural thrombi or diseased valves. Mural thrombi are seen in atrial fibrillation, mitral valve disease, myocardial infarction, left ventricular aneurysm, heart failure of any etiology, and cardiomyopathy, particularly the congestive type. Bacterial infection of diseased mitral or aortic valves **(bacterial endocarditis)** provides a source of septic emboli. Sterile thrombi may form in the valves in certain debilitated states **(marantic endocarditis).** Emboli usually lodge at points where the vessel lumen narrows abruptly—for example, at bifurcations or in the area of an atherosclerotic plaque. The viability of the tissue supplied by the vessel depends on the availability of collateral circulation and on the fate of the embolus. The embolus may propagate locally and lead to a more severe obstruction, or it may fragment and dissolve. **Arterial emboli to the brain cause strokes. In the mesenteric circulation they cause infarction of the bowel,** a complication that presents as an acute abdomen and requires immediate surgery. **Embolism of an artery of the leg leads to sudden pain, absence**

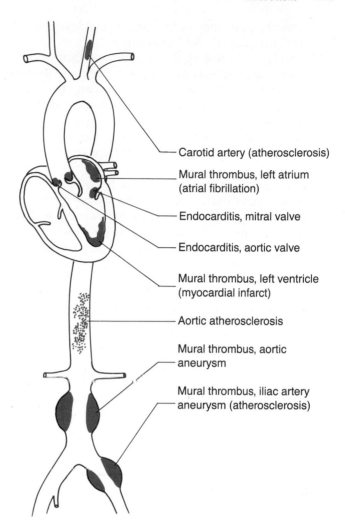

Figure 7-7. Sources of arterial emboli.

Carotid artery (atherosclerosis)

Mural thrombus, left atrium (atrial fibrillation)

Endocarditis, mitral valve

Endocarditis, aortic valve

Mural thrombus, left ventricle (myocardial infarct)

Aortic atherosclerosis

Mural thrombus, aortic aneurysm

Mural thrombus, iliac artery aneurysm (atherosclerosis)

of pulse, and a cold limb. In some cases the limb must be amputated. **Renal artery embolism may infarct the entire kidney but more commonly results in small peripheral infarcts.** The more common sites of infarction are summarized in Figure 7-3.

EMBOLI OTHER THAN THROMBOEMBOLI

Any material introduced into the lumen of an artery or vein may embolize and obstruct the circulation (see Fig. 7-6):

- **Air embolism.** Air may be introduced into the venous circulation through neck wounds, thoracocentesis, punctures of the great veins during invasive procedures, and hemodialysis.

- **Amniotic fluid embolism.** Amniotic fluid embolism is rare, but may be a catastrophic complication of childbirth. The pulmonary emboli are composed of the solid epithelial constituents contained in the amniotic fluid. Of greater importance is the initiation of a potentially fatal consumptive coagulopathy caused by the release of thromboplastic substances.

- **Fat embolism.** Severe trauma to fat-containing tissue, particularly the bone, can release fat emboli into damaged blood vessels. When these emboli lodge in the lung, pulmonary edema may result. Fat emboli may also lodge in the brain, where they produce a change in consciousness.

SHOCK

Shock is a condition characterized by a reduction in tissue perfusion and oxygen delivery below the levels required to meet normal demands. It is ordinarily accompanied by a decreased arterial blood pressure. The term "shock" encompasses all the hemodynamic reactions that occur in response to such alterations of hemodynamic homeostasis.

PATHOGENESIS OF SHOCK

Shock initiates compensatory mechanisms that, for a while, sustain the organism at borderline levels. If the compensatory mechanisms become exhausted, shock is said to enter an irreversible phase. **In the natural course of shock, a rapid circulatory collapse leads to impaired cellular metabolism and death.** Shock is not synonymous with low blood pressure, although hypotension is commonly a part of the shock syndrome. Hypotension is a late sign of shock and indicates failure of compensation. Blood flow is dependent on both perfusion pressure and vascular resistance. Peripheral flow can fall below critical levels, but extreme vasoconstriction can maintain central arterial blood pressure. This distinction between shock and hypotension is important clinically because the rapid restoration of **nutrient blood flow** is the primary goal in treating shock. When blood pressure alone is raised with vasopressive drugs, nutrient flow may actually be diminished.

CARDIOGENIC AND HYPOVOLEMIC SHOCK

Shock is a state in which the perfusion of body tissues is inadequate to meet normal metabolic demands. This decreased perfusion is generally the result of a decreased cardiac output, resulting either from the inability of the heart to pump the normal venous return or from a decreased volume of blood secondary to a decreased venous return. These two mechanisms, which lead to a decreased cardiac output, define the two major types of shock: **cardiogenic** and **hypovolemic** shock (Fig. 7-8). In cardiogenic shock due to myocardial infarction, myocarditis, or pericardial tamponade, a depressed systolic cardiac function (ejection fraction less than 20%) is responsible for the decreased cardiac output and, consequently, for the shock symptoms. In hypovolemic shock, however, a decreased blood volume is reflected in a reduced venous return to the heart, which in turn leads to a decreased cardiac output. A reduction in blood volume results from either **external** or **internal** fluid loss (see Fig. 7-8). Hemorrhage, diarrhea, excessive urine formation, and perspiration are the major mechanisms of external fluid loss; internal fluid loss usually results from an increase in the permeability of the microvasculature caused by endotoxemia, burns, trauma, or anaphylaxis.

In the case of burn or trauma, direct damage to the microcirculation is the mechanism by which vascular permeability is increased. Immunologic mechanisms, coupled to the activation of complement and the release of anaphylotoxins, increase vascular permeability in anaphylaxis.

In both hypovolemic and cardiogenic shock, a decreased cardiac output and resultant decreased tissue perfusion make up the essential pathogenetic mechanisms in the progression from reversible to irreversible shock. Anoxic injury is the common cellular consequence of the initial decrease in tissue perfusion (see Fig. 7-8). A vicious cycle of decreasing tissue perfusion and further cell injury is perpetuated by two mechanisms: (1) Injury to endothelial cells as a result of decreased tissue perfusion increases vascular permeability; in turn, the increased exudation of fluid from the circulation reduces blood volume, decreases venous return, and further decreases cardiac output, thus aggravating anoxic cell injury. (2) Decreased perfusion of the kidneys and skeletal muscles results in metabolic acidosis, which in turn further decreases cardiac output and tissue perfusion; decreased perfusion of the heart injures the myocardial cells and decreases their ability to pump blood, further reducing cardiac output and tissue perfusion.

Septic Shock

Septicemia with gram-negative organisms is the most common condition predisposing a patient to septic shock, but the mechanism for the increase in vascular permeability is not as straightforward. The entry of endotoxin into the blood stream triggers a series of

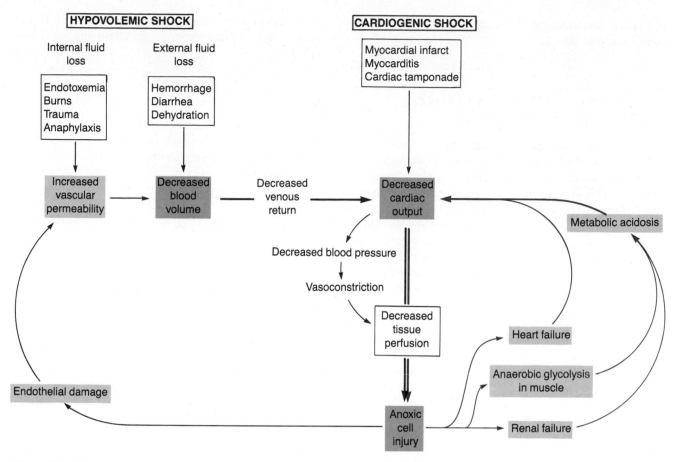

Figure 7-8. The pathogenesis of shock. This graph describes the integration of many factors in the progression of shock. Shock is initiated by one of two principal events: pump failure, or "cardiogenic shock"; and loss of circulatory volume, also called "hypovolemic shock." Hypovolemic shock follows **internal fluid loss,** such as that in endotoxemia, burns, trauma, or anaphylaxis, or **external fluid loss,** such as that caused by hemorrhage, diarrhea, and dehydration. The effect of both events is decreased cardiac output and decreased tissue perfusion. The resulting anoxic cell injury sets into motion several vicious cycles. Metabolic acidosis (renal failure, increased anaerobic glycolysis) and heart failure lead to a further decline in cardiac output. Endothelial damage increases vascular permeability and decreases effective blood volume, reducing venous return and decreasing cardiac output.

reactions that involve leukocytes, platelets, complement, and a number of other blood factors. It is not clear whether endotoxin injures the endothelial cells directly or whether other mediators, such as polymorphonuclear leukocytes and complement, are necessary.

The lipopolysaccharide portion of bacterial endotoxins activates complement by two antibody-independent mechanisms. The lipid region of the lipopolysaccharide molecule (lipid-A) binds directly to C1 and initiates complement activation by the classical pathway. The polysaccharide portion of the molecule activates the alternative pathway by a mechanism that is independent of lipid-A. Complement activation generates potent chemotactic factors that cause leukocytes to

marginate in the microcirculation, an event followed by degranulation and endothelial injury. The neutrophil has therefore been suggested as playing a central role in the pathogenesis of endotoxin-associated injury. Oxygen radicals and neutrophil-derived proteases have, in turn, been implicated in neutrophil-mediated injury to the endothelium. Alternatively, it has been suggested that endotoxin injures endothelial cells directly, and that activated complement and neutrophils only exaggerate the injury by their interactions with the altered endothelium. At present, the many effects of endotoxin on coagulation and complement, platelets, polymorphonuclear leukocytes, endothelial cells, and macrophages/monocytes do not allow a simple explanation of the pathogenesis of microvascular injury that initiates septic shock.

VASCULAR COMPENSATORY MECHANISMS IN SHOCK

Feedback mechanisms maintain blood flow to the vital organs, the heart and the brain, shifting it away from the periphery, skeletal muscle, skin, splanchnic bed, adipose tissue, limbs, and some parenchymal organs. The compensatory mechanisms involve the sympathetic nervous system, the release of endogenous vasoconstrictors and hormonal substances, and local vasoregulation. The integrated regulatory response increases cardiac output by increasing the heart rate and myocardial contractility while constricting the arteries and arterioles.

The **increased sympathetic discharge** also increases the release of catecholamines by the adrenal medulla. The skeletal muscle, splanchnic bed, and skin arterioles respond to this increased sympathetic discharge, while the cardiac and cerebral arterioles are less reactive. In this manner the increased sympathetic tone affects volume regulation. The marked arteriolar vasoconstriction results in reduced capillary hydrostatic pressure and in less fluid shifted into the interstitium, thus permitting an osmotic fluid shift from the interstitium to the vascular system.

The **renin–angiotensin–aldosterone mechanism** also contributes to compensation. Renin converts the circulating angiotensinogen into angiotensin I, which subsequently is transformed to angiotensin II, the most potent endogenous vasoconstrictor. Angiotensin II also stimulates aldosterone secretion, which in turn stimulates sodium and water reabsorption, thus helping to maintain intravascular volume. A similar water-preserving action is provided by the pituitary antidiuretic hormone.

Vascular autoregulation preserves regional blood flow to vital organs, particularly the heart and the brain, by vasodilatation of the coronary and cerebral circulations in response to hypoxia and acidosis. The peripheral circulation of organs such as the skin and skeletal muscles, which are less sensitive to hypoxia, do not display such a tightly controlled autoregulation.

PATHOLOGY OF SHOCK

Shock is associated with a number of specific changes in organs (Fig. 7-9), including acute tubular necrosis,

acute respiratory distress syndrome, liver failure, depression of host defense mechanisms, and heart failure.

HEART

Grossly, the heart shows petechial hemorrhages of the epicardium and of the endocardium, especially the left outflow tract. Microscopically, there are necrotic foci in the myocardium, ranging from the loss of single fibers to large areas of necrosis.

KIDNEY

Acute renal failure has been divided into three phases: the **initiation phase,** from the onset of injury to the beginning of renal failure; the **maintenance phase,** from the onset of renal failure to a stable, reduced renal function; and the **recovery phase.** In survivors, the recovery phase begins about 10 days after an episode of severe systemic shock and lasts up to 8 weeks.

During acute renal failure the kidney is large, swollen, and congested, although the cortex may be pale. Cut section reveals blood pooling in the outer stripe of the medulla. Microscopically, fully developed acute tubular necrosis is manifested by dilatation of the proximal tubules and focal necrosis of cells. Frequently, pigmented casts in the tubular lumina indicate leakage of hemoglobin or myoglobin. Coarse, "ropy" casts are seen in the distal nephron and distal convoluted tubules. Interstitial edema is prominent in the cortex, and mononuclear cells accumulate within the tubules and surrounding interstitium. Renal blood flow is restricted to one-third of normal following the acute ischemic phase, an effect that is even more severe in the outer cortex. The constriction of arterioles reduces the filtration pressure, thus reducing the amount of filtrate and contributing to oliguria. Interstitial edema occurs, possibly through a process termed "backflow." Excessive vasoconstriction is thought to be related to stimulation of the renin–angiotensin system.

LUNG

Following the onset of severe and prolonged shock, injury to the alveolar wall results in focal or generalized interstitial pneumonitis (shock lung). The sequence of changes is mediated by acute inflammatory cells and includes interstitial edema, necrosis of endothelial cells, microthrombi, and necrosis of the alveolar epithelium.

Grossly, the lung is firm and congested. Frothy fluid exudes from the cut surface. Interstitial edema is first

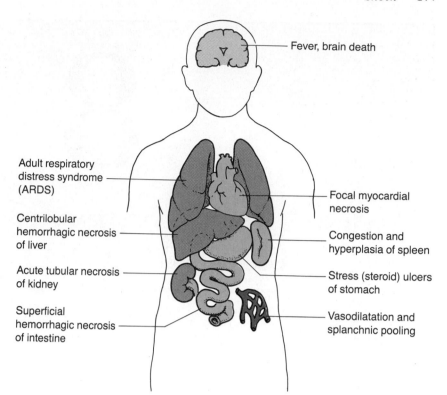

Fever, brain death

Adult respiratory
distress syndrome
(ARDS)

Centrilobular
hemorrhagic necrosis
of liver

Acute tubular necrosis
of kidney

Superficial
hemorrhagic necrosis
of intestine

Focal myocardial
necrosis

Congestion and
hyperplasia of spleen

Stress (steroid) ulcers
of stomach

Vasodilatation and
splanchnic pooling

Figure 7-9. Complications of shock.

seen around peribronchial connective tissue and lymphatics, subsequently filling the interalveolar connective tissue. In this initial period a large fluid volume drains into the pulmonary lymphatics. If removal of this fluid becomes insufficient, or if the balance of forces that keep the fluid in the interstitial space is disturbed, alveolar edema develops.

Edema of the lung is initiated by the loosening of intercellular junctions between the pulmonary capillary endothelial cells, a reaction that occurs at different speeds in different types of shock. It occurs within 2 to 3 minutes following endotoxemia and can be traced to the activation of complement and production of C5, a substance that is chemotactic for polymorphonuclear leukocytes.

A reversible accumulation of platelets in the terminal vascular bed is characteristic of both hemorrhagic and endotoxin shock. Shock-induced lung injury leads to the appearance of hyaline membranes in the alveoli, which are frequently expelled into the alveolar ducts and terminal bronchioles. These lung changes may heal entirely, but in half of the patients the repair processes progress and cause a thickening of the alveolar wall. Type II pneumocytes proliferate and form a picket

line of alveolar lining cells, interfering with gas exchange. Fibrous tissue proliferation also leads to organization of the alveolar exudate.

GASTROINTESTINAL TRACT

Injury to the gastrointestinal tract is one of the more serious consequences of shock, leading to **pancreatitis, erosive gastritis,** and **duodenal ulcer.** Insufficiency of the microcirculation has been thought to be the main cause of intestinal malfunction. Increased circulating catecholamines in shock induce pronounced vasoconstriction and cause mucosal necrosis of varying degrees. Interruption of the barrier function of the intestine may be related to the development of septicemia.

ADRENALS

In severe shock the adrenal glands may exhibit conspicuous hemorrhage in the inner cortex. Frequently, this hemorrhage is only focal, but it can be massive and accompanied by hemorrhagic necrosis of the entire gland, as seen in the **Waterhouse–Friderichsen syndrome.**

8

ENVIRONMENTAL AND NUTRITIONAL PATHOLOGY

EMANUEL RUBIN AND JOHN L. FARBER

Smoking

Alcoholism

Drug Abuse

Environmental Chemicals

Physical Agents

Nutritional Disorders

OKING

king is the single largest preventable cause of
n in the United States. **About 350,000 deaths a
—one-sixth of the total mortality in the United
s—occurs prematurely because of smoking.** Life
ancy is shortened, and overall mortality is pro-
l to the duration of cigarette smoking (Fig. 8-1).
mortality associated with cigarette smoking
r cessation of the habit, and after 15 years
from cigarettes the mortality of ex-
lar to that of those who have never
verall mortality among those who
r pipes is only slightly higher than
ing population.

responsible for the excess mor-
mokers are, in order of fre-
isease, cancer of the lung,
monary disease. Smokers
ce of cancer of the oral
eas, bladder and kid-
and alcohol abuse is
the upper respira-
on, smokers suf-
c aortic aneu-

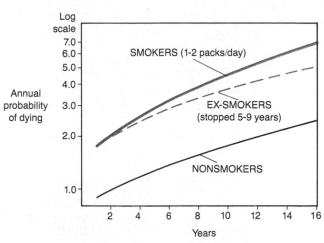

Figure 8-1. The risk of dying in smokers and nonsmokers.
Note that the annual probability of an individual dying, indicated on the ordinate, is a log scale. Individuals who have
smoked for 1 year have a twofold greater probability of
dying than a nonsmoker, while those who have smoked for
more than 15 years have more than a threefold greater
probability of dying.

companing vein, leading to gangrene and amputation
of the lower extremities. Although Buerger's disease is
unquestionably related to smoking, it is rarely seen
today.

CANCER

Cancer of the lung is today the single most common
ncer in both men and women in the United States
8-3). Cigarette tar, the material that is deposited
filter, contains more than 2000 compounds,
which have been identified as carcinogens,
moters and ciliatoxic agents.
l change in the morphologic sequence
cer of the lung is squamous metaplasia of
ucosa. As is often the case in a squa-
he cervix, for example—the meta-
becomes dysplastic and eventually
rcinoma in situ of the bronchial
ement membrane of the epithe-
regional nodes and distant
g lung cancer is directly re-
igarettes smoked (Fig. 8-4).
also an important factor in the
cancer that is associated with cer-
onal exposures, (*e.g.*, uranium or as-

cigar, and pipe
expose the oral
aw tobacco or to-
ngue, **buccal mu-**
in tobacco users.
the esophagus in
Great Britain are be-
ism with the excessive

as likely to die of cancer
s, and 30% to 40% of all
d to smoking.
of the kidney is increased
ers. Men who smoke more
e a five times greater risk of
an in nonsmokers.

TIC DISEASES

t smoking is the principal cause of
s and chronic obstructive lung dis-
n addition, there is a 70% greater
eptic ulcer disease in male cigarette
n nonsmokers.

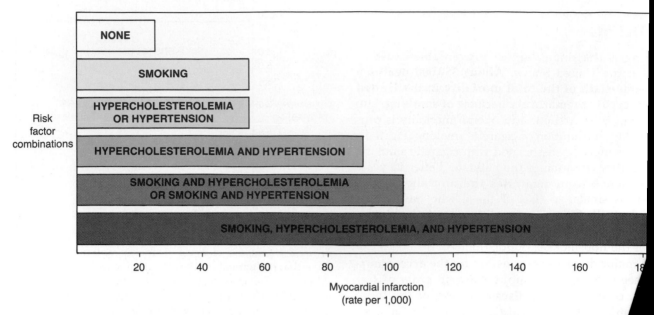

Myocardial infarction
(rate per 1,000)

Figure 8-2. The risk of myocardial infarction in cigarette smokers. Smoking is an independent risk factor and increases the risk of a myocardial infarction to about the same extent as does hypertension or hypercholesterolemia alone. The effects of smoking are additive to those of these other two risk factors.

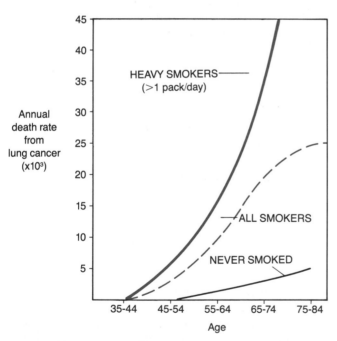

All forms of tobacco use—cigarette smoking, as well as tobacco chewing cavity to the compounds found in bacco smoke. **Cancer of the lip, t cosa, and larynx occur principall**

The risk ratios for **cancer o** smokers in the United States an tween 2 and 9. There is a synerg intake of alcohol.

Cigarette smokers are twice **of the bladder** as nonsmoke bladder cancers are attribute

Primary adenocarcinoma 50% to 100% among smo than two packs a day hav **cancer of the pancreas t**

Figure 8-3. Death rate from lung cancer among smokers and nonsmokers. Nonsmokers exhibit a small, linear rise in the death rate from lung cancer from the age of 50 onward. By contrast, those who smoke more than one pack a day show an exponential rise in the annual death rate from lung cancer starting at about age 35. By age 70, heavy smokers have about a twentyfold greater death rate from lung cancer than nonsmokers.

NON-NEOPLA
IN SMOKERS

It is now clear tha
chronic bronchit
ease (Fig. 8-5).
prevalence of p
smokers than

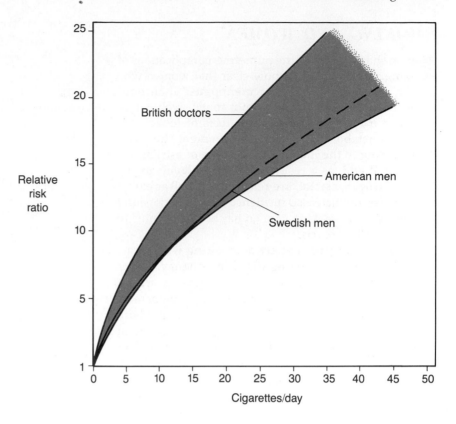

Figure 8-4. Dose-dependent relationship between cigarette smoking and the risk of lung cancer. Prospective studies of three different populations of smokers found a dependence of the risk of lung cancer on the number of cigarettes smoked per day. For example, there is about a threefold greater risk of developing lung cancer in those who smoke 15 cigarettes a day as opposed to those who smoke five. The dashed line is an extrapolation of the data for Swedish men who smoke from 25 to 50 cigarettes a day.

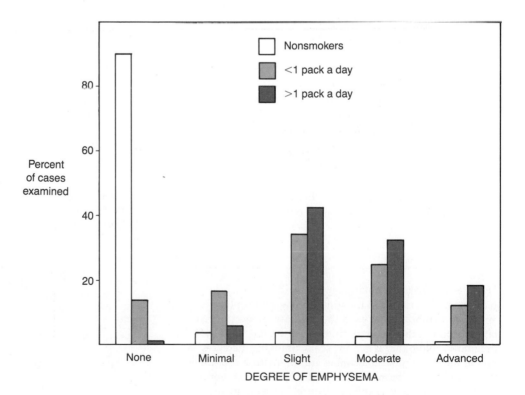

Figure 8-5. The association between cigarette smoking and pulmonary emphysema. Ninety percent of nonsmokers have no detectable emphysema at autopsy. In contrast, virtually all those who smoke more than one pack per day have morphologic evidence of emphysema at autopsy. Emphysema shows a slight dose dependence on the number of cigarettes smoked. Those who smoke less than one pack per day tend to have less severe emphysema, but 85% to 90% of such smokers have some emphysema at autopsy.

SMOKING AND WOMEN

Women share with men the numerous complications of smoking. In addition, it is now clear that women who smoke experience an **earlier menopause** than non-smokers. Although the cause is not conclusively established, it may be related to the effects of tobacco on estrogen metabolism. **In smoking women, the pathway leading to the inactive metabolite of estradiol is stimulated and, as a result, circulating levels of the active estrogen, estriol, are reduced.** As well as earlier menopause, an increased incidence of postmenopausal **osteoporosis** in smoking women has been attributed to decreased estriol levels.

The most dangerous effect of smoking which particularly affects women occurs in pregnancy. Babies born to women who smoke during pregnancy are, on average, 200 g lighter than babies born to comparable women who do not smoke. These infants are not born preterm, but rather are small for gestational age at every stage of pregnancy. Twenty percent to 40% of the incidence of low birth weight can be attributed to maternal cigarette smoking.

The noxious effect of smoking upon the fetus is mirrored by its effect on the uteroplacental unit. Perinatal mortality is increased among the offspring of smokers, the increase ranging from 20% among the progeny of women who smoke less than a pack per day to almost 40% among the offspring of those who smoke more than a pack per day. This excess mortality does not reflect specific abnormalities of the fetus, but rather problems related to the uteroplacental system. The incidences of **abruptio placentae, placenta previa, uterine bleeding, and premature rupture of the membranes** are all increased (Fig. 8-6).

The children of smoking mothers have exhibited measurable deficiencies in physical growth, intellectual maturation, and emotional development that are independent of other known predisposing factors. In the most comprehensive study to date, 17,000 births during one week in Great Britain were studied at ages 7

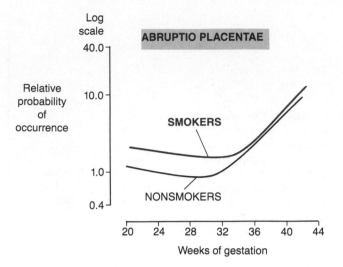

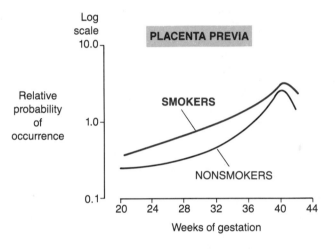

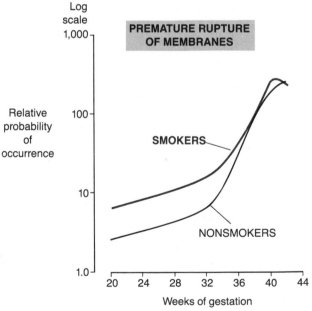

Figure 8-6. Effect of smoking on the incidence of abruptio placentae, placenta previa, and the premature rupture of amniotic membranes. In each the ordinate shows the probability of one of three complications of the third trimester of pregnancy. Note that it is a log scale. Smoking increases the probability of abruptio placentae and premature rupture of the amniotic membranes prior to 34 weeks of gestation, at which time the fetus is still premature. Smoking increases the risk of placenta previa up to 40 weeks of gestation.

and 11 years. The children of mothers who smoked 10 or more cigarettes a year during pregnancy were, on average, 1.0 cm shorter than children of nonsmoking mothers and were 3 to 5 months retarded in reading, mathematics and general intellectual ability.

ALCOHOLISM

It is estimated that there are about 12 million alcoholics in the United States, or about one-tenth of the population at risk. The proportion may be even higher in other countries, particularly those in which wine is consumed in preference to water. Certain ethnic groups—for example, Native Americans and Eskimoes—have notoriously high rates of alcoholism. By contrast, other groups, such as Chinese and Jews, experience little alcoholism. Although this addiction is more common in men, the number of female alcoholics has been rapidly increasing.

The definition of alcoholism is difficult and varies widely with different authors. In view of the large differences in individual susceptibility both to the acute intoxicating effects of alcohol and to the development of alcohol-related disease, it is difficult to derive a simple number for the consumption of ethanol above which a diagnosis of alcoholism is made. It is sufficient that chronic alcoholism be defined as the regular intake of a quantity of alcohol that is enough to injure a person socially, psychologically or physically.

Many of the chronic diseases associated with alcoholism were, at one time, attributed to malnutrition, and it is true that some alcoholics suffer from nutritional deficiencies—for example, thiamin deficiency (Wernicke's encephalopathy) or folate deficiency (megaloblastic anemia). **However, most alcoholics have an adequate diet, and the great majority of alcohol-related disorders should be attributed to a toxic effect of alcohol.**

LIVER

Alcoholic liver disease, the most common medical complication of alcoholism, accounts for a majority of the cases of cirrhosis of the liver in the industrialized countries. (In Asia and Africa, by contrast, most cirrhosis is due to infection with the hepatitis B virus.) the nature of the alcoholic beverage is largely irrelevant; consumed in excess, beer, wine, whiskey, hard cider, and so on all produce cirrhosis. Only the total daily dose (or possibly the lifetime dose) of alcohol is relevant.

PANCREAS

The relationship of acute pancreatitis to alcoholism is unclear, but such episodes are seen with sufficient frequency to suggest that acute pancreatitis is a complication of alcoholism. **Chronic calcifying pancreatitis, on the other hand, is an unquestioned result of alcoholism, and is an important cause of incapacitating pain, pancreatic insufficiency, and pancreatic stones.**

HEART

Chronic alcoholics may suffer from a degenerative disease of the myocardium, termed, **alcoholic cardiomyopathy,** that leads to low-output congestive heart failure. Although the pathogenesis is obscure, it is widely accepted as a toxic effect of ethanol. The alcoholic heart seems also to be more susceptible to arrhythmias, and the occurrence of abnormal cardiac rhythms after an alcoholic binge has been termed the "holiday heart." Many cases of sudden death in alcoholics are probably caused by sudden, fatal arrhythmias.

SKELETAL MUSCLE

A wide range of changes in skeletal muscle is seen in chronic alcoholics, varying from mild alterations in muscle fibers evident only by electron microscopy to a severe, debilitating chronic myopathy, with degeneration of muscle fibers and diffuse fibrosis. On rare occasions, **acute alcoholic rhabdomyolysis**—acute necrosis of muscle fibers and release of myoglobin to the circulation—is seen. This sudden event can be fatal, because of renal failure secondary to myoglobinuria.

ENDOCRINE SYSTEM

The principal endocrine effect of alcoholism in men is on the testis, which are reduced in size. Feminization of chronic alcoholics, together with loss of libido and potency, is common, even in the absence of liver disease. The breasts are enlarged (gynecomastia), body hair is lost and a female distribution of pubic hair (escutcheon) develops. Chronic alcoholism leads to lower levels of circulating testosterone because of a complex interference with the pituitary-gonadal axis, possibly complicated by an accelerated metabolism of testosterone by the liver. Alcohol has also been shown to have a direct toxic effect on the testes.

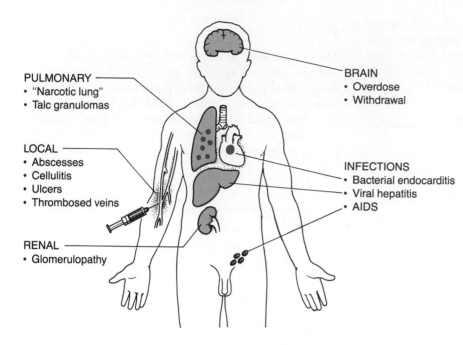

PULMONARY
• "Narcotic lung"
• Talc granulomas

LOCAL
• Abscesses
• Cellulitis
• Ulcers
• Thrombosed veins

RENAL
• Glomerulopathy

BRAIN
• Overdose
• Withdrawal

INFECTIONS
• Bacterial endocarditis
• Viral hepatitis
• AIDS

Figure 8-7. Complications of drug addiction.

GASTROINTESTINAL TRACT

Reflux esophagitis in alcoholics may be particularly painful, and peptic ulcers are also more common in the alcoholic. Violent retching may lead to tears at the esophageal-gastric junction **(Mallory-Weiss syndrome),** sometimes so severe as to result in exsanguinating hemorrhage.

BRAIN

A general cortical atrophy of the brain is common in alcoholics, and may reflect a toxic effect of alcohol. By contrast, most of the characteristic brain diseases in alcoholics are probably a result of nutritional deficiency. **Wernicke's encephalopathy,** caused by thiamine deficiency, is characterized by mental confusion, ataxia, abnormal ocular motility, and polyneuropathy.

The retrograde amnesia and confabulatory symptoms of **Korsakoff's pyschosis,** once thought to be pathognomonic of chronic alcoholism, have now been identified in a number of organic mental syndromes and are considered nonspecific. Alcoholic cerebellar degeneration can be differentiated from other forms of acquired or familial cerebellar degeneration.

DRUG ABUSE

Drug abuse has been defined as "the use of any substance in a manner that deviates from the accepted medical, social, or legal patterns within a given society". For the most part, drug abuse involves agents that affect the higher functions of the brain and are used to alter mood and perception.

The intravenous injection of excessive amounts of heroin and other "street drugs" accounts for more than one-half of all the deaths from drug abuse.

Apart from reactions related to the pharmacologic or physiological effects of substance abuse, the most common complications (15% of direct drug-related deaths) are caused by the introduction of infectious organisms by a parenteral route. The most common infections are local at the site of injection. Among these are cutaneous abscesses, cellulitis, and ulcers (Fig. 8-7). Thrombophlebitis of the veins draining the sites of injection is common. The intravenous introduction of bacteria also leads to septic complications in many organs. Bacterial endocarditis, often involving *Staphylococcus aureus*, occurs on both sides of the heart (Fig. 8-8). Other complications of bacteremia are pulmonary, renal, and intracranial abscesses, meningitis, osteomyelitis, and mycotic aneurysms (Fig. 8-9).

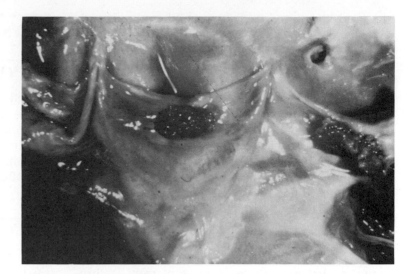

Figure 8-8. Bacterial endocarditis in a drug addict. Two aortic valve cusps display adherent vegetations. A coronary artery ostium is visible in the upper right.

Perhaps the most feared infectious complications today are of viral etiology. Addicts who exchange needles constitute one of the highest risks groups for AIDS and for viral hepatitis. Addicts also suffer from the complications of viral hepatitis, such as chronic active hepatitis, necrotizing angiitis, and glomerulonephritis.

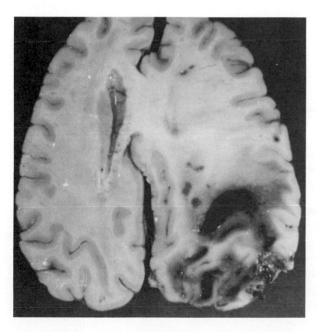

Figure 8-9. Brain abscess (lower right) in an intravenous drug abuser.

ENVIRONMENTAL CHEMICALS

LEAD

Lead poisoning in the United States is mainly a pediatric problem related to pica, the habit of chewing on cribs, toys, furniture, and woodwork, and the eating of painted plaster and fallen paint flakes. In adults occupational exposure to lead occurs primarily among those engaged in the smelting of lead, a process that releases metal fumes and deposits lead oxide dust in the industrial environment. It is still unresolved whether lead-containing automobile exhaust fumes contribute to clinically significant total body lead burdens, despite the clear lowering of mean blood levels in the United States since the introduction of unleaded gasoline.

Lead is absorbed through either the lungs or the gastrointestinal tract. Once in the blood, it rapidly equilibrates with the plasma and red blood cells. A portion of blood lead remains freely diffusible and enters either of two types of tissues. Bones, teeth, nails, and hair represent a tightly bound pool of lead that is not generally regarded as harmful. By contrast, the amount of lead in the brain, liver, kidneys and bone marrow is directly related to its toxic effects. With chronic exposure, 90% of the total body lead burden is in the bones. During metaphyseal bone formation in children, lead and calcium are deposited to produce the increased bone densities ("lead lines") seen radiographically at the metaphysis, thereby providing a simple method of detecting increased body stores of lead in children. Lead is excreted by the kidneys.

Lead toxicity is manifested in the dysfunction of three important organ systems: the nervous system, the kidneys and the hematopoietic system (Fig. 8-10). **The central nervous system is the target of lead toxicity in children; adults usually present with manifestations of peripheral neuropathy.** Children with lead encephalopathy are typically irritable, and ataxic. They may convulse or display altered states of consciousness, from drowsiness to frank coma. The most common manifestation of lead neurotoxicity in the adult is a **peripheral motor neuropathy**, typically affecting the radial and peroneal nerves and resulting in **wrist** and **foot drop** respectively.

Lead intoxication also produces an **anemia** by disrupting heme synthesis in bone marrow erythroblasts, with a resulting microcytic and hypochromic anemia resembling that seen in iron deficiency. The anemia of lead intoxication is also characterized by a prominant **basophilic stippling of the erythrocytes,** related to clustering of ribosomes.

Lead is toxic to the proximal tubular cells of the kidney. The resulting dysfunction is characterized by aminoaciduria, glycosuria and hyperphosphaturia (Franconi's syndrome). Such functional alterations are accompanied by the formation of inclusion bodies in the nuclei of the proximal tubular cells. These inclusions are characteristic of **lead nephropathy** and are composed of a lead-protein complex.

PHYSICAL AGENTS

HYPOTHERMIA

Hypothermia—a decrease in body temperature below 35°C—can result in systemic or focal injury, the latter exemplified by **trenchfoot** or **immersion foot.** In localized hypothermia of these types, actual tissue freezing does not occur. **Frostbite,** by contrast, involves the crystallization of tissue water.

LOCALIZED HYPERTHERMIA

Cutaneous burns are the most frequent form of localized hyperthermia. Both the elevated temperature and the rate of temperature change are important in determining the pattern of the tissue response. A temperature of 70°C or higher for several seconds causes necrosis of the entire dermal epithelium, whereas a temperature of 50°C may be sustained for 10 minutes or more without killing the cells.

Cutaneous burns have been separated into three categories of severity: first-, second- and third-degree burns (Fig. 8-11). A more contemporary classification refers to full thickness (third-degree) and partial thickness (first- and second-degree) burns. First-degree burns, such as a mild sunburn, are recognized by congestion and pain, but are not associated with necrosis.

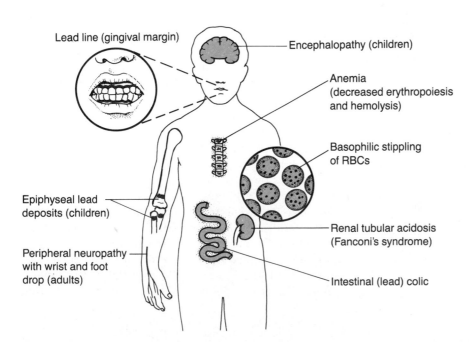

Lead line (gingival margin)

Encephalopathy (children)

Anemia (decreased erythropoiesis and hemolysis)

Basophilic stippling of RBCs

Epiphyseal lead deposits (children)

Peripheral neuropathy with wrist and foot drop (adults)

Renal tubular acidosis (Fanconi's syndrome)

Intestinal (lead) colic

Figure 8-10. Complications of lead intoxication.

FIRST DEGREE

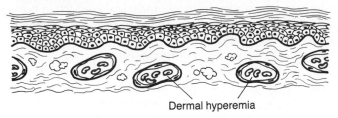

Dermal hyperemia

SECOND DEGREE

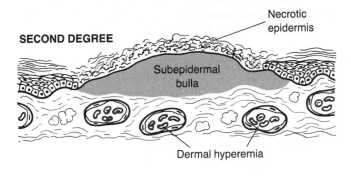

Necrotic
epidermis

Subepidermal
bulla

Dermal hyperemia

THIRD DEGREE

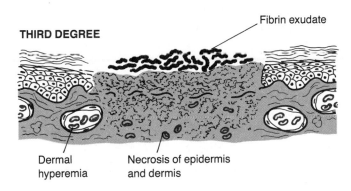

Fibrin exudate

Dermal
hyperemia

Necrosis of epidermis
and dermis

Figure 8-11. The pathology of cutaneous burns. A first-degree skin burn exhibits only dilatation of the dermal blood vessels. In a second-degree burn there is necrosis of the epidermis, and subepidermal edema collects under the necrotic epidermis to form a bulla. In a third-degree burn, both the epidermis and dermis are necrotic.

Mild endothelial injury produces vasodilatation, increased vascular permeability and slight edema. Burns that cause necrosis of the epithelium but spare the dermis are termed second-degree burns. Clinically, these are recognized by blisters, in which the epithelium is separated from the dermis. Third-degree burns char both the epithelium and the underlying dermis. Histologically, the epidermis and the dermis are carbonized and the cellular structure is lost.

The healing of cutaneous burns is related to the extent of the tissue destruction. First-degree burns, by definition, display little if any cell loss, and healing requires only repair or replacement of the injured endothelial cells. Second-degree burns also heal without a scar because the basal cells of the epidermis are not destroyed and serve as a source of regenerating cells for the epithelium. Third-degree burns, in which there is destruction of the entire thickness of the epidermis, usually heal by scarring.

CONTUSIONS

A force with sufficient energy may disrupt capillaries and venules within an organ by physical means alone. If this occurs in the skin, a loss of blood into the tissue space occurs. The resultant altered coloration identifies a **contusion,** namely, a localized area of mechanical injury with focal hemorrhage. The presence of a discrete blood pool within the tissue is termed a **hematoma.** Initially the deoxygenated blood renders the area blue to blue-black, as in the classical "black-eye." Macrophages ingest the red blood cells and convert the hemoglobin to bilirubin, thus changing the color from blue to yellow. Both mobilization of the pigment by macrophages and further metabolism of bilirubin cause the yellow to fade to yellowish green and then to disappear.

LACERATIONS

Should the force be greater, and should the tangential impact be stronger, the epithelium can split and tear, resulting in a **laceration.** Lacerations are usually the result of unidirectional displacement, but they may have crushed margins, in which case they are termed **abraded lacerations.**

IRRADIATION

We can define radiation simply as the emission of energy by one body, its transmission through an intervening medium, and its absorption by another body. Alpha particles, such as the radiation emitted by phosphorus-32, and the beta particles of elements such as tritium and carbon-14 pose few hazards for man. High-energy radiation, in the form of gamma or x-rays, is the mediator of most of the biologic effects discussed here.

Radiation is quantitated in a number of ways. The emission of radiant energy from a source is measured in

roentgens, units that refer to the amount of ionization produced in air. The absorption of radiant energy—biologically, the more important parameter—is measured in terms of the **rad,** the unit that defines the ergs of energy absorbed by a tissue. A newer international unit is the **Gray,** which corresponds to 100 rad. Because low-energy particles produce more biological damage than gamma or x-rays, the **rem** unit was introduced to describe the biological effect produced by a rad of high-energy radiation. For the practical purposes of this discussion of radiation-induced pathology, the roentgen, rad, and rem are comparable.

At the cellular level, radiation essentially has two effects: a somatic effect, associated with acute cell killing, and the induction of genetic damage. Radiation-induced cell death as discussed in Chapter 1, is attributed to the acute effects of the radiolysis of water. The production of activated oxygen species results in lipid peroxidation, membrane injury, and possibly an interaction with macromolecules of the cell. Genetic damage to the cell, whether caused by direct absorption of energy by DNA (target theory) or caused indirectly by a reaction of DNA with oxygen radicals, is expressed either as mutation or as reproductive failure. Both mutations and reproductive failure may lead to delayed cell death, and the former is incriminated in the development of radiation-induced neoplasia.

The vulnerability of a tissue to radiation-induced damage depends on its proliferative rate, which in turn correlates with the natural life span of the constituent cells. Damage to the DNA of a long-lived, nonproliferating cell does not necessarily pose a threat to its function or viability, because the reproductive and metabolic functions of the cell are distinct. By contrast, a short-lived, proliferating cell, for instance an intestinal crypt cell or a hematopoietic precursor, must be rapidly replaced by division of the stem cells and the committed precursor. When radiation-induced DNA damage precludes mitosis of these cells, the mature elements are no longer replaced and the tissue can no longer function.

WHOLE BODY IRRADIATION

Fortunately, there have been very few instances of human disease caused by whole-body radiation, and most of our information has been derived from studies of Japanese atom bomb casualties.

The development of the different acute radiation syndromes reflects only the dissimilarities in vulnerability of the target tissues (Fig. 8-12). At a dose of approximately 300 rad, a syndrome characterized by **hematopoietic failure** develops within 2 weeks. Since all hematopoietic precursor elements are highly sensitive

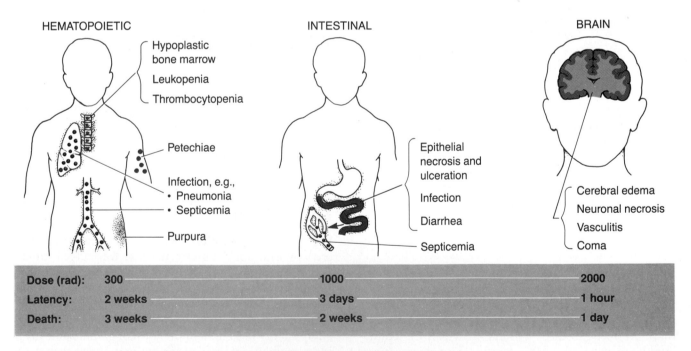

Figure 8-12. Acute radiation syndromes. At a dose of approximately 300 rad of whole body radiation, a syndrome characterized by hematopoietic failure develops within 2 weeks. In the vicinity of 1,000 rad, a gastrointestinal syndrome with a latency of only 3 days is seen. With doses of whole body radiation of 2,000 rad or greater, disease of the central nervous system appears within 1 hour, and death ensues rapidly.

to radiant energy, a pancytopenia typically characterizes the hematopoietic whole-body radiation syndrome. With more intense radiation, in the vicinity of 1000 rad, the principal cause of death is related to the **gastrointestinal system.** Severe destruction of the entire epithelium of the gastrointestinal tract occurs within 3 days, the time that corresponds to the normal life span of the villous and crypt cells. As a result the fluid homeostasis of the bowel is disrupted, and severe diarrhea and dehydration ensue. Moreover, the epithelial barrier to intestinal bacteria is breached, and bacteria invade and disseminate throughout the body. Shock and septicemia kill the victim.

With exposure to whole-body doses of 2000 rad and greater, central nervous system damage causes death within hours. In most cases, endothelial injury, resulting in cerebral edema and loss of the integrity of the blood-brain barrier, predominates, but with extreme doses radiation necrosis of neurons can be expected. Convulsions, coma, and death follow.

The effects of whole-body irradiation on the human fetus have been documented in studies of the survivors of the atom bomb explosions in Japan. Pregnant women exposed to doses of 25 rad or greater gave birth to infants with reduced head size, diminished overall growth, and mental retardation. Other effects of irradiation in utero include hydrocephaly, microphthalmia, chorioretinitis, blindness, spina bifida, cleft palate, club feet, and genital abnormalities.

The survivors of Hiroshima and Nagasaki have failed to manifest evidence of genetic damage in the form of either congenital abnormalities or hereditary diseases in subsequent offspring or their descendants. The risk of genetic damage to future generations from radiation therefore appears inconsequential.

The finding that rodents exposed to whole-body irradiation have a shortened life span has led to the suggestion that radiation accelerates the aging process. A mortality study of the survivors of the atom bomb explosions in Japan has not disclosed any excess mortality not attributable to neoplasia. Nor is there any evidence of acceleration in disease among the survivors in any part of the age range. **Thus, the effects of ionizing radiation on mortality are specific and focal, and there is no reason to believe that premature aging in humans or radiation-induced carcinogenesis is due to a general acceleration of aging.**

LOCALIZED RADIATION INJURY ASSOCIATED WITH RADIOTHERAPY

In the course of radiotherapy for malignant neoplasms, some normal tissue is inevitably included in the radiation field. While almost any organ can be damaged by radiation, the clinically important tissues are the skin,

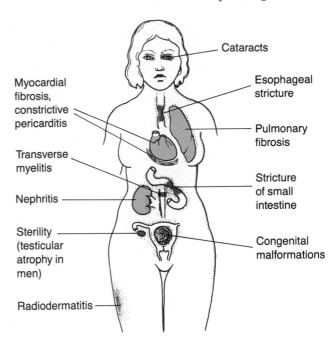

Figure 8-13. The non-neoplastic complications of radiation.

lungs, heart, kidney, bladder, and intestine—organs that are difficult to shield (Fig. 8-13). Localized damage to the bone marrow is clearly of little functional consequence because of the immense reserve capacity of the hematopoietic system.

Radiation-induced tissue injury predominantly affects small arteries and arterioles. Persistent damage to radiation-exposed tissue can be attributed to two major factors: compromise of the vascular supply and a fibrotic repair reaction to the acute necrosis and chronic ischemia. Chronic disease is characterized by **interstitial fibrosis** in the heart and lungs, **strictures** in the esophagus and small intestine, and **constrictive pericarditis.** Chronic **radiation nephritis,** which simulates malignant nephrosclerosis, is primarily a vascular disease characterized by severe hypertension and progressive renal insufficiency. Since all radiotherapy inevitably traverses the skin, it often leads to **radiodermatitis**.

Like other tissues that depend upon continuous cell cycling, the **gonads,** both testes and ovaries, are exquisitely radiosensitive. Also, should the eye lie in the path of the radiation beam, lenticular opacities—that is, **cataracts,**—may result. The spinal cord is unavoidably irradiated during treatment of certain thoracic or abdominal tumors, and the vascular damage in the cord may bring about localized ischemia which can result in a **transverse myelitis** and paraplegia.

RADIATION AND CANCER

High doses of radiation cause cancer. The evidence is incontrovertible and comes both from animal experi-

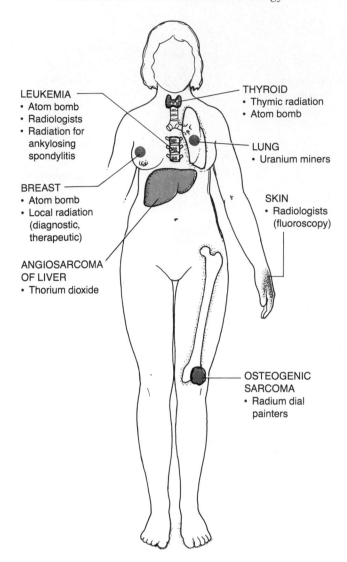

LEUKEMIA
• Atom bomb
• Radiologists
• Radiation for ankylosing spondylitis

BREAST
• Atom bomb
• Local radiation (diagnostic, therapeutic)

ANGIOSARCOMA OF LIVER
• Thorium dioxide

THYROID
• Thymic radiation
• Atom bomb

LUNG
• Uranium miners

SKIN
• Radiologists (fluoroscopy)

OSTEOGENIC SARCOMA
• Radium dial painters

Figure 8-14. Radiation-induced cancers.

ments and from studies of the effects of occupational exposure, radiotherapy for non-neoplastic conditions, the diagnostic use of certain radioisotopes, and the atom bomb explosions (Fig. 8-14).

With respect to **low-dose irradiation,,** the data currently available from radiation studies of cancer induction in animals, chromosomal damage in human cell cultures, malignant transformation of mammalian cells in vitro, and populations exposed to radiation show that the estimates of risk derived from a linear extrapolation from risk at high doses exaggerate the risk, perhaps by an order of magnitude. On the other hand, the data do not by any means show that the risk of radiogenic cancer from low-level radiation is zero. **When the data from atom bomb survivors are subjected to a linear-quadratic analysis, the lifetime risk from 1**

rad of whole-body x or gamma irradiation is 1 excess cancer death per 10,000 persons.

NUTRITIONAL DISORDERS

OBESITY

If one defines obesity as beginning at 20% above the mean adiposity, then 20% of middle-aged American men and 40% of middle-aged American women are obese. Obesity results from a chronic excess of caloric intake relative to the expenditure of energy. There are two general types of obesity: that which begins in childhood and is lifelong, and that which begins in the adult.

Lifelong obesity is associated with a larger number of adipocytes, presumably a genetically determined phenomenon. By contrast, the obesity which begins in adult life develops against a background of larger—that is, hypertrophied—adipocytes, the number remaining the same.

In adult-onset obesity fat is deposited principally on the trunk—that is, the hips and buttocks in women and the abdomen (pot belly) in men. In the type that begins in childhood, weight gain is distributed more peripherally, and is readily measured as an increase in the skinfold thickness over the triceps muscle or in the subscapular area.

Numerous theories of obesity, invoking hormonal changes, alterations in enzymes associated with fat metabolism, and decreased thermogenesis, have been proposed, but none has been substantiated.

The most important consequence of obesity (Fig. 8-15) is maturity-onset (Type II) diabetes, which is associated with normal or high levels of circulating insulin and peripheral resistance to insulin's action. In the United States, more than 80% of Type II diabetes occurs in obese individuals. Weight reduction usually ameliorates the glucose intolerance of Type II diabetes, presumably owing to a decrease in the stimulus for insulin secretion by the pancreatic beta cells. This subject is more fully discussed in Chapter 22.

Obesity has also been linked to atherosclerosis and myocardial infarction. It is noteworthy that obesity is associated with all the major risk factors for myocardial infarction, including hypercholesterolemia, low levels of high-density lipoproteins (HDL), diabetes and hypertension. **Obesity and hypercholesterolemia are also linked to an increased incidence of gallstones, particularly in women.**

Obesity has an important effect on the female reproductive system. **Oligomenorrhea and amenorrhea are**

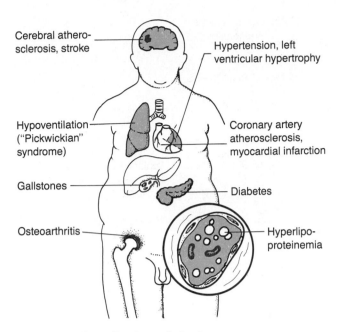

Figure 8-15. Complications of obesity.

KWASHIORKOR

One of the most common diseases of infancy and childhood in the nonindustrialized world is **kwashiorkor** (Fig. 8-16), a syndrome which results from **a deficiency of protein in a diet relatively high in carbohydrates.** As in the case of marasmus, the disorder commonly occurs after the baby is weaned, at which time a protein-poor diet, consisting principally of staple carbohydrates, replaces the mother's milk. Although there is generalized growth failure and muscle wasting, as in marasmus, the subcutaneous fat is normal, owing to the adequate caloric intake. Extreme apathy is a notable feature, in contrast to children with marasmus, who may be alert. Also in contrast to marasmus, severe edema, hepatomegaly, depigmentation of the skin and dermatoses are usual. The "flaky paint" lesions of the skin, which are located on the face, extremities, and perineum, are dry and hyperkeratotic. The hair becomes a sandy or reddish color; a characteristic linear depigmentation of the hair ("flag sign") provides evi-

common in premenopausal obese women. Pregnant obese women have a higher incidence of toxemia of pregnancy. Postmenopausal obese women have higher rates of endometrial carcinoma and uterine fibroids. It has been postulated that the increased body fat provides a larger storage space for estrogens and that the conversion of adrenal androgens to compounds with estrongenic activity is increased. Such mechanisms might lead to greater hormonal stimulation of the endometrium and myometrium.

PROTEIN-CALORIE MALNUTRITION

MARASMUS

Global starvation—that is, a deficiency of all elements of the diet—leads to marasmus. The condition is common throughout the nonindustrialized world, particularly when breast feeding is stopped and a child must subsist on a calorically inadequate diet. The pathologic changes are similar to those in starving adults, and consist of decreased body weight, diminished subcutaneous fat, a protuberant abdomen, muscle wasting and a wrinkled face. In general, the child is a "shrunken old person." An important consequence of marasmus is growth failure. If these children are not provided with an adequate diet during childhood, they will not reach their full potential stature as adults.

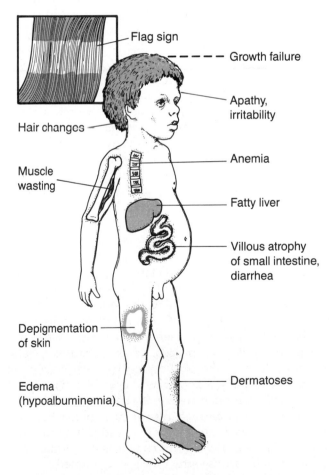

Figure 8-16. Complications of kwashiorkor.

dence of particularly severe periods of protein deficiency. The abdomen is distended because of flaccid abdominal muscles, hepatomegaly and ascites. Along with generalized atrophy of the viscera, villous atrophy of the intestine may interfere with nutrient absorption, and diarrhea is common. Anemia is a usual feature, although not generally life-threatening. Microscopically, the liver of kwashiorkor is conspicuously fatty, and the accumulation of lipid within the cytoplasm of the hepatocyte displaces the nucleus to the periphery of the cell. The adequacy of dietary carbohydrate provides the lipid to the hepatocyte, but the inadequate protein stores do not permit the synthesis of enough apoprotein carrier to transport the lipid from the liver cell. The changes are fully reversible when sufficient protein is made available.

VITAMIN DEFICIENCIES

"Vitamin" is a general term for a number of unrelated organic catalysts that are not endogenously synthesized but are necessary for normal metabolic functions. **The body is therefore totally dependent on dietary sources for these crucial substances.** Critical to the definition of a vitamin is the demonstration that a lack of this compound results in a clearly definable disease. Vitamins A, D, and K are fat soluble, a property which allows for their storage in the liver, and which also accounts for their malabsorption in diseases which interfere with lipid absorption, such as pancreatic disease, biliary obstruction and primary disease of the small bowel (sprue). Because, the water-soluble vitamins—vitamin B complex and vitamin C—are not stored as efficiently as the fat-soluble vitamins, deficiency states occur more rapidly after deprivation of dietary sources.

VITAMIN A DEFICIENCY

Vitamin A, a fat-soluble substance, is important for the maintenance of a number of specialized epithelial linings, skeletal maturation, and the structure of the cell membranes. In addition, it is an important constituent of the photosensitive pigments in the retina. Vitamin A occurs naturally as retinoids, or as a precursor, beta-carotene. The source of the precursor, carotene, is in plants, principally leafy, green vegetables. Fish livers are a particularly rich source of vitamin A itself.

The lack of vitamin A results principally in squamous metaplasia, especially in glandular epithelium (Fig. 8-17). One effect of this change is the formation of an epithelium whose structure is not adapted to functional needs. Stratified squamous epithelium keratinizes, and the keratin debris blocks sweat and tear

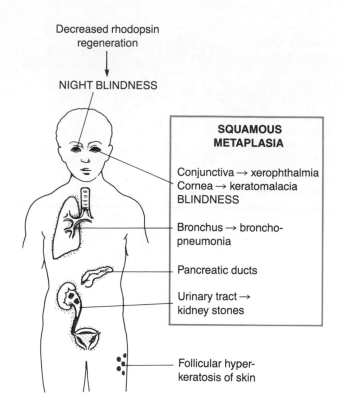

Figure 8-17. Complications of vitamin A deficiency.

glands. Squamous metaplasia is common in the trachea and the bronchi; bronchopneumonia is a frequent cause of death. The lining epithelia of the renal pelvis, pancreatic ducts, uterus, and salivary glands are also commonly affected. Epithelial changes in the renal pelvis are occasionally associated with kidney stones. With further diminution of vitamin A stores, squamous metaplasia of the epithelial cells of the conjunctiva and tear ducts occurs, which leads to **xerophthalmia,** a dryness and wrinkling of the cornea. The cornea becomes softened **(keratomalacia)** and is vulnerable to ulceration and bacterial infection, complications which may lead to blindness. **Follicular hyperkeratosis,** a skin disorder that results from occluded sebaceous glands, is also a feature of this disease.

The earliest sign of vitamin A deficiency often is diminished vision in dim light. Vitamin A is a necessary component in the pigment of the retinal rods and is active in light transduction.

VITAMIN B COMPLEX

Vitamins in the B group of water-soluble vitamins are numbered 1 through 12, but most are not distinct vitamins. The members of the complex which are currently recognized as true vitamins are vitamin B_1 (thiamine), B_2 (riboflavin), niacin, nicotinic acid, B_6 (pyridoxine), and B_{12} (cyanocobalamin).

Deficiencies of thiamine, riboflavin, and niacin are unusual in the industrialized countries because bread and cereals are fortified with these vitamins.

Thiamine Deficiency

With the exception of vitamin B_{12}, which is derived only from animal sources, the vitamins of the B complex, although chemically distinct, are found principally in leafy green vegetables, milk, and liver.

In Western countries, clinical thiamine deficiency (beri-beri) occurs in alcoholics, neglected people with poor overall nutrition, and food faddists. **The cardinal symptoms of thiamine deficiency are polyneuropathy, edema, and cardiac failure** (Fig. 8-18).

The deficiency syndrome is classically divided into **dry beri-beri,** with symptoms referable to the neuromuscular system, and **wet beri-beri,** in which the symptoms of cardiac failure, including generalized edema, predominate. The basic lesion in wet beri-beri is an uncontrolled, generalized vasodilatation and sig-

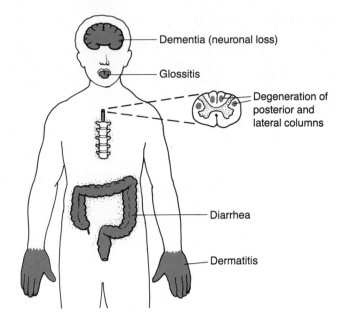

Figure 8-19. Complications of niacin deficiency (pellagra).

nificant peripheral arteriovenous shunting. This combination leads to a compensatory increase in cardiac output, and eventually to a large dilated heart and congestive heart failure. Thiamine deficiency in chronic alcoholics may be manifested by involvement of the brain in the form of **Wernicke's syndrome,** in which progressive **dementia, ataxia** and **ophthalmoplegia** (paralysis of the extraocular muscles) are prominent.

The most reliable diagnostic test for thiamine deficiency is an **immediate and dramatic response to parenteral thiamine.**

Niacin Deficiency

Niacin refers to two chemically distinct compounds: nicotinic acid and nicotinamide. These biologically active components are derived from dietary niacin or are biosynthesized from available tryptophan. Niacin plays a major role in the formation of nicotinamide adenine dinucleotide (NAD) and its phosphate (NADP), compounds important in intermediary metabolism and a wide variety of oxidation-reduction reactions. Animal protein, as found in meat, eggs, and milk, is high in tryptophan, and is therefore a good source of endogenously synthesized niacin. Niacin itself is available in many types of grain. Like other deficiencies of the B vitamins, clinical niacin deficiency, called **pellagra,** is uncommon today; it is seen principally in patients who have been weakened by other diseases and in malnourished alcoholics.

Pellagra (Italian, "rough skin") is characterized by the **three Ds of niacin deficiency: dermatitis, diarrhea, and dementia** (Fig. 8-19).

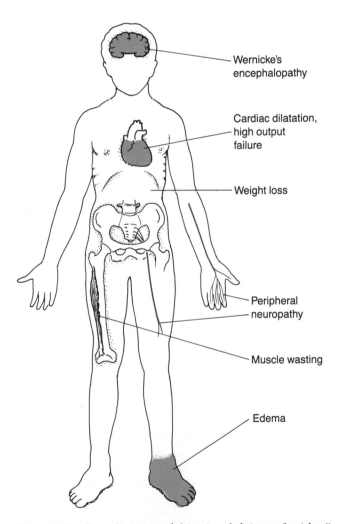

Figure 8-18. Complications of thiamine deficiency (beri-beri).

Riboflavin Deficiency

Riboflavin, a vitamin derived from many plant and animal sources, is important for the synthesis of flavin nucleotides, which play an important role in electron transport and other reactions in which the transfer of energy is crucial.

Riboflavin deficiency is manifested principally by lesions of the facial skin and the corneal epithelium. **Cheilosis,** a term used for fissures in the skin at the angles of the mouth, is a characteristic feature (Fig. 8-20). **Serborrheic dermatitis** involves the cheeks and the areas behind the ears. The tongue is smooth and a purplish (magenta) color, owing to atrophy of the mucosa. The most troubling lesion may be an **interstitial keratitis of the cornea.**

Pyridoxine Deficiency

Vitamin B_6 activity is found in three related, naturally occurring compounds: pyridoxine, pyridoxal and pyridoxamine. For the sake of convenience, they are all grouped under the heading pyridoxine. These compounds are widely distributed in vegetable and animal foods.

Pyridoxine is converted to pyridoxal phosphate, a coenzyme for many enzymes, such as transaminases and carboxylases. Pyridoxine deficiency is rarely caused by an inadequate diet, although infants who have been fed a poorly prepared powdered formula in which the pyridoxine has been destroyed during preparation have suffered convulsions. A higher demand for the vitamin, such as may occur in pregnancy, may lead to a secondary deficiency state. Of particular concern is the deficiency of pyridoxine which follows prolonged medication with a number of drugs, particularly isoniazid, cycloserine and penicillamine. A deficiency state is occasionally seen in alcoholics.

The primary expression of the disease is in the central nervous system, a feature consistent with the role of this vitamin in the formation of pyridoxal-dependent decarboxylase of the neurotransmitter gamma aminobutyric acid (GABA).

Vitamin B_{12} and Folic Acid Deficiencies

A deficiency of vitamin B_{12} is almost always seen in cases of pernicious anemia and results from the lack of secretion of intrinsic factor in the stomach, which prevents absorption of the vitamin in the ileum. Since vitamin B_{12} is found in almost all animal protein, including meat, milk, and eggs, dietary deficiency is seen only in rare cases of extreme vegetarianism, and that only after many years of a restricted diet.

Deficiency of folic acid, the trivial name for pteroyl-monoglutamic acid, is commonly of dietary origin. Leafy vegetables, liver, kidney, and yeast are rich sources of folic acid. However, excessive cooking destroys much of the folic acid in foods. Dietary folic acid deficiency is usually accompanied by multiple vitamin deficiencies. Pregnancy increases the requirement for folic acid fivefold to tenfold. It has been estimated that **two-thirds of anemic pregnant women are folate deficient,** although this may be combined with iron deficiency. Folic acid is absorbed principally in the upper third of the small intestine, and therefore folate deficiency is common in certain diseases of malabsorption, notably nontropical and tropical sprue. The latter condition is responsive to folic acid treatment.

Deficiencies of both vitamin B_{12} and folic acid are associated with **megaloblastic anemia.** In addition, pernicious anemia is complicated by a neurologic condition called **subacute combined degeneration of the spinal cord.** A comprehensive discussion of vitamin B_{12} and folic acid deficiencies is found in Chapter 20, which deals with hematologic disorders, and Chapter 28, which is devoted to neuropathology.

VITAMIN C (ASCORBIC ACID) DEFICIENCY

Ascorbic acid is a powerful biological reducing agent that is involved in numerous oxidation-reduction reac-

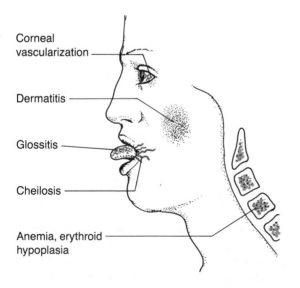

Corneal vascularization

Dermatitis

Glossitis

Cheilosis

Anemia, erythroid hypoplasia

Figure 8-20. Complications of riboflavin deficiency.

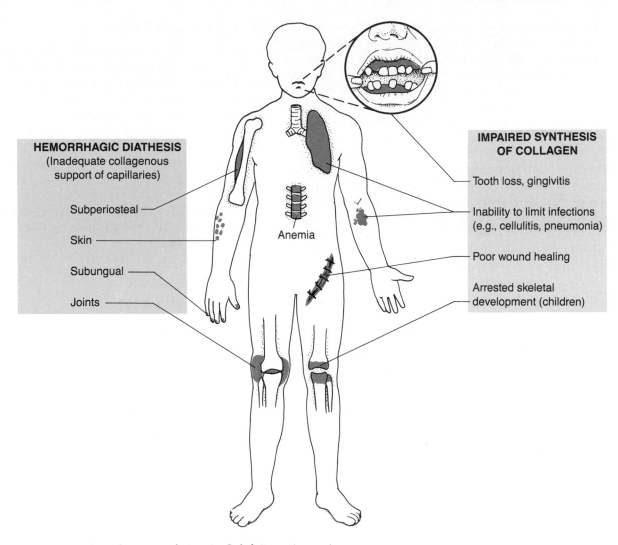

HEMORRHAGIC DIATHESIS
(Inadequate collagenous
support of capillaries)

Subperiosteal

Skin

Subungual

Joints

Anemia

IMPAIRED SYNTHESIS
OF COLLAGEN

Tooth loss, gingivitis

Inability to limit infections
(e.g., cellulitis, pneumonia)

Poor wound healing

Arrested skeletal
development (children)

Figure 8-21. Complications of vitamin C deficiency (scurvy).

tions and the transfer of protons. This vitamin is important in the synthesis of chondroitin sulphate and in the hydroxylation of proline to form the hydroxyproline of collagen. It serves many other important functions, such as preventing the oxidation of tetrahydrofolate and augmenting the absorption of iron from the gut. Without vitamin C the biosynthesis of certain neurotransmitters is impaired because of a reduction in the activity of dopamine-beta-hydroxylase. Wound healing and immune functions are also under the the influence of ascorbic acid. The best dietary sources of vitamin C are citrus fruits, green vegetables, and tomatoes. Man and the guinea pig lack the ability to make ascorbic acid, an incapacity which can be explained as an evolutionary quirk.

The clinical vitamin C deficiency state is termed **scurvy.** Scurvy is uncommon in the Western world, but is often seen in nonindustrialized countries in which other forms of malnutrition are prevalent. In the industrialized countries, scurvy is now a disease of people afflicted with chronic diseases who do not eat well, the neglected aged, and malnourished alcoholics.

Most of the events associated with scurvy are caused by the formation of abnormal collagen that lacks tensile strength (Fig. 8-21). Within 1 to 3 months, subperiosteal hemorrhages lead to pain in the bones and joints. Petechial hemorrhages, ecchymoses and purpura are common, particularly after mild trauma or at pressure points. Perifollicular hemorrhages in the skin are particularly typical of scurvy. In advanced cases, swollen, bleeding gums are a classical finding. Alveolar bone resorption results in loosening and loss of teeth. Wound healing is poor, and dehiscence of previously healed wounds occurs. Anemia may result from prolonged bleeding, impaired iron absorption, or an associated folic acid deficiency. In children, vitamin C deficiency leads to growth failure, and collagen-rich structures such as the teeth, bones, and blood vessels develop abnormally. The effects on developing bone are conspicuous and relate principally to impaired calcification. The effects of scurvy on bone are discussed in greater detail in Chapter 26, which deals with bone pathology. In addition to poor wound healing, scorbutic individuals have difficulty in walling off an infection to form an abscess, and infections therefore spread more easily.

VITAMIN D DEFICIENCY

Vitamin D is a fat-soluble steroid hormone found in two forms: vitamin D_3 (cholecalciferol) and vitamin D_2 (ergocalciferol), both of which have equal biological potency in man. Vitamin D_3 is produced in the skin, and vitamin D_2 is derived from plant ergosterol. **To achieve biological potency, vitamin D must be hydroxylated to active metabolites in the liver and kidney. The active form of the vitamin promotes calcium and phosphate absorption from the small intestine.**

Vitamin D deficiency results from insufficient vitamin D in the diet, insufficient production of vitamin D in the skin because of limited sunlight exposure as a result of occupation or dress, inadequate absorption of vitamin D from the diet (as in the fat malabsorption syndromes), or abnormal conversion of vitamin D to its bioactive metabolites. The last occurs in liver disease and chronic renal failure. **In children, vitamin D deficiency causes rickets; in adults osteomalacia is seen.**

VITAMIN E DEFICIENCY

Vitamin E is an antioxidant that, experimentally at least, protects membrane phospholipids against lipid peroxidation by free radicals formed by cellular metabolism. The activity of this fat-soluble vitamin is found in a number of dietary constituents, principally in alpha-trocopherol. Corn and soy beans are particularly rich in vitamin E. A dietary deficiency of vitamin E is rare, except among the individuals receiving total parenteral nutrition, and a clearly definable syndrome associated with vitamin E deficiency has not been identified in adults. In premature infants, hemolytic anemia, thrombocytosis, and edema have been associated with a deficiency of vitamin E.

VITAMIN K DEFICIENCY

Vitamin K, a fat-soluble material, occurs in two forms: vitamin K_1, from plants, and vitamin K_2, which is principally synthesized by the normal intestinal bacteria. Green leafy vegetables are rich in vitamin K, and liver and dairy products contain smaller amounts. Dietary deficiency of vitamin K is very uncommon in the United States. Most cases are associated with other disorders. However, vitamin K deficiency is common in severe fat malabsorption, as seen in sprue and biliary tract obstruction. The destruction of intestinal flora by antibiotics may also result in vitamin K deficiency. Newborn infants frequently exhibit vitamin K deficiency, because the vitamin is not transported well across the placenta, and the sterile gut of the newborn does not have bacteria to produce it. Vitamin K, which confers calcium-binding properties to certain proteins, is important for the activity of four clotting factors: prothrombin, factor VII, factor IX and factor X. Deficiency of vitamin K can be serious, because it can lead to catastrophic bleeding.

9

INFECTIOUS AND PARASITIC DISEASES

DANIEL H. CONNOR AND DEAN W. GIBSON

DISEASES CAUSED BY VIRUSES

YELLOW FEVER

Yellow fever is an acute viral hemorrhagic fever caused by a flavivirus of the family Togaviridae and characterized by jaundice and renal damage. It is primarily a zoonosis of simians that is transmitted by mosquitoes. The virus is restricted to certain regions of Africa and South America, including both jungle and urban settings. The usual reservoir is tree-dwelling monkeys, the virus being passed among them in the forest canopy by *Aedes* mosquitoes.

In yellow fever there is usually a short incubation period (3 to 6 days), followed by sudden onset of high fever, chills, headache, and myalgia (lasting 3 to 4 days). A second stage consists of hepatic failure, renal failure, bleeding diathesis, leukopenia, and hypotension. Yellow fever tends to heal without sequelae, and mortality is less than 5%.

The major pathologic changes are in the liver and kidney. The liver is bile-stained and has an accentuated lobular pattern caused by midzonal necrosis. Microscopically, there are three characteristic changes: **midzonal necrosis, Councilman bodies, and microvesicular fat.** Councilman bodies are intensely eosinophilic oval bodies that represent necrotic parenchymal cells that have lost their nuclei and have been extruded from the liver cell plate.

DENGUE FEVER

Uncomplicated dengue fever (breakbone fever), a disease of densely populated areas, is a benign, self-limited, febrile disease that affects muscles and joints. By contrast, dengue hemorrhagic fever, a severe and potentially fatal variant, is characterized by high fever, cutaneous and intestinal hemorrhage, thrombocytopenia, shock, and neurologic disturbances. It is a disease of children throughout Southeast Asia, Indonesia, and Pakistan; there was an outbreak in Cuba in 1981. Transmission is highest during and after the rainy season, when mosquitoes are most numerous.

ARTHROPOD-BORNE VIRAL ENCEPHALITIS (ARBOVIRUS ENCEPHALITIS)

Arthropod-borne viruses (arboviruses) are a large, heterogeneous group of viruses transmitted between vertebrates by blood-sucking arthropod vectors, such as mosquitoes and ticks. There are eight arboviruses that cause meningoencephalitis in man, and each of the arthropod-borne viral encephalitides is confined to a particular geographic area and a specific vector.

Clinical symptoms range from a mild grippe-like illness to fulminating and fatal encephalitis. The encephalitis usually begins abruptly, with fever, headache, disturbed consciousness and sometimes signs of meningitis, convulsions, or paralysis. The clinical course is usually short, not chronic as in some other viral infections.

The histologic findings in these encephalitides are usually confined to the central nervous system and are similar for all types. The lesions range from a mild meningitis with scattered lymphocytes to more severe inflammation of the gray matter, mainly around neurons, to prominent necrosis. Perivascular cuffing appears in the acute phase.

EASTERN EQUINE ENCEPHALITIS

Eastern equine encephalitis (EEE) is encountered primarily in the eastern and north central United States and adjoining provinces of Canada. The reservoir is birds and mosquitoes are the vector. EEE occurs primarily during summer in temperate zones.

WESTERN EQUINE ENCEPHALITIS

Western equine encephalitis (WEE) is encountered primarily in the western and central United States and Canada. The reservoir is birds, and mosquitoes are the vector. WEE occurs primarily in May to September.

ST. LOUIS ENCEPHALITIS

St. Louis encephalitis **is the most important arbovirus infection in North America.** It occurs throughout the United States (except New England), in Ontario, Canada, and less frequently in scattered areas in the Caribbean and Central and South America. The reservoir is birds; mosquitoes are the vector. The disease occurs during late summer and early fall.

POLIOMYELITIS

Poliomyelitis is an acute infection by polioviruses. Most infections are asymptomatic, but when the virus invades the central nervous system it destroys lower motor neurons, causing paralysis. Sporadic infections

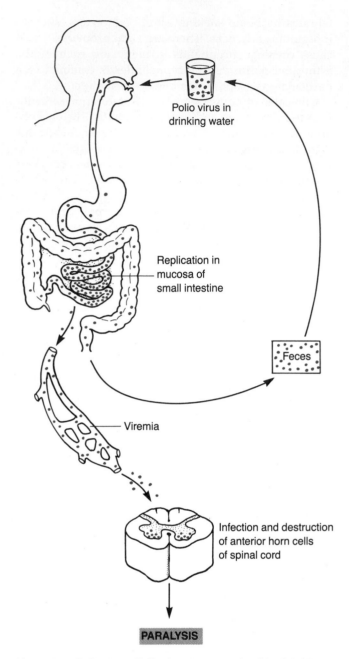

Figure 9-1. Poliovirus. Poliovirus is transmitted in drinking water contaminated with feces. Virions replicate in the mucosa of the small intestine, and some pass into the feces to contaminate water and complete the cycle. Others enter the circulation, invade the spinal cord, and destroy the anterior horn cells, causing paralysis of the lower motor neuron.

may be seen at any time, but outbreaks occur mostly in the summer. More recent epidemics have stricken adults as well as children.

Poliovirus is transmitted in drinking water contaminated with feces (Fig. 9-1). The virus replicates in the mucosa of the small intestine. Some virions pass from there into the feces, contaminating water and completing the cycle. Others enter the bloodstream (viremia) and extend to the spinal cord, where they infect and destroy the anterior horn cells, causing paralysis.

SMALLPOX (VARIOLA)

Before its eradication, smallpox (variola) was an acute, highly contagious, exanthematous viral infection. The virus contains double-stranded DNA and produces a typical plaque, or "pock," when cultured on the choriollantoic membrane of embryonated chicken eggs. Smallpox was transmitted in respiratory droplets and almost always involved face-to-face contact.

The characteristic eruption of smallpox evolved through several stages, beginning as macules, then progressing over a 1- to 2-week period through papules, vesicles, and pustules. The pustules umbilicated within 2 weeks, and desiccated ("crusted") to form scabs. The scabs, which contained the smallpox virus, usually sloughed from the skin, thereby creating fresh, pitted scars.

HERPESVIRUS INFECTIONS

Five herpesviruses infect man: varicella-zoster virus; herpes simplex virus, types 1 and 2; cytomegalovirus; and Epstein-Barr virus (EBV). Varicella-zoster virus causes chickenpox in nonimmune persons and shingles in those who have had chickenpox. Herpes simplex viruses 1 and 2 cause "fever blisters" and genital lesions, respectively. Cytomegalovirus is the agent of cytomegalic inclusion disease, and Epstein-Barr virus causes infectious mononucleosis. Each of these viruses may disseminate and kill patients with defective or suppressed immunity.

Herpesviruses are enveloped double-stranded DNA viruses with similar ultrastructural features. **A principal histologic feature is the formation of Cowdry type A intranuclear inclusions in epithelial and other cells of the host.** These acidophilic (red with eosin) inclusions have a diameter that exceeds half the diameter of the nucleus and are surrounded by a clear zone ("halo") of vacant nucleoplasm.

VARICELLA (CHICKENPOX)— VARICELLA-ZOSTER VIRUS

Varicella (chickenpox) is an acute vesicular exanthem caused by the varicella-zoster virus, an agent that has a worldwide distribution and for which humans are the

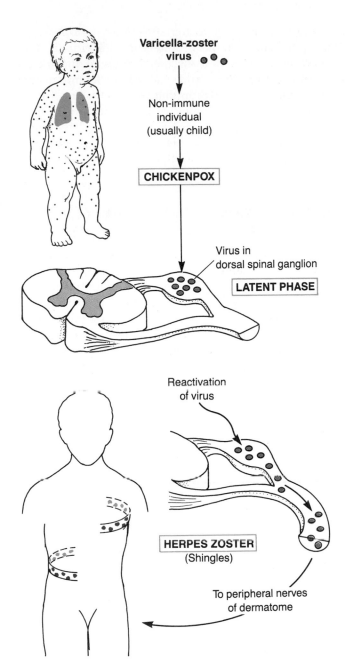

only known host. Although all age groups are susceptible, in temperate zones chickenpox affects mostly children and in the tropics mostly young adults. The virus, which is spread through inhalation of droplets or by direct contact, is highly contagious from about 24 hours before the initial eruption to a week or more thereafter. Although infection with varicella-zoster virus establishes lifelong immunity and chickenpox does not recur, the latent viral genome may be activated years later to cause shingles.

Nonimmune persons (usually children) are susceptible to primary infection with varicella-zoster virus. A red maculopapular eruption develops, usually on the upper trunk and face. The papules rapidly become clear vesicles, which eventually heal without scarring. Complications include pneumonia, encephalitis, hepatitis, carditis, keratitis, orchitis, arthritis, hemorrhages, and acute encephalopathy with fat accumulation in the viscera (Reye's syndrome).

HERPES ZOSTER (SHINGLES)—VARICELLA-ZOSTER VIRUS

Herpes zoster (shingles) is a recurrent, painful, erythematous vesicular eruption caused by the reactivation of latent varicella-zoster virus in an individual who had chickenpox years earlier. Adults with shingles may transmit the virus to children and cause chickenpox. During the latent phase, the virus resides in the dorsal root spinal ganglion or the cranial nerve ganglion (see Fig. 9-2). On reactivation, the virus spreads from the ganglia along sensory nerves to peripheral nerves of the sensory dermatomes. Attacks of shingles produce cutaneous lesions that resemble varicella. In shingles, however, the eruptions are limited to one or more sensory dermatomes, and the vesicles or bullae may be few. Shingles is painful, especially in older people, in contrast to the painless vesicles of children with chickenpox. Eventually the scales over the vesicles slough, and symptoms remit until another attack.

HERPES SIMPLEX—HERPES SIMPLEX VIRUS TYPE 1

Herpes simplex virus type 1 is responsible for a spectrum of vesicular and necrotizing lesions, principally on the skin, lips, and mucous membranes. Neonates and immunodeficient patients may have disseminated infections, with involvement of many organs, including the liver, lung, and brain.

Those without debilitating disease or immunodeficiency, and infants older than 1 month, have a mild infection, lesions being localized to the oral cavity, lips,

Figure 9-2. Varicella (chickenpox) and herpes zoster (shingles).

Varicella (chickenpox). Varicella-zoster virus (VZV) in droplets is inhaled by a nonimmune person (usually a child) and initially causes a "silent" infection of the nasopharynx. This progresses to viremia, seeding of reticuloendothelial cells, and dissemination of VZV to skin and viscera. The VZV resides in a dorsal spinal ganglion, where it remains dormant for many years.

Herpes zoster (shingles). Latent VZV is reactivated and spreads from ganglia along the sensory nerves to the peripheral nerves of sensory dermatomes.

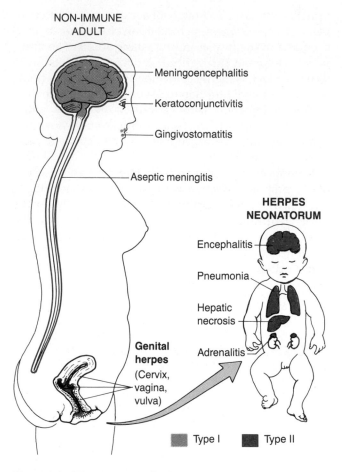

NON-IMMUNE
ADULT

Meningoencephalitis

Keratoconjunctivitis

Gingivostomatitis

Aseptic meningitis

**HERPES
NEONATORUM**

Encephalitis

Pneumonia

Hepatic
necrosis

**Genital
herpes**
(Cervix,
vagina,
vulva)

Adrenalitis

Type I   Type II

Figure 9-3. Herpesvirus infections.
Herpes simplex. Herpes simplex virus type 1 (HSV-1) infects a nonimmune adult, causing gingivostomatitis ("fever blister" or "cold sore"), keratoconjunctivitis, meningoencephalitis, and aseptic spinal meningitis.
Genital herpes. Herpes simplex virus type 2 (HSV-2) infects the genitalia of a nonimmune adult, involving the cervix, vagina, and vulva.
Herpes neonatorum. HSV-2 infects the fetus as it passes through the birth canal of an infected mother. The infant's lack of a mature immune system results in disseminated infection with HSV-2. The infection is often fatal, involving lung, liver, adrenal glands, and central nervous system.

eyes, and skin. In addition to dissemination, complications include gingivostomatitis—commonly known as a "fever blister" or "cold sore"—keratoconjunctivitis, meningoencephalitis, and aseptic spinal meningitis (Fig. 9-3).

During acute gingivostomatitis or asymptomatic primary infection of the oropharynx, the virus invades nerve endings in mucous membranes of the mouth, ascends within axons, and establishes a latent infection in the trigeminal ganglion that persists for life. Various stimuli—e.g., fever, exposure to actinic light, respiratory infections, and stress—reactivate the latent virus. It then descends within the axon to peripheral nerve twigs, reinfects the lip or adjacent mucous membrane, and causes recurrent blisters.

GENITAL HERPES—HERPES SIMPLEX VIRUS TYPE 2

Genital herpes, caused by herpes simplex-virus type 2, is sexually transmitted and produces a spectrum of vesicular and necrotizing lesions on or about the genitalia (see Fig. 9-3). As with herpes simplex virus type 1, primary lesions develop in those without previous exposure and without antibodies, and recurrent lesions are common. **Neonates are especially susceptible to disseminated herpes simplex virus type 2.** Normal adults and infants older than 1 month have mild infections that present as vesicles on the mucous membranes of the genitalia and on the external genitalia. Latent infections are established in a manner analogous to that for the type 1 virus. Months or years later, nonspecific stimuli, including menses and sexual intercourse, reactivate the virus, which descends within axons to the genital mucosa or skin and causes a recurrent genital herpetic lesion.

CYTOMEGALIC INCLUSION DISEASE— CYTOMEGALOVIRUS

Cytomegalic inclusion disease, an infection with cytomegalovirus, may be congenital; perinatal; postnatal in infants after loss of maternal antibodies; "classic" in older adolescents and adults with "normal" immunity; or a disseminated, possibly lethal, opportunistic infection in immunodeficient persons, including those with lymphomas, leukemias, and AIDS. The general population has a high incidence of exposure to this virus, as indicated by seropositivity rates of 50% to 80% among adults. There is special concern for infection in pregnant women because cytomegalovirus may be transmitted to the fetus or infant.

The modes of transmission are the following: (1) intrauterine, from the placenta and maternal circulation; (2) perinatal, as the fetus passes through the birth canal; (3) venereal, from semen or vaginal fluid; (4) mammary, from mother's milk; (5) respiratory, from inhalation of contaminated droplets; (6) transfusional, from latent virus in circulating leukocytes; and (7) transplantational, from grafts taken from donors with latent infections.

The target organs and severity vary with the mode of transmission. Infections in utero damage the brain, sometimes causing mental retardation or death of the fetus. Infants with congenital infections may be premature and exhibit anemia, thrombocytopenia, jaundice, purpura, hepatosplenomegaly (from extramedullary hematopoiesis), and interstitial pneumonitis. Most congenital infections produce no clinically apparent lesions at birth. However, even asymptomatic congenital infections may enter the latent phase and be reactivated years later to cause more serious disease.

The most prominent feature of classic cytomegalic inclusion disease in neonates is the one for which it is named, **the cytomegalic inclusion.** Compared to epithelial cells without inclusions, those that contain inclusions are greatly enlarged. These inclusions, which are more characteristic than any of the other viral inclusions, are typically intranuclear, but may also be intracytoplasmic. The nucleus is enlarged and the chromatin marginated. The round nuclear inclusion is large, sharply outlined, and either amphophilic or eosinophilic. The cytoplasmic inclusions, when present, tend to be amphophilic and of variable shape.

INFECTIOUS MONONUCLEOSIS— EPSTEIN-BARR VIRUS

Infectious mononucleosis, a benign, self-limited disease, results from infection with the Epstein-Barr virus. It is characterized by intense proliferation of lymphoid cells in the spleen, lymph nodes, and blood. Patients have "heterophile antibody" (agglutinin) in their serum. Epstein-Barr virus has the appearance of herpesvirus, but it does not have significant serologic cross-reactivity with other viruses of the herpes group. Many people in western countries are asymptomatic carriers.

In most of the world, primary infection with Epstein-Barr virus is an asymptomatic childhood illness. On the other hand, infectious mononucleosis usually occurs in late adolescence in the upper socioeconomic classes—that is, among those who are unlikely to be exposed in childhood. The virus is commonly transmitted by kissing. In a seronegative person, the virus replicates within the salivary glands or pharyngeal epithelium and is shed into the saliva and respiratory secretions (Fig. 9-4). The virus then infects B-lympho-

cytes, which have receptors for the virus. Polyclonal activation of infected B cells leads to transformed B cells that activate two types of lymphocytes: T_K ("killer") lymphocytes, which kill B cells, and T_s ("suppressor") lymphocytes, which suppress polyclonal immunoglobulin production by B cells. **The activated T cells are the so-called atypical lymphocytes characteristic of infectious mononucleosis.**

The clinical features of infectious mononucleosis include **the triad of fever, sore throat and lymphadenopathy, atypical T_K ("killer") and B lymphocytes in the blood, and heterophile agglutinin in the serum.** In the blood there is an absolute increase in lymphocytes and monocytes, with more than 10% atypical lymphocytes. Splenomegaly is also a common feature. Ninety percent of patients have abnormal liver function, half have variable degrees of thrombocytopenia —some with petechiae—and 40% have hemolytic anemia caused by cold agglutinins.

Epstein-Barr virus was discovered during ultrastructural studies of endemic Burkitt's lymphoma in Africa. There is now evidence that the virus causes two cancers—endemic Burkitt's lymphoma in Africa (Fig. 9-5) and nasopharyngeal carcinoma, especially in the Orient.

MEASLES (RUBEOLA)

Measles (rubeola) is an acute, highly contagious, systemic infection of childhood caused by the measles (rubeola) virus. Humans are the only reservoir. Measles is most commonly transmitted by inhalation.

The prodrome, which lasts 3 to 5 days, is characterized by fever, conjunctivitis, a prominent dry cough, coryza, and **Koplik's spots**—red, irregular macules, 1 to 3 mm in diameter, with a central white speck, located on the buccal mucosa. It recedes with the appearance of the blotchy, erythematous rash of measles. The rash begins as pink macules behind the ears, quickly becomes maculopapular and rapidly spreads over the face and down the neck, trunk, and limbs. The nonproductive cough increases as the rash develops. The rash lasts a few days and then clears.

Measles is usually benign in children with normal immunity, but can have serious or catastrophic complications in the malnourished, in the immunosuppressed, in neonates, and in the elderly. Complications and sequelae include otitis media, pneumonia (either measles virus or secondary bacterial pneumonia), measles encephalitis, subacute sclerosing panencephalitis, juvenile diabetes mellitus and thrombocytopenic purpura.

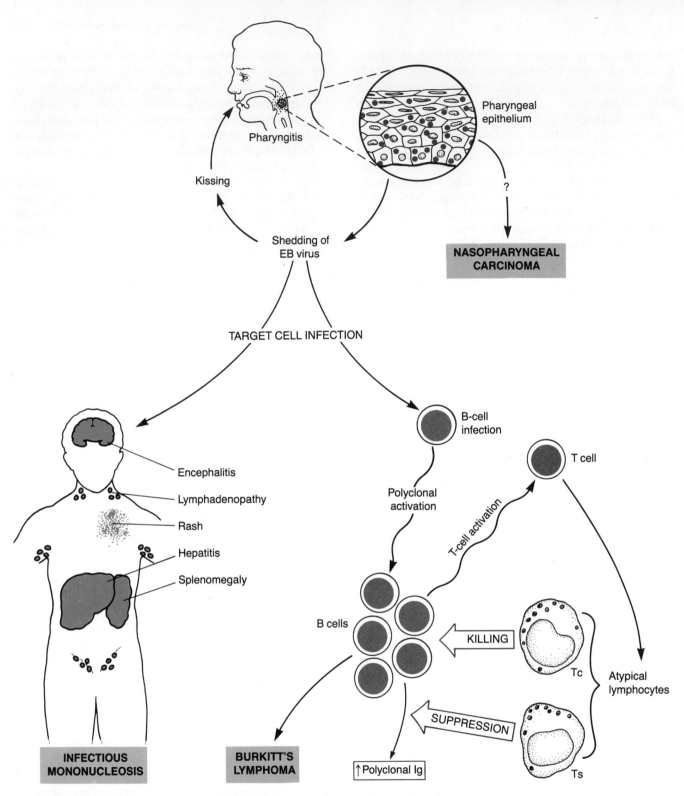

Figure 9-4. Role of Epstein-Barr virus (EBV) in infectious mononucleosis, nasopharyngeal carcinoma, and Burkitt's lymphoma. EBV invades and replicates within the salivary glands or pharyngeal epithelium, and is shed into the saliva and respiratory secretions. In some people, the virus transforms pharyngeal epithelial cells, leading to nasopharyngeal carcinoma. In people who are not immune from childhood exposure, EBV causes infectious mononucleosis. EBV infects B lymphocytes, which undergo polyclonal activation. These B cells stimulate the production of T_k and T_s lymphocytes in the blood of patients with infectious mononucleosis. Some infected B cells are transformed into immature malignant lymphocytes of Burkitt's lymphoma.

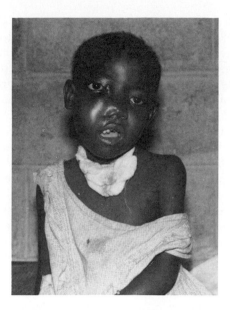

Figure 9-5. Burkitt's lymphoma involving the right maxilla and right mandible of a young African from eastern Zaire.

GERMAN MEASLES (RUBELLA)

German measles, or rubella, is a mild, systemic illness of childhood caused by rubella virus. The disease is characterized by measles-like rash, low-grade fever, and swollen posterior auricular and occipital lymph nodes. Subclinical infections are common. The mild rash and other symptoms resolve within 3 days. Initially, swollen, nontender posterior auricular and occipital lymph nodes appear. A day or two later the nonpruritic rash begins on the face and rapidly spreads over the rest of the body, sparing the palms and soles.

The virus is very contagious and is shed from the nasopharynx. **The virus is also transmitted through the placenta, and rubella infections in pregnant women are a serious public health concern because intrauterine infection causes spontaneous abortion, fetal death, and a variety of congenital abnormalities.** Infection during the first trimester is most serious. The principal congenital abnormalities are patent ductus arteriosus, pulmonary and aortic stenosis, coarctation of the aorta, defects of the atrial or ventricular septum, ocular lesions (cataracts, glaucoma, and chorioretinitis), deafness, microcephaly, mental retardation, and retarded growth.

MUMPS

Mumps is an acute but usually mild viral infection of childhood characterized by swollen and inflamed sali-vary glands, most often the parotids. Less often the virus attacks the pancreas, ovaries, testes, and other organs. Mumps virus is a highly contagious paramyxovirus that is commonly transmitted in respiratory droplets. Mumps is usually diagnosed clinically from swollen salivary glands and confirmed by finding rising titers of mumps virus in the serum of convalescent patients.

The most common complication is a painful orchitis with parenchymal hemorrhage. The tunica albuginea tightly contains the swollen testis, which may result in necrosis of seminiferous tubules, local hemorrhages, and microinfarctions, sometimes leaving permanent fibrous scars. Mumps orchitis is usually unilateral and thus rarely causes male sterility. Infection of the pancreas leads to pancreatitis, characterized by necrosis of pancreatic and fat cells.

RESPIRATORY VIRUSES (VIRAL PNEUMONIAS)

Respiratory disorders are caused by a wide variety of viruses, of different families, species, and serotypes. These include orthomyxoviruses (influenza A, B, and C), paramyxoviruses (respiratory syncytial virus), parainfluenza viruses, measles virus, adenoviruses, herpesviruses (varicella-zoster virus), cytomegalovirus, and herpes simplex virus (HSV), picornaviruses (rhinoviruses, echoviruses, and coxsackieviruses), and human respiratory coronaviruses.

ORTHOMYXOVIRUSES (INFLUENZA)

Influenza viruses are highly contagious and afflict people of all ages. They are transmitted by aerosols generated by coughing and sneezing. Influenza A virus, the most common cause of viral pneumonia in adults, produces pandemics. Influenza B virus causes epidemics, and is associated with Reye's syndrome in children and pneumonitis and croup in infants. Influenza C virus causes sporadic upper respiratory infections, but not epidemic influenza.

The histopathologic features of influenza viruses include a necrotizing bronchitis and diffuse hemorrhagic necrotizing pneumonitis with pulmonary edema. Ciliated epithelial cells are destroyed and goblet cells and mucous glands disrupted. Bronchioles become thickened, distended, and infiltrated with mononuclear cells. There is often severe inflammatory edema, and a fluid exudate in the alveolar spaces has a hyaline appearance.

RESPIRATORY SYNCYTIAL VIRUS

The respiratory syncytial virus is the most common cause of viral pneumonia in children under 2 years of age and is a common cause of death in infants aged 1 to 6 months. Susceptibility is also increased in elderly or immunocompromised patients. This agent accounts for about one-third of hospital admissions for pneumonia and for up to 90% of those for bronchiolitis. Histopathologic features include necrotizing bronchitis, bronchiolitis, and interstitial pneumonia.

PARAINFLUENZA VIRUSES (TYPES 1-4B)

Type 3 parainfluenza is the most prevalent of the parainfluenzas, occurring endemically throughout the year. Infants are especially susceptible. Parainfluenza viruses are spread principally by direct contact or by large droplets (in contrast to the spread of influenza virus by inhalation of small droplets). Histopathologic features include necrotizing bronchitis, bronchiolitis, and interstitial pneumonia.

MEASLES VIRUS (RUBEOLA) PNEUMONIA

Measles pneumonia occurs in up to half of patients with measles, usually within 5 days of development of the rash. The histopathologic appearance varies from pure interstitial (viral) pneumonia to lobar (bacterial) pneumonia. There are often pathognomonic multinucleated giant cells (Warthin-Finkeldey cells), intranuclear and intracytoplasmic inclusions, and hyperplasia of distal bronchial cells. In immunocompromised patients measles pneumonia may occur without rash and is often fatal.

ADENOVIRUS PNEUMONIA

Adenoviruses are common causes of acute respiratory disease, and adenovirus pneumonia is seen in military recruits coming together for the first time for basic training. Adenoviruses are also important causes of chronic pulmonary disease in infants and young children. Histopathologic features of adenovirus pneumonitis include necrotizing bronchitis and bronchiolitis, with necrosis and desquamation of the epithelium.

PICORNAVIRUS PNEUMONIAS

Picornaviruses are animal viruses named for their small size and single-stranded RNA. Pneumonias may be a complication of some infections with three classes of picornavirus: rhinoviruses, echoviruses, and coxsackieviruses.

Rhinoviruses, of which there are more than 100 species, are transmitted by direct contact with infected secretions, rather than by inhalation of aerosols. **These agents replicate in the epithelial cells of the nasal mucosa and are shed primarily from the nose. They are the most common cause of the "common cold."**

Echoviruses and coxsackieviruses are enteroviruses that infect man primarily through the ingestion of fecally contaminated material. After replicating in lymph nodes they may enter the bloodstream, replicate further in the reticuloendothelial system, and disseminate in the bloodstream, a process that infrequently results in respiratory disorders.

Human respiratory coronaviruses, which contain single-stranded RNA, are the second most common causes of the "common cold." They characteristically cause a profuse nasal discharge, but have little or no effect on the lower respiratory tract.

DISEASES CAUSED BY MYCOPLASMAS

Mycoplasma pneumoniae causes tracheobronchitis and "primary atypical pneumonias," most frequently affecting children and adolescents. Infections are worldwide and account for about 20% of all cases of peneumonia in some cities. Most infections occur in small groups of people who have frequent close contact, for example, families, college fraternities, military units, and closed institutions. The organism is spread by aerosol transmission from person to person over a period of several months, with an attack rate of greater than 50% within the group. Clinical features are an initial nonproductive cough followed by the production of watery or mucoid sputum, fever, rhinorrhea, chest pain, and generalized myalgia. The symptoms and signs usually abate within 10 to 14 days, and recovery is hastened by treatment with broad-spectrum antibiotics.

DISEASES CAUSED BY CHLAMYDIAE

Chlamydiae are obligate intracellular gram-negative bacteria. Chlamydial infections are widespread among birds and mammals, and perhaps 20% of the human population is infected. **Chlamydial diseases in humans include trachoma, inclusion conjunctivitis,** psittacosis, lymphogranuloma venereum, infections of the urethra, cervix, and salpinx, and neonatal pneumonitis. Chlamydial cervicitis and urethritis are the most common sexually transmitted diseases in North America.

PSITTACOSIS (PARROT FEVER, ORNITHOSIS)

Psittacosis, a disease of birds that is transmissible to man, is an acute infection caused by *Chlamydia psittaci*. *C. psittaci* is harbored by many birds, including chickens, turkeys, pigeons, and sea gulls, and by many mammals. Man usually acquires the disease by contacting infected birds.

C. psittaci causes systemic disease in man, but pulmonary involvement is most prominent. The organisms are inhaled with dust-born contaminated excreta or aerosolized droplets. The organisms are carried to the reticuloendothelial cells of the liver and spleen, proliferate, and disseminate to the lungs and other organs.

The disease ranges in severity from subclinical to fatal. A persistent dry hacking cough, fine crepitant rales, and tachypnea are typical.

Psittacosis begins as an inflammatory process in the lung and progresses to consolidation, primarily lobular but occasionally lobar. It progresses through a sequence of congestion, edema, and red and gray hepatization. Histopathologically, fibrin, erythrocytes, and neutrophils appear early in the alveolar exudate. Later the alveoli contain large mononuclear cells and epithelial cells. Interstitial infiltration is not present in early stages, but as the disease progresses lymphocytes and monocytes invade the alveolar walls. Hyperplasia of alveolar type 2 pneumocytes is typical.

TRACHOMA

Trachoma is a chronic progressive infection of the conjunctiva and cornea that may cause partial or total blindness. **Infection with *Chlamydia trachomatis* is the leading cause of preventable blindness in the world.** The disease is worldwide, associated with poverty, and most prevalent in dry or sandy regions.

In endemic areas infection is acquired early in childhood, becomes chronic, and eventually progresses to blindness. An abrupt onset of palpebral and conjunctivitis, and photophobia. As chronic inflammation progresses over months and years, there is scarring of the upper tarsal plate and corneal keratitis, with the for-

mation of a vascular pannus. Scarring, trichiasis, and entropion eventually interfere with normal ocular function.

LYMPHOGRANULOMA VENEREUM

Lymphogranuloma venereum, a sexually transmitted disease of man caused by *C. trachomatis*, is characterized by a transient primary cutaneous or mucosal lesion and regional lymphadenitis. Although the disease is present worldwide, the highest prevalence is in the tropics and subtropics: it accounts for up to 6% of sexually transmitted disease in Africa, Southeast Asia, and India. In North America and Europe, lymphogranuloma venereum is now primarily a disease of homosexual men.

A primary lesion, which is painless and herpetiform, develops at the site of infection. It usually occurs on the penis, vagina, or cervix, but lips, tongue, and fingers are other primary sites. Before the primary lesion appears, *C. trachomatis* is carried in the lymphatics to regional lymph nodes, which then enlarge. Any group may be involved and enlargement may be unilateral or bilateral. Over the next few weeks the nodes become tender and fluctuant, and frequently ulcerate and discharge pus. Lymphadenopathy and drainage may persist for several weeks or months. Primary anorectal lymphogranuloma venereum, usually in homosexual men, causes severe proctocolitis, accompanied by ten-

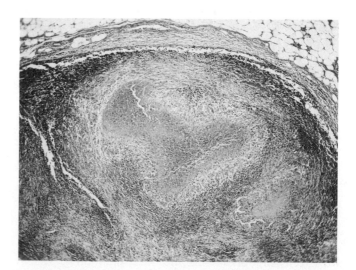

Figure 9-6. Lymphogranuloma venereum. The necrotic central area of this lymph node is surrounded by a granulomatous zone with palisading epithelioid cells, macrophages, and occasional giant cells surrounded, in turn, by a wide zone of lymphocytes and plasma cells.

esmus, diarrhea, bleeding, fever and weight loss. Lymphatic obstruction develops in 10% to 20% of untreated patients and can cause genital elephantiasis in women.

The primary cutaneous lesion is a superficial ulcer without specific features. **The lymph nodes contain characteristic multiple, coalescing abscesses, which have the appearance of granulomas.** There are neutrophils and necrotic debris in the center, surrounded by a zone of palisaded epithelioid cells, macrophages, and occasional giant cells. In turn, this zone is surrounded by lymphocytes, plasma cells, and fibrous tissue (Fig. 9-6). Healing is by fibrosis with effacement of the normal architecture of the node.

CHLAMYDIAL INFECTIONS OF THE GENITAL TRACT

C. trachomatis causes urethritis, epididymitis, and proctitis in men and cervicitis, salpingitis, urethritis, and proctitis in women. **In adults, these infections are sexually transmitted; they have surpassed gonorrhea as the leading cause of sexually contracted disease in North America.**

DISEASES CAUSED BY RICKETTSIAE

EPIDEMIC TYPHUS (LOUSE-BORNE TYPHUS)

Epidemic typhus (louse-borne typhus) is caused by *Rickettsia prowazekii*. This disease is widely distributed in some regions of Africa, Asia, Europe, and the western hemisphere. Its devastating epidemics were associated with cold climates, poor sanitation, and crowding during natural disasters, famine, or war. Epidemic typhus may kill 60% or more of the untreated aged, but kills only about 10% of untreated children.

R. prowazekii is a small gram-negative bacillus (rickettsia) that has a man-louse-man life cycle (Fig. 9-7). These rickettsiae infect and multiply in human endothelial cells. Infected endothelial cells detach and rupture, releasing organisms into the circulation (rickettsemia). A louse taking a blood meal becomes infected with rickettsiae, after which the organisms enter the epithelial cells of its midgut, multiply, and rupture the cells within 3 to 5 days. Large numbers of rickettsiae are released into the lumen of the louse intestine. The

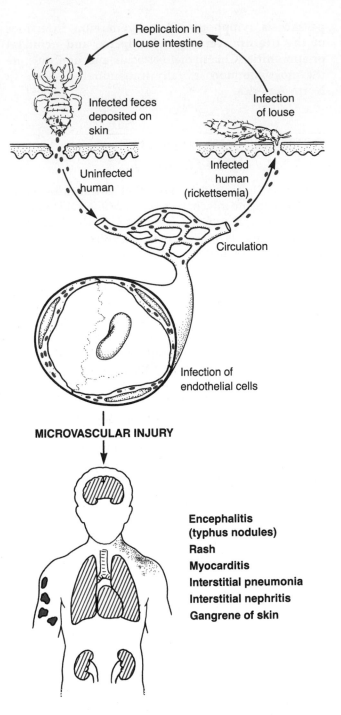

Encephalitis
(typhus nodules)
Rash
Myocarditis
Interstitial pneumonia
Interstitial nephritis
Gangrene of skin

Figure 9-7. Epidemic typhus (louse-borne typhus). *R. prowazekii* has a man–louse–man life cycle. The organism multiplies in endothelial cells, which detach, rupture, and release organisms into the circulation (rickettsemia). A louse taking a blood meal becomes infected with rickettsiae, which enter the epithelial cells of its midgut, multiply, and rupture the cells, thereby releasing rickettsiae into the lumen of the louse intestine. Contaminated feces are deposited on the skin or clothing of a second host and penetrate an abrasion or are inhaled. The rickettsiae then enter endothelial cells, multiply, and rupture the cells, thus completing the cycle.

louse deposits its contaminated feces on the skin or clothing of a second host, where the feces may remain infectious for more than 3 months. A person becomes infected when the contaminated louse feces penetrate an abrasion or scratch in the skin or when the person inhales airborne rickettsiae from clothing containing louse feces. After penetrating the skin or nasal mucous membrane, the rickettsiae enter the person's endothelial cells, multiply, and rupture the cells, thus completing the cycle.

About 4 to 6 days after the onset of fever, the patient develops a maculopapular rash on the back, chest, and abdomen. Dying patients may exhibit encephalitis, myocarditis, interstitial rickettsial pneumonia, interstitial nephritis, and shock (see Fig. 9-7). Although rickettsiae do not produce local lesions on entering the skin or respiratory tract, they do cause a generalized vasculitis of minute blood vessels as they multiply within endothelial cells, and fibrin thrombi often form in capillaries, especially those of the brain, skin, and heart.

ROCKY MOUNTAIN SPOTTED FEVER

Rocky mountain spotted fever is a severe, sometimes fatal systemic infection caused by [2]Rickettsia rickettsii and transmitted by ticks.

The rash, which appears 2 to 6 days after the onset of fever, begins on the wrists and ankles before extending rapidly over the body to include the palms of the hands and the soles of the feet. Cough, nausea, vomiting, abdominal pain, stupor, meningismus, or ataxia are evidence of serious systemic spread.

R. rickettsii is a minute gram-negative bacillus that invades blood vessels, especially the endothelial cells of the kidney, meninges, skin, and heart. In fatal infections the endothelial cells lift away from the vessel, leaving the internal elastic lamella bare. Thrombi form at these sites, platelet counts drop to below 100,000 per microliter, and disseminated intravascular coagulation is a terminal complication.

DISEASES CAUSED BY SPIROCHETES

SYPHILIS (LUES)

Syphilis is a sexually transmitted disease caused by the spirochete [c2]Treponema pallidum. **The disease is divided into three stages (Fig. 9-8):** primary (the chancre), secondary (disseminated), and tertiary (with lesions of deep organs following a latent period of 2 to 20 years or more). Congenital syphilis, acquired in

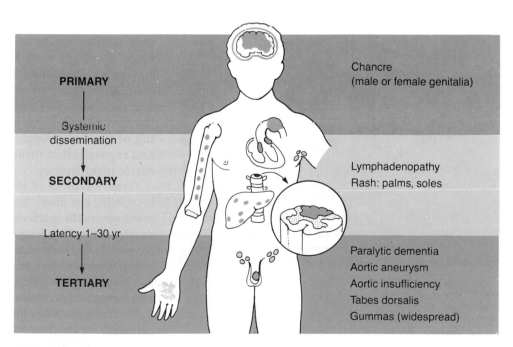

Figure 9-8. Clinical characteristics of the stages of syphilis.

ruptures, leaving a ragged, firm crater with dark, leathery base. In most patients the infection remains localized and subsides. Pulmonary anthrax, sometimes called "wool sorters' disease," is a hazard of handling contaminated raw wool, and develops when spores of *B. antracis* are inhaled. The patient usually dies in an acute toxic stage. Septicemia more commonly follows pulmonary anthrax than malignant pustule. Anthrax of the gastrointestinal tract is rare and is probably acquired by eating contaminated meat.

SALMONELLOSIS (GASTROENTERITIS AND SEPTICEMIA)

The genus *Salmonella* comprises a large, heterogenous group of motile gram-negative bacilli that infect many animals an man. As a group, they are enteroinvasive and enteropathogenic and cause enteric fevers. Three species, associated with three distinct clinical entities, are identified; namely *Salmonella enteritidis* (salmonella enteritis), *Salmonella choleraesuis* (salmonella septicemia), and *Salmonella typhi* (typhoid fever).

Gastroenteritis, caused by *S. enteritidis*, is an acute, self-limited infection of the small bowel, lasting 2 to 5 days. Septicemia, usually caused by *S. choleraesuis*, is characterized by prolonged fever and anemia. Focal suppurative lesions in many tissues and organs include osteomyelitis, pneumonia, pulmonary abscess, meningitis, and endocarditis. There are no gastrointestinal symptoms and the organisms are not cultured from the stools.

TYPHOID FEVER

Typhoid fever, the most serious human salmonellosis, is characterized by prolonged fever, bacteremia, and multiplication of the organisms within mononuclear phagocytic cells of the liver, spleen, lymph nodes, and Peyer's patches.

Humans are the only natural reservoir for *S. typhi*, and typhoid fever therefore must be acquired from convalescing patients or from chronic carriers—especially older women with gallstones or biliary scarring, in whom *S. typhi* may colonize the gallbladder or biliary tree. Typhoid fever is spread primarily through ingestion of contaminated water and food (especially dairy products and shellfish), and much less commonly by direct finger-to-mouth contact with feces, urine, or other secretions.

Untreated typhoid fever progresses through the following five stages: incubation (10 to 14 days); active invasion/bacteremia (1 week); fastigium (1 week); lysis (1 week); and convalescence (several weeks). Bacilli attach preferentially to the tips of villi in the small intestine, invade the mucosa immediately, or multiply in the lumen for several days before penetrating the mucosa (Fig. 9-11). The bacilli then pass to the lymphoid follicles of the intestine and the draining mesenteric lymph nodes. Some organisms pass into the systemic circulation and are phagocytosed by reticuloendothelial cells of liver and spleen. Bacilli invade and proliferate further within the phagocytic cells of the intestinal lymphoid follicles, mesenteric lymph nodes, liver, and spleen. During this initial incubation period, therefore, the bacilli are primarily sequestered in the intracellular habitat of the intestinal and mesenteric lymphoid system.

Figure 9-11. Stages of typhoid fever.
Incubation (10 to 14 days). Water or food contaminated with *S. typhi* is ingested. Bacilli attach to the villi in the small intestine, invade the mucosa, and pass to the intestinal lymphoid follicles and draining mesenteric lymph nodes. The organisms proliferate further within mononuclear phagocytic cells of the lymphoid follicles, lymph nodes, liver, and spleen. Bacilli are sequestered intracellularly in the intestinal and mesenteric lymphatic system.
Active invasion/bacteremia (1 week). Organisms are released and produce a transient bacteremia. The intestinal mucosa becomes enlarged and necrotic, forming characteristic mucosal lesions. The intestinal lymphoid tissues become hyperplastic and contain "typhoid nodules"—aggregates of macrophages ("typhoid cells") that phagocytose bacteria, erythrocytes, and degenerated lymphocytes. Bacilli proliferate in several organs, reappear in the intestine, are excreted in stool, and may reinvade through the intestinal wall.
Fastigium (1 week). Dying bacilli release endotoxins that cause systemic toxemia.
Lysis (1 week). Necrotic intestinal mucosa sloughs, producing ulcers, which hemorrhage or perforate into the peritoneal cavity.

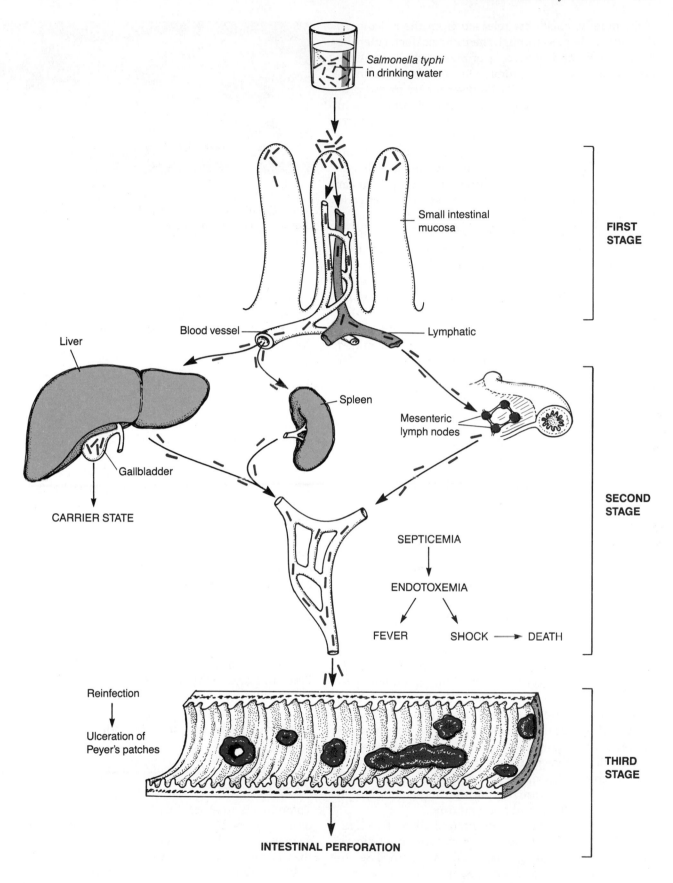

Salmonella typhi in drinking water

Small intestinal mucosa

FIRST STAGE

Blood vessel

Lymphatic

Liver

Spleen

Mesenteric lymph nodes

Gallbladder

CARRIER STATE

SECOND STAGE

SEPTICEMIA

ENDOTOXEMIA

FEVER

SHOCK ⟶ DEATH

Reinfection

Ulceration of Peyer's patches

THIRD STAGE

INTESTINAL PERFORATION

Eventually, bacilli are released from the reticuloendothelial cells, pass through the thoracic duct, enter the bloodstream, and produce a primary transient bacteremia and clinical symptoms. During this active invasion/bacteremic phase, bacilli disseminate to and proliferate in many organs, but are most numerous in organs that possess significant phagocytic activity, namely the liver, spleen, and bone marrow. The Peyer's patches of the terminal ileum and the gallbladder are also hospitable sites. Bacilli invade the gallbladder from either blood or bile, after which they reappear in the intestine, are excreted in the stool, or reinvade the wall of the intestine.

Clinically, patients develop fever, diarrhea or constipation, vomiting, abdominal distention, myocarditis, splenomegaly, leukopenia, and mental changes. Infection of Peyer's patches leads to lymphoid hyperplasia, which can resolve without scarring or can progress to capillary thrombosis, with necrosis and ulceration. *S. typhi* in the blood during the second or third week of illness initiates prolonged bacteremia, often heralded by the transient appearances of "rose spots"—macular lesions on the limbs, lower abdomen, and chest that resemble petechial hemorrhages, but are actually foci of hyperemia (capillary atony).

The patient's temperature follows a characteristic pattern. It remains normal during the incubation period, undergoes daily stepwise elevations during active invasion, remains high during fastigium, falls slowly (with fluctuations) during lysis, and remains normal during convalescence.

In the final phase, usually 3 to 5 weeks after onset, the patient is febrile and exhausted, but recovers if there are no complications. **The most frequent and severe complication is intestinal perforation with peritonitis.** The mortality ranges from 2% to 10% without treatment.

Pathologic changes are apparent throughout the stages of typhoid fever. As the salmonellae pass to lymphoid follicles of the intestine, there is diffuse enterocolitis and hypertrophy of Peyer's patches. This is followed by necrosis of intestinal and mesenteric lymphoid tissues, focal granulomas in the liver and spleen, and characteristic mononuclear inflammatory cells ("typhoid nodules") in many organs. Typhoid nodules are primarily aggregates of altered macrophages—"typhoid cells"—that phagocytose bacteria, erythrocytes, and degenerated lymphocytes. The most common sites for typhoid nodules are the intestine, mesenteric lymph nodes, spleen, liver, and bone marrow.

While bacilli continue to proliferate, dying bacilli release endotoxins that cause toxemia, beginning during invasion and becoming maximal in fastigium. The necrotic intestinal mucosa sloughs, usually during lysis,

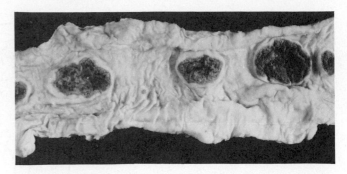

Figure 9-12. Ulcers of the terminal ileum in fatal typhoid fever. The ulcers have a longitudinal orientation because they are over hyperplastic and necrotic Peyer's patches.

producing ulcers that conform to Peyer's patches and are concentrated along the antimesenteric border (Fig. 9-12). The ulcers may bleed or perforate, usually during lysis.

PLAGUE

Plague is caused by *Yersinia pestis*, a plump, bipolar staining, coccobacillus. The Americas, Africa, and Asia are endemic areas. Wild rodents such as squirrels, chipmunks, mice, wood rats, and rabbits are reservoirs. Transmission from animal to animal is by fleas. Infected domestic animals bring the disease to humans by direct contact or flea bites.

Two to eight days after the flea bite, bubonic plague begins with chills, fever, nausea, vomiting, and rapid respiration and pulse. A painful lymph node (bubo) enlarges in the area drained by the bite. The architecture of the lymph node, including the capsule and perinodal fat, is obliterated by necrosis, hemorrhage, and finely granular material. This material comprises solid masses of gram-negative coccobacilli, the plague bacillus. Blood cultures are positive in 50% of patients. **Petechiae and ecchymoses lead to the "black death,"** 60% to 90% of those affected dying within 24 hours if untreated. Toxemia may kill even when antibiotics have arrested the growth of bacteria.

TULAREMIA

Tularemia is an acute, febrile, granulomatous, zoonotic disease caused by *Francisella tularensis*. The organism is a small (0.2 by 0.5 μm), aerobic, gram-negative bacillus that is not motile, encapsulated, or spore-forming. Rabbits and rodents are the most important reservoirs, but many other wild and domestic animals are infected. Humans become infected through broken skin or intact mucosa by handling infected animals and carcasses; by ingesting contaminated food and water; by inhaling bacteria; or by being bitten by infected insects, including ticks, deer flies, and mosquitoes.

Tularemia has four clinical presentations: ulceroglandular, oculoglandular, pneumonic, and typhoidal. Pneumonia may complicate any one of the types. The duration of illness is 1 week to 3 months, but may be shortened by prompt treatment. The most common form is tularemia, **ulceroglandular,** begins as a tender erythematous papule at the site of inoculation, usually on a limb. This develops into a pustule, which ulcerates. The regional lymph nodes become large and tender, and may suppurate and drain through sinus tracts. The initial bacteremia is followed in a week by generalized lymphadenopathy and splenomegaly. Symptoms include fever, headache, myalgia, and occasionally prostration. The most serious infections are complicated by a secondary pneumonia and endotoxic shock, in which case the prognosis is grave.

In **oculoglandular** tularemia the primary lesion is a papule in the conjunctiva, which becomes a pustule or ulcerates. Severe ulceration may penetrate the sclera, allowing organisms to enter the eye and infect the optic nerve, causing blindness. In **glandular tularemia** generalized lymphadenopathy is the first manifestation. A diagnosis of the **typhoid form** is made when fever, hepatosplenomegaly, and toxemia, resembling salmonella sepsis, are the presenting features. The mortality from untreated tularemia ranges from 5% for ulceroglandular tularemia to 30% for the typhoidal and pneumonic forms.

HAEMOPHILUS INFLUENZAE INFECTION

Haemophilus influenzae is a gram-negative, pleomorphic, aerobic bacillus that is nonmotile and does not form spores. It is a strict parasite of humans, and causes pneumonia, meningitis, epiglottitis, pericarditis, bacteremia, cellulitis, pyarthrosis, and "pink eye"—an acute, purulent conjunctivitis. *H. influenzae* type b causes more than 90% of human infections and is **the most common cause of bacterial meningitis in the United States.** *H. influenzae* is recovered from 80% of healthy adults. By 5 years of age, all children have *H. influenzae* in their nasopharynx.

Meningitis in children that is caused by *H. influenzae* usually follows otitis, sinusitis, pneumonia, or impaired immunity. An early symptom is pain when the child sits up or is diapered. Upper respiratory symptoms,

fever, vomiting, irritability, and lethargy accompany the meningitis, and 5% to 10% die within 48 hours. Neurologic deficits are permanent in one-third of those who survive. Bacteria, neutrophils, and fibrin form an exudate in the leptomeninges. The exudate extends from the basal portion of the subarachnoid space into the brain along the vessels. The typical gram-negative coccobacilli are in neutrophils in the exudate around the meningeal blood vessels.

Infection of lung by *H. influenzae* produces fever, cough, purulent sputum, dyspnea, and either bronchopneumonia or lobar pneumonia. The pneumonia usually complicates chronic lung disease and in half of the patients follows a viral infection of the respiratory tract. The alveoli are filled with neutrophils, macrophages containing bacilli, and fibrin. The bronchial epithelium is necrotic and is replaced by macrophages. Bacilli are in macrophages, and short and long filamentous bacilli are packed together in extracellular foci.

The onset of epiglottitis is sudden; fever, dysphagia, accumulation of oropharyngeal secretions, tachypnea, and retraction precede obstruction of the trachea.

WHOOPING COUGH (PERTUSSIS)

Whooping cough is caused by *Bordetella pertussis,* a nonmotile, gram-negative coccobacillus that forms a capsule in its virulent state. *B. pertussis* has a remarkable ability, probably enhanced by its pili, to attach to ciliated bronchial epithelium. Here the organisms proliferate, remain on the surface epithelium, and accumulate in great numbers. The bacteria stimulate the bronchial cells to produce a profuse, tenacious mucus that slows ciliary action and inhibits the bronchopulmonary toilet. Secondary bacterial infections and epithelial necrosis follow.

Cough progresses to severe paroxysms terminating in a gasping, strident, inspiratory effort. During inspiration, air is forcibly drawn through a narrow glottis, giving the characteristic "whoop."

CHANCROID

Chancroid, the "third veneral disease", is an acute, sexually transmitted bacterial infection caused by *Haemophilus ducreyi,* a short gram-negative bacillus. The bacillus is highly infectious and invades on contact, through the skin or mucous membranes. Chancroid is most common in tropical and subtropical regions and especially in the Far East.

The lesions are located on the skin and mucous membranes of the genitalia. A papule develops 1 to 14 days after contact, becomes pustular, and ulcerates. Seven to 10 days after the appearance of the primary lesion, half of the patients develop unilateral, painful, suppurative, inguinal lymphadenitis (a bubo). The skin becomes inflamed, breaks down, and drains pus from the underlying node.

LEGIONELLOSIS (LEGIONNAIRES' DISEASE)

Legionellosis is a severe, necrotizing pneumonia caused by a minute, gram-negative bacillus, *Legionella pneumophila*. Legionnaires' disease occurs sporadically, as epidemics, and as nosocomial infections, especially in patients with compromised immunity. Those who abuse alcohol and smoke heavily are also at increased risk. Common source exposure is frequent. The organism has been recovered from soil, ponds, water systems, and air conditioning systems.

The disease presents as a rapidly progressive pneumonia, accompanied by fever, nonproductive cough, and myalgias. The onset is abrupt, after an incubation period of 2 to 10 days. Within 2 days, most patients develop a persistent high fever and respiratory rales. Radiograms of the chest reveal unilateral, diffuse, patchy bronchopneumonia, progressing to widespread nodular consolidation, usually without cavitation. Toxic symptoms, hypoxia, and obtundation may be prominent, and death may follow in a few days. In those who survive, convalescence is prolonged.

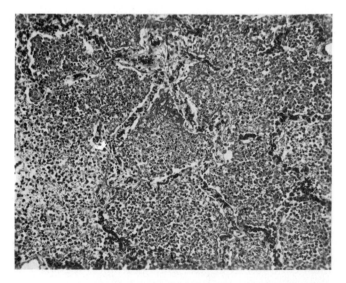

Figure 9-13. Fatal legionellosis, section of consolidated lung. The alveoli are packed with an exudate composed of histiocytes and fibrin.

The main changes in the lung include consolidation, necrosis, and acute congestion. Microscopically, the alveoli are packed with an exudate composed of histiocytes and fibrin (Fig. 9-13). The alveolar walls become necrotic and are destroyed.

CHOLERA

Cholera is caused by an enterotoxin elaborated by *Vibrio cholerae*, a gram-negative bacillus (Fig. 9-14). The organism proliferates in the lumen of the small intestine and causes profuse watery diarrhea, rapid dehydration, and (if fluids are not restored) shock and death within 24 hours of the onset of symptoms.

V. cholerae enters humans via contaminated drinking water and food prepared with contaminated water (see Fig. 9-14). Vibrios enter the small intestine and propagate. **They remain in the lumen and do not invade the intestinal mucosa.** They do, however, elaborate an enterotoxin.

Symptoms begin when the massive secretion of water and sodium in the small intestine, a consequence of the activation of cyclic AMP, exceeds the resorptive capacity of the colon. The small intestine, however, is not damaged morphologically either by the vibrios or by the enterotoxin. Treatment is prompt rehydration. With this treatment, most patients survive.

SHIGELLOSIS

Shigellosis is an acute bacterial dysentery caused by species of *Shigella*. *Shigella* enteritis ranges from mild diarrhea to incapacitating and life-threatening dysentery, the latter caused primarily by *Shigella dysenteriae* (the Shiga bacillus). The enteric lesions, limited to the colon, are destructive, as evidenced by the bloody mucoid stools characteristic of shigellosis.

The shigellae are found worldwide and are most important and conspicuous in tropical and developing countries, where they are a major cause of morbidity and mortality. Unlike the salmonellae, which also invade and colonize the intestinal mucosa, shigellae have no significant animal reservoir. Nor do shigellae survive well outside the stool, being transmitted mainly by direct fecal-oral contamination. Endemic shigellosis, therefore, tends to strike communities with poor standards of hygiene and sanitation. Shigellosis is also spread in closed communities, such as hospitals, barracks, and households.

Symptoms appear 2 to 5 days after the ingestion of bacteria. Milder infections are characterized by the onset of profuse diarrhea before other acute symptoms.

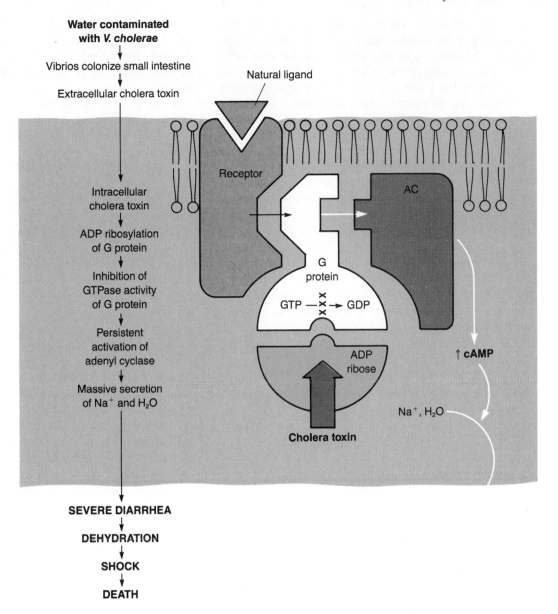

**Water contaminated
with *V. cholerae***

↓

Vibrios colonize small intestine

↓

Extracellular cholera toxin

↓

Intracellular
cholera toxin

↓

ADP ribosylation
of G protein

↓

Inhibition of
GTPase activity
of G protein

↓

Persistent
activation of
adenyl cyclase

↓

Massive secretion
of Na^+ and H_2O

↓

SEVERE DIARRHEA

↓

DEHYDRATION

↓

SHOCK

↓

DEATH

Natural ligand

Receptor

AC

G
protein

$GTP \longrightarrow GDP$

ADP
ribose

Cholera toxin

↑ **cAMP**

Na^+, H_2O

Figure 9-14. Cholera. Infection comes from water contaminated with *Vibrio cholerae* or food prepared with contaminated water. The vibrios traverse the stomach, enter the small intestine, and propagate. Although they do not invade the intestinal mucosa, the vibrios elaborate a potent toxin that induces a massive outpouring of water and electrolytes. Severe diarrhea ("ricewater stool") leads to dehydration and hypovolemic shock.

Early onset of fever, diarrhea, abdominal pain, and tenesmus is more serious and may be life-threatening. Diffuse involvement of the colon is associated with high fever, shaking chills, toxemia, and shock.

The key to the pathogenicity of *Shigella* is its ability to invade and multiply in the epithelium and lamina propria of the terminal ileum and colon. The mucosa becomes edematous and hyperemic, and is covered by pus and mucus. The ulcerated mucosa becomes covered with a granular, dirty-yellow pseudomembrane, consisting of necrotic mucosa, neutrophils, fibrin, and erythrocytes. Sloughed pseudomembrane, together with blood-tinged mucus, comprise the characteristic dysenteric stool of shigellosis. Epithelial regeneration is rapid, and healing is complete in 2 weeks. Endotoxin probably adds to necrosis, but the role of enterotoxin produced by some species of *Shigella* in the pathogenesis of dysentery is uncertain. While clearly secondary to invasion, Shiga toxin probably contributes to the profuse diarrhea that precedes dysentery in some patients. This enterotoxin, which is related antigenically to the enterotoxin of enteropathogenic *Escherichia coli*, activates membrane-associated adenyl cyclase. Thus, shiga toxin, like cholera toxin and *E. coli* enterotoxin, induces hypersecretion of fluid and electrolytes from the mucosa of the terminal ileum.

ESCHERICHIA COLI *INFECTION*

Escherichia coli causes at least three patterns of human enteric diseases: enterotoxigenic, enteroinvasive, and enteroadherent. **Enterotoxigenic** *E. coli* causes a diarrheal disease by elaborating two plasmid-mediated enterotoxins. The heat-labile toxin is antigenically, structurally, and functionally related to the cholera toxin, although the toxin of *E. coli* is less potent than that of cholera. The heat-labile toxin also binds to GM_1 ganglioside on the intestinal epithelial cells. As in cholera, the resulting activation of adenyl cyclase produces a hypersecretory diarrhea. The heat-stable toxin of *E. coli* is different from cholera toxin and apparently acts to impair sodium and chloride absorption and to reduce the motility of the small intestine through a mechanism dependent on cyclic GMP. Dehydration and electrolyte imbalance is a significant cause of morbidity and mortality when appropriate rehydration is lacking—a common combination among infants in less developed countries. Enterotoxigenic *E. coli* is also responsible for 50% of traveller's diarrhea.

Enteroinvasive *E. coli* produces a dysentery-like disease resembling shigellosis. It invades the intestinal mucosa and causes local tissue destruction and sloughing of necrotic mucosa.

Enteroadhesive *E. coli* has only recently been associated with diarrheal diseases. Enteroadhesiveness is plasmid-dependent and is apparently mediated by pili, which bind tightly to receptors on the intestinal epithelial cells.

About 80% of all infections of the urinary tract in humans, ranging from mild cystitis to fatal pyelonephritis, are caused by *E. coli*. In addition, *E. coli* is the etiologic agent in many cases of nosocomial pneumonia, most often in elderly patients with underlying chronic disease. Empyema is a common complication, especially in patients with disease lasting more than a week.

Only rarely does *E. coli* cause meningitis in adults, but it is a **major cause of neonatal meningitis.** Between 40% and 80% of infants with *E. coli* meningitis die, and the survivors frequently suffer from neurologic or developmental anomalies.

CAMPYLOBACTER *ENTERITIS*

Campylobacter species have emerged as the leading cause of acute bacterial enteritis. Formerly identified as vibrios, these flagellated, comma-shaped, gram-negative bacteria cause up to 11% of all infectious dysentery in U.S. hospitals, thus causing more enteritis than *Salmonella* species. *Campylobacter* enteritis is acquired by eating improperly cleaned and cooked food, usually poultry, contaminated by *Campylobacter jejuni*, an organism that colonizes poultry.

C. jejuni, like *Salmonella*, are enteroinvasive and produce a spectrum of disease ranging from subclinical infection to severe dysentery. Illness appears 2 to 5 days after ingestion of contaminated food and lasts about 5 days. Symptoms include abdominal pain, diarrhea, nausea, vomiting, fever, and myalgia. Stools are malodorous and frequently bloody. Inflammation involves the gastrointestinal tract from jejunum to anus. Most patients have colonic crypt abscesses and ulcers resembling those in ulcerative colitis. Microscopically, the small bowel is edematous and hyperemic and is infiltrated with neutrophils, lymphocytes, and plasma cells. Comma-shaped organisms are seen in the intestinal mucosa and lamina propria. The disease is generally benign and self-limited. There is evidence that *Campylobacter pylori* may be involved in the pathogenesis of peptic ulcer disease and gastritis.

BRUCELLOSIS

Brucellosis, a zoonotic disease caused by several species of the genus *Brucella*, may present as an acute severe systemic disease or as a subacute or chronic malady. *Brucella* are small, nonmotile, nonsporulating, gramnegative coccobacilli, which may or may not be encapsulated. Four species infect humans, each from its own animal reservoir. *Brucella melitensis* infects sheep and goats; *Brucella abortus*, cattle; *Brucella suis*, swine; and *Brucella canis*, dogs. The disease is encountered worldwide and in all climates. Virtually every type of domestic animal and many wild ones are affected. The prevalence in humans relates to occupational exposure, cultural or socioeconomic conditions resulting in close contact with animals, and consumption of contaminated milk or milk products. In the United States brucellosis is an occupational disease of farmers, employees of abattoirs, and veterinarians. In much of the world the most common cause of infection is unpasteurized dairy products.

The incubation period is 5 days to several months. The onset of symptoms may be abrupt or insidious. The three clinical types of brucellosis are acute malignant, recurrent, and chronic (intermittent). The presenting features of acute malignant brucellosis resemble those of influenza, and include the sudden onset of high fever, chills, prostration, and somatic aches and pains. Lymphadenopathy and a palpable spleen and liver are the only localized findings. Death may be sudden, within a few days of onset, or after a few weeks of delirium and coma. Recurrent brucellosis **(undulant fever)** is characterized by influenza-like signs and symptoms that recur in wavelike relapses. The cycles may persist for weeks, gradually decreasing in severity. Chronic (intermittent) brucellosis is caused primarily by *B. abortus*.

The most common complications of brucellosis involve the bones and joints and include spondylitis of the intervertebral area of the lumbar spine and localized suppuration in large joints. In addition, peripheral neuritis, meningitis, orchitis, suppurative endocarditis, and pulmonary lesions may develop.

Bacteria enter through skin abrasions, the conjunctiva, oropharynx, or lung and spread in the bloodstream to the liver, spleen, lymph nodes, and bone marrow, where they multiply in phagocytic cells. A generalized histiocytic hyperplasia ensues, with conspicuous noncaseating granulomas, causing lymphadenopathy and hepatosplenomegaly.

CLOSTRIDIAL DISEASES

Clostridia are gram-positive, spore-forming bacilli that are obligate anaerobes. The vegetative bacilli are found in the gastrointestinal tract of herbivorous animals and man. Anaerobic conditions promote vegetative division, while aerobic conditions promote sporulation (Fig. 9-15). Spores pass in the animal feces, contaminate the soil and plants, and can survive unfavorable environmental condition. Under anaerobic conditions the spores revert to vegetative cells, thus completing the cycle. During sporulation, the vegetative cells degenerate, and their plasmids produce a variety of specific toxins that cause widely different clostridial diseases, depending on the species. **Food poisoning and necrotizing enteritis ("pig bel") are caused by the enterotoxins of *Clostridium perfringens*; gas gangrene by the myotoxins of *Clostridium perfringens*, *Clostridium novyi*, *Clostridium septicum*, and others; tetanus by the neurotoxin of *Clostridium tetani*; and botulism by the neurotoxin of *Clostridium botulinum*.**

FOOD POISONING

C. perfringens has five serotypes (A-E). Types A and C produce a toxin, alpha-enterotoxin, that causes food poisoning (see Fig. 9-15). *C. perfringens* is ubiquitous, and is the most widely disseminated of all pathogenic bacteria, typically being 10 to 100 times more numerous than *E. coli* in stool. Type A serotype is the only one commonly found in the colonic flora of animals and humans. It is also omnipresent in the environment, contaminating soil, water, and air samples, clothing, dust, and meat.

Most of the food poisoning is from contaminated beef, gravy, and other meat products. When contaminated food is consumed, the ingested *C. perfringens* reach the intestine, where alpha-enterotoxin is produced during sporulation.

Symptoms may develop within 2 to 4 hours, but 8 to 12 hours is usual. Symptoms include cramping abdominal pain, sudden vomiting, and frequent episodes of watery diarrhea. The patient usually recovers within 2 days.

NECROTIZING ENTERITIS

C. perfringens type C also produces beta-enterotoxin, which causes a necrotizing enteritis. This disorder is seen in malnourished persons who have sudden dietary overindulgence, as was seen, for example, in impoverished children immediately after World War II. Necrotizing enteritis is endemic in the highlands of New Guinea, especially in children who have participated in pig feasts (whence the pidgin term, "pig bel").

The usual incubation period is 48 hours after ingestion of contaminated meat. The presenting symptoms include severe abdominal pain and distention, vomit-

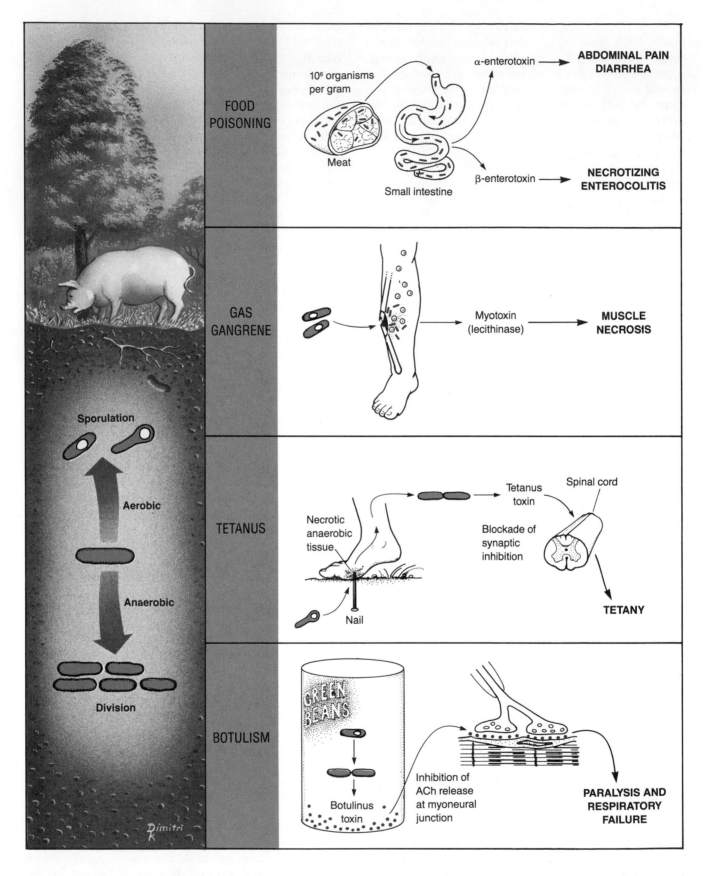

FOOD POISONING

10^6 organisms per gram

Meat

Small intestine

α-enterotoxin → **ABDOMINAL PAIN DIARRHEA**

β-enterotoxin → **NECROTIZING ENTEROCOLITIS**

GAS GANGRENE

Myotoxin (lecithinase) → **MUSCLE NECROSIS**

TETANUS

Necrotic anaerobic tissue

Nail

Tetanus toxin

Spinal cord

Blockade of synaptic inhibition

→ **TETANY**

BOTULISM

GREEN BEANS

Botulinus toxin

Inhibition of ACh release at myoneural junction

→ **PARALYSIS AND RESPIRATORY FAILURE**

Sporulation

Aerobic

Anaerobic

Division

Dimitri K

ing, and passage of bloody or black stools. Patients with fulminating pig bel may die within 24 hours of onset. Half of the patients require surgery.

Necrotizing enteritis is a segmental disease that may be restricted to a few centimeters or may involve the entire small intestine. Green, necrotic pseudomembranes are seen in segmental areas of necrosis and peritonitis. More advanced lesions may perforate the bowel wall. Histologic sections reveal infarction of the mucosa, with edema, hemorrhage, and suppurative infiltrate that extends transmurally. The pseudomembrane is composed of necrotic epithelium containing gram-positive bacilli.

CLOSTRIDIAL MYONECROSIS (GAS GANGRENE)

Gas gangrene is a rapidly progressive, life-threatening illness, in which necrosis of previously healthy skeletal muscle is caused by myotoxins elaborated by a few species of clostridia. *C. perfringens* type A is the most common source of myotoxin (80% to 90% of cases). Myonecrosis usually follows traumatic wounds or surgical procedures in which the site of the wound becomes contaminated with clostridia (see Fig. 9-15).

Under anaerobic conditions clostridia grow rapidly and elaborate the myotoxin(s). The most important exotoxin identified from the species causing gangrene is alpha-toxin, produced by *C. perfringens* type A (and four other causative species). Alpha-toxin is a lecithinase that destroys cell membranes.

The incubation period is commonly 2 to 4 days after wounding, surgery, or abortion. Sudden, severe pain occurs at the site of injury, which is tender and edematous. The skin darkens because of hemorrhage and cutaneous necrosis. The lesion develops a thick, serosanguineous discharge that has a fragrant odor and may contain gas bubbles. Clinically, sweating, low-grade fever, and disproportionate tachycardia give way rapidly to hemolytic anemia, hypotension, and renal failure. In the terminal stages, coma, jaundice, and shock supervene. **Gas gangrene is characterized histologically by necrosis of muscle and overlying soft tissues, with little inflammatory cell reaction.**

TETANUS

Tetanus (lockjaw) is a severe, acute neurologic syndrome of humans and warm-blooded animals. It is

---

Figure 9-15. Clostridial diseases. Clostridia in the vegetative form (bacilli) inhabit the gastrointestinal tract of humans and animals. Spores pass in the feces, contaminate soil and plant materials, and are ingested or enter sites of penetrating wounds. Under anaerobic conditions they revert to vegetative forms. Plasmids in the vegetative forms elaborate toxins that cause several clostridial diseases.
Food poisoning and necrotizing enteritis. Meat dishes left to cool at room temperature grow large numbers of clostridia (more than 10^6 organisms per gram). When contaminated meat is ingested, *C. perfringens* types A and C produce alpha-enterotoxin in the small intestine during sporulation, causing abdominal pain and diarrhea. Type C also produces beta-enterotoxin.
Gas gangrene. Clostridia are widespread and may contaminate a traumatic wound or surgical operation. *C. perfringens* type A elaborates a myotoxin (alpha-toxin), a lecithinase that destroys cell membranes, alters capillary permeability, and causes severe hemolysis following intravenous injection. The toxin causes necrosis of previously healthy skeletal muscle.
Tetanus. Spores of *C. tetani* are in soil and enter the site of an accidental wound. Necrotic tissue at the wound site causes spores to revert to the vegetative form (bacilli). Autolysis of vegetative forms releases tetanus toxin. The toxin is transported in peripheral nerves and (retrograde) through axons to the anterior horn cells of the spinal cord. The toxin blocks synaptic inhibition, and the accumulation of acetylcholine in damaged synapses leads to rigidity and spasms of the skeletal musculature (tetany).
Botulism. Improperly canned food is contaminated by the vegetative form of *C. botulinum*, which proliferates under aerobic conditions and elaborates a neurotoxin. After the food is ingested, the neurotoxin is absorbed from the small intestine and eventually reaches the myoneural junction, where it inhibits the release of acetylcholine. The result is a symmetric descending paralysis of cranial nerves, trunk, and limbs, with eventual respiratory paralysis and death.

caused by tetanus toxin (tetanospasmin), a neurotoxic exotoxin elaborated by plasmids of *Clostridium tetani.*

The vegetative cells of *C. tetani* inhabit the intestine of animals (especially horses and other herbivores) and man. The bacillus has terminal spherical spores, giving the organism a "drumstick" appearance. After sporulation, the spores pass with the feces and contaminate the soil, where they survive for years if not exposed to sunlight. Spores enter the site of a traumatic, penetrating wound—for instance, a wound incurred from stepping on a nail (see Fig. 9-15) or a battle wound. Neonatal tetanus, a disease most prevalent in less developed countries, results when soil or dung contaminates the stump of the umbilical cord.

At the site of injury, necrotic tissue and suppuration contribute to the creation of an anaerobic environment, a condition that causes spores to revert to vegetative cells. Tetanus toxin, one of the most potent toxins known, is released from autolyzed vegetative cells and binds to ganglioside receptors on neuronal cell membranes, thereby causing discharge of local peripheral nerves and spasm of muscles. Although the clostridial infection remains localized, the neurotoxin then undergoes retrograde transport (via intra- and peri-axonal transport) through the ventral roots of peripheral nerves to the anterior horn cells of the spinal cord. There the toxin crosses the synapse and interacts with presynaptic terminals on motor neurons in the ventral horns, blocking release of inhibitory neurotransmitters. This causes uninhibited neural stimulation and sustained contraction of skeletal musculature (tetany) (see Fig 9-15). Blockage of the inhibitory transmitters also induces acceleration of the heart rate, hypertension, and cardiovascular instability.

Clinical manifestations of tetanus include generalized hypertonia (less frequently, localized hypertonia) of the skeletal musculature, accompanied by paroxysmal clonic muscular spasms. The incubation period is 1 to 3 weeks. An early symptom is difficulty in opening the jaw ("lockjaw" or trismus). As the disease progresses, increasing rigidity of the musculature leads to rigidity of the facial muscles (risus sardonicus) and those of the neck, abdominal wall, back, lower limbs, and other sites. Rigidity of the muscles of the back may produce backward arching (opisthotonos). Prolonged spasms of the respiratory and laryngeal musculature lead to death.

BOTULISM

Botulism is a paralyzing, often fatal, illness that follows the ingestion of food containing the neurotoxins of *Clostridium botulinum.* The spores of *C. botulinum* are widely distributed in soil and animals, and contaminate many foods. The spores survive unfavorable conditions, and are especially resistant to drying and boiling. **In the United States the toxin is most commonly present in vegetables or other foods that have been improperly home-canned and stored without refrigeration, conditions that provide suitable anaerobic conditions for growth of the vegetative cells that elaborate the neurotoxins (A-G).**

After food containing neurotoxin is ingested, the toxin resists gastric digestion and is readily absorbed into the blood from the upper portions of the small intestine. Toxin in the circulation eventually reaches the cholinergic nerve endings at the myoneural junction. The toxin binds to membrane receptors (gangliosides) of the synaptic vesicles and inhibits release of acteylcholine, thus causing paralysis and respiratory failure.

The symptoms of botulism begin 12 to 36 hours after the ingestion of food containing toxin. Since the neurotoxin is performed, there is no true "incubation" period for growth of organisms.

The neurotoxin produces a symmetric, descending pattern of weakness or paralysis of the cranial nerves (especially nerve VI), limbs, and trunk. These symptoms may be accompanied by diplopia, dysarthria, dysphagia, and in severe cases, respiratory paralysis.

DIPHTHERIA

Diphtheria is an acute disease that results from a localized infection and a systemic toxemia caused by exotoxin-producing strains of *Corynebacterium diphtheriae.*

The organism is a pleomorphic, nonmotile, grampositive club-shaped bacillus. Its pathogenicity depends on the presence of a toxin-producing, lysogenic bacteriophage. **The exotoxin is one of the most toxic substances known, and a single molecule is sufficient to kill a cell.** It inactivates protein synthesis by modifying elongation factor 2, thus preventing elongation of the nascent protein chain at the ribosome.

The infection spreads from person to person by infected droplets or exudates. Humans are the only significant reservoir and most people are asymptomatic carriers.

Pharyngeal diphtheria is the most common presentation. After an incubation period of 1 to 7 days, during which the corynebacteria proliferate at the site of implantation, the patient experiences fever, sore throat, malaise, and sometimes nausea and vomiting. A graygreen membrane adheres to the underlying epithelium and leaves a bleeding surface when it is peeled away. The membrane may spread over the entire pharynx and in severe infections involves the larynx, trachea, and bronchi, thereby obstructing the airway. The term "bull neck" refers to the edema and cervical adenopathy that obscure the angle of the jaw, the contour of the anterior portion of the neck, and the clavicle. **Absorption of the exotoxin in the nonimmune host causes cardiac enlargement, cardiac arrhythmias, and heart failure.** The exotoxin also causes neuritis, which may progress to paralysis.

Histologically, the membrane is composed of a coagulated fibrinopurulent exudate mixed with necrotic epithelial cells and masses of corynebacteria. The bacilli are concentrated deeply in the lesion beneath the necrotic epithelium. The exotoxin produces diffuse myocarditis, with edema, focal and diffuse degeneration of myocardial fibers, and increased fat within myocytes. The diphtheria exotoxin also cause demyelinization of nerves and interstitial nephritis with proteinuria. Those who survive have no residual effect.

FRIEDLANDER'S BACILLUS (KLEBSIELLA PNEUMONIAE)

Klebsiella pneumoniae, known as Friedlander's bacillus, is a short, encapsulated, gram- negative bacillus that causes a necrotizing lobar pneumonia. This organism also causes 10% of all infections acquired in the hospital, including pneumonia and infections of the urinary tract, the biliary tract, and surgical wounds. Hospital personnel present a special hazard as carriers, especially when resistant strains of *K. pneumoniae* colonize their mouths, throats, and intestines. Predisposing factors to infection with Friedlander's bacillus are indwelling catheters and endotracheal tubes, old age, alcoholism, immunosuppression, diabetes, congestive heart failure, obstructive pulmonary disease, and other debilitating conditions. Secondary *Klebsiella* pneumonias may complicate influenza or other viral infections of the respiratory tract. **The combined mortality rate of primary and secondary *Klebsiella* pneumonias is about 50%.**

Clinically, the pneumonia has a sudden onset, characterized by fever, pleuritic pain, cough, and **thick mucoid sputum.** When infection is severe these symptoms progress to shortness of breath, cyanosis, and death in 2 to 3 days.

Pneumonia develops when the bacilli invade and multiply within the alveolar spaces. The pulmonary parenchyma becomes consolidated, and the mucoid exudate that fills the alveoli is dominated by macrophages, fibrin, and edema fluid. Neutrophils are inhibited by a neutral polysaccharide in the capsule of *K. pneumoniae*, and are not a significant part of the early exudate. Numerous encapsulated gram-negative bacilli

appear free in the exudate and in alveolar macrophages. As the exudate accumulates the alveolar walls become compressed and then necrotic. Numerous small abscesses may coalesce and lead to cavitation.

GRANULOMA INGUINALE

Granuloma inguinale is a sexually transmitted, chronic, superficial ulceration of the genitalia and inguinal and perianal regions caused by *Calymmatobacterium granulomatis*, a small, encapsulated, nonsporulating, nonmotile, gram-negative bacillus.

The incubation period varies from 1 week to 6 months, 2 to 4 weeks being the average. The initial lesion may be a papule, a subcutaneous nodule, or an ulcer. The lesions develops within several weeks into a raised, soft, painless, beefy-red, superficial ulcer. The exuberant granulation tissue resembles a fleshy mass herniating through the skin. In heterosexual men, early ulceration of the penoscrotal skin commonly extends to genitocrural and inguinal folds. In women ulcerations spread to the perineal and perianal skin. In homosexual men the lesions are perianal and anal. Untreated granuloma inguinale follows an indolent, relapsing course, often healing with an atrophic scar. Massive cicatrization of the dermis and subcutis causes genital elephantiasis, probably by lymphatic obstruction.

Microscopically, there is epithelial hyperplasia of the ulcer margin. The dermis and subcutis are infiltrated by

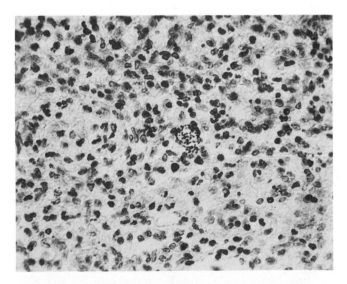

Figure 9-16. Granuloma inguinale, skin, showing *Calymmatobacterium granulomatis* (Donovan bodies) clustered in a large histiocyte. Intense silvering by the Warthin–Starry technique makes the organisms large, black, and easily seen.

numerous histiocytes and plasma cells and by fewer neutrophils and lymphocytes. The neutrophils in the ulcer bed are clustered into poorly defined microabscesses. Interspersed histiocytes contain many bacteria, which are called Donovan bodies (Fig. 9-16).

STAPHYLOCOCCAL INFECTIONS

Staphylococcal infections are caused by species of the genus *Staphylococcus*. These gram-positive cocci are ubiquitous, colonizing the skin and the anterior nasal vestibule of children and adults, and the umbilicus, stool, and perineum of neonates. Three species are pathogenic in humans: *Staphylococcus aureus*, *Staphylococcus epidermidis*, and *Staphylococcus saprophyticus*. About 20% to 40% of adults are nasal carriers of *S. aureus*, and many become carriers while in the hospital, perhaps because medical personnel are more frequent carriers than the general population.

Most staphylococcal infections are caused by *S. aureus*, which grows especially well on skin and mucous membranes, but can infect any part of the body. *S. aureus* causes a wide variety of suppurative diseases, including, among others, **abscesses of the skin** (impetigo, boils, styes, carbuncles, breast abscesses, botryomycosis), **abscesses of bone** (osteomyelitis) and other deep organs, **infections of burns and surgical and other wounds, infections of the upper and lower respiratory tracts** (pharyngitis, bronchopneumonia, empyema), **purulent arthritis, septicemia, acute endocarditis,** and **meningitis.** *S. aureus* releases several exotoxins; enterotoxins (enteritis and food poisoning); exfoliative toxin (exfoliative skin disease); and pyrogenic toxin (toxic shock syndrome).

INFECTIONS OF SKIN

Impetigo is a skin infection that is caused by staphylococci (and by streptococci). Staphylococcal impetigo frequently afflicts school children who have a nasal discharge. Macular and pustular lesions begin around the nose and spread over the face, forming honey-yellow crusts, the hallmark of impetigo.

Furuncles (boils) are deep-seated infections with *S. aureus* in and around hair follicles, often in a nasal carrier. They occur only on hairy surfaces, such as the neck, thighs, and buttocks of men, and the axilla, pubic area, and eyelids of both sexes. The boil begins as a nodule at the base of the hair follicle, followed by a pimple that remains painful and red for a few days. A yellow apex forms, and the central core becomes necrotic and fluctuant.

Styes are boils that involve the sebaceus glands around the eyelid.

Carbuncles result from coalescing infections with *S. aureus* around hair follicles; they produce draining sinuses. Most carbuncles are on the neck, but they also occur on the limbs, trunk, face, and scalp. Necrosis spreads deeply into the skin, and some patients develop bacteremia, with a risk to life.

Breast abscesses usually arise within a few weeks after delivery, when staphylococci are transmitted from an infant with neonatal sepsis to the skin glands in the breasts of the nursing mother.

Botryomycosis (a misnomer) is a chronic **bacterial** infection that is caused by staphylococci (as well as by streptococci, *E. coli*, and other common bacteria). Botryomycosis presents as an indurated fibrotic mass with draining sinuses and grains in a purulent exudate. Macroscopically, these grains cannot be distinguished from those of actinomycosis or a mycetoma. Microscopically, however, microcolonies of staphylococci in clusters within the grain are surrounded by an amorphous eosinophilic coating ("Splendore-Heoppli phenomenon").

ABSCESSES OF BONE (OSTEOMYELITIS)

Acute staphylococcal osteomyelitis most commonly afflicts boys between 3 to 10 years of age, most of whom have a history of infection or trauma. The bones of the legs are involved in most patients. Many patients have an underlying bacteremia *(S. aureus)* with systemic symptoms. Osteomyelitis may become chronic if not properly treated.

Adults over 50 years of age are more frequently afflicted with osteomyelitis of the vertebra. The onset of localized back pain is usually abrupt, but may follow staphylococcal infection of the skin or urinary tract, prostatic surgery, infected abortion, puerperal infection, or a surgical procedure, such as pinning a fracture.

ACUTE AND CHRONIC BACTERIAL ARTHRITIS

S. aureus is the causative organism in half of all cases of septic arthritis. Most of those who have the disease are adults, 50 to 70 years old, and usually only a single joint is involved. Rheumatoid arthritis and steroid therapy are common predisposing conditions. The acute onset of staphylococcal arthritis is marked by severe, throbbing pain, often worse at night, which is accompanied by shaking chills and fever. Acute staphylococcal arthritis may be confused with an acute episode of rheumatoid arthritis.

SEPTICEMIA

Septicemia with *S. aureus* afflicts patients with lowered resistance who are in the hospital for other diseases or conditions. Some have underlying staphylococcal infections (for example, osteomyelitis or septic arthritis), some have had surgery (especially transurethral resection of the prostate), and some have infections from an indwelling intravenous catheter. Staphylococcal septicemia is associated with the common symptoms of bacteremia, such as shaking chills and fever. Miliary abscesses and staphylococcal endocarditis are serious complications.

BACTERIAL ENDOCARDITIS

Acute and subacute bacterial endocarditis are complications of septicemia caused by *S. aureus* (as well as by *S. epidermidis*). Endocarditis may develop spontaneously on normal valves or on valves damaged by rheumatic fever. It may also follow insertion of prosthetic valves or other intracardiac surgery. Those who inject illicit drugs intravenously also have an increased risk of endocarditis from infection with *S. aureus*.

TOXINOSES

Staphylococcal **food poisoning** is caused by the ingestion of preformed staphylococcal enterotoxin in prepared food. This commonly involves food eaten in a restaurant (not industrially processed food), especially unrefrigerated meats, milk or custard and other milk products. *S. aureus* has caused more than half of the food poisoning epidemics in which the causative agent has been identified. At least six enterotoxins are produced by some of the coagulase-positive strains of *S. aureus*, and enterotoxins are also produced by a few coagulase-negative strains. Enterotoxins are resistant to heat and withstand cooking for 20 to 60 minutes.

Usually, nausea and vomiting begin within a few hours of ingesting the toxin. In some cases, however, diarrhea and abdominal discomfort are the only symptoms. Patients with more severe food poisoning have bloody mucus in the vomitus and stools, as well as muscle cramps, headache, and sweating. The acute phase commonly lasts 4 to 6 hours, and recovery is complete within 1 or 2 days.

The exfoliative toxin of *S. aureus* causes the **"scalded skin syndrome,"** which afflicts neonates, infants, and young children, typically in the aftermath of conjunctivitis or minor staphylococcal infection. A painful, brick-red rash begins on the face, neck, axilla, and groin, and then becomes generalized. The rash leads to blisters or bullae, and the upper dermis is shed in large sheets.

TOXIC SHOCK SYNDROME (TSS)

The toxic shock syndrome is a sporadic, febrile illness characterized by fever, hypotension, and a desquamating rash. Some of the symptoms resemble those of scarlet fever, a malady caused by the erythrogenic toxin of *Streptococcus pyogenes*. The toxic shock syndrome may progress to renal and pulmonary failure and death. The disease typically afflicts young, menstruating women, in whom it is usually associated with the use of tampons. However, the syndrome may also afflict nonmenstruating women, men, and children, in association with staphylococcal empyema, septic abortions, fasciitis, osteomyelitis, and abscesses.

STREPTOCOCCAL INFECTIONS

Streptococcal infections are caused by species of the genus *Streptococcus*, which includes *Streptococcus pyogenes* (group A), *Streptococcus agalactiae* (group B), *Streptococcus faecalis* (group D), *Streptococcus pneumoniae A* (pneumococcus), and the viridans streptococci group. The streptococcus is gram-positive and is demonstrated in cultures, smears, and tissue sections. Although streptococci elicit suppurative inflammatory responses, there are several nonsuppurative complications that reflect immune responses and deposition of immune complexes.

To acquire infection, an individual must usually be inoculated with millions of streptococci, spread by close contact with a carrier or with someone who has an active infection.

Group A beta-hemolytic streptococci (for example *S. pyogenes)* cause nasopharyngeal and cutaneous lesions, different strains infecting these sites.

Group B streptococci produce infections of the newborn.

Group C, G, and other streptococci are responsible for respiratory infections.

"Untypable" alpha (green) hemolytic streptococci (for instance *Streptococcus viridans)*, are part of the flora of the mouth and cause about one-half of all bacterial endocarditis.

Group D streptococci (e.g., enterococci) are an important cause of infections of the urinary tract, endocarditis, postsurgical infections, septicemia, and other infections.

Pneumococci (*S. pneumoniae*) produce primary bacterial pneumonia, septicemia, meningitis, and other infections.

INFECTIONS OF THE UPPER RESPIRATORY TRACT

Infections of the upper respiratory tract are caused mainly by group A beta-hemolytic streptococci and present as pharyngitis, pneumonia, and pulmonary abscesses (Fig. 9-17). The pharyngitis varies in intensity from mild lesions resembling the common cold to more severe lesions that involve the epiglottis and the tonsillar crypts.

SCARLET FEVER

Scarlet fever, which results from an acute pharyngitis or tonsillitis caused by group A streptococci, is characterized by a rash produced by the erythrogenic toxin. The incubation period of 2 to 5 days is followed by chills and fever, a fiery red pharyngeal mucosa, small crypt abscesses in enlarged tonsils, and a bright red tongue with edematous papillae ("raspberry tongue"). One to 3 days later there appears a diffuse, punctate, erythematous rash, most prominent over the trunk and inner aspects of the limbs, and involving the face, except for a small area around the mouth ("circumoral pallor"). When the pharyngitis and rash subside, near the end of the first week, desquamation begins. Scarlet fever is notorious for late nonsuppurative sequelae, which are prevented by prompt treatment.

ERYSIPELAS

Erysipelas, caused chiefly by beta-hemolytic group A streptococci, is the classic cutaneous streptococcal infection. It is common in warm climates, but is not often seen before the age of 20 years. Erysipelas is an erythematous swelling of the skin that usually begins on the face and spreads rapidly. The maplike area of brawny erythema has a sharp, well-demarcated, serpiginous border. A diffuse, edematous, acute inflammatory reaction in the dermis and epidermis extends into the subcutaneous tissues. The inflammatory infiltrate (mostly neutrophils) is most intense around vessels and adnexae of the skin. Cutaneous microabscesses and small foci of necrosis are not uncommon.

IMPETIGO

Impetigo, another infection of skin that may be caused by streptococci, has increasingly been reported as a cause of post-streptococcal complications in children. Streptococcal and staphylococcal impetigo have similar lesions, including folliculitis, pyoderma, wound infection, lymphatic spread, and sepsis.

PUERPERAL SEPSIS

Puerperal sepsis, a result of infection by group A streptococci from the contaminated hands of attendants at delivery, was formerly common but, with the acceptance of the "germ theory" of disease and improved hygiene, is now rare in the developed countries. Group B streptococcus is an important neonatal pathogen, causing pneumonia, sepsis, and meningitis. Infants acquire the infection from their mothers during delivery, and mortality rates are high (50% or more) if the onset of infection is within 10 days of delivery.

PNEUMOCOCCAL PNEUMONIA AND MENINGITIS

Pneumococcal pneumonia and meningitis result from infection with *S. pneumoniae* (the pneumococcus), an organism that is responsible for **80% of all bacterial pneumonias.** Pneumococci also spread from the nasopharynx through the systemic circulation and seed the meninges. Some patients develop meningitis from primary pneumococcal pneumonia.

BACTERIAL ENDOCARDITIS

Bacterial endocarditis is a complication of streptococcal septicemia, in which the organisms spread from a site of local infection through the circulation to colonize heart valves. The alpha-hemolytic streptococci are a leading cause of subacute bacterial endocarditis, whereas *S. pneumoniae* frequently produces acute bacterial endocarditis.

The nonsuppurative complications of streptococcal infections include **rheumatic fever, acute glomerulonephritis, and erythema nodosum.** These entities are discussed in the chapters dealing with the heart, kidney, and skin, respectively.

MENINGOCOCCAL INFECTIONS

The gram-negative, bean-shaped diplococcus *Neisseria meningitidis* causes a variety of clinical and pathologic manifestations, including pharyngitis, meningitis, and septicemia (Fig. 9-18). *N. meningitidis* may be cultured from the nasopharynx, blood, or cerebrospinal fluid. In the African meningitis belt, the incidence of meningitis is highest in children 5 to 14 years of age, but in developed countries it is highest in children under the age of 5 years.

Meningococci are transmitted from person to person by respiratory droplets. After exposure most people

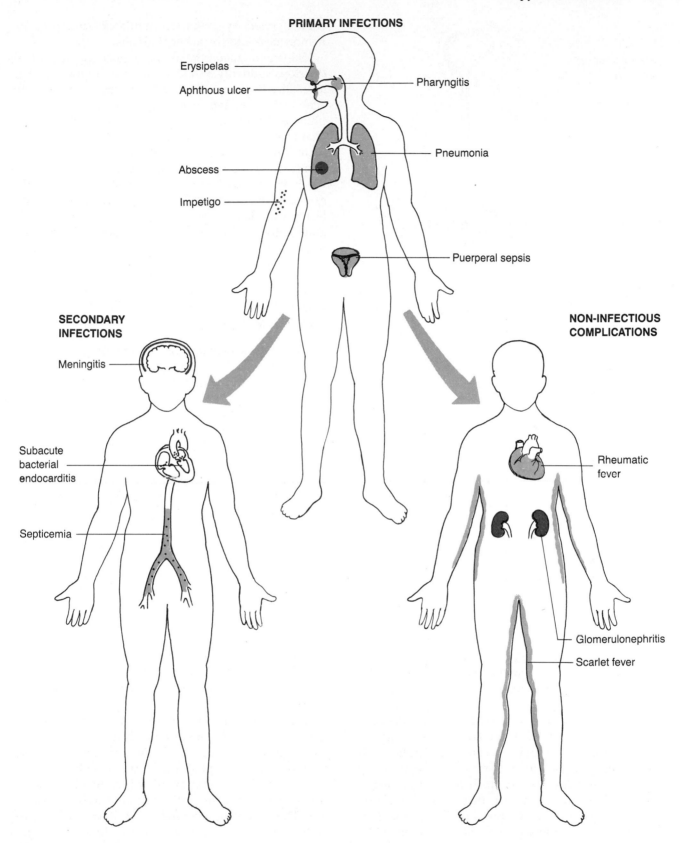

Figure 9-17. Streptococcal diseases.

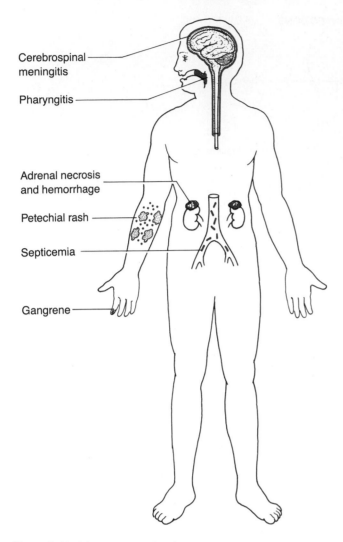

Cerebrospinal meningitis

Pharyngitis

Adrenal necrosis and hemorrhage

Petechial rash

Septicemia

Gangrene

Figure 9-18. Meningococcal infections. Meningococcal infections have a variety of clinical manifestations, including pharyngitis, meningitis, septicemia, and associated complications.

characterized by purpura, circulatory collapse, and hemorrhage into the adrenal glands.

Like meningococcemia, meningococcal meningitis develops suddenly and kills the patient quickly. Characteristically the patient suddenly experiences headache, stiff neck, and fever. Typically there is a neutrophilic leukocytosis and the cerebrospinal fluid shows characteristic changes of acute pyogenic meningitis, including increased white blood cell levels (mainly neutrophils), high protein, and low glucose. At autopsy the brain is covered with thick yellow-gray pus that extends inward along the Virchow-Robin (perivascular) spaces. The exudate, which is composed of fibrin and neutrophils, expands the subarachnoid space, and may also extend to the ventricles.

GONOCOCCAL INFECTIONS (GONORRHEA)

Gonorrhea is a sexually transmitted disease caused by various strains of the gram-negative diplococcus *Neisseria gonorrhoea* (Fig. 9-19). The infection is usually localized to the urogenital tract, most commonly the urethra of men and the endocervix of women. About one-half of infected women have no symptoms. In men, however, infection is usually symptomatic.

Gonorrhea begins as a surface infection of the mucous membranes; that is, a catarrh. The bacteria attach to and spread along the cells of the surface mucous membranes, after which they invade superficially and provoke acute inflammation. The mucous membranes of the urethra, endocervix, and salpinx are characteristic sites. The cell wall of *N. gonorrhoea* lacks a true polysaccharide capsule, but projecting from the cell wall are hairlike extensions called pili. Within the pili is a protease that digests IgA on the surface of the mucous membrane, thus facilitating the attachment of gonococci to the columnar and transitional epithelium of the urogenital tract (see Fig. 9-19).

After an incubation period of 3 to 5 days, men usually have purulent urethral discharge and dysuria. If treatment is not instituted promptly the organisms extend to the prostate, epididymis, and accessory glands, where they cause urethral stricture, epididymitis, orchitis, and sometimes male infertility. Male homosexuals develop pharyngitis and proctitis.

The first manifestation of infection in women is usually endocervicitis, with vaginal discharge or bleeding. There may be urethritis, manifested by dysuria rather than by urethral discharge. In some women (usually during the first menses after exposure), the infection extends to the fallopian tubes, where it produces acute and chronic salpingitis and pelvic inflam-

become carriers but develop no symptoms, except for an occasional mild pharyngitis. Less commonly, organisms invade the bloodstream to cause a fulminating meningococcemia, or to seed the meninges and produce an acute suppurating meningitis. **Thus, the meningococcus is responsible for two distinct fatal lesions: septicemia (meningococcemia) and meningitis.**

Fever, tachycardia, and hypotension are early symptoms of acute meningococcemia. Proliferating meningococci produce an endotoxin that causes circulatory collapse, a characteristic feature of meningococcemia. The toxemia is often sudden and kills the patient within a few hours. Fulminating meningococcemia is also the principal cause of the **Waterhouse-Friderichsen syndrome,** a complication seen mainly in children and

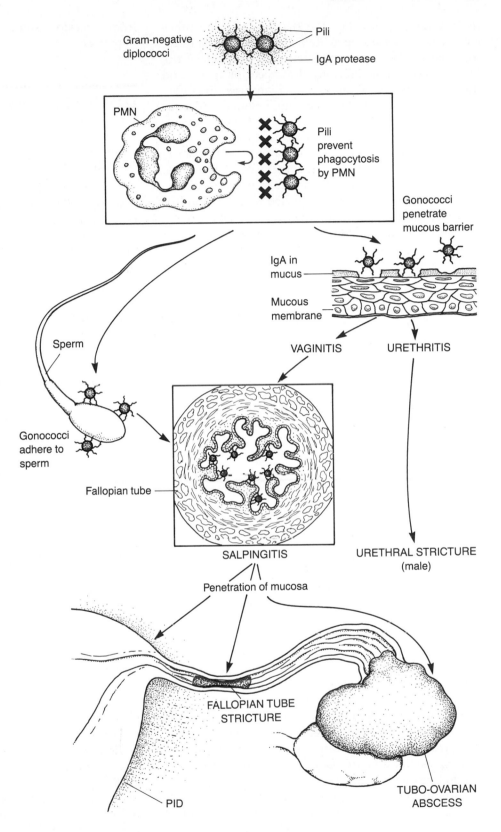

Figure 9-19. Pathogenesis of gonococcal infections. *Neisseria gonorrhoea* is a gram-negative diplococcus whose surface pili form a barrier against phagocytosis by neutrophils. The pili contain an IgA protease that digests IgA on the luminal surface of the mucous membranes of the urethra, endocervix, and fallopian tube, thus facilitating attachment of gonococci. Gonococci cause endocervicitis, vaginitis, and salpingitis. In men, gonococci attached to the mucous membrane of the urethra cause urethritis and, sometimes, urethral stricture. Gonococci may also attach to sperm heads and be carried into the fallopian tube. Penetration of the mucous membrane by gonococci leads to stricture of the fallopian tube, pelvic inflammatory disease (PID), or tuboovarian abscess.

matory disease (see Fig. 9-19). The fallopian tubes swell with pus, causing acute abdominal pain. Infertility occurs when inflammatory adhesions close the tubes at both ends, blocking the ascent of sperm and the descent of ova. From the fallopian tubes the infection may spread to the peritoneum, healing as fine adhesions ("violin string" adhesions) between the capsule of the liver and the parietal peritoneum. Women (and to a lesser extent men) may also develop bacteremia, producing disseminated gonococcal infection, which in turn leads to monarthritis or polyarthritis.

Neonatal infections from infected amniotic fluid or an infected birth canal result in symptoms within a few days after birth. These infections involve the conjunctiva and constitute a major cause of blindness in much of Africa and Asia.

CAT SCRATCH DISEASE

Cat scratch disease is a usually self-limited infection by a gram-negative bacterium that forms filaments up to 10 μm or longer. It has not been cultured but is easily seen in tissue sections of the skin, lymph nodes, and conjunctiva when stained by a silver impregnation technique. The infection begins when the organism is inoculated into the skin by the claws of cats and rarely by other animals, or by thorns or splinters. Infections are more common in children (80%) than adults, and there may be clustering when a stray cat or kitten joins a family.

Most patients have a papule at the site of inoculation, which begins 3 to 14 days after inoculation and may persist for 8 weeks. It is followed by tenderness and enlargement of the regional lymph nodes. The nodes remain enlarged for 3 to 4 months and may drain through the skin. About one-half of the patients have other symptoms, including fever and malaise.

At the site of inoculation the bacteria multiply in the walls of small vessels and about collagen fibers, from which they move through draining lymphatics to regional lymph nodes, where they produce a pyogranulomatous lymphadenitis. In early lesions clusters of bacteria expand and obliterate the walls of small vessels. The lesions in the skin and lymph nodes progress from abscesses to suppurating granulomas and finally to necrosis. Bacteria are abundant in early lesions and rare in late ones.

Without biopsy and the visualization of the characteristic bacteria, the diagnosis is supported when three criteria are met: contact with a cat, a cat scratch, or a primary lesion of the skin or conjunctiva; a positive skin test for cat scratch antigen; and negative results from laboratory studies for other causes of lymphadenopathy.

DISEASES CAUSED BY FILAMENTOUS BACTERIA

ACTINOMYCOSIS

Actinomycosis is a chronic infection characterized by swelling, pain, and draining sinuses that discharge actinomycotic grains. A number of different anaerobic and microaerophilic bacteria cause actinomycosis. These are *Actinomyces israelii, Actinomyces naseslundii, Actinomyces viscosus, Arachnia propionica,* and *Bifidobacterium adolescentis.* The bacteria are long, gram-positive filaments 0.2 to 0.3 μm wide by at least 4.0 μm long. In tissue, actinomyces form round yellow grains, 100 to 300 μm across, which are cemented together by a mucosaccharide-protein matrix.

The actinomycetes are saprophytes and may be part of the normal flora of the oral cavity, the intestine, or the vagina. A break in the epithelial surface and damage to the surrounding tissue allows the actinomycetes to invade and establish infection. Dental extractions, poor oral hygiene, abdominal surgery, appendicitis, and diverticulitis all predispose to actinomycosis. Pulmonary alveoli damaged by aspiration may also become infected by actinomycetes. Women with neglected intrauterine devices have increased actinomycotic flora of the vagina and cervix, and the attached IUD string becomes a nidus for actinomycotic growth. With continued neglect there is a risk of uterine, tubal, or ovarian actinomycosis. Actinomycosis originating in a tooth socket or the tonsils is characterized by swelling of the face and neck, at first painless and fluctuant, but later painful. The infection spreads along tissue planes and by sinus tracts into bone and through the skin. In pulmonary infections sinus tracts may penetrate from lobe to lobe, through the pleura, and into ribs and vertebrae. Night sweats, weight loss, and cough are common and chest radiographs reveal abscesses, particularly at the lung bases. In the abdomen actinomycosis usually begins in the appendix or colon and extends to the abdominal wall, diaphragm, spine, liver, ovaries, kidney, or urinary bladder.

Histopathologically, the grains stain deep purple with hematoxylin and are composed of packed actinomycetes in an eosinophilic matrix (Fig. 9-20). This matrix, also called Splendore-Hoeppli material, coats the actinomycetes projecting from the surface of the grain, giving the perimeter the appearance of radiating clubs.

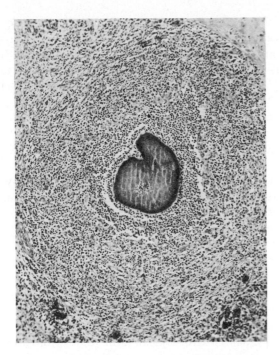

Figure 9-20. Actinomycosis, ovary. A typical grain lies within an abscess surrounded by a fibrogranulomatous reaction.

The grains lie in an abscess surrounded by a granulomatous reaction.

NOCARDIOSIS

Nocardiosis is an infection of the lung that may spread to the brain and skin and, less commonly, to the thyroid, liver, or other organs. The causative organism is *Nocardia asteroides,* a gram-positive, aerobic, branching, filamentous bacillus that is weakly acid fast and belongs to the order Actinomycetales. Debility and immunosuppression predispose to infection. Invasion of the lung causes a bronchopneumonia, which may extend to become lobar.

DISEASES CAUSED BY MYCOBACTERIA

TUBERCULOSIS

Tuberculosis is a chronic communicable disease caused by a variety of tubercle bacilli, especially *Mycobacterium tuberculosis hominis* and *Mycobacterium tuberculosis bovis.* The lungs are the prime target, but any organ may be infected. The characteristic lesion is a spherical granuloma with central caseous necrosis.

M. t. hominis is ordinarily contracted by inhaling contaminated droplets. *M. t. bovis* is contracted through the gastrointestinal tract, from the raw milk of diseased cows. Most people, after exposure, develop a small, limited pulmonary infection. This infection is contained by an inflammatory reaction, and during its course the tuberculin skin test becomes positive. **Thus most tuberculous infections do not progress to clinical disease.**

Distributed throughout the world, tuberculosis is clearly one of the most important bacterial diseases of mankind. Although the risk of infection has been dramatically reduced in developed countries, it remains high for malnourished people in impoverished areas. In the United States, for example, the incidence is 12 per 100,000, and the mortality is one to two per 100,000. In some developing countries, the incidence reaches 450 per 100,000. There are also racial and ethnic differences: Jews, other Caucasians, and Mongolians have greater natural resistance than Africans, Native Americans, and Eskimos. Age may also be a factor. In the United States, tuberculosis is highest among the elderly, possibly a reflection of infections acquired early in life before the decline in the prevalence of the disease.

Tubercle bacilli are slender, beaded nonmotile, acid-fast, and gram-positive bacilli, although their gram-positivity may be difficult to demonstrate. The cell wall is waxy and contains components that confer acid-fastness; that is, the retention of carbolfuchsin after rinsing with acid alcohol. **Tubercle bacilli are strict, obligate aerobes that proliferate within phagocytes.** They grow slowly in culture and require 3 or more weeks to develop colonies. The virulence of tubercle bacilli is associated with a tendency to aggregate and form filaments or cords in liquid media. The organisms resist heat and disinfectants, but are killed quickly by ultraviolet light.

The specific lesions associated with tuberculosis are discussed in Chapter 12, which deals with the lung.

LEPROSY (HANSEN'S DISEASE)

Leprosy (Hansen's disease) is a chronic infection caused by *Mycobacterium leprae.* It affects the cooler parts of the body, especially the nasal mucosa, upper respiratory tract, peripheral nerves, testes, the skin of the ears, and the anterior segment of the eyes. The World Health Organization estimates that worldwide over 15 million persons are infected, most in tropical countries (Fig. 9-21).

Lepra bacilli are slender, weakly acid-fast rods. To date, all attempts to culture the organism have failed or are unsubstantiated. Lepra bacilli multiply in experimental animals at sites with temperatures below that of the internal organs, such as the food pads of mice, and the ear lobes of hamsters, rats, and other rodents. The armadillo is also an experimental model.

Leprosy exhibits a bewildering variety of clinical and pathologic features. The lesions vary from the small, insignificant, and self-healing macules of tuberculoid leprosy to the diffuse, disfiguring, and sometimes fatal lesions of lepromatous leprosy. Ninety-five percent of all people have a natural protective immunity and are not infected, even through intimate and prolonged exposure. In the susceptible 5% who may develop symptomatic infections, a broad immunologic spectrum ranges from anergy to hyperergy. **Anergic patients (i.e., those with little or no resistance) have lepromatous leprosy, whereas hyperergic patients (those with high resistance) develop tuberculoid leprosy.**

Patients with lepromatous leprosy have nodular and diffuse infiltrates of the skin, eye, testes, nerves, and organs of the reticuloendothelial system. The most severe involvement of the skin is in exposed areas; the nodular distortions of the face are called "leonine facies" (see Fig. 9-21). The infiltrates are composed of tumorlike accumulations of histiocytes, each histiocyte containing enormous numbers of lepra bacilli (Fig. 9-22). The epidermis is stretched thinly over the nodules, and beneath it is a narrow, uninvolved "clear zone" of dermis. Rather than destroying the bacilli, the phagocytic cells appear to act as microincubators. Unchecked, these infiltrates expand slowly to distort and disfigure the face, ears, and upper airway and to destroy the eyes, eyebrows and eyelashes, nerves, and testes. Those who are untreated may die of asphyxiation from an obstructed airway or from secondary amyloidosis.

The other end of the spectrum is represented by patients with **tuberculoid leprosy,** a condition characterized by a single lesion or very few lesions of the skin. The hypopigmented macule, with a raised "infiltrated" border, may be hypesthetic or anesthetic. The lesion expands slowly over a period of months or years, and then gradually heals, although the hypesthesia or anesthesia remain. Microscopically, the tuberculoid lesion is a dermatitis, characterized by discrete noncaseating granulomas in the dermis. The granulomas are composed of epithelioid cells and Langhan's giant cells and are associated with varying numbers of lymphocytes and plasma cells. Cutaneous nerves, including the small dermal nerve twigs, are eventually destroyed by the bacilli, which accounts for the sensory deficit.

Figure 9-21. (*A, top*) Lepromatous leprosy. There is diffuse involvement, including a leonine face, loss of eyebrows and eyelashes, and nodular distortions, especially on the face, ears, forearms, and hands—the exposed (cool) parts of the body. (*A, bottom*) The nodular skin lesion of advanced lepromatous leprosy. Swelling has flattened the epidermis (loss of Rete ridges). A characteristic "clear zone" of uninvolved dermis separates the epidermis from tumor-like accumulations of histiocytes, each containing numerous lepra bacilli (*Mycobacterium leprae*). (*B, top*) Tuberculoid leprosy on the cheek, showing a hypopigmented macule with a raised, infiltrated border. The central portion may be hypesthetic or anesthetic. (*B, bottom*) Macular skin lesion of tuberculoid leprosy. Skin from the raised "infiltrated" margin of the plaque contains discrete granulomas that extend to the basal layer of the epidermis (without a clear zone). The granulomas are composed of epithelioid cells and Langhan's giant cells, and are associated with lymphocytes and plasma cells. Lepra bacilli are rare. (*C*) Distribution of leprosy. Prevalence is greatest in tropical regions of Africa, Asia, and Latin America.

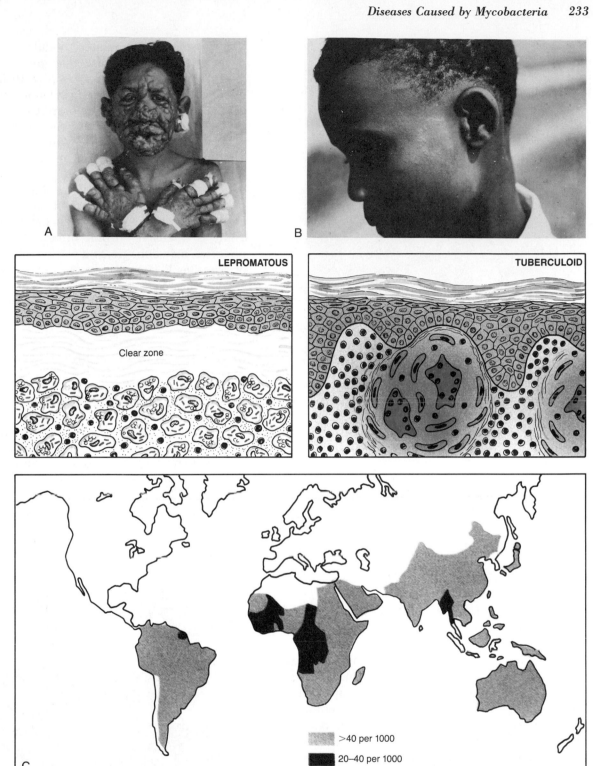

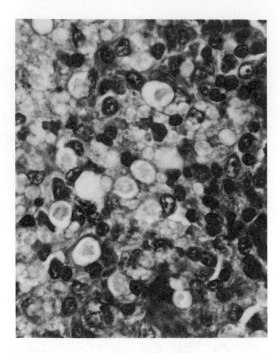

Figure 9-22. Lepromatous leprosy, skin, showing tumorlike mass of histiocytes. The faint masses within the vacuolated histiocytes are enormous numbers of acid-fast bacilli. The histiocytes show no tendency to inhibit proliferation of the lepra bacilli.

DISEASES CAUSED BY PROTOZOANS

CHAGAS' DISEASE

Chagas' disease (American trypanosomiasis), a zoonotic infection by the protozoan *Trypanosoma cruzi*, causes acute, subacute, and chronic parasitemia, with dissemination to many organs, especially the heart, brain, esophagus, and colon. *T. cruzi* infects certain insects and mammals and is commonly transmitted to humans by species of reduviid bugs. American trypanosomiasis exists in every country of Central and South America, but is rarely seen in the United States, Mexico, and the Caribbean islands. Infection is promoted by contact between humans and infected bugs, usually in mud or thatched dwellings of the rural and suburban poor.

ACUTE CHAGAS' DISEASE

In acute Chagas' disease, after an incubation period of about 1 to 2 weeks following inoculation with *T. cruzi*, a subcutaneous inflammatory nodule, the "chagoma," develops at the site. Parasitemia appears 2 to 3 weeks after inoculation and is associated with fever, edema, lymphadenopathy, and hepatosplenomegaly. The dangerous complications are myocarditis (tachycardia, arrhythmia, cardiac failure) and encephalitis.

In fatal cases, the heart is enlarged and dilated, with a pale, focally hemorrhagic myocardium. The liver, lungs, spleen, and intestine are congested, depending on the degree of cardiac failure. Microscopically, numerous parasites are seen in the heart, and amastigotes are evident within pseudocysts in myofibers (Fig. 9-23). There is extensive chronic inflammation, with lymphocytes, macrophages, and plasma cells. Phagocytosis of parasites is conspicuous. Myofibers are destroyed, and the heart shows interstitial edema, endocarditis, pericarditis, and inflammation and parasitization of the sinus node and atrioventricular node.

CHRONIC CHAGAS' DISEASE

Chronic Chagas' disease is the most frequent and most serious consequence of infection by *T. cruzi* and afflicts several million people in Central and South America. The disease develops years or even decades after infection. Chronic Chagas' disease characteristically causes chronic cardiomyopathy, and in some geographic regions (Brazil and Chile), megaesophagus and megacolon. The cardiomyopathy is characterized by a dilated heart, prominent right ventricular outflow tract,

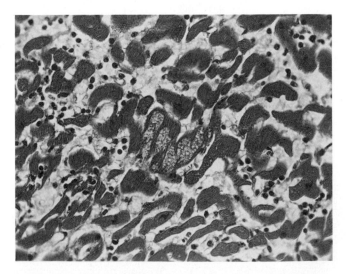

Figure 9-23. Chagas' disease, with myocarditis. The myofibers contain large numbers of amastigotes (leishmanial forms) of *T. cruzi*. There is edema and chronic inflammation.

and dilatation of the valve rings. The interventricular septum is often deviated to the right and may immobilize the adjacent tricuspid leaflet. Microscopically, the myocardium displays focal inflammatory infiltrates (lymphocytes and plasma), interstitial fibrosis, and hypertrophied myofibers. Parasites are difficult to find.

AFRICAN TRYPANOSOMIASIS (SLEEPING SICKNESS)

African trypanosomiasis (sleeping sickness) is a chronic infection with *Trypanosoma brucei gambiense* or an acute one with *Trypanosoma brucei rhodesiense*. These hemoflagellate protozoa are transmitted cyclically by several species of blood-sucking tsetse flies of the genus *Glossina*. The uneven distribution of African trypanosomiasis is related to the habitats of the tsetse flies (Fig. 9-24). In Gambian trypanosomiasis, *T. b. gambiense* is transmitted by tsetse flies of the riverine bush, mainly in focal areas of West and Central Africa. Man in the only important reservoir for *T. b. gambiense*, which causes a chronic infection often lasting more than a year. In Rhodesian trypanosomiasis, *T. b. rhodesiense* is transmitted by tsetse flies of the woodland savanna of East Africa. Antelope, other game animals, and domestic cattle are natural reservoirs of *T. b. rhodesiense*. *T. b. rhodesiense* causes a disabling, acute, and fulminant infection in man, killing the patient in 3 to 6 months.

After an incubation period of 5 to 15 days, the dermal inoculation site develops a primary trypanosomal chancre, a 3- to 4-cm papular swelling in the skin, topped by a central red spot, which subsides spontaneously within 3 weeks. Shortly after the appearance of the chancre (if any), and within 3 weeks after the bite, invasion of the bloodstream is marked by intermittent fever, which lasts up to a week and is often accompanied by splenomegaly and local and generalized lymphadenopathy. Winterbottom's sign—enlargement of the posterior cervical lymph nodes—is characteristic of Gambian trypanosomiasis. In both forms the evolving illness is marked by remittent, irregular fever, headache, joint pains, lethargy, anorexia, muscle wasting, and, in some patients, anemia.

Invasion of the brain (see Fig. 9-24) typically develops early (within weeks or months) in Rhodesian trypanosomiasis, or late (after months or years) in Gambian trypanosomiasis. It results in apathy, irritability, changes in personality, lethargy, daytime somnolence, and sometimes coma. Without treatment African trypanosomiasis is fatal.

LEISHMANIASIS

CUTANEOUS AND MUCOCUTANEOUS LEISHMANIASIS

Cutaneous and mucocutaneous leishmaniasis are caused by three species complexes, *Leishmania tropica*, *Leishmania braziliensis*, and *Leishmania mexicana*. Promastigotes multiply in the gut of the sandfly and, in turn, are injected into the dermis of a vertebrate host (animal or man). The promastigotes invade reticuloendothelial cells, transform into amastigotes, multiply, and invade other reticuloendothelial cells.

The gerbil is the reservoir for *L. tropica major*, which causes cutaneous leishmaniasis ("tropical sore") in moist **rural** environments of the Middle East, Arabia, Russia, India, and sub-subsaharan Africa. Man and dogs are reservoirs for *L. tropica minor*, which causes cutaneous leishmaniasis in dry **urban** environments of the Middle East and the Mediterranean basin. The rock hyrax and tree hyrax (rabbit-like mammals) are reservoirs for *L. tropica aethiopica*, which causes diffuse (anergic) cutaneous leishmaniasis in people whose homesteads encroach on deforested mountain slopes of the Rift Valley in Ethiopia and Kenya.

The primary lesion of cutaneous leishmaniasis is an itching papule, which expands over a period of weeks or months to form a shallow, indolent, slowly expanding ulcer. Histologically, at the site of inoculation the first reaction is an infiltrate of leishmania-containing histiocytes, which expand and proliferate to accommodate the increasing numbers of leishmania. This is followed by an infiltrate of neutrophils, necrosis, and sloughing of large numbers of organisms. Gradually the histiocytes lose their leishmania and become epithelioid cells, after which the reaction matures to a granuloma. During this transition increasing numbers of lymphocytes and plasma cells appear in the exudate. Satellite lesions develop along draining lymphatics. Healing usually begins at 3 to 6 months, but may take a year or longer.

VISCERAL LEISHMANIASIS (KALA-AZAR)

Visceral leishmaniasis (Kala-azar) (Fig. 9-25) is caused by *Leishmania donovani*, which morphologically resembles the leishmania organisms previously described. Leishmania can be identified in smears or tissue specimens of the spleen, lymph nodes, liver, bone marrow, and skin, but splenic aspiration is the surest method of confirming the diagnosis. The life cycle and insect vectors of *L. donovani* are the same as those described for the other *Leishmania* species.

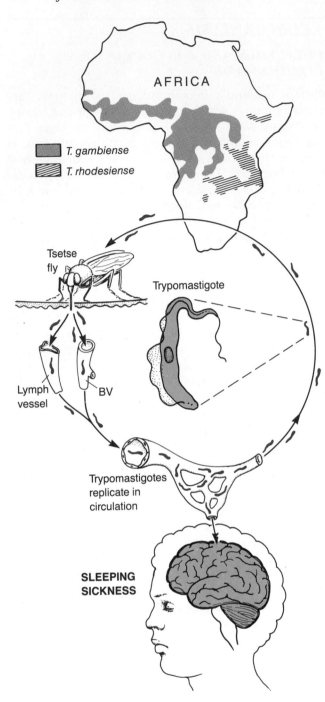

Figure 9-24. African trypanosomiasis (sleeping sickness). The distribution of Gambian and Rhodesian trypanosomiasis is related to the habitats of the vector tsetse flies (*Glossina* sp.). A tsetse fly bites an infected animal or human and ingests trypomastigotes, which multiply into infective, metacyclic trypomastigotes. During another fly bite, these are injected into lymphatic and blood vessels of a new host. A primary chancre develops at the site of the bite (Stage 1a). Trypomastigotes replicate further in the blood and lymph, causing a systemic infection (Stage 1b). Another fly ingests trypomastigotes to complete the cycle. In stage 2, invasion of the central nervous system by trypomastigotes leads to meningoencephalomyelitis and associated symptoms, including lethargy and daytime somnolence. Patients with Rhodesian trypanosomiasis may die within a few months.

Man is the reservoir in India, and foxes in Southern France, Central Italy, and some parts of South America. Jackals are the reservoir for sporadic cases in rural areas of the Middle East and central Asia. Dogs are reservoirs in the Mediterranean basin, China, and some parts of South America. The reservoirs in Africa are incompletely known but may include man, domestic dogs, rats, and other rodents.

Low-grade fever, malaise, and lassitude begin 10 days to 10 months after inoculation. The cardinal features of visceral leishmaniasis are fever, generalized lymphadenopathy, hepatosplenomegaly, panyctopenia, and cachexia. Fair skin turns dark ("kala-azar" is Hindi for "black fever"). Death is often caused by bacterial pneumonia, septicemia, tuberculosis, dysentery, and uncontrolled hemorrhage, or by severe anemia.

Histologically, a granuloma develops at the site of inoculation, and amastigotes spread by the lymph to local lymph nodes and by the blood to the spleen, liver, and bone marrow. Histiocytic cells in the spleen proliferate, replace the parenchyma, and expand the organ. Many amastigotes accumulate in Kupffer cells of the liver and in phagocytic cells of bone marrow. The histiocytes are stuffed with amastigotes and resemble the foamy histiocytes of lepromatous leprosy. The heart, skin, and epididymis also contain numerous leishmania-containing histiocytes.

MALARIA

Human malaria is an acute and chronic protozoal disease caused by any one of a combination of four species of plasmodia, namely *Plasmodium falciparum*, *Plasmodium vivax*, *Plasmodium ovale*, and *Plasmodium malariae*. *P. falciparum* is the most virulent of these and the only one that kills acutely. The other three species are "benign". Infections with *P. ovale* and *P. malariae* are now rare. The plasmodial parasites are transmitted by female mosquitoes of several species of the genus *Anopheles*, and hyperendemic breeding grounds for these mosquitoes are directly related to the prevalence of the disease.

The World Health Organization recognizes malaria as the world's major primary health problem, causing more morbidity and mortality than any other dieseases. Malaria has been eradicated in the United States, Canada, and Europe, but continues to be a scourge in tropical and subtropical areas, especially tropical Africa, parts of South and Central America, India, and Southeast Asia.

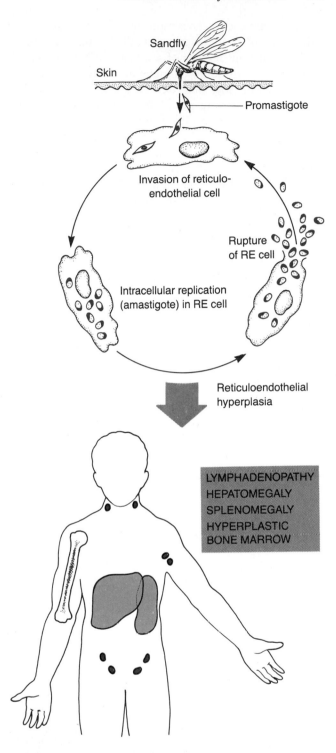

Figure 9-25. Leishmaniasis. Blood-sucking sandflies ingest amastigotes from an infected host. These are transformed in the sandfly gut into promastigotes, which multiply and are injected into the next vertebrate host. There they invade reticuloendothelial cells, revert to the amastigote form, and multiply, eventually rupturing the cell. They then invade other reticuloendothelial cells, thus completing the cycle.

The cardinal clinical symptoms of malaria are cyclic paroxysms of high fever and chills, usually accompanied by varying degrees of anemia and splenomegaly. The major pathologic changes are a consequence of parasitization and destruction of erythrocytes (Fig. 9-26). As succeeding populations of parasites mature within erythrocytes and destroy them, merozoites, malarial pigment, hemoglobin, and cellular debris are released into the bloodstream. Malarial pigment accumulates in phagocytic cells of the reticuloendothelial system, and hemoglobin is absorbed by renal tubular cells. Patients who have massive absorption of hemoglobin by the renal tubules may die with **hemoglobinuric nephrosis** ("blackwater fever").

At autopsy, the spleen and liver in falciparum malaria are enlarged and all organs of the reticuloendothelial system are darkened ("slate gray") by malarial pigment. The gross lesions of the brain—congestion and petechiae—are limited to the white matter, a characteristic feature of cerebral malaria. For reasons that are unclear, parasitized erythrocytes cling to endothelial cells. This "stickiness" has two practical implications. First, parasitized erythrocytes attached to endothelial cells do not circulate, so patients with severe falciparum malaria have few circulating parasites. Second, capillaries of deep organs, especially the brain, become obstructed, leading to hypoxia and death. Phagocytosis of parasitized erythrocytes leads to reticuloendothelial hyperplasia and hepatosplenomegaly. Clusters of parasitized erythrocytes become bound in fibrin thrombi that obstruct small vessels and are associated with microhemorrhages and microinfarcts, if the patient lives long enough for these to develop. Encephalopathy, congestive heart failure, pulmonary edema, and hemoglobinuric nephrosis with renal failure are all fatal complications.

Figure 9-26. Life cycle of malaria. An *Anopheles* mosquito bites an infected person, taking blood that contains micro- and macrogametocytes (sexual forms). In the mosquito, sexual multiplication ("sporogony") produces infective sporozoites in the salivary glands. (1) During the mosquito bite, sporozoites are inoculated into the bloodstream of the vertebrate host. Some sporozoites leave the blood and enter the hepatocytes, where they multiply asexually (exoerythrocytic schizogony), and form thousands of uninucleated merozoites. (2) Rupture of hepatocytes releases merozoites, which penetrate erythrocytes and become trophozoites, which then divide to form numerous schizonts (intraerythrocytic schizogony). Schizonts divide to form more merozoites, which are released on the rupture of erythrocytes and reenter other erythrocytes to begin a new cycle. After several cycles, subpopulations of merozoites develop into micro- and macrogametocytes, which are taken up by another mosquito to complete the cycle. (3) Parasitized erythrocytes obstruct capillaries of the brain, heart, kidney, and other deep organs. Adherence of parasitized erythrocytes to capillary endothelial cells causes fibrin thrombi, which produce microinfarcts. These result in encephalopathy, congestive heart failure, pulmonary edema, and frequently death. Ruptured erythrocytes release hemoglobin, erythrocyte debris, and malarial pigment. (4) Phagocytosis leads to reticuloendothelial hyperplasia and hepatosplenomegaly. (5) Released hemoglobin produces hemoglobinuric nephrosis, which may be fatal.

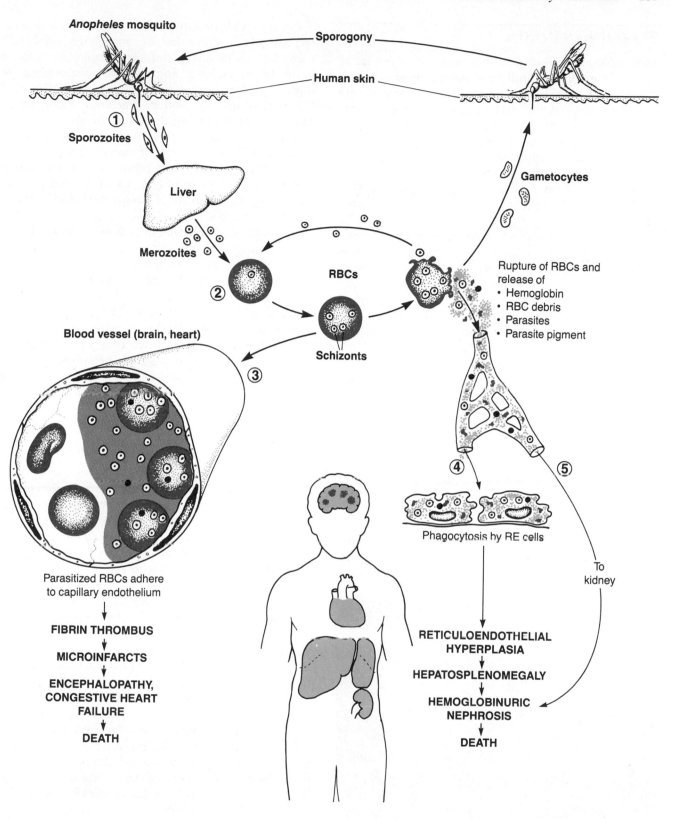

Anopheles mosquito

Sporogony

Human skin

① Sporozoites

Liver

Merozoites

RBCs

Gametocytes

Rupture of RBCs and release of
• Hemoglobin
• RBC debris
• Parasites
• Parasite pigment

②

Schizonts

Blood vessel (brain, heart)

③

④

⑤

Phagocytosis by RE cells

To kidney

Parasitized RBCs adhere
to capillary endothelium
↓
FIBRIN THROMBUS
↓
MICROINFARCTS
↓
**ENCEPHALOPATHY,
CONGESTIVE HEART
FAILURE**
↓
DEATH

**RETICULOENDOTHELIAL
HYPERPLASIA**
↓
HEPATOSPLENOMEGALY
↓
**HEMOGLOBINURIC
NEPHROSIS**
↓
DEATH

TOXOPLASMOSIS

Toxoplasmosis, infection by the protozoan *Toxoplasma gondii*, is worldwide and may be the most common infection of mankind. Most infections, however, are mild or asymptomatic, and clinical disease is uncommon. The final host for infection with *T. gondii* is the cat, which ingests the pathogen in the tissues of an infected mouse or other intermediate host. *T. gondii* is transmitted to humans, other mammals, and birds by oocysts in the feces of cats. Humans ingest the pathogens in food that has contacted feces or contaminated soil.

Toxoplasmosis manifests itself in humans in several ways, including an acute febrile disease, sometimes with pneumonia, myocarditis, and hepatitis; lymphadenopathy; acute or chronic encephalitis in an immunosuppressed host; chronic retinitis; asymptomatic maternal infection and transplacental infection of the fetus; and neonatal infection with jaundice or encephalitis.

In the acute disease the incubation period ranges from 7 to 17 days. The initial symptoms include headache, fever, myalgia, enlarged lymph nodes, and sometimes splenomegaly. Tachyzoites multiply in many tissues, destroy host cells, cause necrosis, and provoke inflammation. Hepatitis, myocarditis, and myositis have been documented.

Toxoplasmic lymphadenitis most commonly involves the posterior cervical lymph nodes, although nodes at other sites may also be affected. Follicular hyperplasia and characteristic small clusters of histiocytes are prominent throughout the parafollicular areas and, sometimes, within the follicles.

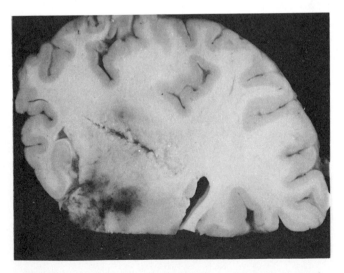

Figure 9-27. Toxoplasmosis, brain. There is a large area of necrosis with focal hemorrhage.

Patients with immunodeficiencies may have acute, recrudescent, necrotic lesions, with huge numbers of tachyzoites, usually in only one organ, such as the brain, heart, or lung. Some immunosuppressed patients develop fatal toxoplasmic encephalitis (Fig. 9-27), in which case scattered areas of infarction are caused by vasculitis and thrombi.

In chronic toxoplasmosis, bradyzoites persist in tissue cysts and cause disease of many organs, especially striated muscle, brain, and retina. The retinal lesions, which may lead to blindness, are often recurrent and are usually the sequelae of congenital infection or exposure in childhood.

Asymptomatic maternal infections, although benign to the mother, are transmitted to the fetus in about a third of cases. The most important lesions in the neonate with congenital toxoplasmosis are in the brain. The lesions progress from small nodules containing tachyzoites through stages of vascular thrombosis, ependymal ulceration, and periventricular lesions with calcification, which may obstruct the aqueduct and kill the infant. Some newborns have hepatitis, with large areas of necrosis and giant cells, and others have adrenal necrosis.

PNEUMOCYSTOSIS

Pneumocystosis is an opportunistic infection of the lungs caused by the protozoan *Pneumocystis carinii*. Two stages, cyst and trophozoite, are both in the pulmonary alveoli. The organism is worldwide, and since 75% of the population have acquired antibodies by 5 years of age, it is reasonable to assume that the organisms are inhaled regularly by all. In healthy people these organisms are killed by the pulmonary macrophages. When phagocytosis is defective, however, organisms remain in the alveoli, proliferate, and eventually fill the alveoli with their carcasses. They do not invade the alveolar walls and provoke little inflammation. Pneumocystosis, therefore, although it may be fatal, is not an infection in the usual sense.

Pneumocystosis afflicts two distinct groups of patients. The first comprises premature and malnourished infants whose immune systems are not yet developed; the second comprises immunodeficient adults. **Pneumocystosis is now recognized as the most common infection of patients with the acquired immunodeficiency syndrome (AIDS).**

The presenting symptom of pneumocystosis is shortness of breath, with or without nonproductive cough, that may progress to respiratory failure and death.

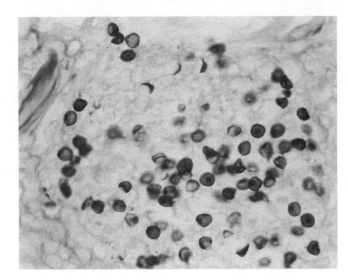

Figure 9-28. Pneumocystosis. The alveoli contain many cysts (*Pneumocystis carinii*). The crescent-shaped organisms are collapsed and degenerated; others have a characteristic dark spot in their wall.

The lungs are consolidated and heavy, but not edematous. Microscopically, the alveoli contain a foamy eosinophilic, honeycombed material, which is composed of alveolar macrophages and cysts and trophozoites of *P. carinii.* There may be hyaline membranes and prominent type 2 alveolar lining cells. In newborns the alveolar septa are thickened by lymphoid cells and histiocytes. Definitive diagnosis requires the identification of the organisms. *P. carinii* is easily seen in sections stained with Gomori's methenamine silver (Fig. 9-28).

AMEBIASIS (ENTAMOEBA HISTOLYTICA)

Amebiasis refers to an infection by the ameba *Entamoeba histolytica*, the most important intestinal ameba of man (Fig. 9-29). Trophozoites invade and ulcerate the colonic mucosa, causing diarrhea, intermittent constipation, abdominal distention, and malodorous flatus. Complications include amebomas of the colon, stricture, amebic abscesses of the liver and lung, and cutaneous amebiasis.

Man is the principal reservoir. Amebiasis is worldwide but is more common and more severe in tropical and subtropical areas, where poor sanitation prevails.

The cysts, found in contaminated water or food, are the infective stage. Ingested cysts pass through the stomach and excyst in the lower ileum. Trophozoites

may colonize any portion of the large bowel, but the area of maximum disease is usually the cecum. Patients with symptomatic amebic colitis usually pass both cysts and trophozoites, but the trophozoites survive only briefly outside the body and are destroyed by gastric secretions.

The incubation period for acute amebic colitis is usually 8 to 10 days. Clinically, gradually increasing abdominal discomfort, tenderness, and cramps are accompanied by chills and fever. Nausea, severe vomiting, malodorous flatus, and intermittent constipation are typical features. Liquid stools (up to 25 a day) contain bloody mucus, and prolonged diarrhea may result in dehydration. Amebic colitis often persists for months or years; between acute attacks there may be recurring cramps; soft, loose stools suggest untreated parasitism. In severe amebic colitis, massive destruction of the colonic mucosa, hemorrhage, perforation, and peritonitis may be fatal complications.

Amebic lesions begin as small foci of necrosis that progress to ulcers. Some lesions remain small and discrete, but others expand. Undermining of the ulcer margin and confluence of one or more expanding ulcers lead to sloughing of the mucosa in broad, irregular geographic patterns. Typically the bed of the ulcer is gray and necrotic, being composed of fibrin and cellular debris. The exudate raises the undermined mucosa, producing chronic amebic ulcers whose shape has been described as resembling a flask, a bottle neck, or a "sea anemone." There is little inflammatory response in early ulcers. However, as the ulcer widens, there is an accumulation of neutrophils, lymphocytes, histiocytes, plasma cells, and sometimes eosinophils.

An **ameboma** is an inflammatory thickening of the wall of the bowel that resembles carcinoma of the colon in location, symptoms, and gross and radiographic appearance. The ameboma tends to form a "napkin-ring" constriction. Histologic sections reveal granulation tissue, fibrosis, chronic inflammatory cells, and clusters of trophozoites.

Intestinal perforation, most often in the cecum, is a feared complication. Patients may have a single or multiple amebic liver "abscesses," which may be large enough to destroy an entire lobe. The so-called amebic abscess contains yellow or gray, opaque, amorphous liquid material that does not contain neutrophils.

GIARDIASIS (GIARDIA LAMBLIA)

Giardiasis, an infection of the small intestine by the protozoan *Giardia lamblia*, has a worldwide distribution, with a prevalence that varies from 1% to more

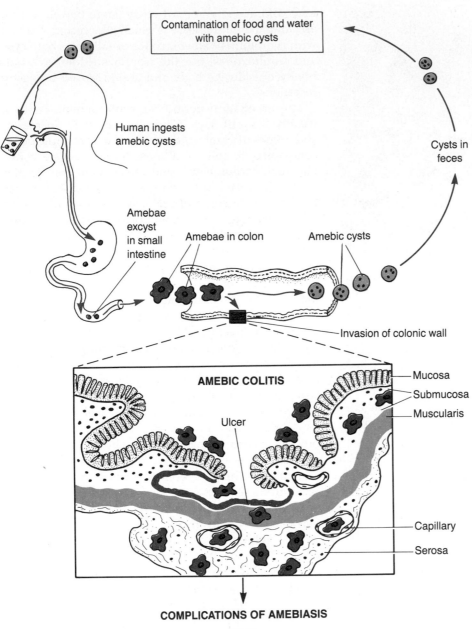

Contamination of food and water
with amebic cysts

Human ingests
amebic cysts

Cysts in
feces

Amebae
excyst
in small
intestine

Amebae in colon

Amebic cysts

Invasion of colonic wall

AMEBIC COLITIS

Mucosa
Submucosa
Muscularis

Ulcer

Capillary

Serosa

Figure 9-29. Amebic colitis results from the ingestion of food or water contaminated with amebic cysts. Cysts are released into the feces, after which fecal contamination of food and water completes the cycle. In the colon the amebae penetrate the mucosa and produce a flask-shaped ulcer of the mucosa and submucosa. The organisms reach the serosa and invade capillaries, thereby disseminating throughout the body and producing local complications.

COMPLICATIONS OF AMEBIASIS

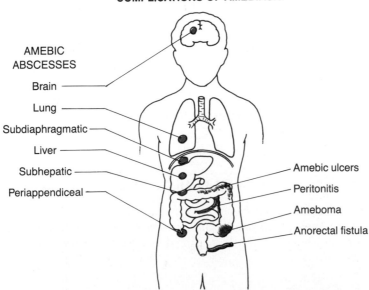

AMEBIC
ABSCESSES

Brain
Lung
Subdiaphragmatic
Liver
Subhepatic
Periappendiceal

Amebic ulcers
Peritonitis
Ameboma
Anorectal fistula

than 25%. The incidence is higher in warmer climates and in crowded, unsanitary environments. Children are about three times more susceptible than adults. Giardia are spread from person to person, or by water and food.

Although the organism is a harmless commensal in most people, it can cause acute or chronic symptoms. Frequent or intermittent diarrhea is the most important clinical complaint.

Biopsy of the small intestine reveals few to many trophozoites attached to the epithelial cells of the intestinal mucosa. The mucosa is essentially normal in many patients, but in others blunting and chronic inflammation of the villi are seen. Tissue invasion is rare.

DISEASES CAUSED BY FUNGI

ASPERGILLOSIS

About 150 species of aspergillus are known, of which only three, *Aspergillus fumigatus, Aspergillus flavus-oryzae,* and *Aspergillus niger* commonly infect man. These fungi are worldwide and ubiquitous. They live in soil as saprophytes, and produce spores in great abundance. Because the spores are constantly inhaled, the lung is the most common site of infection; however, any organ may be invaded, as well as virtually any orifice or surface, including the ear, nose, nasal sinuses, eye, skin, and intestine. Most patients have one or more predisposing conditions, including diabetes, leukemia, lymphoma or other malignant tumors, and treatment with cytotoxic agents, radiation, and broad-spectrum antibiotics.

Aspergillosis may be divided into three categories: aspergilloma, the fungus ball; acute aspergillosis, with or without dissemination, and allergic bronchopulmonary aspergillosis.

Almost all **fungus balls (aspergillomas)** are caused by *A. niger.* Airborne spores or mycelial fragments colonize a cavity or ectatic bronchus caused by prior tuberculosis, bronchiectasis, or histoplasmosis. The fungus ball is a layered compact mass of mycelium and cellular debris, in which the hyphae have a parallel or radial arrangement.

Acute aspergillosis begins in the lung or intestine and spreads in the bloodstream to the brain, heart, kidney, and other organs. *A. fumigatus* is the most virulent of the aspergilli and the most common cause of acute and disseminated infection. Acute aspergillosis is characterized by an abundance of hyphae, which are arranged in a radial pattern and cause a purulent, necrotizing reaction. The hyphae grow along tissue planes,

invade vessels, and cause thrombi and septic infarction. Lesions in the brain are angiocentric and result from septic thrombosis of cerebral arteries and resultant septic infarction.

Patients with **primary allergic bronchopulmonary aspergillosis** are not infected. Rather, owing to sensitization to antigens of *Aspergillus* species, they have an exaggerated humoral response to inhaled spores. *A. fumigatus,* the prevailing saprophytic fungus in some environments, is the common offender. Inhalation of spores is followed by an attack of asthma, with productive cough, fever, malaise, and prostration. Some patients have transient pulmonary infiltrates and high levels of circulating eosinophils. The sputum is purulent and contains eosinophils and fungi. Although fungi are found in the sputum, infection plays no role. The patient recovers within 1 to 2 days.

BLASTOMYCOSIS

Blastomycosis, a chronic infection caused by *Blastomyces dermatitidis,* affects the lungs and skin. Men with outdoor occupations in the basins of the Mississippi, Ohio, Missouri, and St. Lawrence Rivers are most susceptible. The source and route of infection are unproved, but inhalation of conidia from the soil is most likely.

The primary infection is usually in the lung (Fig. 9-30). It may resolve without residue, or it may disseminate to the skin, bone, urogenital organs, and, less commonly, the brain. Symptoms include mild to severe pleuritic pain, fever, productive cough, dyspnea, myalgia, and arthralgia.

The pulmonary infection, which may be solitary or bilateral, results in consolidation of hilar lymphadenopathy. The reaction to the organism is mixed, having suppurative and granulomatous features. Although the lesions usually resolve by scarring, some patients develop progressive miliary lesions or focal consolidation with cavitation.

CANDIDIASIS

Candidiasis is an opportunistic infection caused by *Candida albicans,* and occasionally by *Candida tropicalis* and other species. **One of the most common fungal pathogens of mankind, Candida species are part of the normal flora of the skin and mucocutaneous areas, intestine, and vagina.** Infants are exposed to *Candida* at birth, after which the organisms colonize the intestinal tract and natural immunity develops. Disruption of the balance between the host and the organism leads to the expression of disease. A number

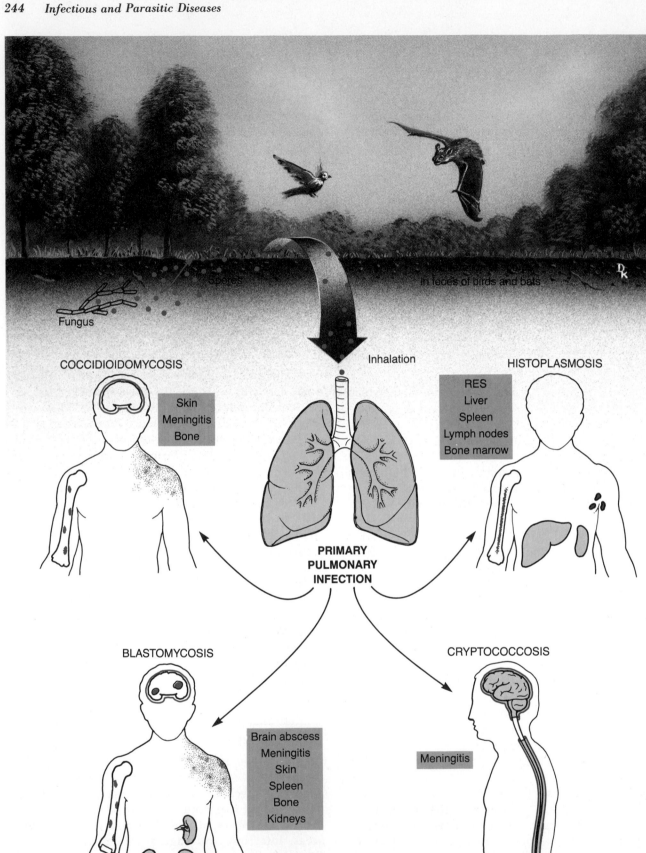

COCCIDIOIDOMYCOSIS

Skin
Meningitis
Bone

Fungus

Spores

Inhalation

in feces of birds and bats

HISTOPLASMOSIS

RES
Liver
Spleen
Lymph nodes
Bone marrow

PRIMARY
PULMONARY
INFECTION

BLASTOMYCOSIS

Brain abscess
Meningitis
Skin
Spleen
Bone
Kidneys

CRYPTOCOCCOSIS

Meningitis

of predisposing factors contribute to infections. Prolonged treatment with antibiotics, particularly with multiple antibiotic therapy, permits an overgrowth of *Candida* by eliminating and impairing the competing bacterial flora that hold *Candida* in check. The lack of a balanced flora predisposes newborns to thrush and diaper rash. During prolonged steroid administration, pregnancy, or endocrine disturbances *Candida* proliferate. In all these situations overgrowth of *Candida* usually resolves without treatment. With impaired immunity, however, superficial candidiasis may progress to mucocutaneous candidiasis and then to systemic infection.

Candida may involve the skin and mucosa or may invade deep organs. **Early in life, oral thrush is the most common form of mucocutaneous candidiasis, and candidal vaginitis during pregnancy predisposes the neonate to infection.** In oral thrush, the lesions begin as small focal areas of colonization of the mucosa that progress into confluent patches. Later, a creamy white pseudomembrane, composed of masses of fungi, covers the tongue, soft palate, and buccal mucosa. When detached, it leaves a reddened inflamed surface, which, in severe disease, may be ulcerated. Vaginal candidiasis is characterized by a thick yellow discharge and by patches of gray-white pseudomembranes on the mucosa. The lesions are pruritic and may extend to involve the vulva and perineum. Systemic candidiasis is rare and is usually a terminal event of an underlying disorder associated with an altered immune system.

COCCIDIOIDOMYCOSIS

Coccidioidomycosis, caused by the inhalation or arthrospores of *Coccidioides immitis*, is a chronic, necrotizing, mycotic infection that clinically and pathologically resembles tuberculosis. Coccidioidomycosis is most prevalent in the western and southwestern United States and is particularly common in the San Joaquin Valley of California, where it is called "valley fever." Coccidioidomycosis also occurs in Mexico and in parts of South America.

Coccidioidomycosis is a disease of protean manifestations, which may vary from a subclinical respiratory infection to one that disseminates and is rapidly fatal. The two most common types of coccidioidomycosis are primary pulmonary and disseminated.

Primary pulmonary coccidioidomycosis is an acute, self-limited infection. The lesion is a solitary grayish focus of consolidation, 2 to 3 cm across, usually in the middle or lower lung fields. Occasionally, a more diffuse pneumonic consolidation or multiple scattered foci of consolidation appear. Hilar lymphadenopathy is usually absent. Symptomatic patients have fever, night sweats, pleuritic pain, dysphagia, cough, and shortness of breath. Histologically, the primary pulmonary nodule is a caseating granuloma.

Cavitation is the most frequent complication of pulmonary coccidioidomycosis. The cavity is usually solitary and may persist for years. In a few patients, progression or reactivation leads to destructive lesions in the lungs or, more seriously, to disseminated lesions throughout the body (see Fig. 9-30).

Disseminated coccidioidomycosis occurs by hematogenous spread of sporangiospores from the lungs into the skin, bones, joints, adrenals, lymph nodes, spleen, liver, and meninges.

CRYPTOCOCCOSIS

Cryptococcosis is a systemic mycosis with worldwide distribution caused by *Cryptococcus neoformans*. The most important lesions are in the lungs and meninges (see Fig. 9-30). Cryptococci are unique among pathogenic fungi in having a mucopolysaccharide capsule, which is essential for their pathogenicity. The main reservoir is pigeon droppings. Clinically significant

Figure 9-30. Pulmonary and disseminated fungal infection. Fungi grow in soil, air, and the feces of birds and bats, and produce spores, some of which are infectious. When inhaled, spores cause primary pulmonary infection. In a few patients the infection disseminates.
Histoplasmosis. Primary infection is in the lung. In susceptible patients, the fungus disseminates to target organs, namely the reticuloendothelial system (liver, spleen, lymph nodes, and bone marrow), and the tongue, mucous membranes of mouth, and adrenals.
Cryptococcosis. Primary infection of the lung disseminates to the meninges.
Blastomycosis. Primary infection of the lung disseminates widely. The principle targets are the brain, meninges, skin, spleen, bone, and kidney.
Coccidioidomycosis. Primary infection of the lung may disseminate widely. The skin, meninges, and bone are common targets.

cryptococcosis is usually an opportunistic infection. People with normal immunity become infected, but the infection is silent and heals spontaneously. People with immunodeficiencies, on the other hand, develop progressive cryptococcal pulmonary infection, with cough, pleuritic pain, malaise, and fever. The lesions are frequently bilateral and localized in the lower lobes, but may involve an entire lobe or lobes and kill the patient quickly. Miliary granulomas, small abscesses, and large solid mucoid lesions are seen.

From the lung the cryptococci spread through the bloodstream to other organs, particularly the central nervous system, where the common presentation is meningitis. The gray mucinous exudate distends the subarachnoid space, especially at the base of the brain and over the cerebral convexities. Untreated cryptococcal meningitis is uniformly fatal.

HISTOPLASMOSIS

Histoplasmosis is a worldwide systemic mycosis caused by *Histoplasma capsulatum*, a dimorphic fungus that grows in humans as a round or oval yeast. The reservoir for *H. capsulatum* is in bird droppings and in the soil. In the Americas, hyperendemic areas are in the eastern and central United States, western Mexico, Central America, the northern countries of South America, and Argentina.

Inhalation of conidia causes a primary pulmonary infection, which in 95% of people is subclinical and transitory. Inhalation of a large number of conidia causes a more aggression infection. The initial infection is followed by a transient fungemia. Symptoms develop in 8 to 15 days and include malaise, cough, and shortness of breath. Most patients abort their infection, leaving residual foci of calcification in the lungs and, sometimes, the spleen. Others develop chronic pulmonary histoplasmosis, which may be confused with tuberculosis because the clinical and pathologic features are similar. (Chronic cough, chest pain, fever, night sweats, malaise, and weight loss are common to both histoplasmosis and tuberculosis.) The lesions may cavitate or heal with a fibrotic scar.

Infants, the elderly, and those with deficient immunity are all prone to disseminated histoplasmosis, a condition characterized by proliferation of the organism in phagocytic cells of the bone marrow, liver, and spleen (see Fig. 9-30). The patient suffers from generalized lymphadenopathy, hepatosplenomegaly, fever, anemia, weight loss, leukopenia, and thrombocytopenia.

DISEASES CAUSED BY FILARIAL NEMATODES

BANCROFTIAN AND MALAYAN FILARIASIS

Bancroftian and Malayan filariasis are infections by *Wuchereria bancrofti* and *Brugia malayi*, respectively. The adult worms inhabit lymphatic vessels, most frequently those in the lymph nodes, testis, and epididymis. Both genera block lymphatic vessels, and they cause similar symptoms and lesions.

Humans are the only definitive host of these worms. Insect vectors, which serve also as intermediate hosts, include at least 80 species of mosquitoes. Bancroftian filariasis is endemic in large regions of Africa, coastal areas of Asia, the western Pacific islands, and coastal areas and islands of the Caribbean basin. Malayan filariasis is endemic in coastal areas of Asia and the western Pacific islands.

Most of those infected remain asymptomatic throughout life. Symptomatic chronic infection is characterized by enlarged lymph nodes, lymphedema, hydrocele, and elephantiasis. Elephantiasis afflicts only a small proportion of patients, and then only after years of infection. Filariasis also causes tropical eosinophilia, which is characterized by cough, wheezing, eosinophilia, and diffuse pulmonary infiltrates.

ONCHOCERCIASIS

Onchocerciasis, infection by the filarial nematode *Onchocerca volvulus*, is one of the world's major endemic disease, afflicting an estimated 40 million people, of whom about 2 million are blind. Man is the only known definitive host. Onchocerciasis is transmitted by several species of blackflies of the genus *Simulium*, which breed in fast-flowing streams. There are endemic regions throughout tropical Africa and in focal areas of Central and South America.

The cardinal manifestations are subcutaneous nodules, dermatitis, sclerosing lymphadenitis, and eye disease. The adult worms live singly and as coiled entangled masses in the deep fascia and the subcutaneous tissues. The worms are detected clinically only when they become encapsulated by a fibrous scar, forming discrete onchocercal nodules (**onchocercomas**) in the deep dermis and subcutaneous tissues. Nodules form over bony prominences of the skull, scapula, rib, iliac crest, trochanter, sacrum, and knee. The adult worms are innocuous, but the gravid female worms produce millions of microfilariae, which migrate from the nodule into the skin, eyes, lymph nodes, and deep organs, thereby causing the corresponding onchocercal lesions. Ocular onchocerciasis results from the migration of microfilariae into all regions of the eye, from the cornea to the optic nerve head, and result in sclerosing keratitis, iridocyclitis, chorioretinitis, and optic atrophy.

DISEASES CAUSED BY OTHER NEMATODES

TRICHINOSIS

Trichinosis, an infection by the nematode *Trichinella spiralis*, is cosmopolitan but is most common in eastern and central Europe, North America, and Central and South America. Although it prevails in areas where pork is eaten, many animals, including dogs, cats, rats, bears, foxes, and wolves, are reservoirs of infection. Humans become infected by eating undercooked or raw meat, mainly pork, containing encysted larvae (Fig. 9-31). The cysts, located in striated muscle, are digested, liberating larvae, which mature to adult worms and attach to the wall of the small intestine. There female worms liberate larvae that invade the intestinal wall, enter the circulation, and penetrate striated muscle, where they encyst and remain viable for years.

In subclinical disease the only sign is eosinophilia. The invasion of muscle by the larvae is associated with muscle pain, swelling of the eyelids, facial edema, eosinophilia, and pronounced fever. Respiratory and neurologic manifestations may appear. Fatal cases are usually attributed to a severe myocarditis. During the chronic phase of the disease the symptoms gradually attenuate.

On invasion of the muscle the larvae cause inflammation and destruction of muscle fibers. A fibrous hyaline layer develops around a single coiled larva. Histiocytes and giant cells may surround the cyst, which eventually calcifies. The most frequently involved muscles are those of the limbs, diaphragm, tongue, jaw, larynx, ribs, and eye. Larvae in other organs, including the heart and brain, cause edema, necrosis, and focal infiltration of neutrophils, eosinophils, and lymphocytes, but they do not encyst.

ANCYLOSTOMIASIS (HOOKWORM)

Ancylostomiasis is an infection of man by one of two hookworms, *Ancylostoma duodenale* or *Necator americanus*. Ancylostomiasis is encountered worldwide and causes serious public health problems across vast areas of the globe. Tropical areas with poor sanitation are ideal for transmission.

On contact with human skin, infective filariform larvae penetrate the epidermis and enter the venous circulation. They are then swept through the right heart and into the pulmonary capillaries. Here they break through vessels into alveolar spaces, migrate to the epiglottis, are coughed up, and then swallowed. They molt in the duodenum, attach to the mucosal wall with toothlike buccal plates, clamp off a section of the villus, and ingest it (Fig. 9-32). Infection causes three main syndromes: a dermatitis when larvae penetrate the skin; a pneumonitis when larvae migrate through the lung; and severe iron deficiency anemia from loss of blood caused by the adult worms biting off bits of intestinal mucosa.

ASCARIASIS

Ascariasis, infection by the large intestinal roundworm *Ascaris lumbricoides*, is cosmopolitan and probably **the most common helminthic infection.** Infection is more common in the tropics, in children, and in crowded rural communities with poor sanitation. Adult worms live in the small intestine, where gravid females discharge eggs that pass in feces. Eggs develop in warm moist soil to become infective in 3 to 4 weeks. The eggs hatch when ingested, and the larvae penetrate the intestinal wall, enter the portal circulation, pass through the liver and heart, reach the lungs, and develop into third-stage larvae. The larvae migrate up the trachea and down the esophagus, reaching the small intestine, where they develop into adult worms. Humans acquire the infection by ingesting infective eggs in contaminated soil, food, or water.

Most patients have few or no symptoms, but heavy infections may cause vomiting, malnutrition, appendicitis, and sometimes intestinal obstruction.

Adult worms in the small intestine usually cause no changes, but when worms migrate into the ampulla of Vater or the pancreatic or biliary ducts, they cause biliary obstruction, acute pancreatitis, suppurative cholangitis, and liver abscesses. *Ascaris* pneumonia, which is occasionally fatal, develops when larvae mi-

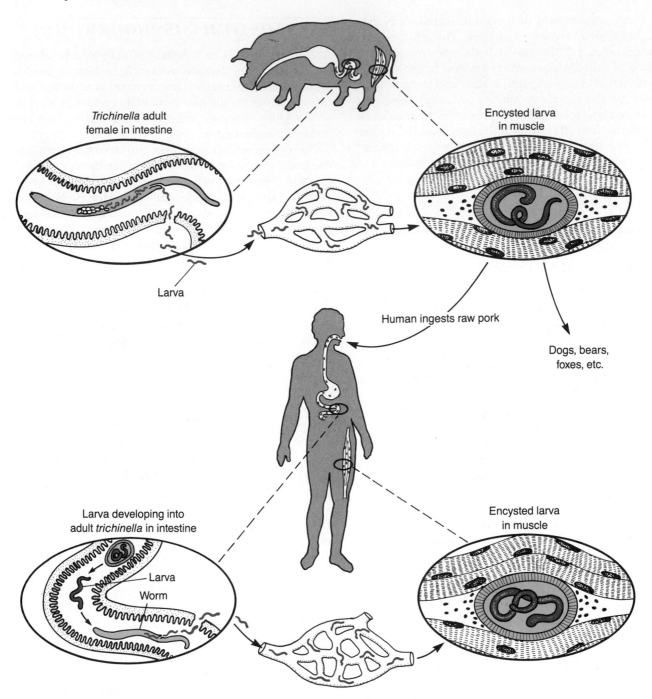

Figure 9-31. Trichinosis. After being ingested by the pig, cysts of *Trichinella* are digested in the gastrointestinal tract, liberating larvae that mature to adult worms. Female worms release larvae that penetrate the intestinal wall, enter the circulation, and lodge in striated muscle, where they encyst. When humans ingest inadequately cooked pork, the cycle is repeated, resulting in the muscle disease characteristic of trichinosis.

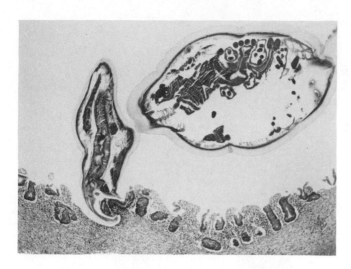

Figure 9-32. Ancylostomiasis of the ileum. Shown are two sections of a single adult worm, *Ancylostoma duodenale,* not connected in this plane of section. A plug of mucosa is in the buccal cavity of the hookworm.

grate within alveolar walls, air sacs, bronchioles, and bronchi.

DISEASES CAUSED BY TREMATODES

SCHISTOSOMIASIS

Schistosomiasis (bilharziasis) is a parasitic infection by flukes (trematodes) of three principal species, namely *Schistosoma haematobium, Schistosoma mansoni,* and *Schistosoma japonicum.* Since the intermediate hosts are freshwater snails, the geographic distribution of schistosomiasis depends on the presence of snails and opportunities for infection of both snail and humans. **Schistosomiasis is increasing in prevalence, affecting about 10% of the world's population and ranking second only to malaria as a cause of morbidity and mortality.** *S. haematobium* is found in large regions of tropical Africa and parts of southwest Asia; *S. mansoni* in much of tropical Africa, parts of southwest Asia, South America, and the Caribbean islands; and *S. japonicum* in parts of Japan, China, the Philippines, India, and several countries in southeast Asia.

A schistosome egg hatches in fresh water, liberating a miracidium that penetrates a snail, where it develops into the final larval stage, the cercaria (Fig. 9-33). The cercaria escapes from the snail into fresh water and penetrates the skin of the human host, becoming a schistosomule. The shistosomule migrates through tissues, penetrates a blood vessel, and is carried to the lung and subsequently to the liver. In hepatic portal venules the schistosomules mature, forming pairs of male and female worms. The "worm pairs" migrate to the small venules, where the female worm deposits immature eggs. *S. mansoni* and *S. japonicum* lay eggs in the intestine, and *S. haematobium,* in the urinary bladder. The eggs pass through the wall of the intestine or the urinary bladder, hatch in fresh water, and liberate miracidia, thus completing the cycle.

The lesions of chronic schistosomiasis vary in severity from insignificant to fatal, the latter occurring in only a small proportion of those infected. The lesions reflect the sites of deposition of the eggs—namely, the bladder with *S. haematobium,* and the intestine and liver with *S. mansoni,* and *S. japonicum.* **The basic lesion is a circumscribed granuloma around an egg, or a diffuse cellular infiltrate around it, composed mainly of eosinophils and neutrophils.**

Eggs that fail to exit the body through the intestine are carried through the portal veins to the liver, where they provoke granulomas and fibrosis (Fig. 9-34) Gradually, broad tracts of portal scar tissue, so-called **pipestem fibrosis,** become obvious on gross examination of the liver. Portal hypertension frequently complicates schistosomal pipestem fibrosis and leads to splenomegaly and hemorrhage from esophageal varices.

Urogenital schistosomiasis is caused by *S. haematobium.* Eggs are most numerous in the bladder, ureters, and seminal vesicles, but they may also reach the lungs, colon, and appendix. Numerous eggs in the urinary bladder and ureters lead to a granulomatous reaction, with evolution of polypoid patches. **There is a high incidence of carcinoma of the bladder in patients with urogenital schistosomiasis.**

CLONORCHIASIS

Humans acquire clonorchiasis—infection by *Clonorchis sinensis* (Chinese liver fluke)—by eating raw or undercooked fish. Adult worms are flat and transparent, live in the bile ducts, and pass eggs to the intestine and the feces. After ingestion by an appropriate snail, the egg hatches in to a miracidium. Cercariae escape from the snail and seek out certain fish, which they penetrate and in which they encyst. When human hosts eat the fish the cercariae emerge in the duodenum, enter the common bile duct through the ampulla of Vater, and mature in the distal bile ducts to an adult fluke.

With massive infection the liver may become up to three times its normal size. Dilated bile ducts are seen through the capsule, and the cut surface is punctuated

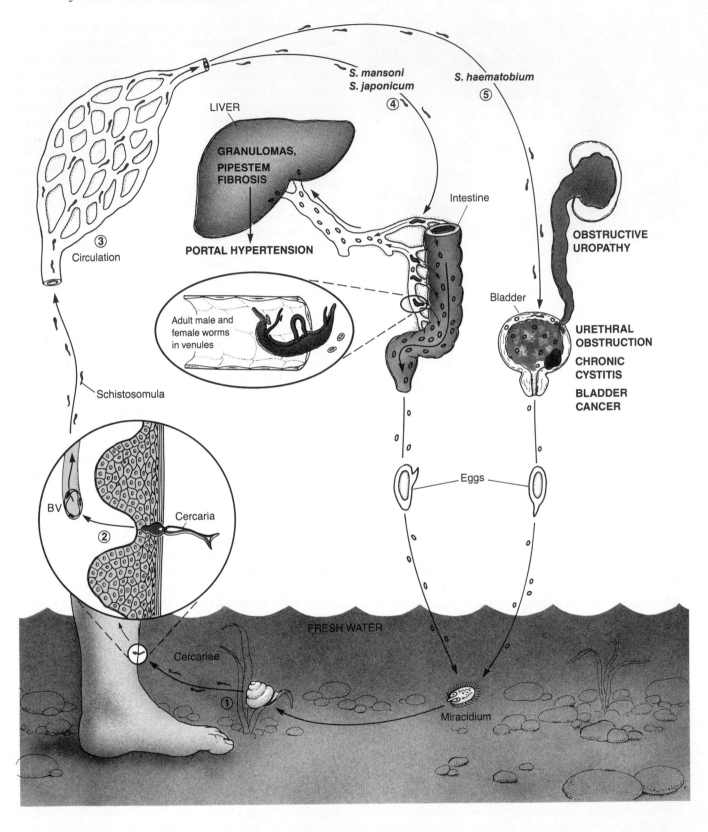

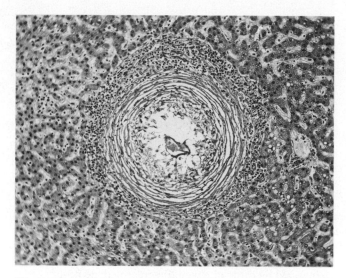

Figure 9-34. Schistosomiasis, liver. A granuloma in a portal tract of the liver surrounds a degenerating egg of *Schistosoma mansoni.*

with thick-walled, dilated bile ducts. Microscopically, the epithelium lining the ducts is initially hyperplastic and then becomes metaplastic.

Patients with clonorchiasis may die from a variety of conditions, including biliary obstruction, bacterial cholangitis and pancreatitis. Cholangiocarcinoma, which may originate in either the intra- or extrahepatic bile ducts, is a complication.

FASCIOLIASIS

Fascioliasis is infection by *Fasciola hepatica*, the sheep liver fluke. Humans may acquire the infection wherever sheep are raised. Humans become infected by eating vegetation, such as watercress, that is contaminated by cysts of *F. hepatica.* In its human host the larvae mature to adults and live in both the intrahepatic and extrahepatic bile ducts. Later, the adult flukes penetrate the wall of the bile ducts and wander back into liver parenchyma, where they feed on liver cells and deposit their eggs. The eggs lead to abscess formation, followed by a granuloma. The worms induce hyperplasia of the lining epithelium of the bile ducts, portal and periductal fibrosis, proliferation of bile ductules, and varying degrees of biliary obstruction.

FASCIOLOPSIASIS

Fasciolopsiasis, an infection by *Fasciolopsis buski*, the giant intestinal fluke, prevails throughout most of the Orient. Humans, the definitive hosts, acquire fasciolopsiasis by eating uncooked aquatic vegetables contaminated with the encysted cercariae of *F. buski.*

The worm is huge (3 x 7 cm) and attaches to the duodenal or jejunal wall. Acute symptoms may be caused by intestinal obstruction or by toxins released by large numbers of worms.

DISEASES CAUSED BY CESTODES

ECHINOCOCCOSIS (HYDATID DISEASE)

Enchinococcosis is a zoonotic infection caused by larval cestodes (tapeworms) of the genus *Echinococcus*. The most common offender is *Echinococcus granulosus* (cystic hydatid disease).

Figure 9-33. Life cycle of *Schistosoma* and clinical features of schistosomiasis. The schistosome egg hatches in water, liberates a miracidium that penetrates a snail, and develops through two stages to sporocyst to form the final larval stage, the cercaria. (1) The cercaria escapes from the snail into water, "swims," and penetrates the skin of a human host. (2) The cercaria loses its forked tail to become a schistosomule, which migrates through tissues, penetrates a blood vessel, and (3) is carried to the lung and later to the liver. In hepatic portal venules the schistosomule becomes sexually mature and forms pairs, each with a male and a female worm, the female worm lying in the gynecophoral canal of the male worm. The organism causes lesions in the liver, including granulomas, portal ("pipestem") fibrosis, and portal hypertension. (4) The female worm deposits immature eggs in small venules of the intestine and rectum (*S. mansoni*, and *S. japonicum*) or (5) of the urinary bladder (*S. haematobium*). The bladder infestation leads to obstructive uropathy, ureteral obstruction, chronic cystitis, and bladder cancer. Embryos develop during passage of the eggs through tissues, and larvae are mature when eggs pass through the wall of the intestine or urinary bladder. Eggs hatch in water and liberate miracidia to complete the cycle.

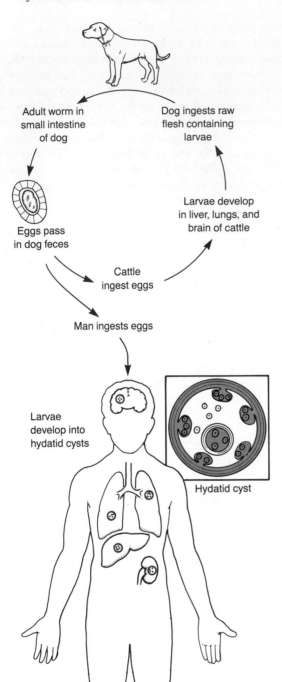

Figure 9-35. Adult worm in small intestine of dog → Eggs pass in dog feces → Cattle ingest eggs → Larvae develop in liver, lungs, and brain of cattle → Dog ingests raw flesh containing larvae. Man ingests eggs → Larvae develop into hydatid cysts. Hydatid cyst.

Figure 9-35. Life cycle of *Echinococcus granulosus* and cystic hydatid disease. The adult cestode lives in the small intestine of a dog (the definitive host). A gravid proglottid ruptures, releasing cestode eggs into the dog's feces. Cestode eggs are ingested by cattle or sheep (the intermediate hosts), hatch in the intestine, and release oncospheres that penetrate the wall of the gut, enter the bloodstream, disseminate to various deep organs, and grow to form hydatid cysts, containing brood capsules and scolices. When another dog ingests raw flesh from the cattle or sheep, the scolices are ingested and develop into mature worms in the dog's intestine to complete the cycle. A person who ingests cestode eggs in contaminated plant material becomes an accidental intermediate host. The larvae increase in size, but the parasite reaches a "dead end" without developing into an adult tapeworm. Hydatid cysts in humans occur predominantly in the liver but may also involve lung, kidney, brain, and other organs.

Figure 9-35 illustrates the life cycle of *E. granulosus*. The adult tapeworms are 2 to 6 mm long and live in the small intestine of a carnivorous host such as the wolf, fox, coyote, jackal, or dog. The terminal, gravid proglottid breaks off and releases eggs, which are eliminated in the feces of the carnivore. Contaminated herbage is then eaten by herbivorous intermediate hosts, such as deer, moose, antelopes, sheep, cattle, and humans. Larvae released from the eggs penetrate the wall of the gut, enter the blood stream, and disseminate to deep organs, where they grow to form hydatid cysts containing brood capsules and scolices. When the flesh of the intermediate host, the herbivore, is eaten raw by a carnivore, the scolices develop into sexually mature worms in the intestine of the definitive host, thereby completing the cycle. Humans become infected by ingesting plant material contaminated by cestode eggs. Cystic hydatid disease (due to *E. granulosus*) is common in sheep- and cattle-raising areas of Australia, New Zealand, and East Africa, many Mediterranean and Middle Eastern countries, and several South American countries.

Echinococcosis is most common in the liver but also involves the lung and, less commonly, the brain, kidney, spleen, muscle, soft tissues, and bone. The larvae enlarge in situ to become cysts, which grow "silently" for years, usually producing no symptoms until they reach a size of 10 cm or more. Because of their size hydatid cysts of the liver often produce hepatomegaly, and since they compress adjacent structures, such as intrahepatic bile ducts, they may lead to obstructive jaundice. Rupture of a cyst may provoke an acute hypersensitivity reaction, including anaphylaxis, to released antigens. A major complication of rupture is the seeding of adjacent tissues with brood capsules and scolices. When these "seeds" grow, they produce many additional cysts, each with the growth potential of the original cyst. Traumatic rupture of hydatid cysts of abdominal organs results in severe diffuse pain resembling that of peritonitis, and a ruptured cyst in the lung may cause pneumothorax and empyema.

OPPORTUNISTIC INFECTIONS IN THE ACQUIRED IMMUNODEFICIENCY SYNDROME (AIDS)

The pandemic of acquired immunodeficiency syndrome (AIDS), which is characterized by a progressive irreversible depletion of T-helper lymphocytes, predisposes its victims to opportunistic infections and unusual cancers. The cause of the immune dysfunction is the human immunodeficiency virus (HIV), which is transmitted by homosexual and, less frequently, heterosexual contact, from mother to child during the perinatal period, and through parenteral exposure to blood or blood products.

Because of the profound defect in cell-mediated immunity, patients with AIDS are susceptible to a wide variety of viral, fungal, bacterial, and parasitic infections (Table 9-1). These opportunistic infections, often numerous and simultaneous, are typically severe, persistent, or relapsing, despite specific therapy.

The pathology of AIDS is divided into three general categories: lymphoid hyperplasia; unusual tumors, most frequently Kaposi's sarcoma or high grade lymphomas; and opportunistic infections.

More than half of the patients develop *Pneumocystis carinii* pneumonia, and this is often the first opportunistic infection detected. Persistent or recurrent diarrhea is common, ranging in severity from several loose stools a day, to copious watery diarrhea that may reach 15 liters a day. Causative agents include *Cryptosporidium, Isospora belli, Entamoeba histolytica, Giardia lamblia, Salmonella, Shigella,* and *Campylobacter.*

Toxoplasma gondii causes acute, subacute, or chronic necrotizing encephalitis in patients with AIDS. Other focal lesions of the brain include lymphomas and infections with mycobacteria, cytomegalovirus, and *Nocardia* species.

Patients with AIDS frequently have clinically significant disseminated cytomegalovirus infections, characterized by pneumonia, enteritis, and chorioretinitis, and other viral diseases, including herpes simplex, herpes zoster, and molluscum contagiosum.

Mycobacterium avium-intracellulare is a ubiquitous environmental saprophyte that rarely caused disseminated infection in adults, regardless of immunologic status, until the AIDS epidemic. In AIDS patients, however, disseminated disease caused by *M. aviumintracellulare* is common.

Table 9-1 *Organisms Causing Opportunistic Infections in Patients With AIDS*

Protozoa

Pneumocystis carinii	*Cryptosporidium* spp.
Entamoeba histolytica	*Giardia lamblia*
Toxoplasma gondii	*Isospora belli*

Viruses

Cytomegalovirus	Epstein-Barr
Herpes simplex	Molluscum contagiosum (poxvirus)
Varicella-zoster	Polyoma

Fungi

Candida spp.	*Histoplasma capsulatum*
Coccidioides immitis	*Histoplasma duboisii*
Cryptococcus neoformans	*Sporothrix schoenckii*

Bacteria and Mycobacteria

Campylobacter spp.	*Mycobacterium avium-intracellulare*
Legionella pneumophila	*Mycobacterium tuberculosis*
Listeria monocytogenes	*Actinomyces* spp.
Salmonella spp.	*Nocardia* spp.
Shigella spp.	

10

BLOOD VESSELS

EARL P. BENDITT AND STEPHEN M. SCHWARTZ

Diseases of Large Blood
  Vessels

Hypertensive Vascular Disease

Inflammatory Disorders of
  Blood Vessels

Aneurysms

Disorders of Veins

Disorders of Lymphatic Vessels

Tumors of Blood Vessels

DISEASES OF LARGE BLOOD VESSELS

ATHEROSCLEROSIS

The complications of atherosclerosis, which include ischemic heart disease, myocardial infarction, stroke, and gangrene of the extremities, account for more than half of the annual mortality in the United States. Ischemic heart disease is by itself the leading cause of death.

There are wide geographic and racial variations in the incidence of ischemic heart disease. For example, the mortality from this condition is eight times higher in Sweden than in Japan.

PATHOGENESIS

The most common acquired abnormality of blood vessels is the atherosclerotic lesion, which develops in the intima against a background of smooth muscle cells, blood-derived white blood cells, and a variable amount of connective tissue. This lesion has two critical features: the proliferation of intimal smooth muscle cells and the accumulation of lipid in the intima. The expansion of this common lesion produces the final clinical result: thrombosis and occlusion of a distributing artery.

At least five hypotheses have been proposed to explain the origins of atherosclerotic plaques. We emphasize that these hypotheses are **not** mutually exclusive. Viewed in this light, most of the controversy lies in individual opinions as to which process is most important in the initiation of the lesions or their progression into clinically significant disease.

Insudation Hypothesis

The insudation hypothesis states that the lipid in atherosclerotic lesions is derived from plasma lipoproteins. The form of lipid in the plasma that has been most closely associated with accelerated atherosclerosis is **low-density lipoprotein (LDL).** Endothelial cells have receptors for LDL and for modified forms of LDL. Transport may occur across intact endothelium either by receptor-mediated uptake of lipoprotein or by nonspecific uptake into micropinocytic channels. Alternatively, lipid may be engulfed by macrophages in the blood and then transported into the vascular wall inside these cells. Recent studies of atherosclerosis in fat-fed animals have demonstrated that macrophages play a major role in the early stages of lipid accumulation. Although the insudation hypothesis explains the source of plaque lipid, it does not provide a complete explanation for the pathogenesis of the atherosclerotic lesion.

Encrustation Hypothesis

The encrustation hypothesis holds that small mural thrombi represent the initial event in atherosclerosis. Organization of these thrombi leads to the formation of plaques, and the expansion of these lesions reflects repeated episodes of thrombosis and organization.

Reaction to Injury Hypothesis

This hypothesis proposes that smooth muscle proliferation in plaques depends on the release of polypeptide growth factors by platelets and monocytes that accumulate at sites of injury. The best known of these is **platelet-derived growth factor (PDGF).** PDGF it not only mitogenic for smooth muscle cells, it is also chemotactic for them. Thus, in addition to stimulating the proliferation of cells already in the intima, PDGF may recruit smooth muscle cells from the media. Platelets, smooth muscle cells, and endothelial cells synthesize growth factors that stimulate the growth of smooth muscle cells.

Monoclonal Hypothesis

The monoclonal concept is also focused on smooth muscle proliferation. It has been established that many plaques are monoclonal—that is, they originate from one or, at most, a few smooth muscle cells. The monoclonality of the fibrous caps of atherosclerotic plaques suggests that some unknown etiologic factor, perhaps circulating mutagens or viruses, might induce plaque formation by altering some genomic features of growth control in the smooth muscle cells of the arterial wall.

Intimal Cell Mass Hypothesis

The third hypothesis that implicates smooth muscle relates the location of atherosclerotic lesions to the focal accumulation of smooth muscle cells in the normal intima at branch points and other sites in the coronary arteries and other vessels. Intimal cell masses are found in infancy, are more pronounced in male infants, and occur in the vessels of people of varying ethnicity and location, irrespective of the incidence of atherosclerosis. The distribution of intimal cell masses in children resembles the distribution of atherosclerotic lesions in adults. This suggests that the intimal cell mass may be either the early lesion of atherosclerosis or a precursor of it.

A Unifying Hypothesis

We can construct a scheme to tie the foregoing hypotheses together:

1. In our hypothetical sequence, the initial lesion is the intimal cell mass, which arises by the trapping of isolated smooth muscle cells in the intima during development or by mutation and migration of pre-existing smooth muscle cells.

2. Lipid accumulation in these foci might depend on properties of the intimal smooth muscle cells. The types of connective tissue synthesized by the cells in the intima may render these sites prone to lipid accumulation.

3. Lipid insudation in these benign accumulations of intimal cells would produce cell injury, thereby leading to the accumulation of macrophages and platelets.

4. In turn, the macrophages and platelets could release growth factors, as proposed in the "reaction to injury" hypothesis. Monocytes would play a central role by participating in lipid accumulation and releasing growth factors, thus stimulating further accumulation of smooth muscle cells.

5. As the lesion progresses, endothelial injury may lead to the loss of the anticoagulant properties of the normal wall. The resulting mural thrombosis would lead to the release of platelet-derived growth factors and further acceleration of smooth muscle proliferation.

Whether or not this particular hypothetical scenario is correct, aspects of these five hypotheses probably do operate as distinct processes during different phases of atherosclerosis. Figure 10-1 shows how these five hypotheses might interact over the course of lesion development.

INITIAL LESION OF ATHEROSCLEROSIS

Two distinct lesions have been proposed as the initial structural abnormality of atherosclerosis. In young children the intima contains focal accumulations of intracellular and extracellular lipid, called **fatty spots** or **fatty streaks.** In these simple focal lesions (Fig. 10-2) cells filled with lipid droplets ("foam cells") accumulate. It has been established that many of the fat-containing cells are modified smooth muscle cells.

Children who die accidentally usually show significant numbers of fatty spots in many parts of the arterial tree, but these do not correspond well to the distribution of atherosclerotic lesions in adults. For example, fatty spots are common in the thoracic aorta in children, but atherosclerosis in adults is typically prominent in the abdominal aorta. Nonetheless, many believe that fatty infiltration represents the initial lesion of atherosclerosis, and that other factors control the distribution of the later, more clinically significant lesions.

As we have already proposed, an alternative candidate for the initial lesion is **intimal thickening** or an **intimal cell mass.** The location of intimal cell masses, particularly in structures called "cushions" located near arterial branch sites, correlates well with the sites of later development of atherosclerotic lesions. However, it should be noted that the concept of the intimal cell mass as the initial lesion is controversial.

Figure 10-1. Unifying hypothesis for the pathogenesis of atherosclerosis. Monoclonality and the intimal cell mass occur very early in plaque development and are good candidates for the initial event. A single smooth muscle cell (*red*) proliferates in the intima, either as a result of a mutation or as part of an "intimal cushion," to form an intimal cell mass. Insudation of plasma lipids into the intimal cell mass occurs by direct passage of LDL across the endothelium and via macrophages that engulf LDL in the blood or in the intima. For reasons that are not clear, the expanding early atherosclerotic lesion is complicated by damage to the endothelium. As a result, platelets adhere to the exposed subendothelial collagen. Platelets and macrophages release growth factors, stimulating a polyclonal proliferation of smooth muscle cells (*green*) to form the characteristic fibrous plaque. The continued insudation of lipid and its release by degenerating macrophages leads to further accumulation of extracellular lipid. Eventually the surface of the plaque ulcerates, and a thrombus forms on the injured luminal surface.

INTIMAL CELL MASS

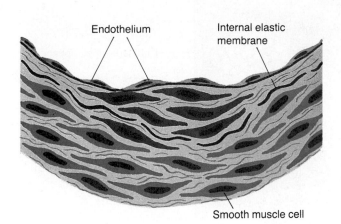

Endothelium

Internal elastic membrane

Smooth muscle cell

INSUDATION

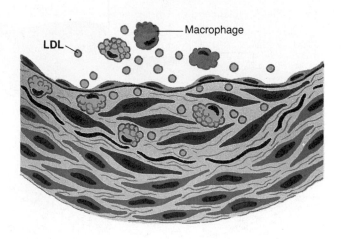

LDL

Macrophage

RESPONSE TO INJURY

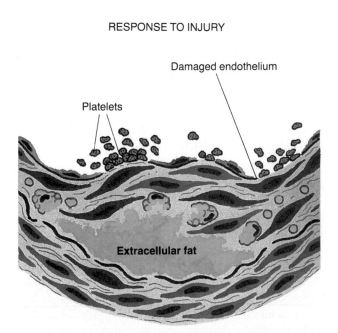

Damaged endothelium

Platelets

Extracellular fat

ENCRUSTATION AND THROMBOSIS

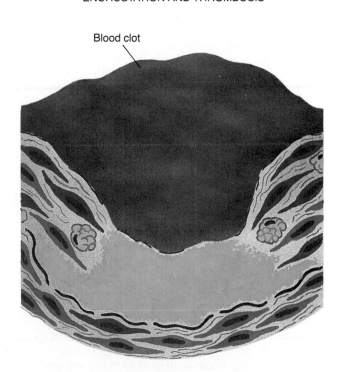

Blood clot

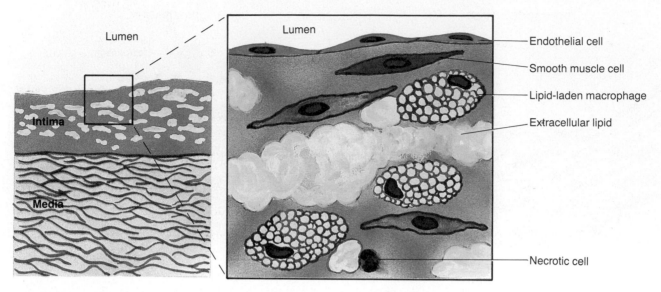

Figure 10-2. Fatty streak of atherosclerosis. The fatty streak, composed largely of foamy macrophages, is presumed to be an early stage in the formation of atherosclerotic lesions. Note the intimal thickening in the left panel and the infiltrating cells in the enlargement on the right.

CHARACTERISTIC LESION OF ATHEROSCLEROSIS

The fibro-fatty lesion characteristic of atherosclerosis consists of two morphologic components (Fig. 10-3). The first, a thick layer of fibrous connective tissue called the **fibrous cap,** is much thicker and less cellular than the normal intima and contains fat-filled macrophages and smooth muscle cells. The second component is the **atheroma,** a necrotic mass of lipid that forms the middle part of the lesion. Virtually all studies show that there is some loss of endothelial continuity during progression to the characteristic lesion of atherosclerosis. Importantly, the characteristic lesion may contain blood-borne cells in addition to monocytes.

COMPLICATED LESIONS OF ATHEROSCLEROSIS

Characteristic lesions of the sort described are of little significance in impairing blood flow. However, their distribution and their similarity to more advanced lesions suggest a progression to the final, clinically significant lesion. The critical changes that characterize complicated lesions are thrombosis, upon and within the fibrous cap; neovascularization of the cap and shoulders of the lesion; thinning of the underlying tunica media; calcification within the atheroma and fibrous cap; and ulceration of the fibrous cap. It is likely that thrombosis on the surface of the final, complicated lesion leads to vascular occlusion and clinical cardiovascular disease.

Progression from the simple characteristic lesion to the more complicated, clinically significant lesion can be found in some people still in their twenties and, in our society, in virtually everyone by age 50 or 60.

MECHANISMS OF LESION PROGRESSION IN ATHEROSCLEROSIS

The characteristic lesion requires as much as 20 to 30 years to form, and the clinically important complicated lesions emerge after several more decades of development (Fig.10-4). The factors that contribute to the progression of simple lesions to complicated ones are not well understood. A prominent factor in lesion progression could be the macrophage, a cell that may play a role even in the earliest events. A large part of the lipid that accumulates in lesions of fat-fed animals is found in the monocyte-macrophage. Once the macrophages are in the lesion, progression may depend on the inflammatory activities of the monocytes. For example, the monocyte synthesizes platelet-derived growth factor, fibroblast growth factor, epidermal growth factor, interleukin-1, tumor necrosis factor, alpha-interferon, and transforming growth factor beta. Each of these can either positively or negatively modulate the growth of smooth muscle or endothelial cells. Interferon and

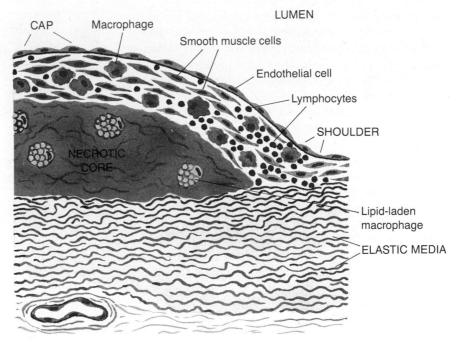

Figure 10-3. Fibrous plaque of athero-sclerosis. In this fully developed fibrous plaque the core contains lipid-filled macrophages and necrotic smooth muscle cell debris. The fibrous cap is composed largely of smooth muscle cells, which produce collagen, small amounts of elastin, and glycosaminoglycans. Also shown are infiltrating macrophages and lymphocytes. Note that the endothelium over the surface of the fibrous cap frequently appears intact.

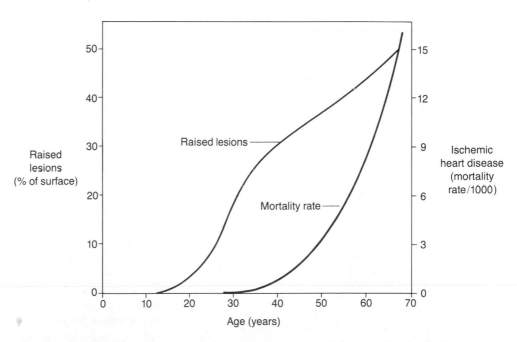

Figure 10-4. Raised lesions in coronary arteries and the mortality rate from ischemic heart disease as a function of age. There is a protracted incubation period of about 25 years between the appearance of raised lesions in the coronary vessels and their lethal complications.

transforming growth factor beta inhibit cell proliferation and could account for the failure of endothelial cells to maintain continuity over the lesion. Alternatively, such growth inhibitors could exert a negative feedback effect in the presence of large amounts of growth stimulatory peptides.

Mediators secreted by monocytes and macrophages are also thought to change the functions of overlying endothelial cells in ways that may be important for lesion progression. Of particular interest is the recent discovery that interleukin-1 and tumor necrosis factor stimulate endothelial cell expression of platelet-activating factor, tissue factor, and plasminogen activator inhibitor. **Thus, the combination of monocytes and endothelial cells may be capable of transforming the normal anticoagulant vascular surface to a procoagulant surface.** A further complication is that atherosclerotic plaques also contain T cells. The expression of HLA-DR antigens on both endothelial cells and smooth

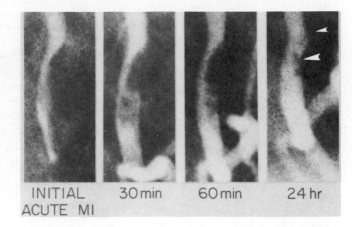

INITIAL ACUTE MI   30 min   60 min   24 hr

Figure 10-6. Dissolution of coronary artery thrombus. These coronary angiograms show a thrombus (*initial*) in the coronary artery of a 48-year-old man, 3 hours after the onset of the symptoms of acute myocardial infarction. He was immediately infused with recombinant human tissue plasminogen activator. Successive frames show stages of dissolution of the thrombus. By 60 minutes after the beginning of infusion, the thrombus is distinctly smaller. The infusion was continued for 6 hours, and at 24 hours the thrombus is almost completely lysed. The lower arrow indicates a small remaining portion of plaque or thrombus; the apparent bulge indicated by the upper arrow is interpreted as an ulceration of the plaque.

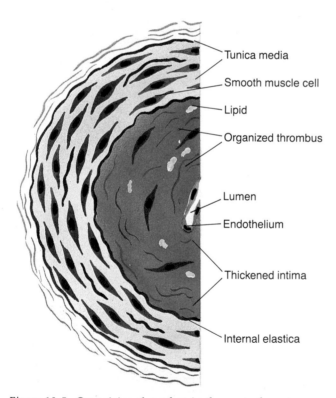

Tunica media
Smooth muscle cell
Lipid
Organized thrombus
Lumen
Endothelium
Thickened intima
Internal elastica

Figure 10-5. Organizing thrombus in the muscular artery. The original platelet mass is augmented by masses of red blood cells and white blood cells. Such a thrombus becomes organized by the ingrowth of endothelial cell sprouts and smooth muscle cells from the intima or inner media. Some lipid and cholesterol crystals may become evident as red blood cells break down.

muscle cells in plaques implies that these cells have undergone some kind of immunologic activation, perhaps in response to gamma interferon released by activated T cells in the plaque. It is possible that these T cells reflect an autoimmune response that is important for the progression of atherosclerotic lesions.

A loss of endothelial continuity is another potential antecedent of plaque progression. The loss of endothelial continuity would (1) increase the permeability of the wall to lipoproteins and, therefore, accelerate lipoprotein accumulation; (2) permit platelet interaction with the vessel wall and the subsequent release of growth factors, resulting in more rapid lesion progression, and (3) allow the formation of a thrombus on the surface of an atherosclerotic lesion. We know from clinical studies that **the formation of a thrombus (Fig. 10-5) is the most common clinical event that leads to myocardial infarction.** An intervention aimed at dissolving such a thrombus can prevent or limit the size of an evolving myocardial infarction. Recent studies have shown that many occlusive thrombi can be dissolved by enzymes capable of activating plasma fibrinolytic activity, including streptokinase and tissue plasminogen activator (Fig. 10-6).

RISK FACTORS

Any factor associated with a doubling in the incidence of ischemic heart disease has been defined as a "risk factor." **The most frequently noted risk factors for ischemic heart disease are hypertension, elevated serum cholesterol levels, cigarette smoking and diabetes (glucose intolerance).** In addition, the rates of myocardial infarction increase with age and are greater for men than for women at all ages, although the rate for the latter rises precipitously after the menopause. Hence, **age and sex are considered risk factors.**

Lipid Metabolism

The insolubility of cholesterol and other lipids (mainly triglycerides) necessitates a special transport system, whose function is subserved by a system of lipoprotein particles (Fig. 10-7). **The major classes of particles are chylomicrons, very-low-density lipoproteins (VLDL), low-density lipoproteins (LDL), and high-density lipoproteins (HDL).** Each of these particles consists of a lipid core with associated proteins, the apolipoproteins. A number of the latter have been described, and each is designated by a letter (and frequently a number).

Lipid Metabolic Pathways, Cholesterol Transport, and Metabolism

The metabolic pathways for lipoproteins containing the B apolipoproteins are two major lipoprotein cascades, one originating from the intestine and the other from the liver (Fig. 10-8). The **exogenous pathway** consists of chylomicrons containing apo B-48 secreted by the intestine. Following secretion, chylomicrons rapidly acquire apo C-II and apo E from HDL. These triglyceride-rich lipoproteins primarily transport lipid from the intestine to the liver. The triglycerides in chylomicrons are hydrolyzed by lipoprotein lipase, which is attached to the endothelial cells of the capillary walls. Apo C-II activates lipoprotein lipase and causes removal of triglycerides. Thus, chylomicrons are converted to "remnants" and finally to intermediate-density lipoproteins (IDL). The chylomicron remnants are removed by the hepatocyte via an apo E-mediated (remnant) receptor process.

The **endogenous pathway** involves triglyceride-rich lipoproteins containing apo B-100 secreted by the liver. As with the chylomicrons, shortly after their secretion the liver VLDL particles acquire apo C-II and apo E from HDL. The triglycerides on VLDL undergo hydrolysis by lipoprotein lipase; the lipoproteins containing apo B-100 are initially converted to IDLs and finally to LDLs. With the conversion of IDL to LDL, most apo

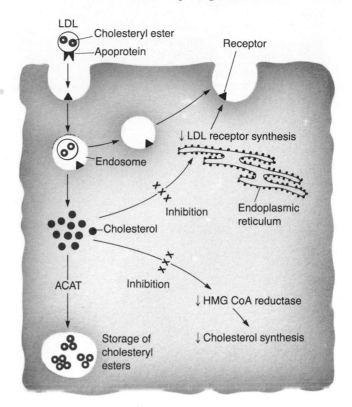

Figure 10-7. The relationship between circulating LDL cholesterol, LDL receptors, and the synthesis of cholesterol. The LDL, which contains cholesteryl esters, is taken up by cells into vesicles by a receptor-mediated pathway to form an endosome. The receptor and lipids are dissociated, and the receptor is returned to the cell surface. The exogenous cholesterol, now in the cytoplasm, causes a reduction in receptor synthesis in the endoplasmic reticulum and inhibits the activity of HMG CoA reductase in the cholesterol synthesizing pathway. Excess cholesterol in the cell is esterified to cholesteryl esters and stored in vacuoles.

C-II and apo E dissociates from the particles and reassociates with HDL. The conversion of IDL to LDL may, in part, be mediated by hepatic lipase, an enzyme that functions both as a triglyceride hydrolase and, more importantly, as a phospholipase. The LDL, which contains apo B-100, interacts with high-affinity receptors on the liver and on the peripheral cells, including smooth muscle cells, fibroblasts, and adrenal cells (see Fig. 10-7). The interaction of LDL with its receptor initiates receptor-mediated endocytosis and the catabolism of LDL.

The HDLs containing apo A-I and apo A-II are synthesized by several pathways, including direct secretion by the intestine and liver and transfer of lipid and apolipoprotein constituents released during the lipolysis of triglyceride-rich lipoproteins that contain apo B.

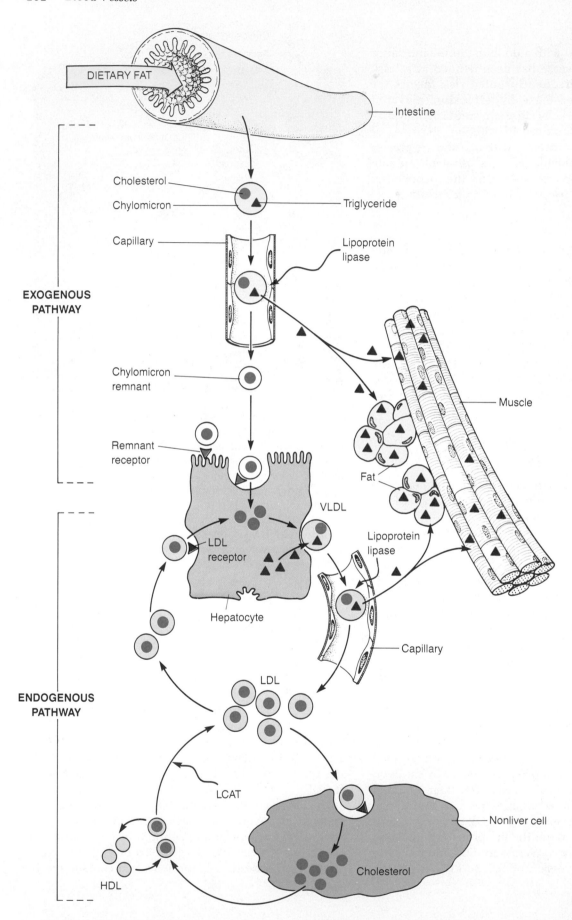

DIETARY FAT

Intestine

Cholesterol
Chylomicron
Triglyceride

Capillary
Lipoprotein lipase

EXOGENOUS PATHWAY

Chylomicron remnant

Muscle

Remnant receptor

Fat

VLDL

LDL receptor
Lipoprotein lipase

Hepatocyte

Capillary

ENDOGENOUS PATHWAY

LDL

LCAT

Nonliver cell

HDL

Cholesterol

HDL has been proposed to have two major functions: serving as a reservoir for apolipoproteins, particularly apo C-II and apo E, and interacting with cells in the uptake and transport of cholesterol from extrahepatic cells to the liver for ultimate removal from the body as cholesterol or bile acids. The latter function has been termed "reverse cholesterol transport." The cholesterol removed from the cells is principally free cholesterol, which rapidly undergoes esterification to cholesteryl esters. Cholesteryl esters are transferred to the core of the lipoprotein particle, or are exchanged to VLDL and LDL. The transfer of cholesteryl esters between lipoprotein particles is mediated by specific transfer proteins. **Defects in cholesteryl ester transfer and exchange lead to dyslipoproteinemias, increased intracellular cholesteryl esters, and premature atherosclerosis.**

Clinical Disorders of Lipoprotein Metabolism

A number of biochemical defects that produce dyslipoproteinemias are now recognized (Table 10-1). Current and evolving knowledge of the biochemical and molecular defects in patients with dyslipoproteinemias forms the basis for a systematic approach to the diagnosis of the disorders.

GENETIC FACTORS IN ATHEROSCLEROSIS

It is now recognized that a defect in LDL receptors is a key factor in certain genetic dyslipoproteinemias. In addition, polymorphisms are present in apo A-I and A-II. Apo E polymorphisms have also been found, accompanied by alterations in LDL levels.

An inverse correlation between ischemic heart disease and HDL cholesterol levels has been established. This has been extended by studies of apoprotein levels and polymorphisms of the principal apoproteins associated with HDL. From these studies emerges the fact that the genes for apo A-I and C-III reside in human chromosome 11 and are physically linked. Polymorphisms of apo A-I have been associated with hypertriglyceridemia and premature atherosclerosis.

VIRUSES AND ATHEROSCLEROSIS

A viral etiology for at least some cases of atherosclerosis is compatible with the importance of cell proliferation in the formation of atheromatous plaques. Furthermore, it could explain several hitherto puzzling features of atherosclerosis and thrombosis, namely (1) intimal cell proliferation in the absence of certain common risk factors, (2) the monoclonal nature of cell pop-

---

Figure 10-8. Exogenous and endogenous cholesterol transport pathway. In the exogenous pathway cholesterol and fatty acids from food are absorbed through the intestinal mucosa. Fatty acid chains are linked to glycerol to form triglycerides. The triglycerides and the cholesterol are packaged into chylomicrons that are returned via the lymph to the blood. In the capillaries (mainly of fat tissue and muscle, but also other tissues) the ester bonds holding the fatty acids in triglycerides are split by lipoprotein lipase. Fatty acids are removed, leaving cholesterol-rich lipoprotein remnants. These bind to special remnant receptors and are taken up by liver cells. The cholesterol of the remnant is either secreted into the intestine, largely as bile acids, or packaged as very low density lipoprotein particles (VLDL), which are then secreted into the circulation. This is the first step in the endogenous cycle. In fat or muscle tissue the triglyceride is removed from the VLDL with the aid of lipoprotein lipase. The intermediate density lipoprotein (IDL) particles (*not shown*) remain in the circulation. Some IDL is immediately taken up by the liver via the mediation of LDL receptors for apo B/E. The remaining IDL in the circulation is either taken up by non-liver cells or converted to low density lipoproteins (LDL). Most of the LDL in the circulation bind to hepatocytes or other cells and are removed from the circulation. High density lipoproteins (HDL) take up cholesterol from cells. This cholesterol is esterified by the enzyme lecithin cholesterol acyltransferase (LCAT), after which the esters are transferred to LDL and taken up by cells.

Table 10-1   Molecular Defects in Patients With Dyslipoproteinemia

	Defect	Clinical Features
Apolipoprotein Defects		
Apo A-I$_{Milano}$	Amino acid change (Arg$_{173}$ → Cys)	Reduced HDL
Apo A-I + apo C-II deficiency (kindred 1)	Rearrangement in apo A-I and apo C-III gene	Virtual absence of HDL, severe atherosclerosis
Apo A-I + apo C-II deficiency (kindred 2)	Unknown	Virtual absence of HDL, severe atherosclerosis
Apo B-100 and apo B-48 absence	Unknown	Ataxia malabsorption, visual defects, hemolytic anemia
Apo B-100 absence	Unknown	Mild ataxia, malabsorption
Apo C-II deficiency	Structural defect in apo C-II	Type I hyperlipidemia, severe hypertriglyceridemia
Apo E$_3$ variants	Apo E$_2$ (Arg$_{158}$ → Cys) Apo E$_2$ (Arg$_{145}$ → Cys) Apo E$_2$ (Lys$_{146}$ → Gln)	Type III hyperlipidemia, elevated plasma cholesterol and triglycerides, premature cardiovascular disease
Enzyme Defects		
Lipoprotein lipase deficiency	Unknown	Type I hyperlipidemia, hypertriglyceridemia
Hepatic lipase deficiency	Unknown	Type IV hyperlipidemia, mild elevations of IDL and HDL
Lecithin cholesterol acyltransferase deficiency	Unknown	Corneal opacities, mild hypertriglyceridemia, and reduced levels of HDL
Receptor defects		
LDL excess	Absence of or defective receptor	Type II hyperlipidemia, severe elevations of LDL, premature atherosclerosis

ulations found in many human atherosclerotic lesions, and (3) the role of certain environmental factors in eliciting vascular occlusive disease.

HEMOSTASIS AND THROMBOSIS

Hemostasis—the arrest of hemorrhage—is a normal response to vascular injury that involves vasoconstriction, tissue turgor, coagulation, and thrombosis. Whereas coagulation can occur in vitro solely as a result of the activation of the clotting cascade, thrombosis (the formation of a blood clot in situ) also involves the adherence and aggregation of platelets, the participation of cellular elements of the monocyte–macrophage system, and endothelial cell functions.

Thrombotic occlusion is frequently the major event leading from atherosclerosis to occlusive cardiovascular disease. Less severe occlusion, in which blood flow is restricted by a gradual increase in the size of an atherosclerotic lesion or by mural thrombosis and organization, can produce ischemia of an organ. Ischemia in the coronary circulation results in **angina pectoris**—chest pain from the heart. Similarly, occlusion of arteries supplying the brain, gut, or legs causes infarction or ischemia. A common form of vaso-occlusive disease in the legs produces muscle pain, termed **intermittent claudication,** on exercise of the leg muscles. Finally, ischemia of one organ can have marked systemic ef-

fects. The best-known example is the result of renal artery narrowing by atherosclerosis. The kidney compensates for poor perfusion by elevating its secretion of renin, an enzyme that elevates blood pressure; the result is "renal" hypertension.

Atherosclerosis also causes tissue injury distal to a plaque by **embolus formation**—that is, loss of parts of a plaque into the circulation, with lodgment of the debris in a critical smaller vessel. Emboli from plaques in the carotid artery are one cause of **cerebral vascular occlusion,** also called **stroke.** The weakened wall of an atherosclerotic vessel may also lead to **aneurysm formation** and subsequent hemorrhage.

The circulating cellular element most intimately involved with injury to the blood vessel is the platelet. When vessels are injured, platelets interact with one another to form a platelet thrombus—that is, an aggregate of activated platelets (Fig. 10-9). These platelet aggregates occlude vessels and prevent the leakage of blood from injured small vessels. The materials released from platelets can stimulate both wound healing and the formation of proliferative lesions in the vessel wall. The latter include both the smooth muscle proliferation seen in the atherosclerotic lesion and, as described below, the proliferative lesions of smooth muscle cells of small vessels in malignant hypertension.

Thrombus formation is normally prevented by blood flow and the anti-thrombotic properties of the endothelium. However, thrombi can form when endothelial

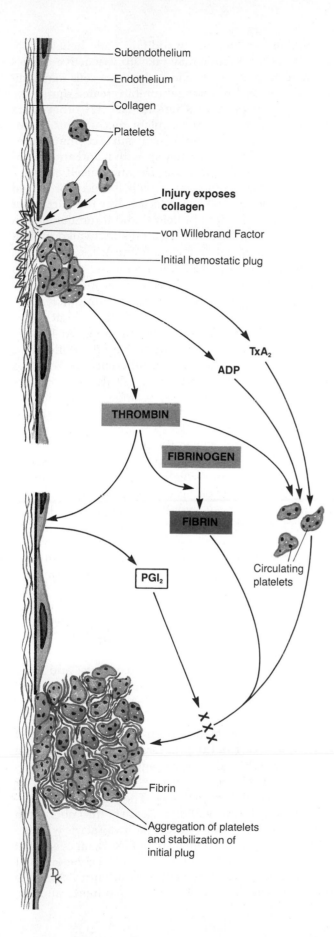

Subendothelium

Endothelium

Collagen

Platelets

Injury exposes collagen

von Willebrand Factor

Initial hemostatic plug

TxA$_2$

ADP

THROMBIN

FIBRINOGEN

FIBRIN

PGI$_2$

Circulating platelets

Fibrin

Aggregation of platelets and stabilization of initial plug

function is altered, when endothelial continuity is lost, or when blood flow is altered or becomes static. **Simple endothelial loss or injury in a vessel with good flow produces platelet pavementing but not thrombosis** (Fig. 10-10). The breakdown of a thrombus may lead to further complications. Fragments of thrombi, called emboli or thromboemboli, may circulate to distal vessels and occlude them. When those fragments originate in the venous circulation, the result is often a pulmonary embolism—a major life-threatening event. Emboli may arise from other sources. For example, the disruption of the fatty part of the atherosclerotic lesion may produce a fat or a cholesterol crystal embolus.

PLATELET AGGREGATION

Thrombosis, the adhesion and aggregation of platelets, is critical to repair at normal wound sites. It is also an important event in any situation in which endothelial integrity and function are lost or blood flow is obstructed. The aggregation of platelets and the activation of the clotting cascade are exquisitely sensitive to alterations in the microenvironment. **The major initiating event for most thrombosis and coagulation in vivo is almost certainly some form of injury to the endothelium (see Fig. 10-9).** Activated platelets in turn release factors that initiate clotting, resulting in the formation of a complex thrombus on the vessel wall (see Figs. 10-5 and 10-9). For thrombosis to occur, endothelial continuity must be disrupted or the endothelial cell surface must change from an anticoagulant to a procoagulant surface. Both processes are believed to occur. The most common denuding endothelial injury is the progressive endothelial disruption of an advancing atherosclerotic lesion.

The endothelium plays an active rather than a passive role in the control of thrombosis. It has been suggested that the major antithrombotic mechanism of the endothelium is the secretion of PGI$_2$, also known as

Figure 10-9. The role of platelets in thrombosis. Following vessel wall injury and alteration in flow, platelets adhere and then aggregate. ADP and thromboxane A$_2$ are released and, along with locally generated thrombin, recruit additional platelets, causing the mass to enlarge. The growing platelet thrombus is stabilized by fibrin. Other elements, including leukocytes and red blood cells, are also incorporated into the thrombus. The release of prostacyclin (PGI$_2$) by endothelial cells regulates the process by inhibiting platelet aggregation.

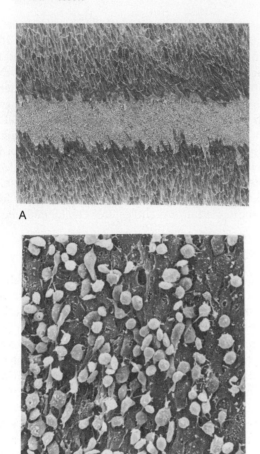

A

B

Figure 10-10. Scanning electron micrograph of the endothelial surface of a rat aorta 1 hour after the endothelial cells were removed by scraping with a nylon filament. (*A*) Intact endothelium and scratched portion. (*B*) Higher-power view of the scratched area showing a pavement of intact platelets that adheres to the underlying connective tissue in the high-velocity arterial stream.

prostacyclin. However, prostacyclin may actually have a minor role; several other features of the endothelium support its antithrombotic activity. Endothelial cells metabolize adenosine diphosphate (ADP). This is important both because ADP is a strong promoter of thrombogenesis and because its metabolites are antithrombogenic. The luminal surface of the endothelium is coated with heparan sulfate. Although there is no direct evidence that this substance participates directly in the inhibition of clotting of blood, as does exogenous heparin, heparan sulfate does bind a number of clotting factors, including the antiprotease alpha-2 macroglobulin. Endothelial cells also synthesize plasminogen activators, and thus may dissolve

some clots as they form. In addition, endothelial cells at the site of thrombosis may take up vasoactive amines released from platelets. Similarly, these cells may limit coagulation by consuming thrombin created during the procoagulant process. There are several other more specific endothelial anticoagulant mechanisms. A cofactor on the endothelial cell surface inactivates thrombin by forming a complex with it and antithrombin 3, a plasma antiprotease. Thrombin itself activates protein C via an interaction with its receptor, called thrombomodulin, which is located on the surface of endothelial cells. Both protein C and thrombomodulin are synthesized by endothelial cells. Activated protein C destroys coagulation factors V and VII.

The presence of these antithrombotic mechanisms on the endothelial surface has raised the intriguing possibility that endothelial dysfunction might lead to thrombosis in vivo. There is also evidence that endothelial cells have prothrombotic functions. At least in culture, endothelial cells synthesize von Willebrand factor, which promotes platelet adherence, and clotting factor V. The cultured endothelial cell also binds factors IX and X, a process that may promote coagulation on the endothelial surface in vivo. Finally, endothelial cells treated with interleukin-1 or tumor necrosis factor present thromboplastin to the plasma, potentially initiating coagulation via the extrinsic pathway. Thus, one can envision that prothrombotic, procoagulant injuries at the surface of blood vessels are produced either by the loss of a normal endothelial function or by the stimulation of an abnormal function.

Once platelets are stimulated to adhere to the vessel wall, their contents are spontaneously released. In turn, these contents promote aggregation with new platelets. Aggregation is enhanced by the release of von Willebrand factor; this substance is adhesive for the GPI_b membrane protein and for fibrinogen. The activated platelets also release ADP and thromboxane A_2, which recruit additional platelets, thereby causing changes in platelet shape, release of granule contents, and more aggregation. The platelet membrane proteins $GP2_b$ and $GP3_a$ adhere to fibrin and fibrinogen, a process that tends to stabilize the forming thrombus.

The generation of thrombin is probably the most important factor in the progression and stabilization of the thrombus through coagulation. Thrombin is generated at the site of injury by either the intrinsic or extrinsic coagulation pathway. The extrinsic coagulation pathway begins with the release of thromboplastin from injured cells. The intrinsic pathway starts with the activation of factor XII (Hageman factor), an event that depends on the binding of this factor to a component of injured cells. Thrombin itself is sufficient to stimulate further release of platelet-granule contents and the subsequent recruitment of new platelets. As coagulation proceeds, fibrin that is formed by the action of thrombin on fibrinogen, forges cross-bridges bound to the GP2$_b$ and GP3$_a$ receptors on platelets. These links stabilize the aggregation of the platelets and their adherence to the underlying denuded surface.

BLOOD COAGULATION AND CLOT LYSIS

Coagulation of blood depends on a cascade of enzyme activations that reflect the sequential actions of proteases (Fig. 10-11). Each coagulation factor acts first as a substrate and then as an enzyme. The net result is a powerful, autocatalytic, biologic amplifier.

Coagulation is initiated by two distinct pathways. In the **intrinsic pathway** the initial event is the interaction of factor XII with any of several biologic surfaces, including products of necrotic cells. The normal endothelium ordinarily prevents factor XII from interacting with such surfaces. The activated form of factor XII, namely factor XII$_a$, is a protease that initiates subsequent interactions among the other factors involved in the intrinsic pathway. These include prekallikrein, factor IX, and factor VIII.

The **extrinsic pathway** begins with tissue factor, also a product of cell injury. Tissue factor is a cell surface protein, the gene for which has recently been cloned. The interaction between tissue factor and circulating factor VII initiates the extrinsic pathway. Activated factor VII and activated factor IX (from the intrinsic pathway) both act on factor X to produce activated factor X (factor X$_a$). In turn, factor X$_a$ interacts with factor V, calcium, and platelet factor 3, a component of the platelet membrane. Platelet factor 3 only becomes available on the platelet surface during platelet activa-

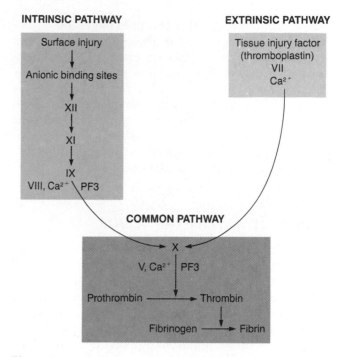

Figure 10-11. Intrinsic and extrinsic pathways for coagulation.

tion. Thus, **coagulation and thrombosis are closely intertwined.** The interaction of factors X$_a$, V, calcium, and platelet factor 3 leads to thrombin formation. Thrombin activates fibrinogen to form fibrin, and the clot is formed.

The combination of platelet thrombus and clot is unstable because of the activation of plasmin, a fibrinolytic enzyme (Fig. 10-12). During clot formation, plasminogen is bound to fibrin and, therefore, is an integral part of the forming platelet mass. Endothelial cells syn-

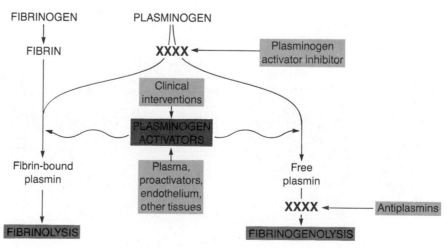

Figure 10-12. Factors and sequences involved in fibrinolysis and points of clinical intervention in thrombolysis therapy.

thesize plasminogen activator, but in larger thombi circulating plasminogen may also be converted to plasmin by products of the coagulation cascade. Plasminogen activator bound to fibrin activates plasmin; in turn, by digesting fibrin, plasmin lyses the clot and disrupts the thrombus. The synthesis of plasminogen activator represents still another antithrombotic mechanism of the endothelial cell. Endothelial cells also synthesize an inhibitor of plasminogen activator. Thus, again this cell possesses pro-and anticoagulant properties.

CORONARY ARTERY OCCLUSION

It is useful to consider the sequence of events that might occur in a 50-year-old man undergoing the initial events in a myocardial infarction. The primary process involves a coronary artery wall that is roughened by the underlying atherosclerotic plaque (Fig. 10-13). At this point the surface is not thrombogenic and the endothelium is intact. **Some change occurs in the lesion to make it thrombogenic.** Perhaps the lesion ulcerates. Possibly, toxic products released by macrophages alter endothelial cell viability, so that the cells are sloughed. Vasa vasorum may hemorrhage into the plaque. Any of these circumstances will lead to exposure of the connective tissue of the vessel wall to the circulating blood.

Alternatively, activated macrophages in the lesion may secrete tumor necrosis factor or interleukin-1, causing endothelial cells to secrete thromboplastin. In any event, platelets are stimulated to interact with collagen, fibronectin, or fibrin on the injured surface, after which they adhere and become activated. The activated platelets stimulate platelet aggregation by releasing thromboxane A_2 and ADP. Von Willebrand factor is liberated from platelet alpha granules and possibly from injured endothelial cells, a process which further accelerates platelet aggregation. The platelet alpha granule contributes to the stabilization of the forming aggregate by liberating fibrinogen and fibronectin. Platelet granules release ADP and vasoactive elements, including histamine, epinephrine, and serotonin. Calcium discharged by the platelets helps to stimulate the coagulation sequence.

Activation of the platelet surface also promotes coagulation by the intrinsic pathway because it leads to binding of factor X, factor V, and calcium. In addition to stimulating platelet aggregation, thromboxane A_2 also provokes constriction of the surrounding vessels, thus worsening the occlusion of the lumen. The initiation of the intrinsic clotting cascade results in the release of thrombin. In addition to stimulating the formation of fibrin, thrombin itself is a powerful promoter of platelet aggregation. Thus, the initial aggregate of platelets becomes converted to a mixture of platelets and thrombus. Injury to surrounding smooth muscle and endothelial cells results in the release of tissue factor, which then initiates the extrinsic coagulation pathway.

The interaction between thrombosis and coagulation results in the formation of layers of fibrin and platelets within arterial thrombi. These layers, which are visible when the thrombus is sectioned, are called **lines of Zahn.** The formation of lines of Zahn depends on a

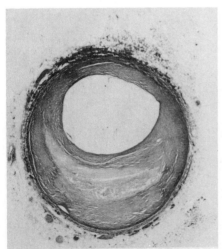
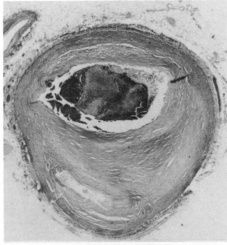

A   B

Figure 10-13. Atherosclerotic coronary occlusion. (*A*) Coronary artery with atherosclerotic plaque in a 54-year-old man. (*B*) Downstream of the plaque is the occluding thrombus that caused the man's death.

high flow rate; thrombi formed in areas of sluggish blood flow, such as veins or atrial appendages, do not show a layered structure. If the thrombus does not progress, it remains attached to the wall and is called a **mural thrombus.** A mural thrombus that becomes sufficiently large occludes the vessel, and is labeled an **occlusive thrombus.**

The organized structure of a thrombus, which reflects a tight interaction between platelets and fibrin, differs in appearance from the **postmortem clot** or the clot formed in a test tube. The lines of Zahn stabilize the thrombus formed during life, whereas the postmortem clot is a more gelatinous structure. Postmortem clots occur in stagnant blood, where gravity fractionates the erythrocytes. The part of the clot that contains many red blood cells is called **currant jelly.** The overlying clot, which represents coagulated plasma without red blood cells, is called **chicken fat** because of its color and consistency.

The mural thrombus overlying an atherosclerotic plaque is a rich source of chemotactic factors and mitogens. These agents stimulate the smooth muscle cells in the plaque to grow, secrete collagen, and convert a labile structure into a more permanent one. The thrombus is invaded by smooth muscle cells and connective tissue, and the resulting **organized thrombus** is a permanent structure. New vessels may invade and provide some blood flow across the organized thrombus, a process called **canalization** of the thrombus. Unfortunately, these new vessels are almost always too small to maintain a clinically significant level of blood flow.

A thrombus over a vascular plaque may propagate and eventually occlude the vessel. The observation is important because this mechanism is probably the most common cause of occlusion of the coronary arteries, and because the recent introduction of thrombolytic therapy has in many cases permitted the reestablishment of the lumen.

The ultimate result of thrombotic vascular occlusion of a coronary artery is myocardial infarction. The same sequence of events occurs in other organs, such as the kidney and brain (Fig. 10-14).

HYPERTENSIVE VASCULAR DISEASE

Hypertension, with its associated atherosclerotic vascular disease, is a common cause of death in the United States. Among black Americans, hypertension is also the most common fatal heritable disease. Most of the disease associated with hypertension is attributed to an increased risk for a variety of cardiovascular disorders. Examples are angina pectoris, sudden death, stroke, and atherothrombotic occlusion of the abdominal aorta or its branches. More than half of the patients with these diseases also have hypertension. More than 70% of patients with dissecting aortic aneurysm, intracerebral hemorrhage, or rupture of the myocardial wall have an elevated blood pressure. Hypertension is a major risk factor for atherosclerosis, as shown in both epidemiologic and experimental studies. In recent years it has become clear that the treatment of hypertension

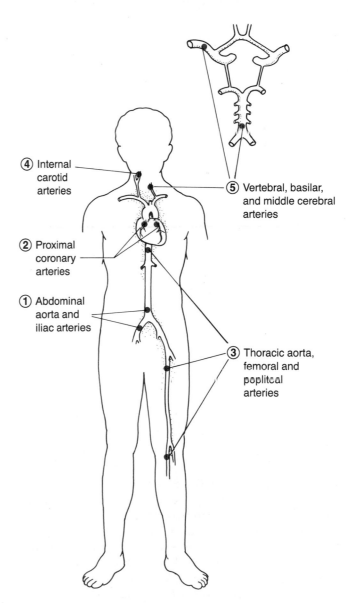

Figure 10-14. Sites of severe atherosclerosis in order of frequency.

can prolong life. It is disturbing to realize that the etiology of most hypertension remains unknown: 95% of patients display no identifiable etiology. Thus, the large majority of hypertensive people are described as having **essential** or **primary hypertension.**

ETIOLOGY

Attempts to identify a single etiology for primary hypertension have been frustrating. We know from family studies that genetic factors are likely to be important; however, no specific genetic defect has been shown to be causal.

The most widespread hypothesis holds that primary hypertension results from an imbalance in the interactions between the mechanisms for controlling cardiac output, renal function, peripheral resistance, and sodium homeostasis (Fig. 10-15). A complex endocrine axis centers on the renin-angiotensin system. Renin is a protease that lyses angiotensinogen to a decapeptide, angiotensin I. In turn, angiotensin I is converted to angiotensin II by angiotensin converting enzyme, a protein found on the surface of the endothelial cell. Although angiotensin II was originally thought of primarily as a vasoconstrictor, it is now recognized that it also has major effects on centers in the central nervous system that control sympathetic outflow and stimulate aldosterone release from the adrenal gland. Aldosterone acts on renal tubules to increase sodium reabsorption. The net effect is an increase in total body fluid volume. Thus, the **renin–angiotensin system** elevates blood pressure by three mechanisms: increased sympathetic output, increased mineralocorticoid secretion, and direct vasoconstriction.

The renin–angiotensin–aldosterone axis is antagonized by a hormone, **atrial natriuretic factor,** secreted by specialized cells in the atria. This factor, acting via its own receptors, increases the urinary excretion of sodium and opposes the vasoconstrictor effects of angiotensin II. Secretion of atrial natriuretic factor may be controlled by atrial distension, a consequence of increased volume, or by as yet undefined endocrine interactions.

There is no clear evidence that a specific defect in the renin-angiotensin axis is the essential lesion of primary hypertension. It has proved difficult to identify a crucial defect in this axis or a critical genetic lesion, because the vascular system responds quickly to changes in the effective rates of flow through tissue beds by **autoregulation** (see Fig. 10-15). **In the case of hypertension, the end result of autoregulation is always increased peripheral resistance.**

The causes of only a small proportion of all cases of hypertension are identifiable. **These include renal artery stenosis, most forms of chronic renal disease, primary elevation of aldosterone, Cushing's syndrome, neoplasms of the adrenal medulla (pheochromocytoma), thyrotoxicosis, coarctation of the aorta, and a few others.** In addition, persons with severe atherosclerosis may have a high systolic pressure because the sclerotic aorta cannot properly absorb the kinetic energy of the pulse wave.

PATHOLOGY

It is important to realize that **the central lesion in most cases of hypertension is a decrease in the size of the lumen in small muscular arteries and arterioles,** the resistance vessels that control the flow of blood through the capillary bed (Fig. 10-16). The lumen may be restricted by active contraction of the vessel wall or an increase in the structural mass of the vessel wall, or both. Changes in the size of the vascular lumen due to active constriction are not detectable morphologically, and the increased resistance is immediately removed by agents that relax smooth muscle contraction. The rapid drop in blood pressure seen when hypertensive animals or people are treated with smooth muscle relaxants suggests that active constriction is very important. However, constriction of a structurally thicker vessel wall would be expected to produce an even more marked narrowing of the lumen than would occur with a normal thinner wall. Thus, some component of hypertension may be attributed to a structural change in the vessel wall.

The morphologic changes associated with moderate elevations of blood pressure are too subtle to be detected by simple histologic studies. On the other hand, severe hypertension produces dramatic changes, particularly at the microvascular level. Segmental constriction and dilatation of the retinal arterioles in severely hypertensive individuals are sufficiently marked to allow the diagnosis of hypertension by ophthalmoscopy.

Small muscular arteries show segmental dilatation as a result of necrosis of smooth muscle cells. Endothelial integrity is lost in these regions, and the increase in vascular permeability leads to the deposition of fibrin and the entry of plasma proteins into the vessel wall. The combination of cell necrosis and deposition of plasma proteins in the vessel wall is termed **fibrinoid necrosis.** The period of acute injury is rapidly followed by smooth muscle proliferation and a striking increase in the number of layers of smooth muscle cells, which yields the so-called **onion-skin** appearance (Fig. 10-17). This form of smooth muscle proliferation may be a response to the release of growth factors derived

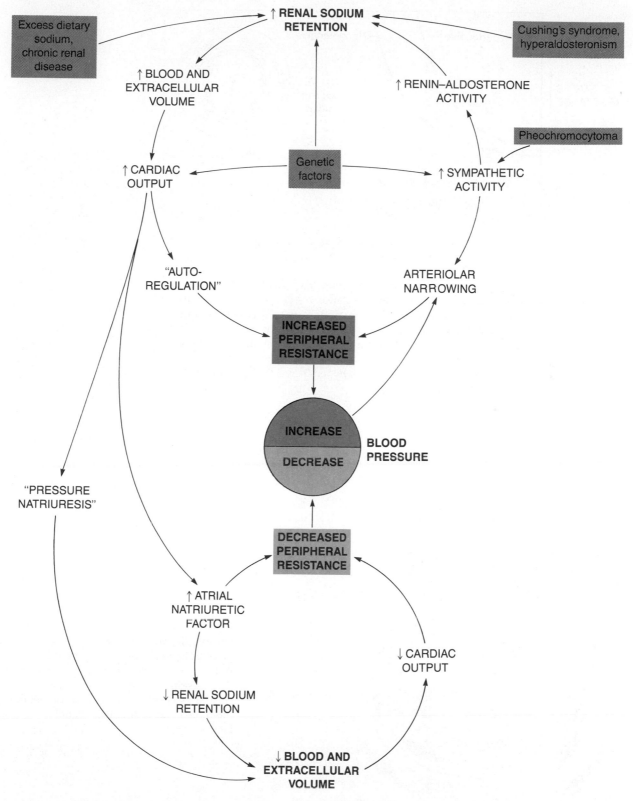

Figure 10-15. Factors contributing to hypertension and the counter-regulatory factors that lower blood pressure. An imbalance in these factors results in the increased peripheral resistance that is responsible for most cases of idiopathic (primary) hypertension. Note the central role of peripheral resistance.

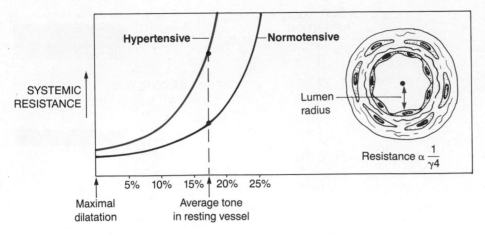

SHORTENING OF MUSCLE CELLS DURING
ARTERIAL CONTRACTION

Figure 10-16. Structural autoregulation of blood pressure. Hypertension, regardless of its primary etiology, increases the ability of the resistance vessel walls to respond to vasoactive stimuli. Resistance is increased even in maximally dilated vessels because the lumen size is decreased in the hypertensive vascular bed. As the smooth muscle cells contract, the increase in vessel wall thickness increases the resistance, which is inversely proportional to the fourth power of the radius of the lumen. Note that at the average resting muscular tone, the resistance in hypertensives is considerably higher than normal.

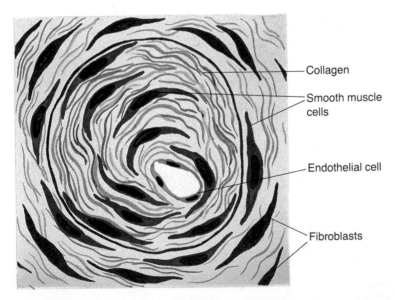

Figure 10-17. Arteriolosclerosis. In cases of hypertension, the arterioles exhibit smooth muscle cell proliferation and increased amounts of intercellular collagen and glycosaminoglycans, resulting in an "onion-skin" appearance. The mass of smooth muscle and associated elements tend to fix the size of the lumen and restrict the arteriole's capacity to dilate.

from platelets and other cells at the sites of vascular injury. Taken together, these changes are labeled **malignant arteriosclerosis** or **malignant arteriolosclerosis,** depending on the size of the vessels affected.

Milder chronic hypertension causes **benign arteriosclerosis,** in which the major change is a variable increase in the thickness of vessel walls. A change typically ascribed to chronic hypertension is called **hyaline arteriolosclerosis.** "Hyaline" refers to the glassy, scarred appearance of blood vessel walls as seen by conventional light microscopy. The vessel wall is thickened by the deposition of connective tissue, particularly collagen, and by the accumulation of plasma proteins. In the small muscular arteries this may be accompanied by the formation of new layers of elastin, presenting as a reduplication of the normal intimal elastic lamina.

Despite the implied association, the finding of hyaline arteriolosclerosis is not diagnostic of hypertension. Hyaline arteriolosclerosis, diffuse intimal thickening of the elastic and large muscular arteries, and the reduplication of the internal elastic lamina in resistance arteries and arterioles are very common changes that occur as part of the aging process. However, hyaline arteriolosclerosis is accelerated in diabetes and in hypertension, diseases that are also associated with accelerated atherosclerosis. Finally, hypertension is a major risk factor for atherosclerosis, although the mechanism by which it operates is not well known.

INFLAMMATORY DISORDERS OF BLOOD VESSELS

Vasculitis, defined as inflammation and necrosis of blood vessels, affects arteries, veins, and capillaries (Table 10-2). Arteries or veins may be damaged by infectious agents, mechanical trauma, radiation, or toxins. However, many cases of vasculitis are without any known specific etiology.

The etiology and pathogenesis of the vasculitic syndromes are thought to involve immune mechanisms, including the deposition of immune complexes, a direct attack on cells by circulating antibodies, and various forms of cell-mediated immunity. Viral antigens have been suspected in experimental animals and in man.

POLYARTERITIS NODOSA

Hepatitis B virus infection is associated with a necrotizing polyarteritis nodosa. In this syndrome, circulating viral antigen-antibody complexes have been demon-

Table 10-2 Inflammatory Disorders of Blood Vessels

Polyarteritis nodosa group of systemic necrotizing vasculitis
  Classic polyarteritis nodosa
  Allergic angiitis and granulomatosis (Churg-Strauss variant)
  "Overlap syndrome" of systemic angiitis
Hypersensitivity vasculitis
  Serum sickness and similar reactions
  Henoch-Schönlein purpura
  Vasculitis associated with connective tissue disorders
  Vasculitis in cases of essential mixed cryoglobulinemia
  Vasculitis associated with other primary disorders
Wegener's granulomatosis
Lymphomatoid granulomatosis
Giant cell arteritis
  Temporal arteritis
  Takayasu's arteritis
Central nervous system vasculitis
Vasculitis associated with cancer
Mucocutaneous lymph node syndrome (Kawasaki's disease)
Thromboangiitis obliterans (Buerger's disease)
Behçet's disease
Miscellaneous vasculitis syndromes

strated, as well as local deposits of viral antigen, immunoglobulins, and complement components in the vascular lesions.

The characteristic lesion of polyarteritis nodosa is patchy and affects mainly the small arteries. However, on occasion it extends into medium-sized arteries, such as the renal, splenic, or coronary arteries. Each lesion, no more than a millimeter in length, may involve the entire circumference of the vessel or only a part of it. At the heart of the lesion is an area of fibrinoid necrosis, in which the medial muscle and adjacent tissues are fused into a structureless eosinophilic mass that stains for fibrin. A vigorous inflammatory response develops around the area of necrosis, usually spreads to involve the entire adventitia (periarteritis), and extends through the other coats of the vessel (Fig. 10-18). Neutrophils, lymphocytes, plasma cells, and macrophages are present in varying proportions, and eosinophils are often conspicuous. As a result of thrombosis in the lumen of an affected segment, infarcts are commonly found in the involved organs. Injury to larger arteries results in the formation of small aneurysms (less than 0.5 cm in diameter), particularly in branches of the renal, coronary, and cerebral arteries. An aneurysm may rupture, and if located in a critical area, fatal hemorrhage ensues.

The clinical manifestations of polyarteritis nodosa are highly variable, depending on the chance occurrence of lesions in different vascular regions. The kidneys, heart, skeletal muscle, skin, and mesentery are most frequently involved, but stomach, bowel, spleen,

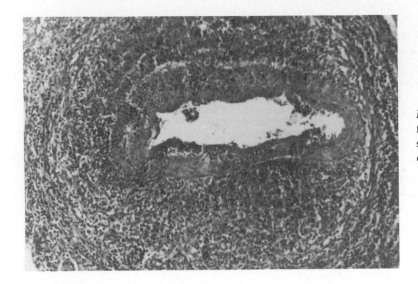

Figure 10-18. Polyarteritis nodosa. The intense inflammatory cell infiltrate in the arterial wall and surrounding connective tissue is associated with disruption of the vessel wall.

pancreas, lungs, liver, nerves, meninges, brain, spinal cord, and endocrine organs may all show lesions. There are characteristic renal glomerular lesions in about two-thirds of the cases. These show florid, patchy, fibrinoid necrosis, accompanied by a periglomerular inflammatory exudate and the typical periarteritic lesions in the renal vessels. Hypertension is a common sequel, and many patients die in renal failure.

GIANT CELL ARTERITIS (TEMPORAL ARTERITIS)

Giant cell arteritis, today perhaps the most common of the vasculitides, is a focal, chronic, granulomatous inflammation of the temporal arteries. Although the disease most often affects the cranial arteries, it can involve the aorta and its branches and occasionally other arteries. The average age of onset is about 70 years; the disease rarely occurs in those under 50 years of age. The incidence rises with age and may reach 1% by age 80 years. Women are affected slightly more often than men. The age of onset helps differentiate this entity from some other vasculitides, such as Takayasu's disease, which occurs in much younger individuals.

The usual onset is with headache and throbbing temporal pain. In other instances there are early symptoms of malaise, fever, anorexia, nausea, and weight loss, followed or accompanied by generalized muscular aching or stiffness in the shoulders and hips. The throbbing and pain over the temporal artery is accom-

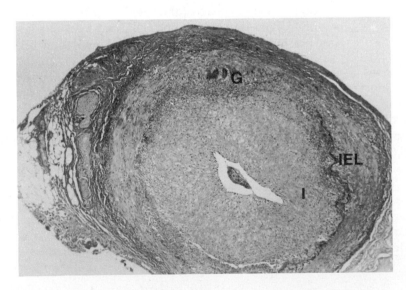

Figure 10-19. Temporal (giant cell) arteritis. A temporal artery shows a fully developed lesion with giant cells in the media (*G*), a thickened intima (*I*), and a few inflammatory cells. *IEL*, internal elastica.

panied by swelling, tenderness, and redness in the skin overlying the vessel. Visual symptoms occur in a minority of patients, but occasionally may proceed from transient to permanent blindness in one or both eyes. The disease in other vessels gives rise to infarcts in the myocardium, brain, or gastrointestinal tract.

The affected artery is cordlike and exhibits nodular thickening. The lumen is reduced to a slit or may be obliterated by a thrombus. The histologic appearance is of granulomatous inflammation of the media and intima consisting of aggregates of histocytes, lymphocytes, and plasma cells, with varying admixtures of eosinophils and neutrophils (Fig. 10-19). Giant cells, though usually conspicuous, vary widely in number, ranging from abundant to scant or absent. Thrombosis may obliterate the lumen, after which organization and canalization occur.

Giant cell arteritis is usually benign and self-limited, the symptoms subsiding in 6 to 12 months. In a minority of cases the disease has serious complications, such as blindness, and may even be fatal. The response to corticosteroid therapy is usually dramatic, with symptoms subsiding in a matter of days.

KAWASAKI'S DISEASE (MUCOCUTANEOUS LYMPH NODE SYNDROME)

Kawasaki's disease is an acute vasculitis of infancy and early childhood characterized by high fever, rash, conjunctival and oral lesions, and lymphadenitis. Acute necrotizing vasculitis of small and medium-sized coronary arteries occurs in as many as 70% of patients and is a cause of death in 1% to 2% of cases. Like many childhood viral diseases, Kawasaki's disease is usually self-limited, and although an infectious cause has been sought, none has been conclusively proved.

THROMBOANGIITIS OBLITERANS (BUERGER'S DISEASE)

Thromboangiitis obliterans occurs almost exclusively in young and middle-aged men who smoke heavily. The symptoms usually start between the ages of 25 and 40 years and take the form of intermittent claudication (cramping pains in muscles following exercise, which are quickly relieved by rest). The blood vessels of the legs are most frequently affected, but those of the arm are not uncommonly involved.

The process appears earliest as an acute inflammation, with infiltration of medium-sized and small arteries by neutrophils (Fig. 10-20). The inflammation extends to involve neighboring veins and nerves. Small microabscesses of the vessel wall distinguish the process from thrombosis associated with atherosclerosis. These abscesses consist of a central area of neutrophils surrounded by fibroblasts and Langhan's giant cells. The early lesions are further complicated by thrombosis of veins and arteries, often severe enough to result in gangrene of the extremity, for which the only treatment is amputation. Late in the course of the disease the thrombi are completely organized and partly canalized.

The etiologic role of smoking in Buerger's disease is emphasized by the observation that cessation of smoking can be followed by a remission, and resumption of smoking by an exacerbation.

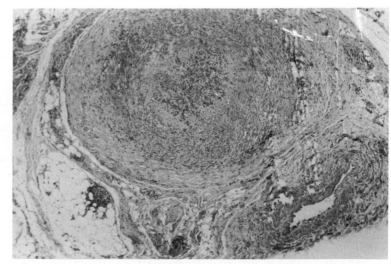

Figure 10-20. Thromboangitis obliterans (Buerger's disease). An artery from an amputated limb of a 55-year-old male cigarette smoker shows an organized thrombus that has completely occluded the artery. Some inflammatory cells are evident in the adventitial fat. In this instance the adjacent vein has been largely spared.

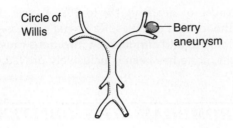

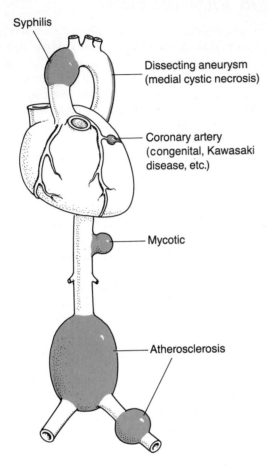

Figure 10-21. The locations of aneurysms. Syphilitic aneurysms are the common variety in the ascending aorta, which is usually spared by the atherosclerotic process. Atherosclerotic aneurysms can occur in the abdominal aorta or muscular arteries, including the coronary and popliteal arteries and other vessels. Berry aneurysms are seen in the circle of Willis, mainly at branch points; their rupture leads to subarachnoid hemorrhage. Mycotic aneurysms occur almost anywhere that bacteria can deposit on vessel walls.

ANEURYSMS

Aneurysms are classified by location, configuration, and etiology (Fig. 10-21). The location refers to the type of vessel involved—artery or vein—and the specific vessel affected, such as the aorta or popliteal artery. The gross appearance of the lesions has led to terms such as **fusiform, saccular,** or **cylindroid.** These conformations are seen in large vessels; smaller aneurysms (berry aneurysms) occur in the brain.

SYPHILITIC ANEURYSMS

Syphilitic (luetic) aneurysms are largely limited to the thoracic aorta, and are caused by inflammation and destruction of the aortic wall. The inflammatory process affects the adventitia, where it involves the lymphatics and the vasa vasorum, and produces an obliterative endarteritis in these small vessels. In severe syphilitic aortitis the wall is slightly thickened and abnormally adherent to surrounding structures. Lesions are usually apparent on the intimal surface. The aorta shows focal depressed scarring, and the roughened intimal surface has a "tree bark" appearance (Fig. 10-22*A*).

Microscopic examination shows endarteritis and periarteritis of the vasa vasorum. These vessels, which arise from branches of the aorta, ramify in the adventitia and penetrate the outer and middle thirds of the aorta, where they become encircled by lymphocytes, plasma cells, and macrophages. Obliterative changes in the vasa vasorum cause foci of necrosis and scarring of the media, with disruption and disorganization of the elastic lamellae (Fig. 10-22*B*). Dense collagen is eventually deposited in the scarred media and intimal patches. These fibrous patches or plaques encircle the orifices of branches of the aorta, including the coronary and intercostal arteries.

ATHEROSCLEROTIC ANEURYSMS

Atherosclerosis weakens the media and is probably the most common cause of aneurysms of the large arteries, particularly the abdominal aorta. Aneurysms of the iliac, femoral, and popliteal arteries also occur, and are often multiple.

Atherosclerotic aneurysms are usually freeform or even cylindrical, but saccular varieties may be seen. Confluent, ulcerated, atheromatous plaques often involve the adjacent arterial intima and extend into the aneurysmal sac. Adherent thrombi are abundant in these aneurysms and may give rise to emboli that occlude distal arteries. Dissection of the aneurysmal ar-

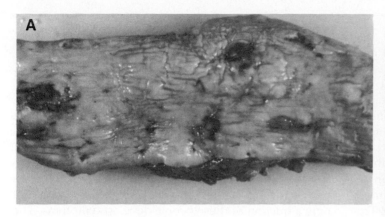

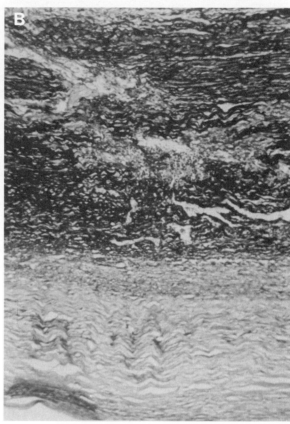

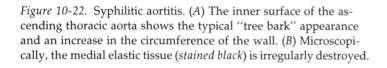

Figure 10-22. Syphilitic aortitis. (*A*) The inner surface of the ascending thoracic aorta shows the typical "tree bark" appearance and an increase in the circumference of the wall. (*B*) Microscopically, the medial elastic tissue (*stained black*) is irregularly destroyed.

tery wall can occur or, as often happens in the aorta, the aneurysm may rupture and allow massive hemorrhage.

MYCOTIC ANEURYSMS

Mycotic aneurysms, which have a tendency to rupture and hemorrhage, result from the weakening of the vessel wall by a bacterial infection. They may develop in the aortic wall or in cerebral vessels during the course of a septicemia or in cases of bacterial endocarditis. Mesenteric, splenic, or renal arteries are also common sites.

ANEURYSMS OF CEREBRAL ARTERIES

Aneurysms of the cerebral arteries are particularly important because of their frequency and dangerous locations. The most common cerebral aneurysm is called

a **berry aneurysm,** because it resembles a berry attached to twigs of the arterial tree. The aneurysms tend to arise at one of the branching angles of the circle of Willis or in one of the arterial branches from it. The most common sites are at the following angles: between the anterior cerebral artery and the anterior communicating artery, between the internal carotid artery and the posterior communicating artery, and between the first main divisions of the middle cerebral artery and the bifurcation of the internal carotid artery. As the aneurysm enlarges, it may become embedded in the brain substance or it may wrap itself around adjacent nerves, arteries, or veins, thereby producing symptoms. Histologically, the neck of a berry aneurysm shows an abrupt cessation of the media at the point of origin of the aneurysm. The internal elastic lamina extends a short way into the wall of the aneurysm but soon disappears, and the wall of the aneurysm then consists merely of a layer of fibrous tissue so thin that it may be transparent. Frequently the dilated aneurysmal sac is filled with a thrombus. Rupture of these aneurysms and resulting subarachnoid hemorrhage is a common complication.

DISSECTING ANEURYSMS

Dissecting aneurysm refers to the entry of blood into the substance of the arterial wall and its extension along the length of the vessel (Fig. 10-23). In effect, the blood is encompassed by a false lumen in the substance of the wall. In fact, although they are conventionally called aneurysms, these lesions are actually a form of hematoma. Dissecting aneurysms most often affect the aorta and its major branches. Men are affected about three times as frequently as women. A dissecting aneurysm may occur at almost any age, but is seen most commonly in the sixth and seventh decades of life. The onset is sudden and often associated with physical exertion. There is a significant association with hypertension.

Commonly, the dissection of the vessel wall starts at the root of the aorta, a centimeter or two above the aortic ring, where a transverse slit in the intima and inner media can be found. The dissection in the media roughly separates the inner two-thirds of the vessel from the outer third. The dissection can involve the coronary arteries, great vessels of the neck, or the renal, mesenteric, or iliac arteries. Rupture into the perivascular space and compression of critical vessels can occur. In dissecting aneurysm of the aorta, the blood within the vessel may occasionally reenter the lumen through a second distal tear. The result is an aorta with a double lumen.

The pathogenesis of dissecting aneurysms in most instances can be traced to a weakening of the aortic media. The changes were originally described as "Erdheim's cystic medial necrosis." Focal loss of elastic and muscle fibers in the media leads to "cystic" spaces filled with metachromatic material (glycosaminoglycans). The causes of the cystic medial necrosis are not known in most cases, but it is often seen in association with Marfan's syndrome, a hereditary collagen disorder.

DISORDERS OF VEINS

VARICOSE VEINS OF THE LEGS

Varicose veins of the legs, one of the most common ailments of man, varies from a trivial knot of dilated vessels to disabling distention of the whole system of veins of the leg, with secondary trophic disturbances. It has been estimated that as much as 10% to 20% of the population has some varicosities in the leg veins, but only a fraction of these people develop symptoms. The incidence of varicose veins rises with age, and may reach 50% in people over the age of 50 years. In the 30- to 50-year-old age group, women are affected more often than men, particularly those women who have experienced pregnancy, because increased venous pressure is associated with the weight of the pregnant uterus on the iliac veins.

There is a strong familial predisposition to varicose veins, possibly owing to inherited configurations and structural weaknesses, either of the walls or the valves of the veins. The pressure in leg veins is five to ten times greater in the erect position than in the recumbent position. Understandably, therefore, the incidence of varicose veins is increased among people whose occupations require them to stand in one place for long periods, such as dentists and sales clerks. Obesity also increases the incidence of varicose veins, possibly because of an increase in intra-abdominal pressure or the poor support to the vessel walls offered by subcutaneous fat. The increase in the incidence of varicose veins with age may reflect degenerative changes of the connective tissues in the vein walls, together with loss of the surrounding supporting fat and connective tissues, loss of muscle tone, and inactivity. Other factors that can augment venous pressure in the legs can cause varicose veins. In addition to the pregnant uterus, pel-

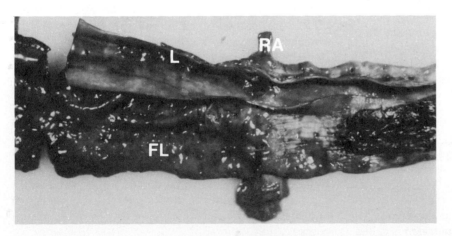

Figure 10-23. Dissecting aneurysm in the abdominal aorta caused by cystic medial necrosis. The aneurysm began in the ascending aorta and dissected from there to the iliac vessels. It tore the renal artery (*RA*), which led to sudden massive hemorrhage. *L*, original lumen; *FL*, false lumen.

vic tumors, congestive heart failure, and thrombotic obstruction of the main venous trunks of the thigh or pelvis cause increased venous pressure.

In the pathogenesis of varicose veins it is not clear whether incompetence of the valves or dilatation of the vessels comes first. Whatever the case, the two reinforce each other. The vein increases both in length and diameter, so that tortuosities develop. Once the process has begun, the varicosity extends progressively throughout the length of the affected vein. As each valve becomes incompetent, a progressively increasing strain is thrown on the vessel and valve below.

The microscopic changes in the wall consist of variations in wall thickness, thinning due to dilatation, and, in other areas, thickening due to muscle hypertrophy, subintimal fibrosis, and incorporation of mural thrombi into the wall. Patchy calcification is frequently seen. Valvular deformities consist of thickening, shortening, and rolling of the cusps.

VARICOSE VEINS AT OTHER SITES

Hemorrhoids, varicose dilatations of the veins of the rectum and anal canal, may occur inside or outside of the anal sphincter. There may be a hereditary predisposition, but the condition is aggravated by constipation and pregnancy. It may also result from venous obstruction by rectal tumors. Hemorrhoids often bleed, which can cause confusion with bleeding rectal cancers. Thrombosed hemorrhoids are exquisitely painful.

Esophageal varices are a complication of portal hypertension caused by cirrhosis of the liver. High portal pressure leads to distention of anastomoses between the portal system and the systemic veins at the lower end of the esophagus. **Hemorrhage from esophageal varices is one of the most common causes of death in cirrhosis.**

A **varicocele** is a palpable mass in the scrotum formed by varicosities of the pampiniform plexus.

PHLEBITIS AND VENOUS THROMBOSIS (PHLEBOTHROMBOSIS)

Inflammation of small veins as part of a local reaction to bacterial infection, termed **phlebitis,** can extend to larger venous channels and cause thrombosis. Venous thrombosis that occurs in the absence of an initiating infection or inflammation is called **phlebothrombosis;** it is associated with prolonged bed rest or reduced car-

diac output and frequently affects the deep leg veins. Such thrombi can be a major threat to life because of embolization to the lung (witness the well-known phenomenon of sudden death occurring upon ambulation after surgery).

DISORDERS OF LYMPHATIC VESSELS

LYMPHANGITIS

On gaining entrance to the lymphatics, bacteria and inflammatory cells are conveyed to the regional lymph nodes. Microscopically the periphery of a focus of inflammation reveals dilated lymphatics filled with fluid exudate, cells, cellular debris, and bacteria.

Almost any virulent pathogen can cause acute lymphangitis, but group A beta-hemolytic streptococci are particularly notorious offenders. The process may extend beyond the lymphatic channels into the surrounding tissues. The draining lymph nodes are regularly enlarged and show changes of lymphadenitis. Clinically, painful subcutaneous red streaking is characteristic of acute lymphangitis.

LYMPHATIC OBSTRUCTION

Lymphatics may be obstructed by scar tissue, tumor cells, pressure from surrounding tumor tissue, plugging with parasites, or traumatic severance. Since collateral lymphatic routes are abundant, lymphedema (distention of tissue by lymph) usually occurs only when major trunks are obstructed, especially in the axilla or groin. For example, dissection of axillary lymph nodes during surgery for carcinoma of the breast frequently disrupts lymphatic channels and leads to lymphedema of the arm. Prolonged lymphatic obstruction causes progressive dilatation of lymphatic vessels, called **lymphangiectasia,** and overgrowth of fibrous tissue. The term **elephantiasis** describes a lymphedematous limb that has become grossly enlarged.

TUMORS OF BLOOD VESSELS

HEMANGIOMAS

Hemangiomas, tumors whose cells tend to form blood vessels, are classified by histologic type and location.

Capillary hemangioma is so designated because it is composed of vascular channels that have the **size and structure of normal capillaries.** Such lesions may be located in any tissue. The most common sites are the skin, subcutaneous tissues, mucous membranes of the lips and mouth, and internal viscera, including the spleen, kidneys, and liver. Capillary hemangiomas vary from a few millimeters to several centimeters in diameter. Their color is bright red to blue, depending on the degree of oxygenation of the blood. In the skin these lesions are known as "birthmarks," "port wine stains," "ruby spots," and so on. The only disability is cosmetic disfiguration.

Juvenile hemangiomas, also called **strawberry type,** are found on the skin of newborns. They grow rapidly in the first few months of life, begin to fade at 1 to 3 years of age, and completely regress in the majority of cases (about 80%) by about 5 years. Histologically, the juvenile hemangioma is composed of packed masses of capillaries separated by a connective tissue stroma. The endothelium-lined channels are usually filled with blood. The growths are not malignant and they do not invade or metastasize.

Cavernous hemangioma is a term reserved for lesions consisting of large vascular channels, frequently interspersed with small, capillary-type vessels. Grossly, the lesion is a red-blue, soft, spongy mass, with a diameter of up to several centimeters. Although the mass is well-defined histologically, it is not encapsulated. Large endothelium-lined, blood-containing spaces are separated by sparse connective tissue. Cavernous hemangiomas can undergo a variety of changes, including thrombosis and fibrosis, cystic cavitation, and intracystic hemorrhages.

These hemangiomas occur in the skin, the mucosal surfaces, and the viscera, including the spleen, liver, and pancreas. Occasionally they are found in the brain, where after long quiescent periods they may slowly enlarge and cause neurologic dysfunction.

Multiple hemangiomatous syndromes, in which a number of hemangiomas are found in a single tissue, are common. Two or more tissues may be involved, such as the skin and the nervous system or the spleen and the liver. Eponym enthusiasts have defined various combinations of sites. For example, Lindau–von Hippel disease is a rare entity in which cavernous hemangiomas occur within the cerebellum or brain stem and the retina. Sturge–Weber disease is characterized by a developmental disturbance of blood vessels in the brain and skin.

Glomangiomas are tumors of the **glomus body,** a convoluted arteriolar-venous anastomosis with a characteristic cellular wall containing a thick layer of cuboidal-epithelium–like cells. The glomus is a neuro-myoarterial receptor that is sensitive to temperature and regulates arteriolar flow. Glomus bodies are widely distributed in the skin but are more frequent in the distal portion of fingers and toes. This pattern is reflected in the distribution of glomangiomas, benign tumors that are characteristically exquisitely painful.

The lesions of glomangiomas are small, usually less than one centimeter in diameter, and many are smaller than a few millimeters. In the skin they are slightly elevated, rounded, red-blue, and firm. The two main components are branching vascular channels in a connective tissue stroma and aggregates or nests of the specialized glomus cells.

The **common cutaneous angioma,** frequently called a "birthmark" or a "port wine stain," is a malformation rather than a neoplasm. Closely related lesions are **plexiform** or **racemose angiomas, cirsoid aneurysms,** and **angiomatous dilatation** of vessels of the central nervous system and elsewhere.

MALIGNANT TUMORS OF BLOOD VESSELS

Malignant angioblastic neoplasms are rare, and only a few arise in preexisting benign angiomas. **Hemangiosarcoma** is marked by single or multiple masses of atypical, neoplastic endothelial cells. These begin as small, painless, sharply demarcated, red nodules and occur in either sex and at any age. The most common locations are skin, breast, and liver. Eventually, most hemangiosarcomas enlarge to become pale gray, fleshy masses without a capsule. Often these tumors undergo central necrosis, with softening and hemorrhage.

Hemangiosarcomas exhibit varying degrees of differentiation, ranging from those mainly composed of recognizable vascular elements with large, anaplastic endothelial cells to undifferentiated tumors with few recognizable blood channels. The latter display frequent mitoses, pleomorphism, and giant cells, and tend to be more malignant. These sarcomas are often difficult to distinguish from other connective tissue sarcomas.

Angiosarcomas of the liver are of special interest because of their association with two known environmental carcinogens: arsenic, which is a component of pesticides, and vinyl chloride, which is used in the production of plastics. Moreover, hepatic angiosarcoma has been associated with the use of Thorotrast (thorium dioxide), a radioactive contrast medium used by radiologists prior to 1950, which is engulfed by the macrophages of the liver sinusoids.

Hemangiopericytoma is a rare, malignant neoplasm presumably arising from pericytes, the smooth muscle

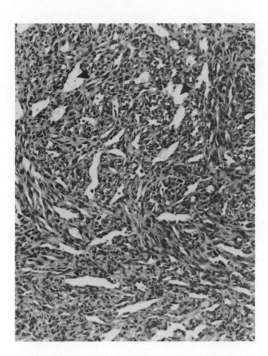

Figure 10-24. Kaposi's sarcoma, showing the characteristic sarcomatous features. Spaces lined with endothelium are evident *(arrows).*

cells that are external to the walls of capillaries and arterioles. These tumors are small and consist of capillary-like channels surrounded by (and frequently enclosed within) nests and masses of round to spindle-shaped cells. The tumor cell type is identified by a characteristic investment of basement membrane, similar to that of its normal counterpart.

Hemangiopericytomas can occur anywhere but are most frequently encountered in the retroperitoneum and lower extremities. They are highly malignant and typically metastasize to lungs, bone, liver, and lymph nodes.

Kaposi's sarcoma was first described as a sporadic tumor that begins as painful purple or brown nodules in the skin that vary from 1 mm to 1 cm in diameter. The tumors occur most often on the hands or feet, but may appear anywhere. The incidence was originally noted to be 10 times higher in men than in women and to occur in the sixth and seventh decades of life. **The disease has now appeared in epidemic form in association with AIDS.**

The histologic appearance of Kaposi's sarcoma shows wide variations. One form, which resembles a simple hemangioma, is characterized by tightly packed clusters of capillaries and scattered hemosiderin-laden macrophages (Fig. 10-24). In other forms of the tumor the lesions are highly cellular and the vascular spaces are less prominent. Such lesions may be difficult to distinguish from fibrosarcomas.

TUMORS OF THE LYMPHATIC SYSTEM

Many histologic and clinical variants of local enlargements of the lymphatics have been described. It is difficult to distinguish among anomalies, proliferations due to stasis, and true neoplasms. In general, the lesions are distinguished by their size and location. The spaces may be small, as in **capillary lymphangiomas,** or large and dilated, as in **cystic or cavernous** lesions. Lymphangiomatous lesions can arise at almost any site, including the skin, mediastinum, retroperitoneum, spleen, and other locations.

Cystic lymphangiomas (or cavernous lymphangiomas) occur most often in the neck and axilla, more rarely in the mediastinum, and occasionally in the retroperitoneum. They may reach a large size—10 to 15 cm in diameter or more. These masses may fill the axilla or distort structures of the neck. The lesions are soft, spongy, and pink, and watery fluid exudes from their cut surfaces. They are composed of endothelium-lined spaces that contain a protein-rich fluid. These spaces are distinguished from blood vessels by their lack of red and white blood cells. An abundance of irregularly distributed smooth muscle and connective tissue cells may be present. These tumors may surround and compress important structures of the neck or mediastinum, thereby causing serious functional problems.

Capillary lymphangiomas, sometimes called "simple lymphangiomas," are usually small, circumscribed, grayish pink, fleshy nodules, which can be single or multiple. They are subcutaneous and usually found in the skin of face, lips, chest, genitalia, or extremities. They are composed of variably sized, thin-walled, endothelium-lined spaces that contain lymph, occasional leukocytes, and, rarely, red blood cells.

11

THE HEART

DONALD B. HACKEL AND ROBERT B. JENNINGS

HEART FAILURE

A common result of various cardiac diseases is heart failure, which is the inability of the heart to pump blood at a rate that is adequate for the body's needs. The functional capacity of the heart to do work can be assessed clinically in a number of ways. For example, one can measure the increased pressure in the venous circulation caused by the heart's inability to propel all of the blood returned to it by the veins. This situation produces the clinical picture of **backward heart failure**.

One can also measure the ability of the heart to propel blood forward. For example, cardiac stroke volume may be decreased, a defect which results in so-called **forward heart failure. Starling's law of the heart states that the stroke volume of the heart is a function of the diastolic fiber length, and that within certain limits, the heart will pump whatever volume of blood is brought to it from the venous circulation.** Thus, cardiac muscle contracts more forcefully when stretched, and an increasing preload (as indicated by elevated end-diastolic ventricular volume) provides a reserve mechanism to augment the performance of the heart.

EFFECTS

The effects of heart failure are seen in all the organs of the body. They become congested and edematous, and show changes of acute and chronic anoxia. A patient who has been in "left-sided heart failure" for a prolonged period will show pulmonary passive congestion, edema, and fibrotic thickening of the alveolar septa. The alveoli contain many hemosiderin-filled macrophages from the phagocytosis of hemoglobin released from red blood cells that have leaked into the alveoli. The edema may be massive, with alveoli being "drowned" in a transudate. Fibrosis results from chronic anoxia, which causes parenchymal damage and subsequent repair. In earlier and more acute episodes of the same process, the findings may consist mainly of massive edema of the lungs (Fig. 11-1) together with acute vascular congestion. The liver of a patient who has had "right-sided heart failure" displays marked congestion. Distended central vein areas stand out as dark red foci against the yellow of the cells in the periphery of the lobule, giving the liver a gross appearance that has been compared to the cut surface of a nutmeg (hence the term "nutmeg liver") (Fig. 11-2).

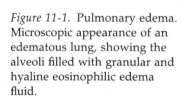

Figure 11-1. Pulmonary edema. Microscopic appearance of an edematous lung, showing the alveoli filled with granular and hyaline eosinophilic edema fluid.

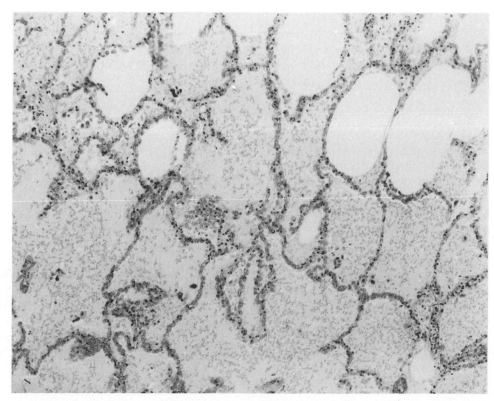

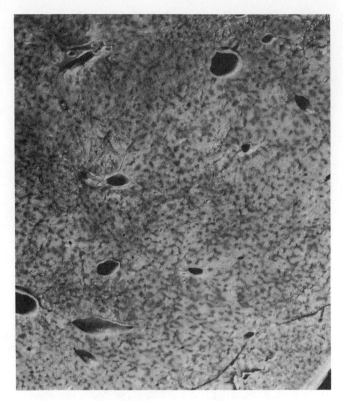

Figure 11-2. Chronic passive congestion of the liver. The gross appearance of the surface of the liver in a patient with congestive heart failure, showing severe passive congestion, with engorged central veins standing out as darker zones ("nutmeg" appearance).

In heart failure the changes in heart are nonspecific. Conspicuous dilatation of the chambers and hypertrophy of the cardiac muscle are usual.

CAUSES

Almost anything that causes the heart to increase its workload for a prolonged period of time or produces anatomical damage, making it more difficult for the heart to function, may eventuate in myocardial failure. The most important of these conditions include:

Congenital heart disease
Ischemic heart disease
Rheumatic heart disease and other "autoimmune" diseases, including
    Lupus erythematosus
    Rheumatoid arthritis
    Scleroderma
Hypertensive heart disease

Inflammatory diseases of the heart
Nutritional, endocrine, and metabolic diseases, including
    Thyrotoxicosis
    Myxedema
    Beriberi
    Carcinoid syndrome
    Storage diseases (lipid, carbohydrate)
    Amyloidosis
Cardiomyopathy

The most common type of heart disease in this list by far is ischemic heart disease, accounting for more than 80% of deaths due to heart disease. Between 1% and 3% of deaths are due to hypertensive heart disease, about 1% are due to rheumatic heart disease, and the remaining types account for less than 1% each.

FACTORS IN THE PRODUCTION OF CONGESTIVE HEART FAILURE

The molecular mechanisms of heart failure remain unknown. However, in the hearts of patients in congestive heart failure there are some changes that may be significant, including a decrease in the beta-adrenergic receptor sites in the myocardium. It has also been demonstrated that the failing heart contains isozymes of myosin with less than normal ATPase activity. Some studies of experimental heart failure have demonstrated decreases in the capacity of the sarcoplasmic reticulum to transport Ca^{2+} (Fig. 11-3).

CONGENITAL HEART DISEASE

INCIDENCE

The incidence of congenital heart disease is usually cited as being between 0.3% and 1% of all live births. A range derived from several sources provides the following figures:

Ventricular septal defect, 25% to 30%
Atrial septal defect, 10% to 15%
Patent ductus arteriosus, 10% to 20%
Tetralogy of Fallot, 6% to 15%
Pulmonic stenosis, 5% to 7%
Coarctation of the aorta, 5% to 7%
Aortic stenosis, 4% to 6%
Complete transposition of the great arteries, 4% to 10%
Truncus arteriosus, 2%
Tricuspid atresia, 1%

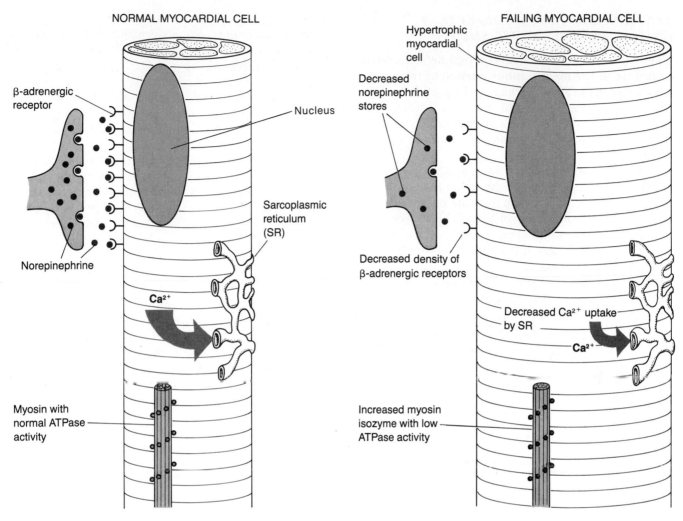

NORMAL MYOCARDIAL CELL

β-adrenergic receptor

Norepinephrine

Nucleus

Sarcoplasmic reticulum (SR)

Ca²⁺

Myosin with normal ATPase activity

FAILING MYOCARDIAL CELL

Hypertrophic myocardial cell

Decreased norepinephrine stores

Decreased density of β-adrenergic receptors

Decreased Ca²⁺ uptake by SR

Ca²⁺

Increased myosin isozyme with low ATPase activity

Figure 11-3. Biochemical characteristics of congestive heart failure.

ETIOLOGY

Whether congenital cardiac defects are genetic or acquired cannot usually be determined. The best evidence for a nongenetic intrauterine influence on the occurrence of congenital cardiac defects relates to maternal infection with rubella virus during the first trimester, especially during the first 4 weeks of gestation. Similarly, thalidomide ingestion early in pregnancy results in a variety of severe congenital lesions, including congenital heart defects in a small number of patients.

CLASSIFICATION

Table 11-1 presents a classification scheme for congenital heart disease.

Table 11-1   Classification of Congenital Heart Disease

Initial Left to Right Shunt

Ventricular septal defect
Atrial septal defect
Patent ductus arteriosus
Persistent truncus arteriosus
Anomalous pulmonary venous drainage

Right to Left Shunt

Tetralogy of Fallot

No Shunt

Complete transposition of the great vessels
Coarctation of the aorta
Pulmonary stenosis
Aortic stenosis
Coronary artery origin from pulmonary artery
Ebstein's malformation
Complete heart block
Endocardial fibroelastosis

VENTRICULAR SEPTAL DEFECTS (INITIAL LEFT-TO-RIGHT SHUNT)

The most common ventricular septal defect is related to failure of the membranous portion of the ventricular septum to form in whole or in part. In addition, there may be defects in the muscular portion of the ventricular septum; these are more common in the anterior region but can occur anywhere in the muscular septum.

Ventricular septal defects vary, and may occur as a small hole in the region of the membranous septum, large defects involving more than the membranous region (perimembranous defects), or complete absence of the muscular septum (leaving a single ventricle).

A small defect may have little functional significance and may actually close spontaneously as the child matures. In larger defects there is an initial left-to-right shunt that produces an increased pulmonary blood flow, eventually resulting in pulmonary arteriolar thickening and increased pulmonary vascular resistance. This resistance may be so great that the direction of the shunt flow is reversed, and goes from right to left **(Eisenmenger's complex).** A patient with this condition displays a late onset of cyanosis (ie., tardive cyanosis).

Complications of ventricular septal defects include heart failure, ventricular hypertrophy, pulmonary hypertension (with reversal of shunt flow and resulting cyanosis), infective endocarditis, paradoxical emboli, brain abscesses, and prolapse of an aortic valve cusp (with resulting aortic valve insufficiency).

ATRIAL SEPTAL DEFECTS

The foramen ovale, an opening in the embryologic atrial septum, persists after birth until it is sealed off by the fusion of the septum primum and septum secundum, after which it is termed "fossa ovalis." However, it remains patent in over 25% of all adults (a "probe-patent foramen ovale"), although it does not normally function as a shunt after birth. The higher pressure in the left atrium normally keeps the valve-like mechanism of the foramen closed.

There are four sites at which the atrial septum may be defective (Fig. 11-4A–E). The first is the upper portion above the fossa ovalis near the entry of the superior vena cava. This uncommon defect, known as a **sinus venosus defect,** occurs in only about 5% of atrial septal defects (Fig. 11-4C). The second site is the middle portion, where the defect is called an **atrial septal defect, ostium secundum type** (Fig 11-4B). **This is by far the most common of the four sites, accounting for about 90% of atrial septal defects.** It varies in size, ranging from a patent foramen ovale (which is recog-

nizable as patent only if tested with a probe) to a large defect of the entire fossa ovalis region. When the defect is only probe patent (25% of adult hearts), it is not normally functional; however, it may become a real shunt if circumstances elevate the right atrial pressure, as can occur with recurrent pulmonary thromboemboli. If this situation develops, a right-to-left shunt will be produced, and particles (e.g., thromboemboli) from the right-sided circulation will pass directly into the systemic circulation. These **paradoxical emboli** can produce infarcts in many parts of the body, most commonly in the brain, heart, spleen, intestines, kidneys and legs. If the atrial septal defect is larger, it may result in an increase in blood flow on the right side of the heart sufficient to dilate and hypertrophy the right atrium and right ventricle.

A variant of the ostium secundum type of atrial septal defect is known as **Lutembacher's syndrome,** an anomaly defined as the combination of mitral stenosis (either congenital or as a result of rheumatic fever) and an ostium secundum type of atrial septal defect.

The third defect site is the region adjacent to the endocardial cushion. This anomaly is termed **atrial septal defect, ostium primum type** (Fig. 11-4D). This condition is also rare, and accounts for about 7% of all atrial septal defects. There are usually clefts in the anterior leaflet of the mitral valve and the septal leaflet of the tricuspid valve, which may be accompanied by an associated defect in the adjacent interventricular septum. The fully developed combined defect is called a **persistent common atrioventricular canal** (also an "endocardial cushion defect", an "atrioventricular septal defect", or an "atrioventricularis communis").

The fourth type of atrial septal defect is the **coronary sinus** type. This rare abnormality is situated in the posteroinferior part of the interatrial septum at the site of the coronary sinus ostium, and is associated with a persistent left superior vena cava, which drains into the roof of the left atrium.

Complications from atrial septal defects include heart failure, right ventricular hypertrophy, pulmonary vascular sclerosis, cyanosis (if shunt reverses from right to left), paradoxical emboli, and brain abscess.

PATENT DUCTUS ARTERIOSUS

Early in its development the embryo supposedly recapitulates an ancestral evolutionary stage, with six aortic arches connecting the ventral and dorsal aortas as part of the branchial cleft system (Fig. 11-5).

The persistence of a patent ductus arteriosus is one of the most common congenital cardiac defects. When present as an isolated anomaly, (rather than as a component of a group of associated anomalies) it can be

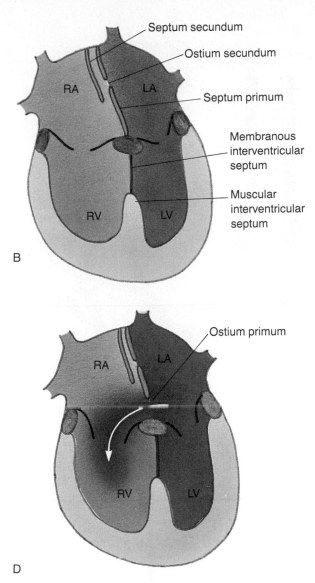

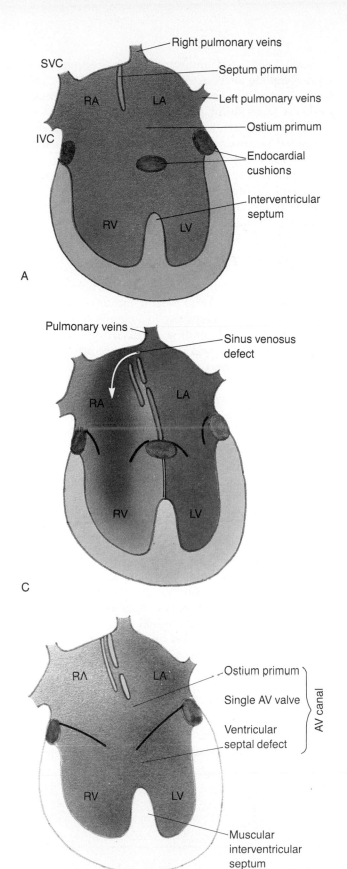

A

- SVC
- RA
- IVC
- LA
- RV
- LV
- Right pulmonary veins
- Septum primum
- Left pulmonary veins
- Ostium primum
- Endocardial cushions
- Interventricular septum

B

- RA
- LA
- RV
- LV
- Septum secundum
- Ostium secundum
- Septum primum
- Membranous interventricular septum
- Muscular interventricular septum

C

- Pulmonary veins
- Sinus venosus defect
- RA
- LA
- RV
- LV

D

- RA
- LA
- RV
- LV
- Ostium primum

E

- RA
- LA
- RV
- LV
- Ostium primum
- Single AV valve
- Ventricular septal defect
- AV canal
- Muscular interventricular septum

Figure 11-4. Pathogenesis of ventricular and atrial septal defects. (*A*) The common atrial chamber is being separated into the right and left atria (*RA* and *LA*) by the septum primum. Because the septum primum has not yet joined the endocardial cushion material, there is an open ostium primum. The ventricular cavity is being divided by a muscular interventricular septum into right and left chambers (*RV* and *LV*). *SVC*, superior vena cava; *IVC*, inferior vena cava. (*B*) The septum primum has joined the endocardial cushions, but at the same time has developed an opening in its mid-portion (the ostium secundum). This opening is partly overlain by the septum secundum, which has now grown down to cover the foramen ovale in part. Simultaneously, the membranous septum joins the muscular interventricular septum to the base of the heart, completely separating the ventricles. (*C*) The sinus venosus type of atrial septal defect is located in the most cephalad region and is adjacent to the inflow of the right pulmonary veins, which thus tend to open into the right atrium. (*D*) The ostium primum defect occurs just above the valve ring, sometimes in the presence of an intact valve ring. It may also, in conjunction with a defect of the valve ring and ventricular septum, form an atrioventricular canal, as shown in *E*. This common opening allows free communication between atria and ventricles.

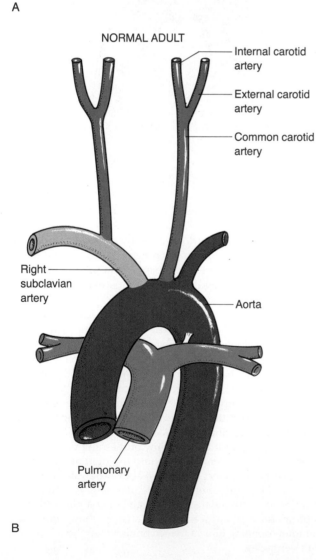

A

B

PRIMITIVE AORTIC ARCHES

Right   Left

1
2
3
4
5
6

NORMAL ADULT

Internal carotid
artery

External carotid
artery

Common carotid
artery

Right
subclavian
artery

Aorta

Pulmonary
artery

clinically diagnosed and surgically corrected, usually with complete success. A small shunt has little long-term effect on the heart and often will close spontaneously. A large shunt, on the other hand, produces a strain on the heart because of the markedly increased workload required to pump the augmented cardiac output. As a consequence, cardiac hypertrophy, a dilated pulmonary artery (with pulmonary hypertension), and eventual heart failure may supervene. Pulmonary hypertension may develop, with a subsequent reversal of shunt flow to a right-to-left direction.

PERSISTENT TRUNCUS ARTERIOSUS

There are several variants of persistent truncus arteriosus. Type 1, which is the most common, consists of a common trunk that gives rise to a common pulmonary artery and to the ascending aorta. In type 2 truncus arteriosus, the right and left pulmonary arteries originate from a common site in the posterior midline of the truncus. In type 3 the separate pulmonary arteries originate laterally from the common trunk. There are other more rare variants (sometimes called type 4) in which there is no pulmonary trunk, and in which the pulmonary circulation is supplied by enlarged bronchial arteries.

In addition to heart failure, ventricular hypertrophy, and pulmonary vascular sclerosis, these patients may exhibit stenosis or insufficiency of the truncus valve.

ANOMALOUS PULMONARY VEIN DRAINAGE

Total anomalous pulmonary vein drainage may occur as an isolated defect, or it may be part of the **asplenia syndrome** (splenic agenesis, congenital heart defects, and situs inversus of abdominal organs). Most commonly the pulmonary veins drain into a common pulmonary venous chamber, and then via a persistent left superior vena cava (the persistent left precardinal vein), into the innominate vein or into the right superior vena cava. A second route for common pulmonary vein drainage is into the coronary sinus.

Heart failure, severe anoxemia, and pulmonary venous obstruction result from this anomaly.

Figure 11-5. Derivatives of the aortic arches. (*A*) Complete primitive aortic arch system. (*B*) In the normal adult the left fourth aortic arch is preserved as the arch of the adult aorta and the left sixth arch is represented by the pulmonary artery and ductus arteriosus.

TETRALOGY OF FALLOT (RIGHT-TO-LEFT SHUNT)

The four anatomic changes that define the tetralogy of Fallot are pulmonary stenosis, ventricular septal defect, dextroposition of the aorta so that it overrides the ventricular septal defect, and right ventricular hypertrophy (Fig. 11-6).

Tetralogy of Fallot is the most common type of cyanotic congenital heart disease in older children and adults, and is usually accompanied by clubbing of the fingers. Pulmonary stenosis is usually due to subpulmonary muscular hypertrophy, with an enlarged infundibular muscle obstructing blood flow into the pulmonary artery. However, in about one-third of these hearts the valve itself is the main cause of the stenosis. The aortic arch is on the right side in about 25% of the cases of tetralogy of Fallot. Patency of the ductus arteriosus is protective, since it provides a source of blood to the otherwise deprived pulmonary vascular bed. Increasing cyanosis and shortness of breath are often signs that this beneficial shunt has spontaneously closed.

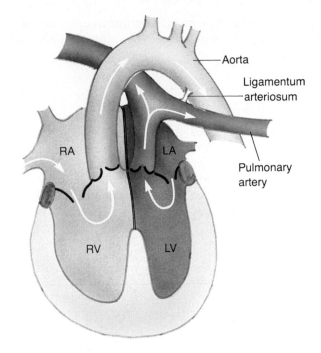

Figure 11-7. Complete transposition of great arteries, regular type. The aorta is anterior to, and to the right of, the pulmonary artery ("D-transposition") and arises from the right ventricle. Since there are no interatrial or interventricular connections and no patent ductus arteriosus, this anomaly is incompatible with life.

Uncorrected tetralogy of Fallot is a fatal disorder, and leads to heart failure, polycythemia, increased blood coagulability, and a thrombotic tendency, which leads to cerebral infarction, infective endocarditis, and brain abscess.

TRANSPOSITION OF THE GREAT ARTERIES (NO SHUNT PRESENT)

The aorta normally curves to the right of the pulmonary artery in its approach to the heart and curves behind the pulmonary artery to reach its cardiac source in a posterior position. In transposition of the great arteries, the aorta is anterior to the pulmonary artery and to its right ("d"-transposition) all the way to its origin (Fig. 11-7). This contrasts with **congenitally corrected transposition,** in which the aorta is anterior to, but passes to the left of, the pulmonary artery ("l"-transposition). This latter anomaly is "corrected" in the sense that there is an inversion of the ventricles relative to the atria. Although the aorta may be anterior to the pulmonary artery and connects with the anatomic right ventricle (which is in the position of the usual left ventricle, and receives the pulmonary venous blood), it still receives the oxygenated blood that is appropriate for it.

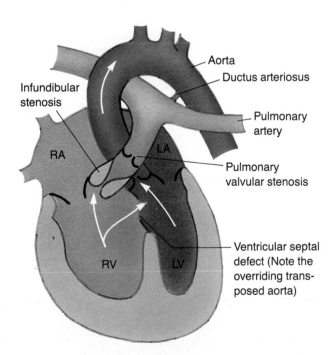

Figure 11-6. Tetralogy of Fallot. Note the pulmonary stenosis, which is due to infundibular hypertrophy as well as to pulmonary valvular stenosis. The ventricular septal defect involves the membranous septum region. Dextroposition of the aorta and right ventricular hypertrophy are shown. Because of the pulmonary obstruction the shunt is from right to left, and the patient is cyanotic.

It is therefore not functionally abnormal at all unless—as is usually the case—there are other complicating anomalies present.

COARCTATION OF THE AORTA

In the developing fetus, the segment of the aorta distal to the origin of the left subclavian artery and proximal to the ductus arteriosus tends to be narrower than the aorta distal to the ductus arteriosus (see Fig. 11-5). If this narrow segment of aorta is so small after birth that it produces a gradient of blood pressure between its

PREDUCTAL COARCTATION OF AORTA

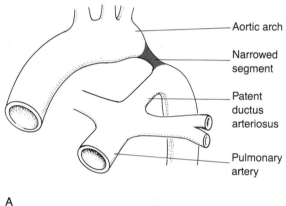

A

POSTDUCTAL COARCTATION OF AORTA

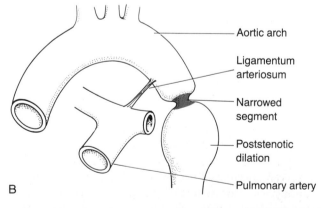

B

Figure 11-8. Coarctation of the aorta. (*A*) Preductal ("infantile") type, showing elongated narrow segment ("tubular hypoplasia") proximal to the widely patent ductus arteriosus. (*B*) Postductal ("adult") type, showing narrowed segment occurring just at or distal to the ductus, which is usually, but not always, closed. A small postcoarctation aneurysm is shown.

proximal and distal segments, it is referred to as a **tubular hypoplastic aorta** or as a **coarctation of the aorta** (Fig. 11-8). A coarctation with this elongated, narrowed segment in the proximal location between the left subclavian artery and the ductus is termed an **infantile (tubular) coarctation,** because this type of defect usually does not permit survival beyond infancy (Fig. 11-8A). More commonly, however, the coarctation is abrupt, and occurs at or immediately distal to the origin of the ductus arteriosus from the aorta (true coarctation). The ductus is usually closed when this so-called **adult coarctation** is present (Fig. 11-8B).

The pressure gradient produced by the coarctation causes hypertension and, occasionally, aortic dilatation proximal to the narrowed focus. The blood pressure measured in the arm is higher than that measured in the leg. Collateral vessels enlarge in an attempt to bridge the gap between the upper and lower aortic segments. Radiologic examination of the chest shows **notching of the inner surfaces of the ribs** due to pressure from the markedly dilated intercostal arteries. Other cardiovascular developmental abnormalities associated with coarctation of the aorta including bicuspid aortic valves and, in the brain, berry aneurysms of the circle of Willis. Renal hepatic cysts are also frequently present.

The prognosis of uncorrected severe coarctation of the aorta is dismal. Complications include heart failure, rupture of a dissecting aneurysm (secondary to cystic medial necrosis of the aorta proximal or distal to the coarctation), infective endarteritis at the point of narrowing or at the site of jet stream impingement on the wall immediately distal to the narrowing, cerebral hemorrhage, and stenosis or infective endocarditis of a bicuspid aortic valve.

PULMONARY STENOSIS (ISOLATED OR "PURE")

Isolated pulmonary stenosis usually involves the valve cusps, which are fused to form an inverted funnel type of constriction. Patients with isolated pulmonary stenosis have clubbing of the fingers and cyanosis, and may suffer from heart failure, right ventricular hypertrophy and dilatation, hypertrophy of the right atrium, patent foramen ovale with right-to-left shunt, polycythemia, and endocardial fibroelastosis.

AORTIC STENOSIS

Three types of aortic stenosis are recognized: valvular, subvalvular, and supravalvular. The most common type, **subvalvular aortic stenosis,** is caused by the abnormal development of a band of subvalvular fibroelastic tissue or a muscular ridge.

Congenital valvular aortic stenosis is usually due to the fusion of two of the three semilunar cusps (the right coronary cusp with the adjacent two cusps), with a resulting bicuspid valve that tends to become calcified over the years. Severe aortic valvular stenosis or atresia may be the main defect underlying the occurrence of the **hypoplastic left heart syndrome,** in which there is hypoplasia of the ascending aorta, the left ventricle, and the mitral valve.

Congenital aortic stenosis is characterized by left ventricular hypertrophy, low blood pressure and consequent fainting spells, endocardial fibroelastosis, and sudden death.

EBSTEIN'S MALFORMATION

In Ebstein's malformation one or more of the tricuspid valve leaflets is abnormal, adhering to the right ventricular wall for a variable distance below the right atrioventricular annulus. There is a downward displacement of the effective tricuspid valve orifice into the ventricle. The ventricle is thus divided by the displaced tricuspid valve into two separate parts: the atrialized ventricle (proximal ventricle) and the functional right ventricle (distal ventricle). Conspicuous dilatation of the functional ventricle occurs in about two-thirds of cases. As a result, the right ventricle is often unable to pump the blood efficiently through the pulmonary arteries. There is also insufficiency of the tricuspid valve, the degree of which depends on the severity and configuration of the defective leaflets.

Ebstein's malformation leads to heart failure, massive right ventricular dilatation, arrhythmias with palpitations and tachycardia, and sudden death.

ENDOCARDIAL FIBROELASTOSIS

Endocardial fibroelastosis occurs in association with other congenital anomalies, especially aortic atresia and coarctation of the aorta, and in patients with an anomalous origin of a coronary artery from the pulmonary artery. However, the isolated occurrence of endocardial fibroelastosis is not uncommon. Hearts showing this condition are dilated and large, weighing two to four times what is expected for the age. The endocardium is porcelain-like, thickened, grayish-white and opaque. The left ventricle is the most commonly involved chamber, although the right ventricle, the left atrium and the mitral and aortic valves occasionally become thickened. The valves may exhibit fusion of their leaflets, and mitral insufficiency is often present.

Patients with isolated fibroelastosis develop cardiac hypertrophy and succumb to heart failure.

ISCHEMIC HEART DISEASE

MANIFESTATIONS

Ischemic heart disease is by far the most common and most important type of heart disease in the United States and other industrialized lands (e.g., Scandinavia, England, Germany). By contrast it is rare in parts of the world that are less well developed, such as, India, Africa, and China. The term, **ischemic heart disease** is applied to **persistent clinical signs and symptoms of myocardial ischemia, when the supply of oxygen in the coronary arterial blood is inadequate to provide for the oxygen demands of the heart.** The major cause of ischemic heart disease is **coronary atherosclerosis,** a condition that narrows the coronary arterial lumen and limits the ability of these arteries to supply blood to the heart.

ANGINA PECTORIS

A typical patient with angina pectoris has recurrent episodes of chest pain, usually brought on by increased physical activity or emotional excitement, although attacks of some types of angina pectoris may also originate during rest or sleep. The pain is of limited duration (1 to 15 minutes) and is usually relieved by decreasing the activity or by taking sublingual nitroglycerine.

MYOCARDIAL INFARCT

A **myocardial infarct** is another important manifestation of ischemic heart disease. **It is defined as a focus of myocardial necrosis having a diameter of more than 2.5 cm. and caused by an insufficient oxygen supply.**

SUDDEN DEATH

It is not uncommon for the initial manifestation of ischemic heart disease to be an unexpected arrhythmia that may result in sudden death. The arrhythmia is most commonly ventricular fibrillation, an irregularity that can often be converted to a normal rhythm by controlled electrical shock, provided that treatment is given quickly. **By far the most common underlying condition of sudden death is coronary atherosclerosis.**

ETIOLOGY

Ischemic heart disease is caused by an imbalance between the oxygen demands of the myocardium and the supply of oxygenated blood (Table 11-2). An understanding of this ratio of supply/demand is important to understanding the various aberrations that can lead to myocardial infarction.

Conditions Influencing the Supply of Blood

ATHEROSCLEROSIS AND THROMBOSIS Atherosclerosis is the most common cause of ischemic heart disease (Fig. 11-9). Its nature and pathogenesis are described in detail in Chapter 10. **The reduction in coronary blood flow caused by atherosclerosis becomes critical when the luminal cross sectional area is decreased by 90% or more. An acute ischemic event is precipitated by the sudden thrombotic occlusion of the narrowed lumen.** The stimulus for this sudden occlusion may be the rupture of an atheromatous plaque and exposure of the underlying collagen, a material which is thrombogenic.

THROMBOEMBOLI Thromboembolism is a rare cause of myocardial infarction and the embolus is usually traced to a cardiac source. For example, it occurs in patients with atrial fibrillation and old rheumatic mitral valve disease who have mural thrombi in the left atrial appendage (Fig. 11-10). Thromboembolism is seen in patients with mural thrombi in the left ventricle secondary to infarction, aneurysm, or conges-

tive cardiomyopathy. The most common sources of thromboembolism from the heart are valvular vegetations, caused either by infectious endocarditis or by nonbacterial thrombotic endocarditis.

CORONARY ARTERY SPASM Myocardial infarction occurs in patients whose coronary arteries are apparently normal, as determined by angiography. In a few of these cases coronary artery spasm has been demonstrated by angiography.

COLLATERAL BLOOD VESSELS The normal coronary arteries function essentially as end-arteries. However, most normal hearts have some intercoronary anastomoses, which may be as large as 40 μm in diameter. Hearts that are chronically ischemic because of coronary atherosclerosis develop extensive collateral connections that protect the myocardium from the effects of acute complete occlusion.

BLOOD PRESSURE, CARDIAC OUTPUT, AND HEART RATE A normal heart accommodates large changes in blood pressure, cardiac output, and heart rate. When the ability of the coronary arteries to dilate is limited by coronary artery sclerosis, however, an increase in heart rate or a sudden decrease in blood pressure or cardiac output may decrease the blood flow through a previously narrowed artery. The region perfused by this artery becomes ischemic and eventually necrotic.

ANEMIA Anemia is a common cause of decreased oxygen supply to the myocardium. Although a heart with normal circulation can survive severe anemia, in the presence of coronary atherosclerosis the capacity to increase coronary blood flow may be limited, and cardiac necrosis may result. An additional problem in patients with anemia is the added burden on the heart of an increased workload, secondary to the increased cardiac output needed to supply the other organs with adequate oxygen.

INCREASED OXYGEN DEMAND

Anything that increases the workload of the heart also increases its need for oxygen. Conditions that **increase the blood pressure or the cardiac output,** such as exercise or pregnancy, result in an increased oxygen demand by the myocardium, and so contribute to angina pectoris or myocardial infarction. Disorders that fall into this category include valvular disease (mitral or aortic insufficiency, or aortic stenosis), infection, and conditions such as hypertension, coarctation of the aorta, idiopathic hypertrophic subaortic stenosis, and luetic aortitis (which results in aortic valve insufficiency). The increased metabolic rate and tachycardia in patients with **hyperthyroidism** are accompanied by an increase in oxygen demand, as well as increase in

---

Table 11-2   Causes of Ischemic Heart Disease

Decreased supply of oxygen
  Conditions that influence the supply of blood
    Atherosclerosis and thrombosis
    Thromboemboli
    Coronary artery spasm
    Collateral blood vessels
    Blood pressure, cardiac output, and heart rate
    Miscellaneous: arteritis (e.g., periarteritis nodosa), dissecting
      aneurysm, luetic aortitis, anomalous origin of coronary
      artery, muscular bridging of coronary artery
  Conditions that influence the availability of oxygen in the blood
    Anemia
    Shift in hemoglobin-oxygen dissociation curve
    CO
    Cyanide
Increased oxygen demand (i.e., increased cardiac work)
  Hypertension
  Valvular stenosis of insufficiency
  Hyperthyroidism
  Fever
  Thiamine deficiency
  Catecholamines
Personality type

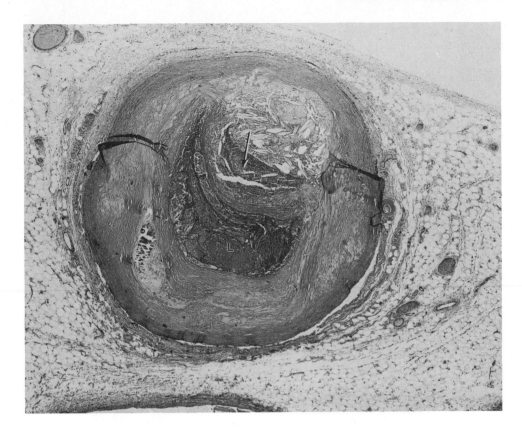

Figure 11-9. Coronary atherosclerosis. Cross section of an epicardial coronary artery showing marked atherosclerosis, with calcium deposits (*lower left, black*), cholesterol clefts (*clear, needlelike spaces, upper right*), hemorrhage (*arrow*) into an intimal plaque, and thrombotic occlusion of the lumen (*L*).

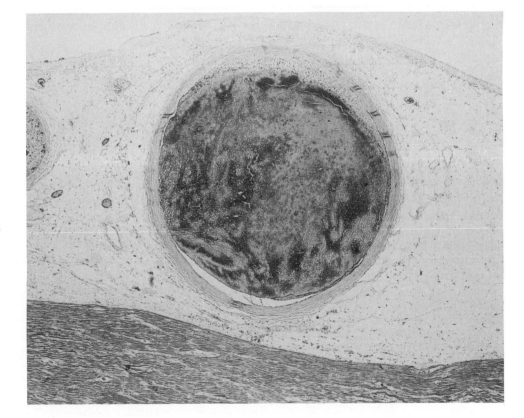

Figure 11-10. Thromboembolus in the left anterior descending coronary artery of a man who suffered from old rheumatic heart disease and who had mitral stenosis and a mural thrombus in the left atrial appendage.

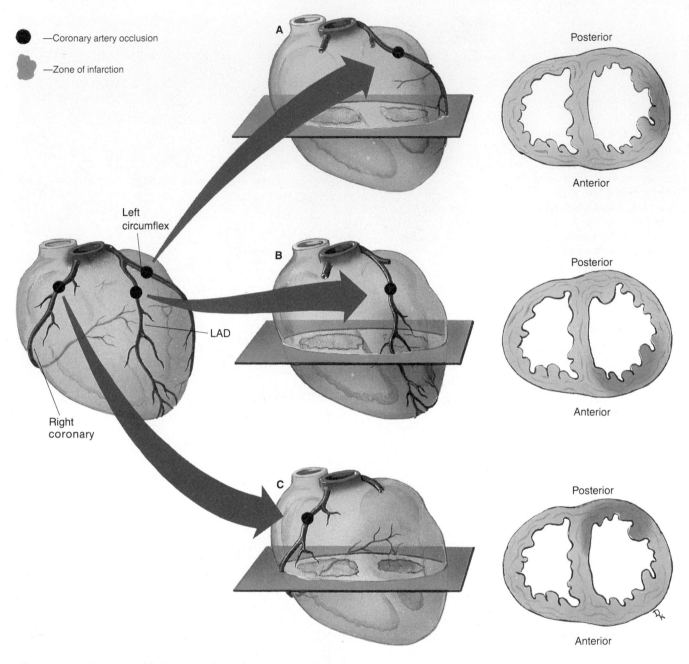

Figure 11-11. Position of left ventricular infarcts resulting from occlusion of each of the three main coronary arteries. (*A*) Posterolateral infarct, which follows an occlusion of the left circumflex artery and is present in the posterolateral wall. (*B*) Anterior infarct, which follows occlusion of the anterior descending branch (*LAD*) of the left coronary artery. The infarct is located in the anterior wall and adjacent two thirds of the septum, in the apical three quarters of the left ventricle. It involves the entire circumference of the wall near the apex. (*C*) Posterior ("inferior" or "diaphragmatic") infarct, which results from occlusion of the right coronary artery and involves the posterior wall, including the posterior third of the interventricular septum and the posterior papillary muscle in the basal half of the ventricle. Note the lateral displacement of the posterior papillary muscle caused by the expansion (i.e., stretching) of the infarct region of the left ventricle.

the workload of the heart, both of which contribute to myocardial ischemia. **Fever also produces an increase in the basal metabolic rate and an increase in cardiac output and heart rate.**

PERSONALITY TYPE

It has been reported that hard-driving, aggressive, time-conscious, executive-type individuals ("type A" personality) have a higher incidence of heart disease than do more easygoing, relaxed people ("type B" personality). However, this relationship is controversial, and some studies have shown no correlation between the two.

PATHOLOGY OF MYOCARDIAL INFARCTION

LOCATION OF INFARCTS

Transmural infarcts are usually located in the distribution of one of the three major coronary arteries (Fig. 11-11). An occlusion of the proximal portion of the right coronary artery results in an infarct of the posterior basal region of the left ventricle and the posterior third of the interventricular septum ("inferior" infarct). An occlusion of the left anterior descending coronary artery produces an infarct of the apical anterior and septal wall of the left ventricle. An occlusion of the left circumflex coronary artery—the least common site—results in the infarct of the lateral wall of the left ventricle.

Table 11-3 Differences Between Subendocardial and Transmural Infarcts

SUBENDOCARDIAL INFARCTS	TRANSMURAL INFARCTS
Multifocal	Unifocal
Patchy	Solid
Circumferential	In distribution of a specific coronary artery
Coronary thrombosis rare	Coronary thrombosis common
Often **result** from hypotension or shock	Often **cause** shock
No epicarditis	Epicarditis common
Do not form aneurysms	May result in aneurysm

Infarcts may involve predominantly the subendocardial portion of the myocardium, or they may be transmural. There are important differences between these two types of infarction (Table 11-3). The subendocardial (nontransmural) infarct is present in the inner one-third to one-half of the ventricle; it is commonly circumferential, so that it is not necessarily in the distribution of any one coronary artery. Coronary artery thrombosis is not usually a cause of subendocardial infarcts. They generally occur as a result of hypoperfusion of the heart in disorders such as aortic stenosis or hemorrhagic shock, or as a result of hypoperfusion during the course of cardiopulmonary bypass. In patients who die, transmural infarcts are more common than subendocardial infarcts.

Infarcts involve the left ventricle much more commonly and extensively than they do the right ventricle. This may be due partly to the greater workload imposed on the left ventricle and the greater thickness of the left ventricular wall. Thus, conditions that tend to increase the work of the right ventricle, such as pulmonary hypertension, are more likely to lead to an infarct of that ventricle.

PATHOLOGY OF INFARCTS

Macroscopically, an acute myocardial infarct is usually not identified less than 12 hours from its time of onset. By 24 hours an infarct can be recognized on the cut surface of the involved ventricle either by its pallor or by a reddish-blue color, the latter reflecting the congestion of blood vessels in the infarcted region. After 3 to 5 days the infarct is mottled and more sharply outlined, with a central pale, yellowish, necrotic region bordered by a hyperemic zone (Fig. 11-12). Occasionally, the infarcted region is hemorrhagic. By 2 to 3 weeks the infarcted region is usually depressed and soft, with a refractile, gelatinous appearance. Older infarcts are firm and have the pale gray appearance of scar tissue (Fig. 11-13).

The earliest microscopic evidence of an infarct is seen best by electron microscopy (Fig. 11-14). At first the myocyte shows some evidence of edema, with swelling of the sarcoplasmic reticulum and mitochondria, and loss of glycogen. After 30 to 60 minutes of ischemia the mitochondria contain amorphous matrix densities, the nucleus shows clumping and margination of chromatin, and there are some discontinuities in the sarcolemma of the myocyte. After 2 to 6 hours of ischemia the cells in the infarcted zone exhibit loss of lactic dehydrogenase, creatin kinase, and other enzymes. At

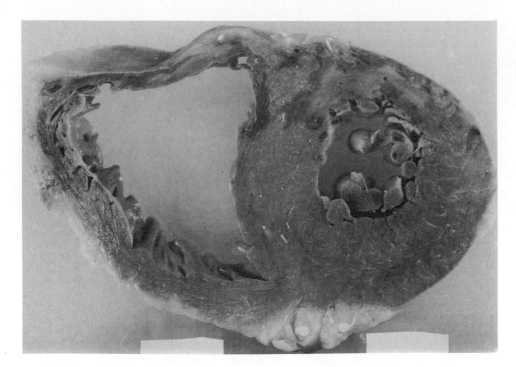

Figure 11-12. Cross section of the ventricles of a man who died 5 days after the onset of chest pain. The infarct is in the posterior and septal regions of both right and left ventricles, is mottled, and has a dark hemorrhagic border. The right coronary artery (*not shown*) was narrowed by severe atherosclerosis and was completely occluded by a recent thrombus. Note the "expansion" of the posterior left ventricular wall, which causes the position of the posterior papillary muscle to become more lateral.

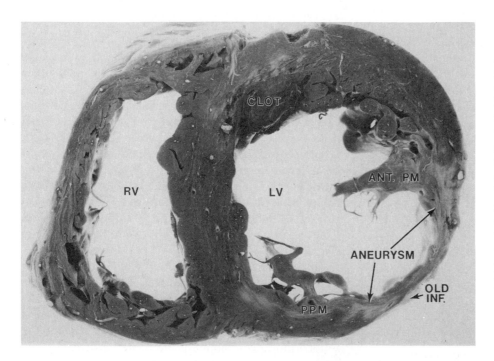

Figure 11-13. Healed myocardial infarct. Cross section of the ventricles of the heart from a man who had long-standing ischemic heart disease. The posterior and lateral left ventricular walls are replaced by scar tissue (*below*). This old transmural infarct (*old inf.*) is thinned and bulges to form an aneurysm. There is an old, patchy, nontransmural infarct in the anterior subendocardial left ventricle (*above*), which has an adherent mural thrombus (*clot*). *Ant. PM*, anterior papillary muscle; *PPM*, posterior papillary muscle.

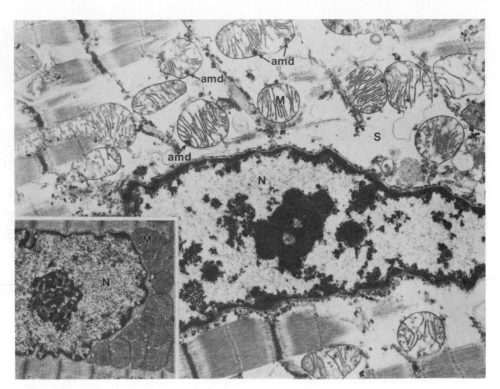

Figure 11-14. Ultrastructure of myocardial ischemia. Electron micrograph of an irreversibly injured myocyte from a dog heart subjected to 40 minutes of low-flow ischemia, induced by proximal occlusion of the circumflex branch of the left coronary artery. A nonischemic control myocyte from the same heart is shown in the insert (also compare Fig. 11-4). The affected myocyte is swollen and has abundant clear sarcoplasm (*S*). The mitochondria (*M*) also are swollen and contain amorphous matrix densities (*amd*), which are characteristic of lethal cell injury. The sarcolemma of this myocyte (*not shown*) exhibited small areas of disruption. The chromatin of the nucleus (*N*) is aggregated peripherally, in contrast to the uniformly distributed chromatin in normal tissue.

about the same time, the tissue potassium concentration decreases, "wavy fibers" can be seen, and contraction bands are demonstrated at the periphery of the infarct. Equivocal alterations in the staining characteristics of the necrotic cells include an increased eosinophilia (Fig. 11-15) and fuchsinophilia and an increase in nonglycogen material stained with the periodic acid-Schiff reaction.

After **1 to 2 days** coagulation necrosis (see Fig. 11-15) leads to an infiltrate of polymorphonuclear leukocytes, interstitial edema, and often hemorrhage. By **2 to 3 days** the muscle cells are more clearly necrotic, nuclei disappear, and striations become less prominent. There are more polymorphonuclear leukocytes, which begin to undergo karyorrhexis. By **5 to 7 days** the acute inflammatory leukocytic response has abated, so that few, if any, polymorphonuclear leukocytes are present. The infarcted region shows clearing of the dead muscle and inflammatory cells, and intercellular edema is prominent. New collagen formation is evident, lymphocytes and monocytes are present, and the number of fibroblasts and small capillaries is increased. This process begins at the periphery of the infarct and gradually extends toward the center. Collagen deposition proceeds, so that by **3 to 4 weeks** there is considerable fibrous tissue. Thereafter, debris is progressively removed and the scar becomes more solid and less cellular.

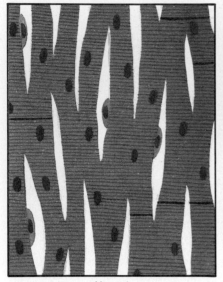
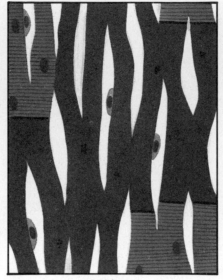
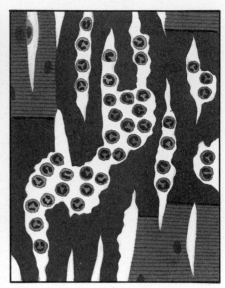

| Normal | 12-18 hours | 1 day |

Figure 11-15. Development of a myocardial infarct. (*A*) Normal myocardium. (*B*) After about 12 to 18 hours the infarcted myocardium shows eosinophilia (red staining) in sections of the heart stained with hematoxylin and eosin. (*C*) About 24 hours after onset of the infarct, polymorphonuclear neutrophils infiltrate around the necrotic myocytes.

CLINICAL FEATURES OF ACUTE MYOCARDIAL INFARCTION

The clinical diagnosis of acute myocardial infarction is based first on the clinical history. The onset may be sudden, with severe crushing pain that is usually substernal or precordial, but which may present as epigastric burning (simulating indigestion). The pain may extend into the jaw or down the inside of either arm. It is often accompanied by sweating, nausea, vomiting, and shortness of breath. About half of the cases of myocardial infarction are clinically silent—that is, they occur without any symptoms and are unrecognized by the patient. Such infarcts are later identified by electrocardiographic changes or at autopsy.

COMPLICATIONS OF MYOCARDIAL INFARCTION

ARRHYTHMIAS

Virtually all patients who have a myocardial infarct suffer from some form of cardiac arrhythmia, a com-

plication which accounts for about half of the deaths from coronary heart disease. Premature ventricular beats, sinus bradycardia, ventricular tachycardia, ventricular fibrillation, paroxysmal atrial tachycardia and partial or complete heart block occur. The heart block is usually transient, especially in patients with posterior infarction.

CARDIOGENIC SHOCK

Cardiogenic shock is most likely to occur when the infarct involves more than 40% of the left ventricle; the mortality rate in these cases is as high as 90%.

RUPTURE

Myocardial rupture may occur within the first 21 days of an acute myocardial infarction, and especially between the second and 10th days, when the infarcted wall is at its weakest. After this time the scar becomes progressively stronger, so that rupture becomes less likely. External rupture of the ventricle produces pericardial tamponade in about 10% of patients with acute myocardial infarction—more commonly in women and in patients with hypertension.

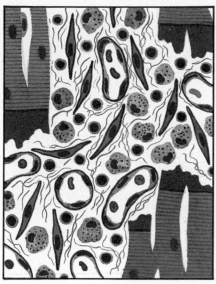
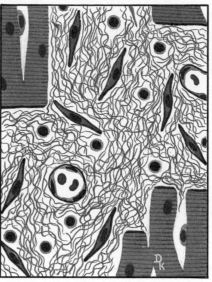

3 weeks   3 months

(*D*) After about 3 weeks the infarct contains granulation tissue with prominent capillaries, fibroblasts, lymphoid cells, and macrophages. The necrotic debris has been largely removed and a small amount of collagen has been laid down. (*E*) After 3 months or more the infarcted region has been replaced by scar tissue.

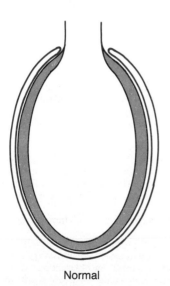
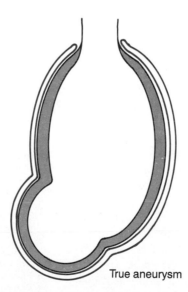
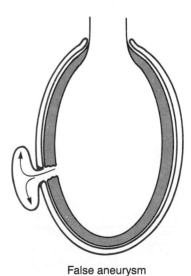

Normal   True aneurysm   False aneurysm

Figure 11-16. True and false aneurysms of the left ventricle. (*Left*) Normal heart. The left ventricular wall (*shaded*) is enclosed by a pericardial sac. (*Center*) True aneurysm shows an intact wall (*black*), which bulges outward. (*Right*) False aneurysm shows a ruptured infarct, which is walled off externally by adherent pericardium. Note that the mouth of the true aneurysm is wider than that of the false aneurysm.

ANEURYSM

Following an acute transmural myocardial infarct, the ventricular wall tends to bulge outward during systole in one-third of all patients. As the infarct matures, the collagenous scar tissue is susceptible to stretching. The occurrence of myocardial thinning and stretching in the region of an acute myocardial infarction is termed "infarct expansion". This is actually an early aneurysm; patients with this condition exhibit an increase in the incidence of myocardial rupture and have a poorer prognosis. Ventricular aneurysms are seen in 12% to 20% of patients with old myocardial infarcts (Fig. 11-16). Intra-aneurysmal thrombi, which are present in half of these cases, are a source of systemic emboli.

MURAL THROMBOSIS AND EMBOLISM

The endocardial damage in an infarct predisposes it to the adhesion of platelets and fibrin deposition, thereby leading to a mural thrombus. Thus, peripheral embolization and infarcts of various organs are a potential hazard after the occurrence of a myocardial infarct, and may justify anticoagulant therapy as a preventive measure.

PERICARDITIS

Pericarditis usually occurs on the area of the heart surface which overlies the necrotic muscle in transmural infarcts. The deposition of fibrin may be limited to the locality of the myocardial necrosis, or may occasionally be diffuse.

METABOLIC AND BIOCHEMICAL EFFECTS OF MYOCARDIAL ISCHEMIA

The heart is exquisitely dependent upon an uninterrupted supply of oxygen. When coronary artery blood flow is inadequate to support the aerobic needs of the heart, or when arterial oxygen content is too low, a series of events leads to depletion of high-energy phosphate compounds (e.g., adenosine triphosphate [ATP]). Unlike skeletal muscle, the heart is unable to develop a significant oxygen debt. When its oxygen supply is suddenly severed, it shifts to anaerobic metabolism, a process that cannot adequately supply the metabolic needs of the working myocardium. The biochemical consequences of sudden coronary artery occlusion include the following conditions that could contribute to cell death: ATP depletion, cellular aci-

dosis, lactate accumulation, activation of intracellular proteases, and elevated intracellular calcium levels.

Table 11-4   Potential Ways to Limit Infarct Size or Prevent Infarct Extension

Decrease energy utilization
Reduce hemodynamic work
- Reduce heart rate—beta blockade, carotid sinus stimulation
- Reduce contractility—beta blockade, Ca^{2+} flux inhibition (verapamil), prostaglandins
- Reduce afterload—intra-aortic balloon counterpulsation
- Reduce preload—nitrates, digitalis (in failing heart)
Reduce cell metabolism directly
- Reduce Ca^{2+} influx—beta blockade, verapamil, nifedipine
- Induce hypothermia
Increase potential energy production
Restore or preserve existing perfusion of ischemic myocardium
- Perform emergency revascularization
- Alter coagulation
    Lyse existing thrombi—streptokinase, urokinase, tissue-type plasminogen activator
    Prevent microthrombi—aspirin, prostaglandins
- Improve or preserve collateral blood flow
    Increase diastolic blood pressure
    Balloon counterpulsation
    Alpha-adrenergic stimulation—methoxamine, norepinephrine
    Vasodilators—verapamil, nifedipine, nitrates, alpha-adrenergic blockade, prostaglandins, dipyridamole
    Decrease diastolic wall tension (reduce preload)—nitrates
    Prevent myocardial edema—osmotic agents (mannitol), hyaluronidase
- Prevent coronary venous retroperfusion or intermittent coronary sinus occlusion
Increase blood oxygen or substrate content despite persistent ischemia
- Increase oxygen—correct hypoxemia and anemia, hyperbaric oxygen
- Increase substrates—glucose-insulin-potassium: hypertonic glucose, ATP, pyruvate, amino acids, ribose, adenosine
- Enhance tissue diffusion—hyaluronidase
Reduce catabolism
- Inhibit adenine nucleotide catabolism—allopurinol
- Inhibit lipolysis—beta-pyridyl carbinol, prostaglandins
- Increase acidosis
- Induce hypothermia
Stabilize cell structure or cytosolic composition
- Reduce electrolyte shifts/prevent cell swelling—beta blockade, Ca^{2+} flux inhibition (verapamil, nifedipine), osmotic agents (mannitol)
- Stabilize cell membranes (plasmalemma, lysosomes)—steroids, prostaglandins
- Prevent free radical production (allopurinol) or introduce free radical scavengers (superoxide dismutase)
Prevent microvascular damage or obstruction
- Prevent endothelial swelling—osmotic agents (mannitol)
- Prevent platelet aggregation—prostaglandins
- Prevent free radical injury—allopurinol, free radical scavengers (superoxide dismutase)
Reduce inflammatory response
- Anti-inflammatory agents—steroids, nonsteroidal anti-inflammatory drugs (ibuprofen)

LIMITATION OF INFARCT SIZE

Experimental studies and clinical trials of strategies to limit infarct size are summarized in Table 11-4.

RISK FACTORS

The major elements which predispose to heart attacks are an elevated blood cholesterol level, hypertension, and cigarette smoking. Any one of these factors significantly increases the risk of heart attacks, and the presence of all three multiplies the risk over sevenfold.

Other risk factors for ischemic heart disease include the following:

- Diabetes mellitus (a fivefold greater risk in women between 30 and 39)
- Obesity (the higher rates of heart attacks may be only indirectly related to obesity; risk may be augmented because obese persons have higher blood pressure, blood fat, and blood sugar levels)
- Age (risk greater with increasing age, up to 80)
- Gender (before age 65, men are more susceptible than women)
- Family history of premature arteriosclerosis
- Use of oral contraceptives
- Sedentary life habits
- Stressful occupation

RHEUMATIC AND OTHER "HYPERSENSITIVITY" DISEASES

RHEUMATIC HEART DISEASE

Rheumatic heart disease is the result of cardiac involvement by rheumatic fever. Rheumatic fever occurs equally in both sexes and at all ages, but it is more common in children, with the peak incidence occurring between the ages 5 and 15. The **clinical diagnosis** of rheumatic fever is made when two major—or one major and two minor—criteria (the "Jones criteria") are met. If this diagnosis is supported by evidence of a preceding streptococcal infection, the probability of rheumatic fever is high.

The **major clinical manifestations** include carditis, (murmurs, cardiomegaly, pericarditis, and congestive heart failure), polyarthritis, chorea, erythema marginatum, and subcutaneous nodules. The **minor manifes-**tations comprise a previous history of rheumatic fever, arthralgia, fever, certain laboratory findings indicative of an inflammatory process (e.g., elevated erythrocyte sedimentation rate, positive test for C-reactive protein, leukocytosis), and electrocardiographic changes.

ANATOMIC FEATURES

Acute Rheumatic Carditis

Acute rheumatic heart disease is a pancarditis, involving all three layers of the heart. The myocardium is most typically involved in the acute stage of the disease. A diffuse nonspecific **myocarditis** is present in some cases, together with a unique type of interstitial inflammation—**the Aschoff body** (Fig. 11-17). The

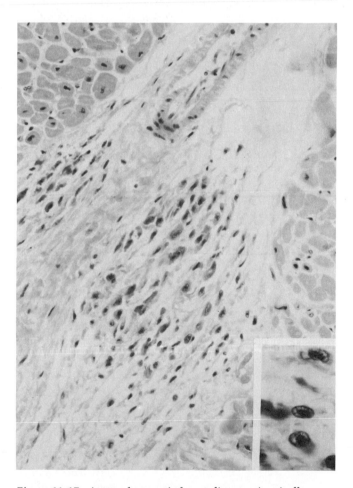

Figure 11-17. Acute rheumatic heart disease. A spindle-shaped Aschoff body is located interstitially in the myocardium. A blood vessel is seen at the top. Within the Aschoff body are noted collagen degeneration, lymphocytes, and Anitschkow cells. (*Inset*) Nuclei of Anitschkow cells, showing "owl eyed" cross sectional appearance and "caterpillar" longitudinal appearance.

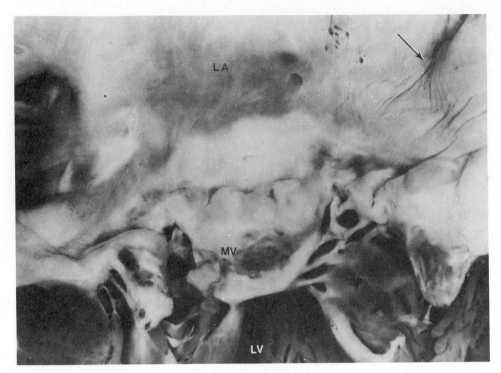

Figure 11-18. Old rheumatic mitral valvulitis. The valve leaflets (*MV*) and chordae tendineae are thickened. This valve was stenotic and also somewhat insufficient. The wrinkled atrial endocardium represents a MacCallum's patch (*arrow*). *MV,* anterior leaflet of mitral valve; *LA,* left atrial cavity; *LV,* left ventricular cavity.

Aschoff body's morphologic feature consists of a perivascular focus of swollen eosinophilic collagen, referred to as showing "fibrinoid necrosis". Surrounding this abnormal collagen are collections of lymphocytes, plasma cells, and monocytes. Also present are **Anitschkow cells,** which are characterized by nuclei which have a central band of chromatin. In cross section these nuclei have an "owl-eye" appearance, and "caterpillar" appearance when cut longitudinally.

The main cause of death in the acute stage of rheumatic heart disease is heart failure from myocarditis.

Also seen during the acute state of the disease is a prominent **pericarditis,** characterized by tenacious deposits of fibrin that resemble the shaggy, irregular surfaces of two slices of buttered bread that have been pulled apart—the so-called bread-and-butter appearance. The pericarditis may be recognized clinically by a friction rub, but the involvement has little functional effect and only rarely leads to constrictive pericarditis. During the acute stage, an **endocarditis** involves mainly the valves, which show a finely nodular "verrucous" appearance at the line of closure. Areas of

Figure 11-19. Etiologic factors in rheumatic heart disease. The upper portion illustrates the initiating beta-hemolytic streptococcal infection of the throat, which introduces the streptococcal antigens into the body and may also activate cytotoxic T-cells. These antigens lead to the production of antibodies to various antigenic components of the streptococcus, which can cross-react with certain cardiac antigens, including those from the myocyte sarcolemma and from the glycoproteins of the valves. This may be the mechanism for the production of the acute inflammation of the heart in acute rheumatic fever that involves all cardiac layers (endocarditis, myocarditis, and pericarditis). This inflammation becomes apparent after a latent period of 2 to 3 weeks. The insult may progress to chronic stenosis or insufficiency of the valves. These lesions involve the mitral, aortic, tricuspid, and pulmonary valves, in that order of frequency.

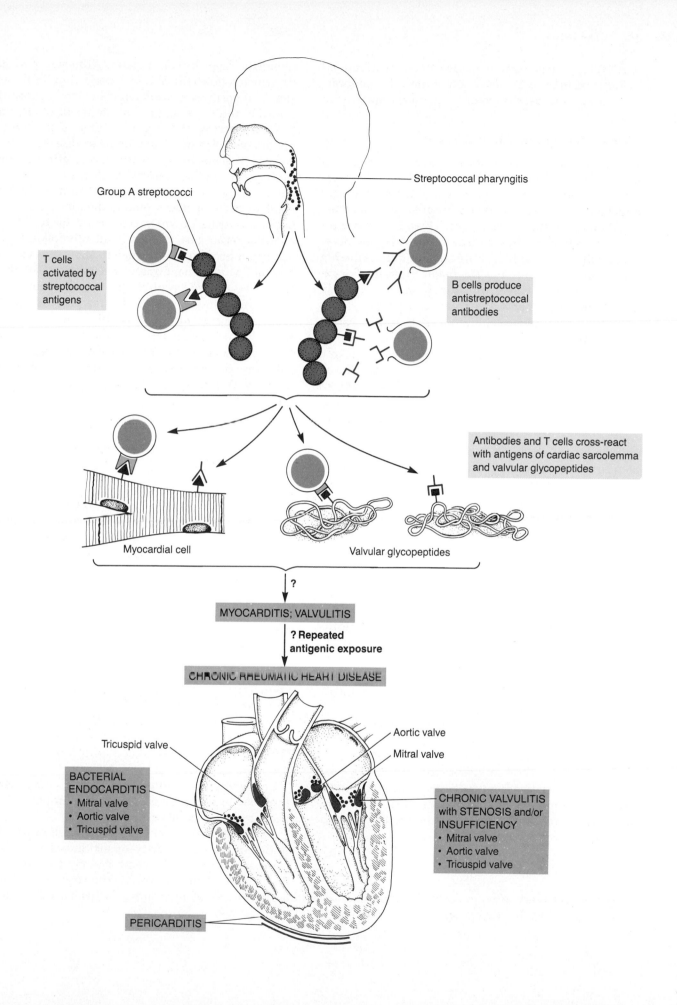

Streptococcal pharyngitis

Group A streptococci

T cells activated by streptococcal antigens

B cells produce antistreptococcal antibodies

Antibodies and T cells cross-react with antigens of cardiac sarcolemma and valvular glycopeptides

Myocardial cell

Valvular glycopeptides

?

MYOCARDITIS; VALVULITIS

? Repeated antigenic exposure

CHRONIC RHEUMATIC HEART DISEASE

Tricuspid valve

Aortic valve

Mitral valve

BACTERIAL ENDOCARDITIS
• Mitral valve
• Aortic valve
• Tricuspid valve

CHRONIC VALVULITIS with STENOSIS and/or INSUFFICIENCY
• Mitral valve
• Aortic valve
• Tricuspid valve

PERICARDITIS

focal collagen degeneration in the valve are surrounded by inflammation, with ulceration of the valve endocardial surface and deposition of fibrin on the surface.

Chronic Rheumatic Heart Disease

A patient who has had an attack of rheumatic fever is more susceptible to recurrent episodes following infections by beta-hemolytic streptococci. **Such recurrent attacks result in repeated and progressively increasing damage to the heart valves. Thus, in chronic recurrent rheumatic heart disease the valve involvement, which was of little clinical significance during the acute attack, becomes the major problem.** For example, the mitral valve, which is the most frequently and severely involved valve, shows conspicuous, irregular thickening and calcification of its leaflets, often with fusion of its commissures and thickening and fusion of the chordae tendineae (Fig. 11-18). As a result, the valve is often severely stenotic and, when viewed from the atrial aspect, has a narrowed orifice described as having a "fish mouth" appearance. The aortic valve, the second most commonly involved valve, shows typical fusion of the commissures and, later, pronounced thickening and calcification of the cusps, with resulting stenosis or insufficiency. The tricuspid valve is similarly involved, although less frequently than the mitral and aortic valves, and the pulmonary valve is the least frequently involved.

ETIOLOGY (FIG. 11-19)

Rheumatic fever occurs after a latent period of 2 to 3 weeks following an infection with a group A beta-hemolytic streptococcus, typically a pharyngitis. Treatment of the initial infection with antibiotics greatly decreases the risk of later rheumatic fever, and prophylactic therapy with penicillin practically eliminates the chance of recurrent rheumatic fever. In some epidemics of group A streptococcal pharyngitis the incidence of rheumatic fever has been as high as 3%, and in patients who have had a previous attack of rheumatic fever without penicillin prophylaxis, the incidence climbs as high as 30%.

Some streptococcal antigens cross-react with heart antigens, an observation which raises the possibility of an autoimmune etiology. There seems to be an additional hereditary factor for susceptibility to rheumatic fever after streptococcal infection.

SEQUELAE

Complete recovery after an acute attack of rheumatic fever is possible. However, certain stigmata of prior rheumatic fever usually remain. **Adhesive pericarditis,** which follows the fibrinous pericarditis of the acute attack, almost never results in constrictive pericarditis. Probably the most significant late result of rheumatic fever is **scarring of the valves.** One of the most important sequelae of rheumatic heart disease is the **increased susceptibility to the localization of infectious agents on the heart valves.** The irregular, scarred nature of these valves provides an attractive environment to bacteria that would ordinarily pass by. The organisms settle down to establish a **bacterial endocarditis.** Because bacteremia frequently follows a tooth extraction or a urethral catheterization, a person who has had a prior diagnosis of rheumatic heart disease should be treated prophylactically with penicillin before performance of either of these procedures. Other sequelae include **mural thrombi,** which can form in the atrial or ventricular chambers and give rise to thromboemboli and infarcts of various organs. Mitral valve disease and congestive heart failure secondary to aortic valve disease lead to congestive changes in the lungs and liver.

HYPERTENSIVE HEART DISEASE

Systemic hypertension is defined, perhaps simplistically, as the persistent presence of blood pressure greater than 140 mm Hg systolic or 90 mm Hg diastolic. The term **hypertensive heart disease** is used when the heart is enlarged in the absence of an apparent cause other than the hypertension.

EFFECTS OF HYPERTENSION ON THE HEART

The main effect of hypertension on the heart is left ventricular hypertrophy, owing to the increased workload imposed on the heart. The left ventricle is thickened and the overall weight of the heart is increased, exceeding 375 g in men and 350 g in women. (The normal heart weight is 300 to 350 g in men and 250 to 300 g in women.)

Left ventricular hypertrophy is a compensatory response to the increased workload imposed on the heart by high blood pressure.

An additional effect of hypertension on the heart is the increased severity of artherosclerosis of the coronary arteries. The combination of increased cardiac workload and narrowed coronary arteries leads to a greater risk of myocardial ischemia, infarction and heart failure.

CAUSES OF DEATH IN PATIENTS WITH HYPERTENSION

The most common cause of death in hypertensive patients is **congestive heart failure,** a complication diagnosed in about 40% of cases. Death may also occur as a result of the previously mentioned coronary arteriosclerosis, dissecting aneurysm of the aorta, or ruptured berry aneurysm of the cerebral circulation. A common cause of death is related to the arteriolar nephrosclerosis that results in **renal failure. Intracerebral hemorrhage** is a frequent fatal complication.

Cor pulmonale is defined as right ventricular hypertrophy that results from a disorder of the lungs. Chronic pulmonary hypertension (and **chronic cor pulmonale)** may be caused by a number of conditions that increase pulmonary vascular resistence, including recurrent pulmonary emboli, pulmonary fibrosis, or chronic lung disease, such as pulmonary emphysema. A small number of cases of cor pulmonale are attributed to "primary pulmonary hypertension", a disorder of unknown etiology.

INFLAMMATORY DISEASES OF THE HEART

INFECTIVE ENDOCARDITIS

ETIOLOGY

The endocardium may develop focal infections of bacteria or fungi in any region, but the valves are the sites most frequently involved by infective endocarditis. The infection may localize on a normal valve if the organism is especially virulent (e.g., *Staphylococcus aureus*) or if the immune system is impaired (e.g., diabetes mellitus, treatment with immunosuppressive agents). Old valvular disease, however, predisposes to the localization of bacteria—especially of the less virulent types, such as alpha-hemolytic streptococci. A prosthetic valve also is a site predisposed to infection. The sources of these organisms are commonly infections of the teeth and gums, urinary tract (including pyelonephritis and acute prostatitis), the skin and the lung.

Other conditions that predispose the heart to localization of organisms include myxomatous degeneration of mitral valve ("floppy valve" or mitral valve prolapse syndrome), nonbacterial thrombotic endocarditis, congenital heart disease (patent ductus arteriosus, tetralogy of Fallot, ventricular septal defect, coarctation of aorta), and intravenous injection of organisms (especially by drug addicts).

ANATOMIC FEATURES (TABLE 11-5)

The mitral valve is most commonly involved with bacterial endocarditis. The vegetations usually form on the atrial surface at the point of closure of the leaflets. The lesions are composed of platelets, fibrin, and masses of organisms. The underlying valve is edematous and inflamed, and may eventually be so damaged that it becomes insufficient. The lesions may vary in size from a small superficial deposit on the valve to exuberant vegetations (Fig. 11-20). **Infected thromboemboli** travel to multiple systemic sites, causing infarcts or abscesses in the brain, kidneys, intestines, spleen, and so forth. The aortic valve is also commonly involved with endocarditis (Fig. 11-20).

NONBACTERIAL THROMBOTIC ENDOCARDITIS (MARANTIC ENDOCARDITIS)

Nonbacterial thrombotic endocarditis is similar in gross appearance to infective endocarditis. However, it does not result in valve perforation, and its microscopic appearance is strikingly different. Infective endocarditis produces a thickened, edematous and inflamed valve, with clumps of bacteria within the vegetation. By contrast, the nonbacterial lesion is bland, and no inflammation or organisms are found.

Table 11-5 *Comparison of Acute and Subacute Bacterial Endocarditis*

FEATURE	ACUTE	SUBACUTE
Duration of clinical symptoms	<6 weeks	>6 weeks
Most common organisms	*Staphylococcus aureus*, beta-streptococci	Alpha-streptococci
Virulence of organism	Highly virulent	Less virulent
Condition of valves	Usually previously normal	Usually previously damaged
	Perforations common	Perforations rare

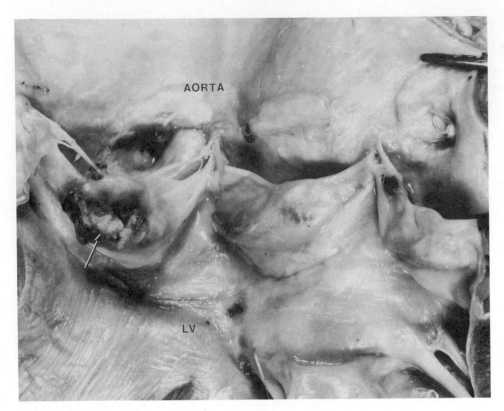

Figure 11-20. Bacterial endocarditis. Aortic valve, with aorta (*above*) and left ventricle (*LV*) (*below*) opened to show a vegetation (*arrow*) on the ventricular surface of the right coronary cusp. The three valve cusps are slightly thickened and have fenestrations (holes) in their free margins, but are otherwise normal. This is from a patient who had bacterial endocarditis caused by *Staphylococcus aureus*. The condition cannot be differentiated grossly from nonbacterial thrombotic endocarditis.

Nonbacterial thrombotic endocarditis usually occurs in a patient with increased blood coagulability. It may be part of the disseminated intravascular coagulation syndrome, and is frequently related to a carcinoma. The endocarditis, therefore, is often a terminal event in patients with wasting diseases, which accounts for the term "marantic". It is clinically manifested by infarcts of the brain, kidney, spleen, intestines, and extremities that result from embolic fragments of the sterile vegetation in the heart.

MYOCARDITIS

ETIOLOGY

Possible causes of myocarditis are listed in Table 11-6.

Table 11-6   Possible Causes of Myocarditis

Idiopathic

- Giant cell myocarditis (Fiedler's myocarditis)

Infectious

- Viral: Coxsackievirus, ECHO, influenza, poliomyelitis
- Rickettsial: Typhus, Rocky Mountain spotted fever
- Bacterial: Diphtheria, staphylococcal, streptococcal, meningococcal, and leptospiral infection
- Fungi and protozoan parasites: Chagas' disease, toxoplasmosis, aspergillosis, cryptococcal and monilial infection
- Metazoan parasites: *Echinococcus*, *Trichina*

Noninfectious

- Hypersensitivity and immunologically related diseases: Rheumatic fever, systemic lupus erythematosus, scleroderma, drug reaction (e.g., to penicillin or sulfonamide), rheumatoid arthritis
- Radiation
- Miscellaneous: Sarcoidosis, uremia

ANATOMIC FEATURES

Myocarditis is suggested grossly by dilatation of the ventricles, an appearance which also characterizes heart failure. Microscopically, interstitial edema is usually seen, along with an infiltrate consisting of lymphocytes, monocytes, and variable numbers of plasma cells, neutrophils and eosinophils. There may be slight to severe myofiber necrosis, and cases of several months duration show considerable interstitial fibrosis. Some cases of myocarditis display a histologic reaction that is better termed "granulomatous". These include cases of tuberculosis of the myocardium (tuberculomas), sarcoidosis, and fungal myocarditis.

PERICARDITIS

Any inflammatory disease of the visceral or parietal pericardium is termed pericarditis. Its causes are similar to those of myocarditis (see Table 11-6) and can be grouped under the same headings (idiopathic, infec-

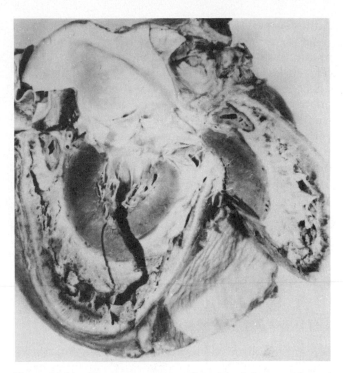

Figure 11-22. Constrictive pericarditis. The left ventricle and aortic valve are illustrated. The atrophic heart (250 g) is solidly encased by a thick, dense, fibrous sheath. The visceral and parietal layers of pericardium are distorted by fibrous and fibrinous bands, and bloody gelatinous material is present in the pericardial sac.

tious and noninfectious). Metastatic neoplasms also may induce a serofibrinous or hemorrhagic exudation and inflammatory reaction when they involve the pericardium. Pericarditis associated with myocardial infarction and rheumatic fever has already been discussed above.

ANATOMIC FEATURES

Pericarditis can be classified according to its gross morphological characteristics. For example, it can be described as being **fibrinous, purulent** (Fig. 11-21), **hemorrhagic, adhesive or constrictive.** Uremia is frequently the cause of the fibrinous type, which has a tendency to become hemorrhagic because of the prominent pericardial granulation tissue. Viral infection also produces a fibrinous pericarditis, as do myocardial infarcts. Pericardial infection by bacteria such as *Staphylococcus aureus* is usually purulent, and may occur secondary to bacterial endocarditis (see Fig. 11-21).

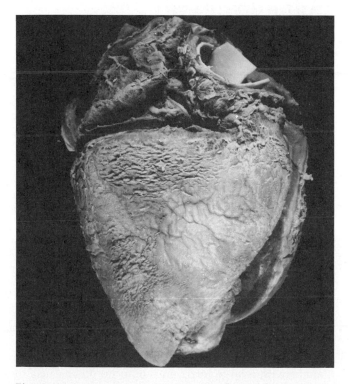

Figure 11-21. Purulent pericarditis. Epicardial surface of right ventricle, showing a shaggy, diffuse fibrinopurulent exudate. The patient was a 25-year-old man who had a bicuspid aortic valve that contained vegetations produced by *Staphylococcus aureus* infection.

Adhesive pericarditis is the sequel of many different types of pericarditis that have healed and left only minor fibrous adhesions. **Constrictive pericarditis** (Fig. 11-22) is rare, and is caused by a previous severe infection that was either purulent or of tuberculous origin. Patients with this type of involvement have a small, quiet heart, in which there is restriction of venous inflow and limitation of diastolic filling. These patients have a high venous pressure, low cardiac output, small pulse pressure and fluid retention, with ascites and peripheral edema.

NUTRITIONAL, ENDOCRINE AND METABOLIC DISEASES OF THE HEART

THYROTOXIC HEART DISEASE

Hyperthyroidism has profound effects on the cardiovascular system. Marked tachycardia and an increased workload, due to the lowered peripheral resistance and increased cardiac output, result in high-output failure.

MYXEDEMA AND THE HEART

Patients with hypothyroidism usually have a decreased cardiac output, decreased heart rate, and decreased myocardial contractility. The hearts of patients with myxedema are usually flabby and dilated. The myocardium exhibits some myofiber swelling, and basophilic (or mucinous) degeneration is common.

THIAMINE DEFICIENCY HEART DISEASE (BERIBERI)

Beriberi has been seen in the Orient in patients whose diet is deficient in vitamins, especially with diets including shelled rice and white bread. In the United States it is occasionally seen in alcoholic patients. Thiamine deficiency results in decreased peripheral vascular resistance and increased cardiac output, a combination that leads to high-output failure.

STORAGE DISEASES

GLYCOGEN STORAGE DISEASE

Of the various forms of glycogen storage disease, types II (Pompe's disease), III (Cori's disease), and IV (Andersen's disease) affect the heart. The most common

and severe cardiac involvement occurs with type II glycogen storage disease. The heart is markedly enlarged (up to seven times normal), and some endocardial fibroelastosis is seen in about 20% of patients. The myofibers are vacuolated by large amounts of stored glycogen. The usual cause of death is cardiac failure.

AMYLOIDOSIS

At autopsy the enlarged heart is firm and rubbery. Amyloid deposits are nodular, waxy, endocardial deposits in the atria; they also cause thickening of the cardiac valves. Amyloid deposits are seen interstitially in the endocardium and in the walls of intramural coronary arteries.

OTHERS

Other storage diseases that may also—directly or indirectly—affect the heart include mucopolysaccharidosis (Hurler's syndrome), sphingolipidoses (Gaucher's and Fabry's disease), and gangliosidosis.

CARDIOMYOPATHY

In **primary** cardiomyopathy the basic and major process involves the myocardium, and the cause is unknown. The **secondary** type is seen in association with another type of heart disease or is secondary to a systemic disease. Cardiomyopathy is classified as congestive (dilated), hypertrophic, or restrictive.

The **congestive cardiomyopathies** include diseases of different etiologies, and it is likely that the initiating event is a viral myocarditis, Chagas' disease, alcoholism, or any one of numerous potential toxins that have not been identified. Anatomic features include cardiomegaly, dilated ventricles, and a high incidence of mural thrombi in the ventricular chambers. The microscopic changes in the myocardium are nonspecific and include myocyte hypertrophy, focal necrosis (usually slight), and myofiber degenerative changes (e.g., fat accumulation).

Many cases of congestive cardiomyopathy occur in chronic alcoholics. Although a specific diagnosis of **alcoholic cardiomyopathy** cannot be made with certainty, it is likely that congestive failure in an alcoholic patient with a large heart, in whom no other cause of heart failure is apparent, is related to the toxic effects on the heart muscle. Other directly toxic effects on the myocardium are produced by various agents, such as cobalt (**beer drinker's cardiomyopathy**) and phenothiazine. The cardiac toxicity of doxorubicin (Adriamycin) limits the dose of this chemotherapeutic drug.

A second common category of cardiomyopathies is **hypertrophic cardiomyopathy,** defined as **a cardiomyopathy which exhibits cardiomegaly but no ventricular dilatation.**

The hearts of such patients show hypertrophy and small ventricular chambers. **Asymmetric septal hypertrophy and myofiber disarray are almost invariable. There is evidence that hypertrophic cardiomyopathy is transmitted as an autosomal dominant genetic trait.**

Restrictive cardiomyopathies are much rarer than the congestive and hypertrophic types. They include those conditions in which there is increased wall stiffness (e.g., amyloidosis), and in which diastolic ventricular volume and stretch are sufficiently impaired to cause a restriction in filling.

LUETIC HEART DISEASE

Tertiary syphilis causes heart disease by two mechanisms.

- Aortic medial scarring may extend to the aortic valve ring and aortic valve cusps. This widens the valve ring and separates the commissures of the cusps, which become thickened and shortened, and display rolled margins. The effect is severe aortic valve insufficiency. The volume workload of the heart is thus increased, an effect which eventually leads to heart failure.
- The changes characteristic of leutic aortitis, which thicken the aortic intima, may extend from the ascending aorta to involve and obstruct the coronary artery ostia, thereby producing myocardial ischemia.

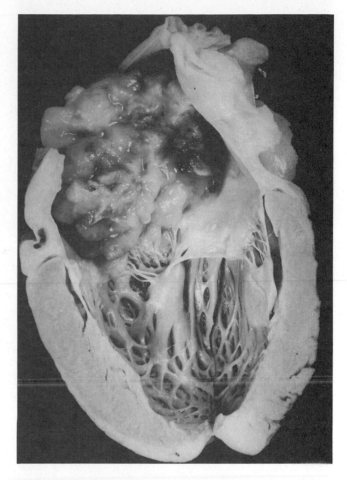

Figure 11-23. Left atrial myxoma. The heart is from a 33-year-old woman who had symptoms of congestive heart failure that had progressively worsened. The clinical diagnosis was "rheumatic mitral stenosis." The woman died after suffering a stroke caused by a tumor embolus. The grapelike gelatinous nodules of the tumor fill the left atrium and obstruct the mitral valve orifice, producing symptoms similar to those of mitral stenosis.

CARDIAC TUMORS

Primary cardiac tumors are rare. The most common primary tumor is the **myxoma** (Fig. 11-23), accounting for 35% to 50% of all primary cardiac tumors. **Most myxomas arise in the left atrium, although they can occur in any cardiac chamber or on a valve.**

Another tumor, which is most common in infants and young children, is the **rhabdomyoma**, which often occurs in association with tuberous sclerosis.

More common than primary heart tumors are metastatic tumors, which derive from melanoma or cancers of the lung, breast and gastrointestinal tract.

12

THE RESPIRATORY SYSTEM

WILLIAM M. THURLBECK

Diseases of the lung are not only important problems for individual patients, but are major public health concerns. Cancer of the lung causes more deaths than any other cancer—over 100,000 a year in the United States. Chronic airflow obstruction represents the single greatest cost of the Veterans Administration. The adult respiratory distress syndrome is responsible for 75,000 deaths a year in the United States. Humble respiratory tract infections, mostly benign and self-limited, are the most common cause of time off from work.

Each day the lung is exposed to harmful environmental agents, the most obvious of which are found in the workplace, where inhalation of such materials as asbestos and silica results in serious disability or death. Air pollution is also a significant factor in lung disease. Although its effects are less serious than those of asbestos or silica, air pollution is more widespread, and may aggravate or help cause other lung conditions. It may have been responsible for such epidemics as that in London in 1952, where smog was associated with some 3000 deaths. Most people spend much of their lives inside the home, where the environment is affected by both the external environment and substances generated in the home (e.g., vapors from gas cooking or urea formaldehyde foam). Both cancer and chronic airflow obstruction are overwhelmingly related to tobacco smoking, primarily cigarette smoking. This unique toxic product has a direct effect on the lung and an indirect effect on other organs, notably those of the cardiovascular system.

Being exposed to air that is usually at a lower temperature than that of the body, of variable humidity, dirty, and laden with infectious agents, the respiratory system possesses effective defense mechanisms. The nose and trachea constitute an efficient air conditioning system, which ensures that the air entering the lung is at body temperature and fully saturated with water. The nose traps almost all particles more than 10 μm in diameter and about half of all particles with an aerodynamic diameter of 3 μm. (Aerodynamic diameter refers to the way particles behave in air rather than to their actual size.) **The airway epithelium is protected by the mucociliary blanket.** The ciliary beat drives the mucous blanket toward the trachea, and particles that land on it are thus removed from the lungs and swallowed or coughed up. The mucociliary blanket is effective in disposing of particles 2 to 10 μm in diameter. **The protector of the alveolar space is the alveolar macrophage.** Alveolar macrophages are derived from the bone marrow, probably undergo a maturation division in the interstitium of the lung, and then enter the alveolar space. Unlike macrophages elsewhere, they depend on oxidative metabolism. They are particularly effective in dealing with particles whose aerodynamic diameter is less than 2 μm. Very small particles behave as a gas and are exhaled.

Although the lung shares with other organs many responses to injuries (e.g., inflammation and neoplasia), we shall emphasize conditions specific to the lung itself:

Chronic airflow obstruction. The major function of the lung is gas exchange; it follows that obstruction to airflow has serious consequences.

Pneumoconiosis (diseases due to respirable inorganic substances). Mining and the processing of minerals require that workers be exposed to minerals and associated dust that produce specific lung lesions.

Restrictive lung disease (infiltrative lung disease). A syndrome referred to as restrictive lung disease is the functional counterpart of infiltrative lung disease. This disorder involves the interstitium of the lung; the tissue around the blood vessels, lymphatics and bronchi; and the airspace walls. The lung becomes stiff and small, with a linear, reticular, or nodular pattern in the chest radiograph.

Infections in the immunocompromised host. Since it handles 5 to 8 liters of air each minute, the lung is exposed to infectious agents more than most organs. Treatment of cancer with immunosuppressive and cytotoxic agents compromises the host's defense mechanisms. In these circumstances lung infections that are often not serious in normal persons may become life-threatening.

PATHOLOGY OF THE LARYNX AND TRACHEA

INFECTIONS OF THE LARYNX AND TRACHEA

Epiglottitis is a serious condition, most commonly caused by *Haemophilus influenzae*, type B. Occurring in infants and young children, it may be a life-threatening emergency. Swelling of the acutely inflamed epiglottis produces obstruction to airflow. Inspiratory stridor (a loud wheezing sound on inspiration) occurs, and the onset of cyanosis may indicate airway obstruction so severe as to require tracheostomy. Similar symptoms may be encountered in viral infections of the larynx and trachea, which are most commonly due to infection with para-influenza viruses.

Epiglottitis and laryngotracheobronchitis in children are associated with **croup,** a syndrome characterized by inspiratory stridor, cough, and hoarseness resulting from varying degrees of laryngeal obstruction. Croup due to laryngotracheobronchitis is a complication of an upper respiratory tract infection and is marked by edema of the larynx.

Both **laryngitis,** which causes hoarseness, and **tracheitis,** associated with cough, are common at all ages. Both are caused by viral infections, varying from the common cold to influenza. The systemic effects of fever and malaise are usually more troublesome to the patient than the respiratory symptoms, and anything other than supportive treatment is ineffective.

TUMORS OF THE LARYNX

Tumors of the larynx are common. A frequently encountered benign lesion, which is **reactive** rather than neoplastic, is the laryngeal nodule **(singer's nodule).** This lesion, usually single but sometimes multiple, consists of a small polypoid structure, with a simple fibrous stroma and squamous mucosa on the true vocal cords. It occurs most commonly in those who use their voice constantly, particularly singers. Changes in timbre of the voice and hoarseness are the main symptoms. Although a trivial biological lesion, such a nodule may jeopardize a singer's career. Surgery is curative, but the quality of the voice may be impaired.

The vast majority of laryngeal cancers are **squamous cell carcinomas,** tumors strongly related to cigarette smoking. Based on the location of the lesion laryngeal carcinomas are divided into four groups, which have relevance to treatment and prognosis:

A **glottic tumor** is a carcinoma limited to one or both true vocal cords. These tumors are slow to metastasize to lymph nodes and have a good prognosis, at least in the early stage.
Transglottic carcinomas, by definition, involve the true and false cords. These tumors are likely to metastasize to lymph nodes and often require total laryngectomy.
Supraglottic carcinomas arise in the ventricle, false cords, or epiglottis and do not, by definition, involve the true cords. Nodal metastases are more common than in glottic tumors. Voice-saving surgical treatment is often possible.
Infraglottic carcinomas either are located below the true cords or involve the true cords, with considerable infraglottic extension. Nodal metastases are common, and total laryngectomy is generally required

FOREIGN BODIES

A lodged foreign body may totally occlude the trachea and result in suffocation. Large pieces of food, often steak, lodge in the trachea, classically in a restaurant when the sufferer has had too much to drink (the "Miami Beach syndrome"). The simplest action is the Heimlich maneuver, in which one stands behind the victim, wraps one's arms around him, makes a double clenched fist over the upper abdomen just below the rib cage, and gives a quick, forceful, upward squeeze. Alternatively, the occluding object may be reached via the pharynx, or an emergency tracheostomy may be necessary.

LESIONS IN CONDUCTING AIRWAYS

INFECTIONS

There is clearly an overlap between infections of the trachea and those of the bronchi, and in many instances the term "tracheobronchitis" is appropriate. Influenza is a characteristic example of tracheobronchitis, and in the occasional patient who dies with this infection, the appearance of the bronchi is dramatic. The surface of the airway is fiery red, reflecting acute inflammation and congestion of the mucosa.

Other infectious agents that involve the intrapulmonary airways usually affect the more peripheral airways (bronchiolitis). The classic examples are adenovirus, measles, and respiratory syncytial virus. All appear most seriously to affect malnourished children and populations not usually exposed to these agents. Severe symptomatic illnesses are usually confined to infants and children, and recovery is the rule. Symptoms include cough, a feeling of tightness in the chest, and, in extreme cases, shortness of breath and even cyanosis. **Adenovirus infection** produces the most serious sequelae, including extensive inflammation of bronchioles and subsequent healing by fibrosis that obliterates bronchioles or occludes them with loose fibrous tissue. Subsequent collapse of the lung (atelectasis) leads to permanent dilatation of the bronchi (bronchiectasis).

IRRITANT GASES

Of the irritant gases in the atmosphere the important ones are oxidants (ozone, oxides of nitrogen) and sulfur dioxide. Oxidants are particularly related to the action of sunlight on automobile exhaust fumes and are notably of importance in major urban areas that experience temperature inversions. Sulfur dioxide is mainly derived from the burning of fossil fuels. Although the precise effects of these agents in low concentration is not certain, and although they clearly have a high nuisance value, it seems likely that they are not a major cause of serious respiratory disease.

BRONCHIAL OBSTRUCTION AND ASPIRATION

ATELECTASIS

Atelectasis refers to the collapse of expanded lung tissue. If the supply of air is obstructed, the transfer of gas from the alveoli to the blood leads to a loss of alveolar air and collapse of the involved region. Atelectasis is an important postoperative complication of abdominal surgery, occurring because of mucous obstruction of a bronchus and diminished respiratory movement resulting from postoperative pain. It is often asymptomatic, but when severe it results in hypoxemia. Another important cause of atelectasis, particularly significant in young children, is aspiration of foreign bodies. Atelectasis may also result from occlusion of a bronchus by a tumor or, less commonly, by lymph nodes containing metastatic cancer.

Although atelectasis is usually caused by bronchial obstruction, it may also result from direct compression of the lung (e.g., hydrothorax or pneumothorax). Such compression, if severe enough, seriously compromises the function of the affected lung.

LUNG ABSCESS

Lung abscess due to aspiration is most often found in alcoholics, especially those with poor dental hygiene (Fig. 12-1). The right side of the lung is more frequently affected than the left, because the right main bronchus follows the direction of the trachea more closely at its bifurcation. The organisms involved are classically anaerobes from the oropharynx, and their effect is compounded by aspiration of vomitus. Acute pneumonia with necrosis of lung tissue ensues. Because of the indolent nature of the process, a fibrous wall forms around the margin. Lung abscesses differ from those elsewhere in their capacity for spontaneous drainage.

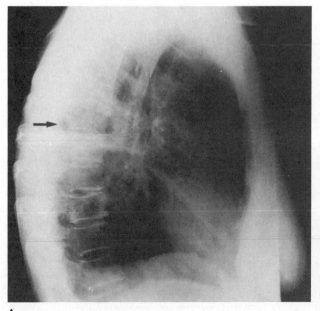
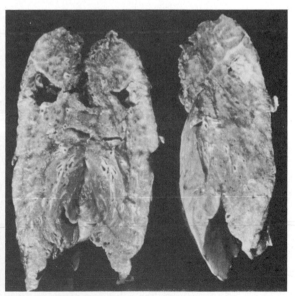

A

B

Figure 12-1. Lung abscess. A 41-year-old alcoholic woman vomited in bed while stuporous. She developed fever and coughed up copious amounts of sputum. (*A*) A lateral chest radiograph shows an abscess in the superior segment of the right lower lobe (*arrow*). A fluid level is apparent. (*B*) The lower lobe was resected and cut into sagittal slices. The walls of the abscess are thin.

NEOPLASIA

PRIMARY CANCER OF THE LUNG

Primary cancer of the lung is the most common cause of death from cancer; more than 100,000 people die each year in the United States from this disease. Regarded as a rare tumor as late as 1945, it now occurs in epidemic proportions. The reason for the enormous increase in lung cancer is tobacco smoking in general, and cigarette smoking in particular. The present epidemic of lung cancer in women reflects the later acceptance of smoking in the female population. There are some occupational causes of lung cancer, notably uranium mining in North America. Asbestos workers who smoke cigarettes exhibit a much higher incidence of lung cancer than similar workers who do not smoke.

COMMON FEATURES OF PRIMARY LUNG CANCER

Lung cancer is more common in men than in women (4:1), except for bronchoalveolar carinomas and carcinoids, in which there are no sex differences. Cancers occur more often on the right side than on the left (52.5% versus 47.5%), reflecting the larger volume of the right lung, and are more common in the upper lobe than in the lower. Metastases occur to the regional intrapulmonary lymph nodes and then to the mediastinal nodes. There are certain sites of predilection for metastasis, notably the adrenals (an unexplained phenomenon), brain, liver, and bone.

TYPES OF PRIMARY LUNG CANCER

Squamous Cell Carcinoma

By light microscopy the diagnosis of squamous cell carcinoma requires the presence of intercellular bridges and keratin formation. Keratin occurs either as pearls (a central, brightly eosinophilic aggregate of keratin surrounded by onion-skin layers of squamous cells) or as individual cell keratinization (the cytoplasm of the cell assumes a glassy, intensely eosinophilic appearance). Ultrastructurally, intercellular bridges are seen as intercellular junctions of the classic desmosome type. The ultrastructural counterpart of keratin is tonofilaments. **Squamous cell carcinomas, characteristically tumors of the major bronchi, are slow-growing** (Fig. 12-2). They present with symptoms related to their bronchial origin: persistent cough, hemoptysis, or bronchial obstruction, the last accompanied by pulmonary infections (recurrent pneumonias, lung abscesses) or atelectasis. Lymph node metastases are often sufficiently limited to allow surgical resection of the tumor.

The histogenesis of squamous cell carcinoma is of interest because respiratory epithelium normally displays no squamous differentiation. Following injury to the epithelium, such as occurs with cigarette smoking, regeneration from the pluripotential basal layer, in the form of squamous metaplasia, commonly occurs. **This squamous metaplastic mucosa follows the same sequence of dysplasia, carcinoma in situ, and invasive tumor as that observed in sites that are normally lined by normal or metaplastic squamous epithelium, such as the cervix, oral cavity, vocal cords, esophagus, and skin** (Fig. 12-3).

Adenocarcinoma

Adenocarcinomas of the lung, characterized by a glandular appearance and the secretion of mucus, are commonly peripheral (i.e., beyond an obvious bronchial origin), but a substantial proportion have a bronchial origin. **Adenocarcinomas metastasize readily, tend to grow more rapidly than squamous cell carcinomas, and have a propensity to invade the pleura.**

Large-Cell Undifferentiated Carcinoma

Large-cell undifferentiated carcinomas are so poorly differentiated that they elude classification as squamous or adenocarcinoma. Many tumors classified as large-cell carcinoma by light microscopy show ultrastructural evidence of squamous or glandular differentiation and should be reclassified. Thus, the frequency of this diagnosis depends on the availability of special diagnostic techniques. The behavior of this category of tumors is similar to that of poorly differentiated adenocarcinoma.

Small-Cell Carcinoma

Small-cell carcinoma, a highly malignant form of lung cancer, is characterized by sheets of small tumor cells and the intermediate cell variant. There is minimal architectural differentiation and a great deal of necrosis. The nuclei are dense and hyperchromatic. There is such scant cytoplasm that the tumor cells are only twice the size of lymphocytes. **These tumors metastasize so early that the lesions are not amenable to surgery.** Chemotherapy is the common treatment, and recent advances have led to a dramatic improvement in prognosis. Small cell carcinomas exhibit **neuroendocrine differentiation** and produce a variety of endocrine peptides. Ultrastructurally, the cells contain scattered dense-core neurosecretory granules.

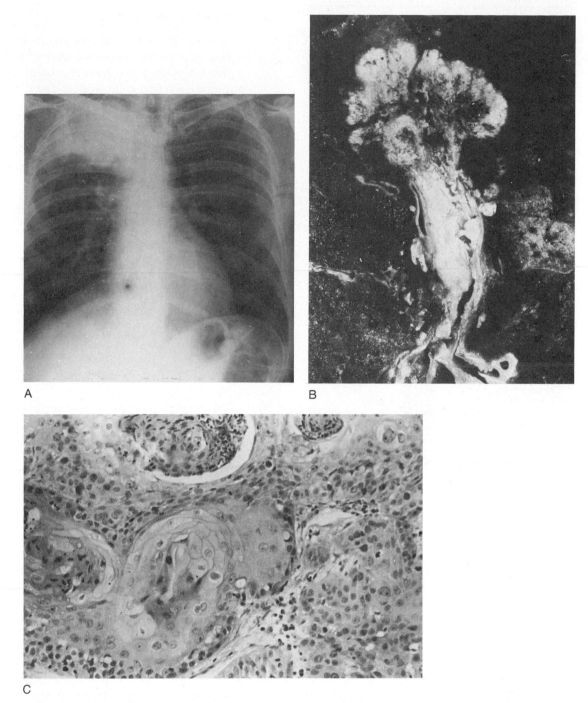

A

B

C

Figure 12-2. Squamous cell carcinoma of the lung. A 62-year-old man had repeated chest infections over a 6-month period. (*A*) A chest radiograph shows a right upper lobe lesion and atelectasis. (*B*) In the resected specimen a large endobronchial tumor is apparent in the right upper lobe bronchus and its segments. This lesion caused the atelectasis. The tumor also invades the lung parenchyma. (*C*) Microscopically, the tumor is a well-differentiated squamous carcinoma.

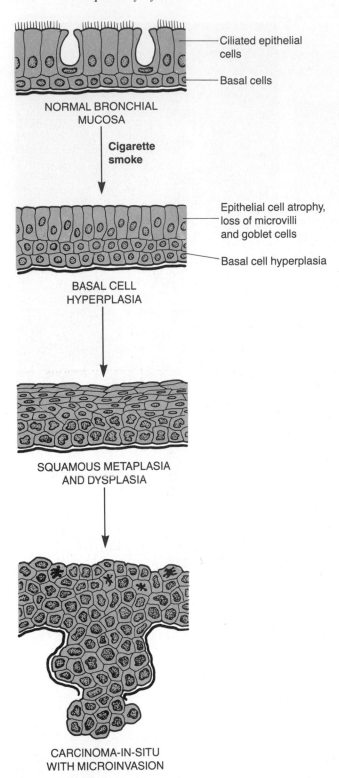

Figure 12-3. The development of squamous cell carcinoma. First, minor changes occur in the bronchial epithelium (basal cell hyperplasia), followed by squamous cell metaplasia with dysplasia. Then carcinoma in situ ensues, first localized to the epithelium and then extending to bronchial glands and penetrating the basement membrane. Extensive invasion and metastases follow.

Bronchoalveolar Tumors

Bronchoalveolar tumors are always peripheral in origin and, as the name indicates, derive from bronchiolar or alveolar epithelium. As such, the tumor may consist of mucus-secreting cells, nonciliated (Clara) cells, or type II pneumocytes. Ciliated cells are not encountered. Bronchoalveolar tumors are well differentiated and characteristically grow along alveolar walls. At their peripheral margins the alveolar architecture is apparent. The important features of bronchoalveolar carcinoma are as follows:

The prognosis, when limited to a single lesion, is good. In the absence of lymph node metastases, the cure rate is more than 50%.

It is impossible to distinguish by light microscopy between a bronchoalveolar tumor and a single metastasis from an adenocarcinoma elsewhere. Statistically, however, solitary metastases almost always occur with a history of a previously excised primary carcinoma, or in a patient with overt symptoms related to the primary cancer.

There is no sex predilection, nor is there a relationship to tobacco smoking.

The usual clinical presentation is as a "coin lesion," a well-circumscribed radiopacity in the periphery of the lung.

In addition to the single peripheral bronchoalveolar tumor, a second gross pattern exists, characterized by multiple bilateral nodules or bilateral infiltrates that grossly and radiographically simulate pneumonia. The ultimate prognosis is hopeless, although the course may be prolonged and the disease may still be limited to the thorax at the time of death. Metastases from other organs, notably the stomach and pancreas, occasionally present with identical pathologic, clinical, and radiologic features.

Carcinoid Tumor

Classically, the carcinoid tumor was classified as a **bronchial adenoma,** a term implying that it is a benign tumor and glandular in appearance. Both of these assumptions are incorrect. **Classic carcinoids resemble small-cell carcinomas in being neuroendocrine tumors, but are much better differentiated.** The nuclei have an open chromatin pattern rather than hyperchromasia, the cytoplasm is more abundant, and there is a definite organoid arrangement of cells in ribbons, tubules, and clusters in a richly vascular stroma. Carcinoids also produce a variety of endocrine peptides and vasoactive amines. The majority of classic carcinoids are central and involve large bronchi; thus, they present with symptoms of obstruction. In contrast to small-cell carcinoma, a substantial proportion of carcinoid tumors occur before the age of 40 years, women are affected as commonly as men, and the tumor is not related to smoking. The malignancy of the tumor is viewed as low grade; death from classic lung carcinoid is unusual.

PARANEOPLASTIC SYNDROMES

As neuroendocrine tumors, small-cell carcinomas secrete a variety of vasoactive amines and polypeptides that are similar or identical to the normal hormones. These are frequently found in the blood of patients with tumors and may become clinically symptomatic. Inappropriate secretion of antidiuretic hormone is characterized by water intoxication and hyponatremia. Cushing's syndrome is a known complication of the secretion of ACTH or ACTH-like substances. Hypercalcemia is caused by parathormone secretion, but unlike the other paraneoplastic syndromes, it is usually associated with squamous cell carcinoma. Clubbing of the fingers is associated with lung cancer of all types, but the reason is not known.

METASTATIC TUMORS

The most common malignant neoplasm of the lung is metastatic tumor. In about a third of all fatal cancers, pulmonary metastases are evident at autopsy. Metastatic tumors in the lung are typically multiple and circumscribed (Fig. 12-4). Single metastases may present a problem in clinical and pathologic diagnosis, particularly when they are adenocarcinomas. Such tumors may resemble primary adenocarcinomas of the lung and may not be distinguishable from them on histologic grounds alone.

LESIONS AFFECTING THE LUNG PARENCHYMA

INFECTIONS

VIRAL INFECTIONS

Viruses are a common cause of airway lesions, but those that primarily affect the airways may also severely affect the lung parenchyma. The best example of

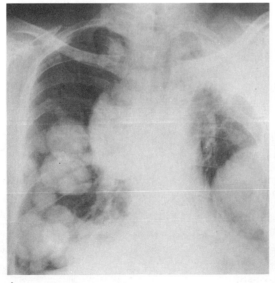
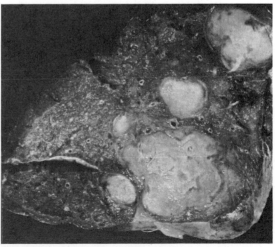

A   B

Figure 12-4. Metastatic tumor in the lung. A 53-year-old man who had a liposarcoma excised from his thigh 2 years previously presented to his physician with shortness of breath. (*A*) A chest radiograph shows multiple discrete masses in both lung fields. (*B*) Gross examination of the lung confirms the discrete nature of the "cannonball" metastases.

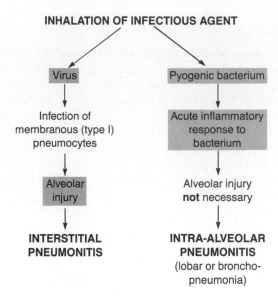

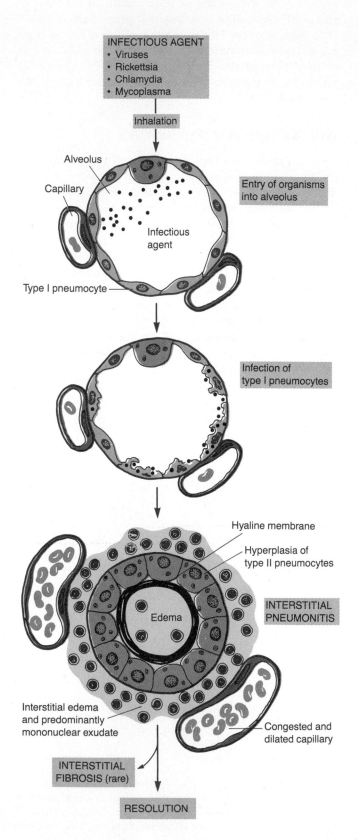

Figure 12-5. Pathogenesis of interstitial and intra-alveolar pneumonitis.

a disease caused by viruses that affect the airways is influenza; the best example of one caused by viruses that affect both is measles. **It is important to note that viral lung infections produce interstitial (rather than alveolar) pneumonia and diffuse alveolar damage.** Initially, viral infection affects the alveolar epithelium and results in a mononuclear infiltrate in the interstitium of the lung (Figs. 12-5, 12-6). Depending on the severity of the insult, there is necrosis of the type I epithelial cells and formation of hyaline membranes, an appearance that is indistinguishable from diffuse alveolar damage due to other causes. In other instances, the alveolar damage may be indolent and may be characterized by hyperplasia of type II cells and interstitial inflammation. This appearance contrasts with that of most bacterial infections, in which an intra-alveolar exudate predominates and in which the interstitium is only incidentally involved (Figs. 12-5, 12-7).

A characteristic interstitial pneumonia is that produced by the **cytomegalovirus.** Initially described in infants, it is now well recognized in the immunocompromised host (e.g., patients treated with cytotoxic agents or those with AIDS). The infected alveolar cells are large ("cytomegalo") and have a dark-blue inclusion within the nucleus, clumps of basophilic material along the nuclear margin, and cytoplasmic basophilic inclusions.

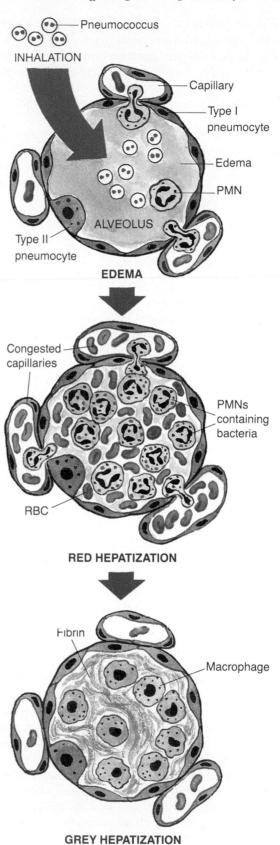

Figure 12-6. (*On opposite page*) Pathogenesis of interstitial pneumonitis. Although interstitial pneumonia is most commonly caused by viruses, other organisms may also cause significant interstitial inflammation. Type I cells are the most sensitive to damage, and loss of their integrity leads to intra-alveolar edema. The proteinaceous exudate and cell debris form hyaline membranes, and type II cells multiply to line the alveoli. Interstitial inflammation is characterized mainly by mononuclear cells. The disease generally resolves completely but occasionally progresses to interstitial fibrosis.

Figure 12-7. Pathogenesis of lobar pneumococcal pneumonia. Pneumococci, characteristically in pairs (diplococci), multiply rapidly in the alveolar spaces and produce extensive edema. They incite an acute inflammatory response, in which polymorphonuclear leukocytes and congestion are prominent (red hepatization). As the inflammatory process progresses, macrophages replace the polymorphonuclear leucocytes and ingest debris (gray hepatization). The process usually resolves, but complications may ensue.

Measles infection, which involves both the airways and the parenchyma, is characterized by the presence of very large (100-μm diameter) multinucleated giant cells that have inclusions in the nucleus. Although interstitial pneumonia is a well-recognized complication of measles, it is rarely fatal, except in immunocompromised, previously unexposed people.

Varicella (both chicken pox and herpes zoster) infection produces disseminated, focally necrotic lesions in the lung, as well as interstitial pneumonia. Pulmonary involvement is usually asymptomatic, except in immunocompromised hosts, in whom it may be fatal.

BACTERIAL INFECTIONS

The traditional pathologic classification of **lobar pneumonia** and **bronchopneumonia** has little clinical relevance. Pulmonary bacterial infection should be classified etiologically, but in reality, this is usually impossible. Pneumococcal pneumonia, the classic example of lobar pneumonia, is characterized by a massive purulent exudate in the alveolar spaces (Fig. 12-7). It is called lobar because a single lobe may be involved, and that involvement may be complete. Bronchopneumonia often occurs in terminally ill patients and is usually found in the dependent (usually posterior) portions of the lung. Scattered irregular foci of pneumonia are centered on bronchioles and respiratory bronchioles. Bronchiolitis and respiratory bronchiolitis are present, with exudation of polymorphonuclear leukocytes into the adjacent alveoli. Large continuous areas of alveolar involvement do not occur. No single bacterial organism is responsible, and several may be present, often ones not regarded as important pathogens. Bronchopneumonia has been referred to as the "old man's friend" because it was regarded as the terminal event that spared prolonged suffering.

Atypical Pneumonia

An important clinical concept is the syndrome of atypical pneumonia. In contrast to lobar pneumonia, the onset is insidious, leukocytosis is absent or slight, and the course is prolonged. Respiratory symptoms may be minimal and the chest radiograph shows a patchy intra-alveolar pneumonia or interstitial infiltrate. The common cause of the syndrome is *Mycoplasma pneumoniae*, but other agents include viruses, chlamydiae, *Coxiella* organisms, and legionellae. It is rarely fatal and is often thought of as a classic example of interstitial pneumonia. Cases that have been examined at autopsy have shown a bronchiolar component, with microatelectasis beyond the bronchiolitis, and interstitial and patchy alveolar pneumonia.

Pneumococcal Pneumonia (Lobar)

Now of diminishing significance because of prompt response to treatment, pneumococcal pneumonia is still a significant illness in industrialized nations; in the nonindustrialized world it is still a major cause of mortality. It is commonly a disease of healthy young to middle-aged adults; it is rare in infants and the elderly and is considerably more common in men than in women. Alcoholics appear to be particularly vulnerable. The onset is acute, with fever and chills. Chest pain due to pleural involvement is common, as is hemoptysis, which is characteristically "rusty," since it is derived from altered blood in alveolar spaces.

Radiologic examination shows alveolar filling in large areas of lung, producing a solid appearance that extends to entire lobes or segments. Before antibiotic therapy the clinical course was characterized by severe fever, dyspnea, debility, and even loss of consciousness. The dramatic event was the "crisis," when the patient, who appeared moribund, would suddenly become afebrile and return from death's door. The satisfactory resolution of the crisis was the result of a good immune response to the infection.

In the earliest stage of pneumococcal pneumonia, protein-rich edema fluid containing numerous organisms (*Streptococcus pneumoniae*) fills the alveoli. Marked congestion of the capillaries is typical. Shortly after this congestion occurs there is a massive outpouring of polymorphonuclear leukocytes, accompanied by intra-alveolar hemorrhage. Many of the red blood cells undergo lysis. These cells, together with polymorphonuclear leukocytes, produce the rusty sputum. Because the firm consistency of the affected lung is reminiscent of the liver, this stage has been aptly named "red hepatization" (see Fig. 12-7).

The next phase, occurring after 2 or more days, depending on the success of treatment, involves the lysis of polymorphonuclear leukocytes and the appearance of macrophages, which phagocytose the fragmented polymorphonuclear leukocytes and other inflammatory debris. The lung is now no longer congested but still remains firm in this stage of "gray hepatization." The alveolar exudate is then removed and the lung gradually returns to normal.

A painful pleuritis is common because the pneumonia often extends to the pleura. Bacteremia is usually present in the early stages and may result in endocarditis or meningitis.

Klebsiella Pneumonia

The only other organism that causes lobar pneumonia with any degree of frequency is *Klebsiella pneumoniae*. The disease is commonly associated with alcoholism and is seen most frequently in middle-aged men. The onset is less dramatic than that of pneumococcal pneumonia, but the prognosis is considerably worse because of the patient's underlying condition and because antibiotic therapy is less effective.

Staphylococcal Pneumonia

Pulmonary infection with *Staphylococcus aureus* commonly occurs as a superinfection following influenzal infections. In the 1957 influenza pandemic it was a major cause of death. Like staphylococcal infection elsewhere, it is characterized by the development of abscesses.

Streptococcal Pneumonia

Streptococcal pneumonia is thought to have been the common superinfection in the 1918–1919 influenza pandemic. It is generally uncommon and was rare in the 1957 pandemic. It usually occurs in debilitated persons and is characterized by a diffuse hemorrhagic pneumonia. Caused by beta-hemolytic streptococci of Lansfield group B, this pneumonia is characteristic of newborn infants, who are infected in the birth canal. The clinical symptoms are similar to those of the infantile respiratory distress syndrome. However, the infants are often full term, have severe toxemia, and die within a few hours.

Gram-Negative Pneumonia

The two common causes of gram-negative pneumonia are *Escherichia coli* and *Pseudomonas aeruginosa*. *E. coli* pneumonia is a recognized complication of gastrointestinal surgery and may be seen in the immunocompromised patient. It presents as a bronchopneumonia and responds poorly to treatment. *Pseudomonas* pneumonia is most often seen in the immunocompromised person, in patients with burns, and in those with cystic fibrosis. In the first two, the infection reaches the lung by the bloodstream. *Pseudomonas* infection is common in cystic fibrosis, probably because of the favorable environment provided by the abnormal bronchial secretions. In cystic fibrosis the infection is airborne and usually produces bronchiolitis, with subsequent bronchial obliteration and bronchiectasis.

Legionella Infections

In 1976 a mysterious respiratory ailment broke out at an American Legion convention in Philadelphia. The infectious agent, whose exact taxonomy is not completely agreed on, was soon identified as a fastidious organism with special cultural characteristics. It then became apparent from serologic studies and from histologic studies of the lung that several previous epidemics had occurred but that the causative agent had not been recognized. The organisms responsible have been dubbed *Legionella pneumophila;* six subtypes are now recognized. Characteristically, outbreaks occur in institutions such as hotels, hospitals, and nursing homes and are due to contamination of air conditioning or heating systems in which the organisms multiply in stagnant water. The onset is usually acute, with malaise, fever, muscle aches and pains, and curiously, abdominal pain. Mortality has been high (10% to 20%), especially in immunocompromised patients. The histologic findings are nonspecific and consist of an alveolar pneumonia.

Tuberculosis

Known since ancient Egypt, tuberculosis became the scourge of nineteenth-century Europe and North America and during that time was the most common cause of death. There has been an exponential decline in the prevalence of tuberculosis throughout much of the twentieth century. The major effect of modern antituberculosis treatment has been to prevent reactivation of the disease, making death from it uncommon.

PATHOGENESIS Tuberculosis is caused by *Mycobacterium tuberculosis,* a slender, acid-fast aerobic organism. Pulmonary tuberculosis is almost always caused by the human strain of *M. tuberculosis*, although atypical mycobacteria may also produce pulmonary infections. The disease has been classically divided into **primary** and **reactivation** tuberculosis; the initial infection is classified as primary tuberculosis and subsequent infections as reactivation tuberculosis.

Primary tuberculosis results from the initial exposure to *M. tuberculosis*, most commonly as a result of inhaling droplet nuclei. These are small particles—2 μm to 10 μm in diameter—produced by coughing, sneezing, and talking. Primary tuberculosis is usually derived from a subject with "open" (cavitary) tuberculosis who coughs up large amounts of organisms. The clinical and pathologic manifestation of primary tuberculosis is the Ghon complex, which consists of a parenchymal component and a prominent lymph node component. The parenchymal lesion can occur almost anywhere but is most commonly found in a subpleural location in the middle and lower lobes of the lung. Gross examination reveals a well-circumscribed nodule. Initially these nodules are centrally necrotic but later they become densely fibrotic and calcified. Histologic examination shows an initial acute inflammation followed by an infiltration of macrophages, which eventually appear as epithelioid cells. Caseous necrosis ensues and the lesion becomes granulomatous, with a peripheral infiltrate of Langhans' giant cells, histiocytes, and lymphocytes, together with a palisaded aggregate of fibroblasts. The lymph node component of the Ghon complex is found in the draining hilar or intrapulmonary nodes and has microscopic features similar to the pulmonary lesions.

TRANSMISSION   Primary infection is associated with the development of both immunity and hypersensitivity, the latter being recognized by a positive tuberculin test. In the past most cases of primary tuberculosis were encountered in children, but the sequence of events that leads to the clinical expression of the disease may occur at any age following the first infection. At present most primary infections occur in adults. A new feature of primary tuberculosis is the occurrence of mini-epidemics in groups living closely together (e.g., submarine crews, teenage groups, and health care workers). This presumably reflects the large proportion of non-immune, tuberculin-negative persons in the community.

COMPLICATIONS   The great majority of primary infections remain localized and heal, but progression or complications do occasionally occur (Table 12-1). **Bacteremia** is probably a common event, and favorite sites of deposition and growth are locations with a high oxygen tension, such as the apices of the lung, growing ends of the long bones, and renal parenchyma. The most serious immediate complication is **miliary tuberculosis,** in which there is invasion of the bloodstream by *M. tuberculosis* and dissemination throughout the body. This occurs when the parenchymal part of the Ghon complex involves a pulmonary artery or vein and discharges its infected contents into the blood. Multiple minute granulomas develop in many organs of the body. The lesions are classically 0.5 to 2 mm in diameter, yellowish white, and evenly distributed through the affected organ. A punctate area of necrosis may be seen in the center. Microscopically, the lesions of miliary tuberculosis consist of small granulomas, usually with a central necrotic portion in which numerous organisms are seen. Few organs are spared; those most often involved are the lung (mainly by recirculation of the organisms), spleen, liver, kidney, meninges, and bone marrow. Miliary tuberculosis used to be found most often in young children, but in industrialized countries it has become more common in the elderly and debilitated, in alcoholics, and in high-risk racial groups, such as native Americans and Eskimos.

On occasion miliary tuberculosis involves only one organ, and that only focally. Almost any organ can be involved, most notably the genitourinary organs and bone (although in the latter case, the disease may be bovine tuberculosis, which has a different pathogenesis). A dreaded complication is tuberculous meningitis. In this disease the parenchymal lesions in the lung may rupture into a bronchus, causing a rapidly developing pneumonia, primarily lobar or segmental in distribution.

The reasons for progression of infection in a minority of those with primary tuberculosis are not known, but several have been suggested. It has long been known that infants, adolescents, and young adults are especially predisposed. Other factors include (1) the dose, with massive inoculation of organisms likely to produce a progressive lesion; (2) poor nonspecific resistance to infection, as occurs in the elderly or in alcoholics; (3) certain diseases, such as silicosis, or drugs, such as corticosteroids; and (4) a racial predilection (notable, for example, in native Americans and very important in populations not previously exposed to tuberculosis). Tuberculosis has classically been more severe in nonwhite populations, who are thought to have been introduced to the disease by whites.

Reactivation tuberculosis represents recurrence of pulmonary disease after sensitization to *M. tuberculosis* during primary infection. The term "reinfection tuberculosis," which has also been used, implies that the

Table 12-1   Natural Course of Untreated Tuberculosis

Complications and Sequelae	Usual Time After Conversion	Frequency in Caucasians
Incubation period 6 weeks (3–8 weeks)		Tuberculin conversion 100%
		Primary illness 30%
		Erythema nodosum 5%
Local spread (epituberculosis)	0–6 weeks	5%–10% in young children
Pleural effusion	2–9 months	5%–10% in adults, adolescents, and older children
Miliary tuberculosis and meningitis	2–8 months	5%–10% of children, later dropping to 1%
Extrapulmonary tuberculosis		
Cervical lymphadenitis	Few weeks to many years later	
Skeletal tuberculosis	First few years	
Genitourinary tuberculosis	Many years later	
Postprimary (reactivation) tuberculosis	At and after puberty	10% in recently infected adolescents, 4% in those infected in early childhood

lesion results from an exogenous reinfection with new organisms. Whether infection occurs from new organisms or old is a contested issue; most believe, however, that the lesions are due to proliferation of preexisting endogenous organisms.

The initial reaction to *M. tuberculosis* is very different in secondary tuberculosis. A cellular immune response occurs after a latent interval and leads to the formation of granulomas and extensive tissue necrosis. Most commonly, the apical and posterior segments of the upper lobe are involved. A diffuse, fibrotic, poorly defined lesion develops that has focal areas of caseous necrosis. Often these foci heal and calcify, but occasionally the material erodes into a bronchus and is coughed up, after which aspiration may lead to tuberculous pneumonia or a walled tuberculous cavity.

Reactivation tuberculosis is associated with constitutional symptoms—classically, fever, weight loss, night sweats, and malaise. Before the introduction of antituberculosis chemotherapy, cavitary tuberculosis had a mortality rate of about 50%, but the outlook is considerably better today. Reactivation tuberculosis is uncommon in North America today, except in selected populations, and the predisposing factors are much the same as those involved in the progression of primary tuberculosis.

Atypical Mycobacteria

A number of organisms closely related to *M. tuberculosis* may cause pulmonary disease. These "atypical" mycobacteria are acid-fast and resemble *M. tuberculosis* morphologically, but their growth rates and growth requirements differ. Disseminated infection with *Mycobacterium avium-intracellulare* is a prominent complication of the acquired immune deficiency syndrome (AIDS).

FUNGAL INFECTIONS

Fungal infections of the lung are now common in North America, indeed more common than tuberculosis, but in healthy people they are rarely serious. However, they may be lethal in those who are immunocompromised or debilitated. The most common pulmonary fungal infections are histoplasmosis and coccidioidomycosis.

Histoplasmosis

Histoplasmosis is classically thought of as a disease of the U.S. Midwest and Southeast in general and of the Mississippi and Ohio valleys in particular, with its epicenter in St. Louis. The causative organism is *Histo-plasma capsulatum*, a small oval yeast about 3 μm in diameter that rarely shows budding. The disease is commonly caused by inhalation of dust infected by bird droppings. The organism is hardy and survives well in soil.

Histoplasmosis has many clinical and pathologic similarities to tuberculosis. The great majority of infections are asymptomatic and result in lesions similar to the Ghon complex, including a parenchymal granuloma and granuloma formation in draining lymph nodes. The condition is usually recognized only on a routine chest radiograph or a positive histoplasmin skin test. The granulomas are particularly prone to calcify, often with a concentric laminar pattern. The acute phase, in which numerous organisms are seen within macrophages, is followed by granulomatous inflammation with central areas of necrosis in the lesions. These characteristically heal by fibrosis and calcification.

In a few cases, the pulmonary lesion progresses or reactivates, which leads to a progressive fibrotic and necrotic lesion that closely resembles reactivation tuberculosis. The lesion has a more fibrotic appearance, and cavitation is less common.

Coccidioidomycosis

Coccidioidomycosis is caused by *Coccidioides immitis*, large (30 to 60 μm) spherical spores that do not bud but that form endospores within the organism. Originally known as San Joaquin Valley fever, where the disease has been endemic for many years, coccidioidomycosis is widely spread through the south-western part of the United States. It shares many of the clinical and pathologic features of histoplasmosis and tuberculosis. In most instances, the lesions are limited to a peripheral parenchymal granuloma, with or without lymph node granulomas, and the disease is recognized by a positive skin test or routine chest radiograph. In a few cases, the lesion is progressive and resembles tuberculosis, although the rate of progression is slow. In dry, dusty conditions the hardy spores that live in the soil are blown into the air and inhaled.

Cryptococcosis

Cryptococcosis is caused by *Cryptococcus neoformans*, a round, budding yeast that varies in size from 2 to 15 μm. It has a thick, mucous gelatinous capsule that shrinks in tissue sections, leaving a halo around the organism. Compared with histoplasmosis and coccidioidomycosis, cryptococcosis is uncommon.

Cryptococcosis results from the inhalation of spores. The organism is frequently encountered in pigeon droppings. A variety of lung lesions is seen, from small parenchymal granulomas to several large granulomatous nodules. Pneumonic consolidation and even cavitation may occur. Most serious pulmonary infections occur in immunocompromised individuals in whom the organisms proliferate extensively within alveolar spaces, with little tissue reaction.

Branching Fungi

Infection by branching fungi is uncommon in healthy people. Aspergillosis and mucormycosis, seen as branching hyphae in tissue sections, are commonly seen only in the lungs of immunocompromised patients.

ASPERGILLOSIS   Aspergillosis, usually caused by *Aspergillus niger* and *Aspergillus fumigatus*, is the most common and important fungal infection of the lung in this category. Aspergillus, a common mold that thrives in cool, wet conditions, is readily recognized with standard hematoxylin and eosin stains but is best seen on silver-stained section. The hyphae are thin (3 to 5 μm) and septate (subdivided by cell walls), and show regular dichotomous branching at a 45-degree angle (Fig. 12-8) **A serious manifestation of aspergillus infection occurs in the immunocompromised person, most commonly in leukemic patients treated with cytotoxic agents.** Extensive blood vessel invasion (usually arterial) results in occlusion, thrombosis, and infarction of lung tissue. The involvement is bilateral and widespread and is not amenable to therapy.

MUCORMYCOSIS   (PHYCOMYCOSIS)   Several closely related organisms—*Mucor, Rhizopus,* and *Nisidia*—may involve the lung in ways identical to those of aspergillus. These infections also occur as angioinvasive pulmonary lesions in an immunocompromised host. **A classic association is with diabetic ketoacidosis. Infection of the nasal sinuses is characteristic of these fungi.** These organisms have the same staining properties as aspergillus, but differ in that the hyphae are not septate and are broader (10 to 15 μm), and they branch by irregular dichotomy, usually at right angles.

CANDIDIASIS (MONILIASIS)   *Candida albicans* is a normal commensal in the oral cavity, gut, and vagina and is best known for infection in these regions and in the skin, often in the immunocompromised host. It also affects the lungs, but usually only the surface epithelium, with noninvasive growth in the airways. Although it may produce surface ulceration, in the lungs it is usually identified only at autopsy in a patient with severe immunosuppression.

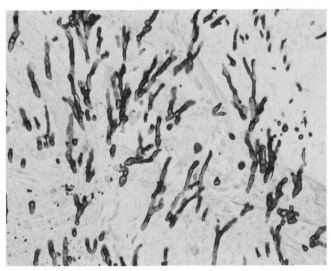

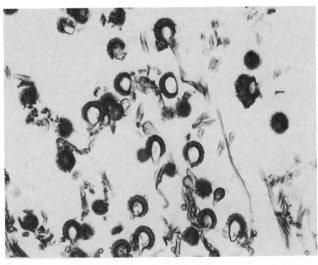

A   B

Figure 12-8. Pulmonary aspergillosis. (*A*) Invasive aspergillosis is apparent in an immunocompromised man with acute myelogenous leukemia treated with cytotoxic drugs. In this tissue section the fungi are septate and show regular dichotomous branching at angles of approximately 45°. (*B*) When cultured at room temperature, aspergilli produce a characteristic spherical fruiting head, as shown here.

PROTOZOAL INFECTIONS

Protozoal infection of the lung is uncommon in industrialized countries, and the only significant one is produced by *Pneumocystis carinii*. Pneumocystic pneumonia came into prominence in North America with the advent of renal transplantation and immunosuppression. Since then it has come to be recognized as a major pulmonary complication of chemotherapy for leukemia and lymphoma and of treatment with steroids. It is now also an important cause of death in patients with AIDS. The organism is ubiquitous, and infection is only expressed in the debilitated and immunocompromised.

Clinically and radiologically, the presentation is variable. At one extreme, symptoms may be minimal; at the other there is rapidly progressive respiratory failure. More usually, there are nonspecific respiratory symptoms, including dyspnea and cough. Infection with pneumocystis should be considered in any pulmonary disease in an immunocompromised patient, particularly since it is sensitive to sulfisoxazole-trimethoprim treatment.

The classic lesion is an interstitial pneumonia, with an infiltrate of plasma cells and lymphocytes, diffuse alveolar damage, and type II cell hyperplasia. The alveoli are filled with a characteristic foamy exudate, the organisms appearing as small "bubbles" in a background of proteinaceous exudate. The organisms are readily recognized by silver stains, which stain the cysts. These are round or indented ("new moon") organisms about 5 μm in diameter (Fig. 12-9). In addition to this classic appearance of pneumocystis pneumonia, the infection may present as acute, diffuse alveolar damage, with hyaline membranes, epithelial necrosis, and even pulmonary fibrosis.

DIFFUSE ALVEOLAR DAMAGE

THE ADULT RESPIRATORY DISTRESS SYNDROME (ARDS)

The most important cause of diffuse alveolar damage is the adult respiratory distress syndrome (ARDS). In this syndrome, (Fig. 12-10) a patient with apparently normal lungs suffers an insult and then develops rapidly progressive respiratory failure, char-

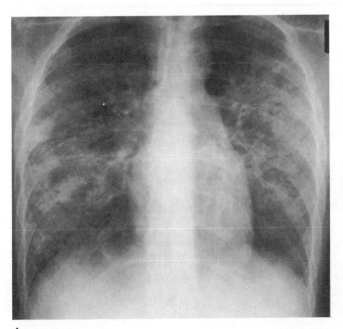

A

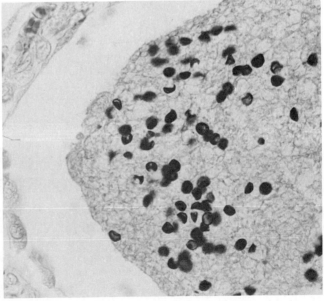

B

Figure 12-9. Pneumocystis carinii infection of the lungs. (*A*) A chest radiograph in a patient with AIDS shows patchy, bilateral, intra-alveolar and interstitial infiltrates. (*B*) A silver stain shows the characteristic features of the *P. carinii* organisms. Some are round and uniform in size, others are irregular and have a crescentic configuration. The alveolar wall is seen on the left; the alveolar space contains a foamy exudate.

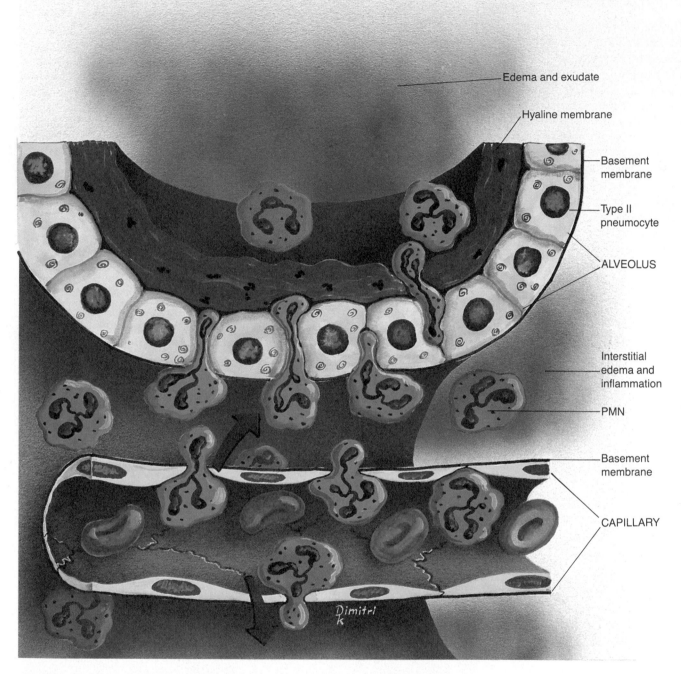

Edema and exudate

Hyaline membrane

Basement membrane

Type II pneumocyte

ALVEOLUS

Interstitial edema and inflammation

PMN

Basement membrane

CAPILLARY

Dimitri K

Figure 12-10. The adult respiratory distress syndrome (ARDS). In ARDS, type I cells die as a result of diffuse alveolar damage. Intra-alveolar edema follows, after which there is formation of hyaline membranes composed of proteinaceous exudate and cell debris. In the acute phase the lungs are markedly congested and heavy. Type II cells multiply to line the alveolar surface. Interstitial inflammation is characteristic. The lesion may heal completely or may progress to interstitial fibrosis.

acterized by hypoxemia and extensive radiologic opacities in both lungs ("white out").

Typically, nonthoracic trauma or infection leads to hemodynamic shock, from which the patient is resuscitated. However, recovery is interrupted by respiratory symptoms—namely, tachypnea, dyspnea, and hypoxemia—and a chest radiograph shows diffuse bilateral infiltrates, which progress to virtually complete opacification. The patient requires ventilatory assistance and increasing amounts of oxygen. The lungs become stiff (decreased compliance), and increasing end-expiratory pressures are required, until the patient needs 100% oxygen to maintain tissue oxygenation. Half of all patients with ARDS die.

The important early event is leakiness of endothelial capillaries, with morphologic loosening of the intercellular junctions. At this stage respiratory failure is not apparent. Then, 24 to 48 hours after the initial insult, pulmonary edema and resultant hypoxemia ensue in the **exudative phase.** The next stage is **diffuse alveolar damage,** in which necrosis of type I epithelial cells and hyaline membranes that line the airspaces are prominent. In the **proliferative phase,** type II cells multiply to reconstitute the alveolar lining and an interstitial inflammatory infiltrate of mononuclear cells is accompanied by proliferation of fibroblasts. All these conditions are present 4 to 7 days after the insult, and the patient usually dies in severe respiratory failure. If the patient survives, the lesions may heal with resorption of the alveolar exudate and hyaline membranes and restitution of the normal alveolar epithelium. Fibroblastic proliferation ceases and the extra collagen is metabolized. It is well documented that patients with ARDS who recover have normal pulmonary function.

The pathogenesis of ARDS is not entirely clear. It is thought that activation of the complement system (e.g., by endotoxin in the case of gram-negative septicemia) results in sequestration of neutrophils in the marginating pool. Only a small proportion, perhaps one-third, of neutrophils actively circulate in the blood; most of the remainder are found in the lung. Normally, the neutrophils cause no damage, but following activation by complement they release oxygen radicals and hydrolytic enzymes (superoxide and hydrogen peroxide) that damage the endothelium of the lung capillaries.

In ARDS produced by the inhalation of toxic gases or near-drowning, the damage occurs primarily at the alveolar epithelial surface. The alveolar epithelial junctions are usually very tight; damage to the epithelium results in exudation of fluid and proteins from the interstitium into the alveolar spaces. Endothelial damage may or may not occur in ARDS that is due to inhalation of toxic substances. However, the sequence of events is similar to that in ARDS that follows trauma or septicemia.

IATROGENIC DIFFUSE ALVEOLAR DAMAGE

Oxygen

Pulmonary lesions have developed in patients with long-term exposure to as little as 28% oxygen, but usually it is safe to breathe 40% oxygen (partial pressure of 300 mm Hg) for long periods of time. The mechanism of oxygen toxicity is related to partially reduced oxygen radicals in the same way as that of ARDS due to other causes.

Radiation Pneumonitis

Radiation pneumonitis is also caused by the generation of oxygen radicals through the radiolysis of water. It is most commonly encountered in irradiation of cancer of the lung, breast, or mediastinum (for lymphoma); the damage is mainly dose-related. The initial lesion is diffuse alveolar damage. The acute phase is measured in terms of weeks or months. The result of healing is varied. In extreme cases, which are now uncommon, the affected lung is shrunken and fibrotic, and the lung architecture is largely lost. More usually, **there is diffuse interstitial fibrosis, general retention of lung structure, and bizarre hyperchromatic nuclei of alveolar type II cells.** Lipid accumulates within the alveolar capillary endothelium to produce foam cells.

Drug-Induced Diffuse Alveolar Damage

The long list of drugs that cause diffuse alveolar damage includes most chemotherapeutic agents. The best known is **bleomycin,** which is used for the treatment of epithelial cancers, but other frequently used agents, such as methotrexate, 5-fluorouracil, busulfan, and cyclophosphamide, are known causes. As a general rule, all cytotoxic agents should be suspected as a cause of diffuse alveolar damage. With bleomycin, an imprecise dose-dependent relationship has been demonstrated, but such an effect is not apparent with most other drugs. **The morphologic features are similar to those of diffuse alveolar damage from other causes.** Bizarre, atypical, hyperchromatic nuclei in type II cells are particularly common in cases of alveolar damage from chemotherapeutic agents. The damage progresses despite withdrawal of the offending agent, although it may be modified by the administration of corticosteroids. Progressive interstitial fibrosis occurs, usually with retention of the lung structure.

PULMONARY HEMORRHAGE: GOODPASTURE'S SYNDROME

Bilateral extensive pulmonary hemorrhage is generally a complication of other diseases, such as mitral stenosis or, rarely, infection. It also occurs in Goodpasture's syndrome, a term applied to the condition of **diffuse bilateral pulmonary hemorrhage accompanied by rapidly progressive glomerulonephritis.**

Goodpasture's syndrome has now become synonymous with the variant of pulmonary hemorrhage associated with circulating antiglomerular basement membrane antibodies. In **anti-glomerular basement membrane antibody disease** antibodies are visualized in the kidneys (and less well in the lung) by immunofluorescence as linear staining of the basement membrane. Although the patients may be adults of any age, they are typically young men and present with hemoptysis, dyspnea, and acute renal disease. Either the renal symptoms or the pulmonary symptoms may come first. The diagnosis is made on the basis of renal biopsy.

Histologically, the alveoli are filled with red blood cells. **The basal laminae of the capillaries in the lungs and the glomeruli are thought to have common antigenic determinants that are targets for antibodies elicited by a primary lung insult or kidney injury.** The resulting damage to the basal laminae produces alveolitis and hemorrhage in the lung and rapidly progressive glomerulonephritis in the kidney. The disease is no longer uniformly fatal.

DISEASE PROCESSES UNIQUE TO THE LUNG

CHRONIC AIRFLOW OBSTRUCTION

Several diseases are grouped together because they have in common an obstruction to airflow in the lungs. The term "chronic airflow obstruction" is no more specific than anemia, jaundice, or fever.

Airflow obstruction has two major causes. Flow has a simple hydraulic basis and can be reduced in only two ways: **by narrowing the tubes or by reducing the pressure to the system. In the lung, narrowed airways produce increased resistance, whereas loss of elastic recoil results in diminished pressure. In simplistic terms, airway narrowing can be thought of as bronchitis, and loss of recoil as emphysema.**

CENTRAL AIRFLOW OBSTRUCTION

The most important causes of central airflow obstruction are chronic bronchitis, asthma, bronchiectasis, and cystic fibrosis. Although all are associated with abnor-

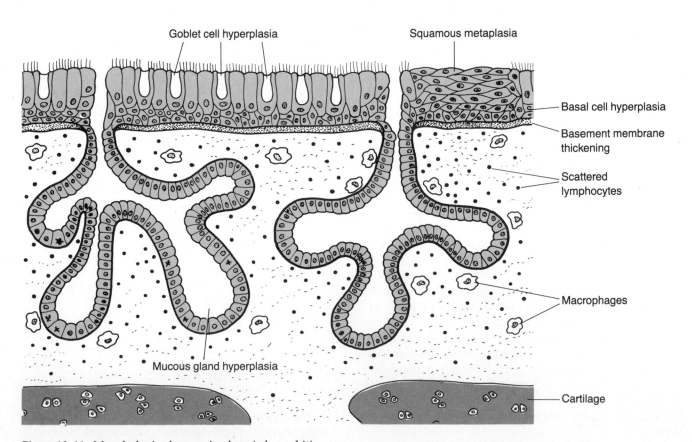

Figure 12-11. Morphologic changes in chronic bronchitis.

malities of the central airways (bronchi), the obstruction to airflow is not necessarily due to these lesions. Chronic bronchitis, a lesion of central airways, may also be associated with peripheral airway narrowing and emphysema. Asthma is primarily a disease of central airways, but in many cases peripheral airway obstruction occurs. In bronchiectasis and cystic fibrosis, the obstruction to flow is actually peripheral to the dilated bronchi. Therefore, these conditions are considered under the rubric of peripheral airway disease.

Chronic Bronchitis

Chronic bronchitis is defined as chronic sputum production and is usually associated with a chronic cough. It is primarily related to tobacco smoking—especially cigarettes; more than 90% of all cases occur in chronic smokers. Dusty occupations, such as coal mining, are also associated with an increase in the frequency of chronic bronchitis.

The morphologic counterpart of chronic bronchitis is an increase in the size of the mucus-secreting apparatus (Fig. 12-11). Most mucus is secreted by the subepithelial tracheobronchial mucous glands, that drain into a duct leading to the epithelial surface. They consist of a series of branched tubules that on cross section look like glands. **Chronic bronchitis is characterized by hyperplasia and hypertrophy of the mucus-secreting cells and an increased proportion of mucous to serous cells.** As a result, both the individual acini and the glands become larger. The increase in size has been measured in a number of ways, but the usual measure is the **Reid index** (Fig. 12-12), that is, the ratio of gland to wall. The normal value is 0.4 or less; in chronic bronchitis it is more than 0.5.

Other morphologic changes are also present in chronic bronchitis, but they have not been as well studied. Of particular importance, **the bronchial wall is thickened, mainly by mucous gland enlargement, but also as a result of edema of the bronchi.** This leads to encroachment on the bronchial lumen. An increase in goblet cells of the central airways is apparent in some cases. Increased amounts of muscle are often present and may reflect bronchial hyperreactivity (see following section on asthma).

Surprisingly, the pathogenesis of chronic bronchitis is not well studied. **The key phenomenon is hypersecretion of mucus in response to chronic injury.** Tracheobronchial glands are under autonomic nervous system (predominantly parasympathetic) control, and disturbances of nervous control may be involved in mucus hypersecretion. Damage to the ciliated cells of the surface epithelium leads to increased mitotic activity of the basal cells, which then preferentially differentiate to mucus-secreting (goblet) cells, the product of which is presumably beneficial. When the insult is suf-

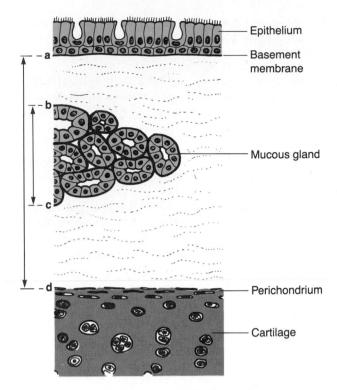

Figure 12-12. Reid index. The Reid index is the ratio of the thickness of the glands (*b–c*) to that of the bronchial wall (basement membrane to inner perichondrium) (*a–d*). It is increased in chronic bronchitis.

ficiently severe, differentiation toward squamous epithelium (squamous metaplasia) occurs (see Fig. 12-11).

Asthma

Most physicians correctly feel that they can recognize asthma with accuracy, but no committee has defined this disease satisfactorily. Although it is imprecise, the following definition is widely used: "asthma refers to a condition of subjects with widespread narrowing of the bronchial airways which changes in severity over short periods of time, either spontaneously or under treatment, and is not due to cardiovascular disease." The following points are worth noting:

Most asthmatic patients, even when apparently well, have persistent airflow obstruction and morphologic lesions.

A substantial proportion of patients with the usual clinical features of chronic airflow obstruction, predominantly middle-aged male smokers with chronic bronchitis and airflow obstruction, frequently also have increased airway reactivity—that is, an asthmatic component.

Although increased airway reactivity also occurs following viral bronchial infection or exposure to a substance such as ozone, no one would refer to such patients as having asthma.

With these provisos, **asthma in most patients is readily recognized as acute attacks of airflow obstruction, often easy to treat. Patients are well between attacks. In addition, many patients with chronic bronchitis have evidence of bronchial reactivity, and some may exhibit a distinct overlap with asthma. Finally, any airway insult may produce bronchial hyperreactivity.**

Asthma is classically divided into **extrinsic asthma** and **intrinsic asthma.** Extrinsic asthma is most commonly an immunologic phenomenon and occurs as a response to inhaled antigens. It is strongly related to allergic skin test reactivity and is usually found in children. The prognosis is good. Intrinsic asthma is a disease of adults and its prognosis is significantly worse. The causative factor may not be apparent and skin reactivity is uncommon.

We can also look at asthma in another way by modifying the preceding into more specific categories (Fig. 12-13):

Antigen-induced asthma is the most common form of asthma. About one-third to one-half of all patients with asthma have known or suspected reactions to allergens. Most allergens are airborne and must be present in the environment for a considerable time to induce hyperreactivity. Common allergens include pollens, animal hair or fur, and insect contamination of house dust. Patients with antigen-induced asthma have classic extrinsic asthma.

Asthma may be associated with inhalation of a number of occupation-related substances. More than 80 different occupations have been identified where such a substance occurs. In some instances, these substances may provoke asthma by obvious hypersensitivity mechanisms (e.g., in animal handlers, bakers, and workers with wood and vegetable dusts, metal salts, pharmaceutical agents, and industrial chemicals). In others, the asthma may be due to release of histamine-like substances, a mechanism postulated in byssinosis ("brown lung"), an occupational lung disease in cotton workers. Occupational exposure may directly affect the autonomic nervous system. For example, organic phosphorous insecticides act as anticholinesterases and produce overactivity of the parasympathetic nervous system. Toluene diisocyanate is thought to have a beta-adrenergic antagonist action.

Environmental pollution is associated with bronchospasm, usually during episodes of massive air pollution. Usually patients with preexisting lung conditions are affected, but new cases of asthma do occur. Sulfur dioxide, oxides of nitrogen, and ozone are commonly implicated environmental pollutants.

Although **drug-induced bronchospasm occurs most commonly in patients with known asthma, the agents themselves may produce asthma. The best-known of these is aspirin,** but several other anti-inflammatory agents have been implicated.

Viral respiratory tract infections trigger attacks in young asthmatics and may cause the first attack. In children under the age of 2 years the respiratory syncytial virus is the usual agent, whereas in older children rhinovirus, influenza, and para-influenza are the common inciting organisms.

Exercise may induce attacks of asthma in patients who already have the disease; some degree of bronchospasm is usual in such subjects. Exercise may also cause the first attack of asthma. Exercise-induced asthma is related to the magnitude of heat loss from the epithelium of the airways to the inspired gas. The more rapid the ventilation (severity of exercise) and the colder and drier the air breathed, the more likely the asthma is to be precipitated.

THE IMPORTANCE OF ASTHMA Asthma is **common, affecting 7% to 10% of children and 5% of adults.** It is most frequent in young children and least common in adolescence; it increases in frequency in adult life. Typically, childhood asthma disappears in adolescence or early adult life and has a good prognosis. Nevertheless, because deaths during acute attacks can occur, acute asthma should be regarded as a medical emergency, and prolonged difficulty in

---

Figure 12-13. Pathogenesis of asthma. (*A*) Immunologically mediated asthma. Allergens interact with IgE on mast cells, either on the surface of the epithelium or, when there is abnormal permeability of the epithelium, in the submucosa. Mediators are released and may react locally or by reflexes mediated through the vagus. (*B*) A variety of other forms of asthma exist that are apparently not immunologically mediated. The morphologic features are the same in the two types of asthma.

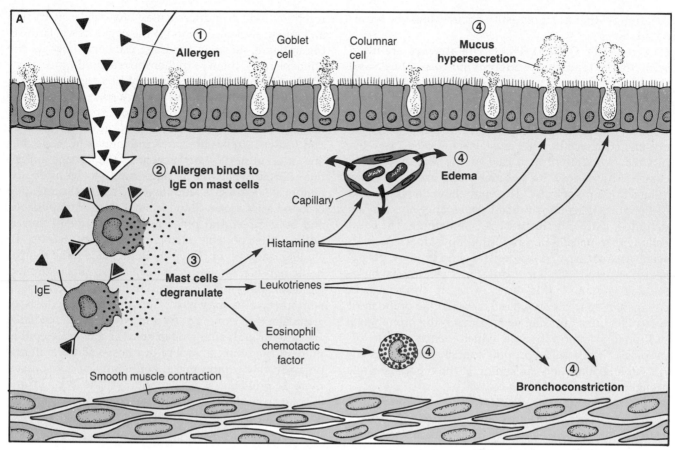

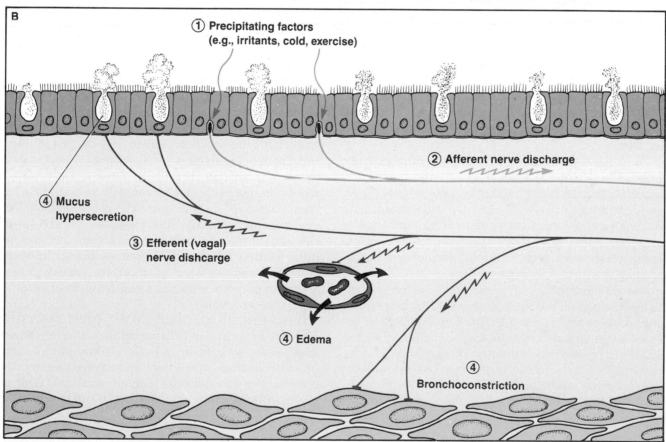

breathing—that is, status asthmaticus—must be terminated.

PATHOLOGY OF ASTHMA   The airways are filled with thick, tenacious adherent mucous plugs, and the lungs are greatly distended with air. Histologic examination shows that the mucous plugs contain strips of epithelium and many eosinophils, the extruded granules of which coalesce to form needlelike crystals (Charcot-Leyden crystals). In some cases the mucoid exudate forms a cast of the airways. These casts, which may be coughed up, are known as "Curschmann's spirals." The epithelium displays a loss of the normal pseudostratified appearance and may be denuded, with only the basal cells remaining. The basal cells are hyperplastic, and squamous metaplasia is seen. An increase in goblet cells (goblet cell metaplasia) is also apparent. Characteristically, the epithelial basement membrane is thickened, owing to an increase in collagen deep to the true basal lamina. One of the most typical features of prolonged asthma is the prominence of bronchial smooth muscle, which reflects muscle hyperplasia. The lamina propria contains numerous eosinophils. Edema and thickening of the bronchial walls are common.

PATHOGENESIS OF ASTHMA   The etiology and pathogenesis of asthma are complex. **The two primary features of asthma—namely bronchial muscle contraction and mucus secretion—are under nervous system control.** Stimulation of the parasympathetic nervous system, represented by the vagus nerve, leads to bronchial constriction and hypersecretion of mucus. The sympathetic nervous system, through beta-adrenergic receptors, mediates bronchial dilatation and, less certainly, diminished mucus secretion. In addition, there is the nonadrenergic (purinergic) inhibitory system that causes relaxation of the airway smooth muscle.

Numerous mediators released from inflammatory cells or from mast cells result in bronchoconstriction, including histamine; bradykinin; leukotrienes C, D, and E; prostaglandins B_2, F_2, and G_2; and thromboxane A_2. Some of these mediators also increase capillary permeability. Other agents are chemoattractants, for example, eosinophil and neutrophil chemotactic factors of anaphylaxis and leukotriene B_4.

The simplest theory of asthma invokes hypersensitivity. The patient becomes sensitized to an antigen, the antibodies to which are IgE of the mast cells. The inhaled antigen binds to its IgE antibody, after which the mast cells release their contents. These in turn produce bronchial smooth muscle contraction, edema, and release of other mediators that amplify the response. In addition, the products of mast cells stimulate irritant receptors, which induces reflex bronchial constriction and mucus hypersecretion via the vagus nerve. How do the antigens sensitize the mast cells and how do the antigens reach them to trigger the reaction? Since bronchial epithelial cells are connected by tight junctions, loosening of the junctions may be a prerequisite for the appearance of asthma. Such loosening may reflect damage caused by infections, environmental irritants, and tobacco smoke-mediated inflammation. Mast cells and afferent nerves are present in the surface epithelium. Thus, when the antigen binds to its antibody, epithelial leakiness is amplified and a reflex stimulation occurs. Easier access to the submucosa is then possible, and both direct and reflex actions on smooth muscle occur. Other possible factors are inherent defects, including leakiness of the epithelium; inadequate sympathetic nervous system inhibitory action (beta-adrenergic blockade); and excessive cholinergic reactivity. In summary, one may envisage the pathogenesis of asthma at two extremes. At one extreme, it is mediated entirely through allergens in spite of a healthy epithelium; at the other, a variety of nonspecific stimuli acts on a severely compromised epithelium. In most cases, there is probably a combination of the two. In any event it seems that there is a final common pathway for all types of asthma, as evidenced by the similarity of lesions.

Bronchiolitis

The terms "small airways," "peripheral airways," and "bronchioles" are often considered synonymous, but they are not. Bronchioles are precisely defined as conducting airways that do not exhibit cartilage in the walls and do not contain gas-exchanging structures (the alveoli). The term "small airways" is used to describe both the smallest bronchi and the bronchioles, and "peripheral airways" has a similar but even less precise connotation. Lesions in these airways play a significant role in chronic airflow obstruction; the term "small airways" disease is used to describe them. **We use the term "bronchiolitis" because it involves specific structures and because the lesions are due to inflammation and its consequences. Bronchiolitis is almost always related to cigarette smoking and occurs in patients with the usual features of chronic airflow obstruction.**

MILD   CHRONIC   AIRFLOW   OBSTRUCTION   Chronic bronchiolar inflammation is the important association with mild chronic airflow obstruction. The inflammation consists of an increased number of lymphocytes (plasma cells with an occasional neutrophil). **Inflammation may induce fibrosis and nar-**

rowing of bronchioles, further compounding airflow obstruction. Goblet cell metaplasia is related to airflow obstruction. Respiratory bronchiolitis is also a significant cause of mild chronic airflow obstruction.

SEVERE CHRONIC AIRFLOW OBSTRUCTION **The consequences of inflammation, notably severe narrowing of the airways with an excess of very small bronchioles (less than 400 μm in diameter), become more important.** Goblet cell metaplasia is also important, but inflammation, fibrosis, and increased muscle are less significant. In patients with severe emphysema, the bronchioles become distorted by irregular narrowing, a condition that results in airway obstruction.

Bronchiectasis

Bronchiectasis **is defined as permanent abnormal dilatation of bronchi.** It is usually thought of as a disease of large airways because this is the location of the obvious lesions. However, the origin in most instances lies in the obliteration of peripheral airways. Often the cause is clearly obstruction of central bronchi by inhaled foreign bodies, tumor, mucus plugs in asthma, and compressive lymphadenopathy. Bronchiectasis is also a feature of cystic fibrosis.

One-half to two-thirds of all cases of bronchiectasis follow a bronchopulmonary infection, hence the term "post-infective bronchiectasis." At present, the most common cause of bronchiectasis is adenovirus infection. The disease is brought about by a severe inflammation of bronchi and bronchioles, which results in destruction of the walls of the central bronchi and obliteration of peripheral bronchi and bronchioles. With the consequent collapse of lung parenchyma (atelectasis), the bronchi dilate. Inflammation in the central airways leads to hypersecretion of mucus and abnormalities of the surface epithelium, including an increased number of goblet cells. A vicious cycle is set up because a pool of mucus is liable to further infection, which leads to progressive destruction of the bronchial walls.

Bronchiectasis is most common in the lower lobes, the left more commonly involved than the right; it is usually bilateral. The dilated bronchi contain thick, mucopurulent secretions. Microscopically, there is destruction of all components of the bronchial wall, chronic inflammation, a disproportionate number of goblet cells, and squamous metaplasia of the epithelium. The distal bronchi and bronchioles are scarred and often obliterated.

Bronchiectasis often complicates **cystic fibrosis,** a heritable disorder affecting mucus secretion and eccrine sweat glands. Pulmonary complications are the most serious manifestation of cystic fibrosis. The bronchial mucus is thick and patients are particularly liable to infection with *Pseudomonas aeruginosa.* The resulting bronchial and bronchiolar obliteration lead to bronchiectasis.

LESIONS IN THE LUNG PARENCHYMA

The acinus is distal to the last conducting airway, the terminal bronchiole (Fig. 12-14). It begins with respiratory bronchioles, which have both alveolated and nonalveolated walls, with progressively more alveoli distally. Respiratory bronchioles are succeeded by conducting structures that are entirely alveolated (alveolar ducts), which then end in the alveolar sacs.

Airflow obstruction results from disease of the acinus, including inflammation of respiratory bronchioles (respiratory bronchiolitis), which may be associated with mild abnormalities of expiratory flow in cigarette smokers.

The most important consequence of involvement of the acinus is emphysema, which has been shown to be the most significant cause of chronic airflow obstruction. Airspace enlargement occurs in conditions other than emphysema, as detailed in Table 12-2.

Emphysema

Emphysema is defined as **a condition of the lung characterized by abnormal permanent enlargement of the airspaces distal to the terminal bronchiole, accompanied by destruction of their walls without obvious fibrosis.** Emphysema is classified in anatomic terms, but the classification should not obscure the fact that **the severity of emphysema is more important than the type.** In practical terms, as emphysema becomes more severe it becomes more difficult to classify, a situation similar to that of endstage renal disease or cirrhosis of the liver. Emphysema is common, being found in about half of all autopsies.

PROXIMAL ACINAR (CENTRIACINAR) EMPHYSEMA The proximal part of the acinus (respiratory bronchioles) is selectively or predominantly involved in centriacinar emphysema, of which there are two forms (see Fig. 12-14). **Centrilobular emphysema** is the common form of emphysema in nonindustrial populations; **focal emphysema** is recognized in dusty occupations, such as coal mining (coal workers' emphysema or simple pneumoconiosis).

Centrilobular emphysema, which involves the proximal part of the acinus, is the form of the disease most frequently encountered and the one usually associated with clinical symptoms (see Fig. 12-14). **It is associated with, and probably due to, tobacco smoking.** The de-

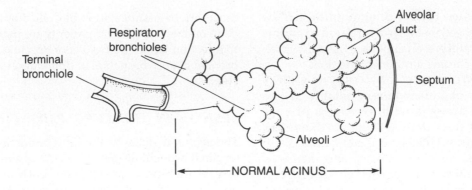

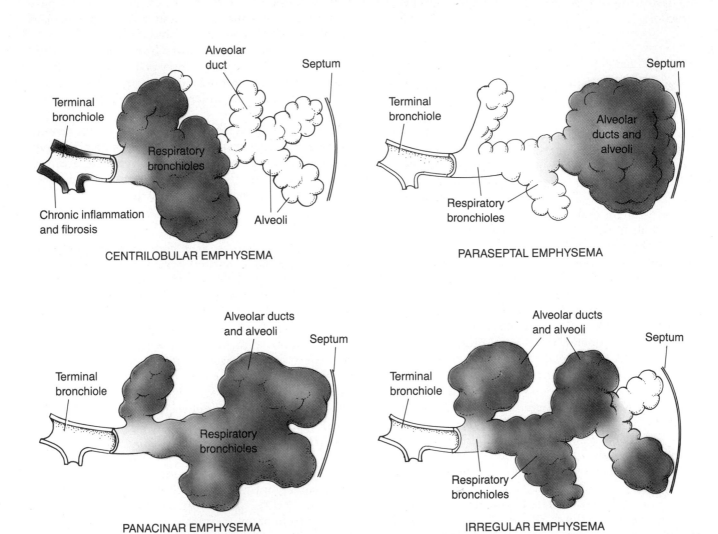

Figure 12-14. Types of emphysema. The acinus is the unit gas-exchanging structure of the lung distal to the terminal bronchiole. It consists of, in order, respiratory bronchioles, alveolar ducts, alveolar sacs, and alveoli. In **centrilobular (proximal acinar) emphysema** the respiratory bronchioles are predominantly involved. In **paraseptal (distal acinar) emphysema** the alveolar ducts are particularly affected. In **panacinar (panlobular) emphysema** the acinus is uniformly damaged. In **irregular emphysema** the acinus is irregularly enlarged and destroyed. There usually is significant fibrosis, so that the condition may be termed **airspace enlargement with fibrosis.**

═══════════════════════════	

Table 12-2 Types of Airspace Enlargement

Simple Airspace Enlargement
Congenital
Acquired

Emphysema (Fig. 12-15)
Proximal acinar (centriacinar) emphysema
Panacinar (panlobular) emphysema
Distal acinar (paraseptal) emphysema

Airspace Enlargement With Fibrosis
Associated with focal scars in the lung
Associated with interstitial pneumonia and honeycombing

stroyed and enlarged respiratory bronchioles form airspaces that are separated from each other and from lobular septa by normal alveolar ducts and sacs. As the lesion progresses, these distal structures may also be involved. The bronchioles proximal to the emphysematous spaces are inflamed and narrowed. **Centrilobular emphysema is most common and most severe in the upper zones of the lung.** It occurs much more often in men than in women and is often associated with chronic bronchitis.

Working with coal, whether as a miner or in other ways, results in an accumulation of coal dust in macrophages in and around respiratory bronchioles. Mild dilatation of respiratory bronchioles results, probably from atrophy of muscle. This condition is called **coal pneumoconiosis. The lesion resembles centrilobular emphysema, but differs in that the enlarged spaces are smaller and more regular, and inflammation of bronchioles is not apparent. Thus, the lesion is primarily distensive rather than destructive.** The anatomic lesion is usually equated with a chest radiograph that shows small nodular densities, although the complete correlation has not been proved. The condition, also referred to as **black lung,** has been considered to cause severe disability. Contemporary evidence, however, suggests that simple coal pneumoconiosis causes only minor impairment of pulmonary function.

PANACINAR EMPHYSEMA The acinus is uniformly involved in panacinar emphysema (see Fig. 12-14). All parts of the acinus are destroyed and in the final stage a lacy network of supporting tissue is left behind (the "cotton candy lung"). Panacinar emphysema occurs in several different situations.

FAMILIAL EMPHYSEMA Familial emphysema is **usually due to a defect in circulating α_1-antiproteinase.** The amount and type of α_1-proteinase is determined by a pair of co-antidominant alleles, referred to

as Pi (proteinase inhibitor). The most common phenotype is PiM (referred to as such since PiMO and PiMM cannot be distinguished). Over 30 different alleles are now recognized. The most serious abnormality is associated with the PiZ allele, which occurs in some 5% of the population. The PiZ allele is most common in those of Scandinavian origin, and is rare in Jews, blacks, and Japanese. The phenotype PiZ (ZZ or ZO) is associated with very low levels of circulating antiproteinase inhibitor, which also has an abnormal electrophoretic mobility. **People with this phenotype often develop cirrhosis of the liver in infancy and emphysema as adults.** The majority of all patients with **clinically** diagnosed emphysema under the age of 40 have α_1-antiproteinase deficiency (PiZ).

PANACINAR EMPHYSEMA IN ASSOCIATION WITH CENTRILOBULAR EMPHYSEMA Panacinar emphysema is often associated with centrilobular emphysema. In such cases, the panacinar form tends to occur in the lower zones of the lung, whereas centrilobular emphysema is seen in the upper ones. The associations are the same as for centrilobular emphysema alone, notably cigarette smoking, chronic bronchitis, and chronic airflow obstruction.

CLINICAL FEATURES OF EMPHYSEMA The frequency of chronic bronchitis increases with the severity of emphysema, and almost all patients with severe emphysema have chronic bronchitis. Although it was once thought that chronic bronchitis leads to emphysema, **it is now recognized that chronic bronchitis and emphysema share a common etiologic agent, namely tobacco smoke.** Patients usually present to their physician between 55 and 60 years of age with dyspnea of insidious onset.

ETIOLOGY AND PATHOGENESIS OF EMPHYSEMA Conclusive evidence now exists that the major cause of emphysema is tobacco smoking, especially cigarette smoking. Moderate to severe emphysema is rarely found in nonsmokers. The dominant hypothesis concerning the pathogenesis of emphysema is the proteolysis-antiproteolysis theory (Fig. 12-15). It is now thought that there is a balance between elastin synthesis and catabolism in the lung. If elastolytic activity increases or antielastolytic activity decreases, emphysema results. Increased numbers of neutrophils, which contain serine elastase, are found in the bronchoalveolar lavage fluid of smokers. Smoking also reduces the α_1-antiproteinase activity in the lung, owing to the oxidation of methionine residues in α_1-antiproteinase. In this way, **unopposed and increased elastolytic activity leads to emphysema.** Although the proteolysis-antiproteolysis theory is attractive, it awaits further confirmation.

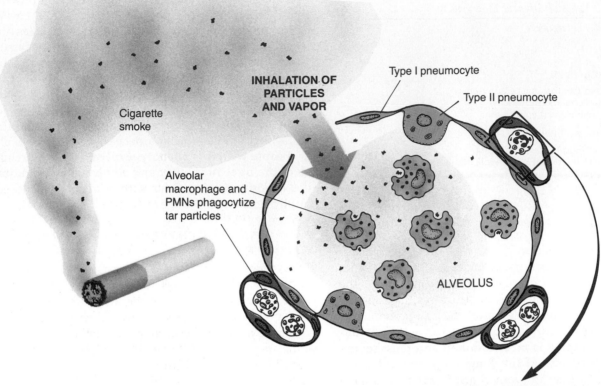

Cigarette smoke

INHALATION OF PARTICLES AND VAPOR

Type I pneumocyte

Type II pneumocyte

Alveolar macrophage and PMNs phagocytize tar particles

ALVEOLUS

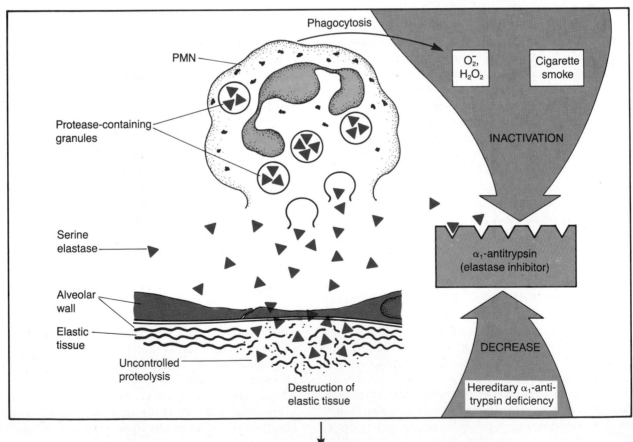

Phagocytosis

PMN

O_2^-, H_2O_2

Cigarette smoke

INACTIVATION

Protease-containing granules

Serine elastase

α_1-antitrypsin (elastase inhibitor)

Alveolar wall

Elastic tissue

Uncontrolled proteolysis

DECREASE

Hereditary α_1-antitrypsin deficiency

Destruction of elastic tissue

EMPHYSEMA

PNEUMOCONIOSIS

The pneumoconioses are diseases caused by the inhalation of inorganic dusts and represent a subset of occupational lung disease, which also includes disorders caused by the inhalation of gases, vapors, and organic material. The many forms of pneumoconiosis have specific names, depending on the substance inhaled (e.g., silicosis, asbestosis, talcosis). In certain instances the offending agent is uncertain and often the occupation is simply cited (e.g., "arc welder's lung"). Historically, occupations were recognized as predisposing to lung disease before an etiologic agent was recognized. Thus the term "knife grinder's lung" was used before this malady was recognized as silicosis.

The most important pathogenetic feature of inhaled dusts, namely their ability to produce fibrosis, is variable (Fig. 12-16). Thus, small amounts of silica or asbestos may produce extensive fibrosis, but coal and iron are weakly fibrogenic at best. In general, lung lesions reflect the dose and size of the particle delivered to the lung. The dose is a function of the amount of dust in the ambient air and the time spent working in the environment. It is important to express size as **aerodynamic particle diameter,** a parameter that describes the way the particle moves in air. The aerodynamic particle diameter determines where the inhaled dusts deposit in the lung (Fig. 12-17), the most dangerous being those that reach the peripheral part of the lung, the smallest bronchioles and the acini. The great majority of large particles (more than 10 μm) are filtered by the nasopharynx and never reach the lower respiratory tract. Most particles 2 to 10 μm in diameter deposit on the bronchi and bronchioles and are removed by the mucociliary escalator.

Whereas the smaller particles terminate in the acinus, the minute ones behave as a gas and are exhaled. The alveolar macrophages, which ingest the inhaled particles, constitute the primary defense mechanism of the alveolar space. Most of these particles ascend to the mucociliary carpet. Others migrate into the interstitium of the lung and then into the lymphatics. A significant number accumulate in the respiratory "sump," in and about respiratory bronchioles and terminal bronchioles.

An important concept in the understanding of pneumoconiosis is that of **individual susceptibility,** which reflects differences in airway anatomy and function, particle clearance, defense mechanisms, and immunologic reactivity.

SILICOSIS

Silicosis is caused by the inhalation of silicon dioxide, of which there are three molecular configurations. The most important is quartz, and the others are crystobalite and trydimite. Silicon dioxide, often referred to as "free silica," has the distinction of producing the best-known and the most widespread pneumoconiosis.

Silicosis is acquired, notoriously, in sandblasting. Mining also involves exposure to silica, as do numerous other occupations, including stone cutting, polishing and sharpening of metals, ceramic manufacturing, foundry work, and the cleaning of boilers.

It was originally thought that the varying degrees of fibrosis associated with different forms of silica reflected differing solubilities. The popular view today is that following the ingestion of silica, macrophages produce a fibroblast stimulating factor. Because of the toxicity of silica, the macrophage dies, thereby releasing the ingested silica and the fibroblast stimulating factor (see Fig. 12-16). The silica is then reingested by macrophages and the process is amplified.

Simple Nodular Silicosis

Simple nodular silicosis is the most common form of silicosis and is almost inevitable in any worker chronically exposed to silica. The lungs contain silicotic nodules (always less than 1 cm in diameter, and usually 2 to 4 mm in diameter) that, on histologic examination, have a characteristic whorled appearance, with concentrically arranged collagen that forms the largest part of the nodule. At the periphery there are aggregates of mononuclear cells, mostly lymphocytes, and fibroblasts. Hilar nodes become enlarged and calcified,

Figure 12-15. The proteolysis-antiproteolysis theory of the pathogenesis of emphysema. Cigarette (tobacco) smoking is closely related to the development of emphysema. Some product in tobacco smoke induces an inflammatory reaction. The serine elastase in polymorphonuclear leukocytes, which is a particularly potent elastolytic agent, injures the elastic tissue of the lung. Normally, this enzyme activity is inhibited by α_1-antitrypsin, but tobacco smoke, directly or through the generation of free radicals, inactivates α_1-antitrypsin (proteinase inhibitor).

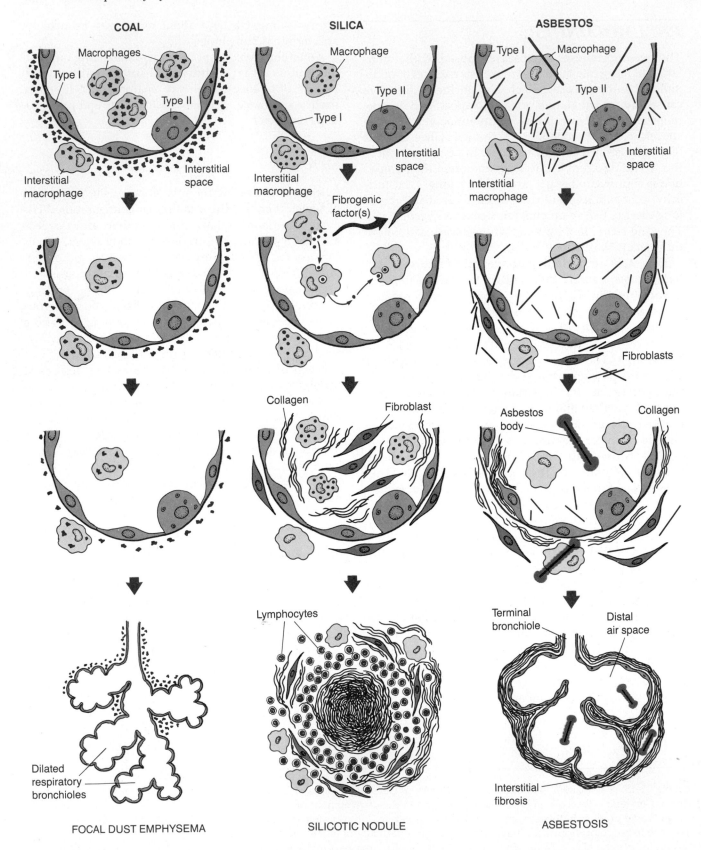

COAL

Macrophages

Type I

Type II

Interstitial macrophage

Interstitial space

SILICA

Macrophage

Type II

Type I

Interstitial macrophage

Interstitial space

Fibrogenic factor(s)

Collagen

Fibroblast

Lymphocytes

ASBESTOS

Type I   Macrophage

Type II

Interstitial macrophage

Interstitial space

Fibroblasts

Asbestos body

Collagen

Terminal bronchiole

Distal air space

Interstitial fibrosis

Dilated respiratory bronchioles

FOCAL DUST EMPHYSEMA

SILICOTIC NODULE

ASBESTOSIS

often at the periphery of the node ("eggshell calcification"). Simple silicosis is not usually associated with significant disability, as assessed by pulmonary function.

Progressive Massive Fibrosis

Progressive massive fibrosis (PMF) is defined radiologically as nodular masses of more than 1 cm diameter in a background of simple silicosis. Most of these lesions are considerably larger than 1 cm (5 to 10 cm) in diameter and are usually located in the upper zones of the lung. Morphologically, the lesions often exhibit central necrosis, although in some instances they consist of aggregates of nodules of simple silicosis ("conglomerate silicosis").

PMF was thought to be due to the combination of silicosis and tuberculosis. However, most observers give less importance to the tuberculous theory of PMF now than was once the case. PMF is now recognized to be related to the amount of silica in the lung. Disability is caused by the destruction of lung tissue that has been incorporated into the nodules.

LUNG DISORDERS IN COAL WORKERS

Simple Coal Pneumoconiosis

Simple coal pneumoconiosis has been discussed in the section on emphysema. Mild, predominantly distensive enlargement of respiratory bronchioles (see Fig. 12-16) is associated with mild abnormalities of pulmonary function. Radiologic examination shows small nodular opacities or linear opacities.

Progressive Massive Fibrosis

Progressive massive fibrosis (PMF) in coal miners has been referred to in the section on silicosis. The size and location of the lesions are similar to those in PMF of

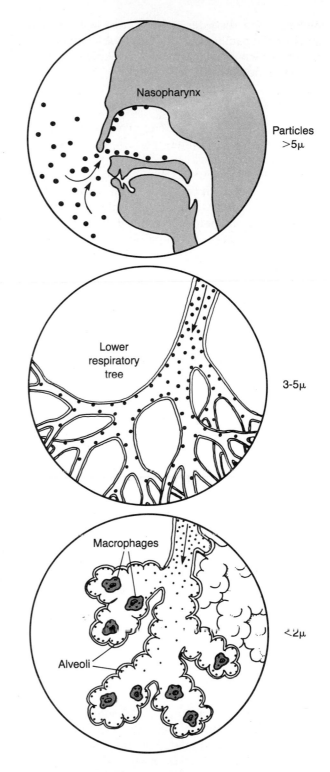

Figure 12-16. Pathogenesis of pneumoconioses. The three most important pneumoconioses are illustrated. In simple **coal pneumoconiosis,** massive amounts of dust are inhaled and engulfed by macrophages. The macrophages pass into the interstitium of the lung and aggregate around the respiratory bronchioles. Subsequently, the bronchioles dilate. In **silicosis,** the silica particles are toxic to macrophages, which die and release a fibrogenic factor. In turn the released silica is again phagocytosed by other macrophages. The result is a dense fibrotic nodule, the silicotic nodule. **Asbestosis** is characterized by little dust and much interstitial fibrosis. Asbestos bodies are the classic feature.

Figure 12-17. Deposition of particles in the respiratory tract. Large particles are trapped in the nose. Intermediate-sized particles deposit on the bronchi and bronchioles and are removed by the mucociliary blanket. Smaller particles terminate in the airspaces and are removed by macrophages. Very small particles behave as a gas and are breathed out.

silicosis. The disorder is associated with significant functional disability, and there is usually an obstructive defect, which may or may not be associated with a restrictive defect.

Pathogenesis of Coal Pneumoconiosis

The role of silica in coal pneumoconiosis has long been controversial. Coal miners are often exposed to substantial amounts of silica, and the term *anthracosilicosis* was widely used. (Anthracite is a form of coal.) It was subsequently shown that those who worked only with coal (e.g., trimmers who loaded only coal) developed only simple coal pneumoconiosis. It has been suggested that the aggregates of coal particles in macrophages in the walls of respiratory bronchioles weaken the respiratory bronchiolar muscle, thus leading to dilatation. Coal miners who have also been exposed to high levels of silica have silicotic nodules in the lung that are heavily pigmented with coal.

ASBESTOS PNEUMOCONIOSIS

Asbestos is a generic term that embraces the silicate minerals that occur as long, thin fibers. They conduct heat poorly and are thus important in insulation. The three major forms of asbestos are crocidolite, which comes mainly from South Africa; chrysotile, the most common form of asbestos, most of which is mined in Quebec; and amosite. **If coal is the classic example of much dust and little fibrosis, asbestos is the prototype of little dust and much fibrosis** (see Fig. 12-16). Most clinically obvious cases occur as a result of the processing and handling of asbestos, rather than in mining, which is a surface operation. Exposure starts with the baggers who package asbestos and continues with those who modify or use it, such as workers who make asbestos products (tiles, cement, insulation material) and those in the construction and shipbuilding industries.

Asbestosis

Classic asbestosis is an interstitial fibrosis of the lung. The features are in general similar to those described in fibrosing alveolitis (usual interstitial pneumonia), as described later. The first lesion is an alveolitis that is directly related to asbestos exposure. Asbestos fibers are long (up to 100 μm) but thin (0.5 to 1 μm), so that their aerodynamic particle diameter is small. They deposit particularly at the bifurcations of alveolar ducts. The smallest particles are engulfed by macrophages, but many submicroscopic particles lie free in the interstitium of the lung. The most diagnostic

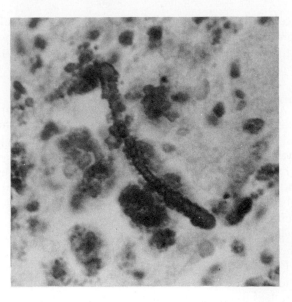

Figure 12-18. Asbestos body. A typical asbestos body has bulbous ends and a beaded body. It is about 75 μm long (for comparison, the visible nuclei are 10 to 15 μm in diameter).

structure is the **asbestos body** (Fig. 12-18), which consists of an asbestos fiber (10 to 50 μm in length) that has beaded aggregates of iron along its length. By light microscopy it is golden brown with hematoxylin and eosin; it stains strongly with the Prussian blue reaction for iron. In the early stages, asbestosis differs from usual interstitial pneumonia in that the fibrosis occurs in and around alveolar ducts, as well as in the periphery of the acinus. As the lesion progresses, honeycombing (end-stage lung) results, as in terminal usual interstitial pneumonia. Asbestosis is usually more severe in the lower zones of the lung. Pleural thickening is often conspicuous.

Pleural Plaques

Pleural plaques are nodular, localized thickenings (2 to 3 mm) of the pleura, most often found in the parietal pleura. The margins are irregular and the size varies from a few millimeters to several centimeters across. Microscopically, they are densely collagenous, with interwoven bands of collagen ("basket-weave" pattern), and are sometimes calcified. Pleural plaques are usually an incidental finding in patients with occupational exposure to substantial amounts of asbestos, but such plaques are not uncommon in people with casual exposure.

Mesothelioma

A clear-cut relationship between asbestos exposure and malignant mesothelioma is now firmly established. Sometimes the exposure is slight, as in the wives of asbestos workers who wash their husbands' clothes. More often mesothelioma is found in workers heavily exposed to asbestos, predominantly of the crocidolite variety. The clinical and pathologic features of this disease are discussed with diseases of the pleura.

Carcinoma of the Lung and Other Organs

Carcinoma of the lung has been reported to be about three to five times more common in nonsmoking asbestos workers than in nonsmoking workers not exposed to asbestos, although this figure remains to be firmly established. In asbestos workers who smoke, the incidence of carcinoma of the lung is vastly increased, the risk being 60 to 80 times greater than in the general nonsmoking population.

OTHER PNEUMOCONIOSES

More than 40 inhaled minerals cause lung lesions and x-ray abnormalities. Most, such as tin, barium, and iron, are relatively innocuous and accumulate in the lung in the same way as coal, but do not produce morphologic or functional abnormalities. Others are the causes of uncommon pneumoconioses, such as beryllosis (beryllium) or talcosis (talc), which may or may not cause disability.

RESTRICTIVE, INFILTRATIVE, OR INTERSTITIAL LUNG DISEASE

More than 100 disorders are conveniently considered together because they have a similar clinical and radiologic presentation. Clinically, the patients present with shortness of breath, often associated with cough. Clubbing of the fingers is common in the advanced stage. Inspiratory crackles ("Velcro" rales) are heard at the bases. Chest radiographs have small linear and punctate opacities (Fig. 12-19). As the condition progresses, cystlike spaces become apparent. Lung volume is reduced because the lung is stiff (decreased compliance). The fibrosis is associated with increased elastic recoil, a condition that makes the airways more patent and is the driving force to increased flow rates. The diffusing capacity for oxygen is decreased and the alveolar-arterial oxygen gradient is increased. Typically, the latter increases further on exercise, hence the older

term "alveolar-arterial capillary block syndrome." Because of the reduction in lung volume, clinicians often refer to the condition as "restrictive lung disease," whereas the radiologic appearance leads radiologists to use the term "interstitial lung disease." Many of the conditions progress to "honeycomb" or "end-stage" lung.

SARCOIDOSIS

Sarcoidosis, a disease that has eluded a satisfactory definition, is characterized by multiple, uniform, discrete, noncaseating granulomas in almost any organ of the body. The lymph nodes and the lung are most commonly involved (Fig. 12-20). The central part of the granuloma is fibrotic and surrounded by palisaded histiocytes. Giant cells at the periphery resemble those of tuberculosis.

Histologically, involvement of both lung and lymph nodes occurs in nearly all instances. Multiple sarcoid nodules are scattered in the interstitium, particularly in relation to lymphatics, that is, in the bronchovascular bundle and in the lobular septa.

In North America sarcoidosis occurs much more frequently in blacks than in whites. It is common in Scandinavian countries. Fever, malaise, and weight loss are characteristic, and erythema nodosum is often seen. Eye complications, such as iridocyclitis and uveitis, also occur. The disease also affects the extrathoracic lymph nodes, spleen, and liver. Despite many theories the etiology of sarcoidosis remains uncertain.

THE INTERSTITIAL PNEUMONIAS

A group of conditions known as the chronic interstitial pneumonias can be regarded as one entity or can be subdivided. Various terms have been used for the group, for example, Hamman-Rich disease, fibrosing alveolitis, idiopathic pulmonary fibrosis, and usual interstitial pneumonia. It is important to note that although the various forms of interstitial pneumonia may be morphologically and, to some extent, clinically distinctive, **they all progress to a nonspecific "honeycomb" or "end-stage" lung.** Because of alveolitis and subsequent fibrosis, the distal part of the acinus shrinks (Fig. 12-21). In a sense the lesion represents a form of atelectasis and is the reverse of emphysema. With shrinkage of the lung parenchyma, the bronchioles dilate. Because of epithelial damage the bronchiolar epithelium grows into the dilated airspaces that may have been proximal respiratory bronchioles but are no longer recognized as such. The end stage is character-

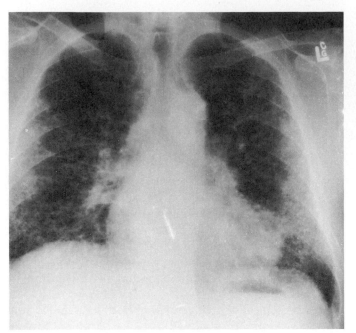

A

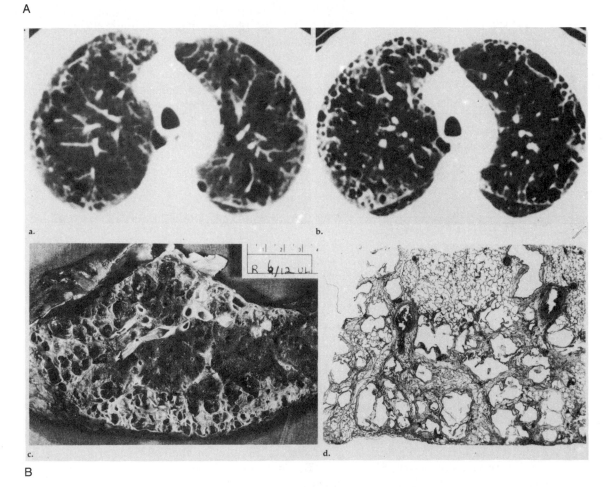

B

Figure 12-19. Usual interstitial pneumonia. A 54-year-old man suffered from worsening shortness of breath on exertion for 5 years. On physical examination he had clubbing of the fingers and late inspiratory crackles. Pulmonary function tests showed severe impairment. (*A*) A chest radiograph shows increased reticulonodular markings and diminished lung volumes. (*B*) A CT scan obtained through the upper lobes shows peripheral honeycombing, as evidenced by the cystic spaces with dense fibrotic (white) walls and minimal involvement of the central lung parenchyma. Changes in the 10-mm collimation scan (a radiographic slice 10 mm thick) (*a*) are more clearly delineated on the 1.5-mm scan (*b*) because the images are not superimposed. The cystic spaces and fibrotic walls can be seen more clearly in *b*. (*c*) A macroscopic specimen of the right upper lobe cut at the level of the CT scan shows dense peripheral honeycombing. (*d*) A low-power microscopic view of the specimen shows irregular subpleural fibrosis, with cysts 2 to 10 mm in diameter.

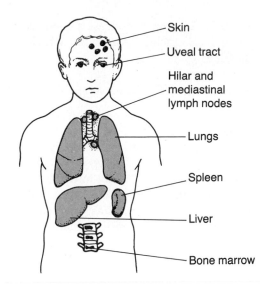

Figure 12-20. Organs commonly affected by sarcoidosis. Sarcoidosis involves many organs, most commonly the lymph nodes and lung.

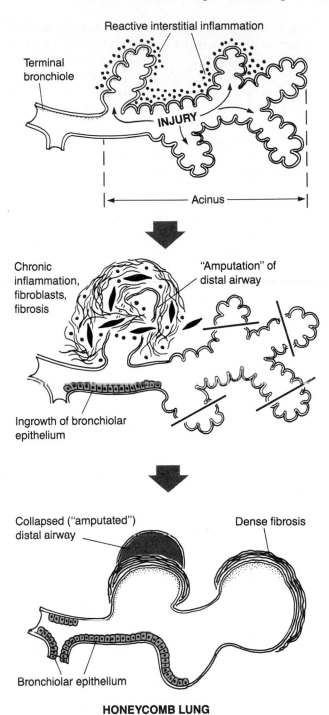

HONEYCOMB LUNG

Figure 12-21. Pathogenesis of honeycomb lung. Honeycomb lung is the end result of a variety of injuries. Interstitial and alveolar inflammation destroys ("amputates") the distal part of the acinus. The proximal parts dilate and become lined by bronchiolar epithelium.

ized by multiple cystlike spaces separated from each other by dense scars (see Figs. 12-19, 12-21). Retraction of the scars, especially of lobular septa, gives the external surface of the lung a hob-nailed appearance, hence the term "pseudocirrhosis."

On histologic examination, the "cysts" (in reality, dilated bronchioles) are found to contain mucus and other debris. Bronchi may also be slightly dilated and irregular. Extensive vascular changes, particularly intimal fibrosis and thickening of the media, are caused by inflammation, fibrosis, and pulmonary hypertension.

Usual Interstitial Pneumonia

Each of the terms **"usual interstitial pneumonia," "cryptogenic fibrosing alveolitis," and "idiopathic pulmonary fibrosis"** stress certain features—the cause is unknown, but alveolar inflammation is an important part of the disease. Fibrosis is the usual sequel, and there may be unusual forms of interstitial pneumonia. The clinical, radiologic, and functional features are those of restrictive lung disease (see Fig 12-19). A useful classification of usual interstitial pneumonia is as follows, but it should be recognized that the morphologic features are the same in each:

Usual interstitial pneumonia associated with collagen vascular diseases. These include rheumatoid arthritis, systemic lupus erythematosus, and progressive systemic sclerosis. About 20% of cases of usual interstitial pneumonia have overt evidence of a connective tissue disease.

Usual interstitial pneumonia associated with serum abnormalities but not with collagen vascular disease. These include cryoglobulinemia, abnormal serum globulins, positive antinuclear antibodies, and positive rheumatoid factor. These abnormalities have been found in up to 40% of cases.

Usual interstitial pneumonia without overt evidence of collagen vascular disease or serum abnormalities.

The key morphologic feature of usual interstitial pneumonia is **heterogeneity of lesions,** that is, different appearances in different parts of the lung, in different lung biopsies, and even in different fields of the same lung biopsy. The variation is so great that in some fields the alveolar walls may actually be entirely normal. Inflammation varies from subtle increased cellularity (mainly lymphocytes) of otherwise apparently normal alveolar walls to diffuse alveolar damage with obvious alveolar wall inflammation and hyperplasia of type II cells. By the time a lung biopsy is performed fibrosis is always present, but its severity varies. Loose granulation tissue in the alveolar spaces leads to alveolar collapse and contraction of fibrous tissue. Eventually the patient is left with "honeycomb" lung.

Interstitial pneumonia is usually diagnosed in the sixth decade. Dyspnea of gradual onset, often over 5 to 10 years, is customary. The prognosis is bleak, with an average survival of 5 years. The response to treatment, usually corticosteroids, is generally poor.

The etiology of usual interstitial pneumonia is not known, but the condition is commonly thought of as an immunologically mediated disorder. Evidence includes (1) the association with collagen-vascular disease and serum protein abnormalities, (2) the presence of circulating immune complexes, (3) the demonstration of immunoglobulins in alveolar walls, and (4) the release of a lymphokine, migration inhibitory factor, when lymphocytes of patients with the disease are exposed to collagen.

According to one theory, macrophages play a central role in the pathogenesis of usual interstitial pneumonia. The initial damage relates to collagen, by an unknown agent. Macrophages engulf collagen fragments and secrete a fibroblast-stimulating factor, thereby leading to fibrosis. They also release a chemotactic factor for polymorphonuclear leukocytes, which then do further damage.

Desquamative Interstitial Pneumonia

Desquamative interstitial pneumonia (DIP) is an uncommon disease characterized by interstitial inflammation and a striking accumulation of macrophages in the alveoli. Opinion is equally divided on whether it is a separate entity or a stage of usual interstitial pneumonia. However, it is important to recognize that desquamative interstitial pneumonia has distinctive clinical features, prognosis, and response to treatment. The patients are younger than those with usual interstitial pneumonia (mean age of 46 years), and the symptoms are of shorter duration (2 to 3 years). Most patients respond to corticosteroid therapy, and survival is at least twice that of usual interstitial pneumonia. On histologic examination, desquamative interstitial pneumonia is diagnosed by the presence of airspaces stuffed with macrophages.

BRONCHIOLITIS OBLITERANS AND ORGANIZING PNEUMONIA

Recently, a clearly defined condition, bronchiolitis obliterans and organizing pneumonia, has been recognized by its histologic features, namely, (1) the presence of bronchiolitis obliterans (i.e., loose granulation tissue in respiratory bronchioles); (2) abundant loose granulation tissue in alveolar ducts and sacs, which resemble the Masson bodies of organizing pneumonia; (3) interstitial pneumonia; (4) diffuse alveolar damage; and (5) interstitial fibrosis of varying severity, but usually mild. Often there is a history of preexisting respiratory infection. This disease entity is important to recognize because its prognosis is good and it responds to corticosteroid treatment.

EXTRINSIC ALLERGIC ALVEOLITIS

Extrinsic allergic alveolitis is a response to inhaled allergens, usually large proteins (Fig. 12-22). The prototype is "farmer's lung," caused by the inhalation of thermophilic actinomycetes. These organisms grow in

Figure 12-22. Extrinsic allergic alveolitis. In extrinsic allergic alveolitis, an antigen-antibody reaction occurs in the acute phase and leads to acute hypersensitivity pneumonitis. If exposure is continued, this is followed by a cellular or subacute phase, with the formation of granulomas and chronic interstitial pneumonitis.

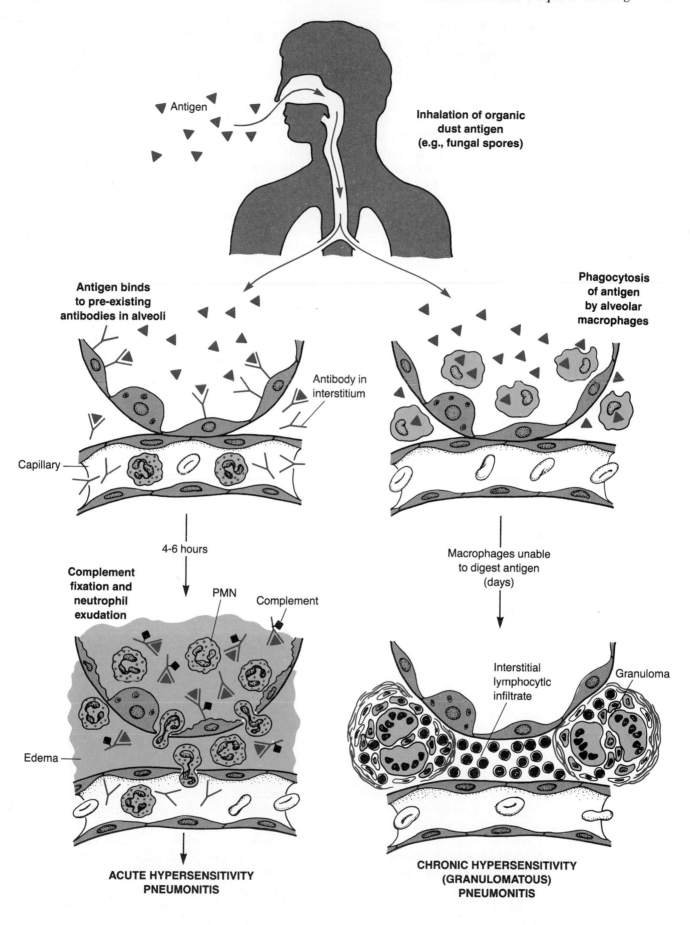

Antigen

Inhalation of organic dust antigen (e.g., fungal spores)

Antigen binds to pre-existing antibodies in alveoli

Phagocytosis of antigen by alveolar macrophages

Antibody in interstitium

Capillary

4-6 hours

Macrophages unable to digest antigen (days)

Complement fixation and neutrophil exudation

PMN   Complement

Interstitial lymphocytic infiltrate

Granuloma

Edema

ACUTE HYPERSENSITIVITY PNEUMONITIS

CHRONIC HYPERSENSITIVITY (GRANULOMATOUS) PNEUMONITIS

moldy hay. Classically, a farmworker enters a barn and in several hours develops tightness in the chest, shortness of breath, cough, and mild fever. The symptoms remit but return on reexposure. With time the symptoms become chronic.

An extensive interstitial pneumonia is characterized by a heavy infiltrate of lymphocytes and a few plasma cells in the alveolar walls. **Most characteristic is the presence of scattered, poorly formed granulomas that contain foreign body giant cells, some of which exhibit doubly refractile material or needlelike clefts.**

Besides material in moldy hay there are more than 20 other substances that produce extrinsic allergic alveolitis. In pigeon breeder's or bird fancier's lung, the antigen is bird protein. The common bird is the parakeet, but chicken handlers also develop the condition. Other rare causes of extrinsic allergic alveolitis include pituitary snuff, fungi in bark (maple bark stripper's lung), cork (suberosis), malt, mushrooms, and detergents. It is important to realize that there may be no apparent antigen exposure and that extrinsic allergic alveolitis may be caused by fungi growing in stagnant water in air conditioners and central heating units. It is essential to distinguish extrinsic allergic alveolitis from usual interstitial pneumonia because removal of the antigen is the only adequate treatment.

WEGENER'S GRANULOMATOSIS

As originally described, Wegener's granulomatosis consisted of a triad of **systemic necrotizing vasculitis, necrotizing granulomas of the respiratory tract, and glomerulonephritis.** It is today regarded as a variant of necrotizing angiitis. Wegener's granulomatosis most commonly affects middle-aged men. The presenting symptoms include sinusitis, middle ear disease, and nonspecific respiratory symptoms. Radiologic examination shows single or, more commonly, multiple intrapulmonary nodules, some of which may cavitate. Ocular and skin lesions are also frequent.

Glomerulonephritis is usual in Wegener's granulomatosis and is generally rapidly progressive. A dramatic improvement in prognosis has resulted from cytotoxic therapy, changing a formerly fatal condition to one with a 90% to 95% remission rate.

The lesions in the respiratory tract show necrotizing granulomas, characteristically with serpiginous margins, in which there are numerous bizarre giant cells. Necrotizing vasculitis involves the branches of the pulmonary arteries or the systemic arteries in the respiratory tract and helps to establish the diagnosis. Focal glomerular necrosis and crescent formation are seen in the kidneys.

DISEASES OF THE PLEURA

PNEUMOTHORAX

Pneumothorax is defined as the presence of air in the pleural cavity. It may be due to traumatic perforation of the pleura or may be spontaneous. Traumatic causes include penetrating wounds of the chest wall (e.g., a stab wound and rib fractures). However, traumatic pneumothorax is most commonly iatrogenic and is seen after aspiration of fluid from the pleura, pleural or lung biopsy, transbronchial biopsy, and assisted ventilation with interstitial emphysema.

Spontaneous pneumothorax is typically encountered in young adults. For example, while exercising vigorously a tall young man develops acute chest pain and shortness of breath. A chest radiograph shows collapse of the lung on the side of the pain and a large collection of air in the pleural space. The condition is due to rupture of emphysematous lesions through the pleura. These lesions are usually placed superficially and superiorly in the lung. In most cases, spontaneous pneumothorax subsides by itself with or without aspiration of the air. In other instances large amounts of air accumulate in the pleural cavity, and there may be a shift of the mediastinum to the opposite side, with compression of the opposite lung. This situation is referred to as "tension pneumothorax" and implies that the pressure is positive in the pleural space. The condition may be life-threatening and must be relieved by immediate drainage. Spontaneous pneumothorax may also complicate widespread emphysema in the middle-aged and, rarely, other lung conditions, such as tumors.

PLEURAL EFFUSION

Normally, only a small amount of fluid in the pleural cavity lubricates the space between the lung and the chest wall. **Pleural effusion** is a term that describes the accumulation of fluid in the pleural cavity. It is subdivided according to the appearance of the effusion. The severity varies, from a few milliliters of fluid detected radiologically only as obliteration of the costophrenic angle to a massive accumulation of fluid that shifts the mediastinum and the trachea to the opposite side (Fig. 12-23).

Hydrothorax refers to an effusion that resembles water and would be regarded as edema elsewhere. It may be due to increased hydrostatic pressure within the capillaries, as is commonly found in patients with heart failure and in any condition that produces systemic or pulmonary edema. In this form of effusion the protein level is less than 3 g/dl, the number of white

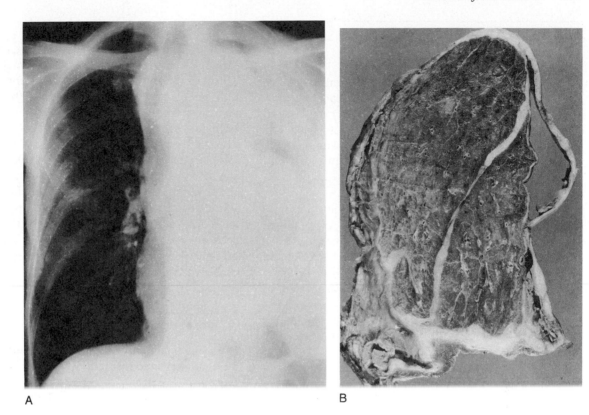

A   B

Figure 12-23. Mesothelioma. A 54-year-old former shipyard worker presented with shortness of breath of 3 months duration. (*A*) A chest radiograph shows a massive left pleural effusion. Note that the trachea and bronchus are displaced to the right, away from the effusion. (*B*) At autopsy extensive mesothelioma surrounds the lung and extends into the major fissure.

cells is low, and the glucose level is close to that of the blood.

Whatever the cause, this type of effusion is referred to as a **transudate.** By contrast, fluid that accumulates in the pleural cavity because of increased capillary permeability is referred to as an **exudate.** The common cause of hydrothorax due to exudation is low-grade inflammation, such as that associated with tumor or tuberculosis. Typically, protein levels are more than 3 g/dl, glucose levels are low, and the cellular content is high. The pleural fluid content of lactate dehydrogenase (LDH) is often used as an indicator of inflammation. **A ratio of pleural fluid: plasma LDH of more than 0.6 is considered indicative of an exudate.**

A turbid effusion that contains many polymorphonuclear leukocytes is referred to as **pyothorax** and results from acute inflammation and infections of the pleura. Commonly, it is a complication of bacterial pneumonia that extends to the pleural surface, the classic example of which is pneumococcal pneumonia. **Empyema** should be thought of as a variant of pyo-

thorax in which the inflammation is both more severe and chronic, with accumulation of thick pus within the pleural cavity, often with loculation and fibrosis. Empyema has the same causes as pyothorax.

Hemothorax is the accumulation of blood in the pleural cavity. This may occur because of trauma and is usually due to bleeding from systemic (intercostal) vessels. Most commonly, a pleural effusion is blood-stained. The common causes are tuberculosis, malignancy involving the pleura, and infarction of the lung.

PLEURITIS

As the name indicates, pleuritis means inflammation of the pleura and is thus frequently associated with pleural effusion. The causes are the same as for pyothorax, but other causes, such as viral infection and pulmonary embolus, are important. Symptoms are usually evident, the most striking being sharp, stabbing chest pain on inspiration.

MESOTHELIOMA

MALIGNANT MESOTHELIOMA

As mentioned earlier, most cases of pleural malignant mesothelioma are related to asbestos exposure. This disease is most commonly encountered in middle-aged men exposed to asbestos, even for a short time. The patient often presents with a pleural effusion (see Fig 12-23A) or a pleural mass, chest pain, dyspnea, and nonspecific symptoms, such as weight loss and malaise.

Characteristically, mesotheliomas exhibit a biphasic histologic appearance. The cells derived from mesothelium form glands and tubules that resemble adenocarcinoma, whereas the malignant cells that originate from the connective tissue deep in the mesothelial surface resemble a fibrosarcoma. On gross examination, the tumor classically encases the lung, extends into fissures and interlobar septa (see Fig. 12-23B), and compresses the lung. Treatment is ineffective and the prognosis is hopeless.

DISEASES OF PULMONARY VASCULATURE

PULMONARY EMBOLISM

The most common lesion of the pulmonary vasculature is pulmonary embolism, and the most common emboli are thrombi derived from the leg veins. Thromboemboli are found in one-quarter to one-third of random autopsies when a thorough search of the pulmonary vasculature is made. They are most common in circumstances in which there is a tendency to increased venous thrombosis, for instance, when venous blood flow is diminished, as in heart failure, prolonged bed rest, or traumatic injury. The most common sources of thromboembolism are the deep veins of the calf, followed by those of the thigh.

SUDDEN DEATH

The most dramatic consequence of pulmonary embolism is sudden death. The classic scenario involves a patient who suddenly drops dead several days after surgery, sometimes while sitting on the toilet. At autopsy a large embolus is commonly found in the main pulmonary artery, occluding both right and left pulmonary arteries (saddle embolus). However, a single pulmonary artery or even a segmental pulmonary artery may be found to be occluded.

INFARCTION OF THE LUNG

As with other organs, occlusion of a pulmonary artery or a branch thereof may result in death of tissue. The lung differs from most other organs in that it has a dual circulation with both systemic (bronchial artery) and nonsystemic (pulmonary artery) contributions. The bronchial arteries supply the airways to about the terminal bronchiolar level, but actual and potential anastomoses exist between the two systems. **As a consequence, pulmonary infarcts are often hemorrhagic in the acute phase because the bronchial artery pumps blood into the infarcted area.** On gross examination, such infarcts are usually pyramidal (triangular in cross section), with the base at the pleura. With the passage of time the blood in the infarct is resorbed and the center of the infarct becomes pale.

PULMONARY EMBOLISM WITHOUT INFARCTION

Pulmonary thromboemboli are frequently found at autopsy without infarcts. Pulmonary embolism without infarction is explained by the bronchial artery collateral circulation, which keeps lung tissue viable.

MULTIPLE RECURRENT PULMONARY THROMBOEMBOLI

Multiple thromboemboli, usually to small pulmonary artery branches, may detach from peripheral veins. They become organized, occlude the pulmonary arterial system, and are a cause of pulmonary hypertension (see later).

FAT EMBOLISM

Fat embolism is the most common form of clinically significant embolism other than thromboembolism. Classically, 12 to 24 hours after the fracture of a long bone, often the femur, the patient becomes short of breath. A chest radiograph reveals a diffuse opacity, which may progress to a "white out" resembling that in the adult respiratory distress syndrome. Indeed, **fat embolism is one of the important causes of the adult respiratory distress syndrome.** Cerebral symptoms (confusion or even coma) can be caused by fat emboli that have passed through the pulmonary artery into the systemic circulation. In fatal cases, the lungs resemble those in the adult respiratory distress syndrome—that is, they are heavy, hemorrhagic, and edematous. Histologic examination shows the capillaries and small vessels to be distended by spherical globules of fat.

Fat embolism is usually thought of as a direct consequence of trauma, with fat entering ruptured capillaries at the site of the fracture.

PULMONARY ARTERIAL HYPERTENSION

In fetal life the pulmonary arterial walls are thick, but after the third day following birth they become thin, mainly because of dilatation (Fig. 12-24). The pressure within the pulmonary arterial system may be increased for one of two reasons—augmented flow or increased resistance within the pulmonary circulation. Whatever the cause, similar morphologic abnormalities result from increased pulmonary arterial pressure. **Pulmonary atherosclerosis is seen in the major vessels.** It should be noted that even mild degrees of atherosclerosis are uncommon when pulmonary arterial pressure is normal. **The walls of the small pulmonary vessels thicken, owing to an increase in muscle in the media and an increase in fibrous tissue in the intima** (see Fig. 12-24). An additional change is the development of muscle in vessels that are normally nonmuscular or partially muscular (arteries generally less than 100 μm in diameter).

Mild structural changes of the pulmonary vasculature are reversible (e.g., with corrective heart surgery). However, severe lesions indicate that pulmonary arterial hypertension is not correctable.

INCREASED FLOW

A shunt from systemic circulation (including the heart) to the pulmonary circulation results in increased flow through the lungs, thereby causing pulmonary hypertension. The great majority of cases represent left-to-right shunts in congenital heart disease. The severity of the lesions in the pulmonary arteries depends on the severity of the pulmonary hypertension.

INCREASED RESISTANCE TO FLOW

Increased resistance to flow may be caused by obstruction proximal to the lung capillary bed (precapillary hypertension), destruction of the capillary bed, or obstruction distal to the capillary bed (postcapillary hypertension).

PRECAPILLARY CAUSES OF PULMONARY HYPERTENSION

PRIMARY PULMONARY HYPERTENSION Primary pulmonary hypertension, of unknown etiology, is caused by increased tone within the pulmonary arteries. It occurs at all ages but is most common in young women in their 20s and 30s. The disorder presents with an insidious onset of dyspnea, and physical signs and radiologic abnormalities are initially slight. As time passes, clinical and radiologic abnormalities become more apparent. Severe morphologic changes of pulmonary hypertension eventually ensue, and the patients die from cor pulmonale and right-sided heart failure. Medical treatment is generally ineffective, and this disease is an indication for heart-lung transplantation.
MULTIPLE RECURRENT PULMONARY EMBOLI Multiple thromboemboli in the smaller pulmonary vessels gradually restrict the pulmonary circulation. The presenting symptoms are often the same as in primary pulmonary hypertension, but some patients have

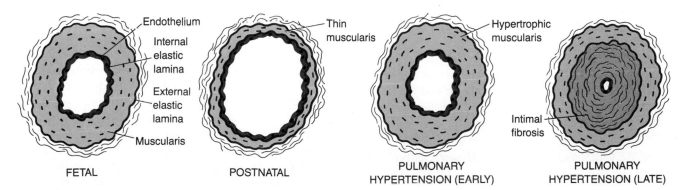

SMALL PULMONARY ARTERIES

FETAL · POSTNATAL · PULMONARY HYPERTENSION (EARLY) · PULMONARY HYPERTENSION (LATE)

Figure 12-24. Histopathology of pulmonary hypertension. In late gestation the pulmonary arteries have thick walls. After birth the vessels dilate and the walls become thin. Mild pulmonary hypertension is characterized by thickening of the media. As pulmonary hypertension becomes more severe, there is extensive intimal fibrosis and muscle thickening.

evidence of peripheral venous thrombosis, usually in the leg veins, or a history of circumstances predisposing to peripheral venous thrombosis. The lesions in the pulmonary vascular system are those of pulmonary hypertension, often severe. Organized thromboemboli are present. Characteristically, these form "webs" in the small pulmonary arteries, being composed of fibrous bands that extend across the lumen of the vessel. **FUNCTIONAL RESISTANCE TO FLOW** The pulmonary circulation is sensitive to hypoxemia, and any condition that produces hypoxemia results in pulmonary hypertension. This is the most common form of pulmonary hypertension and results from constriction of the small pulmonary arteries. Its causes include chronic airflow obstruction due to any condition that is accompanied by hypoxemia—for instance, infiltrative lung disease, living at high altitude, and alveolar hypoventilation. Alveolar hypoventilation may be due to abnormalities of the chest wall that interfere with the mechanics of ventilation, such as severe kyphoscoliosis and extreme obesity, the latter known as the "Pickwickian syndrome."

Capillary Causes of Pulmonary Hypertension

Experimentally, it has been shown that three-fourths of the lung can be removed without ensuing pulmonary hypertension. Pneumonectomy in man does not result in pulmonary hypertension. Emphysema is commonly cited as a cause of pulmonary hypertension, and it is claimed by some that this is due to the loss of capillary bed. **Pulmonary hypertension in emphysema is mainly due to hypoxemia caused by ventilation/perfusion abnormalities, but it may be that this is compounded by a loss of capillary bed.**

Postcapillary Causes of Pulmonary Hypertension

Postcapillary hypertension differs from the other forms of pulmonary hypertension in that there are venous as well as arterial changes, and the parenchyma (alveolar walls) may also be abnormal (chronic passive congestion, see below). Venous changes include intimal fibrosis and thickening, or "arterialization," of veins. Veins normally have little elastic tissue and muscle, but with severe venous hypertension extra elastic laminae and new smooth muscle develop.

Cardiac Causes of Pulmonary Hypertension

Left ventricular failure from any cause increases pulmonary venous pressure and hence pulmonary arterial pressure, but the increase is generally small. By contrast, mitral stenosis produces severe venous hypertension and significant pulmonary arterial hypertension.

Changes in the venous system and parenchyma depend on the severity of the venous hypertension. The parenchymal changes are included under the rubric of **chronic passive congestion** of the lung. The capillaries are dilated and, because of intermittent hemorrhage, red blood cells are seen in alveolar spaces and in the interstitium. Hemosiderosis, resulting from the breakdown of the red blood cells and phagocytosis of their debris, is prominent. Large macrophages loaded with hemosiderin, so-called heart failure cells, often pack the alveoli. In addition, hemosiderin is seen in the interstitium of the lung and may coat blood vessels. On gross examination, the lungs are brown and firm, an appearance that gives rise to the term **brown induration** of the lung.

PULMONARY EDEMA

Pulmonary edema, a common clinical and pathologic condition (Fig. 12-25), is defined as increased water within the lung. The key to understanding it is the Starling equation:

$$\text{Fluid movement} = k[(P_c - \pi_i) - (P_i - \pi_p)]$$

where k is the liquid conductance of the capillary barrier, P is the hydrostatic pressure in the capillary (c) or the interstitium (i) and π is the oncotic pressure of the plasma proteins (p) or interstitial fluid (i).

Although this equation has an admirably scientific appearance, it should be realized that the factors in the equation are not precisely known except for π_p, the capillary oncotic pressure. In more simplistic terms, the outflow of fluid is determined by the difference between the capillary hydrostatic pressure and the interstitial hydrostatic pressure, the hydrostatic pressure being higher. Resorption of fluid is determined by the difference in oncotic pressure between the two compartments. The amount of fluid exuded is modulated by the permeability characteristics of the alveolar capillary membrane. **Thus, there may be hydrostatic, oncotic, or permeability pulmonary edema,** and several forms of edema may be present at the same time.

Pulmonary edema may be interstitial or alveolar. Interstitial edema represents the earliest phase and is an exaggeration of the normal process of fluid filtration. Lymphatics become distended and fluid accumulates in the interstitium of the lobular septa and around veins and the bronchovascular bundle. Radiologic examination reveals a reticulonodular pattern, more marked in the bases of the lung. Lobular septa become edematous and produce linear shadows (**Kerley B lines**). Edema results in the shunting of blood flow from the bases to the upper lobes of the lungs, and increased airflow resistance occurs because of edema of the bronchovascular tree. Patients are often asymptomatic in this early stage.

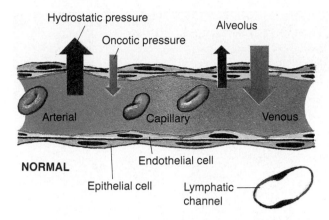

NORMAL

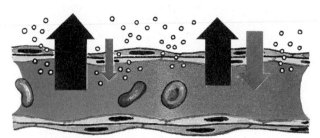

HYDROSTATIC EDEMA
- CONGESTIVE
  HEART FAILURE
- MITRAL STENOSIS

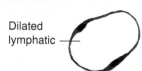

Dilated lymphatic

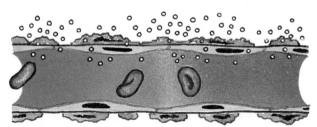

EPITHELIAL DAMAGE
- IRRITANT GASES
- NEAR DROWNING

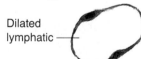

Dilated lymphatic

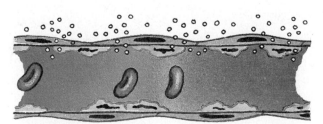

ENDOTHELIAL DAMAGE
- ARDS
- ENDOTOXEMIA
- FAT EMBOLISM

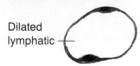

Dilated lymphatic

When the fluid can no longer be contained in the interstitial space, it spills into the alveoli, a condition termed alveolar edema. At this stage an alveolar pattern is seen, usually worst in the central portions of the lung and in the lower zones. The patient becomes acutely short of breath and bubbly rales are heard. In extreme cases, frothy fluid is coughed up or wells up out of the trachea. Histologic examination shows the airspaces to be filled with eosinophilic material.

HYDROSTATIC EDEMA

Hydrostatic edema is due to increased capillary pressure (P_c), usually as a consequence of left-sided heart failure from any cause. Fluid overload during transfusion or resuscitation may also lead to hydrostatic edema.

PERMEABILITY EDEMA

Damage to the endothelium, the epithelium, or both increases capillary permeability. In terms of the Starling equation, the reflection coefficient, Σ, tends toward zero—that is, toward high permeability.

Endothelial damage is probably the initial event in ARDS that is due to trauma or any other condition that leads to the sequestration and adherence of neutrophils. In addition, many chemical and therapeutic agents, and fat embolism, produce edema without affecting neutrophils. Primary epithelial damage results from near drowning, aspiration of gastric contents, inhalation of toxic gases, and viral infections.

ONCOTIC PULMONARY EDEMA

Although systemic edema is a well-recognized complication of low capillary oncotic pressure, notably in starvation or hepatic failure, it is not commonly recognized in the lung, which suggests that the lung tends to keep its interstitium dry. Thus, low capillary osmotic pressure is not often significant in the lung.

Figure 12-25. Pathogenesis of pulmonary edema. There is a balance between hydrostatic forces, which tend to make fluid pass out from the capillaries to the interstitium and alveoli, and oncotic forces, which draw fluid in to the capillary bed from the interstitium. Hydrostatic pressure predominates on the arterial side of the capillary and oncotic pressure on the venous side. In hydrostatic edema, the hydrostatic forces dominate, and the fluid is forced into the interstitium of the lung and alveolar spaces. When epithelial damage occurs, the normal tight junctions of epithelial cells are lost and fluid flows freely into alveolar spaces. When there is endothelial damage, the barrier function of the capillary wall is also impaired.

13

THE GASTROINTESTINAL TRACT

EMANUEL RUBIN AND JOHN L. FARBER

THE ESOPHAGUS

CONGENITAL DISORDERS

The most common esophageal anomaly is the **tracheo-esophageal fistula,** which is frequently combined with some form of **esophageal atresia.** The cause of esophageal atresia is unknown, but in some cases it has been associated with a complex of anomalies identified by the acronym **Vater syndrome** (*v*ertebral defects, *a*nal atresia, *t*racheo-*e*sophageal fistula, and *r*enal dysplasia).

In the most common variety (90%) of tracheo-esophageal fistula the upper portion of the esophagus ends in a blind pouch, and the upper end of the lower segment communicates with the trachea. In this type of atresia the upper blind sac soon fills with mucus, which the infant then aspirates.

Among the remaining 10% of cases, the most common type involves a communication between the proximal esophagus and the trachea; the lower esophageal pouch communicates with the stomach. Infants with this condition develop aspiration immediately after birth. In another variant, termed an H-type fistula, a communication exists between an intact esophagus and an intact trachea.

RINGS AND WEBS

Esophageal webs are thin mucosal membranes that project into the lumen of the esophagus. Usually single, they are occasionally multiple and can be found anywhere in the esophagus. The **Plummer-Vinson (Paterson-Kelly) syndrome** is characterized by a cervical esophageal web, mucosal lesions of the mouth and pharynx, and iron-deficiency anemia. Dysphagia, often associated with aspiration of swallowed food, is the most common clinical manifestation. The Plummer-Vinson syndrome is principally a disease of women (90%). Carcinoma of the oropharynx and upper esophagus is a recognized complication. The prevalence of this syndrome has significantly declined in recent years.

Schatzki's mucosal ring, a common cause of dysphagia, is a lower esophageal narrowing at the junction of the esophageal and gastric mucosae, a few centimeters above the diaphragm. Microscopically, the upper surface of the mucosal ring exhibits stratified squamous epithelium, while the lower is lined by a columnar epithelium. Mild chronic inflammation and fibrosis are common in the submucosa.

ESOPHAGEAL DIVERTICULA

A **true esophageal diverticulum** is an outpouching of the wall that contains all layers of the esophagus. When the sac lacks a muscular layer, it is known as a **false diverticulum.**

The diverticulum that appears high in the esophagus, known as **Zenker's diverticulum,** was once thought to result from luminal pressure exerted in a structurally weak area and was classed as a **pulsion diverticulum.** Today, disordered function of the cricopharyngeus musculature is generally thought to be involved in the pathogenesis of this false diverticulum. Zenker's diverticulum is more common in men and persons over the age of 60 years. The diverticulum can enlarge conspicuously and accumulate a large amount of food. Regurgitation of food eaten some time previously is typical and may lead to recurrent aspiration pneumonia.

Diverticula in the midportion of the esophagus were traditionally termed **traction diverticula** because of their attachment to adjacent mediastinal lymph nodes, usually associated with tuberculous lymphadenitis. However, it is now thought that these pouches more often reflect a disturbance in the motor function of the esophagus. A midesophageal diverticulum usually does not retain food or secretions and remains asymptomatic.

Diverticula immediately above the diaphragm are labeled **epiphrenic diverticula** and are encountered in young persons. Motor disturbances of the esophagus and reflux esophagitis are often found in patients with this true diverticulum. Nocturnal regurgitation of large amounts of fluid stored in the diverticulum during the day is typical.

MOTOR DISORDERS

Any failure of proper muscular function is included in the concept of motor disorders of the esophagus. The hallmark of motor disorders is difficulty in swallowing, termed **dysphagia.** Pain on swallowing is termed **odynophagia.**

ACHALASIA

Achalasia, at one time termed "cardiospasm," is characterized by the absence of peristalsis in the body of the esophagus and failure of the lower esophageal sphincter to relax in response to swallowing. Food is retained within the esophagus, and the organ hyper-

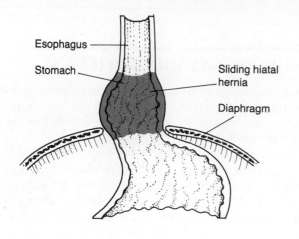

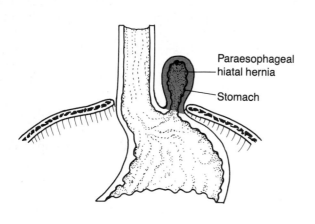

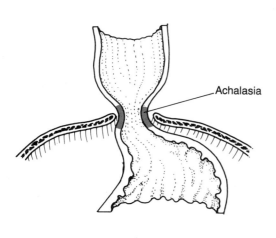

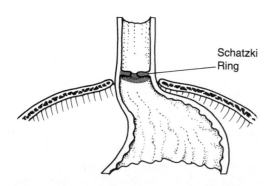

Figure 13-1. Disorders of the esophageal outlet.

trophies and dilates conspicuously. Dysphagia, occasionally odynophagia, and regurgitation of material retained in the esophagus are common.

The cause of achalasia is not well understood, but it is generally agreed that there is a loss or absence of ganglion cells in the myenteric plexus in the area of the lower esophageal sphincter. In Latin America achalasia is a common complication of Chagas' disease, the ganglion cells being destroyed by the organisms of *Trypanosoma cruzi.*

SCHERODERMA (PROGRESSIVE SYSTEMIC SCLEROSIS)

Scleroderma causes fibrosis in many organs and produces a severe abnormality of esophageal muscle function, affecting principally the lower esophageal sphincter. Microscopically, the smooth muscle is atrophied, and submucosal fibrosis and nonspecific inflammatory changes are seen. Intimal fibrosis of the small arteries and arterioles is common.

HIATAL HERNIA

"Hiatal hernia" refers to an acquired herniation of the stomach through an enlarged esophageal hiatus in the diaphragm. **Two basic types are the sliding, or axial, form, which accounts for most hiatal hernias, and the paraesophageal variety (Fig. 13-1).**

In the **sliding hernia** an enlargement of the diaphragmatic hiatus and laxity of the circumferential connective tissue allow a cap of gastric cardia to move upward to a position above the diaphragm. The condition is so common that, upon appropriate manipulation by the radiologist, more than half the population can be demonstrated to have a small sliding hernia.

The **paraesophageal hernia** is characterized by herniation of a portion of the gastric fundus alongside the esophagus through a defect in the diaphragmatic connective tissue membrane that defines the esophageal hiatus (see Fig. 13-1). The hernia progressively enlarges, and the hiatus grows increasingly wide. Most large paraesophageal hernias do not cause significant symptoms.

Symptoms of hiatal hernia, particularly heartburn and regurgitation, are attributed to gastroesophageal reflux. However, evidence suggests that the reflux of gastric contents is independent of the hernia and rather is related to incompetence of the lower esophageal sphincter. Classically, the symptoms are exacerbated when the affected person is in the recumbent position, which facilitates acid reflux. Dysphagia, painful swallowing, and occasionally bleeding may also be troublesome.

ESOPHAGITIS

REFLUX ESOPHAGITIS

Reflux esophagitis, formerly termed "peptic esophagitis," results from the regurgitation of gastric contents into the lower esophagus. By far the most common type of esophagitis, it is commonly seen in conjunction with a sliding hiatal hernia, although it often occurs through an incompetent cardia without any demonstrable anatomic lesion.

The principal barrier to the reflux of gastric contents into the esophagus is the lower esophageal sphincter. Agents that cause a decrease in the pressure of the lower esophageal sphincter (e.g., alcohol, chocolate, fatty foods, cigarette smoke) are associated with reflux. Although acid is damaging to the esophageal mucosa, the combination of acid and pepsin (and possibly refluxed bile) may be particularly injurious.

If reflux is chronic, thickening of the epithelium, termed "leukoplakia," is occasionally seen as irregular greyish white patches. Areas affected by reflux are susceptible to superficial mucosal ulcerations, which appear as vertical linear streaks. Microscopically, the basal layer of the epithelium is thickened, and the rete pegs are elongated and extend toward the surface. Severe reflux esophagitis may lead to **esophageal stricture.**

Barrett's epithelium, defined as replacement of the squamous epithelium in the lower third of the esophagus by columnar epithelium, occurs in response to chronic reflux esophagitis. The metaplastic epithelium may occur in patches or may line the entire lower esophagus. The most common histologic pattern is intestinal metaplasia, characterized by villi lined with intestinal goblet cells and sometimes Paneth cells. In other cases gastric epithelium with parietal and chief cells is found. The two types may coexist. **Barrett's epithelium carries a significant risk of malignant transformation to adenocarcinoma.**

INFECTIOUS ESOPHAGITIS

With the exceptions of **candidiasis** and **herpes simplex,** primary infections of the esophagus are rare. Infection of the esophagus with Candida species has become commonplace because of an increasing number of persons immunocompromised as a result of chemotherapy for malignant disease, immunosuppressive drugs after organ transplantation, or infection with HIV. Dysphagia and severe pain on swallowing are usual, and bleeding from the infected site, sometimes severe, is common.

In severe candidiasis confluent pseudomembranes lie on a hyperemic and edematous mucosa. Microscopically, the candidal pseudomembrane contains fungal mycelia, necrotic debris, and fibrin.

Herpetic esophagitis, often asymptomatic, is most frequently associated with lymphomas and leukemias, but may also occur in apparently healthy people, in whom it often produces severe pain upon swallowing. Herpetic esophagitis is characterized by mucosal ulcers or plaques. Microscopically, the lesions are superficial, and the epithelial cells exhibit typical herpetic inclusions in their nuclei. Monilial and bacterial superinfection results in the formation of pseudomembranes.

CHEMICAL ESOPHAGITIS

Chemical injury to the esophagus is usually a result of accidental poisoning in children or attempted suicide in adults. It is produced by the intake of strong alkaline agents (e.g., lye) or strong acids (e.g., sulphuric or hydrochloric acid) used in various cleaning solutions. Histologically, alkali-induced liquefactive necrosis is accompanied by conspicuous inflammation and saponification of the membrane lipids in the epithelium, submucosa, and muscularis of the esophagus and stomach. Thrombosis of small vessels adds ischemic necrosis to the injury. Strong acids produce immediate coagulation necrosis, which results in a protective eschar that prevents injury and limits penetration. Nevertheless, half of the patients who ingest concentrated hydrochloric or sulphuric acid suffer severe esophageal injury. Severe caustic injury leads to scar formation, which in turn results in esophageal stricture.

LACERATIONS AND PERFORATIONS

Lacerations of the esophagus result from external trauma, such as automobile accidents and falls from

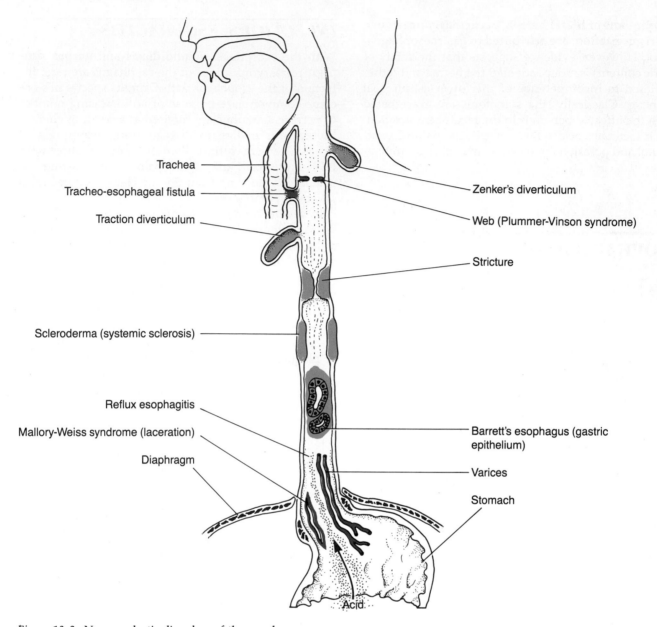

Figure 13-2. Nonneoplastic disorders of the esophagus.

great heights, and from medical instrumentation. However, the most common cause is severe vomiting, during which the intraesophageal pressure may rise as high as 300 torr. In the **Mallory-Weiss syndrome,** severe retching, often associated with alcoholism, leads to mucosal lacerations of the upper stomach and lower esophagus, which result in the vomiting of bright red blood. Bleeding may be so severe as to require the transfusion of many units of blood.

Perforation of the esophagus, whether from trauma or vomiting, can be catastrophic. It is a well-known occurrence in the newborn, in whom it is caused occasionally by suctioning or feeding with a nasogastric tube but in whom it may also occur spontaneously. Rupture of the esophagus as a result of vomiting is known as **Boerhaave's syndrome.**

Figure 13-2 summarizes the major nonneoplastic disorders of the esophagus.

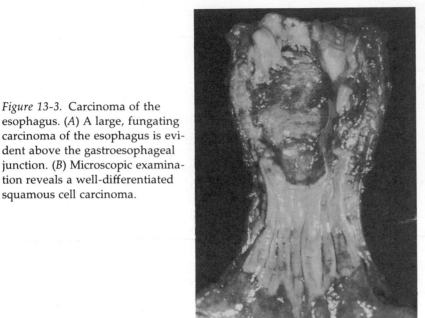

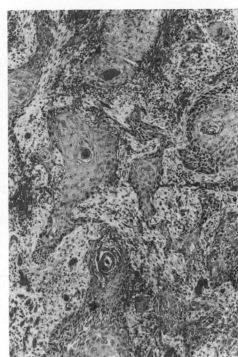

Figure 13-3. Carcinoma of the esophagus. (*A*) A large, fungating carcinoma of the esophagus is evident above the gastroesophageal junction. (*B*) Microscopic examination reveals a well-differentiated squamous cell carcinoma.

A   B

CARCINOMA

EPIDEMIOLOGY

Over 90% of cancers of the esophagus are squamous cell carcinomas (Fig. 13-3). The incidence of this tumor in the United States is low, accounting for 7% of all gastrointestinal cancers. Worldwide, however, there are striking variations. There is an esophageal cancer belt extending across Asia from the Caspian Sea region of Northern Iran and the Soviet Union through Soviet Central Asia and Mongolia to Northern China, where the incidence is 30 to 70 times greater than in the United States. American blacks have a considerably greater incidence than Caucasians, and in the United States urban dwellers are at greater risk than those in rural areas. In the United States there is a male predominance of about 3:1.

ETIOLOGY

The geographic variations in esophageal cancer suggest that **environmental factors contribute strongly to the development of this disease.** In developed countries alcoholism is a risk factor. **Cigarette smoking** is associated with a twofold to fourfold increase in the risk of

esophageal cancer. However, the population in the Caspian littoral of Iran, which has one of the highest rates of esophagal carcinoma in the world, neither consumes alcohol nor smokes cigarettes excessively. **Any condition associated with chronic injury to the esophageal mucosa including chronic esophagitis, achalasia, stricture, webs, rings and diverticula, predisposes to squamous cell carcinoma of the esophagus.**

CLINICAL FEATURES

The most common presenting complaint is dysphagia. Patients with esophageal cancer are almost invariably cachectic, owing to the remote effects of a malignant tumor, anorexia, and difficulty in eating. Surgery and radiotherapy are useful for palliation, but the prognosis remains dismal.

PATHOLOGY

About half the cases of esophageal cancer involve the middle third of the esophagus; the upper and lower thirds each account for one-fourth of the cases. Grossly, the tumors are of three types: **polypoid,** which project into the lumen (see Fig. 13-3*A*); **ulcerating,** which are usually smaller than polypoid; and **infiltrating,** the principal plane of growth of which is in the wall. The bulky polypoid tumors tend to obstruct early, whereas the ulcerated ones are more likely to bleed. The infiltrating tumors gradually narrow the lumen by circumferential compression. Local extension of the tumor is commonly a major problem. Microscopically, the neoplastic squamous cells range from well differentiated, with epithelial "pearls" (see Fig. 13-3*B*), to poorly differentiated.

The rich lymphatic drainage of the esophagus provides a route for most metastases, which are found in thoracic and abdominal lymph nodes. Visceral metastases to the liver and lung are common, and almost any organ may be involved.

Adenocarcinoma of the esophagus accounts for a minority of malignant esophageal tumors. Most adenocarcinomas arise in Barrett's epithelium, but a few originate in mucous glands of the esophagus. The symptoms and clinical course are similar to those of squamous cell carcinoma of the esophagus, but a 20% 5-year survival following radical surgery has been reported.

THE STOMACH

ANATOMY

The interior of the stomach has been divided into five regions (Fig. 13-4): the **cardia,** a small, grossly indistinct zone that extends a short distance from the gastroesophageal junction; the **fundus,** the dome-shaped part of the stomach that is located to the left of the cardia and extends superiorly above a line drawn horizontally through the gastroesophageal junction; the **body,** or **corpus,** which constitutes two-thirds of the entire stomach and descends from the fundus to the most inferior region, where the organ turns right to form the bottom of the J; the **antrum,** the distal third of the stomach, which is positioned horizontally and extends from the body to the pyloric sphincter; and the **pylorus,** the most distal tubular segment of the stomach, which is entirely surrounded by the thick muscular sphincter that governs the passage of food into the duodenum.

The histologic appearance of the gastric mucosa varies according to the anatomic region. The surface mucosa is a mucus-secreting, columnar epithelium perforated by numerous foveolae, or pits, which represent the orifices of millions of branched, tubular glands. The three types of glands are the **cardiac glands,** located in the cardia; the **gastric (oxyntic, parietal) glands,** in the body and fundus of the stomach; and the **pyloric glands,** in the antrum and the pyloric canal.

CONGENITAL DISORDERS

CONGENITAL PYLORIC STENOSIS

Congenital pyloric stenosis, a lesion that obstructs the outlet of the stomach, is the most common indication for abdominal surgery in the initial 6 months of life. It is 4 times more common in males than in females and affects first-born children more often than subsequent ones. It occurs in 1 of 250 to 300 white births but is rare in blacks and Asiatics. The abnormality may have a genetic basis and has been recorded in conjunction with other developmental abnormalities. Embryopathies associated with rubella infection and maternal intake of thalidomide have also been associated with congenital pyloric stenosis.

The symptoms of pyloric stenosis usually become apparent within the first month of life, when the infant manifests **projectile vomiting.** The loss of hydrochloric acid in the vomitus may result in hypochloremic alkalosis, dehydration and wasting. A palpable pyloric "tumor" and visible peristalsis are characteristic of the disorder. The extreme hypertrophy of the circular muscle coat causes concentric enlargement of the pylorus and narrowing of the pyloric canal. Surgical incision of the hypertrophied pyloric muscle is curative.

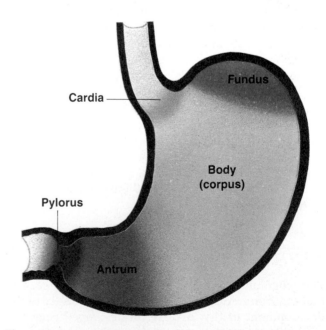

Figure 13-4. Anatomic regions of the stomach.

CONGENITAL DIAPHRAGMATIC HERNIAS

Congenital diaphragmatic hernias, of variable size and location, are associated with defective closure of embryologic foramina or abnormalities of the esophageal hiatus. The stomach, together with other abdominal organs, may eventrate into the thoracic cavity. Congenital diaphragmatic hernias are often associated with congenital malrotations of the intestine. Herniation of the abdominal contents into the thorax may be asymptomatic or may lead to severe respiratory embarrassment, necessitating surgical intervention.

GASTRITIS

EROSIVE GASTRITIS (ACUTE GASTRITIS)

Erosive gastritis is the presence of focal necrosis of the mucosa in an otherwise normal stomach. The erosion of the mucosa may extend into the deeper tissues to form an acute ulcer. The necrosis is accompanied by an acute inflammatory response and often by hemorrhage, which may be so severe as to result in exsanguination.

Erosive gastritis may be associated with the accidental or suicidal ingestion of corrosive substances, such as those that produce erosive esophagitis. However, more commonly the condition is associated with the intake of **alcohol** or certain drugs, particularly **aspirin** and **other nonsteroidal anti-inflammatory agents.** The oral administration of corticosteroids is also occasionally complicated by erosive gastritis.

Gastric erosions are also seen in a variety of other clinical situations, the common factor among which appears to be so-called stress. These **stress ulcers,** long known to occur in severely burned individuals **(Curling's ulcer),** commonly result in bleeding, which is occasionally severe. Another cause of stress ulcers is **trauma to the central nervous system,** either accidental or surgical **(Cushing's ulcer).** These ulcers are characteristically deep and carry a substantial risk of perforation. Severe **trauma,** especially if accompanied by **shock,** prolonged **sepsis,** and **incapacitation** from many debilitating chronic diseases also predispose to the development of erosive gastritis. **The first sign of stress ulcers may be massive, life-threatening hemorrhage.**

Erosive gastritis is characterized by widespread petechial hemorrhages and mucosal lesions of variable size (1–25 mm). Microscopically, patchy mucosal necrosis extending to the submucosa is visualized adjacent to normal mucosa. Healing is usually complete within a few days.

PATHOGENESIS

Stress ulcers have been produced experimentally in rats by restraint, forced exertion, and traumatic or hemorrhagic shock. In rats and other species, burns and neurologic trauma also result in erosive gastritis. Certain types of prolonged psychologic stresses have been reported to produce erosive lesions in the stomach and duodenum. The nonsteroidal anti-inflammatory compounds, corticosteroids, and concentrated ethanol consistently cause gastric erosions in rats.

The role of **hypersecretion of gastric acid** in the pathogenesis of erosive gastritis is not clear. Although some experimental conditions resulting in stress ulcers are accompanied by increased acid secretion, most stress ulcers form without any such increase. Nevertheless, gastric acid may play a permissive role, since inhibition of gastric acid secretion (e.g., with cimetidine) protects against the development of stress ulcers. **Microcirculatory changes in the stomach induced by shock or sepsis may add ischemic injury as a complication of erosive gastritis.**

Since the contents of the stomach would be highly toxic to any tissue outside the gastrointestinal tract, **it is thought that the protective mechanisms of the gastric mucosa are the important defense against mucosal erosion.** It follows that the pathogenesis of erosive gastritis likely involves, at least in part, impairment of these local defensive factors, including (a) decreased mucus production, (b) deficiency of tissue prostaglandins, (c) inhibition of epithelial renewal, and (d) lowering of the intramural pH of the gastric mucosa.

NONEROSIVE GASTRITIS (CHRONIC GASTRITIS)

Nonerosive gastritis is a chronic inflammatory disease of the stomach of unknown cause that ranges from mild superficial involvement to severe atrophy of the gastric mucosa. By itself the disorder gives rise to few if any symptoms. **Nonerosive gastritis should be considered a histologic rather than a clinical entity.**

A cardinal feature of nonerosive gastritis is the progressive **loss of the capacity to secrete acid (achlorhydria),** as a result of the loss of parietal cells in the

FUNDIC MUCOSA WITH
MILD CHRONIC GASTRITIS

INTESTINAL METAPLASIA

Surface mucous cells

Metaplastic
intestinal
cells

Goblet
cells

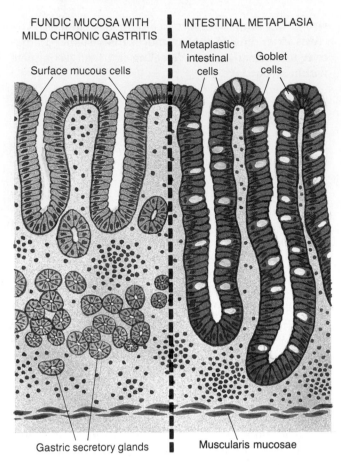

Gastric secretory glands

Muscularis mucosae

Figure 13-5. Schematic representation of the pathology of chronic gastritis. In mild gastritis there is chronic inflammation and a reduction in the number and size of the gastric glands. More severe gastritis is accompanied by intestinal metaplasia, a condition in which the normal gastric epithelium is replaced by a metaplastic intestinal-type epithelium containing enterocytes, goblet cells, and Paneth cells.

body of the stomach. The loss of these cells also leads to a deficiency of intrinsic factor, which is necessary for the absorption of vitamin B_{12} in the ileum. As a consequence, **pernicious anemia** develops.

PATHOLOGY

On the basis of the primary region of the stomach involved, nonerosive gastritis has been divided into **fundal gastritis** and **antral gastritis,** although the lesions characteristically overlap.

Fundal gastritis typically exhibits (a) little or no involvement of the antrum, (b) diffuse gastritis in the body and fundus of the stomach, (c) antibodies to parietal cells, and (d) a significant reduction in or absence of gastric secretion. This form of gastritis may be associated with pernicious anemia, as well as with extragastric "autoimmune" diseases, such as chronic thyroiditis and Addison's disease.

By contrast, antral gastritis, which is considerably more common than fundal gastritis, shows (a) only focal lesions in the body of the stomach, (b) severe involvement of the antrum, (c) a lack of antibodies to parietal cells, and (d) only a modest reduction in gastric secretion. The antral variety of nonerosive gastritis is not associated with pernicious anemia but, like fundal gastritis, carries a significant risk for the development of stomach cancer.

The mildest form of nonerosive gastritis is a **superficial gastritis.** This lesion occasionally reverts to normal but more commonly proceeds to **atrophic gastritis,** a disorder that usually persists indefinitely. In some cases a final stage, **gastric atrophy,** shows few of the inflammatory features of gastritis.

Superficial gastritis typically shows lymphocytes and plasma cells, and occasionally neutrophils, in the lamina propria of the mucosa of the antrum and body of the stomach. Although superficial gastritis does not involve the gastric (parietal) glands, histamine-stimulated secretion of acid and pepsin is impaired.

Atrophic gastritis may evolve from superficial gastritis and, like superficial gastritis, is characterized by prominent chronic inflammation in the lamina propria. Lymphocytes and plasma cells extend into the deepest reaches of the mucosa as far as the muscularis mucosae. Involvement of the gastric glands leads to degenerative changes in their epithelial cells and ultimately a conspicuous reduction in the number of glands; hence the name *atrophic gastritis.* Eventually the inflammatory process may abate, leaving only a thin atrophic mucosa (gastric atrophy).

A common and important histologic feature of nonerosive gastritis is **intestinal metaplasia,** a condition in which the injured gastric mucosa is replaced by an epithelium composed of cells of the intestinal type (Fig. 13-5). Numerous mucin-containing goblet cells and enterocytes line cryptlike glands, and many Paneth cells, which are not normal denizens of the gastric mucosa, are present. However, intestinal villi do not usually form.

PATHOGENESIS AND CONSEQUENCES

The most common determinant of nonerosive gastritis is aging. More than half the population over 40 years of age exhibits superficial gastritis. A decade later the same population is affected by mild or moderate atrophic gastritis.

All individuals subjected to partial gastrectomy develop nonerosive gastritis in the remaining stomach, usually within 2 years. The pattern is typically that of atrophic gastritis with intestinal metaplasia. **Chronic gastric ulcers are always accompanied by superficial and atrophic gastritis of the antrum, usually in association with intestinal metaplasia.**

Pernicious Anemia

Pernicious anemia, a megaloblastic anemia that is associated with complete achlorhydria, is caused by malabsorption of vitamin B_{12} occasioned by a deficiency of intrinsic factor. The stomach invariably displays atrophy of the fundic glands, accompanied by slight chronic inflammation, and intestinal metaplasia may be prominent. Involvement of the antrum may occur but is generally less severe. Although atrophic gastritis is common among the elderly, only a few aged persons develop pernicious anemia.

Pernicious anemia is suspected to be an autoimmune disease, although the pathogenetic significance of autoantibodies is not fully elucidated. Circulating antibodies to parietal cells are found in 40% to 90% of patients with pernicious anemia. In 66%, antibodies to intrinsic factor are present.

Pernicious anemia shows a familial tendency. Ten percent to 15% of first-degree relatives of patients with pernicious anemia demonstrate severe atrophic gastritis and achlorhydria, although they do not suffer from megaloblastic anemia.

Nonerosive Gastritis and Stomach Cancer

It is generally accepted that persons with atrophic gastritis have a higher than normal incidence of carcinoma of the stomach. Patients with pernicious anemia, who invariably suffer from atrophic gastritis, have a threefold to fourfold increased risk of developing gastric cancer. Cancer arises in the antrum several times more frequently than in the body of the stomach. **Intestinal metaplasia of the stomach has been particularly identified as a preneoplastic lesion.**

MENETRIER'S DISEASE (GIANT HYPERTROPHIC GASTRITIS)

Menetrier's disease is an uncommon gastric disorder characterized by giant hypertrophy of the mucosal folds of the stomach. Grossly, the stomach is increased in weight as much as 900 g to 1200 g. **The folds of the greater curvature in the fundus and body of the**

stomach, and occasionally in the antrum, are increased in height and thickness, forming a convoluted surface that has been compared to that of the brain. Microscopically, the disease is restricted to the mucosa. Hyperplasia of the gastric pits results in a conspicuous increase in their depth and a tortuous (corkscrew) structure. The glands are elongated, and many appear cystic. Lymphocytes, plasma cells, and occasional neutrophils are seen in the lamina propria.

Weight loss, sometimes of rapid onset, peripheral edema, and in some cases ascites and cachexia, are related to a **severe loss of plasma proteins (including albumin) from the altered gastric mucosa. Menetrier's disease is considered to be a precancerous condition.**

PEPTIC ULCER DISEASE

"Peptic ulcer disease" refers to breaks in the mucosa of the stomach and small intestine, principally the proximal duodenum, that are produced by the action of gastric secretions. Peptic ulcers of the stomach and duodenum are estimated to afflict 10% of the population of Western industrialized countries at some time during their lives. Many clinical and epidemiologic features distinguish gastric from duodenal ulcers; the common factor that unites them is the gastric secretion of hydrochloric acid. With rare exceptions, **a person who does not secrete acid will not develop a peptic ulcer anywhere.**

The "classic" case of peptic ulcer is characterized by burning epigastric pain that is experienced 1 to 3 hours after a meal or that awakens the patient at night. Both alkali and food are said to relieve the symptoms. However, the majority of patients do not conform to the "classic" presentation. Half do not describe their pain as related to meals, and fewer than half report that the pain is relieved by food or alkali.

EPIDEMIOLOGIC CONSIDERATIONS

Mortality from duodenal ulcers, as well as the number of admissions to hospitals, have fallen. However, newer population studies suggest that **it is inappropriate to draw any firm conclusions regarding trends in the incidence of duodenal ulcer disease.** The incidence of gastric ulcers seems to have remained stationary over the last few decades. The peak incidence of duodenal ulcer disease is between the ages of 30 and 60, although the disorder may occur in persons of any age, even in infants. Gastric ulcers afflict the middle-aged and elderly more than the young. Duodenal ulcers mainly affect men, whereas the incidence of gastric ulcers is the same for men and women.

The common stereotype of the patient with a peptic ulcer is the highly motivated executive operating in a stressful environment. However, careful epidemiologic surveys in the United States and Great Britain have suggested an **inverse relationship between duodenal ulcers and socioeconomic status and education,** although the trends are not marked.

PATHOGENESIS

RISK FACTORS

The evidence to support the contention that the consumption of any food or beverage, including coffee and alcohol, contributes to the development or persistence of peptic ulcers is surprisingly meager. Both prospective and cross-sectional studies indicate that **aspirin** is an important contributing factor in the genesis of duodenal and especially gastric ulcers. Other **nonsteroidal anti-inflammatory agents** and **analgesics** have been incriminated in the production of peptic ulcers. Prolonged treatment with high doses of corticosteroids has been claimed to increase slightly the risk of peptic ulceration. **Cigarette smoking** has been considered a definite risk factor for duodenal and gastric ulcers, particularly gastric ulcers. Recent analysis of the data has weakened, although not eliminated, this association.

GENETIC FACTORS

First-degree relatives of patients with duodenal ulcers have a threefold increased risk of developing a duodenal ulcer but do not have a similar increase in risk of developing a gastric ulcer. Patients with gastric ulcers similarly "breed true."

The risk of duodenal ulcer is about 30% higher in persons with **type O blood** than in A, B, and AB individuals, although patients with gastric ulcers do not exhibit a greater frequency of blood group O. **The quarter of the population that does not secrete blood-group antigens in the saliva and gastric juice is at a 50% increased risk of developing a duodenal ulcer.** The risk of duodenal ulceration is greatly increased (2.5:1) when nonsecretory status is combined with blood group O, a combination that occurs in 10% of the Caucasian population.

Pepsinogen I is secreted by the chief and mucous neck cells of the gastric mucosa and appears in the gastric juice, blood, and urine. Serum levels of this proenzyme correlate with the gastric capacity for acid secretion and are considered a measure of parietal cell mass. **A person with high circulating levels of pepsinogen I is at 5 times the normal risk of developing a duodenal ulcer.** Hyperpepsinogenemia I is present in half of the children of patients with hyperpepsinogenemia and has been attributed to autosomal dominant inheritance. Thus, not only is hyperpepsinogenemia considered a marker for an ulcer diathesis, it is also thought to indicate a genetically predetermined increase in parietal cell mass.

Familial clustering of duodenal ulcers and **rapid gastric emptying** have been demonstrated, and familial **hyperfunction of gastrin-secreting cells (G cells)** in the antrum is also reported.

PSYCHOLOGIC FACTORS

"Stress" has been anecdotally related to peptic ulcers for at least a century, and repressed stress has been considered particularly ulcerogenic. Closer scrutiny of the epidemiologic and experimental evidence supporting these concepts has cast serious doubt on their validity, and many today discount any relationship between stress and ulcers. Whatever the final outcome of this debate may be, **there is no need to incriminate stress in the pathogenesis of peptic ulcers.**

PHYSIOLOGIC FACTORS

The formation and persistence of peptic ulcers in both the stomach and duodenum require the gastric secretion of acid. The gastric secretion of pepsin, which may also play a role in the production of peptic ulcers, parallels that of hydrochloric acid. The maximal capacity for acid production by the stomach is a reflection of total parietal cell mass. Both parietal cell mass and maximal acid secretion are increased up to twofold in patients with duodenal ulcers. However, there is a large overlap with normal values, and **only one third of these patients secrete excess acid.**

The duodenum may also be excessively acidified by the rapid emptying of gastric contents. **Accelerated gastric emptying** has been noted in patients with duodenal ulcers although, as with other factors, there is substantial overlap with normal rates. Normally acidification of the duodenal bulb inhibits further gastric emptying. It has been reported that in most patients with duodenal ulcer this feedback inhibitory mechanism is absent. As mentioned above, rapid gastric emptying may in some cases be an inherited abnormality.

The pH of the duodenal bulb reflects the balance between the delivery of gastric juice and its neutralization by biliary, pancreatic, and duodenal secretions.

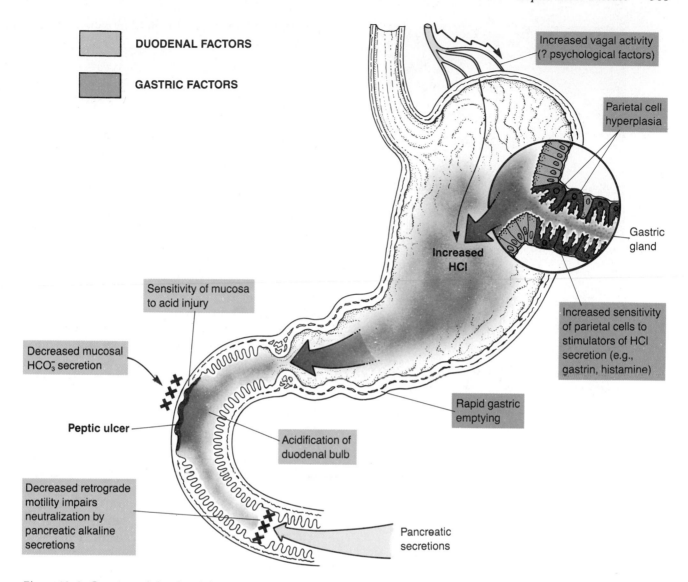

DUODENAL FACTORS

GASTRIC FACTORS

Increased vagal activity
(? psychological factors)

Parietal cell
hyperplasia

Gastric
gland

Increased
HCl

Increased sensitivity
of parietal cells to
stimulators of HCl
secretion (e.g.,
gastrin, histamine)

Sensitivity of mucosa
to acid injury

Decreased mucosal
HCO₃⁻ secretion

Peptic ulcer

Rapid gastric
emptying

Acidification of
duodenal bulb

Decreased retrograde
motility impairs
neutralization by
pancreatic alkaline
secretions

Pancreatic
secretions

Figure 13-6. Gastric and duodenal factors in the pathogenesis of duodenal peptic ulcers.

The production of duodenal ulcers requires an acidic pH in the bulb—that is, an excess of acid over neutralizing secretions. In ulcer patients the duodenal pH following a meal falls to a lower level and remains depressed for a longer time than in normal individuals.

A number of patients with gastric ulcers display hypersecretion of acid, but most secrete not only less gastric acid than patients with duodenal ulcer, but even less than normal people. The occurrence of gastric ulcers in the face of gastric hyposecretion implies the following possibilities: that the gastric mucosa is in some way particularly sensitive to even low concentrations of acid; that some material other than acid damages the mucosa; or that the gastric mucosa is exposed to potentially injurious agents for an unusually long period of time. Gastric ulcers in patients with acid hy-

persecretion are usually near the pylorus and are considered variants of duodenal ulceration.

There is considerable interest in the possibility that peptic ulcer disease may be caused, at least in part, by colonization of the upper gastrointestinal tract by *Campylobacter pylori*. However, the evidence is contradictory, and a role for this organism in the pathogenesis of peptic ulcers remains controversial.

In summary, the pathogenesis of gastric and duodenal peptic ulcers remains poorly understood. The only certainty is that at least some acid is required for both.

The various gastric and duodenal factors that have been implicated as possible mechanisms in the pathogenesis of duodenal ulceration are summarized in Figure 13-6.

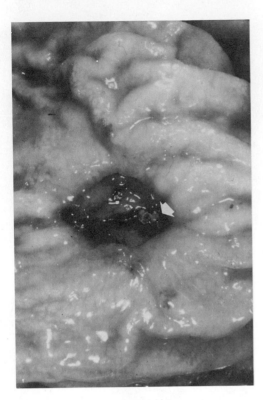

Figure 13-7. Gastric ulcer. A deep peptic ulcer of the stomach has eroded an artery (*arrow*), severe hemorrhage has resulted. The gastric folds converge on the sharply circumscribed ulcer.

ASSOCIATED DISEASES

The incidence of duodenal ulcers in patients with **cirrhosis** is 10 times greater than in normal persons. Patients with **chronic renal failure** maintained on hemodialysis have been reported to be at greater than normal risk for the development of peptic ulcers, although the data are not conclusive. Patients subjected to **renal transplantation** have a substantially increased risk of peptic ulceration.

There is an increased incidence of peptic ulcers in persons with **multiple endocrine neoplasia, type I (MEN I).** The Zollinger-Ellison syndrome (discussed in Chapter 15) is characterized by profound gastric hypersecretion caused by a gastrin-producing islet cell adenoma.

Almost one-third of patients with hereditary **alpha$_1$-antitrypsin deficiency** have peptic ulcers, and this incidence is even higher in patients who have pulmonary disease as well. It has been speculated that in this disorder unopposed proteolytic activity may contribute to peptic ulceration.

Peptic ulcers are found in one-fourth of patients with **chronic lung disease,** and chronic pulmonary disease

is increased twofold to threefold in patients who have peptic ulcers.

PATHOLOGY

A peptic ulcer should be considered chronic when it does not heal readily and when scarring at the base of the ulcer precludes complete restoration of the normal submucosa and muscularis. Most peptic ulcers arise in the lesser curvature, in the antral and prepyloric regions of the stomach, and in the first part of the duodenum. Gastric ulcers (Fig. 13-7) are usually single and less than 2 cm in diameter, although occasionally they reach a diameter of 10 cm or more, particularly if they are on the lesser curvature. The edges are sharply punched out, with overhanging margins. The flat base is grey and indurated and may exhibit clotted blood or an eroded vessel. Scarring of ulcers in the prepyloric region may be severe enough to produce pyloric stenosis.

Duodenal ulcers (Fig. 13-8) are ordinarily located on the anterior or posterior wall of the first part of the duodenum, within a short distance of the pylorus. The lesion is usually solitary, but it is not uncommon to find paired ulcers on both walls—so-called kissing ulcers.

Microscopically, gastric and duodenal ulcers have a similar appearance (see Fig. 13-8). From the lumen outward, the following are noted: a superficial zone of fibrinopurulent exudate; necrotic tissue; granulation tissue; and fibrotic tissue at the base of the ulcer, which exhibits variable degrees of chronic inflammation. The ulceration typically penetrates the muscle layers, thereby causing them to be interrupted by scar tissue. Blood vessels on the margins of the ulcer may be thrombosed or exhibit narrowing of the lumen by initial proliferation. Gastric ulcers are commonly accompanied by nonerosive gastritis, and the tissue surrounding a gastric or duodenal ulcer is often secondarily inflamed.

COMPLICATIONS

Hemorrhage is the most common complication of peptic ulcers, occurring in up to 20% of the patients. In many cases bleeding is occult and, in an otherwise asymptomatic ulcer, may be manifested as iron-deficiency anemia or as occult blood in the stools. Massive life-threatening hemorrhage is a well-recognized danger in patients with active peptic ulcers.

Perforation is a serious complication of peptic ulcer disease that occurs in 5% or less of patients; in one

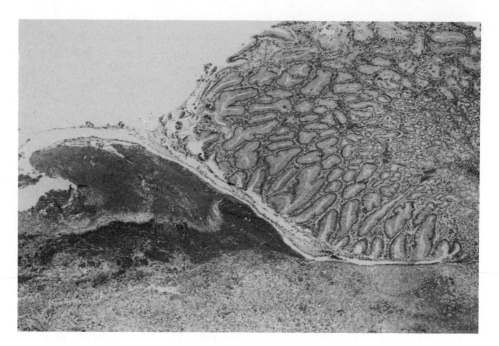

Figure 13-8. Peptic ulcer of the stomach. A photomicrograph demonstrates a sharply demarcated ulcer crater. The bed of the ulcer is covered with a fibrinous and hemorrhagic exudate, below which is inflamed granulation tissue.

third of the cases there are no antecedent symptoms referable to peptic ulcer. Perforations occur more commonly with duodenal than with gastric ulcers, the large majority occurring on the anterior wall of the duodenum. Because the anterior walls of the stomach and duodenum are undefended by contiguous tissue, ulcers in these locations are more likely to be complicated by free perforation, which leads to generalized peritonitis and the accumulation of air in the abdominal cavity, a condition called **pneumoperitoneum.** Posterior gastric ulcers perforate into the lesser peritoneal sac, where the inflammatory reaction may be contained. When ulcers penetrate into the pancreas, liver, or greater omentum, they cause intractable symptoms. Perforated ulcers continue to be associated with a high mortality.

Pyloric obstruction (gastric outlet obstruction) occurs in 5% to 10% of ulcer patients, and peptic ulcer disease is the most common cause of pyloric obstruction in adults. Narrowing of the pyloric lumen by an adjacent peptic ulcer may be caused by muscular spasm, edema, muscular hypertrophy, or contraction of scar tissue. Retention of gastric contents results in epigastric distress, anorexia, early satiety, and eventually obstruction.

In the United States almost half the patients with gastric ulcers also have a duodenal ulcer or an ulcer scar. Individuals with duodenal ulcers are also at higher than normal risk of developing a subsequent gastric ulcer.

Cancers originating in well-recognized benign gastric ulcers probably account for considerably less than 1% of all malignant tumors in the stomach. By contrast, duodenal ulcers never undergo malignant transformation.

NEOPLASMS

BENIGN TUMORS

Leiomyoma, a benign tumor of smooth muscle cells, is the most common tumor of the stomach, occurring in 25% to 50% of the population over 50 years of age. The tumors range in size from barely detectable to large masses more than 20 cm in diameter. Larger tumors may ulcerate and bleed or may cause pain, in which case the disorder is clinically indistinguishable from a peptic ulcer. Grossly, the tumors are submucosal and covered by intact mucosa or, when they project externally, by peritoneum. The cut surface has a whorled appearance and often shows cystic spaces. Microscopically, gastric leiomyomas show variable cellularity and are composed of spindle-shaped smooth muscle cells embedded in a collagenous stroma, like leiomyomas elsewhere.

Epithelial polyps of the stomach, classed as either **hyperplastic** or **adenomatous,** account for almost half of all benign gastric tumors. The large majority of gastric polyps are found in patients with achlorhydria, and both types occur in association with atrophic gastritis and pernicious anemia, as well as in stomachs that harbor carcinoma. Hyperplastic polyps, which represent the majority of polyps, may be single or multiple and present as small pedunculated or sessile lesions. They are not true neoplasms but are probably a result of chronic inflammation and regenerative hyperplasia of the mucosa. Microscopically, the polyps consist of elongated, branched crypts lined by normal foveolar epithelium, beneath which pyloric or gastric glands mingle with collagen and smooth muscle fibers. **Hyperplastic polyps have no malignant potential.**

Adenomatous polyps are true neoplasms. They occur most commonly in the antrum. Grossly, the polyps range from less than 1 cm in diameter to a considerable size, the average being about 4 cm. Most adenomatous polyps are sessile, and they are more often single than multiple. Microscopically, adenomas are composed of villous structures or a combination of tubular and villous glands, usually lined by intestinal or superficial gastric epithelium.

Adenomatous polyps manifest a malignant potential variably reported at 5% to 75%. The malignant potential increases with the size of the polyp and is greatest for lesions larger than 2 cm in diameter. As in the colon, villous adenomas seem to undergo malignant transformation more frequently than tubular adenomas.

MALIGNANT TUMORS

CARCINOMA OF THE STOMACH

As recently as the mid-20th century, carcinoma of the stomach was the most common cause of death from cancer among men in the United States. For reasons that have not been explained, the incidence of gastric carcinoma has steadily decreased. However, it remains the sixth most common cause of cancer death in the United States. The incidence of stomach cancer remains exceedingly high in such countries as Japan and Chile, where the rates are 7 to 8 times that in the United States.

Risk Factors

Dietary factors have been invoked to account for geographic variations in the incidence of gastric cancer, although the issue is still debated. Carcinoma of the stomach is more common among people who eat large amounts of starch, smoked fish and meat, and pickled vegetables. Benzpyrene, a potent carcinogen, has been detected in smoked foods. Attention has also been focused on the possible role of nitrosamines, powerful animal carcinogens, in the pathogenesis of cancer of the stomach. The consumption of whole milk and fresh vegetables rich in vitamin C is inversely related to the occurrence of stomach cancer.

Gastric cancer is uncommon in persons under the age of 30 and shows a sharp peak in incidence in persons over the age of 50 years. However, the age of onset seems to be somewhat lower in Japan, where the disease is endemic. In the United States there is only a slight male predominance, but in countries with a high incidence of this tumor, the male to female ratio is about 2:1. The risk of gastric cancer is particularly high in **low socioeconomic settings,** an observation that has been used to explain the high frequency of the tumor among American blacks and the fact that the incidence of the disease in that population has not declined as rapidly as it has among whites.

Atrophic gastritis, pernicious anemia, subtotal gastrectomy, and **gastric adenomatous polyps** have been discussed above as factors associated with a high risk of stomach cancer.

Two-thirds of patients with stomach cancer have fasting achlorhydria, compared with less than 25% of normal persons of the same age.

Pathology

Adenocarcinoma of the stomach, which accounts for more than 95% of all malignant gastric tumors, originates primarily from mucous cells of the normal superficial epithelium or from areas of intestinal metaplasia. The tumors are most common in the distal stomach, on the lesser curvature of the antrum and prepyloric region. They are rare in the fundus but may occur in any location.

ADVANCED GASTRIC CANCER   By the time most gastric cancers in the Western world are detected, they are advanced—that is, they have penetrated beyond the submucosa into the muscularis and may extend through the serosa. Advanced gastric cancers are divided into three major macroscopic types. First is the **polypoid (fungating) type,** which accounts for about one-third of the cancers. It is a solid mass, up to 10 cm in diameter, that projects into the lumen of the stomach. The surface may be partly ulcerated, and the deeper tissues may or may not be infiltrated. Second is the **ulcerating type,** which constitutes another third of all gastric cancers. Visualized as a shallow ulcer, it varies in size from 1 cm to 10 cm in diameter (Fig. 13-9). The surrounding tissue is firm, raised, and nodular. Characteristically, the lateral margins of the ulcer are irregular and the base is ragged, in contrast to the benign peptic ulcer, which exhibits punched-out margins and a smooth base. The third type of advanced gastric cancer is the **diffuse or infiltrating type,** which constitutes about one-tenth of all stomach cancers. No

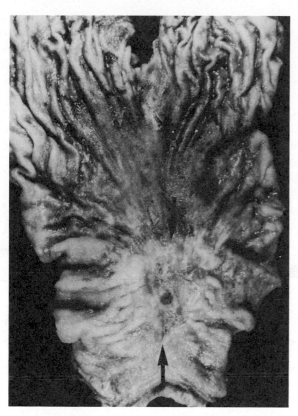

Figure 13-9. Ulcerating carcinoma of the stomach. A centrally ulcerated gastric cancer, characterized by raised, indurated margins (*arrows*), is present in the antrum.

EARLY GASTRIC CANCER In the early 1960s Japanese gastroenterologists, alarmed by the high incidence of stomach cancer in their country, began to screen the adult population endoscopically for early evidence of that disease. They defined **early gastric cancer** as a tumor that is confined to the mucosa or submucosa. (An earlier term, **superficial spreading carcinoma,** should be considered synonymous.) In Japan early gastric cancer accounts for fully one-third of all stomach cancers, whereas in the United States and Europe it constitutes only about 5% of diagnosed cancers.

Early gastric cancer is strictly a pathologic diagnosis; the term does not refer to the duration of the malignant tumor, its size, the presence of symptoms, the absence of metastases, or the curability. In fact, 5% to 20% of early gastric cancers are already metastatic to lymph nodes at the time of detection. Similar to advanced cancer, most early gastric cancers are found in the distal stomach.

Early gastric cancer may be a different disease from advanced cancer, and its more benign course and greater curability may reflect an inherently lower biologic potential for invasion, possibly related to the dif-

true tumor is seen macroscopically; instead, the wall of the stomach is conspicuously thickened and firm. When the entire stomach is involved, the term **linitis plastica (leather-bottle stomach)** (Fig. 13-10) is applied. In the diffuse type of gastric carcinoma, the invading tumor cells induce extensive fibrosis in the submucosa and muscularis. As a result, the wall is stiff and may be more than 2 cm thick.

Microscopically, the histologic pattern of advanced gastric cancer varies from **well-differentiated adenocarcinoma to a totally anaplastic tumor.** The polypoid variant typically contains well-differentiated glands, whereas linitis plastica is characteristically poorly differentiated. Particularly in the ulcerated type of cancer, the tumor cells may be arranged in cords or small foci. Many tumor cells contain clear mucin that displaces the nucleus to the periphery of the cell, resulting in the so-called **signet ring cell.** Extracellular mucinous material may be so prominent that the malignant cells seem to float in a gelatinous matrix, in which case it is called a **colloid** or **mucinous carcinoma.** Tumors that display papillary infoldings are termed **papillary adenocarcinomas,** and those that form solid tumor masses are referred to as **medullary carcinomas.**

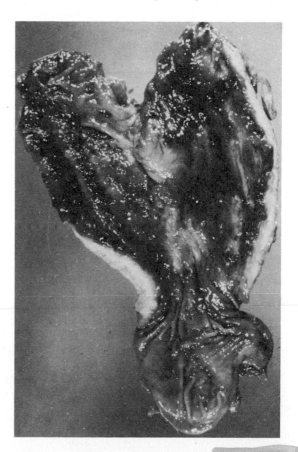

Figure 13-10. Infiltrating gastric carcinoma (linitis plastica). The wall of the stomach is thickened and indurated by diffusely infiltrating cancer.

EARLY GASTRIC CANCER

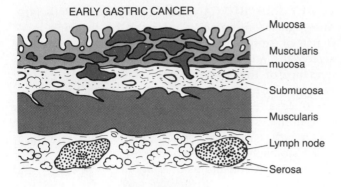

Mucosa

Muscularis mucosa

Submucosa

Muscularis

Lymph node

Serosa

POLYPOID CARCINOMA

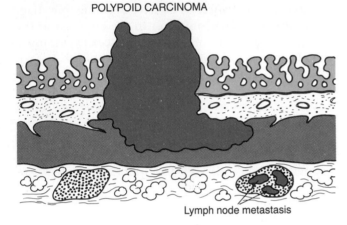

Lymph node metastasis

ULCERATING CARCINOMA

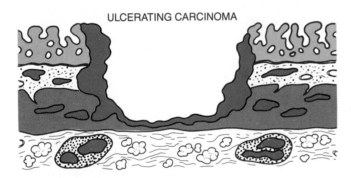

INFILTRATING CARCINOMA (LINITIS PLASTICA)

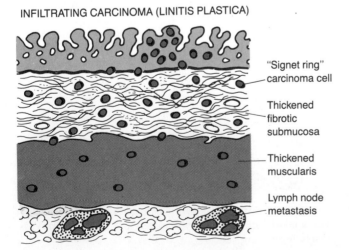

"Signet ring" carcinoma cell

Thickened fibrotic submucosa

Thickened muscularis

Lymph node metastasis

ferences between the intestinal and gastric cell types. Nevertheless, in some cases well-documented early gastric cancer has indeed progressed to advanced cancer. The 10-year survival rate for surgically treated early gastric cancer is about 95%, compared with 20% for advanced gastric cancer.

Gastric cancer metastasizes principally by the lymphatic route to regional lymph nodes of the lesser and greater curvature, the porta hepatis, and the subpyloric region. Distant lymphatic metastases also occur, the most common being an enlarged supraclavicular node, called **Virchow's node** or **sentinal node.** Hematogenous spread may seed any organ, including the liver, lung, or brain. Direct extension to nearby organs is often encountered. Carcinoma of the stomach can also spread to the ovary, where it is termed a **Krukenberg tumor.**

Figure 13-11 schematically depicts the major types of gastric cancer.

GASTRIC LYMPHOMA

Primary lymphoma of the stomach accounts for less than 5% of all malignant stomach tumors, but it is the most common of all extranodal non-Hodgkin's lymphomas, constituting 20% of such neoplasms. **Clinically and radiologically, gastric lymphoma mimics gastric adenocarcinoma.** The age at diagnosis is usually 40 to 65 years, and there is no sex predominance. The histologic varieties are similar to those in primary nodal lymphomas, as described in Chapter 20. The prognosis for gastric lymphoma is considerably better than that for adenocarcinoma. The overall 5-year survival is 40% to 45%.

BEZOARS

Bezoars are foreign bodies in the stomach of animals and humans that are composed of food or hair that has been altered by the digestive process. Phytobezoars are vegetable concretions that are unusual in the normal stomach, except in persons who eat many persimmons or swallow unchewed bubble gum. In the last few decades, phytobezoars have been found principally in patients who display delayed gastric emptying and hypochlorhydria after partial gastrectomy, particularly when the surgery has included vagotomy.

A trichobezoar is a hairball within a gelatinous matrix; it is usually seen in long-haired girls or young women who eat their own hair as a nervous habit.

Figure 13-11. The major types of gastric cancer.

THE SMALL INTESTINE

CONGENITAL DISORDERS

ATRESIA

Intestinal atresia, although rare, is the most frequent cause of neonatal intestinal obstruction. A quarter of the cases are associated with meconium ileus, and cystic fibrosis is discovered in one-tenth of the cases of atresia.

MECKEL'S DIVERTICULUM

Meckel's diverticulum, caused by persistence of the vitelline duct, is the most common and the most clinically significant congenital anomaly of the small intestine (Fig. 13-12). This true diverticulum is found on the antimesenteric border of the ileum 60 cm to 100 cm from the ileocecal valve in the adult. However, 60% of patients are under 2 years of age. The diverticulum is about 5 cm in length, with a diameter slightly less than that of the ileum but considerably larger than that of the appendix.

Most Meckel's diverticula are asymptomatic. Of the minority that become symptomatic, about half contain ectopic gastric, duodenal, pancreatic, biliary, or colonic tissue. **Meckel's diverticulum may be complicated by hemorrhage, intestinal obstruction, diverticulitis, and perforation with peritonitis. The most common complication is bleeding, which is responsible for half of all lower gastrointestinal hemorrhage in children.** Bleeding results from **peptic ulceration** of the ileum adjacent to ectopic gastric mucosa. The diverticulum may act as a lead point for **intussusception** and thus cause intestinal obstruction. Obstruction can also be caused by volvulus around the fibrotic remnant of the vitelline duct. Inflammation of a Meckel's diverticulum—that is, **diverticulitis**—leads to symptoms indistinguishable from those of appendicitis. Perforation, complicated by a rapidly spreading peritonitis, may result from peptic ulceration, either in the diverticulum or in the ileum.

MECONIUM ILEUS

The earliest manifestation of cystic fibrosis is often neonatal intestinal obstruction caused by the accumulation of tenacious meconium in the small intestine. In half of affected infants, meconium ileus is

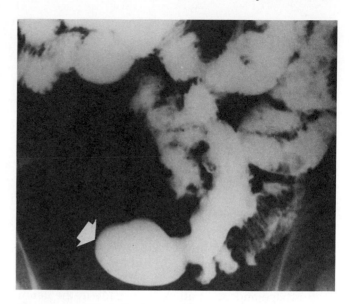

Figure 13-12. Meckel's diverticulum. A contrast radiograph of the small intestine shows a barium-filled diverticulum of the ileum (*arrow*).

complicated by volvulus, perforation with a meconium peritonitis, or intestinal atresia.

INFECTIONS

DIARRHEAL DISEASES

TOXIGENIC DIARRHEA

The prototypic organisms that produce diarrhea by secreting a toxin are *Vibrio cholera* and toxigenic strains of *Escherichia coli*. Toxigenic diarrhea is characterized by the following: damage to the intestinal mucosa is minimal or absent; the organism remains on the mucosal surface, where it secretes its toxin; and, owing to fluid secreted into the small intestine, there is watery diarrhea, which can lead to dehydration, particularly in the case of cholera. Although many organisms have been isolated in so-called **travelers' diarrhea,** the most common pathogen in almost all studies is toxigenic *E. coli*.

DIARRHEA CAUSED BY INVASIVE BACTERIA

Invasive bacteria, as their name implies, cause diarrhea by directly injuring the intestinal mucosa. Among these organisms *Shigella*, *Salmonella*, certain strains of *E. coli*, *Yersinia*, and *Campylobacter* are the most widely recognized. The invasive organisms tend to infect the distal ileum and colon, whereas the toxigenic bacteria mainly involve the upper intestinal tract.

Shigellosis principally affects the colon, although the terminal ileum is occasionally involved. Microscopically, a granular and hemorrhagic mucosa exhibits numerous shallow serpiginous ulcers. The inflammation, which is especially severe in the sigmoid colon and rectum, is usually superficial.

Typhoid fever (salmonella enteritis), today uncommon in the industrialized world, still presents a problem in underdeveloped countries. Necrosis of lymphoid tissue, principally in the terminal ileum, leads to scattered ulcers. Infection of Peyer's patches results in oval ulcers, the longer dimension of which is in the long axis of the intestine. Microscopically, the early lesions of typhoid fever contain large basophilic macrophages filled with typhoid bacilli, erythrocytes, and necrotic debris. Necrosis of lymphoid follicles becomes confluent, and mucosal ulceration follows. Intestinal hemorrhage and perforation, principally in the ileum, are the most feared complications of typhoid fever.

Nontyphoidal salmonellosis, formerly known as "paratyphoid fever," is an enteritis caused by salmonella strains other than *S. typhi* and is generally a far less serious illness than typhoid fever. In addition to causing diarrhea, bacteremia, and fever, there may be hematogenous dissemination from the intestine carrying the infection to bones, joints, and meninges. Interestingly, there seems to be an association between sickle cell anemia and salmonella osteomyelitis.

Yersinia **enterocolitis,** transmitted by pets or contaminated food, is most common in young children. It causes diarrhea, cramps, and fever and lasts 1 to 3 weeks. In addition to causing enterocolitis, *Yersinia* causes acute mesenteric adenitis and pain in the right lower quadrant. Infected children have undergone laparotomy because of a mistaken diagnosis of appendicitis.

Campylobacter **infection** has been recognized only recently as an important cause of gastroenteritis.

FOOD POISONING

Infectious agents can produce gastroenteritis not only by infecting the bowel directly, but also by elaborating enterotoxins in contaminated food, which is then ingested.

Staphylococcus aureus is a common cause of food poisoning. Symptoms result from the ingestion of food contaminated with strains of *Staphylococcus* that produce an exotoxin that damages the epithelium of the gastrointestinal tract. Within 6 hours of the ingestion of tainted food, severe vomiting and abdominal cramps occur, often followed by diarrhea. Most victims recover in 1 to 2 days.

Clostridium perfringens elaborates an enterotoxin that causes vomiting and diarrhea. Watery diarrhea and severe abdominal pain, which begin 8 to 24 hours after ingestion of the contaminated food, last only about 1 day.

VIRAL GASTROENTERITIS

Rotaviruses cause self-limited vomiting and watery diarrhea, principally in children less than 2 years of age.

The **Norwalk viruses** account for one-third of the epidemics of viral gastroenteritis in the United States. The virus targets the upper small intestine, where it causes patchy mucosal lesions and malabsorption. Vomiting and diarrhea are usual, but the symptoms resolve within 2 days.

TUBERCULOSIS

Virtually all cases of intestinal tuberculosis in Western countries are caused by *Mycobacterium tuberculosis*. **Most cases of intestinal tuberculosis are caused either by ingestion of bacteria in food or by the swallowing of infectious sputum.** The bacterium establishes a locus of infection, usually in the ileocecal region. Almost all patients with intestinal tuberculosis complain of chronic abdominal pain, and about two-thirds have a palpable abdominal mass, usually in the right lower quadrant.

Typically, intestinal tuberculosis is characterized by one or more circular or oval ulcers of varying size in the transverse plane of the bowel. As the ulcers heal, reactive fibrosis may cause a circumferential ("napkin ring") stricture of the bowel lumen. Mesenteric lymph nodes are usually enlarged and on cut section display caseous necrosis.

Microscopically, tuberculous granulomas are found in all layers of the bowel wall, particularly in the Peyer's patches and lymphoid follicles, and in the mesenteric lymph nodes. Crohn's disease exhibits virtually all the changes produced by intestinal tuberculosis, and indeed these entities have often been confused by pathologists.

FUNGI

Fungal infection of the gastrointestinal tract occurs almost exclusively in immunocompromised persons or, in the case of actinomycosis, in persons who have suffered trauma to the gut. Suppression of the normal bacterial flora by antibiotics also favors fungal growth.

The most common mycoses are caused by *Candida*, *Mucor* species, and *Histoplasma*. Mucormycosis and candidiasis typically cause mucosal erosions that may progress to larger ulcers. The inflammation is characteristically neutrophilic. Mucormycetes have a tendency to invade blood vessels, but hematogenous dissemination from the intestine is rare. Disseminated histoplasmosis may involve the bowel, where it causes elevated plaques that ulcerate and may even perforate.

VASCULAR OCCLUSION

The sudden occlusion of an artery by thrombosis or embolization leads to infarction of the small bowel before collateral circulation comes into play. Depending on the size of the vessel, infarction may be segmental (Fig. 13-13) or may lead to gangrene of virtually the entire small bowel. About half of the cases of intestinal infarction are caused by **embolic or thrombotic occlusion of the superior mesenteric artery.** About one-quarter are the result of **inferior mesenteric artery occlusion, mesenteric venous thrombosis, or arteritis,** and in the remaining quarter no acute vascular occlusions are demonstrated.

In addition to intrinsic vascular lesions, **volvulus, intussusception,** and **incarceration of the intestine in a hernial sac** may all lead to bowel infarction. Nonocclusive intestinal infarction, which may be extensive, is seen in hypoxic patients with reduced cardiac output as a result of shock or acute myocardial infarction.

Clinically, in mesenteric artery occlusion the abrupt onset of abdominal pain is virtually invariable. Bloody diarrhea, hematemesis, and shock are common, and in untreated cases perforation is frequent. As the infarction progresses, systemic manifestations become more severe, and **death is inevitable without surgical intervention.**

The infarcted bowel is edematous and diffusely purple, and the demarcation between infarcted bowel and normal tissue is usually sharp. Extensive hemorrhage is seen in the mucosa and submucosa, the former becoming necrotic.

Thrombosis of the mesenteric veins occurs under a variety of conditions, including hypercoagulable states, stasis, and inflammation. Almost all thromboses affect the superior mesenteric vein. The collateral flow in the distribution of the superior mesenteric vein is usually sufficient to preclude infarction of the intestine.

Atherosclerotic narrowing of the major splanchnic arteries leads to chronic intestinal ischemia. As in the heart, the result is intermitted abdominal pain, termed **intestinal (abdominal) angina.** Chronic ischemia of

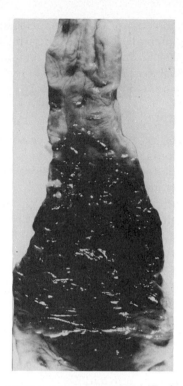

Figure 13-13. Infarct of the small bowel. Occlusion of a branch of the superior mesenteric artery led to hemorrhagic infarction of the small bowel. Note the sharp demarcation between the dilated, infarcted zone and the normal bowel.

the small bowel may lead to fibrosis and the formation of a stricture.

MALABSORPTION

Malabsorption is a general term used to describe a number of clinical conditions in which one or more important nutrients are inadequately absorbed by the gastrointestinal tract. Although some nutrient absorption occurs in the stomach and colon, only absorption from the small intestine, mainly in the proximal portion, is clinically important. The two substances that are preferentially absorbed by the distal small intestine are bile salts and vitamin B_{12}.

Normal intestinal absorption is characterized by a **luminal** phase and an **intestinal** phase. The luminal phase, consisting of those processes that occur within the lumen of the small intestine, alters the physiochemical state of the various nutrients such that they can be taken up by the absorptive cells in the small bowel epithelium. The intestinal phase includes those processes that occur in the cells and transport channels of the intestinal wall.

In the luminal phase of intestinal absorption it is critical that **pancreatic enzymes** and **bile acids** be secreted into the duodenal lumen in adequate amounts and in a normal physiochemical condition.

Luminal-phase malabsorption has four major causes:

1. **Interruption of the normal continuity of the distal stomach and duodenum,** as occurs after gastroduodenal surgery (gastrectomy, antrectomy, pyloroplasty).
2. **Pancreatic dysfunction,** as a result of chronic pancreatitis, pancreatic carcinoma, or cystic fibrosis.
3. **Deficient or ineffective bile salts,** which may result from three possible causes. First is **impaired excretion of bile** because of liver disease. Second is **bacterial overgrowth,** which occurs as a result of a disturbance in the motility of the gut. It is seen in such conditions as blind loop syndrome, multiple diverticula of the small bowel, and muscular or neurogenic defects of the intestinal wall (e.g., amyloidosis, scleroderma, diabetic enteropathy). When gastrointestinal motility is defective, bile salts are deconjugated by the excess small bowel bacteria. The third cause of ineffective or deficient bile salts is **absence or bypass of the distal ileum** caused by surgical excision, surgical anastomoses, fistulas, or ileal disease (e.g., Crohn's disease, lymphoma).
4. **Abnormally low intraduodenal pH,** as seen in patients with hypersecretion secondary to a gastrinoma (Zollinger-Ellison syndrome).

The **intestinal phase** of absorption may be interrupted at four different points:

1. **Microvilli.** The intestinal disaccharidases and oligopeptidases are integrally bound to the microvillous membranes. Abnormal function of the microvilli may be **primary,** as in the primary disaccharidase deficiencies, or **secondary,** when there is damage to the villi, as in celiac disease (sprue).
2. **Absorptive area.** If sufficiently severe, a diminution in the surface area of the small bowel results in malabsorption. The surface area of the small intestinal epithelium may be diminished by small bowel resection (short bowel syndrome), gastrocolic fistulas (bypassing the small intestine), or a number of small intestinal diseases that are associated with mucosal damage (celiac disease, tropical sprue, Whipple's disease).
3. **Metabolic function of the absorptive cells.** Non-specific damage to small intestinal epithelial cells occurs in celiac disease, tropical sprue, Whipple's disease, and gastrinoma. Specific metabolic dysfunction is seen in **abetalipoproteinemia** (associated with acanthocytosis), a disorder in which the absorptive cells are unable to synthesize the apoprotein required for the assembly of lipoproteins and chylomicrons.
4. **Transport.** Impaired transport of nutrients through the capillaries and lymphatic vessels is probably an important factor in the malabsorption associated with Whipple's disease, intestinal lymphoma, and congenital lymphangiectasia.

Figure 13-14 summarizes the major causes of malabsorption.

CELIAC DISEASE (CELIAC SPRUE)

Celiac disease (gluten-sensitive enteropathy, nontropical sprue) is characterized by generalized malabsorption; a typical, but nonspecific, small intestinal mucosal lesion; and a prompt clinical, and slower histologic, response to withdrawal of gluten-containing foods from the diet. Most cases are diagnosed during childhood, although the disease may become clinically apparent for the first time as late as the seventh decade of life. Biopsy studies have indicated that the familial frequency may be over 20%.

ETIOLOGY AND PATHOGENESIS

The clinical features and histologic changes typical of celiac sprue are caused by the ingestion of wheat or wheat products. Both the water-insoluble portion of wheat flour, namely **gluten,** and an alcoholic extract called **gliadin** have the same effect as whole wheat. Approximately 80% of celiac disease patients carry the histocompatibility antigen HLA-B8; a similar frequency has been reported for HLA-DW3.

Celiac disease is occasionally associated with **dermatitis herpetiformis,** a vesicular skin disease that typically affects the extensor surfaces and the exposed parts of the body. Almost all patients with dermatitis herpetiformis have a small bowel mucosal lesion similar to that of celiac disease, although only 10% have overt malabsorption.

CLINICAL FEATURES

Clinically, celiac disease is characterized by generalized malabsorption. Typically, a child comes to medical attention because he ceases to thrive soon after the

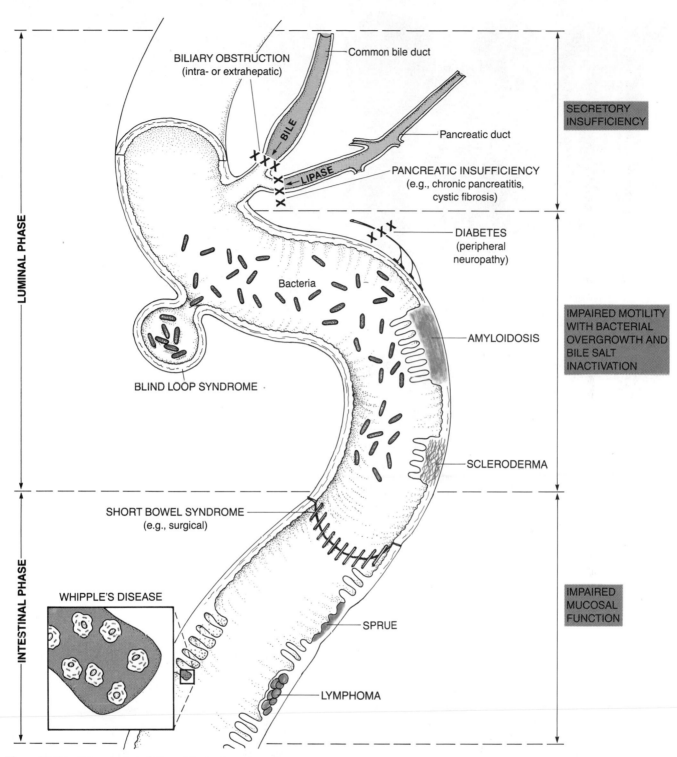

Figure 13-14. Causes of malabsorption.

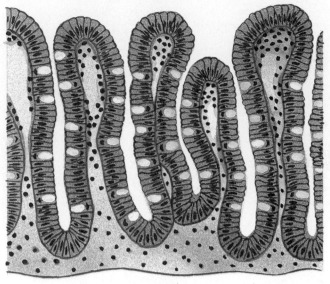

NORMAL

Figure 13-15. Celiac disease. Elongation of the crypts, and chronic inflammation of the lamina propria are characteristic. In complete villous atrophy of longstanding disease the mucosa is flat.

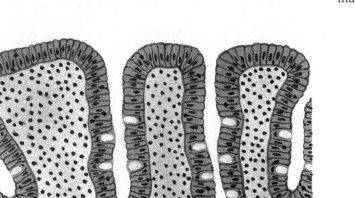

CELIAC DISEASE

introduction of cereals into his diet. Late complications include lymphoma of the small bowel and other malignant diseases of the gastrointestinal tract. Treatment with a strict gluten-free diet is usually followed by a complete and prolonged clinical and histologic remission.

PATHOLOGY

The hallmark of celiac disease is a flat small intestinal mucosa, with blunting or total disappearance of villi, abnormal epithelial cells on the mucosal surface, and increased cellularity of the lamina propria but not of the deeper layers (Fig. 13-15). The numbers of lymphocytes and plasma cells in the lamina propria are markedly increased.

WHIPPLE'S DISEASE

Whipple's disease is a rare systemic disorder in which **the small intestine is consistently involved and malabsorption is the most prominent feature.** It most commonly affects white men in their 30s and 40s.

Whipple's disease typically shows infiltration of the small bowel mucosa by large macrophages that are packed with small, as yet unidentified, rod-shaped bacilli. Dramatic clinical remissions occur with

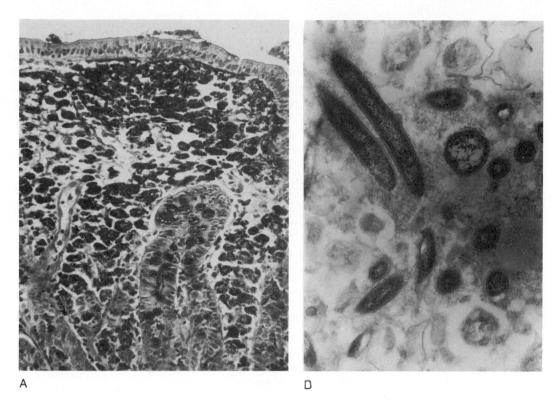

A   B

Figure 13-16. Whipple's disease. (*A*) A photomicrograph of a section of jejunal mucosa, stained by the periodic acid-Schiff (PAS) reaction, shows abundant large macrophages filled with cytoplasmic material. (*B*) An electron micrograph of (*A*) showing small bacilli in a macrophage.

antibiotic therapy. Histologic examination of the small intestine reveals flat, thickened villi and extensive infiltration of the lamina propria with large macrophages (Fig. 13-16). **The cytoplasm of these macrophages is filled with large glycoprotein granules, representing phagocytosed bacteria, that stain strongly with periodic acid-Schiff (PAS).** The lymphatic vessels in the mucosa and submucosa are dilated, and large lipid droplets abound within lymphatics and in extracellular spaces, a finding that suggests obstruction of the lymphatics.

TROPICAL SPRUE

Tropical sprue is a poorly understood disease of obscure cause that is acquired in certain endemic tropical areas (e.g. Caribbean islands and the Far East), and is characterized by progressively severe malabsorption and nutritional deficiency. Cure, or at least amelioration of the symptoms, usually follows treatment with oral tetracycline and folic acid.

Some studies suggest that **long-standing contamination of the bowel with bacteria,** perhaps toxigenic strains of *E. coli,* may be important in causation and that **folate deficiency** may play a role in pepetuating the intestinal lesion. The histologic findings range from mild villous changes to a completely flat mucosa indistinguishable from that seen in celiac sprue.

NEOPLASMS

The small intestine is curiously resistant to neoplasia, despite the fact that it is the longest portion of the alimentary tract. Tumors of the small intestine constitute less than 5% of all gastrointestinal tumors.

BENIGN TUMORS

The most common benign tumors of the small intestine are adenomas, leiomyomas, and lipomas. As in other portions of the gastrointestinal tract, neurogenic tumors, fibromas, angiomas, and hamartomas may be encountered. Although most adenomas remain benign, some, especially the villous type, undergo malignant transformation.

The **Peutz-Jeghers syndrome** is an autosomal dominant hereditary disorder characterized by small intestinal polyps (and occasionally gastric and colonic polyps) and mucocutaneous melanin pigmentation. The polyps in Peutz-Jeghers syndrome are not true neoplasms, but rather **hamartomas.** Histologically, a branching network of smooth muscle fibers continuous with the muscularis mucosa supports the glandular epithelium of the polyp.

MALIGNANT TUMORS

ADENOCARCINOMA

Adenocarcinoma of the small intestine, which accounts for half of all small intestinal cancers, is usually annular; therefore, the symptoms are commonly those of progressive intestinal obstruction. Occult bleeding is common and often leads to iron-deficiency anemia.

A risk factor for adenocarcinoma is inflammatory disease of the small bowel. Patients with Crohn's disease are known to be at a significantly increased risk, perhaps as high as 100-fold. Adenocarcinoma is also a rare complication of celiac disease.

PRIMARY LYMPHOMA

Primary lymphoma, which originates in nodules of lymphoid tissue within the bowel wall, represents the second most common malignant tumor of the small intestine in industrialized countries. By contrast, another type of primary lymphoma comprises more than two thirds of all cancers of the small intestine in underdeveloped countries. The latter type of intestinal lymphoma was originally described in Mediterranean populations, but it is now clear that it is distributed throughout the poorer parts of the world. Because these two types of lymphoma have distinct epidemiologic, clinical, and pathological features, they are labeled, respectively, the "Western" type and the "Mediterranean" variety.

Mediterranean lymphoma typically occurs in poor countries in young men of low socioeconomic status. **This neoplasm has been associated with alpha-chain disease, a proliferative disorder of intestinal B-lymphocytes that secrete IgA.** In fact, Mediterranean lymphoma and alpha-chain disease are thought by some to be the same disorder, termed **immunoproliferative small intestinal disease.**

The Western type of intestinal lymphoma usually affects adults over the age of 40 years and children under the age of 10 years. Microscopically, all varieties of non-Hodgkin's lymphoma are encountered. When the disease is localized and confined to the small intestine, it does not recur after surgical removal in over half the patients. When extraintestinal spread is present, the 5-year survival rate is less than 10%.

An association of the Western type of intestinal lymphoma with celiac disease is well documented, occurring in as many as one tenth of primary lymphoma patients.

CARCINOID TUMOR

Carcinoid tumors of the gastrointestinal tract arise from argentaffin cells, which are part of the neuroendocrine system of the gut, and are located principally in the appendix and the ileum, although they can occur anywhere in the gastrointestinal tract. Although carcinoid tumors constitute less than 1% of all gastrointestinal tumors, **they are the most common benign tumors of the small intestine and account for 20% of all malignant tumors.** In general, the malignant potential of intestinal carcinoid tumors appears to be related to their size. Tumors of less than 1 cm in diameter are rarely malignant, 50% of those between 1 cm and 2 cm in diameter metastasize, and 80% of those larger than 2 cm in diameter metastasize. **For practical purposes carcinoid tumors of the appendix less than 2 cm across do not metastasize.**

Macroscopically, small carcinoid tumors present as yellowish submucosal nodules covered by intact mucosa. Large tumors may grow in a polypoid, intramural, or annular pattern and often undergo secondary ulceration. Microscopically, the neoplasms appear as nests, cords, and rosettes of uniform small, round cells (Fig. 13-17). These neoplasms metastasize first to regional lymph nodes. Subsequently, hematogenous spread leads to metastases at distant sites, particularly the liver.

Carcinoid tumors are marked by a unique clinical condition, termed the **carcinoid syndrome,** that is caused by the release of a variety of active tumor products. Carcinoid tumors are capable of secreting all the peptides and amines produced by their normal counterparts. The most commonly secreted hormone is **serotonin.** Carcinoid syndrome is ordinarily seen only in cases with extensive hepatic metastases. **The classic symptoms of the carcinoid syndrome include diarrhea (often the most distressing symptom), episodic flushing, bronchospasm, cyanosis, telangiectasia, and skin lesions.**

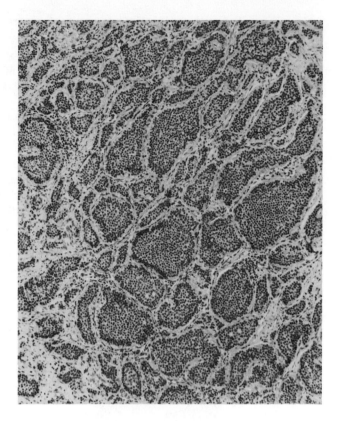

Figure 13-17. Carcinoid tumor of the small intestine. A photomicrograph demonstrates nests and cords of uniform small, round cells.

THE COLON

CONGENITAL MEGACOLON (HIRSCHSPRUNG'S DISEASE)

Hirschsprung's disease is an uncommon, but not rare, familial disorder in which colonic dilatation results from a defect in the innervation of the rectum. **The lesion is a congenital absence of ganglion cells in the wall of the rectum** and sometimes more proximal portions of the colon. The incidence of congenital megacolon is 10 times higher than normal in infants with **Down's syndrome.** The clinical signs are delayed passage of meconium by the neonate and the development of vomiting in 2 to 3 days. In some cases complete intestinal obstruction requires immediate surgical relief. The cure for Hirschsprung's disease is surgical removal of the aganglionic segment.

INFECTIONS

The principal bacterial and parasitic infections that affect the colon, including shigellosis, amebiasis, and tu-

berculosis, have been discussed either in Chapter 9 or above in the context of infectious diarrhea. Most of the remaining infectious diseases are transmitted sexually, principally affect male homosexuals, and primarily involve the anorectal region. These diseases, popularly referred to in medical parlance as the **gay bowel syndrome,** are transmitted by anal intercourse and oral-anal or oral-genital contact. Such diseases include gonorrhea, syphilis, lymphogranuloma venereum, anorectal herpes, and venereal warts (condylomata acuminata). There is also a high incidence of colonic infections, such as amebiasis and shigellosis, among male homosexuals.

PSEUDOMEMBRANOUS COLITIS

Pseudomembranous colitis is an inflammatory disease of the colon characterized by exudative plaques superimposed on a congested and edematous mucosa. *Clostridium difficile,* which has also been implicated in neonatal necrotizing enterocolitis, is the offending organism. *C. difficile* is not invasive, but it produces toxins that damage the colonic mucosa. **Although most cases of pseudomembranous colitis are**

today associated with antibiotic therapy, gastrointestinal surgery remains a risk factor.

Macroscopically, the colon, particularly the rectosigmoid region, exhibits raised yellowish plaques of up to 2 cm in diameter that adhere to the underlying mucosa (Fig. 13-18). In severe cases the plaques coalesce to form extensive pseudomembranes. Microscopic examination of the lesions discloses a loss of the superficial epithelium, thought to be the initial pathologic event. Subsequently, the crypts become disrupted and are expanded by mucin and neutrophils, an appearance similar to that of the crypt abscesses of ulcerative colitis. The pseudomembrane consists of the debris of necrotic epithelial cells, mucus, fibrin, and neutrophils.

DIVERTICULAR DISEASE

Diverticulosis is an acquired herniation (diverticulum) of the mucosa and submucosa through the mus-

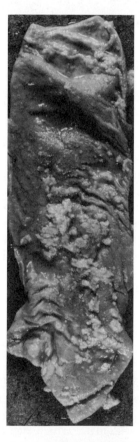

Figure 13-18. Pseudomembranous colitis. The mucosal surface of the colon is covered by raised, irregular plaques composed of necrotic debris and an acute inflammatory exudate.

cular layers of the colon. The presence of necrotizing inflammation in diverticula is called **diverticulitis,** and its complications are included under the rubric of **diverticular disease. Diverticulosis shows a striking geographic variation,** being common in Western societies and infrequent in Asia, Africa, and underdeveloped countries. Diverticulosis is unusual in persons under 40 years of age and increases in frequency with age.

The variation in the prevalence of diverticulosis suggests that environmental factors are primarily responsible for the disease. Western populations consume a diet in which refined carbohydrates and meat have replaced crude cereal grains, and it is widely assumed that the lack of indigestible fibers in some way predisposes to the formation of diverticula.

The abnormal structures that characterize diverticulosis are not true diverticula that contain all layers of the intestinal wall, but rather **pseudodiverticula,** in which only the mucosa and submucosa are herniated through the muscle layers. **The sigmoid colon is affected in 95% of the cases,** but diverticulosis can affect any segment of the colon, including the cecum.

Diverticula vary in number from a few to several hundred (Fig. 13-19A). Most appear in parallel rows between the mesenteric and lateral taeniae. The diverticula, which measure up to 1 cm in greatest dimension, are connected to the intestinal lumen by necks of varying length and caliber. Hardened fecal material is frequently present in the diverticula but does not signify diverticulitis.

Microscopically, a diverticulum characteristically presents as a flasklike structure that extends from the lumen through the muscle layers (Fig. 13-19B). The wall of the diverticulum is in continuity with the surface mucosa and therefore displays an epithelium and a submucosa.

Diverticulosis is generally asymptomatic, and 80% of affected persons remain free of symptoms. However, a significant number of those with diverticulosis complain of episodic colicky abdominal pain. **Sudden, painless, and severe bleeding** from colonic diverticula is a cause of serious lower gastrointestinal hemorrhage in the elderly.

Although the large majority of persons with diverticulosis remain asymptomatic, in 10% to 20% **diverticulitis** supervenes. Low-grade chronic inflammation eventually produces necrosis of the wall of the diverticulum, an event that results in perforation and the release of fecal contents containing bacteria into the peridiverticular tissues. Fibrosis may constrict the lumen of the bowel, thereby causing **intestinal obstruction. Fistulas** may form between the colon and adjacent organs.

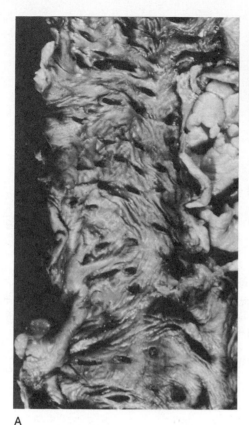

A

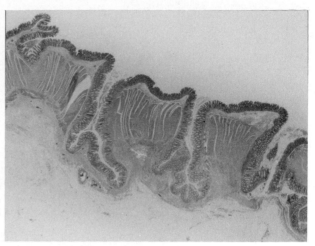

B

Figure 13-19. Diverticulosis of the colon. (*A*) Numerous diverticula open on the mucosal surface of the colon. (*B*) A low-power photomicrograph of (*A*) shows that the mucosa of the diverticula, which extends through the muscle layers, is in continuity with the surface mucosa.

INFLAMMATORY BOWEL DISEASE

"Nonspecific inflammatory bowel disease" is a term that describes two diseases, Crohn's disease (regional enteritis) and ulcerative colitis, which **have different clinical courses and natural histories.**

CROHN'S DISEASE

Crohn's disease occurs throughout the world and usually appears in adolescents or young adults. It is most common among people of European origin, with an apparently higher frequency among Jews. A family history of inflammatory bowel disease (Crohn's disease or ulcerative colitis) has been found in up to 40% of cases. The greatest frequency is among siblings, suggesting that environmental factors play a role. Intensive research since the disease was first described in 1932 has failed to elucidate the etiology and pathogenesis of Crohn's disease.

The most frequent symptoms are abdominal pain, diarrhea, and recurrent fever. In cases of diffuse small intestinal involvement, malabsorption and malnutrition may be the major features. In 10% to 15% of cases the major site of involvement is the anorectal region, and recurrent anorectal fistulas are the presenting sign.

The most common intestinal complications of Crohn's disease are **intestinal obstruction and fistulas. Patients with the disease have a risk of intestinal cancer that is at least threefold higher than normal.** No curative treatment for Crohn's disease is available.

PATHOLOGY

Two major features characterize the pathology of Crohn's disease and serve to differentiate it from other inflammations of the gastrointestinal tract. The inflammation in Crohn's disease usually involves **all** layers of the bowel wall and is therefore referred to as **transmural** inflammatory disease. The inflammation of the intestine is **discontinuous**—that is, segments of inflamed tissue are separated by apparently normal intestine. It is convenient to classify Crohn's disease into four broad macroscopic patterns, although many pa-

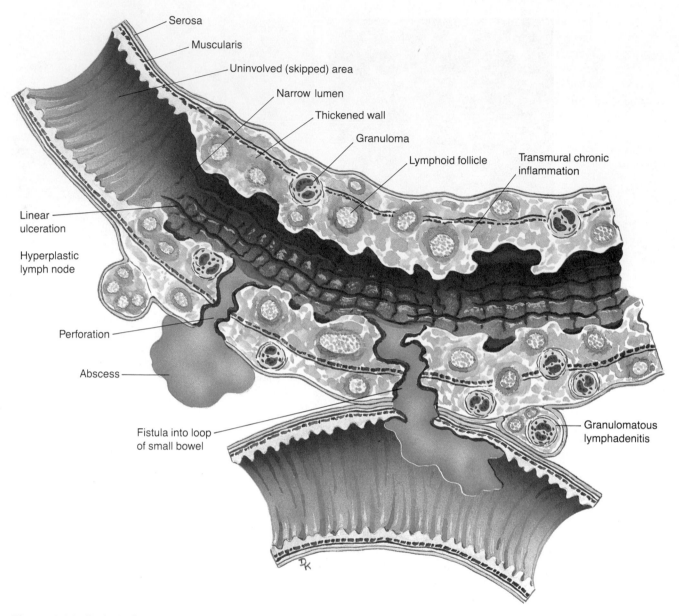

Figure 13-20. Crohn's disease. A schematic representation of the major features of Crohn's disease in the small intestine.

tients do not fit precisely into any one of them: the disease involves mainly the ileum and cecum in 50% of cases, only the small intestine in 15%, only the colon in 20%, and principally the anorectal region in 15%. Crohn's disease is occasionally observed in the duodenum and stomach, and more rarely in the esophagus and oral cavity, almost always in association with small intestinal Crohn's disease.

Macroscopically, the bowel affected by Crohn's disease appears thickened and edematous, as does the adjacent mesentery (Fig. 13-20). Mesenteric lymph nodes are frequently enlarged, firm, and matted together. The lumen is narrowed by edema in early cases and by a combination of edema and fibrosis in longstanding disease. Nodular swelling, fibrosis, and ulceration of the mucosa lead to a "cobblestone" appearance. In early cases the ulcers have an "apthous" or "serpiginous" appearance; later they become deeper and appear as linear clefts or fissures.

Involved loops of bowel often become adherent, and

fistulas between such segments are frequent. These fistulas, presumably a late result of the deep mural ulcers, may also penetrate from the bowel into other organs, including the bladder, uterus, vagina, and skin. Most fistulas end blindly, forming abscess cavities within the peritoneal cavity, in the mesentery, or in retroperitoneal structures. Lesions in the distal rectum may create perianal fistulas.

Microscopically, the disease appears as a **chronic inflammatory process that extends through all layers of the bowel wall**. During early phases of the disease small, superficial mucosal ulcerations are seen. Later, long, deep, fissure-like ulcers are seen. **The microscopic hallmark of Crohn's disease is the appearance of discrete, noncaseating granulomas, mostly in the submucosa. However, the absence of granulomas by no means excludes the diagnosis.**

ULCERATIVE COLITIS

Ulcerative colitis, a disease of unknown etiology in young adults, is characterized by **chronic diarrhea and rectal bleeding.**

The higher than normal incidence of ulcerative colitis in first-degree relatives of patients with the disease (up to 40% familial incidence) points to a possible genetic predisposition. Although abnormal immune responses have been documented, it is possible that they are merely epiphenomena—that is, the result, rather than the cause, of the mucosal damage.

The clinical course and manifestations of ulcerative colitis are highly variable. Most patients (70%) have intermittent attacks, with partial or complete remission between attacks. A small number (less than 10%) have a very long remission (several years) following their first attack. The remaining 20% have continuous symptoms without remission.

Approximately 50% of patients with ulcerative colitis suffer only from rectal bleeding, sometimes accompanied by tenesmus (rectal pressure and discomfort). The disease in these patients is usually limited to the rectum but may extend to the distal sigmoid colon. About 40% of patients suffer from recurrent episodes of loose bloody stools, crampy abdominal pain, low-grade fever and anemia from chronic fecal blood loss. Ten percent of patients have "severe" or "fulminant" ulcerative colitis. These patients have numerous bloody bowel movements daily, frequently accompanied by fever and other systemic manifestations. The loss of blood and fluids rapidly leads to anemia, dehydration, and electrolyte depletion. Massive hemorrhage is occasionally life-threatening. A particularly dangerous compli-

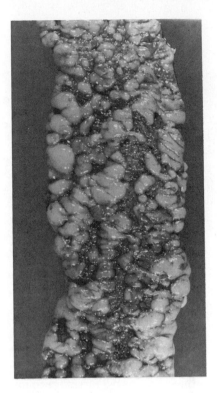

Figure 13-21. Ulcerative colitis. The mucosal surface of the colon exhibits irregular ulcerated areas that surround islands of colonic mucosa.

cation is **"toxic megacolon"**, in which extreme dilatation of the colon occurs. Patients with this condition are at high risk for perforation of the colon, and prompt colectomy may be required.

PATHOLOGY

Three major pathologic features characterize ulcerative colitis and help differentiate it from other inflammatory conditions:

1. Ulcerative colitis is a **diffuse** disease, usually extending from the most distal part of the rectum for a variable distance proximally.
2. The inflammatory process of ulcerative colitis is **limited to the colon.**
3. Histologically, ulcerative colitis is **essentially a disease of the mucosa.**

Macroscopically, the mucosal surface appears raw, red, and granular. Small, superficial ulcers coalesce to form irregular, shallow, ulcerated areas that appear to surround islands of intact mucosa (Fig. 13-21). Subsequently, raised areas of mucosa, corresponding to in-

EARLY

ADVANCED

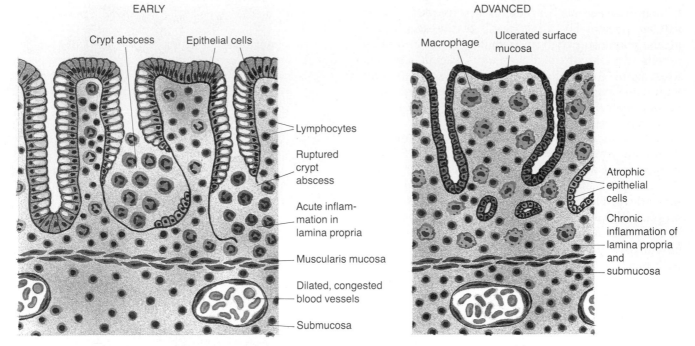

Figure 13-22. Ulcerative colitis. Schematic representation of the major microscopic features of early and advanced ulcerative colitis.

flammatory polyps or "pseudopolyps," can be seen. In cases of toxic megacolon the lumen is widely dilated and the wall is thin and friable.

The early microscopic signs are mucosal congestion, edema, microscopic hemorrhages, a diffuse inflammatory infiltrate in the lamina propria, variable loss of the surface epithelium, and damage to the intestinal crypts, which are often surrounded and infiltrated by neutrophils (Fig. 13-22). Suppurative necrosis of the crypt epithelium gives rise to the characteristic **"crypt abscess"**, which appears as a dilated, degenerated crypt filled with neutrophils. Later in the course of the disease, lateral extension and coalescence of crypt abscesses undermine the mucosa, leaving areas of ulceration adjacent to hanging fragments of mucosa (inflammatory polyps). The fibrosis and strictures characteristic of Crohn's disease are absent. Advanced ulcerative colitis is characterized by mucosal atrophy and a chronic inflammatory infiltrate in the mucosa and submucosa (see Fig. 13-22).

It is generally agreed that **people with long-standing extensive ulcerative colitis have a higher risk of colon cancer than the general population.** In the United States the cumulative risk of colon cancer after 25 years of ulcerative colitis is about 12%.

Epithelial dysplasia is a common finding in the colon and rectum of patients with long-standing ulcerative colitis. The cytologic criteria include variation in the size, shape, and staining qualities of the nuclei; stratification of nuclei; an increase in the number of mitoses; and abnormal goblet cells. It is thought that severe epithelial dysplasia reflects a high probability of cancer elsewhere in the colon or an increased risk for the development of such a cancer.

DIFFERENTIAL DIAGNOSIS

The most important condition to be distinguished from ulcerative colitis is Crohn's disease of the colon (Crohn's colitis, granulomatous colitis). Differences are as follows:

1. Ulcerative colitis is diffuse, whereas Crohn's colitis is a patchy disease, with frequent sparing of the rectum.
2. The inflammation in ulcerative colitis is superficial and acute. Crohn's colitis is transmural and granulomatous.
3. Demarcation of the disease at the ileocecal valve, or in the colon distal to it, favors ulcerative colitis.

Involvement of the terminal ileum, a cobble-stone-like gross appearance, discrete ulcers, and fistulas favor Crohn's colitis.

In approximately 10% of cases a precise diagnosis of ulcerative colitis versus Crohn's colitis cannot be made.

VASCULAR DISEASES

ISCHEMIC COLITIS

Extensive infarction of the colon, unlike the small bowel, is uncommon; chronic segmental ischemic disease is the rule. Some patients present with the symptoms and complications of bowel infarction and require immediate surgical intervention. However, in the majority of patients the acute signs stabilize, and radiographic examination shows only the pattern associated with intramural hemorrhage and edema. Such patients may recover completely or may develop a colonic stricture. **On clinical grounds alone, ischemic colitis often cannot be distinguished from nonspecific ulcerative colitis, Crohn's disease of the colon, or certain forms of infectious colitis.**

ANGIODYSPLASIA (VASCULAR ECTASIA)

Angiodysplasia, a cause of lower intestinal bleeding, is characterized by localized arteriovenous malformations, predominantly in the cecum and ascending colon. The mean age at presentation is 60 years. Younger persons preferentially exhibit lesions at other sites, including the rectum, stomach, and small bowel. Interestingly, angiodysplasia is associated with aortic valve disease in one-quarter of the cases. Patients typically complain of multiple bleeding episodes, although the lesions may also cause chronic occult bleeding. Radiologic studies and examination at laparotomy are usually negative. Thus, the diagnosis is difficult and often requires selective mesenteric arteriography or colonoscopy. Surgical removal of the affected segment is curative.

The resected specimen displays small, often multiple hemangiomatous lesions, usually less than 0.5 cm in diameter. Microscopically, the veins and capillaries of the submucosa are tortuous, thin-walled, and dilated.

HEMORRHOIDS

Hemorrhoids are dilated venous channels of the hemorrhoidal plexuses that result from the downward displacement of the anal cushions. Internal hemorrhoids arise from the superior hemorrhoidal plexus above the pectinate line, whereas **external hemorrhoids** originate from the inferior hemorrhoidal plexus below that line.

Clinically, the salient feature of hemorrhoids is **bleeding,** and chronic blood loss may lead to **iron-deficiency anemia. Rectal prolapse** often develops in patients with hemorrhoids. Prolapsed hemorrhoids may become irreducible, a situation that leads to painful "strangulated" hemorrhoids. **Thrombosis** of external hemorrhoids is exquisitely painful and requires evacuation of the vascular clot.

NEOPLASMS

BENIGN TUMORS
ADENOMATOUS POLYPS

Adenomatous polyps, which arise from the mucosal epithelium, are composed of undifferentiated crypt cells that have accumulated beyond the needs for replacement of the surface cells sloughed into the lumen. The disorder is highest in Western countries, possibly because of a low-fiber, high-fat, diet. In the United States it appears that at least one adenomatous polyp is present in half of the adult population, a figure that rises to more than two thirds among persons over the age of 65 years. In about one quarter of those who harbor at least one polyp, two or more polyps are present. **Almost half of all adenomatous polyps of the colon are located in the rectosigmoid region.**

Tubular adenomas, which constitute two thirds of benign large bowel adenomas, are typically smooth-surfaced spheres; they usually measure less than 2 cm in diameter and are attached to the mucosa by a stalk (Fig. 13-23A). Microscopically, the tubular adenoma exhibits closely packed epithelial tubules, which may be uniform or may be irregular and excessively branched (Fig. 13-23B). The tubules are embedded in a fibrovascular stroma resembling the normal lamina propria. The stalk of the pedunculated tubular adenoma is lined by normal colonic mucosa, and its interior is composed of fibrovascular tissue similar to that of the normal submucosa.

One fifth of tubular adenomas, particularly the

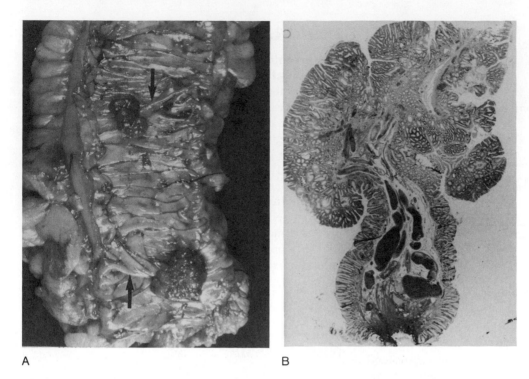

A   B

Figure 13-23. Tubular adenoma of the colon. (*A*) Two pedunculated tubular adenomas are attached to the mucosa by fibrovascular stalks (*arrows*). (*B*) A low-power photomicrograph of a tubular adenoma of the colon shows closely packed epithelial tubules. The fibrous stalk is highly vascular and lined by normal colonic epithelium.

larger tumors, show a range of dysplastic features that vary in severity from mild nuclear pleomorphism to frank invasive carcinoma. **The neoplastic glands must remain superficial to the muscularis mucosae for the polyp to be considered benign.** Penetration of this muscle layer, which is considered evidence of malignant transformation, brings the tumor cells into the region of the lymphatic plexus of the submucosa and thus provides an avenue for metastasis.

Intramucosal lesions that are severely dysplastic are classed by some pathologists as **carcinoma in situ.** They are found in about 10% of resected tubular adenomas. **As long as the dysplastic focus remains superficial to the muscularis mucosae, the lesion is invariably cured by resection of the polyp.**

Villous adenomas, which constitute about one tenth of adenomatous polyps and are found predominantly in the rectosigmoid region, are typically large, broad-based, elevated lesions that grossly display a shaggy, cauliflower-like surface (Fig. 13-24*A*). More than half are greater than 2 cm in diameter and on occasion they reach a size of 10 cm to 15 cm across. Microscopically, villous adenomas are composed of

thin, tall, finger-like processes that superficially resemble the villi of the small intestine; they are lined externally by epithelial cells and supported by a core of fibrovascular connective tissue corresponding to the normal lamina propria (Fig. 13-24*B*). In contrast to tubular adenomas, **villous adenomas commonly contain foci of carcinoma. More than one-third of all resected villous adenomas contain invasive cancer.** Villous adenomas greater than 2 cm in size have a 50% incidence of invasive carcinoma at the time of resection.

The weight of evidence supports the concept that most colon cancers arise in adenomatous polyps.

FAMILIAL POLYPOSIS COLI

Familial polyposis coli, inherited as an autosomal dominant trait, is characterized by the progressive development of innumerable adenomatous polyps of the colon, particularly in the rectosigmoid region. These are mostly tubular adenomas. Carcinoma of the colon is inevitable, nearly always by age 40, unless a

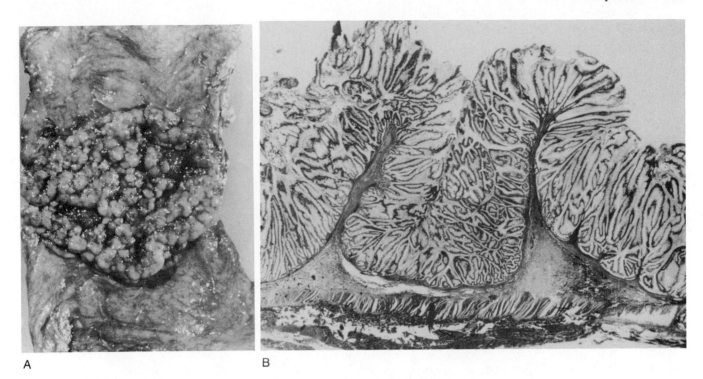

Figure 13-24. Villous adenoma of the colon. (*A*) The colon contains a large, broad-based, elevated lesion that has a cauliflower-like surface. (*B*) A low-power photomicrograph of (*A*) shows finger-like processes that resemble the villi of the small intestine. The villi are supported by cores of fibrovascular connective tissue.

total colectomy is performed. Children of an afflicted parent have an even chance of developing polyposis; other relatives exhibit a 10% risk of manifesting the disease.

NONNEOPLASTIC POLYPS

Hyperplastic Polyps (Metaplastic Polyps)

These polyps, which are particularly frequent in the rectum, present macroscopically as small, sessile, raised mucosal nodules that are usually up to 0.5 cm in diameter but are occasionally larger. Histologically, the crypts of the hyperplastic polyp are elongated and may exhibit cystic dilatation. The epithelium is composed of well-differentiated goblet cells and absorptive cells, without any atypical features. Hyperplastic polyps are not premalignant.

Hyperplastic polyps are remarkably common, being present in 40% of rectal specimens in persons under the age of 40 years and in 75% of older individuals. The association of hyperplastic polyps with rectal cancer is striking; 90% of specimens removed for cancer contain such polyps. Thus, although these asymptomatic lesions are not themselves preneoplastic, they reflect an increased risk of colon cancer.

Juvenile Polyps (Retention Polyps)

Juvenile polyps, as their name implies, are most common in children below the age of 10 years, but about one third occur in adults. Because the lesions are characterized by mucus-filled cysts (hence the name "retention polyp"), and because they do not display epithelial proliferation or atypism, **juvenile polyps are classed as hamartomas.**

Inflammatory Polyps

Inflammatory polyps are not neoplasms, but rather elevated masses of regenerating epithelium and granulation tissue over ulcerations caused by an inflammatory disease of the colon. Such polyps are commonly found in association with ulcerative colitis and Crohn's disease; they are also encountered in cases of amebic colitis and bacterial dysentery.

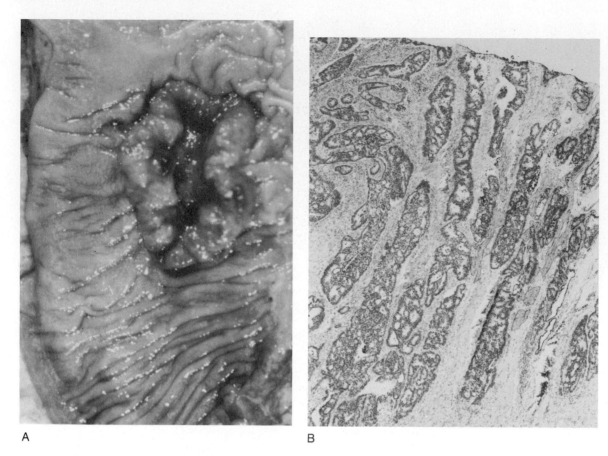

A   B

Figure 13-25. Adenocarcinoma of the colon. (*A*) The opened colon contains an elevated, centrally ulcerated, infiltrating mass. (*B*) A photomicrograph of (*A*) reveals moderately differentiated infiltrating adenocarcinoma extending from the ulcerated mucosal surface.

MALIGNANT TUMORS

ADENOCARCINOMA OF THE COLON AND RECTUM

In Western industrialized societies colorectal cancer is second in incidence only to carcinoma of the lung in men and, except for breast cancer, holds the same rank in women. Overall, in the United States about one third of large bowel cancers occur in the rectum and rectosigmoid regions and an additional one fourth occur in the sigmoid colon.

Risk Factors

The importance of environmental factors in the pathogenesis of colon cancer is emphasized by the high incidence of the disease in industrialized countries and among migrants from low-risk to high-risk regions. **The major environmental risk factor has been sug-** gested to be the diet, specifically a diet low in indigestible fiber and high in animal fat.

Age is probably the single most important risk factor in the general population. The risk is low before age 40 and increases steadily to age 50, after which it doubles with each decade to reach a maximum at age 75. A **prior colorectal cancer** increases the risk of a subsequent tumor. The previously discussed risk of colorectal cancer in **ulcerative colitis** is directly correlated with the duration of this inflammatory disease and its extent within the colon. Recent studies suggest that the risk of colon cancer in patients with Crohn's colitis may be as high as that in patients with ulcerative colitis. Except for Peutz-Jeghers syndrome, the **hereditary polyposis syndromes** are inevitably complicated by colon cancer. Even the Peutz-Jeghers syndrome is not a true exception; its hamartomatous lesions are associated with a higher than normal incidence of adenomatous polyps and, therefore, of colon cancer.

Pathology

The gross appearance of colorectal cancers is similar to that of adenocarcinomas elsewhere in the gastrointestinal tract; they may be **polypoid, ulcerating, or infiltrative, in the last case customarily annular and constrictive** (Fig. 13-25*A*). **The vast majority of colorectal cancers are adenocarcinomas** (Fig. 13-25*B*), which are microscopically similar to their counterparts in other portions of the gastrointestinal tract.

The prognosis of colon cancer is more closely related to the extension of the tumor through the wall of the colon than to its histologic characteristics. Colorectal cancers are usually staged according to the Dukes' classification or its variants (Fig. 13-26). Dukes' A cancer (15%) is confined to the mucosa and submucosa and does not penetrate the muscular layers. Dukes' B classification (35%) refers to a tumor that has penetrated the muscle wall and possibly invaded the periocolic fat but has not metastasized to lymph nodes. A Dukes' C tumor (50%) is similar to Dukes' B but shows lymph node metastases. After the establishment of the Dukes' classification, a D category was added to signify distant metastases. Patients with Dukes' A colon cancer are almost invariably cured by surgical resection. The 5-year survival of patients with Dukes' B tumors is about 60%, while that of patients with stage C disease is about 35%.

Direct spread of colon cancer is commonly observed in resected specimens. Characteristically, **colorectal cancer invades lymphatic channels** and initially involves the lymph nodes immediately underlying the tumor. Venous invasion leads to **blood-borne metastases,** which involve the liver in 75% of patients with metastatic disease.

The tests for carcinoembryonic antigen (CEA) in the serum is usually positive only in advanced cancer; it is therefore not an adequate screening test for early, and hence curable, lesions. Nevertheless, the test is often employed to evaluate patients with metastases of unknown origin and to monitor patients postoperatively for recurrent disease. A positive test for occult blood in the feces with reagent-impregnated paper predicts the presence of a cancer or an adenoma in 40% to 50% of the cases.

CARCINOID TUMORS

Carcinoid tumors of the colon constitute a small proportion of all such tumors in the gastrointestinal tract.

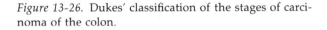

Figure 13-26. Dukes' classification of the stages of carcinoma of the colon.

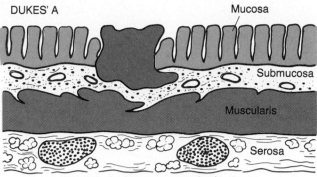

DUKES' A — Mucosa, Submucosa, Muscularis, Serosa

Tumor limited to mucosa and submucosa

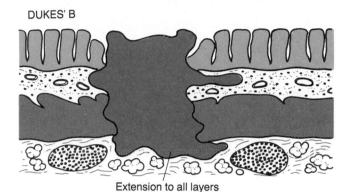

DUKES' B

Extension to all layers

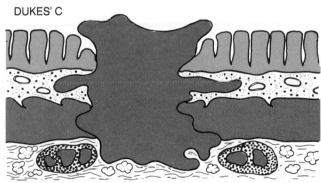

DUKES' C

Metastases to regional lymph nodes

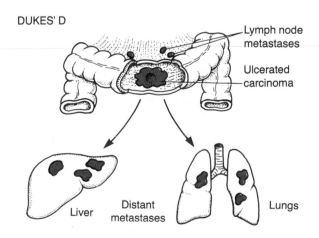

DUKES' D — Lymph node metastases, Ulcerated carcinoma

Liver — Distant metastases — Lungs

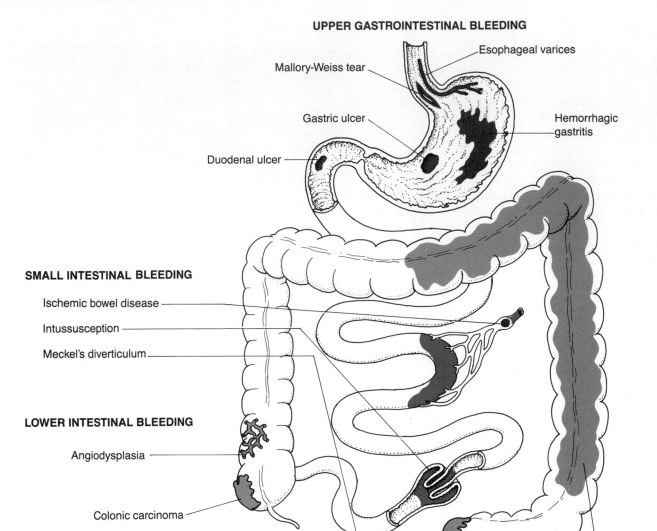

UPPER GASTROINTESTINAL BLEEDING

Esophageal varices

Mallory-Weiss tear

Gastric ulcer

Hemorrhagic gastritis

Duodenal ulcer

SMALL INTESTINAL BLEEDING

Ischemic bowel disease

Intussusception

Meckel's diverticulum

LOWER INTESTINAL BLEEDING

Angiodysplasia

Colonic carcinoma

Rectosigmoid carcinoma

Hemorrhoids

Anal fissure

Inflammatory bowel disease

Diverticulosis

Figure 13-27. Causes of gastrointestinal bleeding.

As with carcinoid tumors of the small intestine, malignancy correlates with size. About half of carcinoid tumors of the colon have metastasized by the time they are discovered.

CANCERS OF THE ANAL CANAL

Carcinomas of the anal canal, which constitute 2% of cancers of the colon, may arise at or above the dentate line. These epithelial neoplams have various histologic patterns, such as **squamous, basaloid,** and **cloacogenic.** There are few clinical differences in behavior among the different tumor types, and they can be conveniently classed as **epidermoid carcinoma.** Carcinoma of the anus penetrates directly into the surrounding tissues; lymphatic spread carries the tumor to the pelvic and inguinal nodes and hematogenous dissemination may lead to distant metastases.

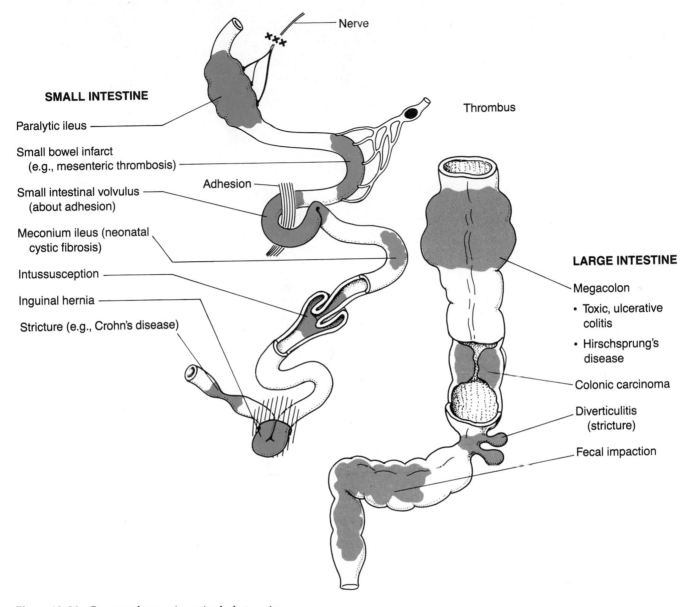

Figure 13-28. Causes of gastrointestinal obstruction.

Figures 13-27 through 13-30 summarize the causes of gastrointestinal bleeding and obstruction and the major benign and malignant tumors of the gastrointestinal tract.

THE APPENDIX

Acute appendicitis, by far the most common disease of the appendix, is the most frequent cause of an abdominal emergency. **The pathogenesis of acute appendicitis is thought to relate to obstruction of its orifice, with secondary distention of the lumen and bacterial invasion of the wall.** Mechanical obstruction by fecaliths or solid fecal material in the cecum is demonstrated in one third of the cases.

As secretions distend the obstructed appendix, the intraluminal pressure rises and eventually exceeds the venous pressure, thereby causing venous stasis and ischemia. As a result, the mucosa ulcerates and permits

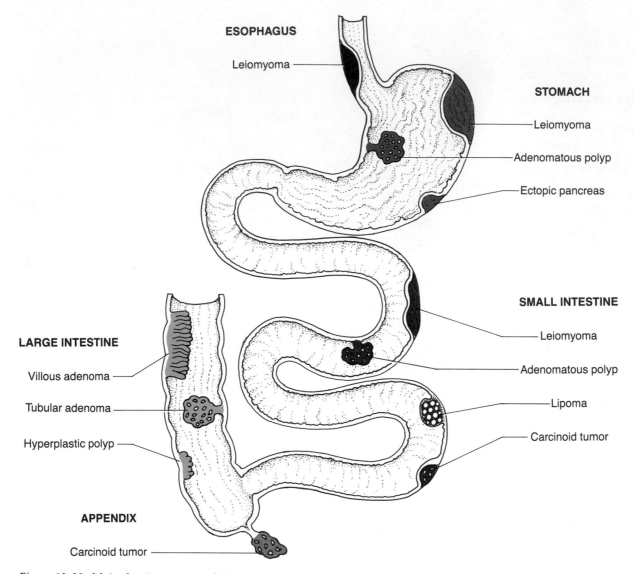

Figure 13-29. Major benign tumors of the gastrointestinal tract.

invasion by intestinal bacteria. The accumulation of neutrophils produces microabscesses, and arterial thromboses aggravate the ischemia. The infected necrotic wall becomes gangrenous and may perforate, often in 24 to 48 hours.

Macroscopically, the resected appendix is congested, tense, and covered by a fibrinous exudate. The lumen often contains purulent material, and a fecalith may be evident (Fig. 13-31). Microscopically, early cases show mucosal microabscesses and a purulent exudate in the lumen. As the infection progresses, the entire wall becomes infiltrated with neutrophils, which eventually reach the serosa. Necrosis of the wall leads to perfora-

tion and release of the luminal contents into the peritoneal cavity.

The complications of appendicitis are principally related to perforation, which is reported to occur in about one third of children and young adults. Almost all children under the age of 2 have a perforated appendix at the time of operation, as do up to three quarters of patients over the age of 60. **Periappendiceal abscesses, fistulous tracts, pylephlebitis** (thrombophlebitis of the intrahepatic portal vein radicals) and **hepatic abscesses** are feared complications. The most common complication of acute appendicitis is **wound infection** following surgery.

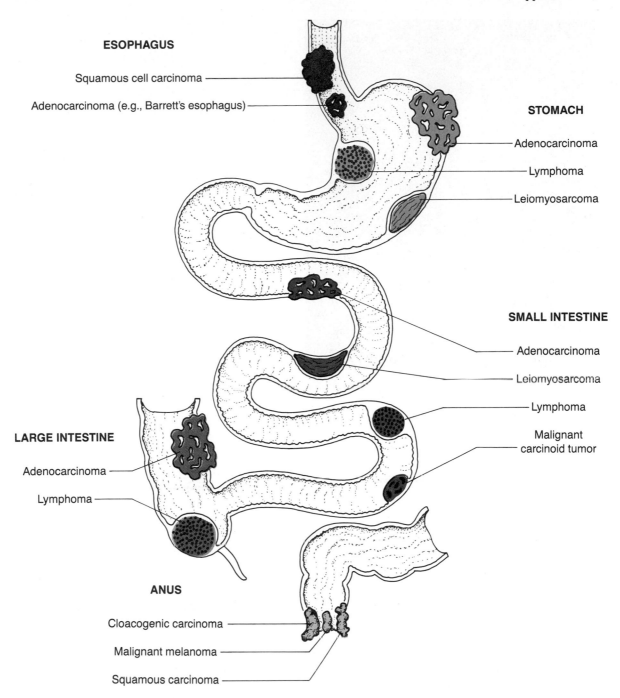

ESOPHAGUS

Squamous cell carcinoma

Adenocarcinoma (e.g., Barrett's esophagus)

STOMACH

Adenocarcinoma

Lymphoma

Leiomyosarcoma

SMALL INTESTINE

Adenocarcinoma

Leiomyosarcoma

Lymphoma

Malignant
carcinoid tumor

LARGE INTESTINE

Adenocarcinoma

Lymphoma

ANUS

Cloacogenic carcinoma

Malignant melanoma

Squamous carcinoma

Figure 13-30. Major malignant tumors of the gastrointestinal tract.

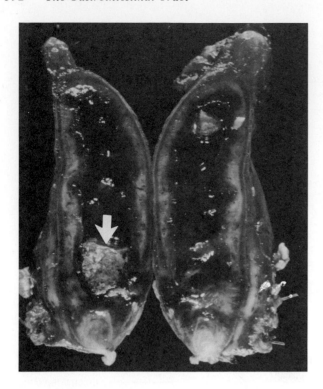

Figure 13-31. Acute appendicitis. The lumen of the appendix is dilated and contains a purulent and hemorrhagic exudate. A fecalith (*arrow*) obstructs the proximal lumen.

THE PERITONEUM

BACTERIAL PERITONITIS

The most common cause of bacterial peritonitis is perforation of an abdominal viscus, as in an inflamed appendix, a peptic ulcer, or a colonic diverticulum. The clinical presentation is often that of an acute abdomen, in which severe abdominal pain and tenderness predominate.

The macroscopic appearance of bacterial peritonitis is similar to that of purulent infection elsewhere. A fibrinopurulent exudate covers the surface of the intestines, and upon organization, fibrinous and fibrous adhesions form between loops of bowel, which become joined to each other. Such adhesions may eventually be lysed, or they may lead to **volvulus** and **intestinal obstruction.** Bacterial salpingitis, usually gonococcal, may lead to pelvic peritonitis and adhesions, a characteristic of **pelvic inflammatory disease.** Chronic **peritoneal dialysis** is today a frequent cause of bacterial peritonitis, owing to contamination of instruments or dialysate.

Spontaneous bacterial peritonitis refers to a perito-

neal infection in the absence of a clear precipitating circumstance, such as a perforated viscus. The disease is not uncommon in children, accounting for 2% of all abdominal emergencies in this age group. Children who develop peritonitis usually suffer from the nephrotic syndrome or from urinary tract infections.

The most common cause of spontaneous peritonitis in adults (occurring in about 10% of such patients) is cirrhosis complicated by portal hypertension and ascites.

CHEMICAL PERITONITIS

The escape of bile into the peritoneum, usually from a perforated gallbladder but sometimes from a needle biopsy of the liver, produces **bile peritonitis,** an insult that may lead to shock. **Hydrochloric acid** from a perforated peptic ulcer of the stomach or duodenum, **hemorrhage,** and **foreign materials,** such as talc, may also elicit an inflammatory reaction in the peritoneum. **Acute pancreatitis** causes the release and activation of potent lipolytic and proteolytic enzymes, which produce a severe peritonitis and fat necrosis. Shock is common and may be lethal unless adequately treated.

14

THE LIVER AND BILIARY SYSTEM

EMANUEL RUBIN AND JOHN L. FARBER

THE LIVER

An understanding of the microscopic structure of the liver is crucial for an appreciation of liver pathology. **The basic unit is the polyhedral lobule** (Figs. 14-1, 14-2), classically depicted as a hexagon. **Portal triads** (or portal tracts) are found peripherally at the angles of the polygon. These portal triads—so named because they contain intrahepatic branches of the **bile ducts, hepatic artery, and portal vein**—are collagenous zones surrounded by an adjacent circumferential layer of hepatocytes called the limiting plate. As its name implies, the **central vein** (also known as the terminal hepatic venule) resides in the center of the lobule. Radiating from it are **one-cell-thick plates of hepatocytes,** which extend to the perimeter of the lobule, where they are continuous with the plates of other lobules. Between the plates of hepatocytes are the hepatic sinusoids, which are lined by endothelial cells, phagocytic Kupffer cells, and fat-storing cells, termed Ito cells.

The classic lobule described above is depicted as arranged around the central vein simply because of the histologic appearance of the liver. However, from the functional point of view, **the lobule can also be thought of as an acinus with its center in the portal tract** (see Fig. 14-2).

The large blood vessels that enter the liver at the porta hepatis eventually divide into the small interlobular branches of the hepatic artery and portal vein in the portal triads. From the portal triads the interlobular vessels distribute blood to the hepatic sinusoids, where it flows centripetally into the central vein. The central veins coalesce to form sublobular veins, which eventually merge into the hepatic veins.

Bile flows in the opposite direction to the blood. Bile is secreted by hepatocytes into the bile canaliculi, formed by the apposed lateral surfaces of contiguous hepatocytes. From the canaliculi the bile flows into the bile ductules (canals of Hering or cholangioles) at the border of the portal tract, and then enters a branch of the intrahepatic bile duct. Within each lobe of the liver,

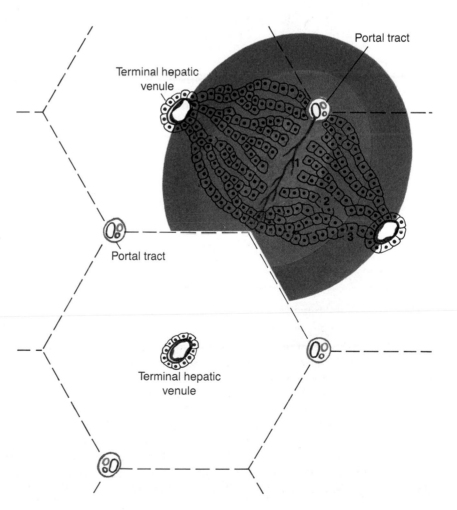

Figure 14-1. Morphologic and functional concepts of the liver lobule. In the classic morphologic liver lobule, the periphery of the hexagonal lobule is anchored in the portal tracts, and the terminal hepatic venule is in the center. The **functional** liver lobule is an acinus derived from the gradients of oxygen and nutrients in the sinusoidal blood. In this scheme the portal tract, with the richest content of oxygen and nutrients, is in the center (*zone 1*). The region most distant from the portal tract (*zone 3*) is poor in oxygen and nutrients and surrounds the terminal hepatic venule.

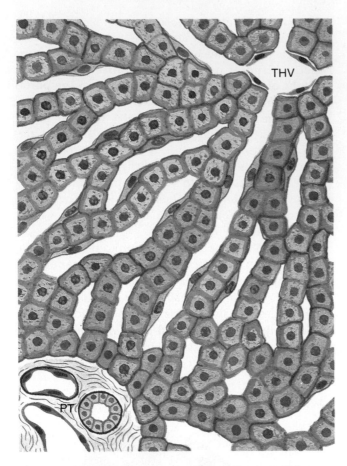

THV

PT

Figure 14-2. Schematic representation of the normal liver lobule. The portal tract (*PT*) contains branches of the hepatic artery, portal vein, and interlobular bile duct. The liver cell plates converge to the terminal hepatic venule (*THV*).

smaller bile ducts progressively merge, eventually forming the right and left hepatic ducts.

MECHANISMS OF JAUNDICE

Bilirubin is the major end product of heme catabolism. An increased concentration of bilirubin in the blood (> 1.0 mg/dl) is termed **hyperbilirubinemia.** When the circulating bilirubin concentration attains levels greater than 2.0 to 2.5 mg/dl, the skin and sclerae become yellow, in which case the condition is known as **jaundice** or **icterus.** As shown in Figure 14-3, many conditions are associated with hyperbilirubinemia. Overproduction of bilirubin, interference with hepatic uptake or intracellular metabolism of bilirubin, and impairment of bile excretion are all causes of jaundice.

OVERPRODUCTION OF BILIRUBIN

An increased production of bilirubin usually results from **increased destruction of red blood cells** (hemolytic anemia), although occasionally ineffective erythropoiesis (dyserythropoiesis) is responsible. The hyperbilirubinemia of uncomplicated hemolytic disease principally involves unconjugated bilirubin, whereas in parenchymal liver disease both conjugated and unconjugated bilirubin participate. Although the unconjugated hyperbilirubinemia of hemolytic disease is of little clinical significance in the adult, in the newborn it may be catastrophic. As discussed in Chapter 6, which deals with genetic and childhood diseases, hemolytic disease of the newborn may result in concentrations of unconjugated bilirubin high enough to cause damage to the brain **(kernicterus).** Kernicterus has generally been associated with bilirubin concentrations over 20 mg/dl, but subtle degrees of psychomotor retardation may follow considerably lower bilirubin concentrations.

DECREASED HEPATIC UPTAKE

Hyperbilirubinemia can result from impaired hepatic uptake of unconjugated bilirubin. Such a situation is seen in generalized liver cell injury, exemplified by viral hepatitis or certain types of drug-induced reactions.

DECREASED BILIRUBIN CONJUGATION

CRIGLER-NAJJAR DISEASE

The condition closest to a pure inherited defect in bilirubin conjugation is **Crigler-Najjar disease.** In this recessively inherited malady, little or no bilirubin is conjugated in the hepatocyte, and the patients suffer from **unremitting unconjugated hyperbilirubinemia.** The defect resides in a **complete absence of UDP-glucuronyltransferase activity.** The liver is histologically normal. Infants with Crigler-Najjar disease invariably develop bilirubin encephalopathy and usually die in the first year of life.

GILBERT'S SYNDROME

Gilbert's syndrome is defined as an **inherited, mild, chronic unconjugated hyperbilirubinemia (< 6 mg/dl) that is caused by impaired clearance of bilirubin in the absence of any detectable functional or**

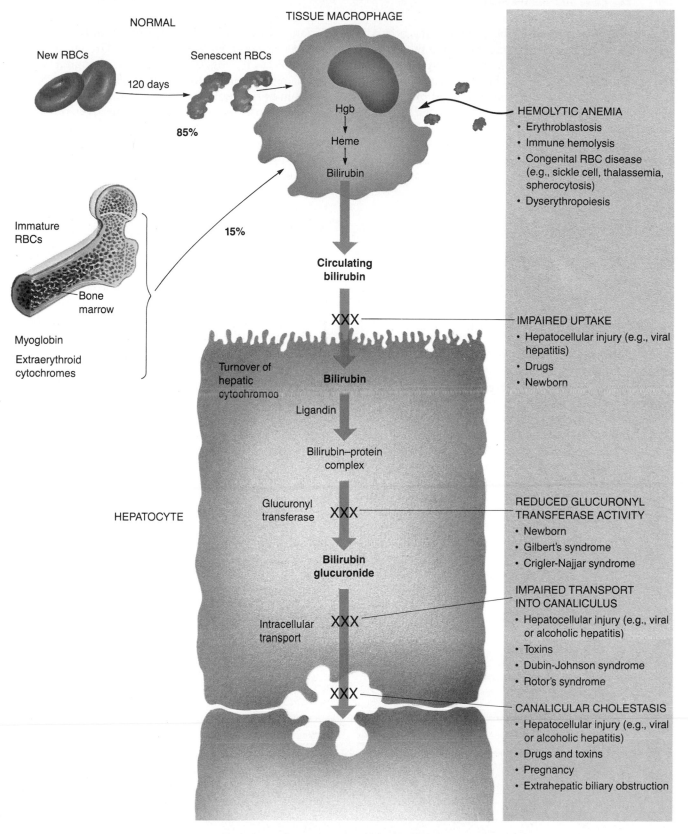

Figure 14-3. Mechanisms of jaundice at the level of the hepatocyte. Bilirubin is derived principally from the senescence of circulating red blood cells, with a smaller contribution from the degradation of erythropoietic elements in the bone marrow, myoglobin, and extraerythroid cytochromes. Jaundice results from overproduction of bilirubin (hemolytic anemia) or defects in its hepatic metabolism. The locations of specific blocks in the metabolic pathway of bilirubin in the hepatocyte are illustrated.

structural liver disease. Gilbert's syndrome occurs in 3% to 7% of the population, more often in men than in women, and is usually recognized after puberty. The precise defect in the hepatic clearance of bilirubin in Gilbert's syndrome has not been defined, but the disease is most likely caused by an **inherited defect in bilirubin conjugation. This hypothesis is strongly buttressed by the observation that UDP-glucuronyltransferase activity is reduced in practically all cases.**

Gilbert's syndrome is, for the most part, asymptomatic, although vague symptoms of lassitude and weakness are common.

DECREASED INTRACELLULAR TRANSPORT OF CONJUGATED BILIRUBIN

DUBIN-JOHNSON SYNDROME

Dubin-Johnson syndrome is a familial disease recognized by chronic or intermittent jaundice, accompanied by a "black" liver. The conjugated hyperbilirubinemia is caused by a defect in the transport of conjugated bilirubin from the hepatocyte to the canalicular lumen. This defect probably reflects a wider impairment of organic anion excretion, since the transhepatic transport of a number of anionic dyes (Bromsulphthalein [BSP], rose bengal, indocyanine green) is also diminished. The color of the liver reflects the accumulation of a **dark-brown pigment in the hepatocytes.**

The syndrome is inherited in an autosomal recessive fashion. Except for mild intermittent jaundice, most patients do not complain of any symptoms; vague, nonspecific complaints are common. The serum bilirubin varies from 2 mg/dl to 5 mg/dl, although it may be much higher transiently. About 60% of the increased bilirubin in the serum is conjugated.

The microscopic appearance of the liver is entirely normal, except for the accumulation of coarse, iron-free, dark-brown lysosomal granules in hepatocytes and Kupffer cells, primarily in the centrilobular zone (Fig. 14-4).

NEONATAL JAUNDICE

In the fetus the transhepatic clearance of bilirubin is negligible; hepatic uptake, conjugation, and biliary excretion are all much lower than in children and adults. Hepatic UDP-glucuronyltransferase activity is only 10% of that in adults. Nevertheless, fetal bilirubin levels remain low because bilirubin traverses the placenta, after which it is conjugated and excreted by the maternal liver.

The liver of the neonate assumes the responsibility for bilirubin clearance before its conjugating and excretory capacities are fully developed. As a consequence **the normal neonate exhibits a transient, physiologic, unconjugated hyperbilirubinemia.** This physiologic jaundice is more pronounced in premature infants, both because the hepatic clearance of bilirubin is less developed and because the turnover of red blood cells is more pronounced than in the term infant. The hepatic bilirubin conjugating capacity reaches adult levels about 2 weeks after birth, and serum bilirubin levels rapidly decline to adult values.

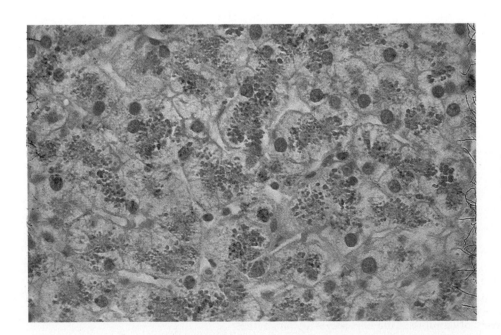

Figure 14-4. Dubin-Johnson syndrome. The hepatocytes contain coarse, iron-free, dark-brown granules.

In cases of maternal-fetal blood group incompatibilities that lead to erythroblastosis fetalis (see Chapter 6), a striking overproduction of bilirubin in the fetus results from immune-mediated hemolysis. Jaundice becomes severe after birth, because maternal metabolism of bilirubin no longer compensates for the immaturity of the neonatal liver.

IMPAIRMENT OF CANALICULAR BILE FLOW

The secretion of bile into the canaliculus and its passage into the biliary collecting system is an active process that depends on a number of factors, including (a) the functional and structural characteristics of canalicular microvilli, (b) the permeability of the canalicular plasma membrane, (c) the intracellular contractile system surrounding the canaliculus (microfilaments, microtubules), and (d) the interaction of bile acids with the secretory apparatus.

Cholestasis is defined by three distinct criteria: morphologic, clinical, and functional. **The pathologist defines cholestasis as the morphologic demonstration of visible biliary pigment within bile canaliculi and hepatocytes (Fig. 14-5).** The clinical diagnosis is based on the accumulation in the blood of materials normally

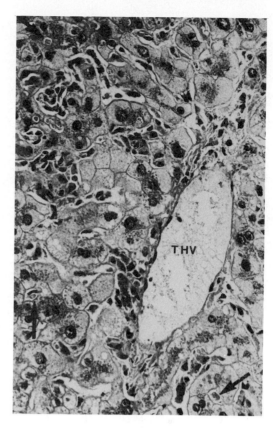

Figure 14-6. Centrilobular cholestasis. A photomicrograph in the area of a terminal hepatic venule (*THV*) shows ballooned hepatocytes that contain prominent bile pigment granules. Bile plugs (*arrows*) in dilated bile canaliculi are evident. Foci of macrophages that have ingested bile are conspicuous.

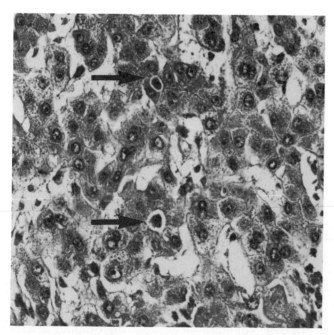

Figure 14-5. Bile stasis. A photomicrograph of liver shows prominent bile plugs (*arrows*) in dilated bile canaliculi. The hepatocytes around the bile plugs are arranged in an acinar fashion.

transferred to the bile, including bilirubin, cholesterol, and bile acids, and the presence in the blood of elevated activities of certain enzymes, typically alkaline phosphatase. **Functionally, cholestasis represents a decrease in bile flow through the canaliculus and a reduction in the secretion of water, bilirubin, and bile acids by the hepatocyte.** Cholestasis may be produced by intrinsic liver disease, in which case the term **intrahepatic cholestasis** is used, or by obstruction of the large bile ducts, a condition known as **extrahepatic cholestasis.** In any event, cholestasis represents a defect in the transport of bile across the canalicular membrane.

Both intrahepatic and extrahepatic cholestasis are characterized by an initially preferential **localization of visible bile pigment in the centrilobular zone** (Fig. 14-6). At the canalicular level, cholestasis may result from (1) damage to the canalicular plasma membrane, (2) alterations in the contractile properties of the canaliculus, or (3) changes in the permeability of the canalicular membrane.

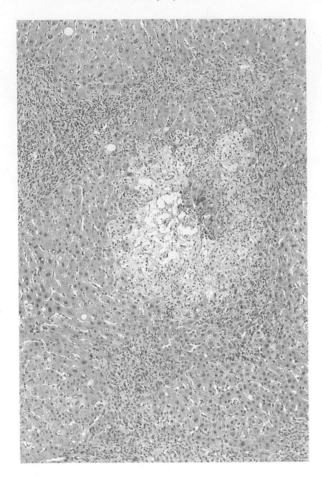

Figure 14-7. Bile infarct (bile lake). A photomicrograph of the liver in a patient with extrahepatic biliary obstruction shows an area of necrosis and the accumulation of extravasated bile.

The invariable presence of bile constituents in the blood of individuals with cholestasis implies a regurgitation from the hepatocyte into the bloodstream. Even in the face of complete bile duct obstruction, the serum bilirubin level rises only as high as 30 mg/dl to 35 mg/dl. Renal excretion of bilirubin prevents further accumulation.

When cholestasis persists, secondary morphologic abnormalities develop. Scattered necrotic hepatocytes probably reflect a toxic effect of excess intracellular bile. Within the sinusoids, macrophages and lymphoid cells appear. The macrophages and resident Kupffer cells contain bile pigment and cellular debris. In general, these changes parallel the severity and duration of the cholestasis. **Whereas early cholestasis is restricted almost exclusively to the central zone, chronic cholestasis is marked by the appearance of bile plugs in the periphery of the lobule as well.**

In longstanding cholestasis (usually the result of extrahepatic biliary obstruction), groups of hepatocytes manifest hydropic swelling accompanied by a diffuse impregnation with bile pigment and a reticulated appearance, a triad termed **feathery degeneration.** The necrosis of such cells, together with the accumulation of extravasated bile in the area, results in a golden-yellow focus of extracellular pigment and debris known as **bile infarct** or **bile lake** (Fig. 14-7).

The sites of obstruction to the flow of bile in the liver are depicted in Figure 14-8.

HEPATIC FAILURE

When either the mass of liver cells is sufficiently diminished or their function is impaired, hepatic failure ensues (Fig. 14-9). For instance, hepatic failure may result from the replacement of liver cells by metastatic carcinoma. By contrast, the liver cell mass is adequate in many cases of cirrhosis, but the associated vascular disorganization and consequent perfusion deficits result in impaired hepatocyte function and liver failure. Thus, the term "hepatic failure" does not refer to one specific morphologic change, but rather to a clinical syndrome that results from inadequate liver function. The consequences of acute and chronic failure are depicted in Figure 14-9, which deals with the complications of cirrhosis, the most common cause of hepatic failure.

JAUNDICE

Hepatic failure is always associated with jaundice as a result of an inadequate clearance of bilirubin by the diseased liver. The hyperbilirubinemia is for the most part conjugated.

HEPATIC ENCEPHALOPATHY

Patients who suffer chronic liver failure, or in whom the portal circulation is diverted, show a variety of neurologic signs and symptoms, collectively termed **hepatic encephalopathy.** With unrelenting liver failure, hepatic encephalopathy may progress as follows: Stage I, sleep disturbance, irritability, or personality changes; Stage II, lethargy and disorientation; Stage III, deep somnolence; Stage IV, coma. This sequence may occur over a period of many months or evolve rapidly in days or weeks in cases of fulminant hepatic failure. Associated neurologic symptoms include a flapping tremor of the hands, called **asterixis,** and hyperactive reflexes

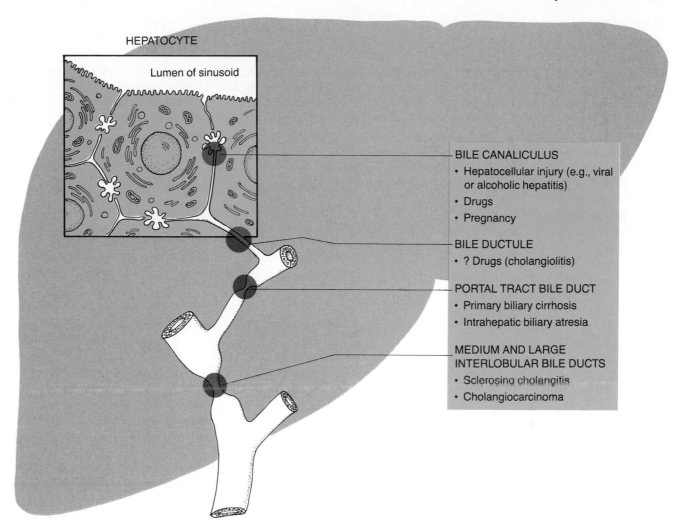

HEPATOCYTE

Lumen of sinusoid

BILE CANALICULUS
• Hepatocellular injury (e.g., viral or alcoholic hepatitis)
• Drugs
• Pregnancy

BILE DUCTULE
• ? Drugs (cholangiolitis)

PORTAL TRACT BILE DUCT
• Primary biliary cirrhosis
• Intrahepatic biliary atresia

MEDIUM AND LARGE INTERLOBULAR BILE DUCTS
• Sclerosing cholangitis
• Cholangiocarcinoma

Figure 14-8. Sites of intrahepatic cholestasis.

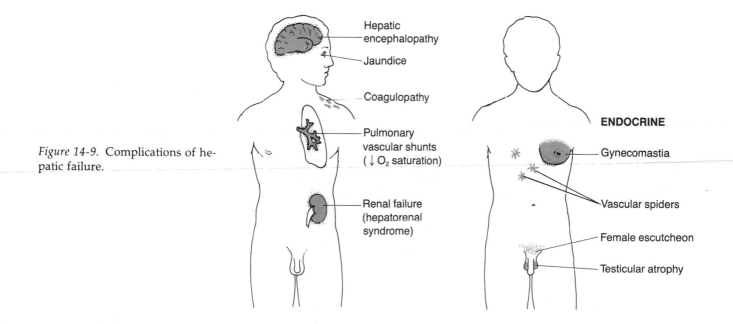

Figure 14-9. Complications of hepatic failure.

Hepatic encephalopathy

Jaundice

Coagulopathy

Pulmonary vascular shunts ($\downarrow O_2$ saturation)

Renal failure (hepatorenal syndrome)

ENDOCRINE

Gynecomastia

Vascular spiders

Female escutcheon

Testicular atrophy

in the earlier stages, extensor toe responses later, and a decerebrate posture in the terminal stages.

The pathogenesis of hepatic encephalopathy remains elusive. It is probable that the encephalopathy is caused in part by toxic compounds absorbed from the intestine that have escaped hepatic detoxification because of hepatocyte dysfunction or the existence of structural or functional vascular shunts. The shunt mechanism is particularly evident after the surgical construction of a portal-systemic anastomosis (portal vein to inferior vena cava or its equivalent) for the relief of portal hypertension, which accounts for the synonym **portasystemic encephalopathy.**

Ammonia levels are usually increased in the blood and brain of patients with hepatic encephalopathy. However, the correlation between the increased concentration of blood ammonia and the severity of hepatic encephalopathy is inexact, and other factors are also thought to play a role.

HEPATORENAL SYNDROME

Acute hepatic failure is commonly marked by an associated renal failure, characterized by azotemia, often with oliguria or anuria. The kidneys appear normal histologically and maintain the ability to function normally. Although no intrinsic renal disease can be demonstrated morphologically, at autopsy jaundiced patients with the hepatorenal syndrome show bile staining of renal tubular cells and bile casts in the lumina: so-called **biliary nephrosis.**

The major determinant of the hepatorenal syndrome seems to be a decrease in renal blood flow and a consequent reduction in glomerular filtration rate.

DEFECTS OF COAGULATION

Bleeding often accompanies hepatic failure, in part because defects in hemostasis parallel the severity of the liver disease. The impairment of hemostasis is caused principally by **reduced hepatic synthesis of coagulation factors and by thrombocytopenia.**

Disseminated intravascular coagulation (DIC) may also occur in liver failure, and at least mild DIC may be universal in severe end-stage liver failure.

A low platelet count (less than $80,000/\mu l^3$) occurs commonly in hepatic failure and is accompanied by qualitative abnormalities in platelet function. The thrombocytopenia may result from hypersplenism, bone marrow depression, or the consumption of circulating platelets by intravascular coagulation.

HYPOALBUMINEMIA

Decreased levels of circulating albumin almost invariably complicate hepatic failure. Hypoalbuminemia is an important factor in the pathogenesis of the edema often seen in chronic liver disease. Impaired synthesis of albumin by the injured liver is the most common cause of hypoalbuminemia.

ENDOCRINE COMPLICATIONS

In assessing endocrine changes associated with chronic hepatic failure, it is important to distinguish between the direct effects of alcohol abuse, a common cause of liver disease, and changes that are better attributed to hepatic dysfunction. Chronic hepatic failure of any etiology in males is associated with feminization, a condition characterized by gynecomastia, a female body habitus, and a female distribution of pubic hair (female escutcheon). In addition, vascular manifestations of hyperestrogenism are common, and include spider angiomas in the territory drained by the superior vena cava (upper trunk and face) and palmar erythema. **Feminization is principally attributed to a reduction in the hepatic catabolism of estrogens and weak androgens, such as androstenedione and dehydroepiandrosterone.** The weak androgens are converted by estrogenic compounds in peripheral tissues, thereby adding to the burden of circulating estrogens.

In addition to feminization, the large majority of chronic alcoholic men also suffer hypogonadism, manifested by testicular atrophy, impotence, and loss of libido. Alcoholic women also exhibit gonadal failure, presenting as oligomenorrhea, amenorrhea, infertility, ovarian atrophy, and loss of secondary sex characteristics. These effects of alcohol on gonadal function in both sexes reflect a direct toxic action of alcohol, independent of chronic liver disease.

ACUTE VIRAL HEPATITIS

Viral hepatitis is defined as a viral infection of hepatocytes that produces necrosis and inflammation of the liver. Many viruses and other infectious agents are capable of producing hepatitis and jaundice (Table 14-1), but in the industrialized world more than 95% of the cases of viral hepatitis involve a limited number of hepatotropic viruses, known as the hepatitis A, hepatitis B, and so-called non-A, non-B hepatitis viruses. Most cases of non-A, non-B hepatitis are caused by a single virus now known as hepatitis C virus (HCV). A fourth virus, found only in association with hepatitis B, is known as the hepatitis D virus.

Table 14-1 Infectious Agents That Cause Hepatitis

Hepatitis A virus
Hepatitis B virus
Non-A, non-B hepatitis virus(es), including hepatitis C virus
Yellow fever virus
Epstein-Barr virus (infectious mononucleosis)
Lassa, Marburg, and Ebola viruses
Rubella virus
Herpes simplex virus
Cytomegalovirus
Enteroviruses other than hepatitis virus A
Leptospires (leptospirosis)
Entamoeba histolytica (amebic hepatitis)

HEPATITIS A

THE HEPATITIS A VIRUS (HAV)

HAV is a small RNA-containing **enterovirus** that is spread by the fecal-oral route. The hepatocyte is the sole site of viral replication, and presumably shedding of progeny virus into the bile accounts for its appearance in the feces.

Following a short incubation period of about a month, patients develop nonspecific symptoms, including fever, malaise, and anorexia. Concomitantly, liver injury is evidenced by a rise in the serum aminotransferase activity (Fig. 14-10). As the activity of ami-

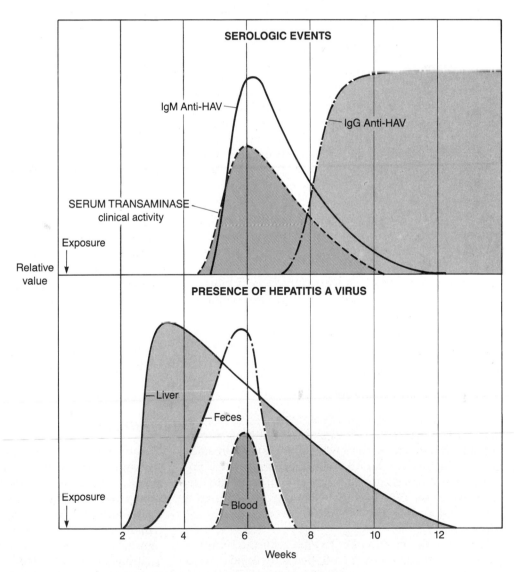

Figure 14-10. Typical serologic events associated with hepatitis A.

notransferase begins to decline, usually 5 to 10 days later, jaundice may appear. It remains evident for an average of 10 days but may persist for more than a month. In most cases the elevated aminotransferase activity returns to normal by the time jaundice has disappeared. **Hepatitis A never pursues a chronic course. There is no carrier state, and infection provides lifelong immunity.** Moreover, virtually all patients recover without hepatic encephalopathy, and fatal fulminant hepatitis occurs only rarely.

The first detectable antibody response to HAV infection is the appearance of IgM anti-HAV in the blood during the acute illness (see Fig. 14-10). The finding of IgM anti-HAV in the serum of a patient with acute hepatitis confirms HAV as the cause. IgG anti-HAV appears as the patient recovers, and it persists for life.

HEPATITIS B

THE HEPATITIS B VIRUS (HBV)

HBV is a hepatotropic DNA virus. The core of the virus contains a DNA polymerase and immunologically reactive elements, called the **core antigen (HBcAg)** and the **"e" antigen (HBeAg).** The core of the virus is enclosed in a coat that contains lipid, protein, and carbohydrate and expresses an antigen termed **hepatitis B surface antigen (HBsAg).**

The surface coat is synthesized by the infected hepatocyte independently from the viral core, and is secreted into the blood in vast amounts. **HBsAg particles are immunogenic, but not infectious. The intact and infectious virus** is also found in the same preparations.

HBV is not directly cytopathic. It has been postulated, but not proved, that the destruction of virus-infected hepatocytes is mediated by immunologic responses.

CLINICAL FEATURES

Acute, Self-Limited Hepatitis B

The acute onset and symptoms of hepatitis B are for the most part similar to those of hepatitis A, although acute hepatitis B tends to be somewhat more severe. In addition, the incubation period is considerably longer. Typically, symptoms do not appear for about 2 to 3 months after exposure, but incubation periods of less than 6 weeks and as long as 6 months are occasionally encountered.

HBsAg is the first marker to appear in the serum of patients with acute hepatitis B, being detected 1 week to 2 months after exposure and 2 weeks to 2 months

before the onset of symptoms (Fig. 14-11). HBsAg disappears from the blood during the convalescent phase in patients who recover rapidly from the acute hepatitis. Simultaneous with or shortly after the disappearance of HBsAg, antibody to HBsAg (anti-HBs) is found in the blood. Its appearance heralds complete recovery, and its presence provides lifelong immunity. Antibody to HBcAg (anti-HBc) appears shortly after anti-HBs, roughly at the time that serum aminotransferase activity begins to rise. HBcAg itself does not circulate freely in the serum of infected persons. Anti-HBc also remains elevated for life and is a useful marker of previous HBV infection, although, unlike anti-HBs, it does not seem to play a role either in clearing the virus or in protecting against reinfection.

HBeAg, the second circulating antigen to appear in hepatitis B, is seen before the onset of clinical disease and after the appearance of HBsAg. HBeAg generally disappears within about 2 weeks, while HBsAg is still present. Anti-HBe appears shortly after the disappearance of the antigen and is detectable for up to 2 years or more after resolution of the hepatitis. The presence of HBeAg in the serum correlates with a period of intense viral replication and, hence, maximal infectivity of the patient.

The Chronic Carrier State

In 5% to 10% of cases of hepatitis B, the patients do not develop anti-Hbs and consequently do not resolve HBs antigenemia. Accordingly, the infection persists, the patients do not recover, and the disease progresses to chronic hepatitis B. **Clinically, HBs antigenemia that is sustained for longer than 6 months, and is accompanied by hepatic dysfunction, indicates chronic hepatitis.** Some of these patients eventually develop anti-Hbs—often after many years—clear the virus, and are restored to full health. Others (no more than 3% of patients with hepatitis B) never develop anti-HBs and suffer from a relentless and progressive chronic hepatitis that may lead to cirrhosis.

The possible outcomes of infection with hepatitis B virus are summarized in Figure 14-12.

EPIDEMIOLOGY

Before the advent of routine screening of blood for HBsAg, chronic HBV carriers posed a public health hazard as a source of post-transfusion hepatitis. The threat of HBV-positive post-transfusion hepatitis has been largely eliminated by routine screening for HBsAg, although 5% to 10% of post-transfusion hepatitis is still attributed to hepatitis B.

It has been suggested that immunosuppressed individuals are more susceptible to persistent HBV infec-

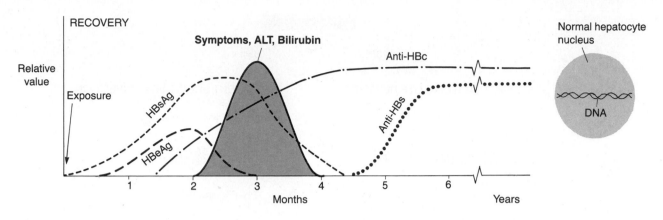

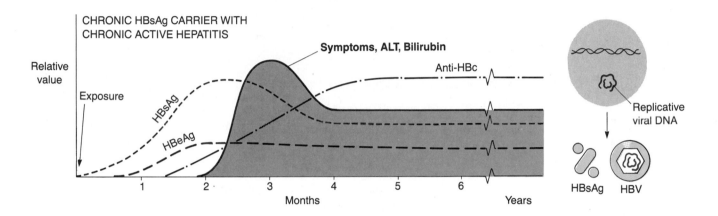

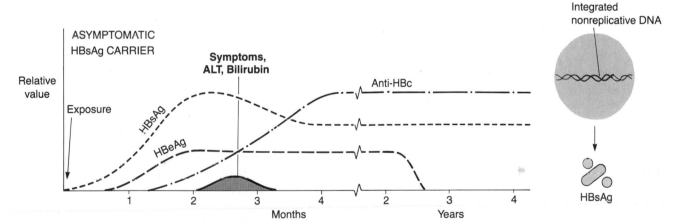

Figure 14-11. Typical serologic events in three distinct outcomes of hepatitis B. (*Top panel*). In most cases the appearance of anti-HBs assures complete **recovery.** Viral DNA disappears from the nucleus of the hepatocyte.

(*Middle panel*) In about 10% of cases of hepatitis B, HBs antigenemia is sustained for longer than 6 months, owing to the absence of anti-HBs. Patients in whom viral replication remains active, as evidenced by sustained high levels of HBeAg in the blood, develop **chronic active hepatitis.** In such cases the viral genome persists in the nucleus but is not integrated into the host DNA.

(*Lower panel*) Patients in whom active viral replication ceases or is attenuated, as reflected in the disappearance of HBeAg from the blood, become **asymptomatic carriers.** In these individuals the HBV genome is often integrated into the host DNA.

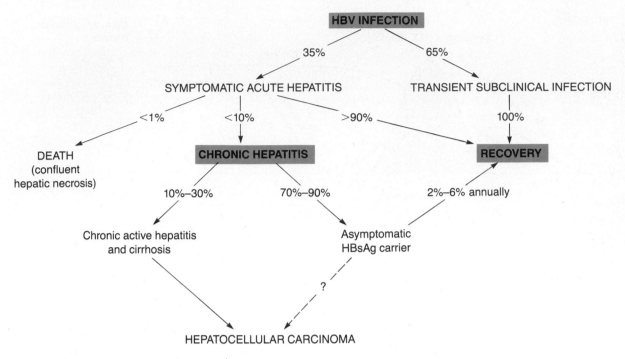

Figure 14-12. Possible outcomes of infection with the hepatitis B virus.

tion, and the carrier state is more common in renal dialysis patients and in persons afflicted with Down's syndrome, leprosy, and chronic lymphocytic leukemia. In the United States chronic HBV carriers are particularly common among male homosexuals, drug addicts, certain health-care workers, and institutionalized mentally retarded children. Of particular public health concern is the fact that paid blood donors are far more likely to harbor HBV than is the general population.

The only significant reservoir of HBV is man. Unlike hepatitis A, hepatitis B is not transmitted by the fecal-oral route, nor does it contaminate food and water supplies. Although HBsAg is found in most secretions, **infectious virus has been demonstrated only in blood, saliva, and semen.** Other than transfusion with contaminated blood, the routes by which contact-transmission occurs are not entirely defined, but it seems probable that a direct transfer of the virus via breaks in the skin or mucous membranes is most common. In this respect, sexual contact, heterosexual or homosexual, is an important mode of transmission.

HEPATITIS D

A distinct hepatotropic virus, hepatitis D virus (HDV, delta agent), is associated exclusively with HBV infection. HDV is likely a defective RNA virus for which HBV is the helper. In cases of HDV infec-

tion, HDV and HBsAg are cleared together, and the clinical course is generally no different from that of the usual acute hepatitis B. However, it has been reported that in some cases the presence of HDV leads to severe, fulminant, and often fatal hepatitis.

NON-A, NON-B HEPATITIS

One form of hepatitis is not associated with HAV or HBV, or any of the serologic markers for these viruses. This form of the disease has been termed *non-A, non-B hepatitis. Today, about 90% of post-transfusion hepatitis in the United States is classed as non-A, non-B* About 20% of sporadic cases of hepatitis (those not associated with a known epidemiologic risk) also represent non-A, non-B hepatitis. It is now thought that there are three or four transmissible agents that produce non-A, non-B hepatitis, although hepatitis C virus (HCV) is now recognized to account for most cases. Although non-A, non-B hepatitis is linked to blood transfusions and the administration of blood products, one non-A, non-B agent is transmitted enterically and is known to cause an epidemic, often water-borne, form of hepatitis in some parts of the world. In the United States the groups at higher risk for hepatitis B seem also to be more likely to contract non-A, non-B hepatitis. Since no serologic markers for the disease exist, non-A, non-B hepatitis remains a diagnosis of exclusion. However, the recent development of a test for anti-HCV promises to change this situation.

The clinical course and mode of transmission of most cases of non-A, non-B hepatitis are similar to those of hepatitis B. Since non-A, non-B hepatitis is associated with the transfusion of blood and blood products, it is clear that a carrier state exists. Chronic liver disease is a more frequent complication in non-A, non-B hepatitis than in hepatitis B. About half of patients with post-transfusion non-A, non-B hepatitis have persistently elevated serum aminotransferase levels for more than 1 year. Up to 20% of these chronic carriers of non-A, non-B hepatitis eventually develop cirrhosis.

CHRONIC HEPATITIS

Chronic hepatitis refers to the presence of inflammation and necrosis in the liver for more than 6 months. The proportion of cases of chronic hepatitis attributable to persistent viral hepatitis is not precisely known, particularly since the diagnosis of non-A, non-B hepatitis has been exclusionary. Only about 15% of patients with chronic hepatitis in the United States display HBs antigenemia, whereas the prevalence in Italy is about 50%, and in parts of Asia it may be even higher. HBsAg-negative chronic hepatitis is probably caused in large part by other viruses, collectively termed non-A, non-B, but it may also result from the use of drugs such as isoniazid and methyldopa. Chronic hepatitis may also be a feature of certain systemic diseases, including Wilson's disease and α_1-antitrypsin deficiency.

A clinically distinct form of chronic hepatitis, termed **"lupoid," or "autoimmune," hepatitis,** occurs in young and middle-aged women and is accompanied by hypergammaglobulinemia, autoantibodies, the lupus erythematosus (LE) cell phenomenon, and multi-system involvement of other organs of a kind commonly attributed to autoimmune mechanisms. Untreated patients, or those who are refractory to therapy, have a high risk of developing liver failure and cirrhosis.

About 90% of patients with **chronic hepatitis B** are male, whereas chronic hepatitis of unknown etiology that has "autoimmune" features shows a female predominance. In chronic hepatitis B the disease characteristically begins as typical acute hepatitis, but in contrast to the usual course of the disease the hepatitis does not resolve within 6 months. However, the large majority of patients who present initially with chronic hepatitis B, with or without cirrhosis, do not have a history of jaundice or acute liver disease. In these cases it is assumed that the episode of acute hepatitis B was clinically inapparent. **Chronic active hepatitis B carries a high risk for the development of cirrhosis. Furthermore, chronic hepatitis B seems to be the** **major predisposing cause of primary hepatocellular carcinoma worldwide.**

In addition to nonspecific constitutional symptoms of anorexia and malaise, patients with chronic hepatitis B display variable degrees of jaundice and hepatosplenomegaly. Serum aminotransferase activity is consistently elevated. HBeAg is more common in patients with chronic active hepatitis B than in asymptomatic carriers and is associated with more severe disease and greater infectivity of the blood.

THE PATHOLOGY OF ACUTE AND CHRONIC HEPATITIS

ACUTE VIRAL HEPATITIS

The morphologic appearance of the liver in acute viral hepatitis is similar in hepatitis A, hepatitis B, and non-A, non-B hepatitis. The hallmark of viral hepatitis is liver cell injury and necrosis (Fig. 14-13). Within the hepatic lobule, scattered necrosis of single

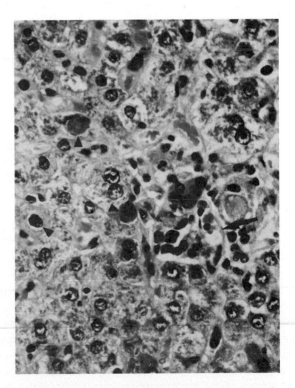

Figure 14-13. Acute viral hepatitis. A photomicrograph shows disarray of liver cell plates, focal drop-out of hepatocytes (*arrow*) and replacement by lymphoid cells, and scattered mononuclear inflammatory cells. The remnants of necrotic hepatocytes have been extruded into the sinusoids, where they appear as acidophilic, or Councilman, bodies (*arrowheads*).

cells or small clusters of hepatocytes is seen. A few necrotic liver cells appear as small, **deeply eosinophilic bodies (Councilman or acidophilic bodies),** sometimes containing pyknotic nuclear material, that have been extruded from the liver cell plate into the sinusoid (see Fig. 14-13). In acute viral hepatitis many liver cells appear normal, but others show varying degrees of hydropic swelling (balloon cells) and differences in size, shape, and staining qualities. Concomitantly, regenerative liver cells, which display a larger nucleus and an expanded basophilic cytoplasm, are also seen. The resulting irregularity of the liver cell plates is termed **lobular disarray.**

Chronic inflammatory cells, principally lymphoid, infiltrate the lobule diffusely, surround individual necrotic liver cells, and accumulate in areas of focal necrosis. In addition to the lymphoid cells, macrophages may be prominent, and eosinophils and polymorphonuclear leukocytes are not uncommon. Cholestasis is sometimes seen, in which case the term **cholestatic hepatitis** is applied.

The portal tracts are almost always enlarged and edematous. As a rule chronic inflammatory cells accumulate within the portal tracts, but the severity of this inflammatory reaction varies from mild to pronounced. All of the pathologic changes are gradually reversed and the normal hepatic architecture is completely restored.

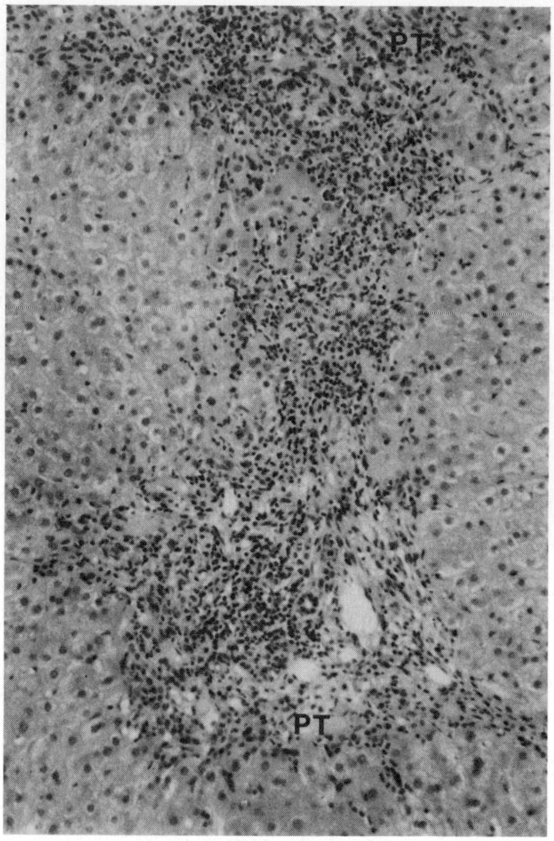

Figure 14-14. Confluent hepatic necrosis. A photomicrograph shows a zone of hepatic necrosis that bridges the portal tracts (*PT*) of adjacent lobules.

CONFLUENT HEPATIC NECROSIS

The term "confluent hepatic necrosis" refers to a severe variant of acute viral hepatitis, which is characterized by the death of a large number of hepatocytes and, in extreme cases, of almost all the liver cells. In contrast to the most common form of acute viral hepatitis described above, in which the necrosis of hepatocytes appears to be random and patchy, **confluent hepatic necrosis typically affects whole regions of the lobule** (Fig. 14-14). At one end of the spectrum of lesions are bands of necrosis **(bridging necrosis),** which stretch between adjacent portal tracts, between adjacent central veins, and between portal tracts and central veins. The death of adjacent plates of hepatocytes results in the collapse of the collagenous stroma to form bands of connective tissue, although increased collagen synthesis also contributes. The presence of bridging necrosis in younger persons (under 30 years of age) has no adverse prognostic significance. However, when this lesion is evident in patients over the age of 40, as many as half eventually die in hepatic failure.

Submassive confluent necrosis defines an even more severe injury involving necrosis of entire lobules or groups of adjacent lobules. Clinically, these patients manifest severe hepatitis, which may rapidly proceed to hepatic failure, in which case the disease is classed as **fulminant hepatitis.** In about one-fifth of the cases that eventually prove fatal, the course is protracted, death from hepatic failure occurring in 2 to 5 months.

Massive hepatic necrosis (acute yellow atrophy), although uncommon, is the most feared variant of acute viral hepatitis, because it is a form of fulminant hepatitis that is almost invariably fatal. Grossly, the liver is shrunken to as little as 500 g (one third of the normal weight). The capsule is wrinkled, and the mottled, red-tan parenchyma is soft and flabby. Microscopic examination reveals that virtually all the hepatocytes are dead (Fig. 14-15), and the hepatic lobule is represented only by the reticulin framework, which in many areas has collapsed. For unknown reasons the massive ne-

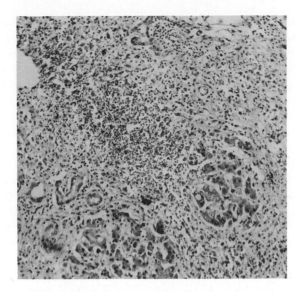

Figure 14-15. Massive hepatic necrosis. A photomicrograph shows the loss of virtually all hepatocytes. The reticulin framework has collapsed, and the area in the center of the field is hemorrhagic. A sparse chronic inflammatory infiltrate is evident throughout the affected lobules.

crosis does not elicit a vigorous inflammatory response in either the parenchyma or the portal tracts.

CHRONIC HEPATITIS

CHRONIC PERSISTENT HEPATITIS

Chronic persistent hepatitis is a mild form of chronic hepatitis that does not progress to more severe disease. About half of those clearly identified as having chronic HBV infection demonstrate **lymphocytic infiltration limited to the portal tracts** (Fig. 14-16). The others, who show little portal change and are often referred to as "normal" or "asymptomatic" HBV carriers, show only minimal or sporadic increases in serum aminotransferase. **Thus, the so-called asymptomatic carrier simply represents the most inactive extreme of the spectrum of persistent viral hepatitis.** Characteristically, the limiting plate is intact. Liver cell necrosis and lobular inflammation are minimal.

CHRONIC ACTIVE HEPATITIS

Chronic active hepatitis is a necrotizing inflammatory disease that often progresses to cirrhosis. Inflammation and focal necrosis early in the course of the

disease are distributed irregularly among the lobules, but later the portal tracts become densely infiltrated by lymphocytes, macrophages, and occasional plasma cells (Fig. 14-17). **The inflammation characteristically penetrates the limiting plate and surrounds individual hepatocytes and groups of hepatocytes on the borders of the portal tracts.**

Strands of connective tissue extend from the portal tracts into the lobules, giving the former a stellate (star-shaped) appearance. Threads of connective tissue also envelop single hepatocytes and groups of cells, particularly adjacent to the portal tracts.

The end stage of chronic active hepatitis is characterized by dense collagenous septa, which destroy the lobular architecture and divide the liver into hepatocellular nodules, an appearance termed cirrhosis (Fig. 14-18).

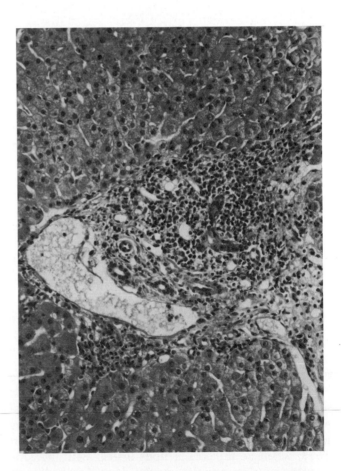

Figure 14-16. Chronic persistent hepatitis. A photomicrograph shows the portal tract infiltrated by mononuclear inflammatory cells. The lobular parenchyma is essentially intact.

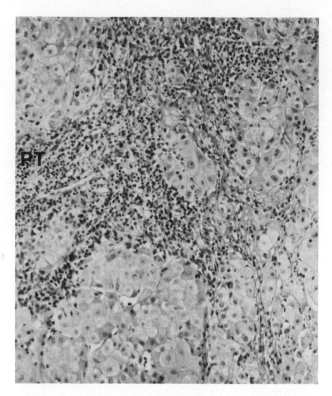

Figure 14-17. Chronic active hepatitis. A photomicrograph shows a mononuclear inflammatory infiltrate in an expanded portal tract (*PT*). The inflammation penetrates the limiting plate and surrounds groups of hepatocytes on the border of the portal tract.

A schematic comparison of the morphologic features of acute and chronic viral hepatitis is shown in Figure 14-19. Table 14-2 compares the major features of the common forms of viral hepatitis.

ALCOHOLIC LIVER DISEASE

The deleterious effects of excess alcohol (ethanol, ethyl alcohol) consumption have been recognized since the early days of recorded history. The prophet Isaiah warned "Woe to him that is mighty to drink wine." The specific association of alcohol abuse and cirrhosis was noted by the English physician Thomas Heberden in 1699, when he linked scirrhous livers" with the consumption of "spirituous liquors." Until the middle of the 20th century, the high incidence of liver disease in alcoholics was generally attributed to a toxic effect of ethanol. Subsequently, however, the similarity between the experimental nutritional liver disease in rats induced by dietary choline deficiency and human alco-

holic liver disease, and the fact that some alcoholics are malnourished, led to the assumption that alcohol per se is not hepatotoxic. Rather, it was thought that the nutritional deficiencies associated with alcohol abuse are responsible for the liver disease commonly seen in alcoholics. This notion was subsequently questioned on clinical grounds, when it became clear that only a very small proportion of all alcoholics are socially deteriorated ("skid row" alcoholics) and that the majority are apparently adequately nourished or even obese. Experiments in which alcohol was given together with nutritionally adequate diets to rats, subhuman primates, and human volunteers demonstrated that alcohol is indeed toxic to the liver, as evidenced by the production of fatty liver and ultrastructural changes in the hepatocytes. Moreover, cirrhosis was produced in baboons fed alcohol with a diet containing all essential nutrients. Thus, today alcohol is again recognized as a direct hepatotoxic agent.

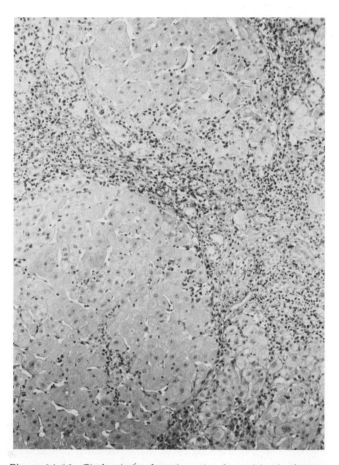

Figure 14-18. Cirrhosis in chronic active hepatitis. A photomicrograph of the liver from a patient with long-standing chronic active hepatitis B shows hepatocellular nodules and chronically inflamed fibrous septa.

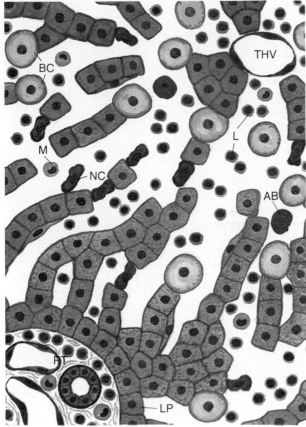

A

Acute viral hepatitis

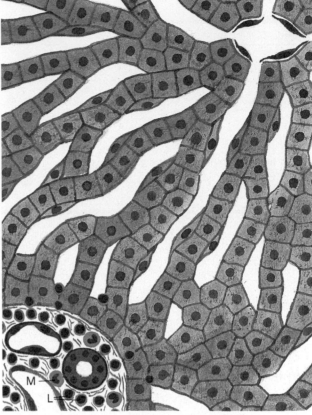

B

Chronic persistent hepatitis

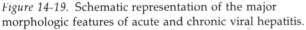

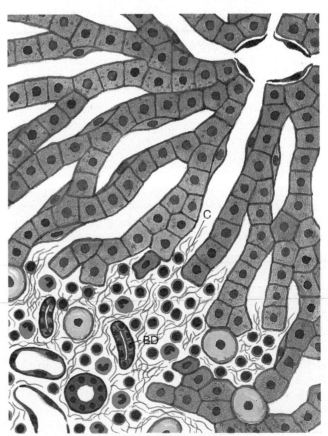

Chronic active hepatitis

C

Figure 14-19. Schematic representation of the major morphologic features of acute and chronic viral hepatitis.

(*A*) **Acute viral hepatitis** is characterized by scattered necrosis of single hepatocytes and small clusters of hepatocytes, ballooned cells (*BC*), necrotic cells (*NC*), and acidophilic bodies (*AB*) free in the sinusoids. The inflammation in the lobules and portal tracts (*PT*) is predominantly lymphocytic (*L*), although a few macrophages (*M*) are also seen. The limiting plate (*LP*) is intact. (*THV*, terminal hepatic venule).

(*B*) In **chronic persistent hepatitis,** chronic inflammation is confined to the portal tracts, and the limiting plate is intact. The lobular parenchyma appears normal.

(*C*) **Chronic active hepatitis** is marked by severe chronic inflammation in the portal tracts. Periportal necrosis of hepatocytes is conspicuous, ballooned cells are present, and the limiting plate is eroded. The inflammation extends into the lobular parenchyma and is accompanied by periportal fibrosis. The expanded portal tracts often display proliferated bile ductules (*BD*). (*C*, collagen)

Table 14-2   Comparative Features of the Common Forms of Viral Hepatitis

FEATURE	HEPATITIS A	HEPATITIS B	NON-A, NON-B HEPATITIS
Genome	RNA	DNA	Unknown
Incubation period	3–6 weeks	6 weeks to 6 months	7–8 weeks (average)
Transmission	Oral	Parenteral	Parenteral (rarely, oral)
Blood	No	Yes	Yes
Feces	Yes	No	Rare
Vertical	No	Yes	Unknown
Fulminant hepatic necrosis	Very rare	Yes	Yes
Chronic hepatitis	No	10%	50%
Carrier state	No	Yes	Yes
Liver cancer	No	Yes	Unknown

LIVER DISEASES PRODUCED BY ALCOHOL CONSUMPTION

FATTY LIVER AND ASSOCIATED LESIONS

Virtually all chronic alcoholics accumulate fat in hepatocytes (steatosis). As a result the liver becomes yellow and enlarged—sometimes massively, to as much as three times the normal weight. Microscopically, the extent of visible fat accumulation varies from minute droplets scattered in the cytoplasm of a few hepatocytes to distention of the entire cytoplasm of most cells by coalesced droplets (Fig. 14-20). In the latter situation, the liver cell is scarcely recognizable as such, and bears a resemblance to an adipocyte, the cytoplasm being represented by a distended clear area, and the nucleus flattened and displaced to the periphery of the cell.

It has been shown that most of the fat deposited in the liver after chronic alcohol consumption is derived from the diet. Within the hepatocyte, ethanol increases fatty acid synthesis, decreases mitochondrial oxidation of fatty acids, increases the production of triglycerides, and impairs the release of lipoproteins (Fig. 14-21). Collectively, these metabolic consequences produce a fatty liver, but the quantitative role for each is not established and may be variable.

Clinically, patients with uncomplicated alcoholic fatty liver have surprisingly few symptoms of liver disease. Despite the striking morphologic change in the liver, alcoholic fatty liver is a fully reversible lesion and does not by itself progress to more severe disease, notably cirrhosis.

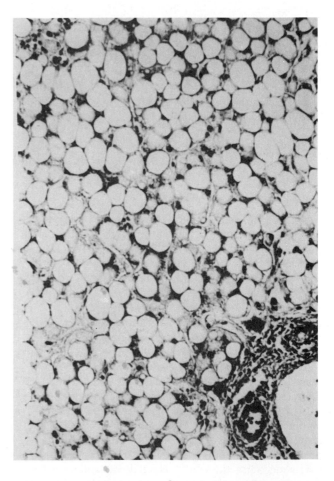

Figure 14-20. Alcoholic fatty liver. A photomicrograph shows the cytoplasm of almost all the hepatocytes to be distended by fat, which displaces the nucleus to the periphery. Note the absence of inflammation and fibrosis.

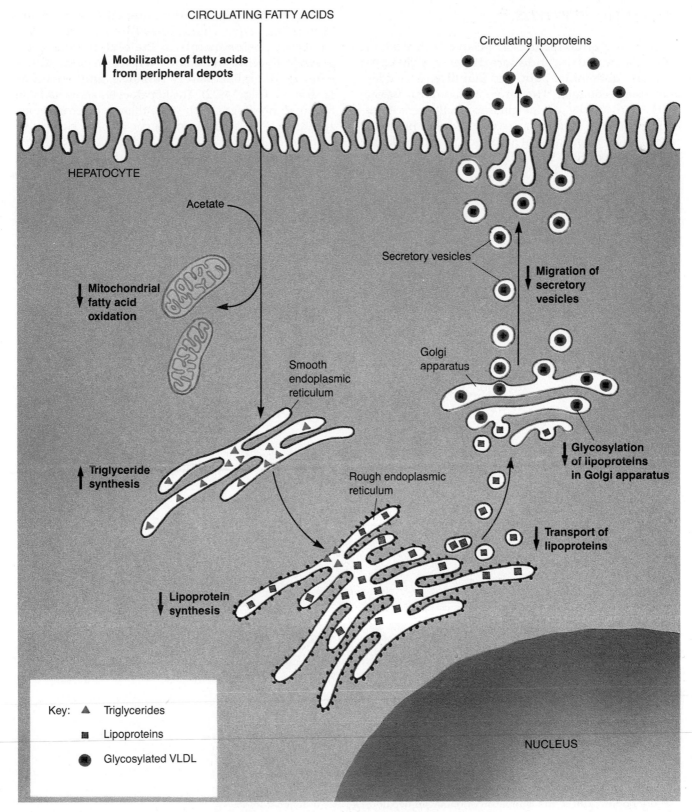

Figure 14-21. Pathogenesis of alcoholic fatty liver.

ALCOHOLIC HEPATITIS

The classic clinical features associated with alcoholic hepatitis are malaise and anorexia, fever, right upper quadrant abdominal pain, and jaundice. A mild leukocytosis is common. The serum aminotransferase activity, particularly that of glutamic-oxaloacetic transaminase (GOT), is moderately elevated, but not to the levels often seen in viral hepatitis. Serum alkaline phosphatase activity is usually increased.

Morphologically, alcoholic hepatitis is an acute necrotizing lesion characterized by necrosis of hepatocytes, predominantly in the central zone, cytoplasmic hyaline inclusions within hepatocytes, a neutrophilic inflammatory response, and perivenular fibrosis (Fig. 14-22). The hepatocytes show variable hydropic swelling, which gives them a heterogeneous appearance. Isolated necrotic liver cells, or clusters of them, exhibit pyknotic nuclei and karyorrhexis. Scattered hepatocytes contain so-called Mallory bodies—

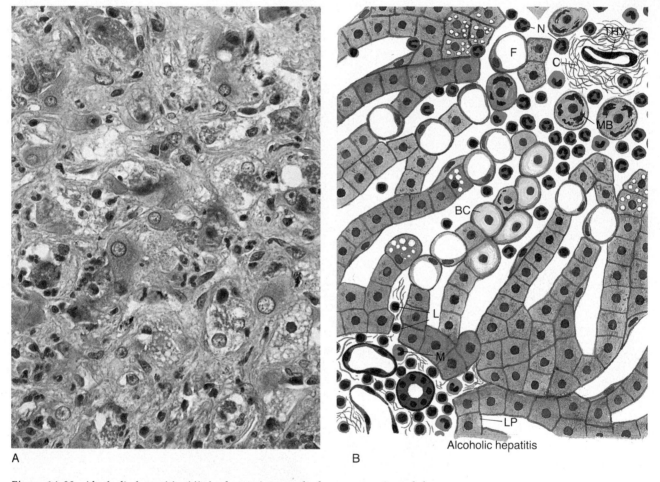

A

B

Alcoholic hepatitis

Figure 14-22. Alcoholic hepatitis. (*A*) A photomicrograph shows necrosis and degeneration of hepatocytes, Mallory bodies (eosinophilic inclusions) in the cytoplasm of injured hepatocytes, and infiltration by neutrophils. (*B*) Schematic representation of the major pathologic features of alcoholic hepatitis. The lesions are predominantly centrilobular, and include necrosis and loss of hepatocytes, ballooned cells (*BC*), and Mallory bodies (*MB*) in the cytoplasm of damaged hepatocytes. The inflammatory infiltrate consists predominantly of neutrophils (*N*), although a few lymphocytes (*L*) and macrophages (*M*) are also present. The central vein, or terminal hepatic venule (*THV*), is encased in connective tissue (*C*) (central sclerosis). Fat-laden hepatocytes (*F*) are evident in the lobule. The portal tract displays moderate chronic inflammation, and the limiting plate (*LP*) is focally breached.

that is, alcoholic hyaline (see Fig. 14-22). These cytoplasmic inclusions, which are more common in visibly damaged, swollen hepatocytes, are visualized as irregular skeins of eosinophilic material or as solid eosinophilic masses, often in a perinuclear location (Fig. 14-23). The damaged, ballooned hepatocytes, particularly those containing Mallory bodies, are surrounded by neutrophils, although a more diffuse, intralobular inflammatory infiltrate is also present. Cholestasis, varying from mild to severe, is present in as many as one-third of the cases. **Alcoholic hepatitis is usually superimposed on an existing fatty liver,** although there is no evidence that fat accumulation predisposes or contributes to the development of alcoholic hepatitis.

Collagen deposition is a constant feature of alcoholic hepatitis, especially around the central vein (terminal hepatic venule). In severe cases the venule and perivenular sinusoids are obliterated and surrounded

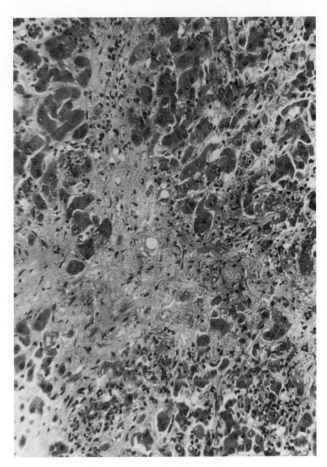

Figure 14-24. Central hyaline sclerosis. A photomicrograph from the liver of a patient with alcoholic liver disease shows the obliteration of the terminal venule by fibrous tissue.

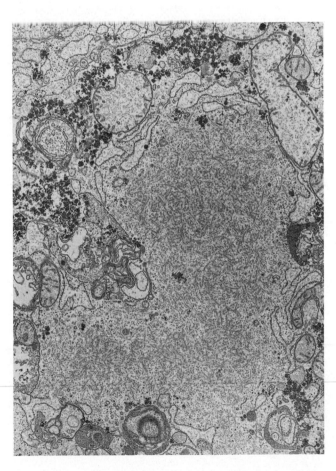

Figure 14-23. Mallory body. An electron micrograph shows an aggregate of filamentous material in the cytoplasm of a hepatocyte. The mass displaces the cytoplasmic organelles peripherally.

by dense fibrous tissue, in which case the lesion has been termed **central hyaline sclerosis** (Fig. 14-24).

The mortality in the acute stage of alcoholic hepatitis ranges from 10% to 30%. If the patient survives and continues to drink, the acute stage may be followed by a persistent alcoholic hepatitis, and more than a third of such patients progress to cirrhosis in only 1 or 2 years. Among those who abstain from alcohol after recovery from acute alcoholic hepatitis, about one in five progresses to cirrhosis.

ALCOHOLIC CIRRHOSIS

In about 15% of alcoholics, hepatocellular necrosis, fibrosis, and regeneration eventually lead to the formation of fibrous septa surrounding hepatocellular nodules, the two features that define cirrhosis (Fig. 14-25). The other lesions of alcoholic liver disease—namely,

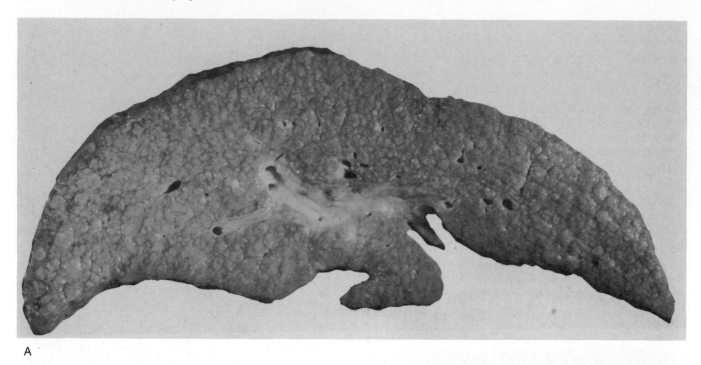

A

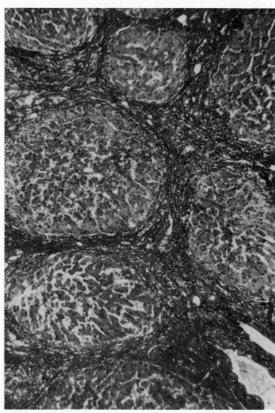

B

Figure 14-25. Alcoholic cirrhosis. (*A*) The cut surface of the liver is divided into innumerable small, regular nodules, separated by connective tissue septa. The pattern is predominantly micronodular. (*B*) A photomicrograph shows small regular nodules surrounded by uniform fibrous septa.

fatty liver and acute or persistent alcoholic hepatitis—are often seen in conjunction with cirrhosis.

PRIMARY BILIARY CIRRHOSIS

Primary biliary cirrhosis is a chronic liver disease that occurs principally in middle-aged women and that is clinically characterized by progressive cholestasis. The use of the term "cirrhosis" in the designation of this malady is misleading, in that the cirrhosis is actually a late complication of the disease. **The basic lesion is a chronic, destructive disease of the intrahepatic bile ducts (nonsuppurative, destructive cholangitis).**

CLINICAL FEATURES

Of those afflicted with primary biliary cirrhosis, 90% to 95% are women, usually between 30 and 65 years of age. In many patients the initial symptoms are fatigue and pruritus without jaundice. On the other hand, a substantial proportion of patients with primary biliary cirrhosis have no symptoms during the early stages of the disease; some of these patients remain asymptomatic and appear to have an excellent prognosis, whereas others ultimately present with advanced cirrhosis and its complications.

In a typical case, a high serum alkaline phosphatase activity is accompanied by a normal or only slightly elevated serum bilirubin level. As the disease advances, most patients have a progressive increase in serum bilirubin level, and the serum cholesterol level is strikingly increased. Cholesterol-laden macrophages accumulate in the subcutaneous tissues, where they appear as localized lesions termed **xanthomas.** Because of the impairment in the excretion of bile into the intestine, severe **steatorrhea** due to fat malabsorption is common. Owing to the associated malabsorption of vitamin D and calcium, **osteomalacia** and **osteoporosis** are important complications of primary biliary cirrhosis. Those patients who eventually develop cirrhosis die in **hepatic failure** or of the complications of **portal hypertension.**

The disease generally pursues an indolent course. Patients who develop cirrhosis usually survive 10 to 15 years, while in those without symptoms life expectancy may not be curtailed.

PATHOLOGY

STAGE I: THE DUCT LESION

Stage I primary biliary cirrhosis is characterized by a unique lesion, namely a **chronic destructive cholan**gitis affecting the intrahepatic small and medium-sized bile ducts (Fig. 14-26). The bile ducts are surrounded principally by lymphocytes, but plasma cells and macrophages are also seen. Characteristically, the bile duct epithelium is irregular and hyperplastic. Foci of necrotic epithelial cells and ulceration of the epithelium are not uncommon. In some portal tracts, lymphoid follicles, occasionally containing germinal centers, are present. Discrete epithelioid granulomas often occur in the portal tracts and may impinge on the bile ducts. In Stage I the lobular parenchyma tends to be normal, but in a minority of cases, mild central cholestasis is present.

STAGE II: SCARRING

As a result of the destructive inflammatory process characteristic of Stage I primary biliary cirrhosis, the small bile ducts virtually disappear, and scarring of medium-sized bile ducts is common. Such scarring constitutes Stage II disease. Proliferation of bile ductules within the portal tracts is usual and may be florid. Relatively acellular collagenous septa extend from the portal tracts into the lobular parenchyma and begin to encircle some lobules. Cholestasis, when present, may be severe.

STAGE III: CIRRHOSIS

The disease terminates as **end-stage liver disease**—that is, **cirrhosis**—characterized by fibrous septa that encompass regenerative nodules. Small bile ducts are scarce and medium-sized ducts conspicuously reduced in number. There is little inflammation within either the fibrous septa or the parenchymal nodules. Importantly, duct lesions may still be apparent in end-stage cirrhosis.

IMMUNOPATHOGENESIS

Primary biliary cirrhosis is associated with many immunologic abnormalities and is, therefore, widely held to be an autoimmune disease. Almost all (85%) patients with primary biliary cirrhosis have at least one other disease usually classed as autoimmune, and almost half (40%) have two or more such ailments. Among these disorders are chronic thyroiditis, rheumatoid arthritis, scleroderma, and Sjögren's syndrome. More than 90% of the patients have circulating antimitochondrial antibodies, a finding commonly used in the diagnosis of primary biliary cirrhosis. The most attractive explanation for the initial destruction of bile ducts in primary biliary cirrhosis is an attack on the biliary epithelial cells by cytotoxic T lymphocytes.

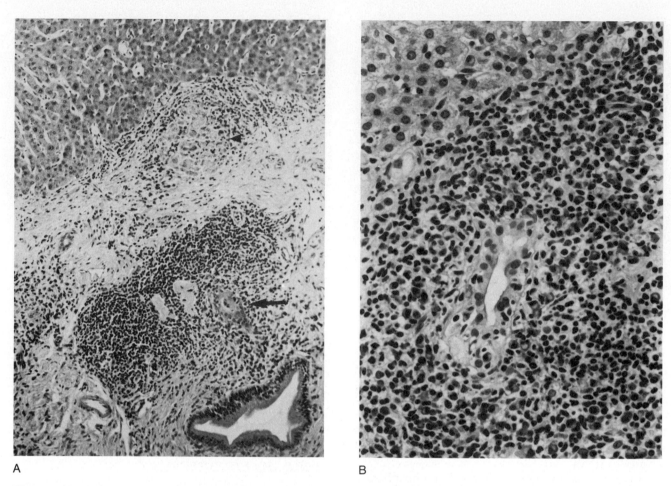

A   B

Figure 14-26. Primary biliary cirrhosis, Stage 1. (*A*) A photomicrograph shows a portal tract expanded by a lymphocytic infiltrate. A large interlobular bile duct (*lower right*) exhibits an irregular and hyperplastic epithelium. A smaller duct (*arrow*) shows severe degenerative changes. An epithelioid granuloma (*arrowhead*) is present within the portal tract. The hepatocytes appear normal. (*B*) A higher-power view of a portal tract shows a dense infiltrate of lymphoid cells surrounding a damaged interlobular bile duct (chronic destructive cholangitis).

CIRRHOSIS

The end stage of chronic liver disease is cirrhosis, defined as the destruction of normal hepatic architecture by fibrous septa that encompass regenerative nodules of hepatocytes.

MORPHOLOGIC CLASSIFICATION

The number of terms applied to the different forms of cirrhosis rivals the number of etiologic agents incriminated in chronic liver disease. Out of this apparent complexity, we can extract a simple spectrum of nodular patterns. At one end of this spectrum, usually in the early evolution of cirrhosis, is the **micronodular** type, characterized by small, uniform nodules separated by thin fibrous septa (see Fig.14-25). At the other end of the spectrum, ordinarily late in the course of the disease, is **macronodular cirrhosis,** in which grossly visible, coarse, irregular nodules are mirrored histologically by large nodules of varying size and shape. These nodules are encircled by bands of connective tissue that also vary conspicuously in width (Fig. 14-27). Between these two extremes are many cases which show features of both types, and for which the term **mixed cirrhosis** is appropriate.

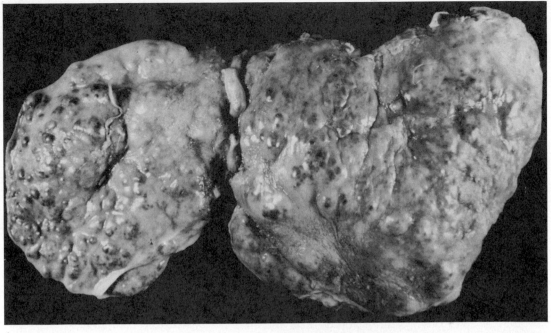

A

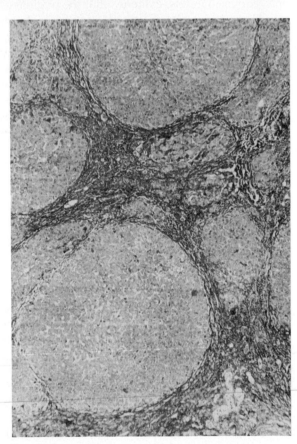

B

Figure 14-27. Macronodular cirrhosis. (*A*) The liver is misshapen and its external surface is studded with irregular nodules and connective septa of varying width. (*B*) A photomicrograph shows nodules of varying size and irregular fibrous septa.

Micronodular cirrhosis was previously termed "Laennec's," "portal," "septal," or "nutritional" cirrhosis. This form of cirrhosis exhibits nodules scarcely larger than a lobule, measuring less than 3 mm in diameter. The micronodules show no landmarks of lobular architecture in the form of portal tracts or central venules. The connective tissue septa separating the nodules are usually thin, but irregular focal collapse of parenchyma may lead to the presence of wider septa. In active stages of the cirrhotic process, numerous mononuclear inflammatory cells and proliferated bile ductules inhabit the septa.

The prototype of micronodular cirrhosis is alcoholic cirrhosis, but this pattern may also be observed in primary and secondary biliary cirrhosis, hemochromatosis, Wilson's disease, chronic obstruction to the venous outflow of the liver (Budd-Chiari syndrome), and certain inherited metabolic disorders.

Macronodular cirrhosis was formerly labeled postnecrotic, posthepatitic, or multilobular cirrhosis. Large, irregular nodules often contain portal tracts and efferent venous channels, evidence that the original process was characterized by multilobular necrosis that healed with the formation of large scars surrounding more than a single lobule. **However, it is now recognized that the micronodular pattern can be converted into a macronodular one by continued regeneration and expansion of existing nodules.** This is particularly the case in alcoholics who manifest micronodular cirrhosis. The connective tissue septa in macronodular cirrhosis are characteristically broad and contain elements of pre-existing portal tracts, mononuclear inflammatory cells, and proliferated bile ductules.

ETIOLOGY

The diseases that lead to cirrhosis are listed in Table 14-3. It is clear that they have little in common except that they are all accompanied by persistent liver cell necrosis. Most cases of cirrhosis are attributable to alcoholism and chronic viral hepatitis. The following discussion will focus on less common causes of cirrhosis.

EXTRAHEPATIC BILIARY OBSTRUCTION

The extrahepatic biliary system may be obstructed by gallstones passing through the cystic duct to lodge in the common bile duct, cancer of the bile duct or surrounding tissues (pancreas or ampulla of Vater), external compression by enlarged neoplastic lymph nodes in

Table 14-3   Causes of Cirrhosis

Alcoholic liver disease
Chronic active hepatitis
Primary biliary cirrhosis
Extrahepatic biliary obstruction
Hemochromatosis
Wilson's disease
Cystic fibrosis
α_1-Antitrypsin deficiency
Glycogen storage disease, Types III and IV
Galactosemia
Hereditary fructose intolerance
Tyrosinemia
Hereditary storage diseases: Gaucher's, Niemann-Pick, Wolman's, mucopolysaccharidoses
Zellweger's syndrome
Indian childhood cirrhosis

the porta hepatis (as in Hodgkin's disease), benign strictures (postoperative or primary sclerosing cholangitis), and congenital biliary atresia (Fig. 14-28).

Initially, centrilobular cholestasis is accompanied by edema of the portal tracts. As obstruction proceeds, mononuclear inflammatory cells infiltrate the portal tracts. Tortuous and distended bile ductules, characterized by a high cuboidal epithelium, proliferate (Fig. 14-29). The cholestasis eventually extends to the periphery of the lobule. Dilated bile ducts may rupture, leading to the formation of pools of extracellular bile, termed **bile lakes, a feature diagnostic of extrahepatic biliary obstruction.** Damaged hepatocytes containing large amounts of bile show **feathery degeneration.** Infection of the obstructed biliary passages often leads to superimposed suppurative cholangitis, intraluminal pus, and even intrahepatic abscesses.

With time the portal tracts become enlarged and fibrotic. Typically, the **periductal fibrosis** is concentric, giving rise to the term **"onion skin" fibrosis.** In about 10% of cases of cirrhosis caused by extrahepatic biliary cirrhosis, septa eventually extend between the portal tracts of contiguous lobules and form a micronodular cirrhosis.

HEMOCHROMATOSIS

Hemochromatosis is defined pathologically as the accumulation of very large amounts of iron in the parenchymal cells of a variety of organs and tissues. The liver is always affected, contains more than 0.5 g iron per 100 g wet weight, and is usually cirrhotic. Siderosis refers to the accumulation of excess iron without tissue injury.

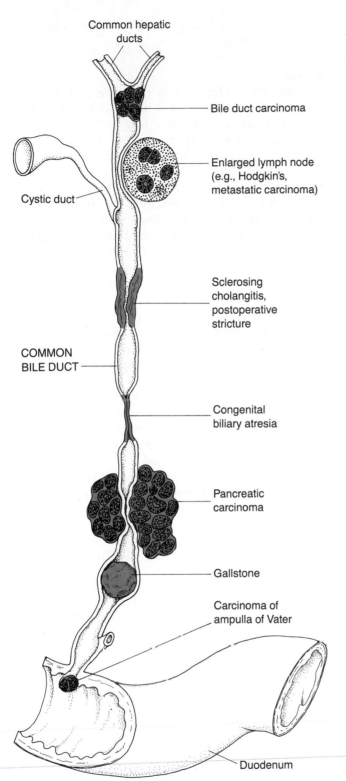

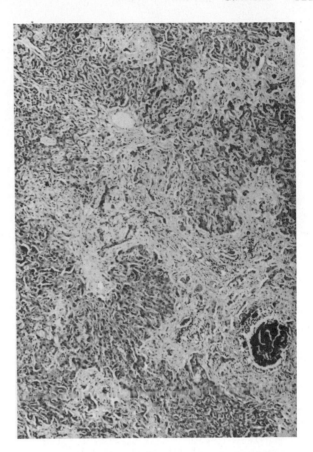

Figure 14-29. Secondary biliary cirrhosis. A photomicrograph of the liver from a patient with carcinoma of the pancreas that obstructed the common bile duct is shown. Irregular fibrous septa extend from an enlarged portal tract (*lower right*). Numerous proliferated bile ductules are seen within the septa. A dilated interlobular bile duct contains a dense biliary concretion.

Figure 14-28. Major causes of extrahepatic biliary obstruction.

Primary Hemochromatosis

In primary hemochromatosis, 20 g to 40 g of iron—that is, up to ten times the normal content—accumulates in the body. **The clinical hallmarks of advanced hemochromatosis are cirrhosis, diabetes, skin pigmentation, and cardiac failure (Fig. 14-30).** The disease is most often manifested clinically in patients between 40 to 60 years of age, and men are afflicted ten times as often as women. This striking male predilection may be attributed to the increased loss of iron in women during the reproductive years. However, given sufficient time to absorb additional iron, postmenopausal women also seem to be at risk for the development of hemochromatosis. The excess iron is located exclusively within the storage compartment, and thus iron stores are in-

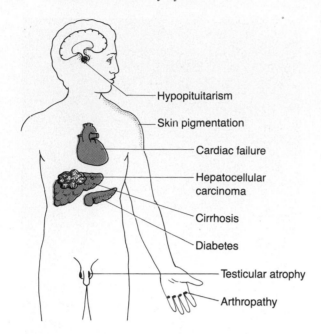

Figure 14-30. Complications of hemochromatosis.

creased up to 50 times normal. The fact that maximum iron absorption is about 4 mg per day explains why hemochromatosis takes years to develop.

Primary hemochromatosis appears to be inherited as an autosomal recessive disorder. The histocompatibility antigens A3, B7, and B14 occur more commonly in patients with hemochromatosis than in the normal population.

The mechanisms underlying the increased deposition of iron in parenchymal organs in primary hemochromatosis are obscure, but it is clear that the absorption of iron is in excess of body needs.

Secondary Hemochromatosis

Hemochromatosis may also occur in persons who do not carry the gene for primary hemochromatosis. Many patients with hemochromatosis (up to 40%) have a long history of alcohol abuse, and it is thought that alcohol may enhance both the accumulation of iron and its associated cell injury.

Massive iron overload occurs in patients with certain anemias such as thalassemia major, sideroblastic anemias, and other anemias associated with ineffective erythropoiesis. As a result **secondary hemochromatosis** may develop even in children and adolescents. The source of the excess iron is the patient's diet or transfused blood. Increased iron absorption occurs despite the saturation of transferrin; the

release of iron by intravascular hemolysis adds a further burden of iron.

Pathology

THE LIVER   The liver in hemochromatosis is enlarged and reddish brown, and exhibits a uniform micronodular cirrhosis (see Fig. 14-30). The hepatocytes and bile duct epithelium are filled with iron granules (Fig. 14-31). Late in the disease, many Kupffer cells contain large deposits of iron derived from the phagocytosis of necrotic hepatocytes. Within the fibrous septa, iron is conspicuous in proliferated bile ductules and macrophages. Eventually, as in micronodular cirrhosis of other causes, the pattern is transformed to that of a macronodular cirrhosis.

Hepatocellular carcinoma is a significant late complication of hemochromatosis, occurring in up to 15% of cases.

EXTRAHEPATIC MANIFESTATIONS   The skin in patients with primary hemochromatosis is typically pigmented, but only half exhibit increased iron deposition in the skin. Most patients display increased melanin in the basal melanocytes.

Diabetes, a common complication of hemochromatosis, results from the **deposition of iron in the pancreas.** Frequently, there is degeneration of acinar cells and a reduction in the number of islets of Langerhans. The combination of pigmented skin and glucose intolerance in patients with hemochromatosis is often referred to as **bronze diabetes.**

Congestive heart failure is a common cause of death in patients with hemochromatosis. Microscopically, the myocardial fibers contain iron pigment. Necrosis of cardiac myocytes and accompanying interstitial fibrosis is common.

Iron is deposited in the pituitary; as a result the release of gonadotropins is impaired. Thus, **testicular atrophy** is seen in a quarter of the male patients, even without iron deposition in the testes. The disturbance in the pituitary-gonadal axis is characterized by loss of libido and amenorrhea in women, and impotence and sparse body hair in men.

Arthropathy, most severe in the fingers and hands, is common in patients with hemochromatosis, but the pathogenesis is unclear.

Laboratory Diagnosis and Treatment

In patients with primary hemochromatosis, the serum iron concentration is more than doubled and transferrin is entirely saturated. Treatment is based on the removal of iron from the body, most effectively by repeated phlebotomy.

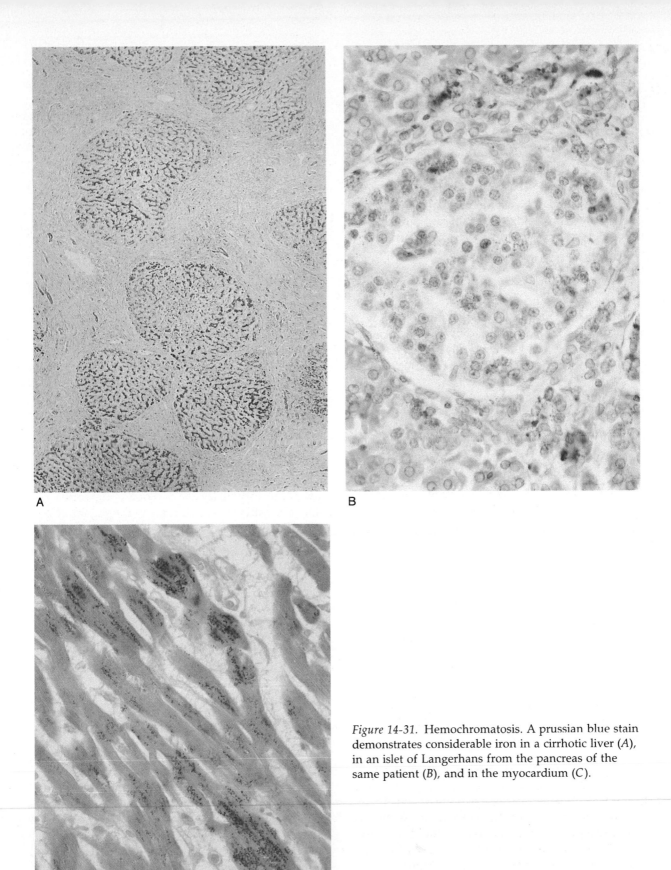

Figure 14-31. Hemochromatosis. A prussian blue stain demonstrates considerable iron in a cirrhotic liver (*A*), in an islet of Langerhans from the pancreas of the same patient (*B*), and in the myocardium (*C*).

HERITABLE DISORDERS ASSOCIATED WITH CIRRHOSIS

WILSON'S DISEASE (HEPATOLENTICULAR DEGENERATION)

Wilson's disease is a hereditary disorder of copper metabolism in which injury to the liver and brain is associated with deposition of excess copper. The disease is transmitted by an autosomal recessive gene.

Biliary excretion of copper is the primary mechanism by which body copper balance is maintained, since negligible amounts of copper are reabsorbed by the intestine. About 90% to 95% of circulating copper is bound to ceruloplasmin, from which it is made available to peripheral tissue as well as returned to the liver.

Wilson's disease is characterized by a striking reduction in the serum levels of ceruloplasmin. However, several observations suggest that hepatic copper overload in Wilson's disease cannot be attributed simply to diminished ceruloplasmin levels alone. It is now clear also that intestinal absorption of copper is unaltered in Wilson's disease. On the other hand, biliary, and therefore fecal, excretion of copper is reduced to about a quarter of the normal rate. Although the primary lesion in Wilson's disease is probably related to defective biliary excretion of copper, the exact pathogenesis remains obscure. The primacy of the liver as the seat of the disease is attested to by its cure with liver transplantation.

Clinical Features

Half of the patients with Wilson's disease display some symptoms by adolescence, and the remainder become ill in their early adult years. The presenting symptoms are referable to chronic liver disease in about half of the patients, while one-third initially present with neurologic complaints, and about one-tenth are seen because of psychiatric manifestations.

The **liver disease** begins insidiously and progresses to chronic liver disease that is indistinguishable from that of other forms of chronic active hepatitis. Eventually chronic hepatitis and cirrhosis result in jaundice, portal hypertension, and hepatic failure. Unlike hemochromatosis, Wilson's disease is not associated with an increased risk of primary hepatocellular carcinoma.

The **neurologic disease** begins with mild incoordination and tremors. In untreated cases dysarthria and dysphagia appear, and in late stages disabling dystonia and spasticity occur.

Ophthalmic manifestations invariably accompany the neurologic disease. The **Kayser-Fleischer ring** is a golden-brown, bilateral discoloration of the cornea, which encircles the periphery of the iris and obscures its muscular pattern. It represents a deposition of copper in Descemet's membrane.

Renal glomerular and tubular dysfunction manifested by proteinuria, lowered glomerular filtration, aminoaciduria, and phosphaturia is common in Wilson's disease. These defects are thought to be secondary to copper deposition in the renal tubules.

Transient **acute hemolytic episodes,** presumably related to a sudden release of free copper from the liver, occur in as many as 15% of patients with Wilson's disease.

Pathology

The disease progresses from mild to severe chronic active hepatitis, with all of the typical histologic features of that disease. Cirrhosis may develop rapidly, even in childhood, and is characterized by the presence of fat, Mallory bodies, hepatocellular necrosis, and cholestasis, a pattern which may lead to an **erroneous diagnosis of alcoholic liver disease.** The liver contains more than 250 μg copper per gram dry weight.

In the brain the corpus striatum and occasionally the subthalamic nuclei display a reddish-brown discoloration. The central white matter of the cerebral or cerebellar hemispheres may manifest spongy softening or cavitation, in which case the overlying cortex is atrophic. The astrocytes proliferate in the putamen, and the number of neurons is decreased.

Treatment

Treatment of Wilson's disease not only prevents the accumulation of tissue copper but also extracts copper that has already been deposited. D-Penicillamine, a copper-chelating agent, augments the excretion of copper in the urine. When D-Penicillamine treatment is initiated during the early, asymptomatic phase, the clinical disease is entirely prevented. Liver transplantation is curative, even after neurologic symptoms have developed.

CYSTIC FIBROSIS

Newborns with cystic fibrosis may present with obstructive jaundice within the first few weeks of life. Biliary obstruction results from the accumulation of tenacious mucous plugs in the intrahepatic biliary tree, and in that sense is analogous to the meconium ileus found in half of these patients. Recovery typically occurs in 1 to 6 months, but some infants die in hepatic failure.

In children who survive to adolescence, clinically symptomatic liver disease develops in as many as 15%, and cirrhosis is found in 10% of patients who

survive beyond the age of 25 years. The pattern of cirrhosis closely resembles that seen with extrahepatic biliary obstruction.

α_1-ANTITRYPSIN DEFICIENCY

The clinical expression of liver disease in α_1-antitrypsin deficiency is highly variable, ranging from a rapidly fatal neonatal hepatitis to an absence of any hepatic dysfunction. **Of those infants with the ZZ genotype —that is, those who are susceptible to the development of clinical disease—about 10% develop neonatal cholestatic jaundice (conjugated hyperbilirubinemia).** This condition is far more common than previously recognized, and accounts for 15% to 30% of all cases of neonatal conjugated hyperbilirubinemia. Most infants recover within 6 months, but a few progress to cirrhosis within 1 to 2 years.

The characteristic feature in the liver of patients with α_1-antitrypsin deficiency is the presence of faintly eosinophilic, PAS-positive cytoplasmic droplets (Fig. 14-32). A definitive diagnosis is made by

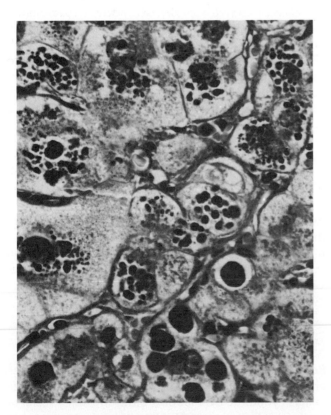

Figure 14-32. α_1-Antitrypsin deficiency. A photomicrograph of a section of liver stained by the periodic acid–Schiff (PAS) reaction shows the presence of numerous cytoplasmic droplets in the hepatocytes.

demonstrating their reactivity with antibody to α_1-antitrypsin.

The cirrhosis of α_1-antitrypsin deficiency is complicated by a very high incidence of hepatocellular carcinoma.

INBORN ERRORS OF CARBOHYDRATE METABOLISM

Glycogen Storage Diseases

The biochemical basis of the glycogen storage diseases has been discussed in Chapter 6. These disorders seem to be inherited as autosomal recessive traits. Only glycogenosis Type IV (brancher deficiency, Andersen's disease) is inevitably complicated by cirrhosis. A slowly developing cirrhosis may be seen in glycogenosis Type III (debrancher deficiency, Cori's disease), but is not inevitable. Glycogenosis Type I (Glucose-6-phosphatase deficiency, von Gierke's disease) is associated with striking hepatomegaly, and Type II (acid maltase deficiency, Pompe's disease) with mild hepatomegaly. Neither is complicated by cirrhosis.

In **Type I disease,** the hepatocytes are distended by large amounts of glycogen, which appears pale in sections stained with hematoxylin and eosin. The PAS stain is heavily positive, and electron microscopy demonstrates masses of glycogen particles in the cytoplasm. Fat accumulation varies from mild to severe, but fibrosis is usually absent.

Type II disease is characterized by only mild distention of hepatocytes, without fat or fibrosis.

Infants with **glycogenosis Type III** show severe hepatomegaly, and morphologically the liver resembles that seen in Type I. Fat is less conspicuous, but fibrosis is present and may progress to cirrhosis.

In **glycogenosis Type IV,** infants present with severe hepatomegaly and die of cirrhosis by the age of 4 years. Sharply circumscribed, PAS-positive inclusions, somewhat resembling those seen in α_1-antitrypsin deficiency by light microscopy, are present in enlarged hepatocytes. Deposits of abnormal glycogen are also found in the heart, skeletal muscle, and brain. Extensive fibrosis eventually progresses to cirrhosis.

Galactosemia

Galactosemia, inherited as an autosomal recessive trait, is caused by a deficiency of galactose-1-phosphate uridyl transferase, the enzyme that catalyzes the second step in the conversion of galactose to glucose. As a result of this metabolic defect, galactose and its metabolites accumulate in the liver and other organs. Infants with this disorder who are fed milk rapidly develop

hepatosplenomegaly, jaundice, and hypoglycemia. Cataracts and mental retardation are common.

Microscopically, within 2 weeks of birth the liver shows **extensive and uniform fat accumulation, and striking proliferation of bile ductules in and around the portal tracts.** Within 6 months the lesion progresses to **cirrhosis.** The institution of a galactose-free diet has been reported to ameliorate the disease and reverse many of the morphologic alterations.

Hereditary Fructose Intolerance

Hereditary fructose intolerance is an autosomal recessive disease caused by a deficiency of fructose-1-phosphate aldolase. When fructose is fed early in infancy, hepatomegaly, jaundice, and ascites develop. **Infants who suffer from liver disease show the changes of neonatal hepatitis**—namely, hepatocellular necrosis, giant hepatocytes, inflammation, ductular proliferation, and cholestasis. Fat accumulation may be marked. **Progressive fibrosis culminates in cirrhosis.**

Tyrosinemia

Tyrosinemia is an autosomal recessive disease that interferes with the catabolism of tyrosine to fumarate and acetoacetate. The disorder occurs in acute and chronic forms. In the acute disease, which begins within a few weeks or months of birth, hepatosplenomegaly is associated with **liver failure and death, usually before the age of 12 months.** The appearance of the liver is remarkably similar to that of galactosemia, including progression to **cirrhosis.** The chronic disease begins in the first year of life, and is characterized by **growth retardation, renal disease, and hepatic failure.** Death usually supervenes before the age of 10 years. The incidence of **hepatocellular carcinoma** associated with tyrosinemia is extraordinarily high.

PORTAL HYPERTENSION

Portal hypertension, defined as a sustained increase in portal venous pressure, is almost always a result of obstruction to blood flow somewhere in the portal circuit. Complications arise from the increased pressure and dilatation of the venous bed behind the obstruction. **The major complications of this increased pressure and the opening of collateral channels are bleeding from gastroesophageal varices, ascites, and splenomegaly.**

For the sake of convenience, obstruction to the flow of portal blood can be pictured as **prehepatic** (occurring before the blood enters the hepatic sinusoids), **intrahepatic** (occurring during transit through the portal tracts and lobules), or **posthepatic** (occurring after exit of the blood from the lobules) (Fig. 14-33). In this scheme the term "hepatic" refers to the lobule rather than the entire liver.

INTRAHEPATIC

By far the most common cause of portal hypertension is cirrhosis. Regenerative nodules impinge upon and deform the **hepatic veins,** thereby obstructing blood flow distal to the lobules. The small **portal veins and venules** are trapped, narrowed, and often obliterated by scarring of the portal tracts. Moreover, blood flow through the hepatic artery is increased, and small **arteriovenous communications** become functional. In this way, portal hypertension due to obstruction of blood flow distal to the sinusoid is augmented by the increase in arterial blood flow.

PREHEPATIC

The classic example of **prehepatic portal hypertension** is **portal thrombosis,** which may be caused by tumors, infections, hypercoagulability states associated with oral contraceptive use and pregnancy, pancreatitis, and surgical trauma. Some cases are without known cause, but **the most common association in portal vein thrombosis is with cirrhosis.** When the portal vein is obstructed by a septic thrombus, bacteria may seed the intrahepatic branches of the portal vein **(suppurative pylephlebitis)** and cause multiple hepatic abscesses.

Worldwide, hepatic schistosomiasis (*Schistosoma mansoni* and *Schistosoma japonicum*) is a major cause of portal hypertension. The ova released from the intestinal veins traverse the portal system and lodge in the portal venules, where they elicit a granulomatous reaction that heals by scarring. Hepatic function is well maintained, but the vascular obstruction leads to severe prehepatic portal hypertension.

POSTHEPATIC

Posthepatic portal hypertension can be defined as any obstruction to blood flow through the hepatic veins beyond the liver lobules, either within or distal to the liver. **Occlusion of the hepatic veins,** commonly known as the **Budd-Chiari syndrome,** occurs in

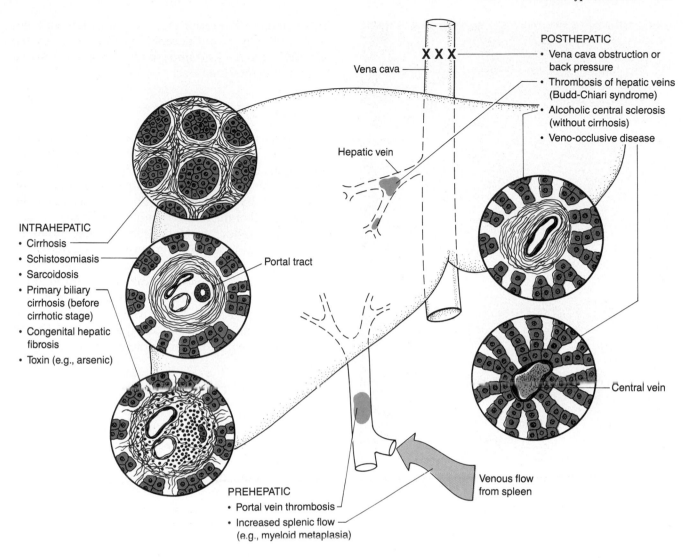

POSTHEPATIC
- Vena cava obstruction or back pressure
- Thrombosis of hepatic veins (Budd-Chiari syndrome)
- Alcoholic central sclerosis (without cirrhosis)
- Veno-occlusive disease

Vena cava

Hepatic vein

INTRAHEPATIC
- Cirrhosis
- Schistosomiasis
- Sarcoidosis
- Primary biliary cirrhosis (before cirrhotic stage)
- Congenital hepatic fibrosis
- Toxin (e.g., arsenic)

Portal tract

Central vein

Venous flow from spleen

PREHEPATIC
- Portal vein thrombosis
- Increased splenic flow (e.g., myeloid metaplasia)

Figure 14-33. Causes of portal hypertension.

venous tributaries of any size, including central hepatic venules. The principal cause of the Budd-Chiari syndrome is thrombosis of the hepatic veins, in association with such diverse conditions as polycythemia vera, hepatocellular carcinoma, tumor metastases from the adrenals and kidneys, bacterial infections, the use of oral contraceptives, pregnancy, and trauma. However, in more than half of the cases, no specific etiology for the Budd-Chiari syndrome is evident.

Thrombosis of the hepatic veins, when total, presents as an acute illness characterized by abdominal pain, enlargement of the liver, ascites, and mild jaundice. Acute hepatic failure and death often occur rapidly. Liver transplantation has been successful in curing the disease.

In the early acute stage of the Budd-Chiari syndrome the hepatic veins display thrombi in varying stages of evolution, from recent clots to well-organized thrombi that have been recanalized (Fig. 14-34). As the acute stage progresses, the sinusoids of the central zone are dilated and packed with red blood cells. The liver cell plates are compressed, and necrosis of centrilobular hepatocytes is accompanied by the deposition of fibrin. Eventually, connective tissue septa link adjacent central zones to form nodules. The fibrosis is usually not severe enough to justify a label of cirrhosis.

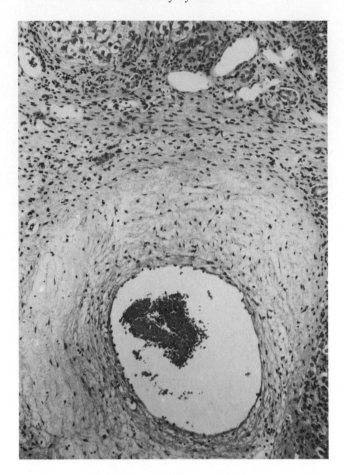

Figure 14-34. Budd-Chiari syndrome. A photomicrograph shows a recanalized hepatic vein. Perivenous fibrosis and a markedly thickened intima are evident.

COMPLICATIONS

ESOPHAGEAL VARICES

The most important complications of portal hypertension arise from the opening of portasystemic collaterals as an adaptation to decompress the portal venous system. The collaterals of most clinical significance are located in the submucosa of the lower esophagus and upper stomach, and represent communications between the portal vein and the gastric coronary vein. One of the most common causes of death in patients with cirrhosis and other disorders associated with portal hypertension is exsanguinating upper gastrointestinal hemorrhage from **bleeding esophageal varices.** The prognosis in cases of bleeding esophageal varices is poor, and the acute mortality may be as high as 40%. Death associated with bleeding esophageal varices is frequently not attributable directly to exsanguination and shock, but rather is the result of **hepatic failure.**

This condition is precipitated by stress, ischemic necrosis of the liver, and encephalopathy caused by the acute nitrogenous load imposed by the exsanguinated blood in the intestinal tract.

SPLENOMEGALY

The spleen in portal hypertension enlarges progressively, and splenomegaly is considered by some the single most important diagnostic sign of portal hypertension. The enlarged spleen often gives rise to the syndrome of **hypersplenism**—that is, a decrease in the life span of all of the formed elements of the blood and, therefore, a reduction in their circulating numbers. Hypersplenism is attributed to an increased rate of removal of red blood cells, white blood cells, and platelets because of the prolonged transit time through the hyperplastic spleen. Grossly, the spleen is firm and enlarged, up to 1000 g. Microscopically, the sinusoids are dilated, and their walls are thickened by fibrous tissue and lined by hyperplastic reticuloendothelial cells.

ASCITES

Ascites, the accumulation of fluid in the peritoneal cavity, often accompanies portal hypertension, most commonly in patients with decompensated cirrhosis. The amount of fluid may be so great—frequently many liters—that is not only distends the abdomen but also interferes with breathing. The onset of ascites in cirrhosis is associated with a poor prognosis.

The pathogenesis of ascites remains a subject of investigation, but it is generally thought that the increased formation of hepatic and intestinal lymph is important (Fig. 14-35). Hypoalbuminemia in patients with cirrhosis also contributes to the formation of ascites, because of the decreased plasma oncotic pressure.

The sequestration of fluid in the peritoneal cavity leads to a decrease in the effective plasma volume, which in turn leads to renal sodium and fluid retention through a number of possible mechanisms, including decreased glomerular filtration, increased aldosterone activity, and increased sodium reabsorption. The increased renal retention of sodium and fluid aggravates ascites formation, and creates a vicious cycle.

TOXIC INJURY

The spectrum of acute chemically induced hepatic injury is so broad that it runs the gamut of liver disease, from clinically trivial, transient cholestasis,

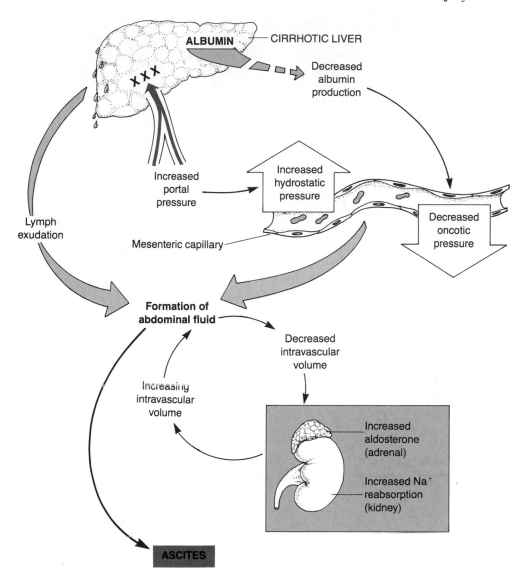

Figure 14-35. Pathogenesis of ascites.

to fatal fulminant hepatitis. Chronic toxic injury to the liver is equally diverse, being expressed, at one extreme, as a mild persistent hepatitis and, at the other, as an active cirrhosis.

In general, certain hepatotoxic chemicals invariably produce liver cell necrosis—that is, their action is entirely **predictable.** The defining characteristics of the liver injury produced by "predictable" hepatotoxins are as follows:

The agent, in sufficiently high doses, always produced liver cell necrosis.

The extent of hepatic injury is dose dependent.

Although exceptions exist, these compounds produce the same lesions in different species.

The liver necrosis is characteristically zonal—often, but not exclusively, centrilobular.

The period between administration of the toxin and the development of liver cell necrosis is brief.

Toxic liver necrosis is, in most (though not all) cases, a consequence of the metabolism of the compound by the mixed-function oxidase system of the liver, by which activated oxygen species and reactive metabolites are produced.

In contrast to the aforementioned classic poisons, **most reactions to drugs are unpredictable** and seem to represent **idiosyncratic** events, i.e., manifestations of unusual sensitivity to a dose-related side effect. Sensitive individuals may be predisposed to idiosyncratic reactions either because they possess metabolic pathways different from those of the general population, or because they are unusually sensitive to a uniform pharmacologic effect of the drug other than the desired therapeutic response. For example, chlorpromazine, a drug administered because of its effects on the central nervous system, reproducibly inhibits bile flow in experimental animals. On the other hand, when chlorpromazine is given chronically to patients in the usually therapeutic dose range, only a small proportion of patients develop cholestatic jaundice. Under these circumstances, it is not clear whether the jaundice in man results from a qualitative difference in the response of the hepatocyte to chlorpromazine or simply reflects an exaggerated inhibition of bile flow.

An immunologic reaction to drugs, their metabolites, or modified liver cells has not been ruled out, although direct evidence is weak. **Drugs that are principally cholestasic do not necessarily depend upon metabolism for their action.**

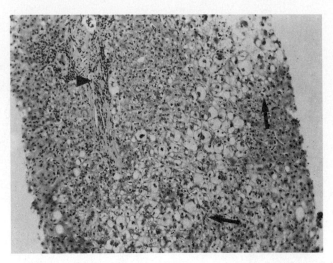

Figure 14-36. Toxic centrilobular necrosis. A liver biopsy specimen from a young woman who had ingested a large amount of acetaminophen in a suicide attempt shows centrilobular ballooning and necrosis of hepatocytes (*arrows*). The area surrounding the portal tract (*arrowhead*) appears normal.

ZONAL HEPATOCELLULAR NECROSIS

Drugs and chemicals that are predictable hepatotoxins and act via their metabolites typically cause centrilobular necrosis (Fig. 14-36), presumably because of the greater activity of drug-metabolizing enzymes in the central zones. Examples of such agents are carbon tetrachloride, acetaminophen, and the toxins of the mushroom *Amanita phalloides*. In the affected zones hepatocytes show coagulative necrosis, hydropic swelling, and variable amounts of fat. Inflammation is often sparse. If the dose of the hepatotoxin is sufficiently large, necrosis may extend to involve the entire lobule. Patients die in acute hepatic failure or recover without sequelae.

FATTY LIVER

The accumulation of triglycerides within the hepatocytes—that is, hepatic steatosis, or fatty liver—occurs in response to a variety of hepatotoxins, generally in a predictable fashion. Although substantial overlap may exist, two morphologic patterns are seen, namely, **macrovesicular and microvesicular steatosis** (Fig. 14-37).

In macrovesicular steatosis, light microscopy shows the cytoplasm of the liver cell to be occupied by fat, seen as a large clear area that distends the cell and displaces the nucleus to the periphery. In the microvesicular variety, small fat vacuoles are dispersed throughout the cytoplasm, and the nucleus retains its central position. In addition to its association with chronic ethanol ingestion, macrovesicular fat results from the experimental administration of, or accidental exposure to, such direct hepatotoxins as carbon tetrachloride and the poisonous constituents of certain mushrooms. Moreover, corticosteroids and some antimetabolites, such as methotrexate, may cause macrovesicular steatosis. There is no reason to believe that the presence of fat, per se, is in any way injurious to the hepatocytes. Rather, its accumulation reflects the underlying liver cell damage. In many, but not all, instances of toxic steatosis, the basis for fat accumulation is impaired secretion of lipoproteins as a consequence of an interference with protein synthesis.

In contrast to macrovesicular steatosis, which by itself is in general clinically inconsequential, microvesicular fatty liver is commonly associated with severe, and sometimes fatal, liver disease, although milder forms are recognized. Perhaps the most common and widely feared example of liver disease associated with microvesicular steatosis is **Reye's syndrome, an acute disease of children characterized by hepatic failure and encephalopathy.**

Under the light microscope, the liver in Reye's syndrome displays a typical microvesicular steatosis

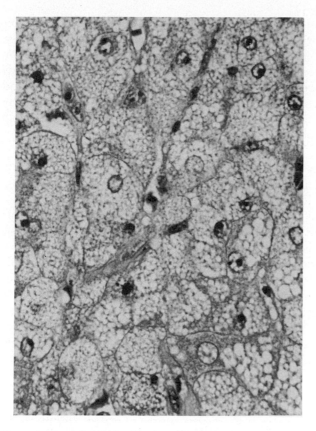

Figure 14-37. Microvesicular fatty liver. A liver biopsy specimen in a case of Reye's syndrome shows small droplets of fat in hepatocytes and a centrally located nucleus.

in the portal tracts, a feature that suggests a hypersensitivity reaction to chlorpromazine or its metabolites.

LESIONS RESEMBLING THOSE OF VIRAL HEPATITIS

All the typical clinical and morphologic features of acute viral hepatitis can be seen after the administration of some drugs that cause idiosyncratic (unpredictable) liver injury. The most widely appreciated examples are the inhalation anesthetic halothane, the anti-tuberculosis agent isoniazid, and the anti-hypertensive drug methyldopa. Although the incidence of these viral hepatitis-like reactions is low, they are far more dangerous than viral hepatitis itself causing more severe disease and a much higher mortality rate. The entire range of acute liver injury, from mild anicteric hepatitis to rapidly fatal fulminant hepatic necrosis, is encountered. It deserves repetition that, for practical purposes, the pattern of liver injury is morphologically indistinguishable from that of documented acute viral hepatitis. As in viral hepatitis, when the offending agent is removed—that is, when the virus is cleared or the drug is withdrawn—complete recovery is the rule.

CHRONIC ACTIVE HEPATITIS

Persistent intake of hepatotoxic drugs can lead to a syndrome indistinguishable from chronic active hepatitis. Like chronic active hepatitis caused by persistent viral infection, drug-induced chronic active hepatitis may progress to cirrhosis. On discontinuation of drug administration, the lesion usually resolves, although this may require many months. Among the drugs incriminated in the production of chronic active hepatitis are the laxative oxyphenisatin, the antihypertensive agent methyl-dopa, the anti-tuberculosis drug isoniazid and certain sulfonamides.

without accompanying hepatocellular necrosis or inflammation. Electron microscopy demonstrates **characteristic alterations in mitochondria of the liver and brain.**

INTRAHEPATIC CHOLESTASIS

Acute intrahepatic cholestasis is one of the most frequent manifestations of idiosyncratic types of drug-induced liver disease. A few drugs, principally sex steroids of the contraceptive or anabolic type, cause **bland centrilobular cholestasis** with virtually no hepatocellular necrosis or inflammation. Except for mild jaundice, pruritus, and an elevated serum alkaline phosphatase level, the patients feel well.

Many other drugs, of which chlorpromazine is the prototype, are associated with **centrilobular cholestasis, slight to moderate inflammation, and mild hepatocellular injury.** Eosinophils are often conspicuous

MISCELLANEOUS DRUG REACTIONS

A number of drugs occasionally associated with hepatotoxicity may also induce noncaseating, "sarcoid-like" granulomas in the portal tracts and the lobular parenchyma. Also, the use of oral contraceptives, and uncommonly anabolic steroids, may be associated with the development of **hepatic adenomas,** benign tumors of hepatocytes whose greatest danger lies in their propensity to rupture and then bleed profusely.

VASCULAR DISORDERS

CONGESTIVE HEART FAILURE

ACUTE PASSIVE CONGESTION

At autopsy it is common for the liver to be acutely congested, presumably because of a failing heart in the agonal period. On cut section, the liver is diffusely speckled with small red foci, which microscopic examination reveals to be centrilobular zones with moderately dilated and congested sinusoids and terminal venules. These changes are not clinically significant.

CHRONIC PASSIVE CONGESTION

In the face of **persistent congestive heart failure,** the pressure in the peripheral venous circulation increases, impeding venous outflow from the liver and producing chronic passive congestion of that organ. Unlike acute congestion, in which it is somewhat enlarged, with chronic congestion the liver is often reduced in size. On gross examination the cut surface of the liver exhibits an accentuated lobular pattern, with a mottled appear-

ance of alternating light and dark areas. Because this pattern is reminiscent of a cut nutmeg, it has been termed **"nutmeg liver"** (Fig. 14-38). In severe cases the centrilobular terminal venules and adjacent sinusoids are conspicuously dilated and filled with red blood cells. The liver cell plates in this zone are thinned by pressure atrophy, and may even be absent, leaving a collapsed reticulin framework.

CARDIAC FIBROSIS OF THE LIVER

In cases of particularly severe and longstanding **right-sided heart failure**—for example, tricuspid valvular disease or constrictive pericarditis—chronic passive congestion progresses to varying degrees of hepatic fibrosis that radiates from the centrilobular zones. In prolonged cases of heart failure, the septa may link adjacent central veins, thereby producing a "reverse lobulation." The older term "cardiac cirrhosis" is inappropriate, since the complete septa and regenerative nodules of true cirrhosis are rarely encountered.

NONVIRAL INFECTIONS

BACTERIAL

Bacterial infections are uncommon causes of liver disease in the industrialized countries, and when seen are for the most part complications of infections elsewhere. **The characteristic reactions in the liver are granulomas, abscesses, and diffuse inflammation.** Infections associated with granulomatous inflammation elsewhere—for instance, tuberculosis, tularemia, and brucellosis—also cause granulomatous hepatitis. Staphylococci, streptococci, and gram-negative enterobacteria produce **pyogenic hepatic abscesses.** It is increasingly recognized that anaerobic inhabitants of the gastrointestinal tract, particularly *Bacteroides* species and microaerophilic streptococci, are a common cause of liver abscesses. Organisms reach the liver in arterial or portal blood or through the biliary tract. Seeding of the liver with organisms from distant sites in cases of septicemia is through the arterial blood. By contrast, intra-abdominal suppuration, as in peritonitis or diverticulitis, is transmitted to the liver in portal blood, where it typically causes **pylephlebitic abscesses.**

Biliary obstruction from any cause is often complicated by bacterial infection of the biliary tree, termed **ascending cholangitis.** The retrograde biliary dissemination of organisms (usually *Escherichia coli*) leads to the formation of **cholangitic abscesses** in the liver (Fig.

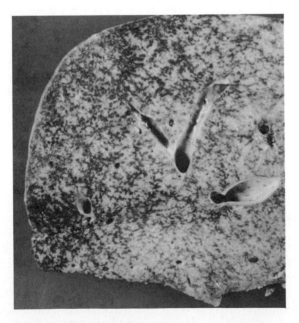

Figure 14-38. Chronic passive congestion of the liver. The surface of the liver exhibits an accentuated lobular pattern, termed "nutmeg" liver.

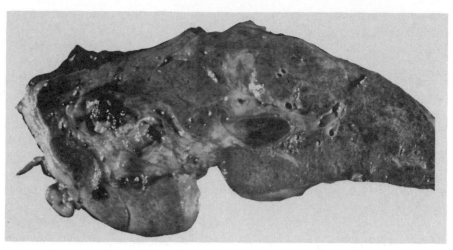

Figure 14-39. Cholangitic abscesses of the liver. The cut surface of the liver shows a large irregular abscess cavity in the right lobe and smaller ones in the other areas. The patient died of pancreatic carcinoma, which had obstructed the common bile duct.

14-39)—today the most common form of hepatic abscess in Western countries. Nevertheless, in about half of all cases of hepatic abscess, the source of infection cannot be demonstrated.

Patients with a hepatic abscess typically present with high fever, rapid weight loss, right upper quadrant abdominal pain, and hepatomegaly. Jaundice occurs in a quarter of the cases, but the serum alkaline phosphatase level is almost always elevated. The mortality from hepatic abscess, even in treated cases, remains high, ranging from 40% to 80%.

PARASITIC

Parasitic infestations of the liver are a serious public health problem worldwide, although they are uncommon in industrialized countries. These diseases are discussed in Chapter 9, which deals with infectious diseases. Here we summarize the major parasitic diseases that involve the liver.

AMEBIASIS

Amebiasis of the liver, the most common extra-intestinal complication, leads to amebic abscesses, which are multiple in about half of the cases (Fig. 14-40). Secondary infection of an amebic abscess with pyogenic organisms is common. If the abscess continues to grow, it may rupture into the peritoneal cavity, where it produces peritonitis, a complication associated with a mortality as high as 40%. The amebae may also invade the blood, in which case abscesses of the brain and lung may ensue.

MALARIA

Hepatic involvement in malaria is a frequent cause of hepatomegaly in endemic areas, and reflects Kupffer cell hypertrophy and hyperplasia. This reaction is secondary to the phagocytosis of the debris resulting from the rupture of parasitized erythrocytes.

VISCERAL LEISHMANIASIS (KALA-AZAR)

As in malaria, the hepatomegaly of chronic visceral leishmaniasis results from reticuloendothelial hyper-

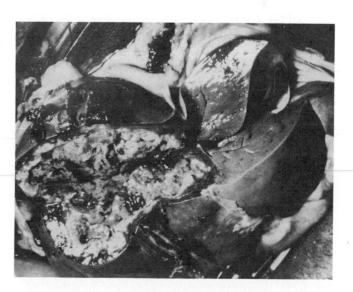

Figure 14-40. Amebic abscess of the liver. The liver has been incised to reveal a large amebic abscess of the right lobe.

plasia in the liver. In leishmaniasis, however, the Kupffer cells ingest the parasitic organisms themselves, which appear as "Donovan bodies."

LIVER FLUKES

The major parasitic flukes that involve the human liver are *Clonorchis sinensis* and *Fasciola hepatica*. Man is the definitive host for *C. sinensis*, whereas sheep and cattle are the principal reservoir of *F. hepatics*. Both parasites lodge in the intrahepatic biliary tree, where they provoke hyperplasia of the biliary epithelium, particularly severe in clonorchiasis. Secondary infection of the bile with *E. coli* causes cholangitis and cholangitic abscesses, common causes of surgical emergencies in some Oriental Countries. Biliary infestation with *C. sinensis* is an etiologic factor in the development of cholangiocarcinoma.

ECHINOCOCCOSIS (CYSTIC HYDATID DISEASE)

Infection with the tapeworms of the genus *Echinococcus*, principally *E. granulosus*, is an important zoonosis that involves the human liver. Larvae, termed *onchospheres*, pass from the intestine into the portal circulation and lodge in the liver, where they encyst. In a few days a germinal membrane develops, from which brood capsules, containing innumerable scolices (the future head of the adult worm), arise. The cyst expands slowly, and produces symptoms only after many years.

SYPHILIS

Congenital syphilis causes neonatal hepatitis, which results in diffuse fibrosis in the portal tracts and around individual liver cells or groups of hepatocytes. Up to 10% of patients with **secondary syphilis** develop a hepatitis that is clinically similar to viral hepatitis. **Tertiary syphilis** is characterized by single or multiple hepatic gummas—focal lesions resembling granulomas, which heal with a dense scar. Retraction of the scars in severe cases with multiple gummas produces deep clefts and a gross pseudolobation of the liver, termed **hepar lobatum,** a condition that should not be confused with cirrhosis.

NEONATAL HEPATITIS

Neonatal hepatitis is a poorly defined clinical and pathologic entity of multiple etiologies. These disorders have in common **prolonged cholestasis, morphologic**

evidence of liver cell injury, and inflammation. In about 50% of all cases of neonatal hepatitis, the cause is discernible (Table 14-4), and about 30% of cases are assigned to α_1-antitrypsin deficiency alone. Most of the other cases with known causes can be attributed to viral hepatitis B and infectious agents such as the TORCH group (toxoplasmosis, rubella, cytomegalovirus, and herpes simplex). A few cases represent hepatic injury associated with metabolic defects, for instance galactosemia or fructose intolerance. The remaining 50% are of unexplained etiology. Most patients who have uncomplicated neonatal hepatitis recover without sequelae.

The characteristic hepatic lesion of neonatal hepatitis is giant cell transformation of hepatocytes, hence the former term "giant cell hepatitis" (Fig. 14-41). The giant cells contain as many as 40 nuclei and may appear detached from other cells in the liver plate. Ballooned hepatocytes, acinar transformation, and acido-

Table 14-4   Causes of Neonatal Hepatitis

Idiopathic

Idiopathic neonatal hepatitis
Prolonged intrahepatic cholestasis
   1. Arteriohepatic dysplasia (Alagille's syndrome)
   2. Paucity of intrahepatic bile ducts not associated with specific syndromes
   3. Zellweger's syndrome (cerebrohepatorenal syndrome)
   4. Byler disease

Mechanical Obstruction of the Intrahepatic Bile Ducts

Congenital hepatic fibrosis
Caroli's disease (cystic dilatation of intrahepatic ducts)

Metabolic Disorders

Defects of carbohydrate metabolism
   1. Galactosemia
   2. Hereditary fructose intolerance
   3. Glycogenosis Type IV
Defects of lipid metabolism
   1. Gaucher's disease
   2. Niemann-Pick disease
   3. Wolman's disease
Tyrosinemia (defect of amino acid metabolism)
α_1-Antitrypsin deficiency
Cystic fibrosis
Parenteral nutrition

Hepatitis

Hepatitis B
TORCH agents
Varicella
Syphilis
Echoviruses
Neonatal sepsis

Chromosomal Abnormalities

Down's syndrome
Trisomy 18

Extrahepatic Biliary Atresia

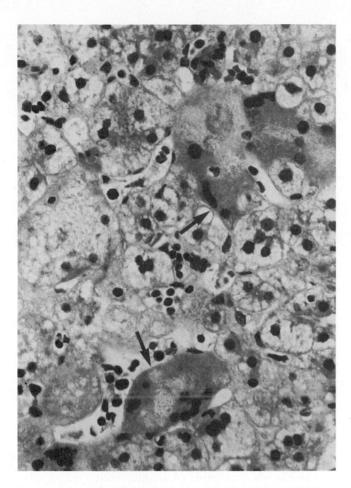

Figure 14-41. Neonatal hepatitis. A photomicrograph shows multinucleated giant hepatocytes (*arrows*), liver cell injury, and a mild chronic inflammatory infiltrate.

philic bodies are also typical of neonatal hepatitis. Pericellular fibrosis around degenerating hepatocytes, singly or in groups, is common, and fibrous tissue septa extend from the portal tracts.

BILIARY ATRESIA

The confusion surrounding the concept of neonatal hepatitis is aggravated by its association with both intrahepatic and extrahepatic biliary atresia. Extrahepatic biliary atresia, like pure intrahepatic biliary atresia, is often associated with full-blown neonatal hepatitis. Thus it has been suggested that biliary atresia in the neonate, whether intrahepatic or extrahepatic, is secondary to neonatal hepatitis. Alternatively, the etiologic agent of neonatal hepatitis may independently cause biliary atresia. Indeed, it may well be true that neonatal hepatitis, intrahepatic biliary atresia, extrahe-

patic biliary atresia, and possibly choledochal cyst **all result from a common inflammatory process** ("infantile obstructive cholangiopathy") and are not true congenital anomalies.

Intrahepatic biliary atresia associated with neonatal hepatitis carries a poor prognosis, and in many children progresses to biliary cirrhosis. Uncorrected extrahepatic biliary atresia invariably results in progressive secondary biliary cirrhosis and is incompatible with survival. While surgical correction has been successful in some anatomically favorable cases, the majority of cases of extrahepatic, as well as intrahepatic, biliary atresia can be cured only by liver transplantation.

NEOPLASMS

BENIGN TUMORS AND TUMOR-LIKE LESIONS

HEPATIC ADENOMA

Hepatic adenomas are benign tumors of hepatocytes that occur almost always in women in the reproductive years, usually as a solitary, sharply demarcated mass up to 40 cm in diameter and 3 kg in weight (Fig. 14-42). In about a third of patients with hepatic adenomas—particularly pregnant women who have previously used oral contraceptives—the tumors bleed into the peritoneal cavity and require treatment as a surgical emergency.

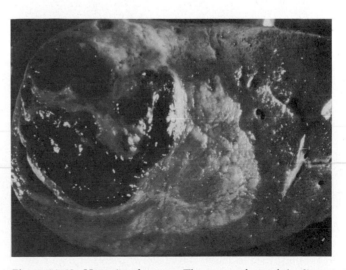

Figure 14-42. Hepatic adenoma. The cut surface of the liver shows a large vascular and hemorrhagic mass in the right lobe.

Microscopically, the neoplastic hepatocytes resemble their nomal counterparts, except that they are not arranged in a lobular architecture (Fig. 14-43). Portal tracts and central venules are not present. The cells composing the adenoma may be very large and eosinophilic, or filled with glycogen, which makes the cytoplasm appear clear.

Hepatic adenomas were exceedingly rare before the availability of oral contraceptives, but since their introduction, many such tumors have been reported. Today they are a well-recognized, although uncommon, complication of oral contraceptives.

FOCAL NODULAR HYPERPLASIA

Focal nodular hyperplasia is a nodular liver mass varying in size from 5 cm to 15 cm in diameter and weighing as much as 700 g. The cut surface exhibits a characteristic central scar from which fibrous septa radiate. Microscopically, hepatocytic nodules are circumscribed

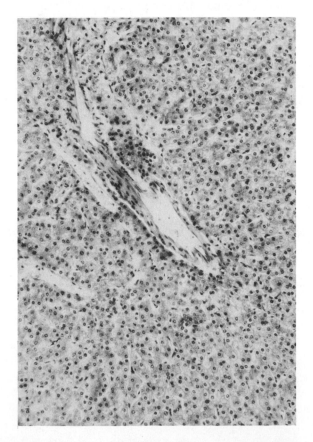

Figure 14-43. Hepatic adenoma. A photomicrograph of the mass illustrated in Figure 14-42 shows plates of highly differentiated, neoplastic hepatocytes without discernible hepatic architecture. A large blood vessel is evident in the center.

by fibrous septa (Fig. 14-44), which contain numerous tortuous bile ducts and mononuclear inflammatory cells. Within the nodules, lobular architecture is absent.

MALIGNANT TUMORS

HEPATOCELLULAR CARCINOMA

Hepatocellular carcinoma occurs in all parts of the world, but its incidence shows a striking geographic variability. In Western industrialized countries the tumor is uncommon, but in sub-Saharan Africa, Southeast Asia, and Japan, the rates are up to 50 times greater.

An association between hepatocellular carcinoma and infection with the hepatitis B virus (HBV) is now clearly established. The geographic incidence of this tumor correlates strongly with the prevalence of the carrier state for HBV. Moreover, in areas of high incidence, HBV infection is documented in 80% to 90% of patients with hepatocellular carcinoma. The carrier state is indeed dangerous, since such individuals are estimated to have as much as a 200-fold increased risk of developing hepatocellular carcinoma. About a quarter of those with chronic hepatitis B acquired at or near birth ultimately develop hepatocellular carcinoma. Further evidence that HBV has an important role in the development of hepatocellular carcinoma comes from the demonstration that in cases of this tumor **the genome of HBV is integrated into the host DNA of both the non-neoplastic liver cells and the tumor cells.**

Various forms of cirrhosis are associated with a high incidence of hepatocellular carcinoma. Liver diseases occurring in conjunction with hemochromatosis and α_1-antritrypsin deficiency carry a substantial risk of hepatocellular carcinoma, and about 10% of patients with hemochromatosis may be expected to develop the tumor.

Hepatocellular carcinoma is considerably more common in men than in women, presumably a reflection of the increased occurrence of the HBV carrier state in men. The tumor usually presents as a painful and enlarging mass in the liver. Ascites, portal vein thrombosis, occlusion of hepatic veins, and hemorrhage from esophageal varices are common. The prognosis is dismal, and patients die of malignant cachexia, rupture of the tumor with catastrophic bleeding into the peritoneal cavity, bleeding esophageal varices, or hepatic failure.

Hepatocellular carcinomas appear grossly as soft and hemorrhagic tan masses in the liver. The tumor has a tendency to grow into portal veins, and may extend to the vena cava, and even the right atrium, through the

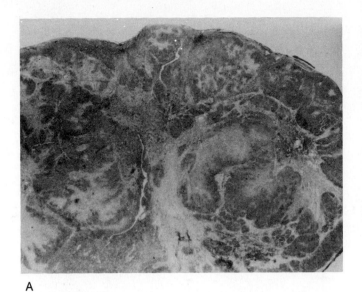

A

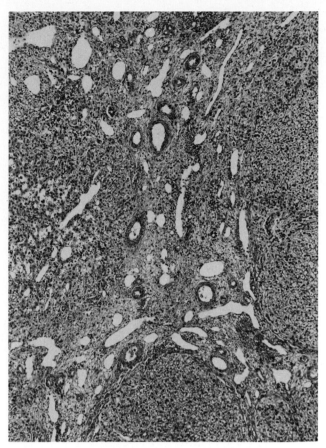

B

Figure 14-44. Focal nodular hyperplasia. (*A*) A low-power photomicrograph reveals irregular fibrous septa and a disorganized hepatic parenchyma. (*B*) A higher-power photomicrograph shows hepatocellular nodules and irregular, highly vascularized, and chronically inflamed fibrous septa.

hepatic veins. A number of histologic patterns are recognized, but no prognostic significance can be attributed to any of them. Most hepatocellular carcinomas exhibit a **trabecular** pattern—that is, the tumor cells are arranged in trabeculae or plates that resemble the normal liver (Fig. 14-45). The plates are separated by endothelium-lined sinusoids, but Kupffer cells are absent.

Hepatocellular carcinomas may reach a large size before metastasizing. Metastases occur widely, the most common sites being the lungs and portal lymph nodes.

CHOLANGIOCARCINOMA (BILE DUCT CARCINOMA)

Cholangiocarcinomas, defined as malignant hepatic tumors of biliary epithelium, arise anywhere from the large intrahepatic bile ducts at the porta hepatis to the smallest bile ductules at the periphery of the hepatic lobule. They are composed of small cuboidal cells arranged in a ductular or glandular configuration (Fig.

14-46). Characteristically, they show substantial fibrosis, and on liver biopsy they may be confused with metastatic scirrhous carcinoma of the breast or pancreas.

Cholangiocarcinomas show a lesser tendency to invade the portal and hepatic veins than hepatocellular carcinomas. They metastasize to a wide variety of extrahepatic sites, and show a greater predilection for the portal lymph nodes than do hepatocellular carcinomas.

METASTATIC CANCER

Metastatic cancers are by far the most common malignant neoplasms of the liver. The liver is involved in a third of all metastatic cancers, including half of those of the gastrointestinal tract, breast, and lung. Other tumors that characteristically metastasize to the liver are pancreatic carcinoma and melanoma. The liver may show only a single nodule of tumor or may be virtually replaced by metastases (Fig. 14-47); liver weights of 5 kg or more are not uncommon. In fact, liver metastases are the most common causes of massive hepatomegaly.

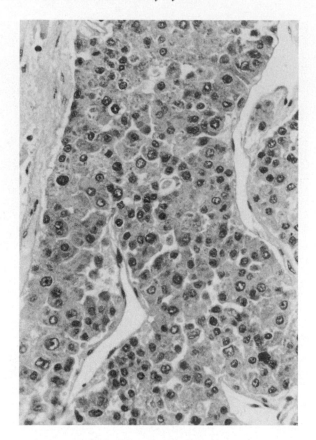

Figure 14-45. Hepatocellular carcinoma. A photomicrograph shows a trabecular pattern of malignant hepatocytes.

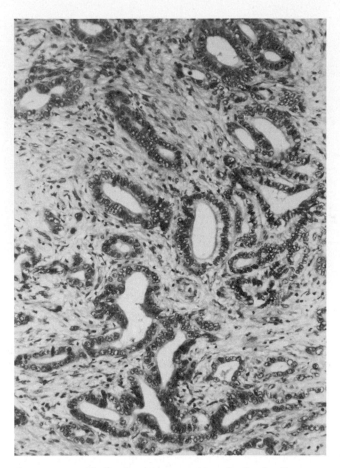

Figure 14-46. Cholangiocarcinoma. Neoplastic glands are embedded in a dense fibrous stroma.

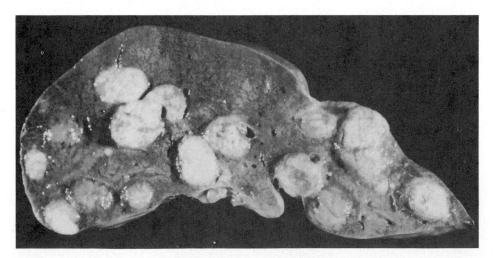

Figure 14-47. Metastatic carcinoma in the liver. The cut surface of the liver shows many firm, pale masses of metastatic colon cancer.

Often the first indication of metastatic tumor in the liver is an unexplained increase in the serum alkaline phosphatase level. The majority of patients die within a year of the diagnosis of liver metastases.

THE GALLBLADDER AND EXTRAHEPATIC BILE DUCTS

CHOLELITHIASIS

Cholelithiasis is defined as the presence of stones within the lumen of the gallbladder or in the extrahepatic biliary tree. In the industrialized countries, about three-quarters of gallstones consist primarily of cholesterol, while the remainder are composed of calcium bilirubinate and other calcium salts (pigment gallstones). Pigment stones predominate in the tropics and the Orient.

CHOLESTEROL STONES

Cholesterol stones are round or faceted, yellow to tan, single or multiple, and vary from 1 mm to 4 cm in greatest dimension (Fig. 14-48). Between 50% and 100% of the stone is composed of cholesterol; the rest consists of calcium salts and mucin. During their reproductive years, **women are three times more likely than men to develop cholesterol gallstones,** the incidence being higher in users of oral contraceptives and in women with several pregnancies.

PATHOGENESIS

The pathogenesis of cholesterol stones relates principally to the composition of the bile (Fig. 14-49). Normally, cholesterol, a compound highly insoluble in water, is secreted by the hepatocytes into the bile, where it is held in solution by the combined action of bile acids and lecithin (phospholipid) and carried in the form of mixed lipid micelles. If the bile contains excess cholesterol or is deficient in bile acids, the bile becomes supersaturated, and under some circumstances the cholesterol precipitates as solid crystals. **The bile of persons afflicted with cholesterol gallstones has more cholesterol as it leaves the liver than that of normal individuals, pointing to the liver, rather than the gallbladder, as the culprit in the genesis of cholesterol stones.** The hepatocytes of patients with cho-

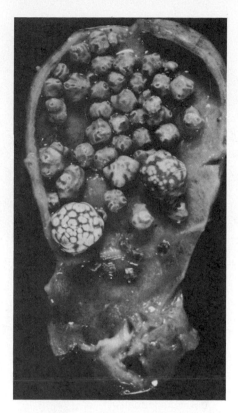

Figure 14-48. Cholesterol gallstones. The gallbladder has been opened to reveal numerous yellow cholesterol gallstones. The gallbladder wall is thickened as a result of chronic cholecystitis.

lesterol gallstones are deficient in 7α-hydroxylase, the enzyme involved in the rate-limiting step by which bile salts are formed from cholesterol. As a result, **the total size of the bile salt pool is reduced.** The resulting decrease in bile salt secretion contributes to the stone-forming (lithogenic) properties of the bile. Furthermore, **in obese people, cholesterol secretion by the liver is augmented,** further adding to the supersaturation of the bile with cholesterol.

Although cholesterol supersaturation of the bile is apparently required for gallstone formation, additional factors are also required. Cholesterol does not precipitate from saturated bile obtained from patients without gallstones, even after prolonged incubation. On the other hand, bile from persons without gallstones, but with properties similar to those in the bile of patients with gallstones, crystallizes without difficulty. It is thought that the mucinous glycoproteins secreted by the gallbladder epithelium provide the necessary nidus for crystallization.

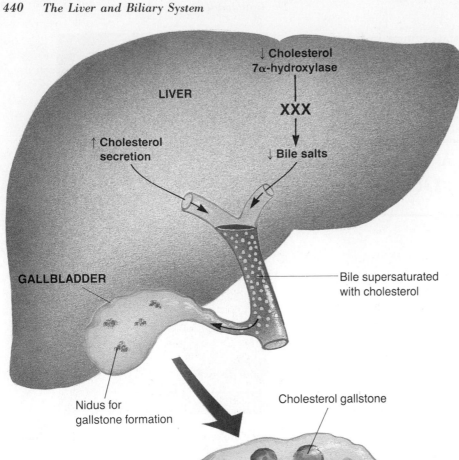

Figure 14-49. Pathogenesis of cholesterol gallstones.

Risk factors associated with increased biliary cholesterol secretion include the following:

Increasing age
Obesity
Certain ethnic groups, including Chilean women and some groups of Northern Europeans
Familial predisposition
Diets high in calories and cholesterol
Certain metabolic abnormalities associated with high blood cholesterol levels, for instance, diabetes, some genetic hyperlipoproteinemias, and primary biliary cirrhosis.

PIGMENT STONES

Pigment stones are classed as **black** or **brown** stones, which have different characteristics. Black stones are irregular and measure less than 1 cm across. On cross section, the surface appears glassy. Black stones contain calcium bilirubinate, bilirubin polymers, calcium salts, and mucin. The incidence of black stones is increased in old and undernourished people, but no correlations with gender, ethnicity, or obesity have been made. **Chronic hemolysis,** such as occurs with sickle cell anemia and thalassemia, predisposes to the development of black pigment stones. **Cirrhosis,** either because it leads to increased hemolysis or because it is linked to damage to liver cells, is also associated with a high incidence of black stones. **However, in most instances no predisposing cause for the formation of black pigment stones is evident.**

The pathogenesis of black pigment stones is related to an increased concentration of unconjugated bilirubin in the bile. When increased amounts are secreted by the hepatocyte, the unconjugated bilirubin precipitates as calcium bilirubinate.

Brown pigment stones are spongy and laminated, and contain principally calcium bilirubinate mixed with cholesterol and calcium soaps of fatty acids. In contrast to the other types of gallstones, brown pigment stones are found more frequently in the intrahepatic and extrahepatic bile ducts than in the gallbladder. These stones are almost always associated with bacterial cholangitis, in which *E. coli* is the predominant organism.

The pathogenesis of brown pigment stones also relates to an increased concentration of unconjugated bilirubin in the bile. It has been proposed that conjugated bilirubin is hydrolyzed to unconjugated bilirubin by the action of bacterial beta-glucuronidase or other hydrolytic enzymes.

CLINICAL COURSE

Most of the complications of cholelithiasis relate to the obstruction of the cystic duct or common bile duct by stones. Gallstones may pass into the common duct **(choledocholithiasis),** where they may lead to obstructive jaundice, cholangitis, and pancreatitis. In fact, in populations where alcoholism is not a factor, gallstones are the most common cause of acute pancreatitis. In obstruction of the cystic duct, with or without acute cholecystitis, the bile in the gallbladder is reabsorbed, to be replaced by a clear mucinous fluid secreted by the gallbladder epithelium. The term **hydrops of the gallbladder (mucocele)** is applied to the distended and palpable gallbladder, which may become secondarily infected.

ACUTE CHOLECYSTITIS

In 90% to 95% of cases acute cholecystitis is associated with the presence of gallstones. The initial symptom of acute cholecystitis is abdominal pain in the right upper quadrant, and most patients have already experienced episodes of biliary colic. Mild jaundice, caused by stones in or edema of the common bile duct, is evident in about 20% of patients. In most cases the acute illness subsides within a week, but persistent pain, fever, leukocytosis, and shaking chills indicate progression of the acute cholecystitis and the need for cholecystectomy.

The external surface of the gallbladder in acute cholecystitis is congested and layered with a fibrinous exudate. The wall is remarkably thickened by edema, and opening the viscus reveals a fiery-red or purple mucosa. Gallstones are usually found within the lumen, and a stone is often seen obstructing the cystic duct. Microscopically, edema and hemorrhage in the wall are striking, but neutrophilic infiltration is ordinarily only modest. Secondary bacterial infection may lead to true suppuration in the gallbladder wall. The mucosa shows focal ulcerations or, in severe cases, widespread necrosis, in which case the term **gangrenous cholecystitis** is applied.

The pathogenesis of acute cholecystitis is related to the presence of concentrated bile and gallstones within the gallbladder. Bacterial infection is secondary to biliary obstruction, rather than a primary event.

CHRONIC CHOLECYSTITIS

Chronic cholecystitis, almost invariably associated with gallstones, is the most common disease of the gallbladder. It may result from repeated attacks of acute cholecystitis, or, more often, from longstanding gallstones.

Grossly, the wall of the gallbladder is thickened and firm, and the serosal surface may show fibrous adhesions to surrounding structures as a result of previous episodes of acute cholecystitis. Gallstones are usually found within the lumen, and the bile often contains "gravel"—that is, fine precipitates of calculous material. The bile is infected with coliform organisms in about half of the cases. The mucosa may be focally ulcerated and atrophic, or may appear intact. Microscopically, the wall is fibrotic and often penetrated by sinuses of Rokitansky-Aschoff. Chronic inflammation of variable degree may be seen in all layers. In longstanding chronic cholecystitis, the wall of the gallbladder may become calcified, in which case the term "porcelain gallbladder" is used.

PRIMARY SCLEROSING CHOLANGITIS

Primary sclerosing cholangitis is an inflammatory and fibrosing process that narrows and eventually obstructs the extrahepatic and intrahepatic bile

ducts. The majority of patients are men under the age of 40 years. Clinically, progressive biliary obstruction leads to persistent obstructive jaundice and eventually to secondary biliary cirrhosis. The cause of primary sclerosing cholangitis is unknown, but about two-thirds of the patients also have ulcerative colitis.

Grossly, the wall of the common bile duct is thickened and the lumen is stenotic, either uniformly or segmentally. When the intrahepatic bile ducts are involved, a segmental pattern is the rule. Microscopically, diffuse fibrosis and moderate chronic inflammation are noted. The mucosa remains normal. The end stage of the disease is characterized by typical secondary biliary cirrhosis.

Primary sclerosing cholangitis has a poor prognosis; the mean survival after the appearance of symptoms is 6 years. Liver transplantation is the most promising treatment.

CARCINOMA OF THE GALLBLADDER

The most common tumor of the gallbladder is **adenocarcinoma** (Fig. 14-50). **Because this cancer is usually associated with cholelithiasis and chronic cholecystitis, it is considerably more common in women than men.** By the time the tumor becomes symptomatic, it is almost invariably incurable, the 5-year survival rate being less than 3%. **The tumor is characteristically an infiltrative, well-differentiated adenocarcinoma.** It is usually **desmoplastic,** and thus the wall of the gallbladder becomes thickened and leathery. The rich lymphatic plexus of the gallbladder provides the most common route of metastasis, but vascular dissemination and direct spread into the liver and contiguous structures occurs.

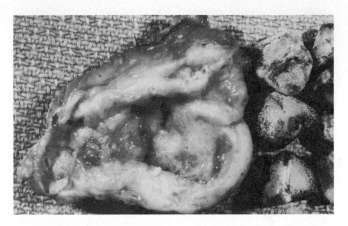

Figure 14-50. Carcinoma of the gallbladder. The gallbladder wall is infiltrated by a firm, greyish-white tumor. The lumen contains cholesterol gallstones.

15

THE PANCREAS

DANTE G. SCARPELLI

Pancreatitis

Adenocarcinoma of the
Exocrine Pancreas

Islet Cell Tumors

PANCREATITIS

Pancreatitis is defined as an inflammatory condition of the exocrine pancreas that results from injury to acinar cells. It ranges from a mild, self-limited disease, consisting of acute inflammation and edema of the stroma with little or no acinar cell necrosis, to the more severe and sometimes fatal acute hemorrhagic pancreatitis with massive necrosis. A debilitating form, chronic **relapsing pancreatitis,** is characterized by recurrent attacks of severe abdominal pain and progressive fibrosis, ultimately leading to pancreatic insufficiency.

ACUTE PANCREATITIS

The mild and presumably reversible form of acute pancreatitis, termed **interstitial** or **edematous pancreatitis,** has not been extensively studied because of its brief and benign clinical course. An infiltrate of polymorphonuclear leukocytes and edema of the connective tissue between lobules of acinar cells constitute the initial lesion. There is no necrosis of acinar cells, fat necrosis, or hemorrhage. **Acute hemorrhagic pancreatitis** is a condition of middle age, with a peak incidence at 60 years. It is often associated with chronic biliary disease and alcohol abuse and erupts abruptly, usually following a heavy meal or excessive alcohol intake. It is more common in men than in women, especially when it is associated with the chronic abuse of alcohol. Clinically, the patient presents with severe epigastric pain that is referred to the upper back and is accompanied by nausea and vomiting. Within a matter of hours catastrophic peripheral vascular collapse and shock ensue. When shock is sustained and profound, pancreatitis may be complicated within the first week of onset by the adult respiratory distress syndrome and acute renal failure, a situation that is fatal in 7% of cases. Early in the disease, pancreatic digestive enzymes are released from injured acinar cells into the blood and the abdominal cavity. Elevations of serum amylase and lipase levels as early as 24 to 72 hours are diagnostic, as are high enzyme levels in the abdominal ascitic fluid.

Acute pancreatitis is usually recognized macroscopically. Initially, the pancreas is edematous and hyperemic. Within a day, pale, gray foci appear, rapidly becoming friable and hemorrhagic. As the disease progresses, **these foci enlarge and become so numerous that most of the pancreas is converted into a large retroperitoneal hematoma, in which pancreatic tissue is barely recognizable** (Fig. 15-1 *A, B*). Yellowwhite areas of fat necrosis appear at the interface between necrotic foci and fat tissue in and around the

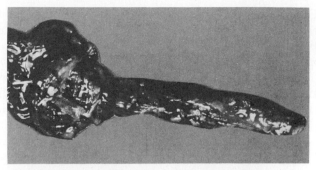

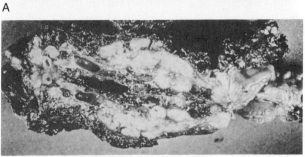

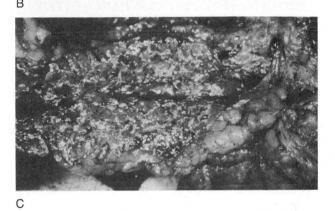

Figure 15-1. Acute hemorrhagic pancreatitis. (*A*) The head, body, and tail of the pancreas are intensely hemorrhagic. (*B*) The longitudinal cut surface shows large areas of confluent hemorrhagic necrosis that are clearly demarcated from pale nodular foci of nonnecrotic pancreas. (C) Numerous yellow-white foci of fat necrosis are present on the surface and in the substance of a necrotic pancreas at a stage somewhat later than that shown in *B*.

pancreas, including the adjacent mesentery (Fig. 15-1 *C*). These nodules of necrotic fat have a pasty consistency, which becomes firmer and chalklike as more calcium and magnesium soaps are produced. Saponification reflects the interaction of cations with free fatty acids released by the action of activated lipase on triglycerides in fat cells. As a result, the level of blood calcium may be depressed—sometimes to the point of causing neuromuscular irritability, such as facial tics.

Extrapancreatic fat necrosis, arising as a consequence of the release of lipase from the injured pancreas into the blood, has been reported in subcutaneous fat, skeletal muscle, and bone marrow.

On microscopic examination **the most prominent tissue alterations in acute pancreatitis are acinar cell necrosis, an intense acute inflammatory reaction** (Fig. 15-2*A*), **and foci of necrotic fat cells** (Fig. 15-2*B*). Late sequelae in patients who survive the shock and its systemic complications include the formation of pancreatic abscesses and **pseudocysts.** In the latter structures, large spaces limited by connective tissue contain degraded blood, debris of necrotic pancreatic tissue, and fluid rich in pancreatic enzymes. Pseudocysts may enlarge enough to compress and obstruct the duodenum. They may become secondarily infected and form an abscess. Rupture of a pseudocyst is a rare complication that leads to a chemical or septic peritonitis, or both.

PATHOGENESIS OF ACUTE PANCREATITIS

Autopsy studies at the turn of the century established the association of chronic cholecystitis and cholelithiasis with acute hemorrhagic pancreatitis. In some cases gallstones were found lodged near the orifice of the common duct beyond the point where it is joined by the pancreatic duct. Since a stone impacted at this site **obstructs both ducts,** it would be expected to cause the reflux of bile into the pancreas. Therefore, it was theorized that such obstruction was the etiologic factor in the development of acute hemorrhagic pancreatitis. This notion was prevalent for many years and gained support from experimental studies in animals in which hemorrhagic pancreatitis was induced by retrograde infusion of a mixture of pancreatic juice and bile into the main pancreatic duct. However, in recent years it has become increasingly apparent that although pancreatitis is often accompanied by conditions that serve to impair normal duct secretion, frank obstruction of the common duct or pancreatic duct is often not present. Increasingly, studies suggest that failure of one or more of the complex systems of physiologic checks and balances existing in the blood, pancreas, and other tissues, whose role it is to prevent the inappropriate activation of pancreatic enzymes and to protect the host from their deleterious effects, may also contribute to the development of acute pancreatitis. **It is clear that a breakdown of intracellular compartmentalization of digestive proenzymes, which are synthesized by the acinar cell, and inappropriate and premature activation of these proenzymes are common to all variants of pancreatitis.**

The pancreas is protected from the harmful effects of its lytic enzymes by a series of highly compartmentalized systems of intracellular membranes. These membranes effectively isolate the pancreatic enzymes, from their synthesis by the rough-surfaced endoplasmic reticulum to their release into the ductular lumen in response to stimulation by the gastrointestinal hormone cholecystokinin. At each step of their formation and secretion the enzymes are totally sequestered in membrane-bound granules. The various potent inhibitors of proteolytic enzymes present in many body fluids and tissues constitute a second line of protection, defending the organism against inappropriate activation of the digestive proenzymes of the pancreas. However, this defense is not total. Four potent protease inhibitors have been identified in human plasma: α_1-antitrypsin, α_2-macroglobulin, C_1 esterase inhibitor, and pancreatic secretory trypsin inhibitor. Although collectively these can inhibit two types of trypsin, in addition to chymotrypsin and elastase, they are without effect on two other potent proteases, carboxypeptidases A and B. Since activated trypsin is also able to activate other pancreatic proenzymes, such as chymotrypsinogen, proelastase, prophospholipase, and procarboxypeptidase, its incomplete inhibition in pancreatic juice and plasma poses a hazard.

Secretion by acinar cells delivers fluid rich in proenzymes to the ductules, where they are activated almost immediately. **Although most of the secretion is discharged into the duct system and enters the duodenum, a small amount diffuses back into the periductular extracellular fluid and eventually the plasma.** This happens because normal ducts contain fluid under some, albeit low, pressure. Thus, any condition that tends to diminish the patency of pancreatic ducts or the easy outflow of exocrine secretion would be expected to exacerbate back-diffusion across the ducts, which can trigger a massive inappropriate activation of digestive proenzymes. If the obstruction is sufficiently severe, this process could even involve the acinar cells. Well-documented causes of pancreatic duct obstruction include gallstones, frequently in association with chronic cholecystitis, and chronic alcohol abuse. Although ethanol is well recognized as a chemical toxin, a direct toxic effect on pancreatic acinar or duct cells has yet to be demonstrated. **However, large amounts of ethanol can adversely affect the pancreas by causing spasm or acute edema of the sphincter of Oddi, especially following an alcoholic binge, and by stimulating the release of secretin from the small intestine, which in turn triggers the exocrine pancreas to secrete pancreatic juice.** When these effects occur together (i.e., enhanced secretion into an obstructed

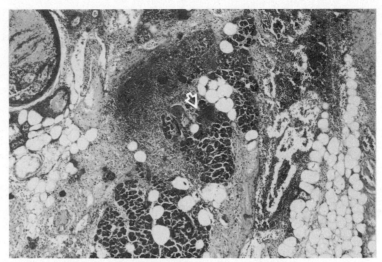

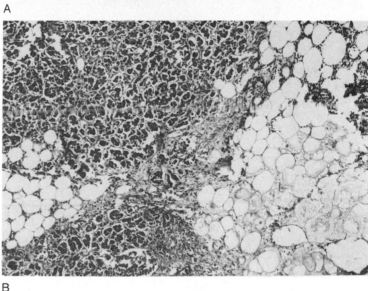

A

B

Figure 15-2. Acute hemorrhagic pancreatitis. (*A*) Hemorrhage is evident in the center and right of the microscopic field. The pancreatic lobule in the center shows a focus of acinar cell necrosis (*arrow*). (*B*) A later stage of acute pancreatitis. A focus of fat necrosis (*right*) can be compared with normal fat tissue (*left*).

duct), the results may be disastrous. The transudation of pancreatic secretion into periductal pancreatic tissue, and eventually into peripancreatic tissue, leads to chemical injury. The activated enzymes digest proteins, lipids, and carbohydrates of cell membranes. Phospholipase A causes lysis of cell membranes, and when mixed with bile converts lecithin to the potent cytotoxin lysolecithin. Damage to the capillaries leads to hemorrhage and local anoxia, which further intensifies and extends tissue damage. Other factors that cause pancreatic acinar cell injury and pancreatitis include viruses, endotoxemia, ischemia, drugs, trauma, hypertriglyceridemia, and hypercalcemia. The pathogenesis of acute hemorrhagic pancreatitis is outlined in Figure 15-3.

CHRONIC PANCREATITIS

Chronic pancreatitis is thought to result from recurrent bouts of acute pancreatitis, which lead to a progressive destruction of acinar cells, followed by healing and fibrosis. As a result, exocrine and endocrine functions are lost. Like acute pancreatitis, chronic pancreatitis may be associated with alcoholism and, less commonly, with biliary tract disease, hypercalcemia, or hyperlipidemia. About one-half of cases are seen in patients without any of these risk factors. In the acute phase, focal pancreatic necrosis is accompanied by a polymorphonuclear infiltrate, which is replaced by lymphocytes and plasma cells. Healing is characterized

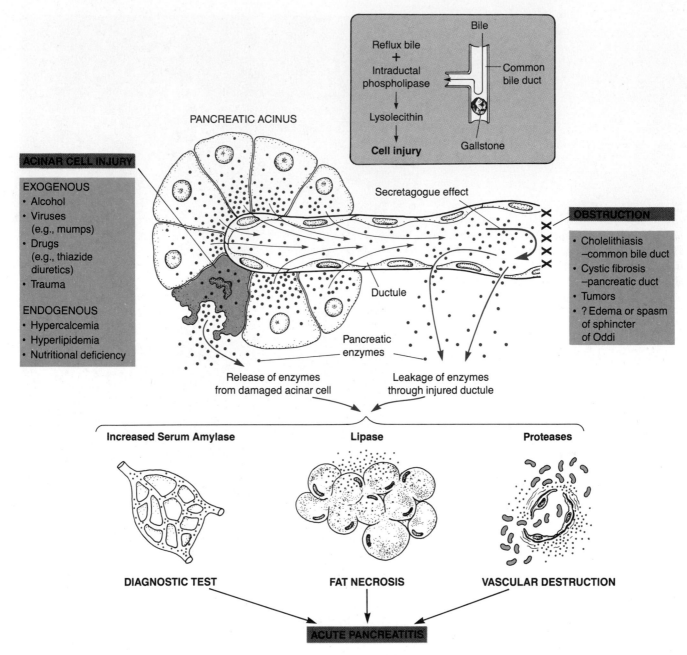

Figure 15-3. The pathogenesis of acute pancreatitis. Injury to the ductules or the acinar cells leads to the release of pancreatic enzymes. Lipase and proteases destroy tissue, thereby causing acute pancreatitis. The release of amylase is the basis for a test for acute pancreatitis.

by the removal of necrotic tissue by macrophages, a proliferation of capillaries and fibroblasts, and finally the deposition of collagen. In advanced cases, large areas of the pancreas are replaced by fibrosis, and the exocrine and endocrine tissues become atrophic.

The most common type of chronic pancreatitis is chronic calcifying pancreatitis, a disorder most frequently associated with alcoholism. In the calcifying type, intraductal protein plugs eventually calcify and lead to the formation of stones in the ducts (Fig. 15-4). In chronic pancreatitis following sustained alcohol abuse, ductules and ducts are so often filled with thick proteinaceous secretion that some have concluded that such secretions may be an important mechanism of obstruction. Since alcohol is a potent secretagogue for the exocrine pancreas, one can visualize a situation of secretion against obstruction. In another form of this disease, chronic obstructive pancreatitis, stenosis of the sphincter of Oddi is associated with gallbladder stones. Although in this condition the pancreatic ducts are filled with thick proteinaceous secretions, they are rarely the focus of calcification or stone formation.

Chronic pancreatitis is more common in men, and in about 10% of cases it is associated with pancreas divisum (incomplete fusion of the ventral and dorsal pancreatic anlage). **Diabetes mellitus, pancreatic insufficiency with its attendant steatorrhea and malabsorption, and pancreatic pseudocysts are frequent complications in the late stages of chronic pancreatitis** (Fig. 15-5).

ADENOCARCINOMA OF THE EXOCRINE PANCREAS

Carcinoma of the exocrine pancreas arises from duct cells and, more rarely, acinar cells. Cancer of the exocrine pancreas has shown a steady increase in the United States over the past 15 years and now ranks as one of the most common tumors. The 5-year survival is less than 2%. Pancreatic carcinoma is a disease of late life, with the greatest incidence in persons over age 60, although its appearance as early as the third decade is not rare. Ductal adenocarcinoma accounts for almost 90% of all pancreatic cancers; only about 1% derive from acinar cells.

Adenocarcinoma arises anywhere in the anatomic segments of the pancreas, with the most frequent focus in the head (60%), followed by the body (13%) and the tail (5%). In the remaining 22% the pancreas is diffusely involved. Tumors in the head cause biliary obstruction by compressing the ampulla of Vater, common bile duct, and duodenum early in their development. The classic **Courvoisier's sign,** consisting of an acute painless dilatation of the gallbladder accompanied by jaundice, is due to obstruction of the common bile duct and is often the first evidence of cancer of the pancreas. Because tumors in the head give early clinical symptoms, they tend to be discovered sooner than those in the more clinically silent body and tail, and thus carry a somewhat better survival. Extensive metastases involve the regional lymph nodes, followed in descending order by liver, lungs, peritoneum, duodenum, adrenals, and stomach.

Patients with carcinoma of the pancreas present with symptoms of anorexia, weight loss, and gnawing pain in the epigastrium that often radiates to the back. Jaundice is present in about half of all patients with cancer localized in the head, and in less than 10% of those in whom the body or tail of the pancreas is the focus of disease. The clinical course of pancreatic cancer is one of progressive deterioration, with intractable pain, cachexia, and death. Ten percent of patients develop a migratory thrombophlebitis, especially when the cancer involves the body and tail of the pancreas. In this condition, also known as **Trousseau's syndrome,** thrombi develop in multiple veins, including the subclavian, saphenous, iliacs, inferior vena cava, portal, and inferior and superior mesenteric. The complications of pancreatic ductal adenocarcinoma are summarized in Figure 15-6.

Grossly, pancreatic carcinoma is a firm, gray, poorly demarcated multinodular mass, often embedded in a dense connective tissue stroma. Carcinoma localized in the head, if extensive, causes atrophy of the body and tail. In the body and tail, the tumors are larger and extend more widely than do those localized in the head. They permeate the retroperitoneal space and may invade the adjacent spleen and the splenic vein, showering the liver with metastases. Intraperitoneal metastases appear as small, grayish, firm nodules in the mesentery and on the surface of intraperitoneal organs.

Most ductal adenocarcinomas of the pancreas are well differentiated, secrete mucin, and stimulate a florid synthesis and deposition of collagen by the host, a process referred to as a desmoplastic reaction (Fig. 15-7).

ETIOLOGY AND PATHOGENESIS

The factors involved in the causation of pancreatic cancer are obscure. **Notable among the host factors is chronic gallbladder disease, particularly that associated with cholesterol gallstones, diabetes mellitus, and chronic hereditary pancreatitis. Environmental factors that have been implicated include cigarette**

(Text continues on p. 452)

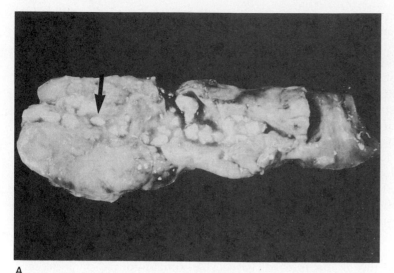

A

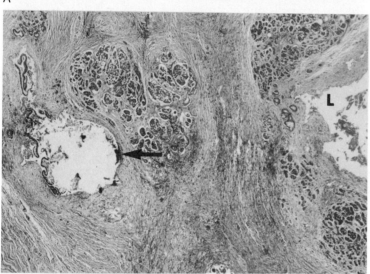

B

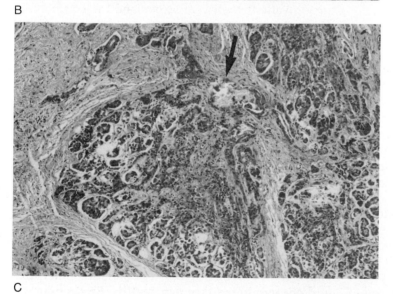

C

Figure 15-4. Chronic calcifying pancreatitis. (*A*) A gross photograph shows numerous calculi in the pancreatic duct (*arrow*). The gross architecture of the organ is severely distorted by fibrosis. (*B*) Atrophic lobules of acinar cells are surrounded by dense fibrous scar tissue infiltrated by lymphocytes. To the right of the lumen (*L*) a major duct contains granular deposits of calcified material, and to the left, a dilated medium-sized duct is partially denuded of its epithelial lining and has dense linear calcific deposits at its periphery (*arrow*). (*C*) At a higher magnification, lymphocytic infiltration and scarring are evident in part of an acinar cell lobule. Calcific material occludes its draining ductule (*arrow*).

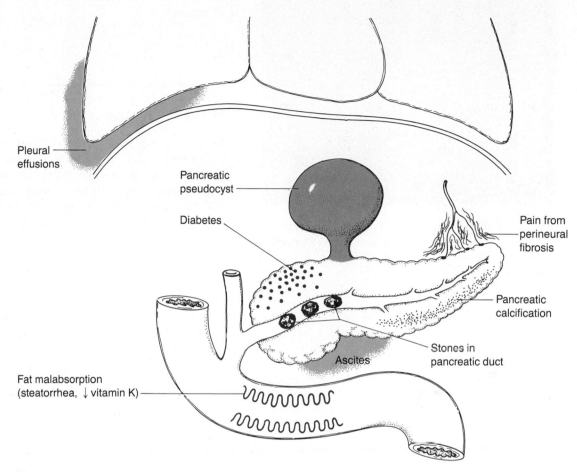

Figure 15-5. Complications of chronic pancreatitis.

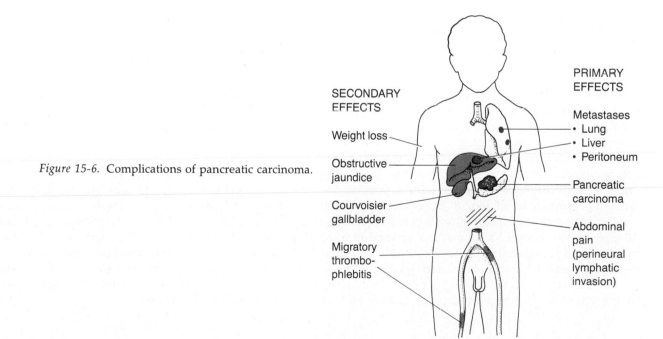

Figure 15-6. Complications of pancreatic carcinoma.

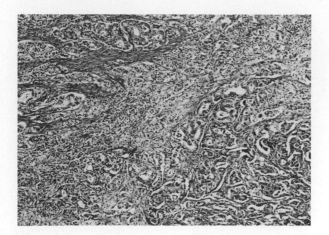

Figure 15-7. Carcinoma of the head of the pancreas. A tissue section of adenocarcinoma of pancreas reveals markedly atypical neoplastic glands that infiltrate the connective tissue of the pancreas.

smoking, diets high in meat and fat, and occupational exposure to chemicals, namely, β-naphthylamine, benzidine, and coal tar derivatives. Diabetes mellitus, especially in women, is an important risk factor for the development of carcinoma of the pancreas, the incidence being two times higher in diabetics than in the rest of the population.

ISLET CELL TUMORS

ALPHA CELL TUMORS (GLUCAGONOMAS)

Glucagon-secreting tumors of the pancreatic islets (glucagonomas) are rare and have been encountered mainly in perimenopausal and postmenopausal women. **These tumors are associated with a syndrome consisting of mild diabetes, a necrotizing, migratory, erythematous rash of the lower body, and anemia.** Late diagnosis, together with a possibly increased propensity for malignant behavior of alpha cell tumors, may serve to explain why more than half of the 40-plus cases reported have been malignant and have metastasized to regional lymph nodes and liver. In patients with alpha cell tumors, plasma glucagon levels are elevated, up to 30 times above normal. In addition to the characteristic hyperglycemia, fasting plasma

amino acid levels are decreased to levels as low as 20% of normal.

BETA CELL TUMORS (INSULINOMAS)

Beta cell tumors are the most common of the islet cell neoplasms. The functional variant releases sufficient insulin to induce severe hypoglycemia (<40 mg/dl) and a syndrome of sweating, nervousness, and hunger, which may progress to confusion, lethargy, and coma. Most tumors produce only a mild hypoglycemia, and in some the tumor is not functional, which may delay the diagnosis. Neoplastic beta cells, unlike their normal counterparts, are not regulated by the blood glucose level and continue to secrete insulin autonomously, even when the level of glucose is very low. **Most beta cell tumors are benign single lesions in the body or tail of the pancreas;** some are as small as 1 mm in diameter. Only 5% demonstrate malignant behavior and in the majority surgical enucleation is accompanied by a rapid disappearance of symptoms. Histologically, the insulinoma cells usually resemble normal beta cells (Fig. 15-8A). The diagnosis is established by the demonstration of high levels of insulin in the blood and in the tumor cells (Fig. 15-8B). Electron microscopy of the tumor usually shows the pleomorphic, paracrystalline cores, typical of insulin stored in normal beta cells, surrounded by a clear halo.

DELTA CELL TUMORS (SOMATOSTATINOMAS)

This rare tumor causes a syndrome consisting of mild diabetes mellitus, gallstones, steatorrhea, indigestion, and hypochlorhydria. These conditions result from the inhibitory actions of somatostatin on other cells of the pancreatic islets and on endocrine cells of the gastrointestinal tract that secrete insulin, cholecystokinin, glucagon, and gastrin. Thus, the levels of insulin and glucagon in blood are decreased. In addition to producing somatostatin, some delta cell tumors also secrete calcitonin or adrenocorticotropic hormone (ACTH). The tumor is usually solitary and slow-growing, and in about one-half of the cases it exhibits malignant behavior with hepatic metastases.

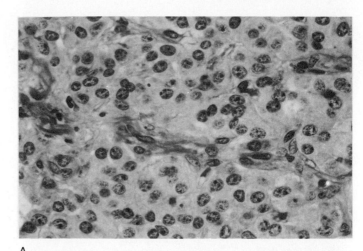

A

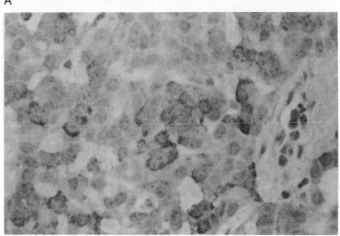

B

Figure 15-8. A functional insulinoma. (*A*) Nests of tumor cells resembling normal islet cells are surrounded by numerous capillaries. (*B*) The cytoplasm of the tumor cells stain with insulin antibody as demonstrated by the immunoperoxidase technique.

D_1 TUMORS (VIPOMAS)

D_1 tumors consist of islet cells that synthesize and secrete vasoactive intestinal polypeptide (VIP). **They give rise to the Verner-Morrison syndrome, which is characterized by explosive and profuse watery diarrhea, accompanied by hypokalemia and hypochlorhydria.** Severe dehydration and debility are frequent complications, which, together with the intractable diarrhea, has led to the term "pancreatic cholera." These profound effects are due to the excessive activation of adenyl cyclase in the mucosal cells of the small intestine by VIP. In turn, high levels of cyclic adenosine monophosphate (cAMP) drive the active secretion of intracellular electrolytes, including potassium and water. D_1 tumors are usually solitary and benign, and there are few reports of malignant behavior.

PANCREATIC GASTRINOMAS (ULCEROGENIC ISLET CELL TUMORS)

Pancreatic gastrinoma is an islet cell tumor consisting of so-called G-cells that synthesize and secrete gastrin, a potent hormonal stimulus for the secretion of gastric acid. The location of this tumor in the pancreas is curious, because **gastrin-containing cells have not been**

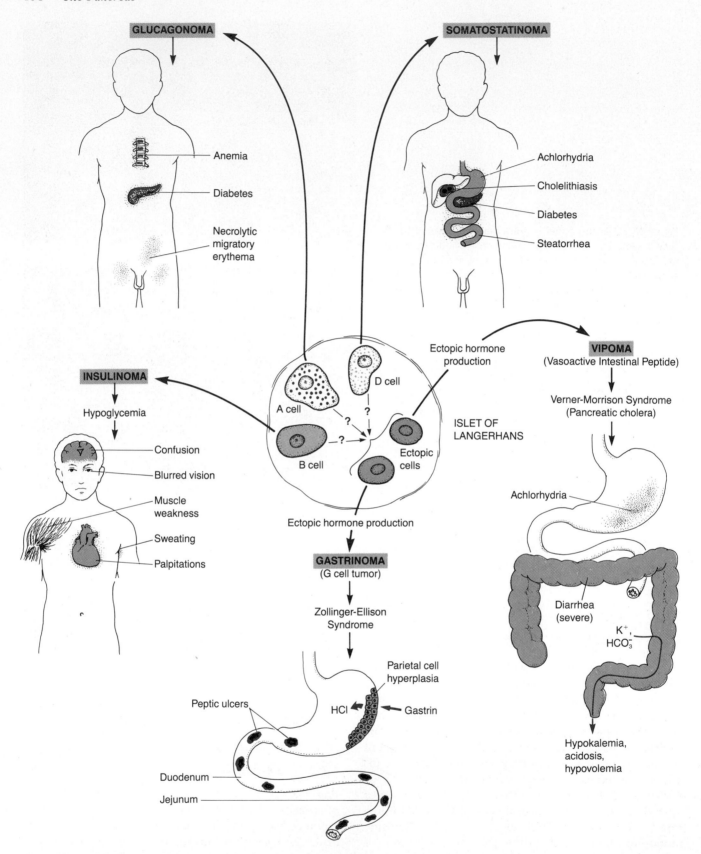

GLUCAGONOMA

- Anemia
- Diabetes
- Necrolytic migratory erythema

SOMATOSTATINOMA

- Achlorhydria
- Cholelithiasis
- Diabetes
- Steatorrhea

INSULINOMA

Hypoglycemia

- Confusion
- Blurred vision
- Muscle weakness
- Sweating
- Palpitations

A cell

D cell

B cell

Ectopic cells

ISLET OF LANGERHANS

Ectopic hormone production

Ectopic hormone production

VIPOMA
(Vasoactive Intestinal Peptide)

Verner-Morrison Syndrome
(Pancreatic cholera)

Achlorhydria

Diarrhea (severe)

K^+, HCO_3^-

Hypokalemia, acidosis, hypovolemia

GASTRINOMA
(G cell tumor)

Zollinger-Ellison Syndrome

Parietal cell hyperplasia

HCl ← Gastrin

Peptic ulcers

Duodenum

Jejunum

Figure 15-9. Syndromes associated with islet cell tumors of the pancreas.

demonstrated in normal islets. The tumor is thought to arise from multipotent endocrine stem cells that have undergone inappropriate differentiation to form gastrin-secreting islet cells (G-cells) in the endocrine pancreas. This tumor was incriminated some 30 years ago as the cause of **intractable gastric hypersecretion and severe peptic ulceration of the duodenum and jejunum, the so-called Zollinger-Ellison syndrome.**

Among islet cell tumors, pancreatic gastrinomas are second in frequency only to insulinomas. Malignant gastrinomas are more common than the benign variant, and multiple adenomas are more frequent than single ones. Metastases to regional lymph nodes and liver are often functional. The syndromes and complications of the major types of islet cell tumors are summarized in Figure 15-9.

16

THE KIDNEY

BENJAMIN H. SPARGO AND JAMES R. TAYLOR

CLINICAL SYNDROMES IN RENAL DISEASE

Traditionally, kidney diseases have been divided into four morphologic components: glomerular, tubular, interstitial and vascular. However, most disease processes will result in changes in more than one component. For example, the nephrotic syndrome, which is characterized by the loss of large amounts of protein in the urine, is almost invariably the result of a glomerular disease. The tubules, interstitium and blood vessels are often entirely normal morphologically, at least early on in the course of the disease. Ultimately, damage in one of the these components results in changes in the others. With progression to advanced disease it may become impossible to ascertain which component was initially involved. Thus, so-called end stage renal disease is the sequel to a broad spectrum of chronic renal diseases. Because diseases involving different components of the kidney have different clinical presentations, several major syndromes have been described.

The **nephrotic syndrome** is characterized by heavy proteinuria, at a rate of 3.5 g or more of protein lost per 24 hours. These patients usually display a low serum albumin level, edema and hypercholesterolemia.

The **nephritic syndrome** is characterized invariably by microscopic hematuria and often by gross blood in the urine. Variable degrees of proteinuria, a decreased glomerular filtration rate, and oliguria are usual. Salt and fluid retention often result in edema and hypertension. A clinicopathologic entity called **rapidly progressive glomerulonephritis** is a severe form of the nephritic syndrome, in which a rapid and progressive decline in renal function is observed clinically. Oliguria is usually severe. Histologically, glomerular crescents are usually seen.

Acute renal failure is characterized by oliguria (a 24-hour urine volume less than 400 ml) and a rapid onset of azotemia, without substantial proteinuria. The cause may be an inadequate perfusion of the kidneys (e.g., prerenal azotemia), intra-renal parenchymal disease, (e.g., acute tubular necrosis, interstitial nephritis), or a postrenal obstruction of the urinary tract. **Chronic renal failure,** which can be the end stage of a number of renal diseases, is characterized by prolonged symptoms and uremia.

Chronic interstitial nephritis is a term used to describe tubular atrophy and renal scarring in association with an inflammatory infiltrate. In patients with this disease, impaired tubular function results in an inability to concentrate the urine, obligatory sodium wasting and reduced acid secretion. A number of disorders, including repeated chronic infections (chronic pyelo-

nephritis), chronic reflux of urine, and chronic exposure to certain drugs (analgesic nephropathy), can lead to this condition.

Hypertension, if longstanding, results in renal parenchymal destruction ("benign" nephrosclerosis and "malignant" nephrosclerosis). Hypertension can also be secondary to acute and chronic renal diseases.

CYSTIC DISEASE OF THE KIDNEY

CYSTIC RENAL DYSPLASIA

Cystic renal dysplasia is defined as an abnormality of differentiation in the kidney, or a part of the kidney, that results in the persistence of abnormal structures, such as cartilage and undifferentiated mesenchyme. This sporadic lesion, which does not exhibit a familial tendency, is usually unilateral, but on occasion is bilateral. **Renal dysplasia is the most common cystic disorder in children and is the most frequent cause of an abdominal mass in newborn infants.**

Grossly, a dysplastic kidney reveals a disorderly mass of cysts that vary in size from microscopic to several centimeters in diameter. Dysplasia is recognized histologically by focally dilated ducts that are lined by a cuboidal or columnar epithelium. These are surrounded by mantles of undifferentiated mesenchyme, which sometimes contain smooth muscle and islands of hyaline cartilage.

POLYCYSTIC KIDNEY DISEASE

ADULT POLYCYSTIC DISEASE

Adult polycystic disease, an important cause of renal failure, is responsible for 8% to 10% of all end-stage kidney disease. It is usually inherited as an autosomal dominant trait, although there is a significant incidence of spontaneous mutation. Patients typically present with symptoms by the fourth decade. These include a sense of heaviness in the loins, the presence of bilateral masses and the passage of blood clots in the urine. Azotemia (elevated blood urea nitrogen) progresses to uremia (clinical renal failure) over a period of several years. Involvement is nearly always bilateral.

Grossly, the kidneys in adult polycystic disease are markedly enlarged bilaterally; each kidney may weigh as much as 4500 grams (Fig. 16-1). The external contour of the kidney is distorted by numerous cysts, which may be as large as 5 cm in diameter. These are usually filled with a clear to straw-yellow fluid, al-

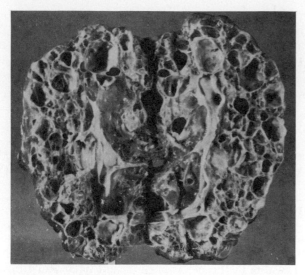

Figure 16-1. Adult polycystic disease. The kidney is strikingly enlarged and the parenchyma almost entirely replaced by cysts of varying size.

though occasionally there is hemorrhage into a cyst. Microscopically, the cysts are lined, for the most part, by a nondescript cuboidal and columnar epithelium. As the cysts progressively expand, they exert pressure on the normal areas, a process which leads to increasing loss of renal parenchyma.

About one third of patients with adult polycystic disease also have hepatic cysts lined by biliary epithelium. Cysts are also seen occasionally in the spleen and pancreas. Fifteen percent of patients have an associated cerebral aneurysm. Subarachnoid hemorrhage is the cause of death in many of these patients.

INFANTILE POLYCYSTIC DISEASE

Infantile polycystic disease is rare, compared to the adult variety. It is found primarily in infants and small children, although exceptional cases present in adults. Inheritance in most cases appears to be autosomal recessive. Two clinical presentations are seen in this condition; the more frequent is in the newborn, who suffers from congenitally enlarged, spongy kidneys and renal insufficiency. Less frequently, older children present with enlarged kidneys that have small cysts, tubular atrophy and interstitial fibrosis. The involvement is invariably bilateral. There are usually associated liver changes, termed *congenital hepatic fibrosis,* which are characterized by enlargement of portal areas, an increase in connective tissue and a proliferation of bile ducts. Most infants with polycystic disease die in the perinatal period, often because the large kidneys compromise expansion of the lungs.

In contrast to adult polycystic disease, the external surface in the infantile disorder is smooth. The kidneys are often so large that the delivery of the infant is impeded. The fusiform cysts are dilatations of cortical and medullary collecting ducts that have a striking radial arrangement. Interstitial fibrosis and tubular atrophy are common, particularly in children who present at an older age.

SIMPLE RENAL CYSTS

Simple renal cysts are very common acquired lesions, found in about half of people over the age of 50 years. They are usually incidental findings and rarely produce clinical symptoms, unless they are very large. These cysts, which may be solitary or multiple, are found in the outer cortex, bulging the capsule, or in the medulla. Microscopically, they are lined by a nondescript flat epithelium. Although the cysts are entirely benign, they may be confused clinically with renal cell carcinoma.

NONINFLAMMATORY LESIONS ASSOCIATED WITH THE NEPHROTIC SYNDROME

EPITHELIAL CELL DISEASE, (MINIMAL CHANGE DISEASE, LIPOID NEPHROSIS)

Epithelial cell disease is predominantly a disorder of children, in whom it is the major cause of the nephrotic syndrome. However, the disorder also occurs in adults with significant frequency (18% of adults with the nephrotic syndrome). Most patients are boys who present initially below the age of 6 years. Although neither the cause nor the pathogenesis of epithelial cell disease is known, there is a significant association between an allergic history and the onset of the nephrotic syndrome, which sometimes follows infection or exposure to allergens.

Most adults and children with epithelial cell disease show complete remission of proteinuria within 8 weeks of initiation of corticosteroid therapy. However, after the withdrawal of corticosteroids about half of the patients suffer intermittent relapses for up to 10 years. Each relapse is responsive to corticosteroid therapy, and **there is no tendency to progress into chronic renal failure.** A subgroup of patients shows only partial remission with corticosteroid therapy and continues to lose protein in the urine, the degree of proteinuria frequently depending on the dosage of steroids. A yet smaller group is totally resistant to corticosteroid therapy. Finally, a small group of patients achieves complete remission without any therapy. A fatal outcome or progression to renal failure is now exceptional.

By light microscopy **the glomeruli in minimal change (epithelial cell) disease appear entirely normal.** In actuality, however, there is often some irregular prominence of epithelial cells, and minor degrees of mesangial enlargement are common.

The lowered oncotic pressure of the plasma leads to increased lipoprotein secretion by the liver and a consequent hyperlipemia. The presence of lipid in the proximal tubular cells and in the urine reflects the loss of lipoproteins through the glomeruli and is responsible for the term *lipoid nephrosis,* which was used previously for this condition.

Characteristically, **electron microscopic examination reveals total effacement of epithelial cell foot processes, the basement membrane being covered by sheets of cytoplasm** (Fig. 16-2). No electron dense deposits are seen (Fig. 16-3). **Since the changes are completely reversible during remission, the diagnosis of epithelial cell disease can only be confirmed when there is significant proteinuria.**

Immunofluorescence studies for antibodies or complement in epithelial cell disease are negative, but weak mesangial reactions for IgM and the C3 component of complement are occasionally seen. This is probably a manifestation of increased mesangial uptake of macro-

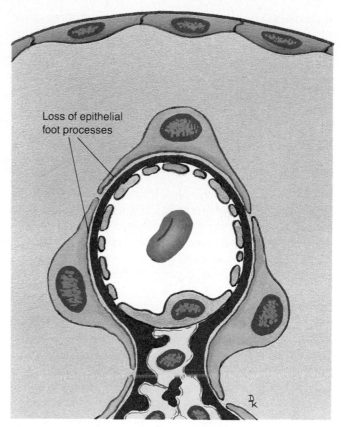

Figure 16-2. Epithelial cell disease. This condition is characterized predominantly by epithelial cell changes, particularly the effacement of the foot processes. All other glomerular structures appear intact.

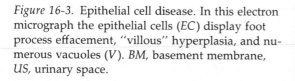

Figure 16-3. Epithelial cell disease. In this electron micrograph the epithelial cells (*EC*) display foot process effacement, "villous" hyperplasia, and numerous vacuoles (*V*). *BM*, basement membrane, *US*, urinary space.

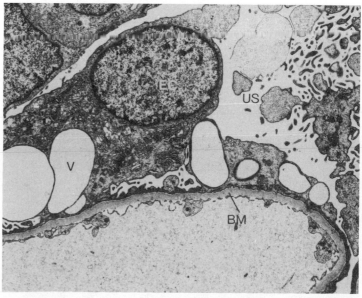

molecules, rather than a localization of immune complexes. The localized deposition of IgM and C3 in glomerular tufts is important, because it may represent the first indication of a focal segmental sclerosing lesion, before it is evident by light microscopy.

FOCAL SEGMENTAL GLOMERULOSCLEROSIS

Focal segmental glomerulosclerosis accounts for 10% of the nephrotic syndrome in children and 10% to 20% in adults, with a slight male predominance. This morphologic pattern is seen in many types of glomerular disease; therefore, it is questionable whether it is a distinct entity. The pathogenesis of this morphologic lesion is obscure.

Most patients with the diagnosis of focal segmental glomerulosclerosis present with the insidious onset of the nephrotic syndrome and a nonselective proteinuria. Many of these patients are hypertensive; microscopic hematuria is also frequent. Corticosteroids are rarely of benefit in adults with an initial biopsy diagnosis of focal segmental glomerulosclerosis, and their effect in children is variable. Most patients suffer a progressive decline in renal function for a period of up to 10 years, although a few, often those with a more severe degree of proteinuria at presentation, progress to end-stage renal failure in fewer than 3 years.

By light microscopy varying numbers of glomeruli show segmental areas of capillary loop collapse (Fig. 16-4) and adjacent synechial adhesions to Bowman's capsule. Lipid-containing foam cells are located in the mesangial area of involved glomeruli. The frequent accumulation of a PAS- positive material in the affected areas produces the lesion referred to as *hyalinosis.* Un-involved glomeruli appear entirely normal, although on occasion a diffuse, global, mesangial hypercellularity is superimposed on all of the glomeruli. By electron microscopy diffuse effacement of the epithelial cell foot processes is identical to the lesion of minimal change nephropathy. In addition, folding and thickening of the basement membrane (Fig. 16-5) and capillary collapse are present in sclerotic glomeruli. Deposits of immune complexes are not found.

Immunofluorescence studies show trapping of IgM or C3 in the segmental areas of sclerosis and hyalinosis. IgG, C4, and Clq are less frequently found. These segmental reactions may precede light microscopic evidence of damage. This trapping of material is nonspecific and presumably is not related to the pathogenetic mechanisms of the disease.

MEMBRANOUS NEPHROPATHY

Membranous nephropathy is the most frequent cause of the nephrotic syndrome in adults (30% of the cases), and is thought to be caused by the deposition of immune complexes.

Most patients have the primary, idiopathic form of membranous nephropathy. However, a number of associated conditions predispose to the development of "secondary" membranous nephropathy. In adults, **one of the most frequent associations is with epithelial neoplasms, which have been found in up to 10% of patients.** Certain drugs, such as gold and penicillamine (used in the treatment of rheumatoid arthritis), can result in the lesion. **Membranous nephropathy has been seen in association with various systemic infections, most frequently hepatitis B. Up to 10% of patients with systemic lupus erythematosus present with a membranous lesion.**

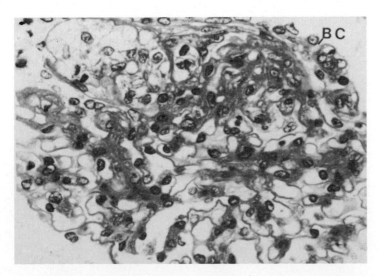

Figure 16-4. Focal segmental glomerulonephritis. Light microscopy shows areas of collapse of the capillary loops with loss of vascular lumina and adjacent adhesions to Bowman's capsule (*BC*).

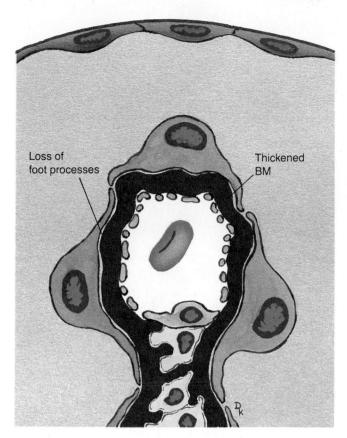

Figure 16-5. Focal segmental glomerulosclerosis. This disorder typically displays epithelial cell change and thickening of the basement membrane. The epithelial cells show effacement of the foot processes and distension of the cytoplasm. The basement membrane is thickened and folded. The glomeruli located deep within the cortex are the earliest to demonstrate these pathognomonic changes, at a time when the other glomeruli may show only the minimal change described in Figure 16-2.

By light microscopy the glomeruli are slightly enlarged, yet normocellular (Fig. 16-6). Depending on the length of time the patient has had the disease, the capillary walls are normal or thickened. In the early stages of the disease silver stains reveal multiple projections, or "spikes", of argyrophilic material on the epithelial surface of the basement membrane. As the disease progresses, there is encroachment on the capillary lumina and eventually glomerular obsolescence. This lesion is classified as noninflammatory because there is no cellular proliferation. However, in advanced disease irregular capillary collapse may result in the erroneous impression of mesangial hypercellularity. Late in the course of the disease, with advanced stages of glomerular sclerosis, this lesion cannot be distinguished from other forms of chronic glomerulonephritis. Tubular loss and focal prominence of the interstitial tissue parallel the degree of glomerular sclerosis.

In the early phase of the disease (Stage I), small granular subepithelial deposits (Fig. 16-7) are seen along the basement membrane. Intracapillary mesangial and subendothelial deposits are not present. Stage II is characterized by protrusion of "spikes" of basement membrane between deposits of electron-dense material (Fig. 16-8). By Stage III, these deposits are incorporated into the widening basement membrane. In Stage IV the basement membrane is markedly distorted, and mobilization of the deposits has imparted a moth-eaten appearance to the membrane. With resolution of the lesion the basement membrane is reconstituted and assumes an essentially normal appearance, except for the increased thickness.

Immunofluorescence reveals peripheral granular staining for IgG and C3 in a membranous pattern. Mesangial deposits are not seen in the idiopathic variety of

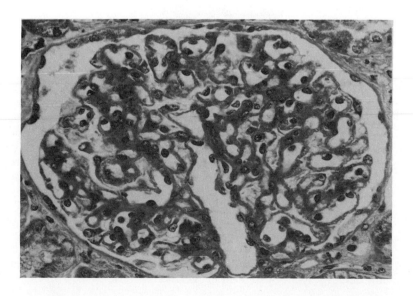

Figure 16-6. Membranous nephropathy, light micrograph. The glomerulus is slightly enlarged and shows slight diffuse thickening of the capillary walls. There is no hypercellularity.

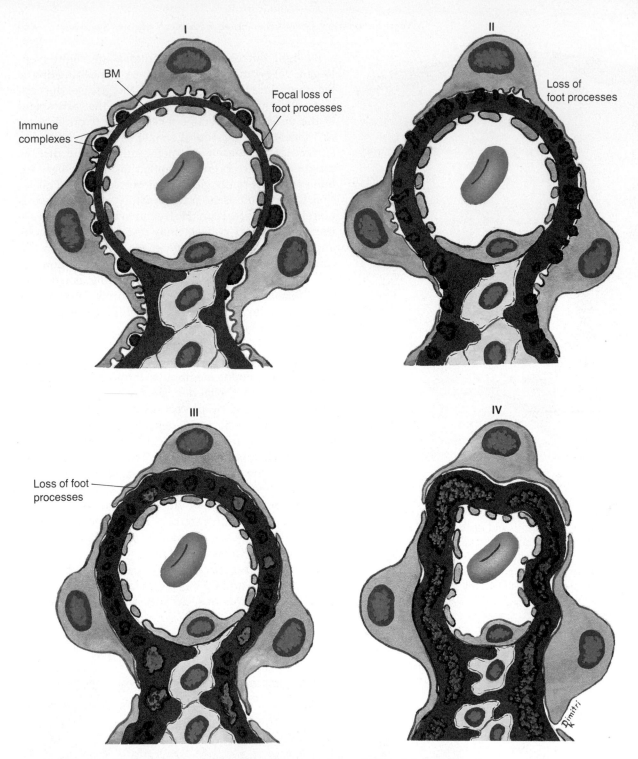

Figure 16-7. **Membranous nephropathy.** Membranous nephropathy is related to the extracapillary deposition of immune complexes and the accompanying changes in the basement membrane. Stage I exhibits marked, diffuse subepithelial deposits in both the peripheral capillaries and the stalk. The outer contour of the basement membrane remains smooth, and foot process effacement is focal. Stage II disease has a spike and dome pattern. The domes are the deposits that gradually extend into the basement membrane. Reactive spikes of newly formed basement membrane tent up the epithelial cells, the foot processes of which are extensively effaced. In Stage III disease newly formed basement membrane has sequestered intramembranous deposits. Variations in density of trapped deposits relate to light areas where the deposit has disappeared, leaving the spongy-appearing and thickened basement membrane. With Stage IV disease there is further loss of deposits and even greater widening of the now diffusely spongy basement membrane.

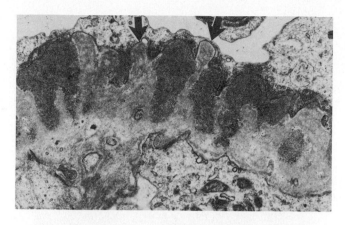

Figure 16-8. Diffuse membranous nephropathy of long duration. An electron micrograph shows deposits of electron-dense material between spikes (*arrows*) of widened glomerular basement membrane.

membranous nephropathy, but they are frequent in the membranous lesion of systemic lupus erythematosus.

The usual course in adults is chronic proteinuria and slow deterioration into renal failure within 10 to 15 years. Recent evidence suggests that corticosteroids are beneficial in patients with idiopathic membranous nephropathy who have begun treatment before there has been deterioration of renal function. Overall the prognosis is better in children, owing to the greater frequency of permanent remission.

DIABETIC GLOMERULOSCLEROSIS

Only the glomerular lesion of diabetes mellitus is discussed here. A more general discussion of diabetes is found in Chapter 22. The term *diabetic glomerulosclerosis* (Kimmelstiel-Wilson syndrome) embraces the glomerular changes seen in diabetes. These alterations are an expression of the diabetic microangiopathy that is seen in many systemic arterial small vessels and capillaries. As in the systemic vessels, glomerular sclerosis is caused by the progressive accumulation of basement membrane material, a deposit that results in an enlargement of the glomeruli. The pathogenesis of the lesion is controversial, but it appears to be related to the severity and duration of hyperglycemia.

The earliest detectable lesion of diabetic glomerulosclerosis is a diffuse widening of mesangial areas by the accumulation of a PAS-positive matrix. With progression the capillary basement membrane appears thicker and the mesangium becomes increasingly prominent (Fig. 16-9). The glomerulus becomes enlarged and may appear hypercellular. **Diffuse glomerulosclerosis,** the term that refers to this state of enlarged glomeruli with diffusely thickened basement membranes, may occur

alone or may be mixed with **nodular glomerulosclerosis.** In the latter condition the nodules in the glomeruli are rounded, homogeneous, eosinophilic masses that appear in centrilobular areas (Fig. 16-10). Insudative changes occur in both the adjacent arterioles and the glomerular tufts. The most prominent lesion is hyaline arteriolosclerosis (Fig. 16-10), which **in diabetics uniquely involves both the afferent and efferent arterioles.**

The thickening of the capillary wall is caused by a widening of the basement membrane, which may be many times its normal width. An accumulation of basement membrane-like stroma in the mesangium parallels the diffuse widening of the basement membrane, and may become nodular and acellular (Fig. 16-11). There are no deposits of immune complexes.

The proteinuria in diabetic glomerulosclerosis is initially mild and may remain so. Patients who have proteinuria in the nephrotic range (> 1g/24 hours) usually progress to renal failure within 6 years.

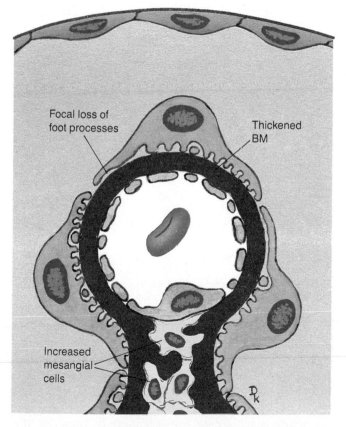

Figure 16-9. Diabetic glomerulosclerosis. The glomerular tuft is enlarged and displays a thickened basement membrane that retains a normal texture and density with smooth inner and outer contours. Focal effacement of the epithelial cell foot processes is common. An accumulation of basement membrane–like stroma in the mesangium parallels the diffuse widening of the basement membrane.

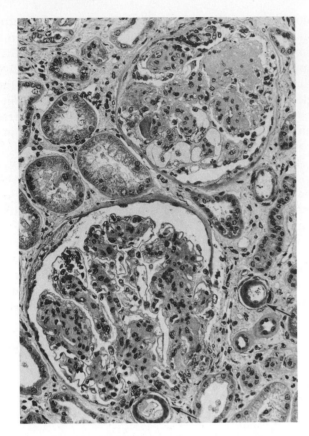

Figure 16-10. Diabetic glomerulosclerosis. A light micrograph shows a prominent increase in the mesangial matrix. Capillary dilatation and the presence of foam cells are conspicuous features. The arrows indicate "hyalinized" arterioles.

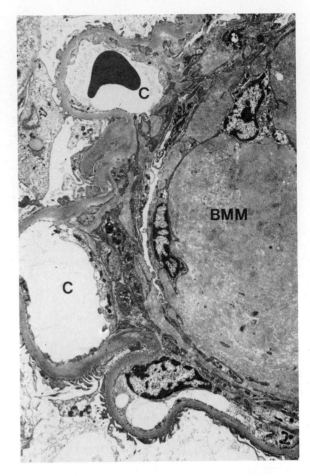

Figure 16-11. Advanced nodular glomerulosclerosis. An electron micrograph shows an aggregate of basement membrane material (*BMM*). The peripheral capillary (*C*) demonstrates diffuse basement membrane widening, but a normal texture.

AMYLOIDOSIS

Amyloidosis is actually a group of diseases, all of them characterized by the extracellular deposition of a proteinaceous material in a variety of tissues (see Chapter 23). The accumulation of this material results in the obliteration of tissue structure and disturbed function. Amyloid is conventionally defined as an eosinophilic, amorphous material by light microscopy that shows a fibrillar ultrastructure and a beta-pleated sheet configuration by x-ray diffraction analysis. By light microscopy, the most secure identification is made by the presence of a characteristic apple-green color in sections stained with Congo red and examined under polarized light.

Renal involvement is frequent in most systemic forms of amyloidosis. The glomeruli are most frequently affected, a situation which results in alterations in permeability and leads to proteinuria. This proteinuria is nonselective and in 60% of patients is severe enough to produce the nephrotic syndrome. Severe infiltration of the glomeruli and renal vasculature results in renal failure. Only glomerular amyloidosis is discussed here.

Amyloid deposition is initially mesangial, producing diffuse widening of axial areas (Fig. 16-12). However, it progressively spreads to obliterate capillary lumina (Fig. 16-13). With increasing deposition of amyloid, the glomeruli become enlarged and the hyaline mesangial pattern becomes nodular. Finally, the glomerular structure is obliterated, and the glomeruli appear as large hyaline balls.

Electron microscopy provides the most secure method for the identification of amyloid. It appears as

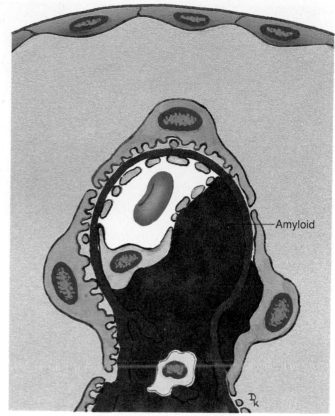

Figure 16-12. Amyloid nephropathy. This disorder is initially associated with the accumulation of characteristic fibrillar deposits in the mesangium. These inert masses, which are fibrillar by electron microscopy, extend along the inner surface of the basement membrane, frequently obstructing the capillary lumen. Focal extension of amyloid through the basement membrane may elevate the epithelial cell, in which case irregular spikes along the outer surface of the basement membrane are seen.

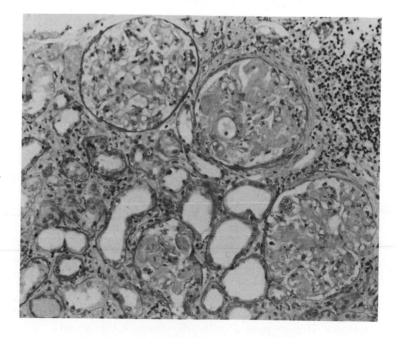

Figure 16-13. Amyloid nephrosis. A light micrograph shows glomeruli that contain irregular deposits of amyloid. There is cellular loss and considerable capillary obstruction.

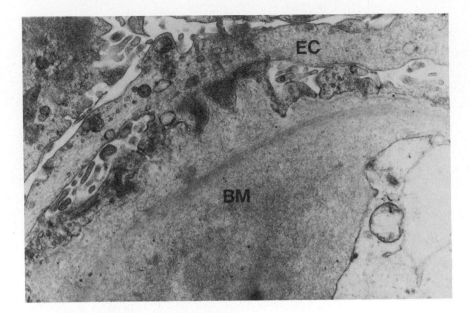

Figure 16-14. Amyloid nephrosis. An electron micrograph demonstrates amyloid fibrils that are deposited in and distort the basement membrane (*BM*). *EC*, epithelial cell.

fibrils composed of randomly arranged non-branching rods, measuring 8 to 10 nm in diameter. The fibrils are seen first in the mesangial areas (Fig. 16-12). The epithelial cell foot processes overlying the basement membrane are obliterated, and the epithelial cells are tented by the amyloid fibrils, which are often arranged perpendicularly to the basement membrane (Fig. 16-14). The severity of the epithelial cell disruption correlates with the degree of proteinuria.

INFLAMMATORY GLOMERULAR LESIONS

Inflammation of the glomeruli is termed glomerulonephritis and is a frequent cause of end-stage renal disease. Clinically, inflammatory lesions of the glomeruli are most frequently associated with the nephritic syndrome.

A number of distinct patterns of glomerular injury exist. Involvement of all or nearly all of the glomeruli is called **diffuse.** When only some of the glomeruli are affected the distribution is termed **focal.** The distribution within individual glomeruli can be identified as **global,** or **generalized,** when the entire glomerulus is involved, or **segmental** when it is not.

A proliferation of cells that results in a hypercellular appearance is the hallmark of an inflamed glomerulus. This increased cellularity may be due to an increase in mesangial cells, in which case the process is called mesangioproliferative. Proliferation of the endothelial cells occurs frequently and is nearly always associated with mesangial proliferation.

Severe glomerular inflammation leads to a proliferation of both the visceral and parietal epithelial cells, which results in the formation of **crescents.** In addition to the epithelial cells, circulating monocytes contribute to the cellularity of these crescents. Neutrophils are found in large numbers within the glomerular tuft in certain types of glomerulonephritis, particularly in children. In these circumstances the lesion is called an **exudative glomerulonephritis.**

Immune complexes are seen in mesangial, subendothelial, subepithelial and membranous (or epimembranous) locations. **Mesangial deposits** are found within the mesangial area, frequently separating the basement membrane from the mesangial cells. **Subendothelial deposits,** found between the endothelium and the inner aspect of the capillary basement membrane, frequently represent an extension of a mesangial deposit. A deposit between the epithelial cells and the outer aspect of the basement membrane is called **subepithelial,** a term commonly used for a deposit first seen at the junction of the outer surface of the basement membrane and the epithelial cell cytoplasm. In time this deposit works its way into the lamina densa. Mesangial and subendothelial deposits are called **intracapillary deposits** because they are seen inside the basement membrane.

PATHOGENETIC MECHANISMS

Four basic types of immunologic injury are recognized: (1) trapping of circulating immune complexes, (2) in situ immune complex formation, (3) activation of the alternate pathway of complement and (4) cell-mediated processes.

In *circulating immune complex nephritis* glomerular injury is caused by the trapping of circulating antigen-antibody complexes. The aggregates of immune complexes penetrate the glomerular basement membrane and are trapped in a subepithelial position. Their presence is confirmed electron microscopically by finding subepithelial "humps". With immunofluorescence a peripheral granular staining with antisera directed against IgG and C3 is noted.

Examples of immune complex nephritis induced by exogenous antigens include **bacterial antigens** in the glomerulonephritis associated with streptococcal infections and bacterial endocarditis, and **viral antigens** in glomerulonephritis induced by hepatitis B. **DNA** acts as an endogenous antigen in the pathogenesis of lupus nephritis. **Tumor-associated antigens** have been implicated in the development of some cases of glomerulonephritis.

The glomerulus may also be damaged by the binding of circulating antibody to an antigen that has already deposited in the glomerular basement membrane **(in situ immune complex formation).** The best-known example is Goodpasture's syndrome, in which the basement membrane acts as an endogenous antigen to which circulating antibasement membrane antibodies bind. Immunofluorescence shows a linear localization of IgG along the basement membrane. The combination of antigen with antibody results in the activation of complement, and a rapidly progressive glomerulonephritis usually results.

The **alternate complement pathway** is important in the pathogenesis of a lesion called **membranoproliferative glomerulonephritis.** In some forms of this disease, only complement C3 is found in the glomeruli by immunofluorescence, and immunoglobulins are absent. The alterante pathway for complement activation is also important in focal glomerulonephritis due to IgA depositon.

Once immune complexes have localized within a glomerulus, a number of secondary pathogenetic mechanisms appear to play a role in effecting immunologic injury. These include the complement-neutrophil system, monocytes and macrophages, and the coagulation system. The role of complement activation in the recruitment of polymorphonuclear leukocytes is well established, and neutrophils are conspicuous in many glomerular diseases. Monocytes and macrophages infiltrate the glomerulus in many forms of renal disease and contribute to the cellularity of the glomerular tufts and the surrounding crescents. Activated macrophages release a number of biologically active molecules that are probably important in tissue damage. Fibrin can usually be demonstrated in Bowman's space early in the formation of crescents and is probably partially responsible for subsequent epithelial cell proliferation and crescent formation. Finally, platelets may be activated by sensitized mast cells and basophils upon exposure to antigens or immune complexes.

ACUTE GLOMERULONEPHRITIS (POSTINFECTIOUS GLOMERULONEPHRITIS)

Although acute glomerulonephritis has been documented as a sequel to a variety of infectious agents—such as staphylococci, pneumococci, spirochetes, and viruses—the most frequent association is with **group A streptococci.** Although not seen as frequently now as in the past, this disorder still represents one of the most common renal diseases in childhood. The exact mechanism by which the infection brings about the characteristic proliferative changes is still not completely characterized. Only certain strains of group A streptococci are nephritogenic. The primary infections may be in either the pharynx or, especially in hot and humid environments, the skin. Because the organisms may not be recoverable at the time of the nephritis, the diagnosis depends on the serologic evidence of a rise in titers to streptococcal products. The disease most commonly affects children. The nephritic syndrome typically begins abruptly with oliguria, hematuria, facial edema, and hypertension. Usually there is a depression of serum C3 during the acute syndrome. This returns to normal within 1 to 2 weeks, as does the clinical condition of most patients. However, in a minority of patients an abnormal urinary sediment persists for years after the acute episode. Exacerbations of the disease may occur on reinfection with another nephritogenic organism.

By light microscopy, a diffuse enlargement and hypercellularity of the glomeruli is present if the biopsy is taken within the first 3 weeks of the onset of acute glomerulonephritis (Fig. 16-15). The hypercellularity is due to the proliferation of both endothelial and mesangial cells (Fig. 16-16), and to infiltration of neutrophils. The proliferation of mesangial cells results in an exaggeration of the normal lobular pattern. Tubulointerstitial damage and inflammation occur in parallel with the glomerular changes.

The characteristic ultrastructural features of acute postinfectious glomerulonephritis are the subepithelial "humps." These deposits are invariably accompanied by intracapillary, mesangial and subendothelial deposits, although the latter two may be much more difficult to find in the acute phase. The humps are variably sized, dome-shaped deposits, which are situated on the epithelial aspect of the basement membrane (Figs. 16-16 and 16-17). The deposits result in peripheral granular reaction for IgG and C3 by immunofluorescence.

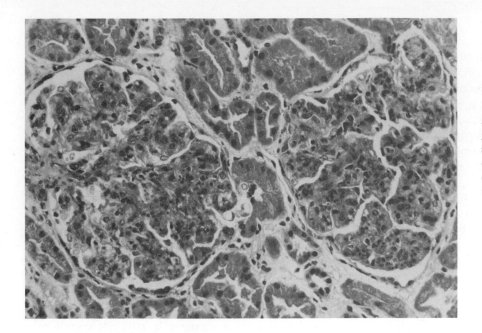

Figure 16-15. Acute poststreptococcal glomerulonephritis. A light micrograph shows enlarged glomerular tufts and obstructed capillaries. Mesangial and endothelial cells are proliferated. Scattered neutrophils are present.

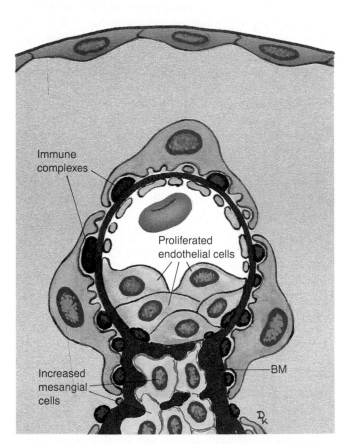

Immune complexes

Proliferated endothelial cells

Increased mesangial cells

BM

Figure 16-16. Postinfectious glomerulonephritis. Trapping of immune complexes in a subepithelial pattern ("lumpy-bumpy") is seen, together with focal effacement of foot processes. Less prominent subendothelial immune complexes are associated with endothelial cell proliferation and are related to increased capillary permeability and narrowing of the lumen. Frequently, proliferation of mesangial cells and a thickened mesangial basement membrane result in widening of the stalk and conspicuous trapping of immune complexes.

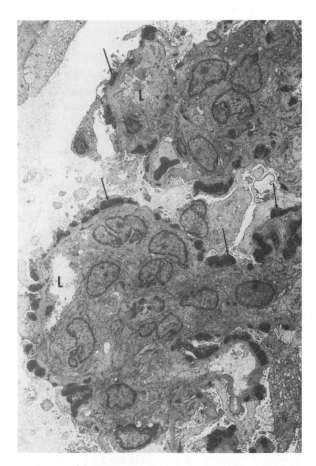

Figure 16-17. Postinfectious glomerulonephritis. An electron micrograph demonstrates numerous subepithelial humps (*arrows*). The capillary lumina (*L*) are markedly narrowed.

The typical morphologic features of acute inflammation usually have resolved by 8 weeks from the onset of the nephritis. Although some degree of caution remains with respect to the long-term prognosis of renal function, most data suggest that complete recovery, particularly in children, is the rule. Generally, those patients who recover completely will have done so both clinically and histologically by 3 years from onset. A few patients present with an unusually severe lesion that displays many crescents and progresses quickly to renal failure, a condition termed **rapidly progressive glomerulonephritis.**

CRESCENTIC GLOMERULONEPHRITIS

Crescentic glomerulonephritis is an ominous morphologic pattern (Fig. 16-18) in which the majority of glomeruli are surrounded by an accumulation of cells in Bowman's space. The crescent is an expression of fulminant glomerular damage and always leaves severe residual scarring. Crescentic glomerulonephritis is associated with a number of underlying conditions and should always prompt a search for other diagnostic features that allow a sub-classification (Table 16-l).

Clinically, most patients with a substantial number of crescents suffer a rapid and progressive decline in renal function. Irreversible renal failure with severe oliguria or anuria occurs within weeks unless adequate therapy is administered.

The escape of fibrin into Bowman's space seems to be important for the formation of glomerular crescents. **Fibrin can invariably be demonstrated by immunofluorescence in active crescentic glomerulonephritis.** Recent evidence suggests that macrophages contribute to the cellularity of young "cellular" crescents at least as much as epithelial cells.

Crescents range from small groups of cells filling only a segment of Bowman's space (Fig. 16-19) to circumferential masses of cells that completely surround the glomerulus. They evolve from a cellular to a fibrocellular form; eventually they scar and form the foundation of a fibrous crescent. Later, segmental crescents become incorporated in Bowman's capsule as a segmental fibrous collar, or in the glomerulus as a segmental glomerular scar. Circumferential crescents result in globally scarred glomeruli. Assignment into one of the specific entities listed in Table 16-1 requires careful examination of the glomerular lesions in crescentic glomerulonephritis.

Idiopathic crescentic glomerulonephritis is essentially a diagnosis of exclusion that is made when there

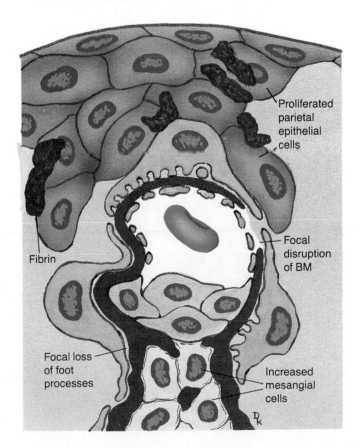

Figure 16-18. Crescentic (rapidly progressive) glomerulonephritis. This severe variety of glomerulonephritis shows not only changes in the glomerular tuft but also conspicuous proliferation of parietal epithelial cells, the latter forming the "crescent." Fibrin is often prominent between the proliferating epithelial cells. White blood cells may also be present in active cellular crescents. Focal disruption of the peripheral capillary basement membrane may result in red blood cells in Bowman's space. Crescentic glomerulonephritis is not a specific diagnostic entity, but describes the morphologic counterpart of a maximally active process, as, for example, crescentic poststreptococcal, crescentic IgA, and crescentic lupus glomerulonephritis.

Table 16-1   Differential Diagnosis of Crescentic Glomerulonephritis

Condition	Light Microscopy	Electron Microscopy	Immunofluorescence
Idiopathic crescentic glomerulonephritis	Crescents and tuft proliferation	Negative	Negative
Anti-glomerular basement membrane disease	Crescents and segmental tuft proliferation	Negative	Linear IgG and C3
Poststreptococcal glomerulonephritis	Crescents, tuft proliferation, exudative changes	Intracapillary deposits, subepithelial "humps"	Peripheral, granular IgG and C3
Membranoproliferative glomerulonephritis	Crescents, lobular distortion of the tuft, mesangial interpositioning	Subendothelial deposits, mesangial interpositioning	Peripheral, granular C3, properdin
IgA nephropathy/Henoch–Schönlein purpura	Crescents, tuft proliferation	Mesangial deposits	Mesangial IgA, with variable C3, IgG IgM
Systemic lupus erythematosus	Crescents, wire loops, hematoxylin bodies	Subendothelial and mesangial deposits, "fingerprinting" of deposits, peritubular deposits	"Full house" pattern of both mesangial and peripheral IgG, IgA, IgM, C3, C4, C1q
Systemic vasculitis	Crescents, focal arteritis	Negative	Negative

is no ultrastructural or immunohistochemical evidence of immune complex localization or vasculitis. Specific systemic diseases that can cause crescentic glomerulonephritis are streptococcal infections, membranoproliferative glomerulonephritis, IgA nephropathy, Henoch-Schonlein purpura, systemic small vessel arteritis, and systemic lupus erythematosus.

Anti-glomerular basement membrane disease is a rare condition in which the patient develops an antibody directed against his own glomerular basememt membrane. This immune attack results in a rapidly progressive, crescentic glomerulonephritis. Eighty percent of these patients are male, with an average age of 29 years at the onset of disease. Many simultaneously suffer from pulmonary hemorrhages and recurrent hemoptysis—sometimes severe enough to be life threatening—because of a cross reactivity of the antibodies with the alveolar basement membranes. When both the lungs and kidneys are involved, the eponym *Goodpasture's syndrome* is used. Anti-glomerular basement membrane antibody is revealed by the presence of a linear binding of IgG and C3 with immunofluorescence and by the identification of circulating anti-basement membrane antibodies.

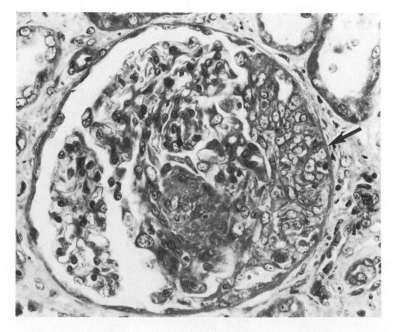

Figure 16-19. Crescentic glomerulonephritis. A light micrograph shows prominent sheets of proliferating epithelial cells (*arrow*) that fill much of Bowman's space.

MEMBRANOPROLIFERATIVE LESIONS

Membranoproliferative lesions are inflammatory lesions whose name comes from the **characteristic combination of basement membrane thickening and endothelial and mesangial cell proliferation.** In the initial description, children and young adults presented with either the nephrotic or nephritic syndrome and persistently low levels of the third component of complement (C3). The patients did not have poststreptococcal glomerulonephritis or other systemic inflammatory conditions that could account for the hypocomplementemia. The vast majority of these patients progressed to end-state renal failure. It is now clear that not all patients with this group of diseases have low complement levels, and this is no longer a required feature for diagnosis. Furthermore, although the light microscopic appearance of the renal lesion in the majority of these patients is very similar, there are sufficient distinctions, both ultrastructurally and immunologically, to warrant the division of the disease into two predominant groups. These are called membranoproliferative type I and type II.

Type I membranoproliferative glomerulonephritis (also called membranoproliferative glomerulonephritis with subendothelial deposits) (Fig. 16-20) has been associated with a number of conditions, including, most importantly, hepatitis B antigenemia, infection of ventriculoatrial shunts (for the treatment of hydrocephalus), bacterial endocarditis, streptococcal infections and cancer. **However, the great majority of cases are idiopathic.** By light microscopy, marked centrilobular, mesangial cell proliferation in diffusely enlarged glomeruli, produces a lobular distortion to the glomeruli (Fig. 16-21). Silver stains characteristically show a double contour to the peripheral basement membrane in this disease. This feature, which has been erroneously described previously as "splitting" of the basement membrane, is a consequence of the marked inflammatory expansion of the mesangial area. As a result, the cytoplasm and matrix of the mesangium are forced peripherally into the capillary loops and insinuate themselves between the endothelial cells and the basement membrane. This process is called **mesangial interpositioning** and is characteristic of, but not limited to, the membranoproliferative lesions. Typically, there is a continuous layer of mesangial cytoplasm around the entire capillary. Subendothelial and mesan-

Figure 16-20. Membranoproliferative glomerulonephritis, type I. In this disease the glomeruli are enlarged. Hypercellular tufts and narrowing or obstruction of the capillary lumen are seen. Large subendothelial deposits of immune complexes extend along the inner border of the basement membrane. The mesangial cells proliferate and migrate peripherally into the capillary. Basement membrane material accumulates in a linear fashion parallel to the basement membrane in a subendothelial position. The interposition of mesangial cells and basement membrane between the endothelial cells and the original basement membrane creates a double-contour effect. The accumulation of mesangial cells and stroma in the tufts narrows the capillary lumen. The stalk is also widened by the proliferation of mesangial cells and the accumulation of basement membrane stroma. The entire process leads progressively to lobulation of the glomerulus, consolidation of the lobules, and eventually a "cannonball" effect. Note the proliferation of endothelial cells and focal effacement of foot processes.

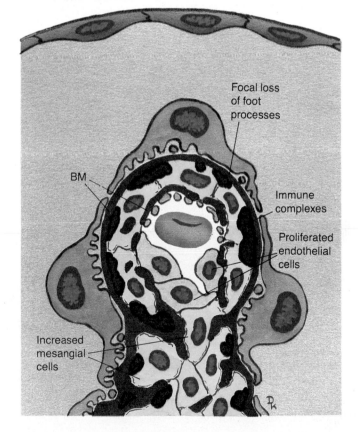

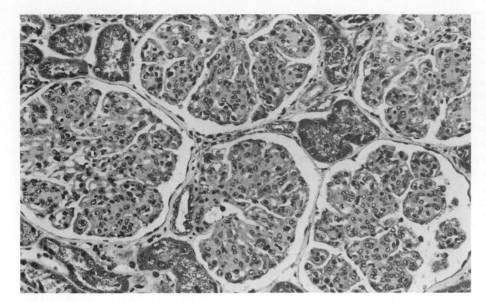

Figure 16-21. Membranoproliferative glomerulonephritis, type I. A light micrograph shows glomerular lobulation and diffuse mesangial proliferation. Peripheral extension of mesangial matrix material obstructs the lumina and widens the capillary walls.

gial electron-dense deposits are present in type I disease (see Fig. 16-20). Subepithelial humps may also be seen. Immunoglobulins and complement are demonstrated in the majority of cases by immunofluorescence.

Another term for **type II membranoproliferative glomerulonephritis** is **dense deposit disease.** The clinical presentation and course are similar to type I membranoproliferative glomerulonephritis. Nearly all patients have a circulating immunoglobulin of the IgG class (C3 nephritis factor) that causes continued activation of the alternative complement pathway by altering the delicate balance between activator and inactivator enzymes.

The light microscopic appearance of type II disease is identical to that of type I, although the degree of cellularity may be more variable between glomeruli. The pathognomonic feature of this form of the disease is the characteristic ribbonlike zone of increased density located centrally within the thickened basement membrane (Fig. 16-22). In contrast to type I disease, immunofluorescence shows only weak, discontinuous reactions for C3 along the basement membrane. Immunoglobulins are not found.

FOCAL GLOMERULONEPHRITIS

Focal glomerulonephritis is a morphologic term that is used when only some of the glomeruli are involved. In conditions which produce this lesion, the inflammation is frequently also limited to segmental

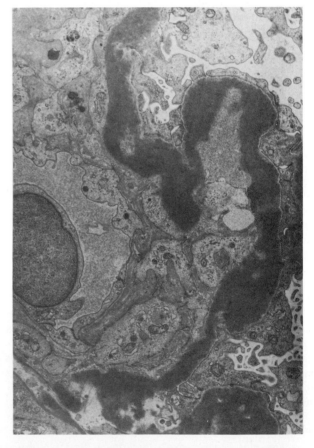

Figure 16-22. Membranoproliferative glomerulonephritis, type II (dense deposit disease). An electron micrograph demonstrates thickening of the basement membrane and increased density of the lamina densa.

Table 16-2 Differential Diagnosis of Focal Glomerulonephritis

Condition	Light Microscopy	Electron Microscopy	Immuno-fluorescence	Other
Idiopathic focal glomerulonephritis	Focal glomerulonephritis, often segmental	Negative	Negative	—
IgA nephropathy	Mesangial cell proliferation	Mesangial deposits	Mesangial IgA, C3	Intermittent hematuria
Henoch–Schönlein glomerulonephritis	Mesangial cell proliferation, frequently crescentic	Mesangial deposits	Mesangial IgA, C3	Purpura, arthritis, abdominal pain
Anti-glomerular basement membrane disease	Frequently segmental, often necrotizing	Negative	Linear IgG and C3	± pulmonary hemorrhage
Lupus glomerulonephritis	Mesangial and endothelial proliferation	Various deposits, "fingerprinting" of deposits, tubulo-vesicular bodies	"Full house" pattern of immune complex deposits	± systemic syndrome, anti-nuclear factor, etc.
Bacterial endocarditis	Mesangial and endothelial proliferation, segmental	Variable	Variable	Cardiac murmur, fever
Systemic vasculitis	Often crescentic, segmental necrosis, focal arteritis	Negative	Negative	Systemic symptoms

portions of the glomerular tufts. This disorder must be distinguished from the focal sclerosing lesions seen in focal segmental glomerulosclerosis. Focal glomerulonephritis may occur as an early or mild manifestation of a systemic disease that usually affects all glomeruli, or as a primary glomerulonephritis. Thus, as in crescentic glomerulonephritis, the light microscopic appearance of focal glomerulonephritis may be produced by a number of conditions (Table 16-2). The lesion is subclassified by immunofluorescence and electron microscopy (see Table 16-2).

IgA nephropathy (also known as **Berger's disease) is the most common type of adult primary glomerulonephritis in many parts of the world, accounting for over 20% of cases in France, Italy, Australia, Japan and Singapore.** In the United States the incidence is lower, ranging from 3% to 10%. IgA nephropathy is primarily a disease of young men, with a peak age of 15 to 30 years. The pathogenesis of this lesion is not understood. **Up to 20% of these patients develop end-stage renal failure.** Once diagnosed, the lesion does not spontaneously resolve and is unresponsive to therapy. IgA nephropathy (Fig. 16-23) is a mesangial proliferative lesion, meaning that mesangial cell proliferation is the sole or predominant abnormality in many of the cases. Frequently, hyaline material, representing mesangial deposits, can be seen, particularly in those patients destined to progress to renal failure, who exhibit segmental necrosis of the glomerular tufts, crescents and scarring. Ultrastructural examination reveals a variable amount of finely granular, electron dense

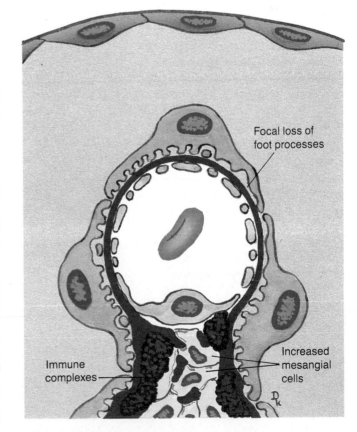

Focal loss of foot processes

Immune complexes

Increased mesangial cells

Figure 16-23. IgA nephropathy. Significant accumulation of IgA is seen in the stalk, most commonly between the mesangial cells and the basement membrane. The disease is associated with a variable inflammatory reaction.

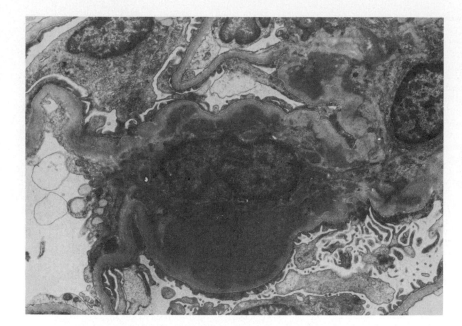

Figure 16-24. IgA nephropathy. An electron micrograph demonstrates prominent IgA deposits in the widened mesangial stalk.

deposits, located primarily in the mesangium (Fig. 16-24). Immunofluorescence microscopy, which is pivotal in the diagnosis of this entity, reliably shows a diffuse mesangial reaction with IgA, usually accompanied by IgG, IgM, and C3.

A close relationship exists between IgA nephropathy and the renal lesion of **Henoch-Schonlein (allergic purpura) nephritis.** The latter, however, usually presents with a more severe degree of inflammation.

RENAL DISEASES ASSOCIATED WITH SYSTEMIC DISORDERS

SYSTEMIC LUPUS ERYTHEMATOSUS

Systemic lupus erythematosus is an autoimmune disorder that primarily affects young women. As many as 70% develop clinically significant renal disease.

Systemic lupus erythematosus is the prototypic example of a human immune complex disease. There is a generalized hyperactivity of the B-cell system, with an outpouring of antibodies to a variety of nuclear and nonnuclear antigens, including native, double-stranded and single-stranded DNA, RNA and nucleoproteins. In contrast to the increased B-cell activity, T-cell function is diminished. The trapping of circulating immune complexes, probably those containing double-stranded DNA, is responsible for much of the renal damage in this disease. A more detailed discussion of systemic lupus erythematosus is found in Chapter 4.

A description of the morphologic alterations in lupus nephritis centers on the glomeruli, because they bear the brunt of the immunologic assault. Cellular proliferation in lupus glomerulonephritis is typically mesangial and often irregular. Mild glomerular involvement is characterized by diffuse mesangial expansion, with or without hypercellularity, and there is often a superimposed, segmental endothelial cell proliferation. More severe inflammation is manifested by enlarged, hypercellular glomeruli; enhanced lobulation; segmental areas of tuft necrosis; karyorrhexis; polymorphonuclear cell infiltration; and crescent formation (Fig. 16-25). Immune complexes, which are particularly prominent in this disease and may display unusual crystalline patterns, localize in mesangial, subendothelial or epimembranous areas (see Fig. 16-25). Often IgG, IgA and IgM and C3, C4 and Clq, are present in the same glomerulus—the so-called "full house" pattern. Heavy subendothelial deposits can usually be recognized at the light microscopic level by a marked thickening of the involved capillary wall, which results in a characteristic formation that has been called a "wire loop" (Fig. 16-26). In areas of segmental necrosis, "hematoxylin bodies," which are lilac-tinged fragmented nuclei, may be found. **The hematoxylin bodies are considered to be the only pathognomonic light microscopic feature of tissue damage of lupus erythematosus in the kidney and other organs.**

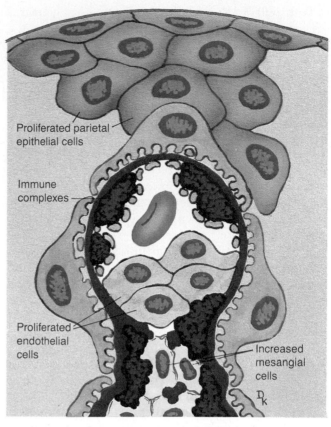

Figure 16-25. The glomerulonephritis of systemic lupus erythematosus. The glomerulus in this disease is characterized by conspicuous intercapillary immune complexes. The mesangial deposits separate the basement membrane from the proliferating mesangial cells and extend into the peripheral capillary as subendothelial deposits. Severe cases not only show changes in the glomerular tuft but also exhibit conspicuous proliferation of capsular epithelial cells and formation of cellular crescents.

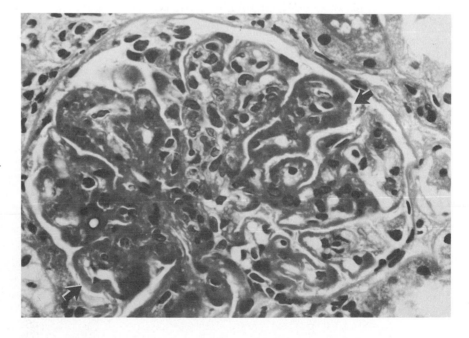

Figure 16-26. Systemic lupus erythematosus. In this light micrograph "wire loops" (*arrows*) represent marked subendothelial widening caused by the deposition of immune complexes.

Both inflammatory and noninflammatory glomerular lesions are manifested in this disease. There is a correlation between the pattern of glomerular injury and the localization of immune complex deposits as demonstrated by immunofluorescence and electron microscopy. Patients with no immune complex deposits or deposits limited to the mesangium may have normal-appearing glomeruli or may show only mild mesangial cell proliferation. Inflammatory changes are associated with extension of deposits into the subendothelial area. Finally, 10% of patients show a localization of deposits primarily in the epimembranous area. The glomeruli then resemble those in the idiopathic membranous lesion without cellular inflammatory changes.

Some degree of interstitial inflammation is almost invariable in significant lupus glomerulonephritis and is related to the extraglomerular deposition of immune complexes. **On occasion, the interstitial involvement may be a major morphologic feature, while the glomerular changes are only minor.** A necrotizing arteritis is occasionally found in lupus nephritis, usually in association with a florid, diffuse, proliferative glomerulonephritis with crescents. The presence of a vascular lesion is associated with a poor overall prognosis.

Renal disease is one of the major prognostic determinants in patients with systemic lupus erythematosus, and renal failure is the cause of death in over a third of the patients. There is a good correlation with the WHO classification and prognosis for the renal disease. Generally the mesangial proliferative (Class II) and membranous (Class V) nephropathies have the most benign course. The degree of glomerular and interstitial scarring is a better prognostic indicator than the intensity of the acute inflammation.

mary amyloidosis, Waldenstrom's macroglobulinemia and cryoglobulinemia.

Multiple myeloma is a disease of the immunoglobulin-producing B lymphocyte that occurs predominantly in the fifth decade and later. More than half of all multiple myeloma patients have renal involvement at some point in the course of their disease. In addition to the circulating paraproteins, other factors, such as hypercalcemia, hyperuricemia and frequent renal infections, also contribute to the incidence of renal failure in these patients. The renal lesions of multiple myeloma comprise two major types: that associated with the excretion of large amounts of light chains (called Bence-Jones proteins), in which there is primarily tubular destruction, and the deposition of immunoglobulin fragments in the form of amyloid fibrils.

"Myeloma cast nephropathy" is the term used to describe the renal lesion associated with the excretion of large amounts of light chains. **The characteristic lesions consist of multiple, dense, lamellated and fractured casts in the distal and collecting tubules** (Fig. 16-27). These casts are brightly eosinophilic and refractile and are frequently surrounded by multinucleated giant cells. Immunohistochemical staining of this material shows that they are usually composed of kappa light chains.

The more common type of tissue deposition of immunoglobulin fragments is in the form of **amyloid fibrils.** The nature and staining properties of these fibrils, which are composed in part of immunoglobulin light chains, is described in the section on the nephrotic syndrome and in Chapter 23. Lambda light chains are demonstrated more frequently than kappa chains in amyloid deposits.

DIABETES MELLITUS

Diabetes mellitus is a major cause of morbidity from renal disease; as many as 30% of juvenile diabetics eventually develop end stage disease. The lesions of diffuse and nodular glomerulosclerosis, which have already been discussed, are the major causes of renal insufficiency in diabetes. However, the diabetic state also affects the renal vasculature (arteriolar sclerosis) and the tubules, and increases the susceptibility of the kidney to pyelonephritis and papillary necrosis.

KIDNEY LESIONS ASSOCIATED WITH PARAPROTEINEMIA

Diseases in which paraproteins are frequently associated with renal damage are multiple myeloma, pri-

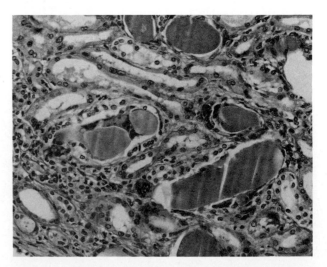

Figure 16-27. Myeloma of the kidney. A light micrograph shows the broad casts and multinucleated giant cells that are characteristic of obstructive light chain nephropathy.

HEREDITARY NEPHRITIS

A hereditary form of glomerulonephritis is referred to by the eponym **Alport's syndrome.** The disease affects both sexes, but is more severe in men, who usually die of renal failure before the age of 40. Even though affected women show signs of the disease, and some die prematurely, others live a normal life span. Variable proteinuria and hematuria are the rule, and the nephrotic syndrome complicates the course of the disease. Thirty percent to 50% of patients exhibit high frequency nerve deafness, and some suffer from abnormalities of the eyes, including disorders of the lens and the macula.

By light microscopy the glomerulonephritis is patchy and its severity varies across the entire spectrum of glomerular disease, from a mild focal proliferative form to a full-blown crescentic glomerulonephritis. Focal loss of tubules and interstitial fibrosis accompany the glomerular lesions. By electron microscopy the basement membrane is thickened by a splitting of the lamina densa into interlacing lamella that surround electron-lucent domains.

A defect in the chemical composition of basement membranes remains a likely basis of the renal disease as well as of the abnormalities occurring in the eye and ear in Alport's syndrome.

TUBULOINTERSTITIAL DISEASES

Renal diseases which are initially limited to the tubules and interstitium are usually grouped together. The clinico-pathologic entity of **chronic interstitial nephritis,** a term that describes marked tubular atrophy with interstitial fibrosis, is the result of a number of pathologic processes.

PYELONEPHRITIS AND URINARY TRACT INFECTION

Infection is a major cause of tubulointerstitial disorders. Pyelonephritis—defined as a combined inflammation of the parenchyma, calyces, and renal pelvis—occurs in two forms: acute pyelonephritis, which is always a result of a bacterial infection of the kidney, and chronic pyelonephritis, the pathogenesis of which is controversial.

ACUTE PYELONEPHRITIS

The development of ascending acute pyelonephritis depends upon four factors: (1) a source of pathogenic microorganisms, (2) infection of the urine, (3) reflux of the infected urine up the ureters into the renal pelvis and calyces, and (4) entry of the bacteria through the papillae into the renal parenchyma.

In some women who seem to be unusually vulnerable to recurrent attacks of acute pyelonephritis, the normal flora of the distal urethra are replaced by organisms from the gastrointestinal tract, which gain entry to the urethra from the perineum and vestibule of the vagina. Thus, **the most common offending organism is *Escherichia coli*.** Bacteria in the bladder urine usually do not gain access to the kidneys. The ureter commonly inserts into the bladder wall at a steep angle (Fig. 16–28) and courses parallel to the bladder wall between the mucosa and muscularis in its most distal portion. The intravesicular pressure produced by micturition occludes the distal lumen of the ureter, thereby preventing reflux of urine. In many individuals who are particularly susceptible to ascending pyelonephritis, an abnormally short passage of the ureter within the bladder wall is associated with an angle of insertion that is more perpendicular to the mucosal surface of the bladder. Thus, on micturition, rather than occluding the lumen, intravesicular pressure forces urine into the patent ureter. This reflux is sufficiently powerful to force the urine into the renal pelvis and calyces.

Even when present in the calyces, bacteria are not necessarily carried into the renal parenchyma by the reflux pressure. The simple papillae of the central calyces are convex and do not readily admit reflux urine (see Fig. 16–28). By contrast, the concave shape of the peripheral compound papillae allows easier access to the collecting system. However, if the pressure is prolonged, as in obstructive uropathy, even the simple papillae are eventually rendered vulnerable to retrograde entry of urine. From the collecting tubules the bacteria gain access to the interstitial tissue of the kidney.

The vast majority of cases of acute pyelonephritis stem from ascending infection, but under some circumstances and with certain organisms, blood-borne pathogens can become resident in the kidney. For example, gram-positive organisms, such as staphylococci, can disseminate from the infected valve of a bacterial endocarditis and establish a focus of infection in the kidney. In such cases, the cortex is more commonly the site of the infection than the medulla and pyramids, and abscesses are more likely to be seen than in ascending pyelonephritis.

Symptoms of acute pyelonephritis include costovertebral angle tenderness and systemic evidence of infection, such as fever and malaise. The peripheral white blood cell count is often elevated. The differentiation of upper from lower urinary tract infection is often clinically difficult but the finding of white blood cell casts in the urine is diagnostic of pyelonephritis.

Grossly, the kidneys of acute pyelonephritis may have small abscesses on the subcapsular surface. In

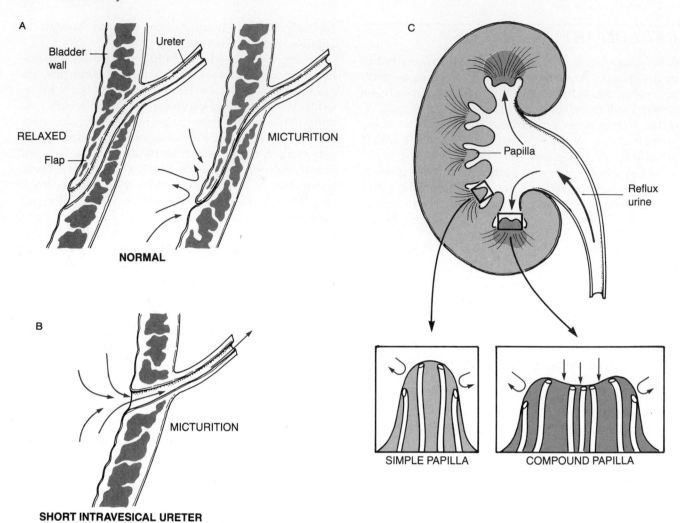

Figure 16-28. Anatomic features of the bladder and kidney in pyelonephritis caused by ureterovesical reflux. **Bladder.** (*A*) In the normal bladder the distal portion of the intravesical ureter courses between the mucosa and the muscularis of the bladder. A mucosal flap is thus formed. On micturition the elevated intravesicular pressure compresses the flap against the bladder wall, thereby occluding the lumen. (*B*) Persons with a congenitally short intravesical ureter have no mucosal flap, because the entry of the ureter into the bladder approaches a right angle. Thus, micturition forces urine into the ureter. **Kidney.** (*C*) The so-called simple papillae of the central calyces are convex and do not readily allow reflux of urine. By contrast the peripheral compound papillae are concave and permit entry of refluxed urine.

areas where there has been severe reflux or obstruction, the cortex is thinned and the papillae blunted. Most infections involve only one or two papillary systems. The parenchyma, particularly the cortex, may be extensively destroyed by the acute inflammatory process (Fig. 16-29), although vessels and glomeruli often show some resistance to infection. A modest number of polymorphonuclear leukocytes may also be seen. In severe cases, necrosis of the papillary tip may occur. Acute pyelonephritis and chronic pyelonephritis are focal diseases and much of the kidney often appears normal.

CHRONIC PYELONEPHRITIS

Chronic pyelonephritis is a chronic tubulointerstitial disorder in which there is gross, irregular and often asymmetric scarring, together with deformation of the calyces and the overlying parenchyma. It often progresses to so-called end-stage kidney—that is, a shrunken and fibrotic kidney that is insufficient to maintain renal function. In fact, about 15% of patients referred for renal dialysis or transplants suffer from chronic pyelonephritis. **The relationship of the tubulointerstitial damage to the calyx in this disease can**

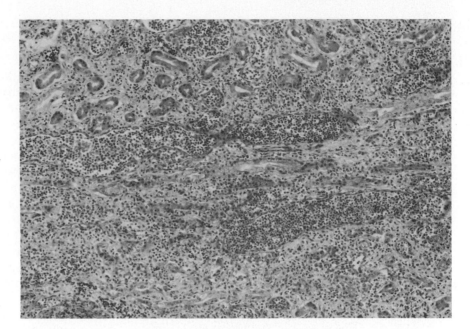

Figure 16-29. Acute pyelonephritis. A light micrograph shows an extensive infiltrate of neutrophils in the collecting tubules and interstitial tissue.

not be overemphasized. Tubular atrophy and interstitial fibrosis result from a number of conditions, but only chronic pyelonephritis and analgesic nephropathy (see later) produce this combination of calyceal deformity with overlying corticomedullary scarring. The role of bacterial infection in chronic pyelonephritis is less secure than in the acute form of the disease, although in most cases infection is thought to play a role.

Chronic pyelonephritis is divided into cases with some form of obstruction and those without (Fig. 16-30). The vast majority of cases without obstruction are associated with vesicoureteral reflux (so called **reflux nephropathy**). In cases with mechanical obstruction, the pathologic changes are due to a combination of obstruction and infection; all of the calyces and the renal pelvis are dilated and the parenchyma is uni-

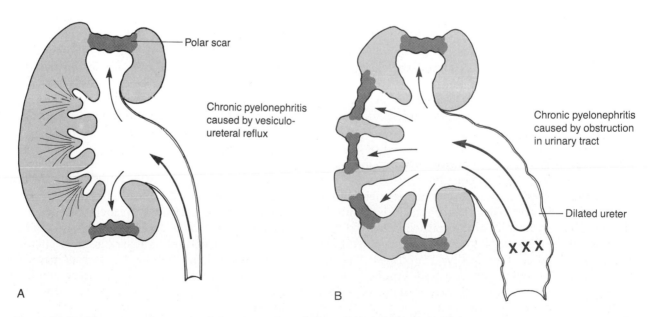

Polar scar

Chronic pyelonephritis caused by vesiculo-ureteral reflux

Chronic pyelonephritis caused by obstruction in urinary tract

Dilated ureter

A

B

Figure 16-30. The two major types of chronic pyelonephritis. (*A*) Vesicoureteral reflux causes infection of the peripheral compound papillae and, therefore, scars in the poles of the kidney. (*B*) Obstruction of the urinary tract leads to high-pressure back-flow of urine that causes infection of all papillae and diffuse scarring of the kidney and thinning of the cortex.

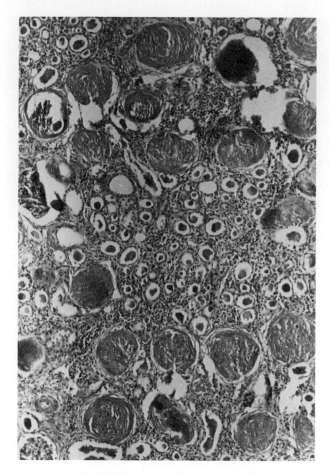

Figure 16-31. Chronic pyelonephritis. A light micrograph illustrates a cluster of atrophic tubules containing casts in their lumina (so-called thyroidization), surrounded by sclerotic glomeruli.

formly thinned. In cases associated with vesicoureteral reflux, the calyces at the poles of the kidney are preferentially expanded and are associated with overlying discrete, coarse scars that cause an indentation of the renal surface.

Microscopically, the scars are composed of atrophic dilated tubules, which are surrounded by interstitial fibrous tissue (Fig. 16-31). The glomeruli may be completely uninvolved, may have periglomerular fibrosis, or may be sclerotic. The most characteristic tubular change is severe atrophy of the epithelium with diffuse eosinophilic hyaline casts. In cross section such tubules resemble colloid-containing thyroid follicles. The pattern is called thyroidization. A mixed lymphocytic and histiocytic inflammatory infiltrate is seen, especially early in the course of the disease.

TUBULOINTERSTITIAL NEPHRITIS CAUSED BY DRUGS

Acute drug-induced tubulointerstitial nephritis of the hypersensitivity type is now a well-recognized clinicopathologic reaction to an increasing number of drugs. It is characterized clinically by acute renal insufficiency, microscopic or macroscopic hematuria, fever, nausea, vomiting, and an elevated erythrocyte sedimentation rate. It has most frequently been associated with synthetic penicillins (methicillin, ampicillin), but other antibiotics, diuretics and nonsteroidal anti-inflammatory agents have also been implicated. The symptoms typically begin about 2 weeks after drug administration has begun. The histologic findings, which are not specific, include a lymphohistiocytic inflammatory widening of the interstitium and interstitial edema. Granulomas may be seen, especially when the lesion is associated with the use of sulfonamides or methicillin. The glomeruli are generally uninvolved.

Antibiotics, such as the aminoglycoside gentamicin, and antifungal agents, such as amphotericin B, often cause renal insufficiency by a direct nephrotoxic effect. They produce an acute tubular necrosis that is indistinguishable from that seen in shock or mercuric chloride poisoning. This type of injury, which is limited to the tubules and the interstitium, is usually dose related.

Chronic tubulointerstitial renal disease can be caused by the heavy usage of analgesic compounds that contain phenacetin. Symptoms, which tend to occur only in the late stages of the disease, include premature aging, a brownish discoloration of the skin, an inability to concentrate the urine, metabolic acidosis and anemia. Sloughing of necrotic papillary tips into the renal pelvis may result in renal colic.

In advanced stages of chronic tubulointerstitial disease caused by analgesic abuse, both kidneys are shrunken equally. Retracted cortical scars overlie necrotic papillae. Early microscopic changes, which are confined to the papillae and the inner medulla, consist of patchy necrosis of the cells of the loops of Henle and focal widening of the interstitium. These necrotic areas eventually become confluent and extend to the corticomedullary junction, after which the collecting ducts become involved. There are characteristically few inflammatory cells around the necrotic foci. Eventually the entire papilla becomes necrotic, often remaining in place as a structureless mass. In such circumstances, dystrophic calcification of the necrotic papilla is common. There is an associated secondary tubular atrophy in the overlying cortex, as well as diffuse interstitial fibrosis.

URATE NEPHROPATHY

Any condition associated with elevated levels of uric acid in the blood may lead to a urate nephropathy. The classic disease in this category is primary gout, in which the biochemical basis of the hyperuricemia has not been established. At least as common today are those disorders in which hyperuricemia reflects an increased cell turnover (e.g., leukemia and polycythemia). Chemotherapy for malignant tumors can result in a sudden increase in blood uric acid, owing to the massive necrosis of cancer cells and consequent breakdown of DNA nucleotides. Diseases that interfere with the excretion of uric acid can also result in hyperuricemia, as after the chronic intake of certain diuretics.

Urate nephropathy can present as either acute renal failure or as chronic tubulointerstitial disease. Acute renal failure reflects the obstruction of the collecting ducts by precipitated crystals of uric acid. Histologically, the tubular deposits appear as amorphic, but in frozen sections the crystalline structure is apparent. Some collecting ducts are penetrated by uric acid crystals, which provoke a foreign body giant cell reaction.

Chronic gout can result in chronic tubulointerstitial nephropathy caused by the tubular and interstitial deposition of crystalline monosodium urate. The basic disease process is similar to that of acute urate nephropathy, but the prolonged course results in a more substantial deposition of urate crystals in the interstitium, interstitial fibrosis, and cortical atrophy. Uric acid stones occur in 20% of patients with chronic gout and 40% of those with acute hyperuricemia. Uric acid stones are not uncommon, accounting for one tenth of all cases of urolithiasis.

NEPHROCALCINOSIS

Calcium deposits in the kidney are not uncommon, having been reported in as many as one fifth of kidneys at autopsy and in many renal biopsies, particularly in children. These incidental deposits are usually insignificant morphologically and are not associated with any functional alterations. By contrast, significant degrees of calcification are seen in conditions associated with hypercalcemia or with injury localized to the kidney (Table 16-3).

In the face of severe hypercalcemia, typified by primary hyperparathyroidism, gross examination characteristically reveals wedge-shaped scars adjacent to normal renal tissue. These scars do not result from vascular obstruction, but reflect tubular atrophy and dila-

Table 16-3   *Causes of Nephrocalcinosis*
Increased Resorption of Calcium From Bone
Primary hyperparathyroidism
Multiple myeloma
Bone metastases
Paraneoplastic hypercalcemia (bronchogenic carcinoma, renal cell carcinoma)
Increased Absorption of Calcium From the Gastrointestinal Tract
Sarcoidosis
Hypervitaminosis D
Milk-alkali syndrome
Idiopathic hypercalcemia
Renal Osteodystrophy
Dystrophic Calcification
Previous toxic renal injury
Previous acute vascular injury (cortical necrosis, acute tubular necrosis)
Renal tubular acidosis

tion, with interstitial fibrosis secondary to the obstruction of the larger collecting ducts. Microscopically, there is also a striking calcification of the basement membranes of the renal tubules. Surrounding the tubules the interstitial tissue also displays calcium deposits. Scattered glomeruli show calcification of Bowman's capsule, and the walls of the intrarenal arteries may be similarly affected. The calcification seen after necrosis caused by drugs or vascular insults is probably due to dystrophic calcification of necrotic tissue.

ACUTE TUBULAR NECROSIS

Acute tubular necrosis is the most frequent cause of the clinical syndrome of acute renal failure. In the majority of patients it results in a rapid deterioration of renal function, characterized by oliguria that may last from 4 days to 4 weeks. This is followed by a diuretic stage, in which there is relief of the oliguria, but persistent severe tubular dysfunction. Any event which precipitates shock, either hypovolemic or endotoxic shock, often results in ischemic acute tubular necrosis. Such events include trauma, hemorrhage, burns, dehydration, and sepsis.

Most of the tubular changes, which may be patchy, are seen in the border zone between the outer medulla and the cortex. Both the straight terminal portion of the proximal convoluted tubule and the medullary thick ascending limb of Henle's loop show morphologic changes. These alterations include shedding and ne-

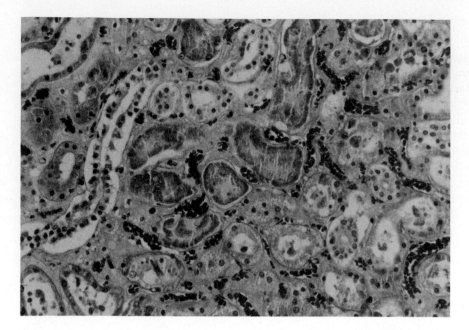

Figure 16-32. Acute tubular necrosis. A light micrograph illustrates early necrosis with a pattern of variable nuclear disruption. The casts in the lumina are disrupted cells.

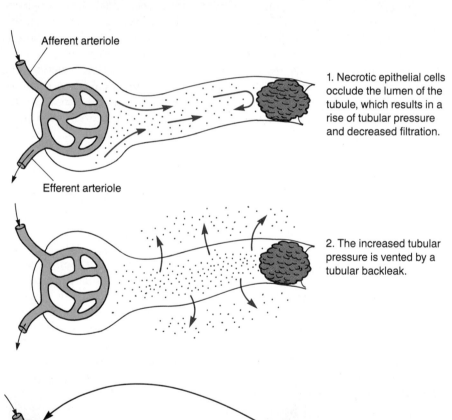

Afferent arteriole

Efferent arteriole

1. Necrotic epithelial cells occlude the lumen of the tubule, which results in a rise of tubular pressure and decreased filtration.

2. The increased tubular pressure is vented by a tubular backleak.

Figure 16-33. Pathogenesis of oliguria in acute tubular necrosis.

3. A tubulo-glomerular feedback mechanism results in a prolonged afferent arteriolar vasoconstriction, which further decreases filtration.

crosis of epithelial cells (Fig. 16-32) and sloughing of cellular debris into the tubular lumina, which results in the formation of hyaline and granular casts in the distal tubules and the collecting ducts of the papillae. Later in the development of the lesion, re-epithelialization of the tubules is manifested by a flat, cuboidal epithelial lining that has frequent mitotic figures. Since this regenerated epithelium is functional, therapy is directed toward supporting the vital functions of the patient until this stage is reached.

The cause of the decreased renal function and oliguria in acute tubular necrosis is not well understood. In all probability a combination of the following is important: leakage of tubular fluid back through the damaged epithelial lining, tubular obstruction due to sloughing of necrotic epithelial cells, and arteriolar vasoconstriction, which shunts blood away from the cortex (Fig. 16-33).

VASCULAR DISEASES

HYPERTENSION

Hypertension is separated into benign and malignant forms. The pathologic changes of benign nephrosclerosis relate to the consequences of ischemia. Ischemic glomeruli display irregular changes that are distinctly different from those of intrinsic glomerular disease (i.e., glomerulonephritis). Moreover, totally obliterated glomeruli may be located beside completely normal ones. Initially, the glomerular capillaries are thickened and shriveled. Cells of the glomerular tuft are progressively lost, and collagen and matrix material are deposited within Bowman's space, most prominently, distant from the hilus. Eventually, the glomerular tuft is represented by a dense, eosinophilic globular mass enclosed in a scar, all within Bowman's capsule. Tubular atrophy, a consequence of the obsolescence of the glomerulus, is associated with fibrosis of the related interstitium. The pattern of change in the blood vessels depends on the size of the involved vessels. Large arteries down to the size of the arcuate arteries show arteriosclerotic changes of the intima, splitting of the internal elastic lamina, and partial replacement of the muscular coat with fibrous tissue. In addition to similar changes interlobular arteries show medial hypertrophy. Arterioles display hyaline thickening of the entire wall.

Malignant hypertension occurs more frequently in men than in women, typically about the age of 40. Blacks are particularly susceptible to this lesion. The diastolic pressure is generally above 115 Hg. Headache and unusual mental disturbances occur frequently, as does a characteristic retinopathy. Acute and chronic renal failure are common.

Malignant nephrosclerosis, the morphologic counterpart of malignant hypertension, shows many of the same sclerotic changes described previously. In addition the glomeruli frequently exhibit fibrinoid necrosis, sometimes in continuity with a necrotizing lesion of the preglomerular arterioles. The arterioles exhibit fibrinoid necrosis, whereas in the larger arteries the lumen is markedly reduced in size by profuse intimal thickening, owing to cellular proliferation and the accumulation of a myxoid matrix (Fig. 16-34).

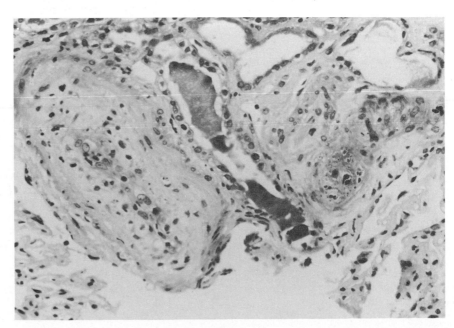

Figure 16-34. Malignant hypertension. A light micrograph illustrates interlobular arteries that show a near-obliteration of the lumina with marked intimal thickening. There is a prominent fluid and cellular exudate in the vessel wall.

HEMOLYTIC UREMIC SYNDROME

Historically, the hemolytic uremic syndrome was considered to affect infants and children. Shortly after a nonspecific respiratory or gastrointestinal illness, the child suddenly develops anemia, bleeding, renal failure, neurologic abnormalities and cardiovascular symptoms. No specific etiologic agent has been demonstrated. A major factor in the pathogenesis of this syndrome is endothelial damage associated with a deficiency of prostacyclin activator, which is a vasodilator and a potent inhibitor of platelet aggregation. Another important factor is intravascular coagulation, which also may relate to endothelial damage. In this respect thrombi composed of varying combinations of fibrin and platelets are often found within glomerular capillaries, arterioles, and small arteries. Since the original descriptions, the disease has been reported in adults, commonly in women who have used oral contraceptives or who suffer acute renal failure in the postpartum period. Treatment with drugs such as mitomycin and cyclosporin has also been implicated.

The glomerulus appears to be the principal site of damage in the kidney. Endothelial swelling is prominent, and foci of epithelial cell proliferation and even crescents appear. By electron microscopy, a clear area of subendothelial widening, a foamy mesangial matrix, and some aneurysmal capillary dilatation are prominent. Thrombi are variably present in glomeruli. The preglomerular arterioles display focal damage, with insudation of fibrin and red blood cells, and thrombosis.

The infantile and childhood type, which frequently has only glomerular lesions, is associated with complete recovery in the large majority of cases, and a mortality of less than 5%. The adult and postpartum type usually presents with involvement of glomeruli, afferent arterioles, and interlobular arteries. The prognosis is more guarded, and a fatal outcome is seen in 60% of the cases.

SYSTEMIC SCLERODERMA (PROGRESSIVE SYSTEMIC SCLEROSIS)

Systemic scleroderma is a disease in which there is deposition of collagen, typically in the skin, but also in other organs, such as the gastrointestinal tract, lungs, and heart. Vascular changes, particularly in the fingers (Raynaud's phenomenon) and the kidney, virtually always develop. Azotemia followed by severe hyper-

tension and renal failure are common and indicate a grave prognosis.

The smaller arterial vessels—namely, the interlobular arteries and afferent arterioles—show luminal narrowing by loose fibrous tissue, in which the cells are disposed in a concentric fashion. The proliferated tissue shows a mucinous appearance, which reflects the presence of hyaluronic acid. Fibrin is deposited within the thickened intima, and small fibrin thrombi are occasionally seen in the lumen. In advanced cases conspicuous fibrin deposition, severe enough to be termed fibrinoid necrosis, is seen in the afferent arterioles. These vascular changes may result in small infarcts. Some glomeruli are intensely congested and even infarcted, whereas other glomeruli appear normal.

RENOVASCULAR HYPERTENSION

The total occlusion of a main renal artery produces a type of hypertension which is potentially curable by reconstitution of the arterial lumen. The initial experiments that led to the understanding of this syndrome were carried out a half century ago by Goldblatt, and since that time the kidney totally deprived of vascular supply has been known as the Goldblatt kidney. Ninety percent to 95% of the cases are caused by lesions of atherosclerosis. The other major lesion that produces this syndrome is fibromuscular dysplasia of the renal arteries. The lesion consists of a fibrous and fibromuscular stenosis of the renal artery that is not atherosclerotic, is more common in women, and occurs at a younger age (average age 35 years).

Whether vascular occlusion is caused by atherosclerosis or by fibromuscular dysplasia, the involved kidney typically is reduced only slightly in size. The glomeruli, the arteries and the arterioles all appear normal. Focal tubular atrophy is often noted. The juxtaglomerular apparatus is prominent and demonstrates hyperplasia, increased granularity, and a greater length.

The pathogenesis of hypertension in cases of renal artery stenosis relates to the hyperplasia of the juxtaglomerular apparatus and the resulting increase in the production of renin, angiotensin II and aldosterone.

RENAL INFARCTS

Renal infarcts for the most part are caused by arterial obstruction, and the majority represent embolization to branches of the main renal artery. Common sources of emboli include mural thrombi overlying myocardial infarcts or, in longstanding fibrillation, located on the atrial wall; infected valves in bacterial endocarditis; and complicated atherosclerotic plaques in the aorta.

Variably sized, wedge-shaped areas of ischemic necrosis, with the base on the capsular surface, are typical. All structures within the affected zone are necrotic. Acute infarcts are bordered by a hemorrhagic zone. Healed infarcts are sharply circumscribed, and depressed cortical scars contain obliterated glomeruli, atrophic tubules, interstitial fibrosis, and a mild chronic inflammatory infiltrate. Dystrophic calcification is occasionally encountered in old infarcts. At the margins of a healed infarct, the viable tissue resembles that seen in chronic ischemia or in chronic pyelonephritis.

Recurrent infarction may lead to a shrunken end-stage kidney difficult to distinguish from that of chronic pyelonephritis. If enough renal parenchyma is lost, hypertension and renal failure ensue.

HYDRONEPHROSIS

Hydronephrosis is defined as dilatation of the renal pelvis and calyces, flattening of the papillae, and atrophy of the renal cortex. **Hydronephrosis is always the result of urinary tract obstruction,** whether from tumors, stones, vesicoureteral reflux, or other obstruction. The causes of urinary tract obstruction are discussed in detail in the chapter on urologic pathology (Chapter 17).

In early hydronephrosis, the most prominent finding is dilatation of the collecting ducts, followed by dilatation of the proximal and distal convoluted tubules. Eventually the proximal tubules become widely dilated, and loss of tubules is common. Interestingly, the glomeruli are usually spared. The hydronephrotic kidney is more susceptible to pyelonephritis.

Left untreated, renal atrophy and chronic renal failure are inevitable in bilateral hydronephrosis. Unilateral obstruction is frequently missed clinically because of the lack of symptoms.

RENAL STONES

The pelvis and calyces of the kidney are common sites for the formation and accumulation of calculi. Stones vary in composition, depending on individual factors, geography, metabolic alterations, and the presence of infection. For unknown reasons, renal stones are more common in men than in women. They vary in size from gravel, in which the stones may be less than a millimeter in diameter, to a large stone that dilates the entire renal pelvis.

The most common stone contains calcium complexed with oxalate or phosphate, or a mixture of these anions. In the presence of infection with urea-splitting bacteria, the resulting alkaline urine favors the precipitation of magnesium ammonium phosphate (struvite) stones. Formerly termed infection stones, these vary in consistency from hard to soft and friable. Struvite stones occasionally fill the pelvis and calyces to form a cast of these spaces, in which case they are referred to as staghorn calculi. Uric acid stones occur in 25% of patients with gout.

In most cases, the presence of a renal stone is associated with an increased blood level and urinary excretion of its principal component. This is clearly the case with uric acid stones. However, in many patients with calcium stones, hypercalciuria is found in the absence of hypercalcemia. The mechanism underlying this **idiopathic hypercalciuria** is not firmly established, but has been linked to increased intestinal absorption and a decrease in proximal tubular reabsorption of calcium.

Kidney stones may be well tolerated, but in some cases they lead to severe hydronephrosis and pyelonephritis. Moreover, they can erode the mucosa and cause hematuria. The passage of a stone into the ureter causes excruciating flank pain, termed renal colic. Although until recently most kidney stones required surgery for their removal, ultrasonic disintegration (lithotripsy) is now an effective alternative.

TUMORS OF THE KIDNEY

NEPHROBLASTOMA (WILMS' TUMOR)

Renal nephroblastoma, one of the most common solid tumors in very young children, usually presents before the age of 4 years, although it is occasionally seen in adults. Most children present with a large abdominal mass, occasionally accompanied by abdominal pain or intestinal obstruction.

Grossly, the tumors are usually large, with a bulging, pale-tan surface enclosed within a thin rim of renal cortex and capsule. Histologically, the tumor is composed of three elements: (1) metanephric blastema (which is the counterpart of normal embryonic tissue), (2) immature stroma, and (3) immature epithelial ele-

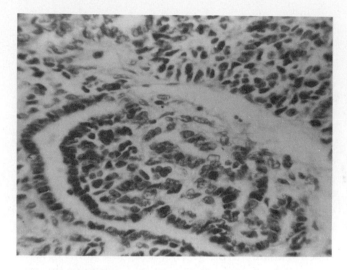

Figure 16-35. Wilms' tumor. A light micrograph illustrates a glomerulus-like structure.

ments. Morphologically, the component corresponding to blastema is composed of small ovoid cells, with a scanty cytoplasm, growing in nests and trabeculae. The epithelial component presents as small tubules, and occasionally immature structures resembling glomeruli are found (Fig. 16-35). The stroma between the other elements is composed of undifferentiated spindle cells, although occasionally distinct fibroblastic and striated

muscle differentiation is seen. Bone cartilage, adipocytes, and smooth muscle cells are occasionally encountered.

Chemotherapy and radiotherapy, combined with surgical resection, have dramatically improved the outlook of patients with this tumor, and many centers now report long-term survival rate of more than 90%.

MALIGNANT TUMORS OF THE KIDNEY IN ADULTS

RENAL CELL CARCINOMA

The most important neoplasm of the kidney is renal cell adenocarcinoma, which accounts for 90% of malignant renal tumors in adults. The incidence of this tumor peaks in the sixth decade. Hematuria is the single most frequent presenting sign; the **classic triad of hematuria, flank pain, and a palpable abdominal mass** is found in less than 10% of patients.

Grossly, these protruding tumors are yellow-orange and show conspicuous focal hemorrhage and necrosis, often in the background of a cystic pattern (Fig. 16-36). The histologic patterns are variable, and solid, alveolar, and tubular patterns of growth are common. The **most frequent and characteristic neoplastic cell has an unusually clear cytoplasm** (Fig. 16-37), owing to the removal of glycogen and lipids by the water and solvents used in the preparation of the tissue. Frequently, there is little cellular or nuclear pleomorphism, although an-

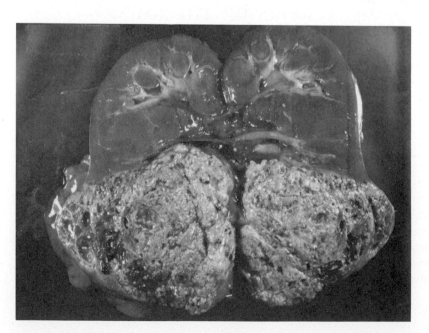

Figure 16-36. Renal cell carcinoma. The large tumor shows necrosis and hemorrhage.

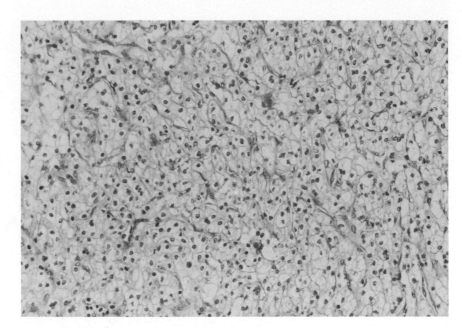

Figure 16-37. Renal cell carcinoma. A light micrograph shows characteristic large clear cells.

aplastic, sarcomatoid variants do occur. Renal cell adenocarcinoma derives from the lining cell of the proximal convoluted tubule.

The overall survival for this tumor is approximately 40% at 5 years. Distant metastases are found most frequently in the lung and the bones. The treatment is essentially limited to complete operative removal.

Small tumors that appear microscopically to be well-differentiated renal cortical carcinomas but that are less than 3 cm in diameter are referred to by some authors as **renal cell adenomas.** However, distant metastases have been documented on occasion from tumors with a diameter as small as 2 cm. It is, therefore, generally thought that all such tumors should be considered potentially malignant.

TRANSITIONAL CELL CARCINOMA OF THE RENAL PELVIS

Between 5% to 10% of tumors of the kidney are transitional cell carcinomas of the renal pelvis. These are morphologically identical to the more frequent bladder transitional cell carcinomas and are associated with them in half of the cases. A further discussion of this tumor is given in the chapter on urologic pathology (Chapter 17).

17

THE URINARY TRACT AND MALE REPRODUCTIVE SYSTEM

ROBERT O. PETERSEN

Renal Pelvis and Ureter

Urinary Bladder

Urethra

Testis

Testicular Adnexa

Prostate

Penis

Scrotum

RENAL PELVIS AND URETER

INFLAMMATORY DISORDERS

Inflammatory disorders of the renal pelvis and ureter are most commonly associated with ascending infection, often as a complication of partial ureteral obstruction or associated with lithiasis. Frequently, inflammatory changes of the ipsilateral kidney (pyelonephritis) are observed, especially in association with intrapelvic lithiasis. In most instances gram-negative organisms are implicated. The histologic findings are usually nonspecific and include a chronic inflammatory cell infiltrate of variable intensity in the lamina propria of the affected urinary tract segment. On occasion, mucosal ulceration is observed.

FIBROEPITHELIAL POLYPS

Fibroepithelial polyps are usually observed at the ureteropelvic junction or in the proximal one-third of the ureter. They have been variously regarded as congenital, inflammatory, hamartomatous, or neoplastic; synonyms include inflammatory polyp, fibroma, and hamartoma.

Fibroepithelial polyps are smooth nodules or, alternatively, filiform projections, varying in size from a few millimeters to several centimeters. Histologically, the urothelium covering the centrally edematous stromal stalk is either normal or hyperplastic. The stroma contains collagen fibers, variable numbers of small blood vessels, and, on occasion, smooth muscle fibers. Acute and chronic inflammatory cells, focal hyalinization of the stroma, and calcification are all inconstant features.

NEOPLASMS

Most neoplasms of the renal pelvis and ureter are carcinomas. Mesenchymal tumors, both benign and malignant, are distinctly rare. Benign transitional cell papillomas in the urinary tract are currently regarded as uncommon.

CARCINOMA

Carcinoma of the upper urinary tract is of the transitional cell variety in 90% of cases. Of the remainder, squamous cell carcinomas far outnumber primary adenocarcinomas of the renal pelvis and ureter. All histologic types of renal pelvic and ureteral carcinomas show a definite male predilection, with a peak frequency in the sixth and seventh decades of life.

The gross and microscopic features of each of the three histologic types of carcinoma affecting the renal pelvis and ureter allow for a specific diagnosis. Transitional cell carcinomas are usually exophytic, with papillary projections evident on gross examination. The extent of invasion of the underlying wall of the renal pelvis or ureter is variable at the time of surgical excision. Squamous cell carcinomas tend to be more infiltrative and exhibit a lesser exophytic component. Surface ulceration and an association with lithiasis are also more frequent with squamous cell carcinomas. Adenocarcinomas are characteristically mucinous, a feature detected on gross inspection of the opened specimen.

The World Health Organization classification of transitional cell carcinoma comprises three grades. Grade 1 carcinoma is composed of papillary projections lined by neoplastic transitional cells that show minimal nuclear pleomorphism and mitotic activity. The papillae are long and delicate, and fusion of papillae is focal and limited. Grade 3 carcinoma is characterized by significant nuclear pleomorphism, frequent mitoses, and fusion of the papillae. Occasional bizarre cells may be present, and focal sites of squamous differentiation are often seen. The histologic and cytologic features of grade 2 transitional cell carcinomas are intermediate between those of grade 1 (the best differentiated) and grade 3 (the most poorly differentiated).

Squamous cell carcinomas are identified by the presence of widespread and uniform squamous differentiation; adenocarcinomas are characterized by gland formation, frequently with abundant mucin production.

Metaplastic and dysplastic changes in the urothelium adjacent to the overt neoplasm may include foci of sufficient atypism to be labeled carcinoma in situ. Such changes may be observed in association with urothelial tumors of all three histologic types.

The development of multiple similar urothelial neoplasms is integral to the natural history of transitional cell carcinomas, but not the other types. Patients with transitional cell carcinomas of the renal pelvis show similar ureteral tumors in 20% of cases, and 13% suffer from simultaneous tumors in the urinary bladder. Moreover, an additional 20% develop independent transitional cell carcinomas of the bladder after removal of the original tumor by radical nephrectomy. A similar multiplicity of urothelial neoplasms is observed with primary tumors of the ureter: 10% of patients show simultaneous bladder transitional cell carcinomas, and an additional 27% develop these neoplasms in the bladder following primary surgical treatment for the ureteral tumor. From these figures it becomes clear that close long-term follow-up is obligatory for patients with previously diagnosed transitional cell carcinomas in any part of the urinary tract.

The ultimate survival of patients with primary transitional cell carcinomas of the renal pelvis and ureter is closely related to both the stage and grade of the tumor. Neoplasms confined to the mucosa, as well as those in which invasion is limited to the lamina propria, have a good prognosis. A progressive decrease in survival at 5 years is observed with all tumors that show greater local infiltration. Few patients with local invasion beyond the ureter or with distant metastases survive 5 years. The poor survival rates observed with primary renal pelvic or ureteral squamous cell carcinomas and adenocarcinomas are attributable to the consistently higher stage of these tumors at the time of primary surgical therapy.

URINARY BLADDER

CONGENITAL MALFORMATION OF THE URINARY BLADDER

Uncommon congenital malformations of the urinary bladder include agenesis, complete and incomplete duplication, hourglass deformity, and diverticulum. Two disorders are of major clinical significance: exstrophy and complications of persistent urachus.

EXSTROPHY

Exstrophy is a congenital vesicocutaneous fistula that remains after the incomplete closure of the anterior abdominal wall and the underlying anterior bladder wall, and results from an overgrowth of the cloacal membrane. The normal mesodermal structures develop around the central diversion, which ultimately ruptures, exposing the bladder mucosa to the exterior around and through the defect of the anterior abdominal wall. Abrasion by clothing and the continuous escape of urine result in chronic infection of the involved area.

The externalized bladder mucosa exhibits acute and chronic inflammation and metaplastic changes, most frequently squamous and glandular metaplasia. Fibrosis and chronic inflammation are present in the muscularis in all patients older than 1 year.

The condition of the patient with an uncorrected exstrophic bladder is lamentable. There is continuous leakage of urine, persistent or recurrent local infection, and an increased risk of ascending urinary tract infection. Moreover, there is an increased risk of neoplastic transformation of the metaplastic urothelium, with resultant adenocarcinoma, squamous cell carcinoma, and, least frequently, transitional cell carcinoma.

BLADDER DIVERTICULUM

Bladder diverticula are common and require surgical excision only infrequently. Some studies indicate that diverticula are produced by increased intravesical pressure secondary to bladder outlet obstruction, while some regard bladder diverticula as congenital. The majority are observed in men older than 50 years and are commonly associated with obstruction secondary to prostatism. Diverticula occasionally are encountered in infants and children who have no evidence of obstruction. The most common location is the vicinity of the ureteral orifices. Progressive enlargement of the diverticulum leads to stagnation of urine, infection, and the formation of bladder stones—conditions that indicate a need for surgical intervention.

The excised bladder diverticulum has a narrow orifice that opens into a larger cavity. The diverticulum distorts the outside contour of the urinary bladder. The narrow intramural neck is found between bundles of the inner layer of the bladder muscle. The distended wall of the diverticulum contains attenuated muscle fibers, which are most commonly observed in young patients.

The most serious complication of a bladder diverticulum, fortunately rare, is the development of cancer within it. Transitional cell and squamous cell carcinomas are the most frequently encountered types.

PERSISTENT URACHUS

The urachus is a tapered cephalic extension of the urogenital sinus (which later becomes the urinary bladder) that is contiguous with the allantois. Following birth, this tubular structure normally undergoes progressive fibrous atrophy as it descends caudally with the urinary bladder, to which it remains attached. The point of attachment is most commonly in the vesical dome. The regressive changes that result in closure of the cephalad end at the umbilicus and the caudal end at the bladder wall obliterate the intervening segment and convert it to a solid fibrous cord.

The clinical disorders associated with persistent urachus relate to the extent and location of the urachus that remains patent. Persistence of the entire urachus from the bladder to the umbilicus results in drainage of urine from the umbilicus, and supervening infection is common. Alternatively, incomplete persistence of the urachus forms a blind pouch, open either to the skin at the umbilicus or to the urinary bladder. Segmental persistence of the lumen with closure at both ends leads to a urachal cyst. The least common—but most serious—complication of persistent urachal segments is cancer: 90% are adenocarcinomas, although transitional and squamous cell carcinomas are encountered.

PROLIFERATIVE AND METAPLASTIC VARIANTS OF BLADDER CANCER

A spectrum of hyperplastic and metaplastic changes of the urothelium is commonly observed in the urinary bladder. Indeed, these same mucosal changes are observed throughout the urinary tract.

The hyperplastic urothelial changes include simple hyperplasia of the surface urothelium, focal proliferative mucosal invaginations—termed Brunn's buds or Brunn's nests, and cystitis cystica. The metaplastic proliferations include cystitis glandularis, squamous metaplasia, and nephrogenic metaplasia. **These alterations are observed in circumstances characterized by urothelial inflammation, including urinary tract infections, bladder stones, neurogenic bladders, and exstrophy.**

Although squamous metaplasia has traditionally been attributed to reactive urothelial proliferations associated with inflammation, apparently spontaneous squamous metaplasia is seen in about half of normal bladders in adult women and in approximately 10% of those in adult men. The question of whether there is an increased risk or neoplastic conversion of this metaplastic squamous cell population remains problematic.

INFLAMMATORY DISORDERS

POLYPOID CYSTITIS

Polypoid cystitis is a reversible inflammatory lesion of the bladder mucosa characterized by papillary, polypoid, exophytic mucosal projections. Histologically, there is vascular congestion, stromal edema, and an inflammatory cell infiltrate within the lamina propria. Most cases of polypoid cystitis are associated with indwelling catheters, an association that explains the disease's predilection for the posterior wall and dome of the bladder.

CHRONIC INTERSTITIAL CYSTITIS (HUNNER'S ULCER)

Chronic interstitial cystitis, an inflammatory disorder of unknown etiology, is classically associated with a mucosal ulcer (Hunner's ulcer), although it is not required for the diagnosis. Typically the disease is chronic and involves middle-aged women, but the lesion has been observed in adult men and, rarely, in children. The most common symptoms are long-standing suprapubic pain, frequency, and urgency, with or without hematuria. At cystoscopy, mucosal edema, focal petechiae, and irregular hemorrhagic areas are characteristic. The lesions are most prevalent in the dome and posterior wall. The negative urine cultures are both characteristic and confounding when attempting to determine the underlying cause.

Histologically, the mucosal ulcer displays an intense acute inflammatory reaction. The predominant findings in the lamina propria are vascular dilatation and edema, but importantly, a chronic inflammatory cell infiltrate composed of lymphocytes and mast cells is commonly observed within the muscularis, which frequently also shows fibrosis.

MALACOPLAKIA

Malacoplakia, an inflammatory disorder of unknown cause, was originally described in the gastrointestinal tract, but more recently has been reported in a wide variety of organs. **The inflammatory lesions are characterized by a predominance of histiocytes,** the so-called von Hansemann cells, which have diagnostic intracytoplasmic inclusions, the Michaelis-Gutmann bodies (Fig. 17-1).

The urinary bladder is the single most common site of this enigmatic disorder. There is a marked preponderance of cases in women, regardless of the site of occurrence. A clinical background of intercurrent disease, including immunosuppression, chronic infectious disorders, and cancer, is not uncommon. An acquired functional impairment of monocytes is currently considered a likely cause of malacoplakia.

IATROGENIC CYSTITIS

Cystitis as a complication of radiation therapy or chemotherapy, most commonly treatment with cyclophosphamide, has received increasing attention. The typical features of all radiation-induced lesions—endothelial proliferation, subendothelial accumulation of histiocytes, and atypical fibroblasts within the stroma—are also seen in the bladder. The histologic changes associated with cyclophosphamide produce a form of hemorrhagic cystitis, commonly in association with cytologic atypia of the urothelial cells. The bladder lesions result not from cyclophosphamide itself, but from its metabolic breakdown products in the urine.

ENDOMETRIOSIS

The urinary bladder is the most common site of endometriosis of the urinary tract. Patients present with pelvic pain, frequency, and urgency. Hematuria is reported in only one-fourth of the patients. The fact that about 60% of the patients have a history of pelvic sur-

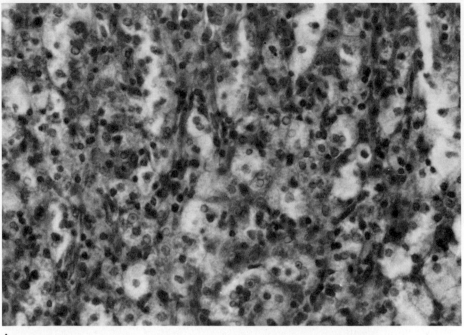

A

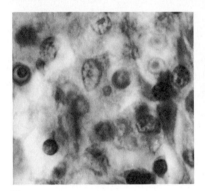
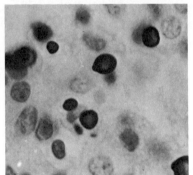

B

Figure 17-1. Malacoplakia. (*A*) Numerous Michaelis-Gutmann bodies are seen as well-defined spherical structures, some of which have a central inclusion. The background inflammatory cells are composed principally of histiocytes, with fewer lymphocytes. (*B*) Michaelis-Gutmann bodies are seen at high magnification following special staining procedures.

gery suggests an implantation pathogenesis. The cause of endometriosis in the absence of prior surgery remains controversial.

The diagnosis of vesical endometriosis requires the identification of endometrial glandular epithelium in association with endometrial stromal cells (Fig. 17-2). Past hemorrhage is identified by the presence of hemosiderin in the stromal tissue.

NEOPLASTIC DISORDERS

The urinary bladder is the site of origin of benign or malignant epithelial and mesenchymal neoplasms. **Epithelial neoplasms, virtually all of which are transitional cell carcinomas, comprise more than 98% of all primary tumors.** Benign epithelial tumors and all mesenchymal neoplasms are rare.

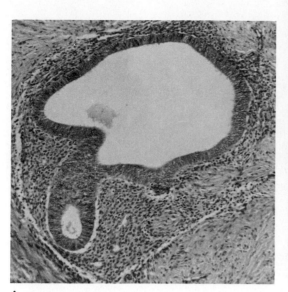
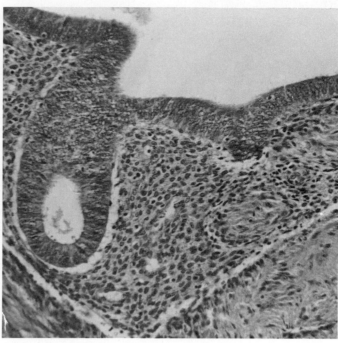

A   B

Figure 17-2. Endometriosis of the bladder. (*A*) Endometrial glandular epithelium with associated endometrial stromal cells within the muscularis layer of the bladder is diagnostic. (*B*) Higher magnification of (*A*).

BENIGN EPITHELIAL NEOPLASMS OF THE URINARY BLADDER

Transitional cell papillomas of the urinary bladder exhibit a normal urothelial mucosal epithelium seven layers thick or less. They comprise 2% to 3% of bladder epithelial neoplasms and occur most frequently in men over the age of 50 years. The majority of cases show single lesions 2 to 5 cm in diameter, but multiple lesions are not unusual. **"Recurrences" are common (70% of patients) and the development of invasive carcinoma occurs in about 7% of patients.**

PAPILLARY TRANSITIONAL CELL CARCINOMA

The association of bladder cancer with occupational exposure to certain organic chemicals has been known since its original observation in 1895. Occupational exposure to carcinogens with an increased risk of bladder cancer has been identified in the leather, rubber, paint, and organic chemical industries.

Transitional cell carcinoma of the bladder typically presents with sudden hematuria. The histologic patterns display a range of appearances, from small, delicate papillary lesions that are apparently limited to the surface, to larger, solid, invasive masses that frequently show surface ulceration. Transitional cell carcinomas of the bladder show growth patterns that are exophytic and papillary, infiltrating, or both. The lower grade (more differentiated) neoplasms tend to be predominantly, if not exclusively, papillary and exophytic; the predominantly infiltrating neoplasms are more typically high grade—that is, less differentiated.

The extent of transitional cell carcinoma is described according to a staging classification (Fig. 17-3). Tumors that are limited to the mucosa, without evidence of invasion, are regarded as stage O. Stage A tumors are those that invade the lamina propria. Invasion of muscle is designated as stage B. If only superficial muscle invasion is noted, the stage is termed B1; if the invasion is deep, it is classified B2. Perivesical invasion is considered stage C, and metastatic tumors are regarded as stage D. **At the time of initial presentation, 85% of patients have tumor confined to the urinary bladder (stages O to C), and 15% have regional or distant metastases (stages D1 and D2, respectively).**

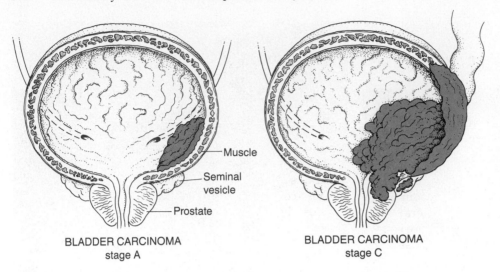

BLADDER CARCINOMA
stage A

BLADDER CARCINOMA
stage C

Muscle

Seminal
vesicle

Prostate

Figure 17-3. Clinical staging of bladder carcinoma. Carcinoma of the bladder, stage A, is restricted to the mucosa and lamina propria. Advanced carcinoma, stage C, exhibits a larger intravesical mass and invasion of the bladder wall, where it may obstruct the ureter and produce hydroureter. In this stage the tumor extends beyond the bladder to the prostate and seminal vesicles.

An increased probability of tumor progression and subsequent recurrences is associated with a number of factors, including:

- large tumor size
- high-stage tumor
- high-grade tumor
- the presence of multiple tumors
- vascular or lymphatic invasion
- urothelial dysplasia, including carcinoma in situ

Overall, tumor progression has been reported in as many as 30% of patients who initially present with superficially invasive or noninvasive neoplasms.

Metastases of bladder carcinoma are most frequent in regional lymph nodes and periaortic lymph nodes, liver, lung, and bone, in order of decreasing frequency.

UNCOMMON HISTOLOGIC TYPES OF BLADDER CARCINOMA

Squamous Cell Carcinoma

In the United States, squamous cell carcinoma of the urinary bladder is distinctly uncommon. By contrast, the frequency of this histologic type is significantly higher in the Middle East, where it is epidemiologically related to the prevalence of schistosomiasis. **At the time of initial presentation, virtually all patients with squamous cell carcinoma demonstrate invasion of the bladder wall, and therefore have a poorer prognosis than those with transitional cell carcinoma.** Squamous metaplasia of the nontumorous vesical urothelium is common in cases of squamous cell carcinoma.

Adenocarcinoma

Adenocarcinoma is the third most frequent histologic type of bladder carcinoma, but is not often encountered. The diagnosis of this neoplasm requires its differentiation from those adenocarcinomas of either urachal or metastatic origin. Rare examples of primary vesical carcinoid tumor, small undifferentiated carcinomas, and malignant melanomas have been observed. Equally uncommon are mesenchymal neoplasms, most which are of smooth muscle origin. The urinary bladder is an infrequent site of metastatic tumor.

URETHRA

CONGENITAL DISORDERS

Congenital disorders of the urethra are uncommon, and include abnormalities of the location of the external urethral orifice: in **hypospadias** the urethra opens on the underside of the penis; in **epispadias** the urethra opens on the upper side of the penis.

INFLAMMATORY DISORDERS

Among the most frequently seen and clinically important inflammatory disorders of the urethra are those caused by *Neisseria gonorrhoeae* and *Chlamydia trachomatis*. The pathogenesis and pathologic features of these infections are discussed in Chapters 9 and 18.

CARUNCLES

Urethral caruncles are inflammatory lesions near the urethral meatus that produce pain and bleeding. They occur exclusively in women, most frequently after menopause. The etiology and pathogenesis are unclear, but prolapse of the urethral mucosa and associated chronic inflammation have been suggested.

The constant features of caruncles are intense acute and chronic inflammation involving the mucosa and lamina propria. The severe inflammation and associated stromal edema produce an exophytic polypoid mass. There is no evidence that a caruncle leads to subsequent urethral cancer.

EPITHELIAL NEOPLASMS

Carcinoma of the urethra is unusual, with a female predominance of 2:1. In order of decreasing frequency, squamous cell carcinoma, transitional cell carcinoma, adenocarcinoma, and malignant melanoma have been reported in the urethra.

The histologic type of urethral carcinoma can often be related to its site of origin. Transitional cell carcinomas tend to arise in the proximal urethra, squamous cell carcinomas in the distal urethra, and adenocarcinomas in the mid-urethra.

The majority of carcinomas of the urethra originate in the distal or anterior portion or, alternatively, involve the entire urethra at the time of presentation. In spite of the accessible location and associated symptoms of these neoplasms, the majority of urethral tumors have spread to adjacent tissues or metastasized to regional lymph nodes at the time of initial presentation.

TESTIS

CONGENITAL DISORDERS

Congenital disorders of the male gonads include abnormalities of location, number, and structure. With the exception of cryptorchidism, all are rare. Disorders of sexual differentiation are discussed in Chapter 6, which deals with genetic diseases.

CRYPTORCHIDISM

The failure of the testes to descend completely into their normal position within the scrotum is termed cryptorchidism. At term, 4% of male newborns demonstrate one or more cryptorchid testes. Spontaneous descent of the testis occurs in the vast majority of these infants within the first year of life. Cryptorchidism is most commonly unilateral and is usually an isolated anomaly. **It is associated with infertility and germ cell neoplasms** (Fig. 17-4), **and therefore requires therapy.**

The histologic changes observed in the cryptorchid testis are related to age. If orchiopexy (therapeutic repositioning of the testis) is delayed beyond puberty, a decreased number of germ cells, stromal fibrosis, and infertility are observed (Fig. 17-5). The earliest changes in the malpositioned testis, from birth to 5 years of age, are reduced diameters of the seminiferous tubules and decreased numbers of germ cells. Indeed, complete absence of germ cells has been observed in patients as young as 3 years of age.

The risk of developing germ cell tumors (most commonly seminomas and embryonal carcinomas) in cryptorchid testes is increased 35-fold. Virtually all patients who have developed germ cell tumors after orchiopexy had that operation postponed to age 10 years or later. Germ cell tumors have not been reported in patients in whom orchiopexy was performed before age 5.

INFERTILITY

Male infertility is broadly classified into pretesticular, testicular, and post-testicular causes. Primary testicular disorders are the most common, and post-testicular disorders the least common. Among the pretesticular causes are primary genetic, pituitary, and systemic metabolic disorders, including uremia, cirrhosis, and diabetes. Primary testicular disorders include Klinefelter's syndrome, varicocele, orchitis, and a variety of injurious physical and chemical agents, including heat, radiation, and exogenous drugs. Post-testicular causes of male infertility involve congenital and therapeutic obliteration of the epididymis or vas deferens, and retrograde ejaculation as a result of transurethral prostatic resection.

Infertile males may exhibit structural immaturity of the seminiferous tubules, hypospermatogenesis, germ cell maturation arrest, intratubular sloughing of germ cells, and peritubular or tubular fibrosis (see Fig. 17-5).

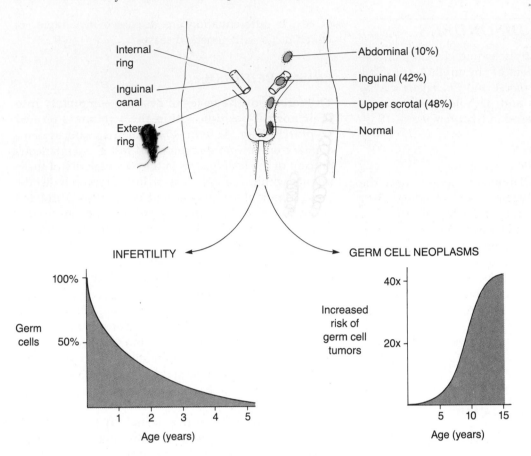

Figure 17-4. Cryptorchidism and associated complications. There is a 50% reduction in germ cell number after the first year of life and virtually a complete loss by 4 to 5 years of age. After age 5 the risk of germ cell tumors increases steeply.

Not uncommonly, mixed patterns of testicular abnormalities are observed. Alternatively, morphologic changes in the testis may be enigmatically absent.

INFLAMMATORY DISORDERS

Clinically, orchitis takes the form of acute and chronic inflammation, frequently in association with concurrent involvement of the ipsilateral epididymis. Most cases have an underlying gram-negative bacterial infection, frequently in association with urinary tract infection. Orchitis due to viral, fungal, or rickettsial organisms is less common. Testicular involvement by spirochetes in syphilis is discussed in Chapter 9.

The most common viral orchitis is caused by **mumps** and presents with pain and gonadal swelling, most often unilateral.

Chronic orchitis is uncommon, although gonadal involvement in tertiary syphilis, tuberculosis and a number of fungal infections is well documented.

TESTICULAR NEOPLASMS

GERM CELL NEOPLASMS

The histogenesis of germ cell neoplasms has been largely clarified as a result of experimental and morphologic studies. Cytologic atypism of germ cells in the context of cryptorchidism progresses to germ cell carcinoma in situ within the seminiferous tubules, an event followed by microinvasion.

The neoplastic transformation of a germ cell gives rise to either a seminoma (an undifferentiated germ cell neoplasm) or an embryonal carcinoma (a neo-

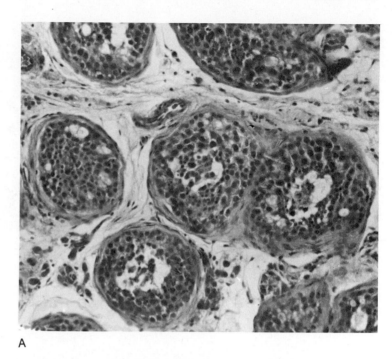

A

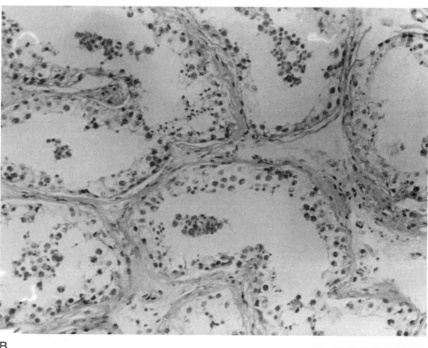

B

Figure 17-5. Histopathology of the testis in infertility. (*A*) Maturation arrest. The tubules contain only early stage germ cells. There is a complete absence of spermatids and spermatozoa. (*B*) Hypospermia. The number of germ cells is markedly reduced.

plasm of totipotential cells). **Embryonal carcinoma may undergo somatic differentiation and become a teratoma. Alternatively, extraembryonic differentiation results in a yolk sac tumor (entodermal sinus tumor) or a choriocarcinoma.** Direct transformation of cytologically malignant intratubular germ cells to each of these histologic types of germ cell neoplasms has been reported.

Three peak age groups for testicular germ cell tumors are observed: infants and children, men in the third and fourth decades, and men older than 50 years. **Infants and children are most commonly afflicted with yolk sac tumors and teratomas. Choriocarcinomas are more frequent in the second and third decades, embryonal carcinoma in the third decade, and seminoma in the fourth decade.**

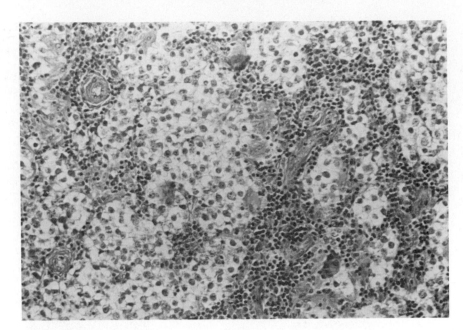

Figure 17-6. Classic seminoma. Nests of tumor cells are confined by fibrous septa containing numerous lymphocytes.

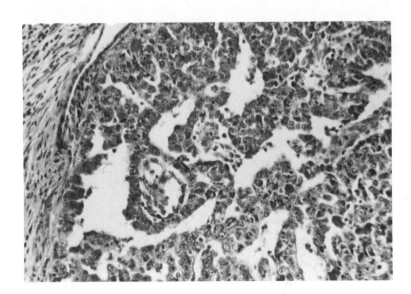

Figure 17-7. Embryonal carcinoma. A cystic space is lined and almost filled with carcinoma cells that lack distinct cell membranes.

Elevations of serum chorionic gonadotropin are typically found in patients with choriocarcinoma, while patients with elevations of α-fetoprotein are generally found to have yolk sac tumors or embryonal carcinomas with yolk sac components. Following orchiectomy, a fall in the serum levels of these tumor markers is observed, and tumor recurrences are frequently associated with a return of elevated serum levels of these same markers.

The clinical evolution of germ cell tumors is characterized by contiguous infiltration of the epididymis and metastatic spread, primarily to regional lymph nodes and subsequently to the lungs. In contrast to other germ cell tumors, choriocarcinoma disseminates primarily by hematogenous routes to the lung. In order of decreasing frequency, the retroperitoneal lymph nodes, lungs, liver, and mediastinal lymph nodes are most commonly involved by germ cell tumor metastases. Distant metastases are most often observed in the first 2 years following the initial diagnosis and surgical therapy. The histologic features of the metastatic tumor may be divergent from those observed in the primary gonadal neoplasm.

Germ cell neoplasms are solid intratesticular growths that tend to bulge from cut surface. Areas of cystic change are not prominent, except in teratomas. Variable amounts of necrosis, commonly with hemorrhage, are observed in virtually all germ cell tumors, especially the largest ones. In choriocarcinoma, hemorrhagic necrosis involves even small tumors. Germ cell tumors may invade the epididymis.

Seminomas display solid nests or cords of proliferating cells between randomly scattered, thin, fibrovascular trabeculae (Fig. 17-6). A lymphocytic infiltrate is usual in the septa, and noncaseating granulomas are occasionally present. The tumor cells, which have well-defined borders and clear cytoplasm, typically occur in solid sheets and show no tendency to form tubular, papillary, or grandular structures.

Embryonal Carcinomas

Embryonal carcinomas typically show variable histologic patterns, such as acinar, tubular, and papillary forms (Fig. 17-7). The cell borders are ill-defined, and the nuclei have prominent nucleoli and coarse chromatin. Variably extensive hemorrhage and necrosis are usual.

Teratomas

Teratomas are identified by the random admixture of tissues derived from the ectoderm, entoderm, and mesoderm (Fig. 17-8). Squamous epithelial mucosa is admixed with gastrointestinal or respiratory epithelium. Occasionally, thyroid and neural elements are also present. The background stroma may contain foci of cartilage, bone, and fat. **The morphologic features of teratomatous germ cell tumors are not directly related to their natural history.** Specifically, morphologically mature teratomas, which would ordinarily be interpreted as benign, commonly behave in a malignant manner and metastasize. By contrast, teratomas in infants and children, including those with foci of undifferentiated cells, are uniformly benign.

Yolk Sac Neoplasms

Yolk sac neoplasms, the most common germ cell tumor of infants, display a reticulated pattern of tumor cells with multiple microcysts and papillary clusters, all in a background of myxoid stroma. The tumor cells surround a characteristic structure, the Schiller-Duval body, which consists of a microcyst with a glomerulus-like structure containing a central fibrovascular core (Fig. 17-9). Immunoperoxidase stains identify α-fetoprotein within tumor cells. The descriptive names "entodermal sinus tumor" and "yolk sac tumor" reflect the histologic similarity of this neoplasm to the structure of the rat placenta.

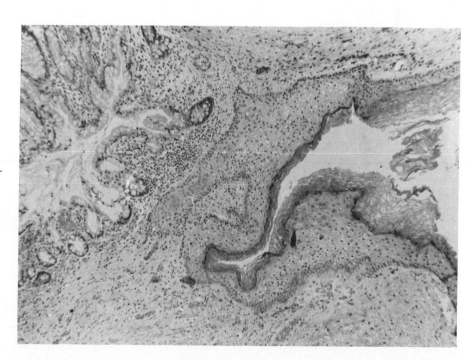

Figure 17-8. Teratoma. A cyst lined by well-differentiated squamous epithelium is in proximity to a focus of entodermal glands that resemble colonic mucosa.

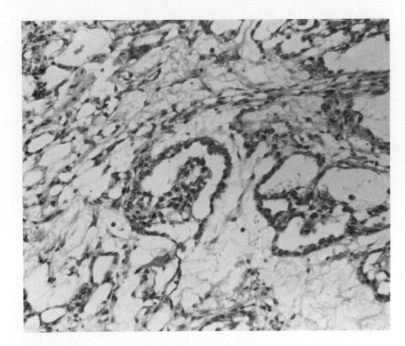

Figure 17-9. Yolk sac (entodermal sinus) tumor. The tumor is composed of dilated tubular spaces lined by flattened cells with an edematous stroma. A glomerulus-like structure is present at the center.

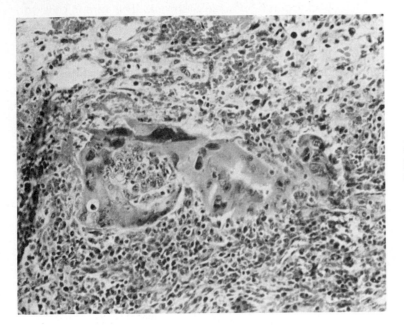

Figure 17-10. Choriocarcinoma. The syncytiotrophoblast cells surround a cluster of cytotrophoblast cells. Hemorrhage is evident in the adjacent tissue.

Choriocarcinomas

Choriocarcinomas, representing germ cell differentiation to an extraembryonic structure, namely the placenta, are composed of neoplastic syncytiotrophoblasts and cytotrophoblasts (Fig. 17-10). These tumors usually occur as a component of a mixed germ cell neoplasm. The characteristic multinucleated syncytiotrophoblasts are intimately admixed with clusters of cytotrophoblasts. Syncytiotrophoblasts stain positively for chorionic gonadotropin. The tumor cells are typically found in areas of extensive hemorrhage and necrosis.

Mixed Germ Cell Tumors

Mixed germ cell tumors, which exhibit more than one type of neoplastic germ cell, are common. There are more than a dozen possible combinations, but the most frequent are teratoma with embryonal carcinoma (teratocarcinoma) and teratoma with embryonal carcinoma and seminoma.

GONADAL STROMAL/SEX CORD TUMORS

Primary neoplasms of Sertoli, Leydig, granulosa, and theca cells constitute 5% to 6% of testicular tumors. These tumors may occur in "pure" form or as mixtures of neoplastic Sertoli and Leydig cells.

Leydig Cell Tumors

Leydig cell tumors are rare and occur in two age groups: boys younger than four years of age and men in the third to sixth decades. The endocrine effects from these interstitial cell (Leydig cell-derived) tumors in prepubertal children lead to precocious physical and sexual development. By contrast, feminization, such as gynecomastia, is observed in some adults with this tumor. Most cases (90%) are clinically benign.

Leydig cell tumors are well-circumscribed, and some appear encapsulated. The cut surface is yellow to brown. Microscopically, the tumor reveals sheets of polygonal cells with variably abundant eosinophilic or vacuolated cytoplasm

Sertoli Cell Tumors

Neoplasms of Sertoli cells are even more infrequent than those of Leydig cells, and 20% have been malignant. These tumors usually develop in the first four decades of life.

Sertoli cell neoplasms are well-circumscribed, solid, and yellow-gray. Microscopically, they demonstrate a tubular arrangement, with solid cords of cells and a fibrous trabecular framework.

TESTICULAR ADNEXA

TESTICULAR TUNICS

The most common cause of scrotal swelling is hydrocele, a collection of serous fluid in the scrotal sac (Fig. 17-11). Hydroceles are either congenital and associated with a patent processus vaginalis or acquired because of an inflammatory disorder, usually one that involves the epididymis and the testis. The complications of hydrocele include infection (vaginalitis) and hemorrhage (hematocele). Hydroceles are differentiated from **spermatoceles** (cystic enlargements of the epididymis) by the presence of sperm in the cyst fluid of the latter. **Varicoceles** are dilatations of tributaries of testicular veins, a disorder that may have a deleterious effect on fertility.

EPIDIDYMIS

Most cases of epididymitis in men younger than 35 years of age are due to *Neisseria gonorrhoeae* **and** *Chlamydia trachomatis;* **in older men** *Escherichia coli* **from associated urinary tract infections serves as the most common etiologic agent. Epididymal inflammation caused by** *N. gonorrhoeae* **is a common cause of male infertility.**

Spermatic granulomas result from an intense inflammatory response to sperm that have gained entrance to the interstitium of the epididymis. Histologically, a mixed inflammatory cell infiltrate is associated with numerous extravasated sperm fragments and phagocytosis of sperm by histiocytes. Ultimately the inflammatory process results in interstitial fibrosis and ductal obstruction.

PROSTATE

PROSTATITIS

Acute prostatitis characteristically presents as intense discomfort on urination and is associated with fever, chills, and perineal pain. Gram-negative bacteria, especially *E. coli,* are the most common etiologic agents. The pathogenesis of most prostatic infections is thought to involve reflux of the infected urine into the prostatic ducts.

CHRONIC PROSTATITIS

Beyond the impression that chronic prostatitis represents a failure of acute prostatitis to resolve, the understanding of this disorder is limited. It is most common in men older than 50 years, but has been reported in virtually all age groups. Gram-negative cocci are implicated most frequently, but some investigators have claimed gram-positive cocci to be the most common etiologic agents. The pathogenesis of chronic prostatitis involves reflux of infected urine into the prostatic ducts. Additional factors such as prostatic calculi, local prostatic duct obstruction, and regional vascular abnormalities may all contribute to the perpetuation of the infection.

NONSPECIFIC GRANULOMATOUS PROSTATITIS

The symptoms of chronic nonspecific granulomatous prostatitis are vague, and the diagnosis is made histologically. The pathogenesis is not understood but may involve an inflammatory reaction to inspissated secre-

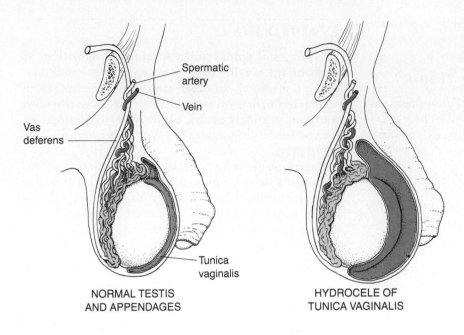

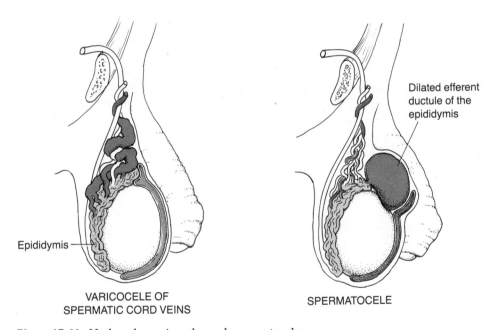

Figure 17-11. Hydrocele, varicocele, and spermatocele.

tions or bacterial products, reflecting localized prostatic duct obstruction. Histologically, noncaseating granulomas are associated with localized destruction of prostatic ducts and acini.

NODULAR PROSTATIC HYPERPLASIA

INCIDENCE AND EPIDEMIOLOGY

Three epidemiologic factors—geography, race, and age—are related to the incidence of prostatic hyperplasia. Prostatic hyperplasia is least frequent in the Orient and most frequent in Western Europe. The prevalence of this disorder in the United States is intermediate between these two extremes, with a higher frequency among American blacks than whites. The peak age of patients with **clinical** prostatism is the seventh decade. By contrast, autopsy studies show no such peak in the age distribution, but rather a progressive increase in frequency with age. The incidence of prostatic hyperplasia in all age groups is far greater at autopsy than is suggested by clinically apparent prostatism (Fig. 17-12). **About 75% of men 80 years of age or older have prostatic hyperplasia, but the disorder is rarely observed in men younger than 40 years of age.**

PATHOGENESIS

It has been postulated that stromal–epithelial interactions ultimately give rise to the hyperplastic nodules, although it is not clear whether the stroma induces the epithelial proliferation or vice versa. Pure stromal hyperplasia in a nodular configuration and virtually pure epithelial nodules are both observed, and a relationship between the two remains speculative.

Although the role of testosterone in the hormonal regulation of prostatic growth is well documented, its role in the pathogenesis of prostatic hyperplasia is less clear. Exogenous testosterone has no observable effect on the histologic appearance of hyperplastic nodules. On the other hand, prostatic hyperplasia has been produced in dogs by the administration of dihydrotestosterone. Serum levels of estrogen increase with advancing age in men, but its role, if any, in the production of prostatic hyperplasia is not understood.

PATHOLOGY

Early nodular hyperplasia occurs in the periurethral submucosa of the proximal urethra, recently described as the transitional zone. The developing nodules distort and compress the centrally located urethral lumen and the more peripherally located normal prostate. In examples of well developed nodular hyperplasia, the normal prostate is limited to an attenuated rim of tissue beneath the prostatic capsule. Each nodule is clearly demarcated from adjacent nodules and from normal prostate by an enveloping fibrous pseudocapsule. On cut section, secondary changes of focal hemorrhage and infarction may be present, especially in the larger nodules. The secondary changes resulting from prostatism are related to bladder outlet obstruction (Fig. 17-13).

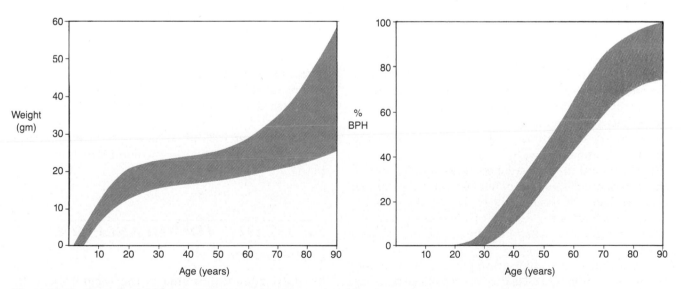

Figure 17-12. Growth of the prostate (*left*) and frequency of nodular hyperplasia (*right*). By 80 years of age, most men have benign prostatic hyperplasia.

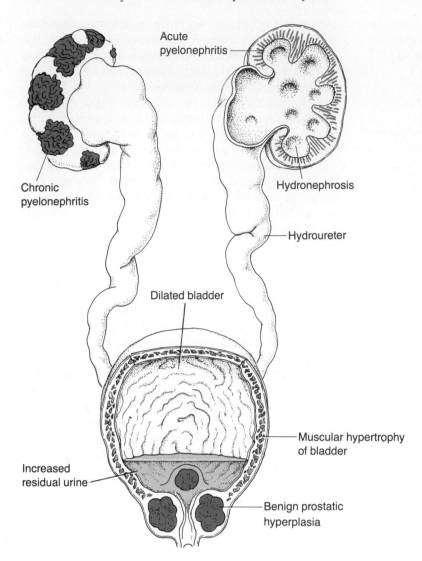

Figure 17-13. Complications of benign prostatic hyperplasia.

Histologically, nodular hyperplasia reflects the proliferation of epithelial cells of the acini and ductules, the smooth muscle cells, and the stromal fibroblasts— all in variable proportions. Five types of nodules have been described: stromal (fibrous), fibromuscular, muscular, fibroadenomatous, and fibromyoadenomatous (the most common type).

In the typical fibromyoadenomatous nodule, the epithelial (adenomatous) component reveals tall columnar cells overlying the basal cell layer. This epithelium lines acini of various sizes—some of microcystic proportions. Intraglandular papillary hyperplasia is characteristic.

The stroma of each type of nodule differs in composition, but common to all is the absence of elastic tissue. The proportion of stroma and glandular epithelium varies over a wide spectrum, with some nodules com-

posed exclusively of fibrous tissue and intermixed smooth muscle. The glands of the uninvolved peripheral region of the prostate are frequently atrophic and compressed by the expanding nodules.

Incidental foci of prostatic adenocarcinoma are found in about 10% of surgical specimens submitted with the preoperative diagnosis of prostatic hyperplasia.

PROSTATIC ADENOCARCINOMA

EPIDEMIOLOGY

Prostatic adenocarcinoma is the second most frequent cancer in American men, among whom it causes an estimated 26,000 deaths yearly. The effect of age, geography, and race on the frequency of prostatic carcinoma has been extensively documented. **It is a disease of elderly men; patients younger than 50 years of age constitute less than 1% of cases of prostatic carcinoma in the United States.** At the age of 50 years the estimated lifetime probability of developing clinically apparent prostatic carcinoma is about 10% for American men. **The mortality rate from prostatic carcinoma among black American men is among the highest observed in the world, significantly exceeding that of white Americans.** Approximately 75% of all patients with clinically diagnosed prostatic carcinoma are 60 to 79 years old. The true frequency of prostatic carcinoma is significantly higher than that indicated by the clinical frequency and is shown in autopsy studies. The term "latent carcinoma" has been applied to clinically undetected carcinomas, which constitute 67% to 94% of all prostatic carcinomas. **The incidence of prostatic carcinoma at autopsy progressively increases, rising from less than 10% among men 40 to 50 years of age to between one-third and one-half of men over the age of 80 years.**

ETIOLOGY AND PATHOGENESIS

The etiology of prostatic adenocarcinoma is unknown, but the principal focus of research interest is directed toward endocrine influences. The hormonal (testosterone) control of normal prostatic growth and the responsiveness of primary and metastatic carcinomas to therapeutic castration and exogenous estrogens provide supportive evidence for a role of hormones in the production of prostatic adenocarcinoma. Unfortunately, despite considerable research, these empirical observations are not matched by a corresponding increase in our understanding of the role of hormones. Attempts to demonstrate higher levels of serum androgens in patients with prostatic carcinoma have not yielded consistent results. Elevated urinary estrone/androsterone ratios have been reported in patients with prostatic carcinoma.

HISTOGENESIS

Currently, most investigators believe that the most probable source of prostatic adenocarcinoma resides in foci of hyperplastic acinar cells in otherwise atrophic peripheral glands. Occasionally, such hyperplastic foci demonstrate atypical cytologic features.

PATHOLOGY

Prostatic adenocarcinomas, which account for 98% of all primary prostatic tumors, are most commonly lo- **cated in the peripheral zones.** These neoplasms are commonly multicentric. The cut surface of the prostate characteristically shows irregular, yellow-white, indurated subcapsular nodules. Characteristically, the best-differentiated tumors show uniform medium- or small-sized glands (Fig. 17-14). **Most glands are lined by a single layer of uniform neoplastic epithelial cells.** Progressive loss of differentiation of prostatic adenocarcinomas is characterized by increasing variability of gland size and configuration and by intraglandular patterns of epithelial proliferation. The majority of prostatic adenocarcinomas of acinar origin are well-differentiated.

The spectrum of differentiation is expressed in a grading system that has prognostic value and is based primarily on an assessment of the degree of differentiation of the tumor glands. Cytologic features, which are not included in the criteria for grading, also exhibit a spectrum, from minimal to marked nuclear pleomorphism and hyperchromatism. One or two prominent nucleoli in the background of chromatin clumped near the nuclear membrane is the most frequent nuclear feature. The cytoplasm may be vacuolated and may simulate the clear cell variety of renal cell carcinoma, or it may stain as lightly eosinophilic. Cell borders are distinct in the better-differentiated tumors, but are indistinct in the more poorly differentiated examples. **A single layer of cuboidal cells in neoplastic acini is, from a practical standpoint, the most frequently employed criterion to establish the diagnosis of prostatic adenocarcinoma.**

EXTRAPROSTATIC SPREAD OF PROSTATIC ADENOCARCINOMA

The high frequency of invasion of the prostatic capsule observed with adenocarcinoma is related to the high frequency of its subcapsular location. In both intraprostatic and periprostatic locations, **perineural invasion by this neoplasm is usual.**

Contiguous invasion of the seminal vesicles by direct extension is common. Direct invasion of the urinary bladder is less frequent until late in the clinical course.

Wide dissemination of prostatic carcinoma is characteristic at the time of death. Accumulating evidence from surgical staging procedures suggests that the earliest metastases occur in the obturator lymph node. Subsequent lymphatic dissemination involves the iliac and periaortic lymph nodes. Metastases to the lung result from further lymphatic spread through the thoracic duct and, independently, through venous dissemination via the prostatic venous plexus and the inferior vena cava.

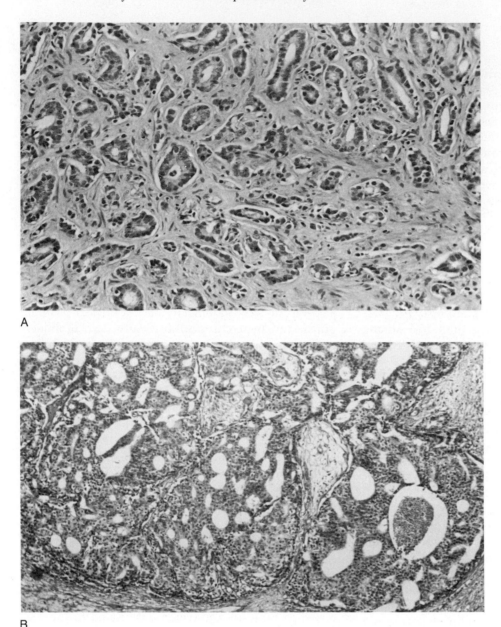

A

B

Figure 17-14. Adenocarcinoma of the prostate. (*A*) Neoplastic glands lined by a single layer of tumor cells are separated by stroma infiltrated by tumor cells. (*B*) Large nests of tumor cells have a cribriform arrangement.

NATURAL HISTORY

Stage A carcinomas are detected as incidental microscopic foci in clinically benign specimens of prostatic tissue (Fig. 17-15). Substage A1 is the appropriate designation when the tumor foci are focal; if a high proportion of prostatic chips contain tumor, it is designated stage A2. Tumor associated with clinically palpable nodules but still confined to the prostate is termed clinical stage B. Again, focal lesions are stage B1, and if more than one lobe of the prostate is involved, the stage is B2. Stage C is the term applied to prostatic neoplasms that demonstrate local invasion beyond the prostatic capsule, but in which there are no metastases to regional lymph nodes or distant sites. Stage D represents those cases that have metastasized to regional pelvic lymph nodes (D1) or exhibit distant metastases (D2). **About 25% of prostatic carcinomas are detected at the time of microscopic examination of clinically benign prostate tissue (stage A). An additional 30% of patients present with a clinically detectable prostatic nodule identified by rectal examination.** About 15% of patients have clinical evidence of local spread (stage C) at the time of initial presentation, and the remaining 30% suffer from regional or distant metastases.

Understaging a diagnosis of prostatic carcinoma is a much more common problem than the reverse. It is difficult to detect intraprostatic carcinoma by rectal examination. Furthermore, the ability to detect extraprostatic spread (stage C) by rectal examination has been only recently surpassed by radiologic evaluation (CT scan). The more recently developed bone scanning techniques have significantly improved the accuracy of staging of patients with bone metastases.

At the time of autopsy, metastases of prostatic carcinoma are observed in the lymph nodes, bones, lung, and liver, in order of frequency. Widespread dissemination of the tumor (carcinomatosis), frequently with terminal pneumonia or sepsis, is the most common cause of death.

PENIS

The disorders of the penis of greatest clinical frequency are sexually transmitted inflammatory disorders and

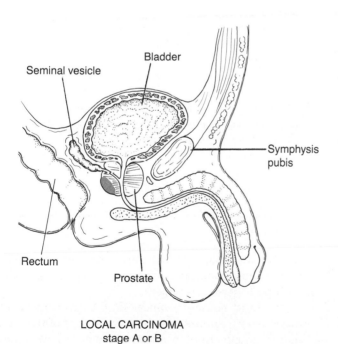

LOCAL CARCINOMA
stage A or B

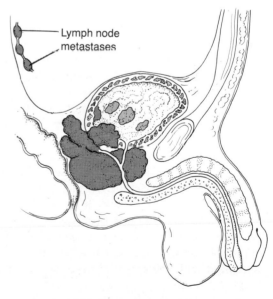

EXTENSIVE CARCINOMA
stage C or D

Figure 17-15. Clinical staging of prostatic carcinoma. In stages A and B the tumor is confined to the prostate. In stage C the carcinoma has extended beyond the prostatic capsule to involve adjacent structures. Lymph node or distant metastases are present in stage D.

epithelial neoplasms, principally squamous cell carcinoma in the latter category. Balanoposthitis (inflammation of the glans and prepuce) is usually associated with congenital or acquired **phimosis,** which is the inability to retract the prepuce because of an abnormally small preputial orifice. Circumcision is effective therapy for phimosis and the complication of balanoposthitis.

SEXUALLY TRANSMITTED INFLAMMATORY LESIONS

Sexually transmitted inflammatory lesions of the penis include syphilis, chancroid, granuloma inguinale, lymphogranuloma inguinale, and genital herpes. The causative agents, pathogenesis, and histologic features are discussed in detail in Chapter 9.

The vesicular lesions caused by herpesvirus type II contrast with the epithelial proliferative lesion—wart-like exophytic proliferations—caused by the human papillomavirus in cases of condyloma acuminatum.

NEOPLASTIC DISORDERS

Squamous cell carcinoma in situ has been described in three clinical pathologic variants: Bowen's disease, erythroplasia of Queyrat, and the more recently described Bowenoid papulosis. Whether Bowen's disease and erythroplasia of Queyrat indeed represent two separate nosologic entities remains a matter of debate. The clinical distinctiveness of Bowenoid papulosis is unquestioned.

In contrast to the average age of 50 years of Bowen's disease and erythroplasia of Queyrat, Bowenoid papulosis occurs in men two decades younger. In addition, Bowenoid papulosis presents as multiple violet papules in the penile shaft. Bowen's disease and erythroplasia of Queyrat usually involve the glans penis.

The frequency with which Bowen's disease and erythroplasia of Queyrat progress to invasive squamous cell carcinoma remains unsettled. To date no examples of invasive squamous cell carcinoma have been associated with the reported cases of Bowenoid papulosis.

SQUAMOUS CELL CARCINOMA OF THE PENIS

The frequency of penile squamous cell carcinoma shows a marked geographic variation, with the highest incidence observed in Asian countries, Africa, and Central America. The lesion is uncommon in the United States. This variation in frequency has been associated with personal, social, and religious practices, including personal hygiene and the practice of circumcision. Fewer than 10 cases of penile cancer have been reported in men who were circumcised at birth. The average age of patients is approximately 60 years.

The etiology of this skin cancer remains unknown. Possible contributions of viruses or smegma in the causation of penile cancer are currently unknown.

Clinically, squamous cell carcinoma of the penis is found on the glans or the prepuce, and presents as an ulcerated and hemorrhagic mass. The typical squamous cell carcinoma of the glans penis may evidence both exophytic and infiltrating characteristics. Microscopically, the typical features of a well-differentiated, focally keratinizing squamous cell carcinoma are observed. An invasive tumor is associated with a dense, chronic inflammatory cell infiltrate in the adjacent dermis, which may show dysplastic changes. The tumor may invade deeply and extensively along the penile shaft.

The ultimate prognosis is closely related to the extent of tumor growth at the time of primary surgical excision and to the presence of lymphatic or vascular invasion. Although most penile squamous cell carcinomas are confined to the penis at the time of initial presentation, occult metastases to inguinal lymph nodes are not uncommon. Conversely, half of the patients with clinically enlarged regional lymph nodes have no nodal metastases, but rather reactive changes secondary to the inflammation associated with the primary penile tumor.

The natural history of penile squamous cell carcinoma is dissemination to the inguinal lymph nodes, followed by further spread to the iliac lymph nodes, and ultimately widespread distant metastases. The overall 5-year survival is 65% to 75%.

SCROTUM

Inflammatory disorders of the scrotum are generally of minor clinical significance and are usually associated with poor personal hygiene.

The most common cancer of the scrotum is squamous cell carcinoma. The high frequency of this malignancy among chimney sweeps was originally reported in 1775 by Sir Percival Pott, who is considered by many to be the father of occupational medicine. Pott implicated constant exposure to soot as the causative agent of the scrotal skin tumors. That coal miners did not show the high frequency of scrotal carcinoma observed among chimney sweeps suggested that the carcinogen was produced in the combustion of coal. Indeed, numerous carcinogens were subsequently identified in soot.

Squamous cell carcinoma of the scrotum is most frequently seen in men in their sixth and seventh decades. The lesion is usually single and limited to one side of the scrotal sac, commonly the anterior inferior surface. Typically, the lesion is well-differentiated. At the time of initial clinical presentation, many patients demonstrate invasion and metastases beyond the scrotum, principally to the regional inguinal or ilioinguinal lymph nodes.

18

GYNECOLOGIC PATHOLOGY

STANLEY J. ROBBOY, MAIRE A. DUGGAN,
ROBERT J. KURMAN

INFECTIOUS DISORDERS

Infectious disorders of the female genital tract are common and caused by a wide variety of pathogenic organisms (Table 18-1). Most of these pathogens are acquired during sexual intercourse, and collectively the resulting diseases are called "sexually transmitted diseases."

SEXUALLY TRANSMITTED DISEASES

BACTERIA

Gardnerella Infection (G. vaginalis)

G. vaginalis, **a sexually transmitted, gram-negative coccobacillus, accounts for 90% of cases of nonspe-** **cific vaginitis.** A biopsy specimen is usually normal, because the organism neither penetrates the mucosa nor elicits an inflammatory reaction.

Gonorrhea (Neisseria gonorrhoeae)

N. gonorrhoeae, a fastidious, gram-negative diplococcus, is the causative organism of gonorrhea. **It is a frequent cause of acute salpingitis and pelvic inflammatory disease.**

The organism adheres to the mucous membranes of the lower genital tract and reaches the tubal lumen directly by ascending the cervical and endometrial cavities (Fig. 18-1) In the fallopian tube the organism elicits a pronounced, acute, fibrinous, inflammatory reaction. The infection may spread to involve the ovary, a course that results in a tubo-ovarian abscess. It may also spread more widely to involve the pelvic and abdominal cavities, with the formation of subdiaphragmatic

Table 18-1   Infectious Diseases of the Female Genital Tract

Organism	Disease	Distinctive Feature
Sexually Transmitted Diseases		
GRAM-NEGATIVE RODS AND COCCI		
Calymmatobacterium granulomatis	Granuloma inguinale	Donovan body
Gardnerella vaginalis	Gardnerella infection	Clue cell
Haemophilus ducreyi	Chancroid (soft chancre)	
Neisseria gonorrhoeae	Gonorrhea	
THE SPIROCHETES		
Treponema pallidum	Syphilis	
THE MYCOPLASMAS		
Mycoplasma hominis	Nonspecific vaginitis	
Ureaplasma urealyticum	Nonspecific vaginitis	
THE RICKETTSIAS		
Chlamydia trachomatis, types D-K	Various forms of PID*	
Chlamydia trachomatis, type L (1–23)	Lymphogranuloma venereum	
VIRUSES		
Papilloma virus	Condyloma acuminatum	Koilocyte
Herpes simplex, type 2	Herpes infection	Multicleate giant cell
Molluscum contagiosum	Molluscum infection	Molluscum body
Cytomegalovirus	Cytomegalic inclusion disease	
PROTOZOA		
Trichomonas vaginalis	Trichomoniasis	
Selected Non-Sexually Transmitted Diseases		
GRAM-POSITIVE BACTERIA		
Staphylococcus aureus	Toxic shock syndrome	
THE ACTINOMYCES AND RELATED ORGANISMS		
Actinomyces israelii	PID (one of many organisms)	Sulfur granules
Mycobacterium tuberculosis	Tuberculosis	Necrotizing granulomas
FUNGI		
Candida albicans	Candidiasis	

* PID, pelvic inflammatory disease.

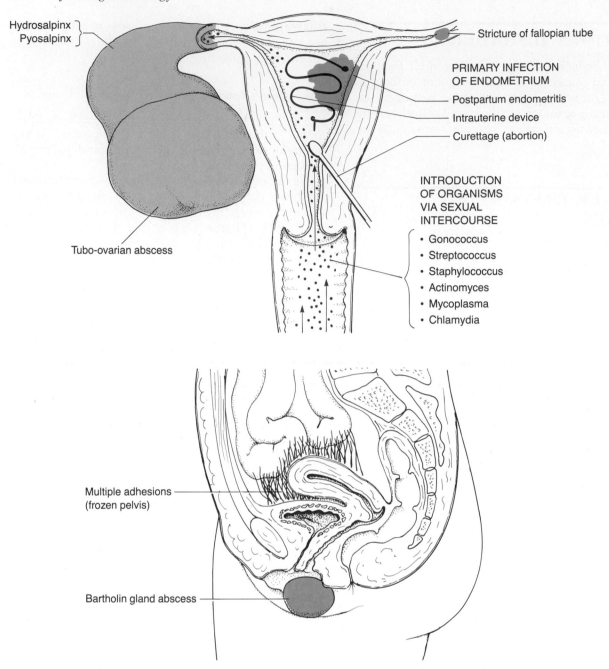

Figure 18-1. Pelvic inflammatory disease.

and pelvic abscesses. **Healing, with distortion and destruction of the tubal epithelium, often leads to sterility.**

THE SPIROCHETES

Syphilis (Treponema pallidum)

Syphilis is a venereal disease caused by *T. pallidum*, a thin, motile, spiral-shaped (spirochete) bacterium. It is acquired through sexual contact with an infected indi-

vidual or *in utero* (congenital syphilis). Untreated syphilis may progress through three stages: primary, secondary, and tertiary (early, infectious, and late syphilis, respectively).

The initial manifestation, the chancre, usually appears at the portal of entry after an incubation period of about 3 weeks. Initially, this lesion is a painless, indurated papule, 1 cm to 2 cm in diameter, surrounded by an inflammatory cuff, which breaks down to form an ulcer. The chancre may persist for 2 to 6 weeks and then heals spontaneously. The secondary stage, which appears after a latent period of several weeks to several months, is characterized by low-grade fever, headache, malaise, lymphadenopathy, and the reappearance of highly contagious syphilitic lesions called condylomata lata (syphilitic warts). After 2 to 6 weeks, the secondary infectious lesions heal and the symptoms disappear spontaneously. Any time thereafter, the tertiary stage, complicated by cardiovascular and nervous system involvement, may develop.

RICKETTSIA

Chlamydia

C. trachomatis, a rickettsial organism, is a common venereally transmitted organism. In genital infections, the cervical mucosa is inflamed and the endocervical metaplastic squamous cells reveal small inclusion bodies. Complications include ascending infection of the endometrium, fallopian tube, and ovary, with consequent pelvic inflammatory disease, tubal occlusion, and infertility.

VIRUSES

Condyloma Acuminatum (Human Papilloma Virus)

The human papilloma virus is a DNA virus. Over 40 types are recognized, five of which are associated with genital tract disease. Types 6 and 11 are usually seen with **condyloma acuminatum** (veneral warts), lesions that are being increasingly recognized as a **common form of sexually transmitted disease**. Of particular concern with these diseases is their **association with and possible etiologic role in the development of cervical dysplasia, carcinoma in situ, and squamous cell carcinoma.** Types 16, 18, and 31 have been found in the vast majority of high-grade precancerous lesions and invasive carcinomas (see below).

Condylomas, which are entirely benign, occur on the vulva, perianal region, perineum, vagina, and cervix, and may involve the distal urethra and rectum. They grow as papules, plaques, or nodules and eventually as spiked or cauliflower-like excrescences. The most striking finding on microscopic examination is a papillomatous proliferation of squamous epithelium. The characteristic epithelial cell is the koilocyte, a cell with a wrinkled nucleus that contains viral particles and a prominent, perinuclear clear space. The morpholgic changes of condyloma are common in dysplastic epithelial cells of the lower genital tract. The presence of viral DNA sequences in the preneoplastic lesions, in cancers, and even in the metastases of squamous cell cancers provides strong evidence of an etiologic role of the **papilloma virus in the development of cancer of the cervix, vagina, and vulva** (see below).

Herpes Simplex (H. Simplex, Type 2)

Herpes simplex, serotype 2, an intranuclear, double-stranded DNA virus, is a common cause of sexually transmitted, genital infection. After an incubation period of 1 to 3 weeks, many small vesicles develop on the vulva, vagina, and cervix. The vesicles develop into painful ulcers. In the latent state the virus remains in the sacral ganglia. Characteristic cytologic features include multinucleated giant cells and, occasionally, large nuclei with eosinophilic inclusions. Intraepithelial vesicles show ballooning degeneration of the adjacent epithelial cells, many of which contain large nuclei with eosinophilic inclusions. Complications include a **possible oncogenic role in the development of cervical cancer** (see below) and transmission of the virus to the neonate during birth. **Neonatal infection is often fatal.**

PROTOZOA

Trichomoniasis (Trichomonas vaginalis)

T. vaginalis is a large, pear-shaped, flagellated protozoan that is **a common cause of vaginitis.** The disease is sexually transmitted; about 25% of women are asymptomatic carriers. The infection presents as a heavy, yellow-gray, thick, foamy discharge accompanied by severe itching, dyspareunia (painful intercourse), and dysuria (painful urination).

DISEASES NOT TRANSMITTED SEXUALLY

BACTERIA

Toxic Shock Syndrome (Staphylococcus aureus)

The toxic shock syndrome was first identified in 1978 in women using tampons. Symptoms include high fever, vomiting, diarrhea, a diffuse rash, and shock. At the peak incidence of the disease in 1980, 90% occurred in women at the time of menstruation. The fatality rate is about 6%. *S. aureus* colonizes the damaged vaginal mucosa and releases exotoxins that are responsible for the major manifestation of the syndrome. Pathologic features include perivasculitis in many organs and changes associated with shock.

FUNGI

Candidiasis (Candida albicans)

Approximately 10% of women are asymptomatic carriers of vulvovaginal fungi, *C. albicans* being the most common. About 1% to 2% of nonpregnant and 5% to 10% of pregnant women present with clinically apparent vulvovaginitis. Pregnancy, diabetes mellitus, and the use of oral contraceptives promote vaginal candidiasis.

DISEASES OF MULTIPLE CAUSES (POLYMICROBIAL)

PELVIC INFLAMMATORY DISEASE

Pelvic inflammatory disease (PID) describes an infectious process of the pelvis and pelvic organs that usually follows extension of bacteria present in the vagina at the time of the menses (see Fig. 18-2). *N. gonorrhoeae* is the principal single organism causing PID, but most infections are polymicrobial. Infection with chlamydia, which is typically silent, is one of the most common infectious causes of infertility due to tubal damage. In the later stages of PID, the ovaries may become involved with abscess formation. Rupture of a tubo-ovarian abscess is a life-threatening complication.

VULVA

DYSTROPHY

Dystrophy, a term that refers to a group of lesions **without malignant potential,** is defined as a disorder of epithelial growth that often presents as a white lesion of the vulva.

Hyperplastic dystrophy is characterized by a proliferation of squamous epithelium (acanthosis) that results in enlargement and confluence of the epidermal rete ridges. Commonly, the thickened epithelium displays a marked increase in superficial keratin, a condition called hyperkeratosis. Biopsy is required to distinguish hyperplastic dystrophy, which is benign, from dysplasia and carcinoma.

Lichen sclerosis is characterized by hyperkeratosis, blunting or loss of rete ridges, and a homogeneous, acellular, subepithelial zone. This acellular zone results from swelling and splitting of the collagen bundles into individual fibers and fibrils, which become enveloped by a gel-like matrix. A band of chronic inflammatory cells typically lies beneath this layer. Itching is the most common symptom, and dyspareunia is often troublesome. There is no association with cancer.

CYSTS

BARTHOLIN'S GLAND CYST The paired Bartholin's glands produce a clear mucoid secretion that continuously lubricates the vestibular surface. The ducts are prone to obstruction and consequent cyst formation. The cysts may become infected, which leads to the formation of abscesses.

MALIGNANT TUMORS AND PREMALIGNANT CONDITIONS

SQUAMOUS CELL LESIONS

Dysplasia and Carcinoma in Situ

The epidemiologic characteristics of patients with vulvar intraepithelial neoplasia and cancer are similar to those of women with cervical intraepithelial neoplasia and cancer, an association that suggests that a venereally transmitted agent may play a role in the genesis of squamous neoplasia in both sites. Papilloma virus, usually HPV-16, is found in over 80% of the lesions of vulvar intraepithelial neoplasia. Following local excision, dysplasia often persists or recurs (25%) or progresses to invasive carcinoma involving the vulva, vagina, or anus (20%).

Squamous Cell Carcinoma

Squamous cell carcinoma of the vulva (Fig. 18-2) accounts for 3% of all genital cancers in women and is **the most common primary malignant neoplasm of the vulva (90%).** The tumors grow slowly, extend to the contiguous skin, vagina, and rectum, and metastasize to inguinal, femoral, and pelvic lymph nodes.

Patients with involvement of the pelvic lymph nodes have a 5-year survival rate of less than 25%. When only the inguinal nodes are involved, the survival rate is 65%. The survival rate approaches 90% when the nodes are uninvolved.

Tumors invasive to less than 5 mm have an 11% rate of metastasis. Tumors with a depth of invasion of 1 mm or less have virtually no metastatic potential.

Verrucous carcinoma is a distinct variety of squamous cell carcinoma that presents a large fungating mass, resembling a giant condyloma acuminatum. The tumor is usually well differentiated, being composed of large nests of squamous cells with copious cytoplasm and relatively small, bland nuclei. Squamous pearls are uncommon and mitoses are rare. **This**

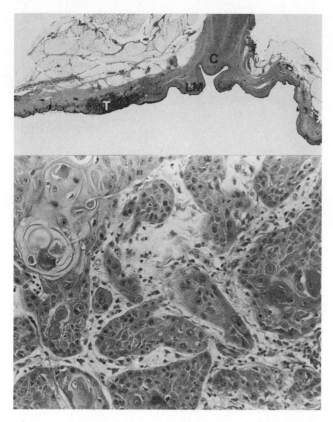

Figure 18-2. Squamous cell carcinoma of the vulva. (*Top*) A 1-cm tumor (*T*) confined to the dermis. The specimen shows left and right halves of the perineum, including the labia minora (*LM*) and clitoris (*C*). (*Bottom*) Small nests of neoplastic squamous cells, some with keratin pearls, invade the stroma.

cancer typically invades locally but does not metastasize. Wide local surgical excision is the treatment of choice.

PAGET'S DISEASE

Paget's disease is primarily an integumentary neoplasm found in the milk line, from the axilla to the vulva. It occurs most often in the nipple, where it is almost always associated with an underlying ductal adenocarcinoma. In the vulva, Paget cells arise de novo in the epidermis or in epidermally derived adnexal structures, but the exact cell origin is still unknown. Paget's disease of the vulva is an intraepithelial neoplasm that may become invasive. Paget cells are usually confined to the epidermis and appear as large single cells or, less commonly, as clusters of cells that lack intercellular bridges and have a pale, vacuolated cytoplasm. **Paget's disease is often far more extensive than is apparent on preoperative biopsy. Treatment requires wide local excision with generous borders or simple vulvectomy.**

VAGINA

NON-NEOPLASTIC CONDITIONS

SENILE ATROPHIC VAGINITIS

Senile atrophic vaginitis is a superimposed **secondary infection of an atrophic squamous epithelium, a consequence of postmenopausal estrogen deficiency.** The epithelium becomes thin and, as a result, a poor barrier to infection or abrasion. Common symptoms are dyspareunia or vaginal spotting.

VAGINAL ADENOSIS AND SQUAMOUS METAPLASIA (DES-RELATED CHANGES)

Exposure during prenatal life to diethylstilbesterol (DES) is associated with the subsequent development of clear cell adenocarcinoma of the vagina, adenosis (presence of glandular tissue in the vagina), squamous metaplasia, cervical ectropion, gross structural changes in both the vagina and cervix, and upper genital tract abnormalities. It has been estimated that up to two million women were exposed *in utero* between 1940 and 1971; the vast majority were exposed during the 1940s and 1950s. In addition to the DES-related cases, adenosis has been also found on occasion in older women who were born before the DES era.

The lesions of adenosis are composed of one of two types of cells: mucinous columnar cells that resemble the normal cells lining the endocervix, and cells that resemble the normal ones lining the endometrium or fallopian tube (Fig. 18-3).

BENIGN TUMORS AND TUMOR-LIKE CONDITIONS

MALIGNANT TUMORS

Primary malignant tumors of the vagina are rare, constituting less than 2% of all genital tract tumors. Most

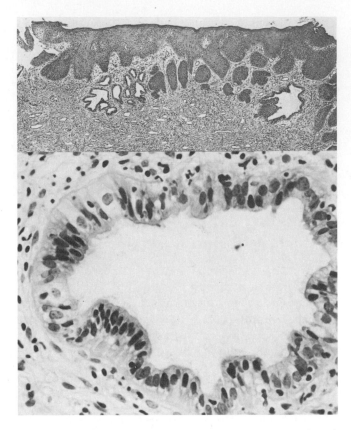

Figure 18-3. Vaginal adenosis. (*Top*) Glands lined by ciliated dark cells resembling tubal or endometrial epithelium are present in the inflamed lamina propria. In areas outside the photograph they merge with the squamous pegs. The surface epithelium is composed of glycogen-free squamous cells, which account for the abnormal iodine staining. (*Bottom*) Higher-power view of the epithelial cells.

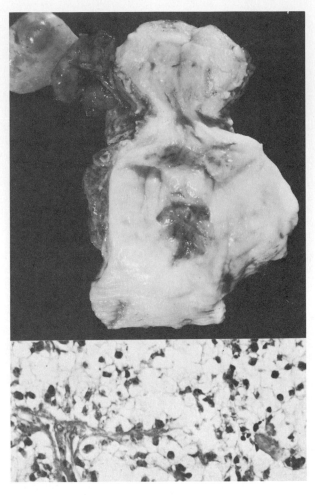

Figure 18-4. Clear cell adenocarcinoma of the vagina (*top*). Microscopic pattern of clear cell tumor (*bottom*).

are squamous cell carcinomas, and the prognosis is related to the clinical stage of the tumor. It is a disease of older women, the peak incidence lying between the ages of 60 and 70 years.

Clear Cell Adenocarcinoma

Approximately 0.1% of women exposed *in utero* to DES develop **clear cell adenocarcinoma,** most frequently on the anterior wall of the upper third of the vagina (Fig. 18-4). The tumor rarely appears before age 13 and is most common between ages 17 and 22. **Although almost all clear cell adenocarcinomas are associated with vaginal adenosis, very few women with adenosis develop this cancer.**

CERVIX

INFLAMMATORY DISEASE

Acute and chronic cervicitis result from infection by any number of microorganisms, particularly *Streptococcus, Staphylococcus,* or *Enterococcus,* and, less commonly, *Neisseria gonorrhoeae* and *Chlamydia trachomatis.* Some of these microorganisms are sexually transmitted, whereas others may be introduced by foreign bodies, such as residual fragments of tampons and pessaries. Purulent, malodorous vaginal discharge is a clinical sign of acute cervicitis.

BENIGN TUMORS AND TUMORLIKE CONDITIONS

ENDOCERVICAL POLYP

The endocervical polyp is the most common cervical growth. It often presents with vaginal bleeding or discharge and appears as a single, smooth, or lobulated mass, typically less than 3 cm in diameter. The lining epithelium is mucinous, with varying degrees of squamous metaplasia. The stroma is edematous and contains thick-walled blood vessels. Carcinoma rarely arises in polyps (0.2% of cases).

MALIGNANT AND PREMALIGNANT NEOPLASMS

SQUAMOUS CELL DISEASE

Dysplasia and Carcinoma in Situ

Dysplasia and carcinoma in situ are encompassed in the classification of **cervical intraepithelial neoplasia (CIN). CIN is defined as a spectrum of intraepithelial change that begins with minimal overall atypia and progresses through stages of more marked intraepithelial abnormality to invasive squamous cell carcinoma.** *Dysplasia,***which means abnormal growth, implies an alteration in the morphologic and constitutional character of a cell such that it has acquired the potential for malignant transformation.** *Carcinoma in situ,* **abbreviated CIS, refers to a malignant lesion that is confined to the epithelium—that is, one that has not invaded the underlying stroma.** The following classification has been adopted: CIN I, mild dysplasia; CIN II moderate dysplasia; CIN III severe dysplasia and carcinoma in situ.

It is believed that half of all dysplasias regress. Only 10% progress to carcinoma in situ, and fewer than 2% progress to invasive cancer. The rate of progression to a higher grade depends on the degree of preexisting dysplasia: higher degrees of dysplasia require shorter transit times to carcinoma in situ. It is thought that the average time for all dysplasias to progress to carcinoma in situ is on the order of ten years.

EPIDEMIOLOGY AND ETIOLOGY Multiple sexual partners and early age of first coitus are the most important factors that correlate with the development of CIN. As a consequence, dysplasia and carcinoma in situ are considered within the context of sexually transmitted diseases. **Most investigative work points to a virus in association with a cocarcinogen as the responsible agent.** The most frequently implicated viruses are the herpes simplex virus, type 2 (HSV 2), and the human papillomavirus (HPV).

HUMAN PAPILLOMAVIRUS Human papillomavirus has recently been recognized as a likely etiologic agent for cervical squamous carcinoma. Although only a small percentage of women infected with the virus develop CIN, **80% of early dysplastic lesions demonstrate cytologic features of HPV infection. Moreover, epithelial cells in almost all grades of CIN and invasive carcinoma contain HPV DNA.**

The classic benign condyloma contains either HPV 6 or HPV 11; these are regarded as low-risk HPV types. By contrast, cells in the vast majority of severe dysplasias and invasive cancer contain HPV 16, 18, or 31; these are therefore considered to be high-risk HPV types. The lower grades of dysplasia contain a heterogeneous distribution of all HPV types.

HISTOLOGY (Fig. 18-5) In mild dysplasia (CIN I), the most pronounced changes are in the basal third of the epithelium. Generally, substantial cytoplasmic differentiation occurs in cells in the upper two-thirds of the epithelium. In moderate dysplasia (CIN II), the most profound changes are found in the lower and middle thirds of the epithelium. Cytodifferentiation occurs in cells in the upper third but is less than in mild dysplasia. In severe dysplasia and carcinoma in situ (CIN III), the nuclear changes involve all layers of the epithelium, and cytodifferentiation is minimal.

Microinvasive Squamous Cell Carcinoma

Microinvasive carcinoma is an early stage in the spectrum of cervical cancer (Stage IA), and is characterized by **minimal invasion of the stroma by neoplastic cells.** Small clusters of cells or solid lesions invasive to less than 3 mm without vascular invasion are not associated with lymph node metastases. Therefore, such lesions do not require radical treatment. Therapy consists of a simple hysterectomy.

Squamous Cell Carcinoma

Squamous cell carcinoma of the cervix has become an uncommon disease in the United States, where the incidence is 15 new cases annually per 100,000 women. In Central and South America, parts of Asia, and Africa, it remains a leading cause of cancer death. In some high-risk areas, the incidence has reached 1 new case per 1000 women a year. The age of presentation

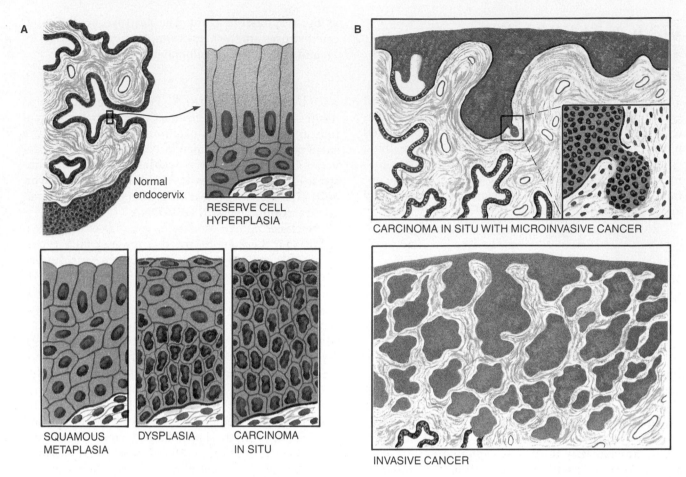

A Normal endocervix

RESERVE CELL HYPERPLASIA

SQUAMOUS METAPLASIA   DYSPLASIA   CARCINOMA IN SITU

B CARCINOMA IN SITU WITH MICROINVASIVE CANCER

INVASIVE CANCER

Figure 18-5. Pathologic sequence of states leading to squamous cell carcinoma of the cervix. (*Upper left*) Reserve cell hyperplasia in an endocervical gland in the region of the squamocolumnar junction. (*Lower left*) The reserve cell hyperplasia becomes more extensive and is called squamous metaplasia. The metaplastic cells undergo changes leading to mild abnormalities (mild dysplasia) and more severe changes (carcinoma in situ). (*Upper right*) Focus of microinvasive (early invasive) cancer arising in carcinoma in situ. (*Lower right*) Invasive squamous cell carcinoma.

peaks at 51 years, or about 10 to 20 years after the peak of carcinoma in situ. Invasive carcinoma and CIN share similar epidemiologic factors.

Three main microscopic patterns occur. **Large cell nonkeratinizing carcinoma,** accounting for two thirds of the cases, is characterized by solid nests of large malignant epithelial cells with no more than individual cell keratinization. **Large cell keratinizing carcinoma** shows nests of keratinized cells organized in concentric whorls—the so-called keratin pearls. The third and least common pattern, **small cell carcinoma,** is composed of infiltrating masses of small, cohesive, malignant cells without evidence of keratinization. The prognosis is similar for the different tumor patterns.

Cervical cancer spreads by direct extension and via lymphatic vessels, and only rarely by the hematogenous route. Local extension into surrounding tissues results in ureteral compression; the corresponding clinical complications are hydroureter, hydronephrosis, and renal failure, the last being the most common cause of death (50% of patients). Bladder and rectal involvement lead to fistula formation. Metastasis to regional lymph nodes involves the paracervical, hypogastric, and external iliac nodes.

The clinical stage of the tumor is the best prognostic indicator of survival (Table 18-2, Fig. 18-6). The overall 5-year survival rate for all tumors combined is 60%. Survival rates are as follows: Stage I,

Table 18-2 *Clinical Staging of Carcinoma of the Cervix Uteri*

STAGE	DESCRIPTION
0	Carcinoma in situ (cervical intraepithelial neoplasia III)
I	Carcinoma confined to cervix (corpus extension disregarded).
Ia	Preclinical carcinoma (diagnosed by microscopy only)
Ia1	Minimal microscopic stromal invasion
Ia2	Measurable lesions detected microscopically (Max 5 mm)
Ib	All lesions greater than Stage Ia2
II	Invasive carcinoma extending beyond the cervix but not reaching lateral pelvic wall; involvement of vagina limited to upper two-thirds.
IIA	Paracervical extension not suspected.
IIB	Paracervical extension suspected.
III	Invasive carcinoma extending to lateral pelvic wall or lower third of vagina.
IIIA	No extension to the pelvic wall.
IIIB	Extension to pelvic wall, hydronephrosis, or nonfunctioning kidney.
IV	Extended spread involving:
IVA	Mucosa of urinary bladder or rectum.
IVB	Extension beyond true pelvis.

90%; Stage II, 75%; Stage III, 35%; and Stage IV, 10%. Approximately 15% of patients will develop recurrences on the vaginal wall, bladder, pelvis, or rectum within 2 years of therapy.

ADENOCARCINOMA

Endocervical adenocarcinoma has increased in frequency in recent years and now accounts for about 10% of cervical malignant tumors. The mean age at presentation is 56 years. Most adenocarcinomas are of the endocervical cell (mucinous) type. On gross examination they have a fungating polypoid or papillary appearance. The tumor spreads in a fashion similar to squamous cell carcinoma of the cervix, and the overall 5-year survival rate is about 50%.

BODY OF UTERUS AND ENDOMETRIUM

PHYSIOLOGIC CHANGES

PREGNANCY

Under the progestational influence of the corpus luteum of pregnancy, the endometrial stroma undergoes a marked decidual change. The endometrial glands become hypersecretory and exhibit widely dilated glands lined by cells with abundant glycogen. Even if the pregnancy is ectopic or trophoblastic disease is present, an exaggerated hypersecretory response may occur. The changes can persist for up to 8 weeks after delivery.

INFLAMMATORY CHANGES

ACUTE ENDOMETRITIS

Acute endometritis, characterized by the presence of polymorphonuclear leukocytes, results when an infection ascends from the cervix. The usually impervious cervical barrier is compromised by abortion, delivery, and instrumentation. Curettage is both diagnostic and curative because it removes the necrotic tissue that serves as the nidus of infection.

CHRONIC ENDOMETRITIS

Chronic endometritis is diagnosed by the identification of plasma cells in the endometrium. Lymphocytes and lymphoid follicles are normally found scattered in the normal endometrium, but their presence is not considered diagnostic of chronic endometritis. Chronic endometritis is associated with IUD use, pelvic inflammatory disease, and retained products of conception after an abortion or delivery. The condition is generally self-limited.

DYSFUNCTIONAL BLEEDING

Dysfunctional uterine bleeding is defined as abnormal bleeding in the absence of an organic lesion of the endometrium. The bleeding may be due to anovulatory cycles related to excessive and prolonged estrogenic stimulation. Without ovulation, a corpus luteum does not develop and progesterone is not secreted. The endometrium, therefore, fails to proceed through the normal secretory phase, and an abnormal menstrual cycle results.

ANOVULATORY BLEEDING

Anovulatory bleeding is the most common form of dysfunctional uterine bleeding, particularly during adolescence and the climacteric period. Estrogen maintains the stromal fluid turgescence that supports the blood vessels. Anovulatory bleeding is caused by a fall in estrogen levels, which results in loss of fluid from the stroma and hence loss of vascular support. The vascular collapse leads to compression of the vessels, which in turn leads to stasis, thrombosis, infarction, and hemorrhage.

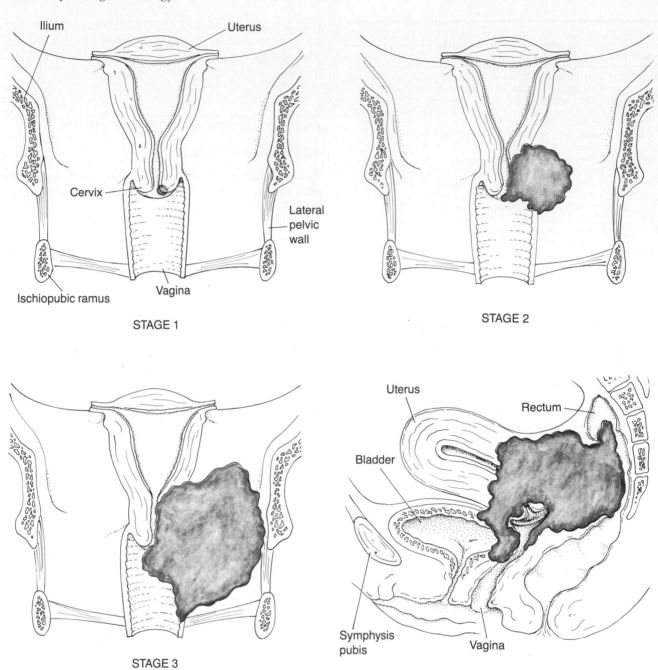

Figure 18-6. Stages of cervical cancer. (*Upper left*) Stage I: tumor is confined to the cervix. (*Upper right*) Stage II: tumor involves upper vagina. (*Lower left*) Stage III: tumor is fixed to the bones of the pelvic sidewall. (*Lower right*) Stage IV: tumor involves the mucosa of the bladder and rectum.

PHYSICALLY INDUCED ENDOMETRIAL LESIONS

ADENOMYOSIS

Adenomyosis is defined as the presence of endometrial glands and stroma within the myometrium. It affects parous women of reproductive age and regresses after menopause. Patients usually present with varying degrees of dysfunctional uterine bleeding and dysmenorrhea.

Adenomyosis is believed to develop as a consequence of endometrial implantation during uterine trauma caused by parturition, myomectomy, or curettage. Occasionally, it is found in nulliparous women who have had no instrumentation. In these cases the foci may develop as a consequence of metaplasia of uncommitted mesenchymal cells.

The uterus becomes enlarged because of smooth-muscle hypertrophy around the endometrial foci. On gross examination the myometrium contains small, soft, red areas, some of which are cystic. Microscopic examination reveals glands lined by mildly proliferative to inactive endometrium and surrounded by endometrial stroma.

INFERTILITY

Approximately 15% of couples in the United States are involuntarily infertile. In women, fertility can be impaired by a wide range of anatomic and structural abnormalities, such as congenital anomalies, tumors, pelvic inflammation, and endometriosis. Fertility is also reduced by various physiologic and endocrine disturbances of reproductive tract function, some of which are discussed elsewhere in this chapter. Representative causes are depicted in Figure 18-7.

ABNORMAL PROLIFERATIONS OF ENDOMETRIAL GLANDS AND STROMA

POLYPS

Endometrial polyps are more common after menopause and typically present with bleeding. Polyps vary in size from several millimeters to large enough to fill and even expand the entire endometrial cavity (Fig 18-8). Microscopic examination reveals endometrial glands admixed with a normal to fibromatous endo-

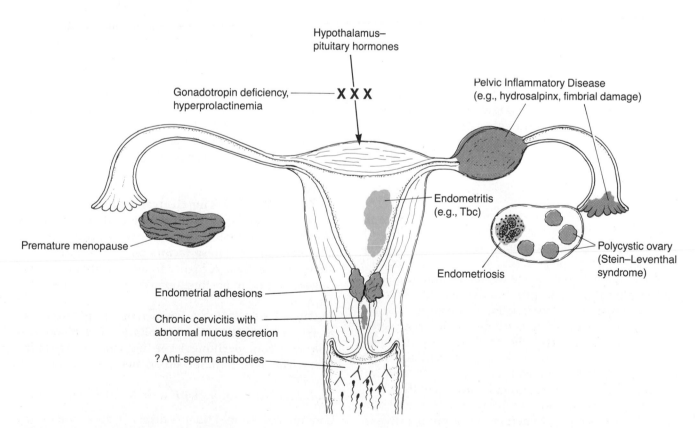

Figure 18-7. Causes of acquired infertility.

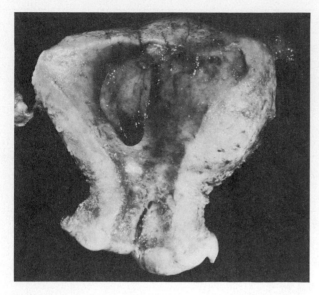

Figure 18-8. Endometrial polyp. Bleeding resulted from the necrotic tip.

metrial stroma and covered by endometrial epithelium. Approximately 0.5% to 3.0% of polyps contain adenocarcinoma.

ENDOMETRIAL HYPERPLASIA AND ADENOCARCINOMA

A broad **spectrum of proliferative disease, constituting a morphologic and biologic continuum, begins with hyperplasia of endometrial glands and ends with adenocarcinoma.** Endometrial hyperplasias and adenocarcinomas are frequently associated with exogenous or endogenous estrogen excess.

Hyperplasias

Cystic hyperplasia, at the low end of the proliferative spectrum, is the most common form of hyperplasia. Dilated glands of varying size are lined by columnar epithelium and exhibit some degree of mitotic activity and stratification. The proliferative activity helps to distinguish it from cystic (senile) atrophy—the so-called Swiss cheese endometrium—which is a regressive change. **The more advanced degrees of hyperplasia, which border on early adenocarcinoma, have been called "adenomatous hyperplasia," "atypical hyperplasia," and "carcinoma in situ,"** but their variable definitions preclude comparison.

"Mild" or "simple" hyperplasia is a proliferative lesion that displays no evidence of cytologic atypia and minimal glandular complexity and crowding (Fig. 18-9). About 1% of such lesions progress to adenocarcinoma.

"Moderate" or "complex" hyperplasia, or "simple hyperplasia with atypicality," is a proliferative lesion with cytologic atypia or marked glandular crowding. About 5% of such lesions progress to adenocarcinoma.

"Severe" or "complex atypical" hyperplasia is characterized by a proliferative lesion with cytologic atypia and marked glandular crowding, generally as back-to-back glands. About 30% of such lesions progress to adenocarcinoma.

The duration of progression from the milder degrees of hyperplasia to cancer is about 10 years. The duration from more advanced hyperplasia with cytologic atypia is about 4 years.

Adenocarcinoma

ADENOCARCINOMA of the endometrium has several morphologic patterns, each with a different prognosis. **The most common type, accounting for approximately 60% of all endometrial carcinomas, is the pure adenocarcinoma, which is composed entirely of glandular cells.** Adenocarcinomas of the endometrium are divided into three grades: well differentiated (grade 1), moderately differentiated (grade 2), or poorly differentiated (grade 3) (Fig. 18-10).

The second most common type of carcinoma contains squamous cells in addition to the glandular element. If the **squamous element is well differentiated,** exhibiting minimal atypia, the tumor is called **adenoacanthoma.** If it is **poorly differentiated,** the tumor is called **adenosquamous carcinoma and has a poor prognosis.**

SURVIVAL   The actuarial survival rate of all patients with endometrial cancer following treatment (regardless of history of estrogen usage) is 80% after the second year, 73% after the fifth year, and 64% after 10 years.

PATHOGENESIS   The clinical features associated with endometrial cancer include diabetes mellitus, obesity, hypertension, breast cancer, nulliparity, and late menopause. These factors point to an increased estrogenic milieu. A higher frequency of endometrial cancer is found in postmenopausal women treated with estrogens.

CLINICAL COURSE   Adenocarcinoma of the endometrium spreads by the lymphatics, the blood vessels, and transperitoneal seeding via the fallopian tubes. The most common site of metastasis is the lung.

Endometrial Tumors with a Stromal Component

Endometrial stromal tumors display a spectrum of malignant behavior that can be correlated with their histo-

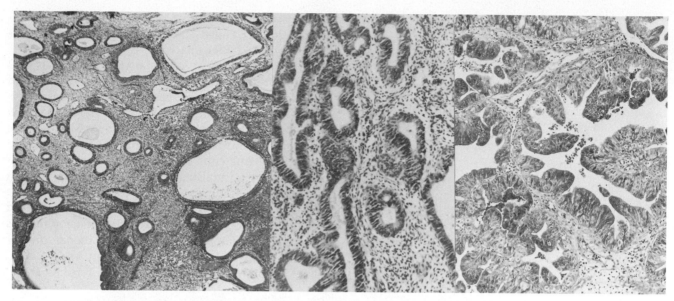

Figure 18-9. Hyperplasia of the endometrium: Mild (*left*), moderate (*middle*), and severe, or markedly atypical (*right*). The glands in mild hyperplasia are dilated, and the lining epithelium is proliferative and has occasional mitoses. Moderate hyperplasia is characterized by more closely packed glands. Severely atypical hyperplasia displays closely packed glands with highly proliferative epithelium and marked architectural abnormality.

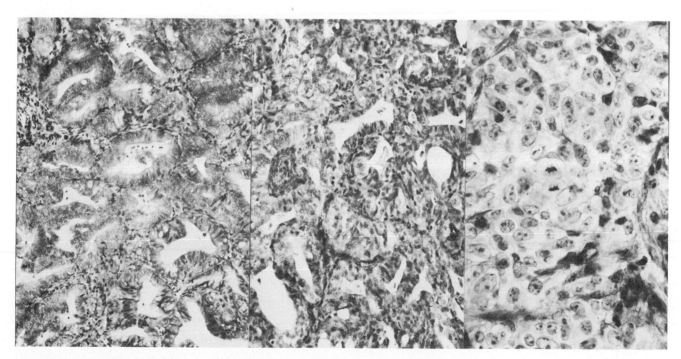

Figure 18-10. Adenocarcinoma of endometrium, grades 1–3. Grade 1 (*left*): well-differentiated tumor composed entirely of glands. Grade 2 (*middle*): moderately differentiated tumor characterized architecturally by both glands and solid sheets of cells. Grade 3 (*right*): poorly differentiated tumor composed entirely of sheets of cells; no glands are present.

Table 18-3   Nomenclature of Uterine Tumors

TUMOR	EPITHELIUM	MESENCHYME
Epithelium and Stroma		
Endometrial hyperplasia	Hyperplastic	—
Endometrial adenocarcinoma	Malignant	—
Endometrial stromal nodule	—	Benign
Endometrial stromal sarcoma		
Low-grade	—	Malignant
High-grade	—	Malignant
Adenosarcoma	Benign	Malignant
Carcinosarcoma	Malignant	Malignant
Malignant mixed	Malignant	Malignant
mesodermal tumor		(heterologous)
Smooth Muscle		
Leiomyoma	—	Benign
Cellular leiomyoma	—	Benign
Intravenous leiomyomatosis	—	Benign
Leiomyosarcoma	—	Malignant

logic features (Table 18-3). The low-grade sarcomas have also been called **endolymphatic stromal myosis** and **endometrial stromatosis**.

CARCINOSARCOMA AND MALIGNANT MIXED MESODERMAL TUMORS "Carcinosarcoma" and "malignant mixed mesodermal tumor" are terms applied to mesenchymal tumors of the uterus in which the epithelial and stromal components, which are derived from multipotential stromal cells, are malignant. If heterologous elements—**mesenchymal components not normally found in the uterus,** such as striated muscle, bone, osteoid, cartilage or fat—are present, the tumor is designated a **malignant mixed mesodermal tumor.** If the mesenchymal component is a nonspecific sarcoma, the term **carcinosarcoma** is used. A history of prior irradiation can be elicited in about 5% of these patients. The overall 5-year actuarial

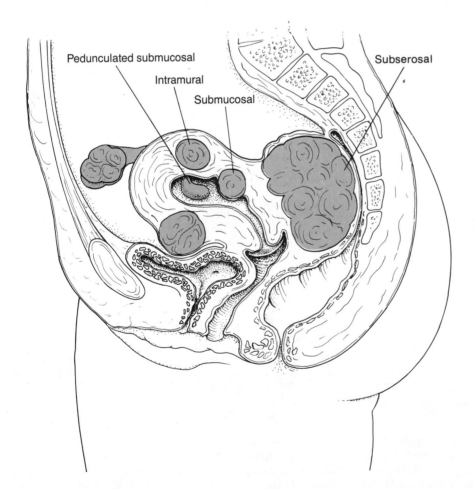

Figure 18-11. Leiomyomas of the uterus. The leiomyomas are intramural; submucosal, with a pedunculated one appearing in the form of an endometrial polyp; subserosal, with one compressing the bladder and the other the rectum.

survival is about 25%. Although earlier reports indicated a difference in survival rates between carcinosarcoma and mixed mesodermal tumors, more recent studies do not substantiate this claim.

NEOPLASMS OF MYOMETRIAL SMOOTH MUSCLE

LEIOMYOMA

The most common uterine tumor is the leiomyoma, also known colloquially as "myoma" or "fibroid" (Fig. 18-11). Leiomyomas occur in 25% of women older than 30 years of age and are rare before age 20; most regress after menopause. Although estrogens seem to influence the growth of leiomyomas, it has not been established that they initiate these tumors.

Grossly, the tumors are firm, pale gray, whorled, and unencapsulated. The masses, which are composed of interlacing bundles of smooth muscle (Fig. 18-12), may be small as 1 mm or as large as 30 cm in diameter. Most

are intramural, but some are subserosal or pedunculated. Submucosal leiomyomas may cause bleeding, an effect due to ulceration of the thinned, overlying endometrium or to dilated and thrombosed venules. Leiomyomas may be symptomatic simply because of sheer bulk. Cramping may be caused by their entrapment in the endocervical canal. Large leiomyomas may affect bowel or bladder function. Leiomyomas usually grow slowly, but occasionally they increase rapidly in size during pregnancy. Leiomyomas with low mitotic activity have little or no malignant potential.

LEIOMYOSARCOMA

The single best criterion for predicting the behavior of smooth-muscle tumors is mitotic activity. On this basis, smooth-muscle tumors with no mitotic activity are **leiomyomas** and those with five or more mitoses per 10 high-power fields are **sarcomas** (Fig. 18-13). It is believed that only a rare leiomyoma (<0.01%) undergoes malignant transformation. Women with leiomyosarcomas are, on average, a decade older than women

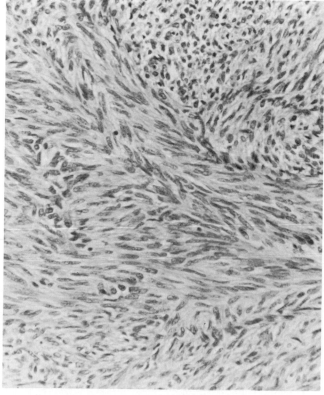

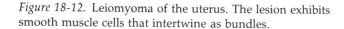

Figure 18-12. Leiomyoma of the uterus. The lesion exhibits smooth muscle cells that intertwine as bundles.

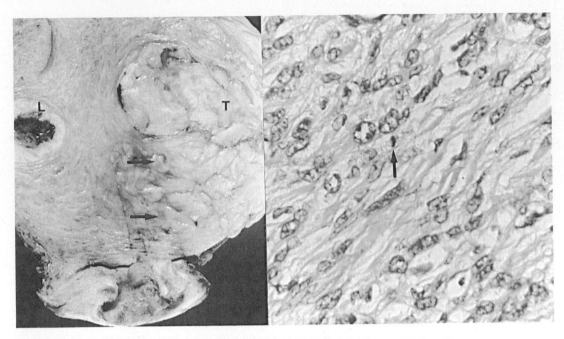

Figure 18-13. Leiomyosarcoma of the uterus. (*Left*) The malignant tumor (*T*) is soft and tan, has irregular borders (*arrows*), and invades into the surrounding myometrium. A small leiomyoma (note smooth border) with a hemorrhagic infarcted center is present for comparison (*L*). (*Right*) The cells of the leiomyosarcoma are moderately disorganized in arrangement, irregular in shape, and display mitoses (*arrow*).

with leiomyomas, and the tumors are larger. Leiomyosarcoma should be suspected if on gross examination the neoplasm is soft and has irregular borders. These tumors are highly malignant and usually fatal.

FALLOPIAN TUBE

INFECTIONS

Acute salpingitis usually results from an ascending infection from the lower genital tract. The most common causative organisms are *E. coli, N. gonorrhoeae, Chlamydia,* and *Mycoplasma. Clostridia perfringens* and various other anaerobes are less commonly encountered. **A fallopian tube damaged by prior infection is particularly susceptible to reinfection** Typically, the infection is polymicrobial.

CHRONIC SALPINGITIS

Chronic salpingitis usually results from repeated episodes of acute salpingitis. The acute episodes, particularly those associated with chlamydial infection, may be asymptomatic. Complications may be caused

by either destruction of epithelium or deposition of fibrin on the mucosal plicae; the fibrin bridges cause the plicae to adhere to one another. Ovarian involvement leads to the formation of a **tubo-ovarian abscess.** The consequence of the blocked lumen may be **hydrosalpinx** or **pyosalpinx.** Because of destruction of the tubal epithelium and fibrosis, chronic salpingitis may lead to **infertility** and **ectopic pregnancy.**

TUBERCULOUS SALPINGITIS

Tuberculosis should always be considered a possible cause of chronic granulomatous salpingitis. Tuberculous salpingitis is found in 1% of infertile women in the United States and in more than 10% of such women in less developed countries, where pulmonary tuberculosis is more common. The route of infection is hematogenous from a primary locus elsewhere in the body, usually the lung.

ECTOPIC PREGNANCY

Ectopic pregnancy, which occurs in 1 in 200 live births in the United States, refers to any gestation that develops outside the endometrium. Over 95%

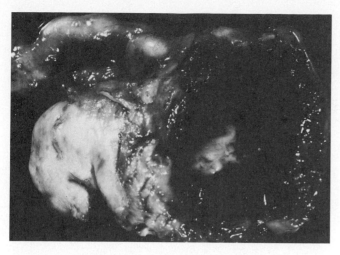

Figure 18-14. Ectopic pregnancy with remains of fetus.

occur in the tube, mostly in the distal and middle thirds (Fig. 18-14). Tubal rupture with subsequent hemorrhage is a life-threatening complication. Ectopic pregnancy results when the passage of the conceptus along the fallopian tube is impeded—for example, by mucosal adhesions or abnormal tubal motility secondary to inflammatory disease or endometriosis. The trophoblast readily penetrates the mucosa and wall, a situation which results in an abnormal implantation. **As a consequence, bleeding occurs at the implantation site and blood enters the peritoneal cavity, causing abdominal pain. The wall of the fallopian tube is thin, and unless the ectopic pregnancy is discovered, the wall usually ruptures by the 12th week of gestation.**

As in intrauterine pregnancies, the syncytiotrophoblast in ectopic pregnancies secretes hCG, the basis of a useful test in the diagnosis of pregnancy. The hCG, possibly through its activity on the corpus luteum, also stimulates the endometrium to become hypersecretory, a state characteristic of pregnancy.

OVARY

NON-NEOPLASTIC CONDITIONS

CYSTS

Non-neoplastic ovarian cysts are the most common cause of enlarged ovaries. Their presence is often indicated by menstrual irregularities (due to an imbalance of estrogen and progesterone) and abdominal pain. Neoplasms, in contrast, are usually asymptomatic until they become large enough to cause mechanical symp-

toms. Non-neoplastic cysts are subdivided into hormonally functional and nonfunctional types.

Nonfunctional Cysts

SEROUS INCLUSION CYST Serous cysts in the superficial or deep cortex of the ovary are common and arise by invagination of the surface epithelium, which becomes pinched off. The cysts are limited by low cuboidal, endometrial, or tubal type epithelium (serous epithelium). Most are less than 1 cm in diameter, but occasionally a cyst may attain a diameter of several centimeters. The cysts are believed to be the site of origin of common epithelial tumors.

Functional Cysts

FOLLICLE CYST Follicle cysts of the ovary may be single, multiple, or bilateral. **Since they arise from follicles undergoing atresia, they lack an ovum. The cyst rarely exceeds 5 cm in diameter and is thin, smooth-walled, and lined by granulosa cells, with an external layer of theca interna.** In an unstimulated state, the granulosa cells have uniform, round nuclei and little cytoplasm. The thecal cells are small and spindle-shaped. Occasionally, the layers may be luteinized, in which case the lumen contains fluid with a high estrogen content. If the cyst persists, the hormonal output can lead to precocious puberty in a child and menstrual irregularities in the adult. Complications include intraperitoneal rupture and intracystic hemorrhage.

CORPUS LUTEUM CYST Formation of a corpus luteum cyst results from delayed resolution of the central cavity of a corpus luteum following ovulation. The cystic cavity is lined by a thin layer of fibrous tissue, which is surrounded by a **scalloped shell of luteinized granulosa cells.** Continued progesterone synthesis leads to menstrual irregularities. A corpus luteum cyst can also cause hemorrhage into the abdominal cavity.

POLYCYSTIC OVARY SYNDROME (STEIN-LEVENTHAL SYNDROME) The syndrome refers to a triad of **obesity, hirsutism, and secondary amenorrhea,** together with a characteristic histologic appearance of the ovary. **It is one of the most common causes of infertility.** The current name, **polycystic ovary syndrome,** recognizes the inclusion of a subset of women with chronic anovulatory syndrome. The polycystic ovary syndrome is thought to result from excessive secretion of luteinizing hormone releasing factor by a locus in the hypothalamus. This results in excessive ovarian synthesis of androgen and peripheral conversion of androgens to estrone. A positive feedback effect on the central nervous system results in more luteinizing hormone being released. **Both ovaries are enlarged** and the capsule is thick and smooth, an appearance that reflects an absence of ovulation. **Nu-**

merous cystic subcapsular follicles are lined by thick zones of theca interna, some cells of which may be luteinized. The follicles may also be separated by hyperplastic stroma, which also may contain luteinized cells **(hyperthecosis).**

OVARIAN TUMORS

Cancer of the ovary is the third most frequent gynecologic malignancy after those of the cervix and endometrium. It carries a higher mortality rate (more than 10,000 per year) than all other genital cancer death combined.

The broad range of histologic features encountered in ovarian tumors reflects the diversity of cell types present in the normal gonad (Fig. 18-15). Most tumors are categorized into one of three broad groups: **tumors of the surface epithelium, germ cell tumors, and sex cord stromal tumors.** Metastatic tumors to the ovary account for a small proportion of all ovarian malignancies. The most common metastasis is from cancer of the colon. **The term "Krukenberg tumor" connotes a mucin-forming adenocarcinoma, usually metastatic from stomach cancer.**

EPIDEMIOLOGY

Serous adenocarcinoma is associated with factors believed to disrupt the epithelial surface, such as repeated ovulation. The tumors occur most commonly in women who are nulliparous, and conversely, occur least often in women in whom ovulation is suppressed (as a result of pregnancy or oral contraceptive use).

TUMORS OF EPITHELIAL ORIGIN

In order of frequency of occurrence, the four major types of ovarian tumors, which all resemble tissues of müllerian origin, are: **serous** (cells resembling those

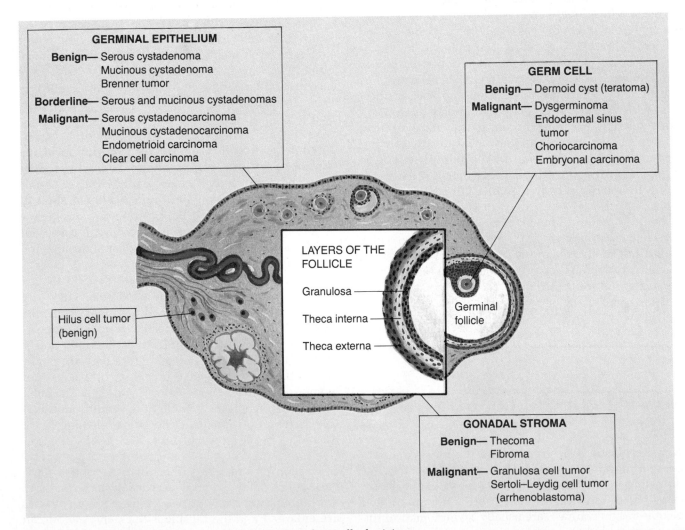

Figure 18-15. Classification of ovarian neoplasms based on cell of origin.

lining the fallopian tube, Fig. 18-16), **mucinous** (mucinous cells resembling the lining of the endocervix, Fig. 18-17), **endometrioid** (columnar cells resembling the lining of the endometrium), and **clear cell** (glycogen-rich cells resembling the lining of the endometrial glands in pregnancy).

General Features

BENIGN TUMORS Cystadenomas (cystomas, adenomas) generally occur in women under the age of 40 years. They may be of any size, and a third are bilateral. Serous tumors tend to be unilocular, and mucinous tumors multilocular. On microscopic examination cystadenomas are lined by a single layer of epithelium.

TUMORS OF LOW MALIGNANT POTENTIAL Tumors of low malignant potential—the so-called borderline carcinomas—generally occur in women between the ages of 20 to 45 years. Because mucinous lesions are slow-growing, they can achieve gigantic proportions. About a third are bilateral. When a large cyst is opened, it is common to find a small cluster of grapelike structures arising from one segment of the wall. These tumors microscopically display papillary fronds, in which a thick fibrovascular core is covered by a mantle of atypical, stratified neoplastic cells.

MALIGNANT TUMORS (INVASIVE CARCINOMAS) Frankly malignant tumors of the ovary are rare in women under the age of 40 years. They may be of any size, although by the time a tumor becomes 10 cm to 15 cm in diameter, it often has already spread beyond the ovary and seeded the peritoneum. Serous adenocarcinomas are commonly bilateral. On macroscopic examination the malignant lesions often present as a solid mass. Microscopically, they are characterized by stromal invasion.

METASTATIC SPREAD Ovarian tumors spread by surface seeding ("peritoneal carcinomas") and lymph node metastasis. Growth outside the abdominal cavity is unusual.

SURVIVAL AND BIOLOGICAL BEHAVIOR The treatment of ovarian cancer is influenced by clinical staging (Table 18-4). Patients with tumors of low malignant potential have an excellent prognosis even if the tumors are of an advanced stage. Low-grade tumors that are already in the peritoneal cavity at diagnosis are still associated with an 80% 5-year survival, a figure

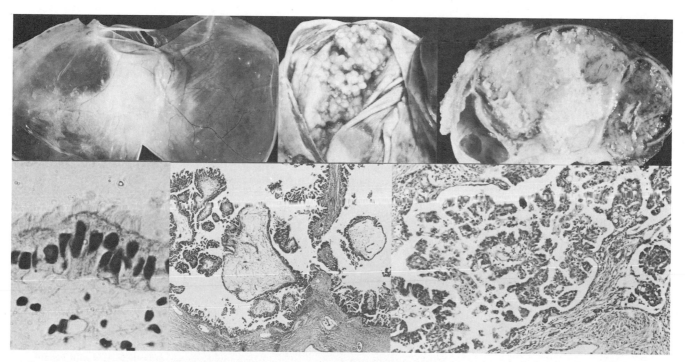

Figure 18-16. Serous tumors of the ovary. (*Left*) Serous cystadenoma, in which the opened unilocular cyst is 20 cm in greatest dimension, has a paper-thin wall, and is lined by a single layer of highly ciliated serous cells. (*Middle*) Serous tumors of low malignant potential are characterized by a protuberance resembling a bunch of grapes arising from the wall of the unilocular cyst. Each grapelike structure is composed of a fibrovascular center covered by atypical serous cells one to several cells thick. (*Right*) Serous adenocarcinoma is a solid mass of focally necrotic tumor. The tumor is highly papillary and extensively invades the stroma.

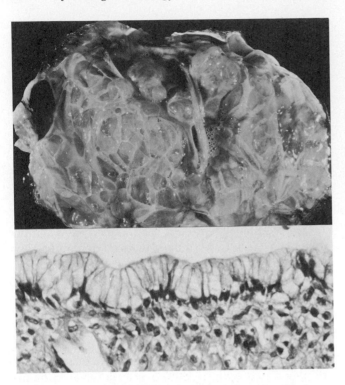

Figure 18-17. Mucinous cystadenoma of the ovary. Each cyst in the multilocular tumor (*top*) is lined by a single layer of mucinous epithelial cells (*bottom*).

toneal cavity, a condition known as **pseudomyxoma peritonei.**

ENDOMETRIOID ADENOCARCINOMAS Endometrioid adenocarcinomas are often miscategorized as serous tumors, which accounts for their overall low rate of reported frequency. In contrast to serous and mucinous neoplasms, **almost all endometrioid tumors are malignant.**

CLEAR CELL ADENOCARCINOMA Clear cell adenocarcinoma, which is thought to be closely related to endometrioid adenocarcinoma, is often found in association with endometriosis.

BRENNER TUMOR Brenner tumor, unlike the other common epithelial tumors, has two components. The tumor itself, when benign, is composed of solid nests of urothelium-like cells encased in a dense, fibrous stroma. The most superficial epithelial cells may exhibit mucinous differentiation. A small number of cases are of low malignant potential (so-called proliferative Brenner tumor) or frankly malignant.

TUMORS OF SEX CORD-STROMA

Tumors of sex cord-stroma range from benign to malignant, and differentiate toward female or male struc-

that contrasts with a 20% survival rate if the tumor is frankly malignant histologically (e.g., serous adenocarcinoma).

Selected Features of Common Epithelial Tumors

SEROUS TUMORS **Serous cystadenoma is the most common benign epithelial tumor.** Serous tumors of low malignant potential account for 15% of all ovarian malignancies. **Serous adenocarcinoma is the most common malignant ovarian tumor,** accounting for 25% of the total. Laminated calcified concretions, referred to as psammoma bodies, are often associated with serous tumors.

MUCINOUS TUMORS **Mucinous tumors can grow to an extremely large size, some to more than 40 lbs.** Whether they are benign, of low malignant potential, or frankly malignant, the tumors are usually multilocular. **Unlike the serous tumor, which may secrete some mucin, mucinous tumors exhibit extensive mucin throughout the cytoplasm.** The tumors may be bilateral, but this occurs less frequently than in the case of serous tumors. Mucinous adenomas of low malignant potential may excrete pools of mucin into the peri-

Table 18-4   Clinical Staging of Carcinoma of the Ovary*

STAGE	DESCRIPTION
I	Tumor limited to ovaries
IA	Tumor limited to one ovary; no ascites
IA(i)	No tumor on external surface; capsule intact
IA(ii)	Tumor on external surface and/or capsule ruptured
IB	Tumor limited to both ovaries; no ascites
IB(i)	No tumor on external surface; capsule intact
IB(ii)	Tumor on the external surface and/or capsule ruptured
IC	Tumor either IA or IB, but with ascites or positive peritoneal washings
II	Tumor involving one or both ovaries with pelvic extension
IIA	Extension and/or metastases to uterus and/or tubes
IIB	Extension to other pelvic tissues
IIC	Tumor either IIA or IIB, but with ascites or positive peritoneal washings
III	Tumor involving one or both ovaries with intraperitoneal metastases outside the pelvis, and/or positive retroperitoneal nodes. Tumor limited to true pelvis with histologically proven malignant extension to small bowel or omentum
IV	Tumor involving one or both ovaries with distant metastases. If pleural effusion, positive cytology required. Liver metastases must be parenchymal.

* Staging is based on clinical examination, surgical exploration, and microscopic tissue findings.

tures. As a group, they account for less than 10% of all ovarian tumors.

Granulosa-Stromal Cell Tumors

Granulosa cell tumors can occur at any age, but are unusual before puberty. They display an array of patterns, the most characteristic being the macro- and microfollicular patterns **(Call-Exner bodies)** (Fig. 18-18). Poorly differentiated tumors commonly have a sarcomatous appearance. **About a quarter of the tumors are functional and secrete estrogens; about 20% of affected women have associated endometrial hyperplasia or cancer.**

Thecoma-Fibroma Group

Fibromas are typically white, firm, and pearly and composed of fibrous tissue. When the cells are partially or largely filled with lipid, the tumor is called a thecoma. **Thecomas are often estrogenic and cause the endometrium to proliferate and become hyperplastic. Theca cell tumors are rarely malignant.** Tumors with conspicuous mitotic activity are termed fibrosarcoma and are highly malignant.

Sertoli-Leydig Cell Tumors

The Sertoli-Leydig cell tumor (previously called arrhenoblastoma or androblastoma) is a tumor of low malignant potential that has structures resembling those of the testis. The most characteristic features are Leydig cells and fine trabeculae of sex cords. The tumor generally occurs in young women (ages 15 to 40), **is frequently associated with virilization,** is almost always unilateral, and usually does not recur after removal. **The marked virilization is caused by the secretion of testosterone or other androgenic hormones by the neoplasm.**

GERM CELL TUMORS

GERM CELL TUMORS constitute 20% of all ovarian tumors. Most are benign, and they account for only 3% of all malignant neoplasms of the ovary. **However, they are the most common ovarian cancers in children** (accounting for 60% of all ovarian tumors and 30% of malignant ovarian tumors in this age group). Germ cell tumors are rare after menopause. The neoplastic germ cell may follow one of several lines of differentiation (Fig. 18-19). The tumor may proliferate as undifferentiated neoplastic germ cells—that is, as a germinoma—in which case we speak of **dysgerminomas** in women and **seminomas** in men. (The tumor in an extragonadal location is called germinoma, regardless of the patient's sex.) If the tumor exhibits embryonic tissues, it is called **teratoma.** Extraembryonic structures lend the names of **entodermal sinus tumor (yolk sac carcinoma)** or **choriocarcinoma.**

The age of the patient provides a clue as to the type of tumor that develops. Tumors of infants tend to be solid and immature—for instance, entodermal sinus tumor, embryonal carcinoma, and immature teratoma. Tumors in women who are somewhat older (15 to 30) tend to show greater differentiation (cystic teratoma). Germ cell tumors in women over 40 years of age are usually a result of malignant transformation of a component of a benign cystic teratoma. These include carcinoid tumor, struma ovarii, and squamous cell cancer.

In general, the malignant germ cell tumors are highly aggressive. Until the advent of adjuvant chemotherapy, the solid germ cell tumors were uniformly

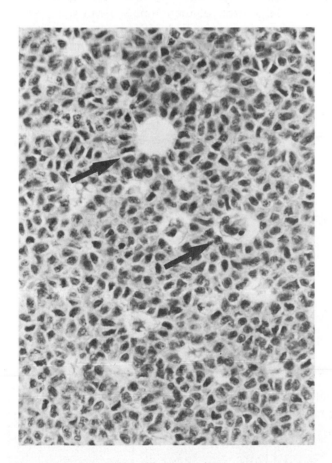

Figure 18-18. Granulosa cell tumor of the ovary, microfollicular pattern. Call-Exner bodies (*arrows*) are formed by granulosa cells with haphazardly oriented nuclei abutting the central space.

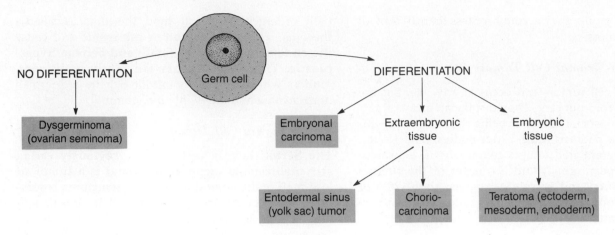

Figure 18-19. Classification of germ cell tumors of the ovary.

fatal. Now, the survival rate of many germ cell tumors exceeds 80%.

Dysgerminoma

Dysgerminoma is the ovarian counterpart of the testicular seminoma. It accounts for 1% of all ovarian tumors and for 10% of tumors in women under the age of 20 years. Most patients are between 10 and 30 years of age. The tumors are often large and firm and have a bosselated external surface. Microscopic examination reveals large nests of monotonous germ cells, which have clear cytoplasm filled with glycogen and irregularly flattened central nuclei. Dysgerminoma is highly radiosensitive, and 5-year survival rates exceed 90%.

Teratoma

MATURE TERATOMA (MATURE CYSTIC TERATOMA, DERMOID CYST)   The most common germ

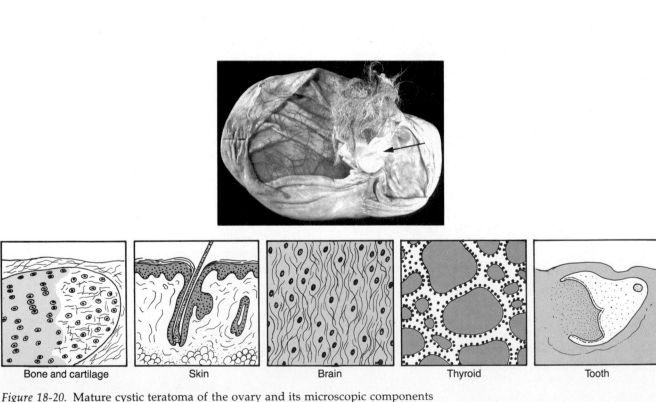

Figure 18-20. Mature cystic teratoma of the ovary and its microscopic components differentiating toward well-differentiated tissues.

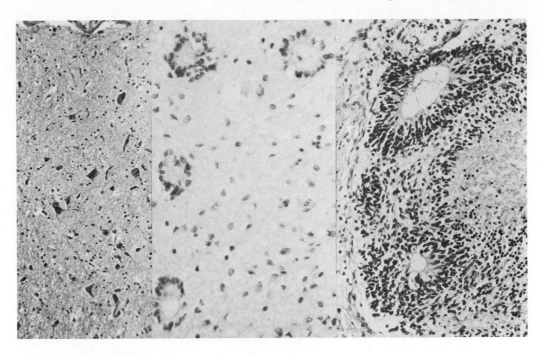

Figure 18-21. Teratoma of the ovary with neuroepithelial tissues of differing degrees of differentiation. Mature neural tissue (*left*) shows neurons and glia of normal cellularity. (*Middle*) Epithelial rosettes are lined by a single layer of epithelium. Malignant neural tissue (*right*) exhibits rosettes with multilayered nuclei; embryonal glia display densely packed atypical nuclei.

cell tumor, **the mature cystic teratoma (dermoid cyst), accounts for approximately 25% of all ovarian tumors.** The peak incidence occurs in women between 20 and 30 years of age. This tumor develops by parthenogenesis—that is, the diploid tumor cells develop from a haploid germ cell. The tumor is cystic, and contains hair and sebum. There is often a small nodule along one margin of the cyst wall that contains tissue elements of all three germ-cell layers, namely, ectoderm (skin and glia), mesoderm (cartilage), and entoderm (gut) (Figs. 18-20 and 18-21).

Dermoid cysts rarely undergo malignant transformation.

IMMATURE TERATOMA Immature teratoma is an ovarian cancer composed of embryonal tissues that almost always is in the form of a solid teratoma. Although uncommon, it accounts for 20% of malignant tumors of the ovary in women under the age of 20 years.

Choriocarcinoma

Choriocarcinoma, a rare tumor, has two possible origins. A **derivation from germ cells** is assumed if it arises before puberty or in combination with another form of germ cell tumor. In women of reproductive age, it may be of **gestational origin,** either as a metastasis or from an ovarian pregnancy. The patients are almost always young and have complaints of precocious sexual development, menstrual irregularities, or rapid breast enlargement. **The tumor is unilateral, solid, and highly hemorrhagic.** Microscopically, it is composed of an **admixture of malignant cytotrophoblastic and syncytiotrophoblastic cells.** The syncytial cells secrete hCG, which accounts for the frequent finding of a positive pregnancy test. In addition to being useful in diagnosis, serial determination of serum hCG levels is useful in follow-up. The tumor is highly aggressive but responsive to chemotherapy.

PLACENTA AND GESTATIONAL TROPHOBLASTIC DISEASE

DISTURBANCES OF CIRCULATION

INFARCTS AND RETROPLACENTAL HEMATOMAS

Infarcts and retroplacental hematomas have clinical significance when they diminish the placenta's reserve

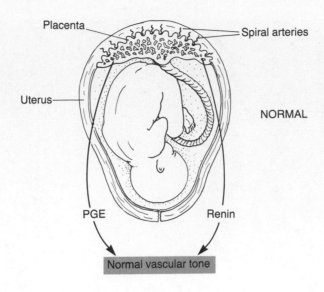

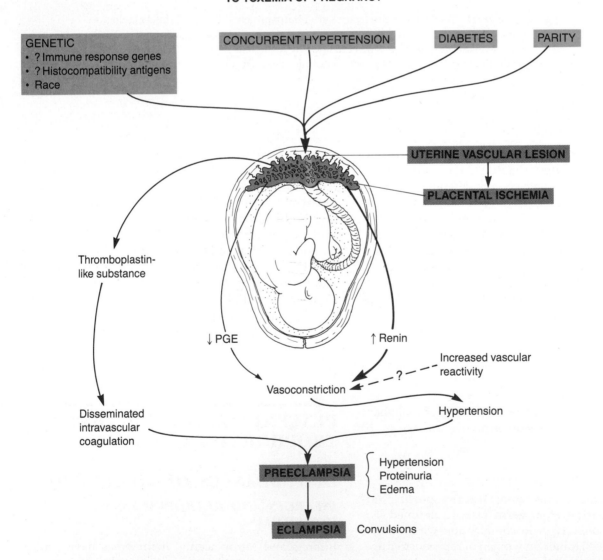

capacity. Although infarcts occur in 20% of uncomplicated term pregnancies, few are extensive enough to impair placental function.

Retroplacental hematomas consist of blood between the basal plate of the placenta and the uterine wall. Hemorrhage usually results from the rupture of a maternal artery but may be due to premature placental separation. Retroplacental bleeding is commonly associated with abruptio placentae (premature separation of the placenta) and is a significant complication of preeclampsia (pregnancy-induced hypertension). Small retroplacental hematomas generally have no clinical consequence, but hematomas involving one-third or more of the maternal surface can result in fetal death.

TOXEMIA

During the late trimester of pregnancy, a triad of hypertension, proteinuria, and edema may develop. This condition is labeled "preeclampsia" (Fig. 18-22). Some of those affected have a history of prior renal disease or hypertension. **The disease is called "eclampsia" when convulsive seizures appear.** Toxins are not produced with this disease—the name toxemia, therefore, is a misnomer. The disorder is characterized by hypertension associated with vasospasm. **Fibrin thrombi** are found in liver, brain, and kidneys. It is believed that the initiating factor lies in the placenta and is a result of ischemia. Except for the consequences of cerebral hemorrhage, the systemic changes are reversible.

SPONTANEOUS ABORTION

The term spontaneous abortion applies to any pregnancy that terminates before the fetus is viable. Approximately 15% of recognized pregnancies spontaneously abort and an additional 30% of women abort without being aware that they are pregnant. **Thus, the overall spontaneous abortion rate is estimated to be 45%.** The known etiologic factors responsible for abortion are infection early in pregnancy; physical factors, such as submucous uterine fibroids or cervical incompetence; endocrinologic factors, such as inadequate progesterone production; immunologic factors; congenital abnormalities, such as neural tube defects; and chromosomal abnormalities.

INFECTION

Infection of the placenta and its membranes may be hematogenous or may result from direct spread from the endometrium. **The most common and clinically significant route is ascending infection from the maternal birth canal.** In this type of infection the inflammatory process affects the membranes (chorioamnionitis) rather than the placental tissue. Microscopic examination reveals varying numbers of neutrophils, with or without fibrin. A direct relationship exists between prolonged rupture of membranes and the presence of chorioamnionitis. Microorganisms cultured from placentas with chorioamnionitis are *E. coli*, coagulase-positive staphylococci, *Gardnerella vaginalis*, streptococci, *Proteus mirabilis*, *Klebsiella*, and *Pseudomonas*. The main risk to the fetus is infection.

Chorioamnionitis does not usually result in complications for the fetus, but frequently the mother develops intrapartum fever.

GESTATIONAL TROPHOBLASTIC DISEASE

The clinical term "gestational trophoblastic disease" embraces hydatidiform mole (complete or partial mole), invasive mole, gestational choriocarcinoma, and placental site trophoblastic tumor (Fig. 18-23).

HYDATIDIFORM MOLE

Complete

In complete hydatidiform mole, **grossly swollen chorionic villi, which resemble a bunch of grapes, show varying degrees of trophoblastic proliferation.** There is no embryo. Complete mole results from fertilization of an egg in which the maternal chromosomal material has been lost or inactivated by a single sperm with a 23X set of chromosomes, which duplicates to 46XX.

The risk for development of hydatidiform mole is related to the age of the patient and has two peaks. **Girls under 15 years of age have a twenty times higher risk than women who are between 20 and 35 years old. The risk increases progressively for women over the age of 40 years. Women over 50 years of age have a risk 200 times greater than between 20 and 50 years.** The risk of hydatidiform mole

Figure 18-22. Toxemia of pregnancy. In a normal pregnancy the vasodilatory effects of prostaglandin E released from the placenta are balanced by the vasoconstrictor effects of renin from the kidney. With placental ischemia, a decrease in PGE and an increase in renin favor vasoconstriction, with resulting hypertension. Concomitantly, a release of thromboplastin-like substance from the ischemic placenta produces intravascular coagulation.

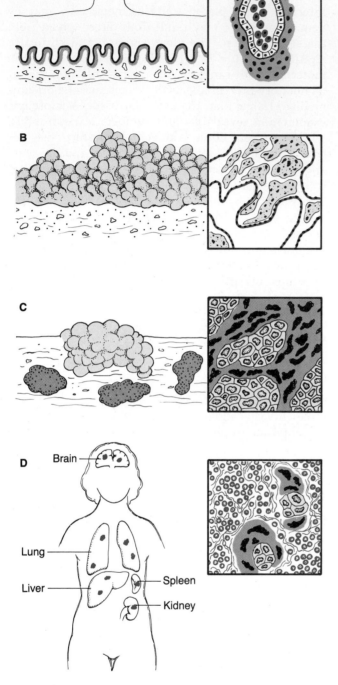

is many times higher in Oriental women than among Caucasians, reaching an incidence in Taiwan that is twenty-five times greater than in the United States. **Women who have had a previous hydatidiform mole are at a 20 to 40 times greater risk than the general population.**

Complications of complete hydatidiform mole include uterine hemorrhage, coagulopathy, uterine perforation, trophoblastic embolism, and infection. **The most important complication is the development of choriocarcinoma.**

Treatment consists of suction curettage of the uterus and subsequent monitoring of serum hCG levels. Levels that plateau or rise suggest persistent or progressive disease, for which chemotherapy is administered. With such management, the rate of survival approaches 100%.

CHORIOCARCINOMA

Choriocarcinoma is composed of a dimorphic population of cytotrophoblast and syncytiotrophoblast, with varying degrees of intermediate trophoblast also present. Typically, the tumor undergoes central hemorrhage with necrosis, viable tumor being confined to the periphery of the mass immediately adjacent to underlying normal tissue. **The tumor metastasizes widely by the hematogenous route to any site, but especially to lung, brain, gastrointestinal tract, and liver.** hCG is localized within the syncytiotrophoblastic element. **In Caucasians 25% of choriocarcinomas arise from term deliveries, 25% from spontaneous abortions, and 50% from hydatidiform moles.** The risk that a hydatidiform mole will develop into a choriocarcinoma is small, about 2%. **Overall, however, the risk of choriocarcinoma is 1000 times higher after a hydatidiform mole than after a normal term delivery.** As with the hydatidiform mole and the placental site trophoblastic tumor, serial serum hCG levels are used to monitor the effectiveness of chemotherapy.

Figure 18-23. Proliferative disorders of the trophoblast. (*A*) Normal chorionic villus of 8-week fetus, with blood vessel containing nucleated red blood cells. (*B*) Hydatidiform mole with hydropic villi. The villi are enlarged by an edematous stroma devoid of blood vessels. The trophoblastic epithelium is hyperplastic and exhibits variable anaplasia. (*C*) Choriocarcinoma with admixed malignant syncytiotrophoblastic and cytotrophoblastic elements. (*D*) Common sites of metastasis from choriocarcinoma.

ENDOMETRIOSIS

Endometriosis is defined as the presence of benign endometrial glands and stroma outside the uterus (Figs. 18-24 and 18-25). The sites most frequently affected, in order of decreasing frequency, are ovary (80% of all pelvic endometriosis), fallopian tube, uterus, cul-de-sac of Douglas, uterosacral ligaments, gastrointestinal tract, and, rarely, distant areas such as lungs, pleura, and extremities. **Endometriosis is a disease of women of reproductive age and regresses following natural or artificial menopause.** Dysmenorrhea, the most common complaint, is related to implants on the uterosacral ligaments, which swell just

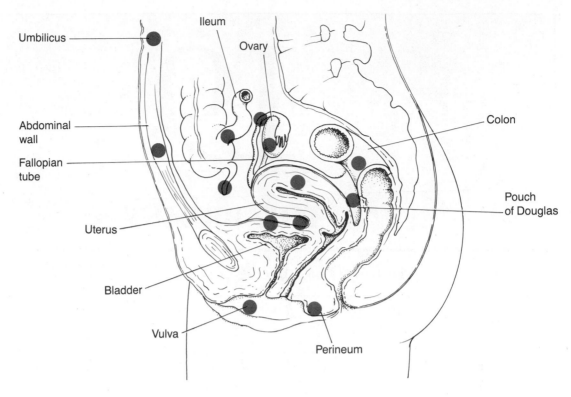

Figure 18-24. Sites of endometriosis.

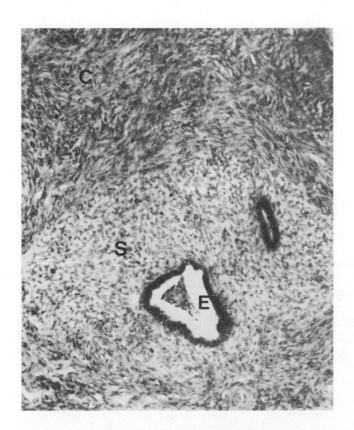

Figure 18-25. Endometriosis of the ovary. A nodule of endometrial-type glands (*E*) and stroma (*S*) lies in the ovarian cortex (*C*).

before or during menstruation. Infertility is the primary complaint in a third of cases. Dyspareunia and gastrointestinal abdominal pain are other symptoms. The periodic nature of the pelvic pain is attributed to bleeding with the foci and secondary irritation of the peritoneum that is hormonally related and therefore cyclical. Reactive fibrosis of the hemorrhagic areas results in the scarring responsible for much of the subsequent symptomatology.

The pathogenesis of endometriosis has long been controversial. The most widely accepted theory holds that **foci of menstrual endometrium regurgitate through the fallopian tubes and implant on the various pelvic organs. Since the fimbrial openings are in the posterior area of the pelvis, most deposits from the menstrual "spill" implant on structures located in the posterior pelvis.**

Early lesions involving the ovary vary from 1 mm to 5 mm in size and appear as red or bluish nodules. With repeated hemorrhage, they enlarge. Occasionally, the foci become cystic and the lumen fills with clotted blood, for which reason the cysts are called **chocolate cysts.** Some attain a size of 20 cm.

The microscopic diagnosis of endometriosis depends on the identification of endometrial glands and stroma. The glandular epithelium is usually endometrioid in type but may be tubal. Less than 1% of endometriotic foci undergo malignant change.

19

THE BREAST

SUE A. BARTOW AND CECILIA FENOGLIO-PREISER

NON-NEOPLASTIC DISEASES

JUVENILE HYPERTROPHY AND GYNECOMASTIA

Abnormal **hypertrophy** of the breast may occur at any age, but it is most commonly identified in the neonatal and peripubertal periods. **Neonatal hypertrophy** is induced by maternal hormones and resolves as levels of these hormones fall after birth. **Pubertal** or **juvenile hypertrophy** may occur in both females and males, and may be bilateral or unilateral.

Morphologically, hypertrophy and hyperplasia involve the tissues of the adolescent breast, that is, the fibrous stroma and the ducts. Lobules are not yet formed and so do not participate in the hyperplastic process.

In some instances, hypertrophy may be secondary to abnormally high hormone levels, such as in functioning ovarian, adrenocortical, or pituitary tumors. If the hormone levels are lowered, the hypertrophy resolves. In other instances the etiology is inapparent. It usually presents no major problem, except to the psyche of the adolescent girl or boy, and will usually regress as puberty advances. Occasionally, however, the process becomes severe and fails to regress. Surgical correction is then appropriate.

Gynecomastia (Fig. 19-1) refers to enlargement of the male breast and is morphologically similar to juvenile hypertrophy. The two terms, in fact, may be used interchangeably when the process occurs in a young, pubertal male; however, in the adult male it is always called gynecomastia. In the adult, although it may be idiopathic, it is often seen in a setting of abnormally increased estrogens or as a paraneoplastic manifestation. Thus, gynecomastia in the adult male commonly is associated with liver disease (which results in inappropriate metabolism of estrogens) or with carcinoma of the lung. It is also seen in association with Klinefelter's syndrome and in rare instances of feminizing testicular tumors. Gynecomastia has also been associated with the intake of a number of illicit drugs, including marijuana, amphetamines, and heroin.

ACUTE MASTITIS AND ABSCESS

Acute bacterial mastitis may be seen at any age; however, by far the most common setting is the postpartum involuting or lactating breast. It is usually secondary to obstruction of the duct system by inspissated secretions that cause stasis of the secretory products of the breast. The most common organisms isolated are *Staphylococcus* and *Streptococcus*. The acute inflammatory process may progress to abscess formation, an outcome that

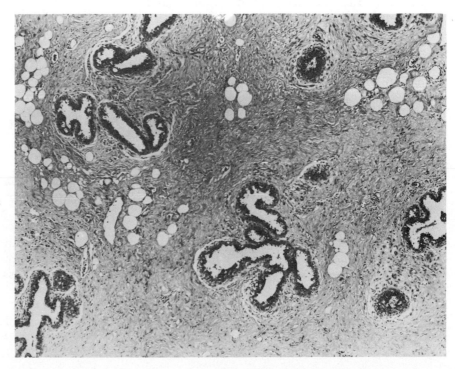

Figure 19-1. Gynecomastia. There is proliferation of branching intermediate size ducts. The epithelium lining the ducts is hyperplastic. Epithelial mitoses may be seen. A concomitant increase in the surrounding fibrous connective tissue causes a palpable mass.

TERMINAL DUCT LOBULAR UNIT

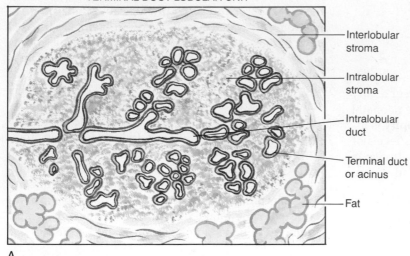

— Interlobular stroma

— Intralobular stroma

— Intralobular duct

— Terminal duct or acinus

— Fat

A

Figure 19-2. Schematic representation of benign breast lesions. (*A*) The normal terminal duct lobular unit.

requires surgical intervention. After the diffuse inflammatory process resolves, a firm, healed, nontender abscess may be mistaken for cancer.

DUCT ECTASIA

Duct ectasia, or focal dilatation, is the result of chronic obstruction or stasis of breast secretions. The disease commonly involves the large collecting ducts immediately under the areola. It usually affects older, multiparous women who have had repeated and/or prolonged episodes of breast feeding. In younger women the peripheral, intermediate-sized ducts may be involved. The cause of the obstruction in this setting is unknown. Although the peripheral form is less common, it is more often subjected to biopsy because of the difficulty of clinically distinguishing this condition from carcinoma.

Morphologically, the involved ducts are markedly dilated and contain acellular debris, along with foamy macrophages. Grossly this debris has a characteristic toothpastelike consistency. As a secondary process, these dilated ducts not infrequently rupture and incite a chronic, sometimes granulomatous, inflammatory cell response in the surrounding stroma. Because many of the infiltrating cells are plasma cells, the diagnosis of **plasma cell mastitis** is sometimes made. The terms "plasma cell mastitis" and "duct ectasia" are commonly used interchangeably.

FAT NECROSIS

A history of trauma usually precedes cases of fat necrosis. Initially the lesion consists of hemorrhage with an infiltrate of inflammatory cells and histiocytes that phagocytose the lipid debris. Subsequently, granulation tissue grows into the area. As the more acute process resolves, there may be a marked increase in fibroblastic proliferation, and foamy (xanthomatous) histiocytes are present. The healing, fibrosing process can send fingers of fibrous scar tissue into adjacent normal breast. **As a result, an irregular, fixed, and hard mass may be the presenting picture. Dystrophic calcifications, detected radiographically, may also occur. Because these features are also characteristic of carcinoma, these lesions are often examined by biopsy.**

FIBROCYSTIC DISEASE

Fibrocystic disease is a common and complex entity. To the woman (and to the physician examining her breasts), the term may be synonymous with increased breast lumpiness and pain in the second half of the menstrual cycle. To the radiologist, it indicates dense parenchyma occupying more than 25% of the total breast volume. To the pathologist, it is a morphologic constellation of features seen grossly as well as micro-

Figure 19-2 (continued). (*B*) Fibrocystic change. Cystic dilatation of the terminal ducts with varying degrees of apocrine metaplasia and fibrous stroma is depicted. Proliferative lesions that involve the epithelium of the terminal duct lobular unit in fibrocystic disease include the histologic patterns of (*C*) ductal type hyperplasia and (*D*) lobular type hyperplasia. (*E*) Fibrocystic change is occasionally accompanied by a proliferation of small ducts in association with deposition of connective tissue. This is termed "sclerosing adenosis." (*F*) A benign tumor that originates from the terminal duct lobular unit is the fibroadenoma, in which proliferated stroma contains secondarily increased and distorted ductal structures.

FIBROCYSTIC CHANGE

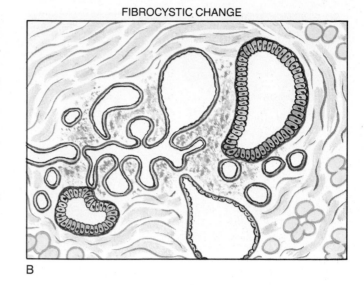

B

INTRADUCTAL EPITHELIAL HYPERPLASIA

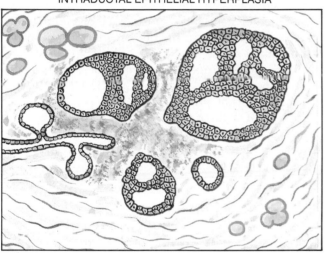

C

ATYPICAL LOBULAR HYPERPLASIA

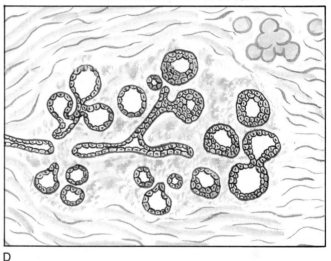

D

SCLEROSING ADENOSIS

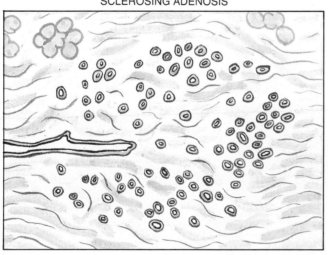

E

FIBROADENOMA

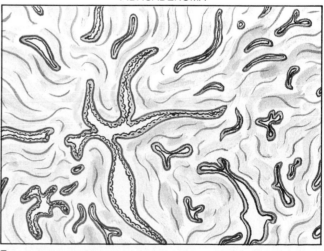

F

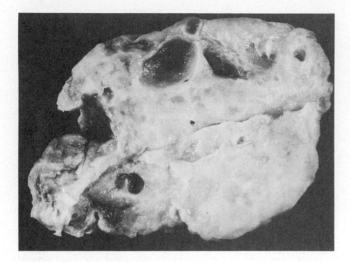

Figure 19-3. Fibrocystic disease. Cysts of various sizes are dispersed in dense fibrous connective tissue.

scopically. **A common denominator is the presence of excess fibrous tissue in the breast parenchyma relative to a "normal" woman of the same age.** It is important to realize that the criteria for this diagnosis are age-related. Most women up to about age 20 have predominantly dense, fibrous breasts, while those over age 80 have mostly fatty breasts. **Fibrocystic disease is** usually diagnosed in women in their late twenties to middle forties.

The most common morphologic finding in fibrocystic disease is an abundance of dense, fibrous stroma (Fig. 19-2). This is almost always accompanied by some degree of **cystic dilatation of the terminal ductules** (see Fig. 19-2*B*). A frequent concomitant of simple dilatation is an alteration of the epithelial lining, termed **apocrine metaplasia.** The metaplastic cells are larger and more eosinophilic than the cells usually lining the ducts. Histologically and ultrastructurally these cells resemble apocrine sweat gland epithelium. **Apocrine metaplasia is not per se a premalignant change** and may be focally present in breasts without any fibrocystic changes.

Commonly, cystic changes are minor and not the cause of discrete masses. However, occasionally cystic dilatation of the terminal ducts is so severe as to cause a prominent mass in the breast (Fig. 19-3). The large cysts often contain dark, serosanguineous fluid, which imparts a blue color to the unopened cysts—so-called **blue-domed cysts.**

Fibrocystic change is always present in multiple areas of both breasts. Therefore, treatment of fibrocystic change is not primarily surgical. To the surgeon, palpation of a discrete mass raises the possibility of breast cancer arising in a background of fibrocystic disease. Such a concern often leads to biopsy in women with fibrocystic disease.

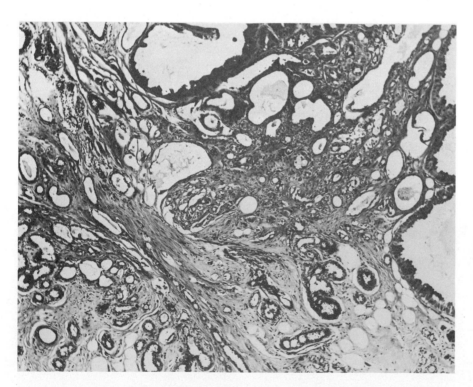

Figure 19-4. Fibrocystic disease with epithelial proliferative components. The terminal duct lobular unit is grotesquely distorted by cystic change, sclerosis, and adenosis. Apocrine metaplasia is seen in the more dilated ducts. Duct epithelial hyperplasia is seen in less dilated ducts in the lower half of the field.

The histologic features of fibrocystic disease are complicated by a subset of epithelial proliferative changes in the terminal duct lobular unit (Fig. 19-4). The most commonly seen change is an increase in the number of cells lining the terminal ductules, referred to as **ductal epithelial hyperplasia** (see Fig. 19-2C). It may also be termed **epitheliosis** or **papillomatosis**. The latter term was coined because the proliferation can at times become exuberant and form papillomatous structures within the lumen of the distended ductule.

The second—and much less common—form of hyperplasia also involves the cells lining the terminal ducts, but it has a different histologic and cytologic appearance; it has been termed **lobular hyperplasia** (see Fig. 19-2D).

These epithelial proliferative lesions in fibrocystic disease originate from the same epithelial structures that give rise to carcinoma of the breast. In fact, there appears to be a morphologic spectrum that extends from minor degrees of hyperplasia, through exuberant—but cytologically benign—hyperplasia, to cytologic atypia and other histologic features characterized as carcinoma in situ. When some, but not all, of the features of malignancy are present in these proliferating lesions, the diagnosis of "atypical" ductal or lobular hyperplasia is made. These two forms of atypical hyperplasia have their counterparts in the classification of breast carcinoma, which will be discussed later.

The atypical proliferative lesions increase the risk for the subsequent development of carcinoma of the
breast (Table 19-1). The lesions may be multifocal and bilateral, and the risk of subsequent carcinoma is equal in both breasts. Epithelial hyperplasia, with or without atypia, is a microscopic finding, and does not by itself cause a clinically perceived mass.

A less common subset of epithelial proliferative change is termed **adenosis** or **sclerosing adenosis** (see Fig. 19-2E). This is almost always associated with simple fibrocystic change, as well as with ductal epithelial hyperplasia. **The term "adenosis" is used when there is a proliferation of small ducts and myoepithelial cells reminiscent of the normal terminal ductules.** Because this lesion commonly has a fibrous connective tissue component, the term "sclerosing adenosis" is often used. Sclerosing adenosis has no apparent atypical counterpart and is not associated with an increased risk for carcinoma. **Sclerosing adenosis, usually a microscopic finding, is occasionally so florid that it gives rise to a distinct mass that can be mistaken clinically for carcinoma.**

NEOPLASIA

FIBROADENOMA

The most common benign neoplasm of the breast is the fibroadenoma. As its name implies, it is composed of a **mixture of fibrous connective tissue and epithelial ductal structures.** Although it may vary in size from a microscopic lesion to a large tumor, it is usually 2 to 4 cm in diameter. A smooth, round, firm, rubbery tumor, it is sharply delineated from the surrounding breast tissue, and thus freely movable (Fig. 19-5A).

The histologic features of fibroadenomas are distinctive (Fig. 19-5B). In these lesions, ducts are situated within the fibrous stroma, varying from simple, small structures to an elongated and branching network. The site of origin of fibroadenoma is the terminal duct lobular unit (see Fig. 19-2F).

Fibroadenomas usually are seen in patients between the ages of 20 and 35. They also occur in adolescent girls. A minority in this group have a different pathologic and clinical presentation, warranting the diagnosis **juvenile fibroadenoma.** Because some of these juvenile fibroadenomas attain great size, they have been described as **giant fibroadenomas.**

INTRADUCTAL PAPILLOMA

The intraductal papilloma is a distinct neoplasm that displays a papillary histologic pattern and occurs in the

Table 19-1   Risk Factors for Carcinoma of the Breast

FACTOR	RELATIVE RISK (%)
Family History	
Primary relative	1.2–3.0
Postmenopausal unilateral	1.5
Premenopausal bilateral	8.5–9.0
Menstrual History	
Age at menarche < 12 years	1.3
Age at menopause > 55 years	1.48–2.0
Pregnancy	
First child after 35	2.0–3.0
Nulliparous	3.0
Other Breast Disease	
Fibrocystic change without epithelial hyperplasia	0.9
Moderate or severe epithelial hyperplasia without atypia	1.5–2.0
Atypical ductal or lobular hyperplasia	4.0–5.0
Ductal or lobular carcinoma in situ	8.0–10.0

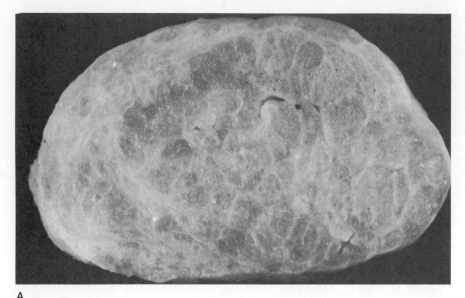

A

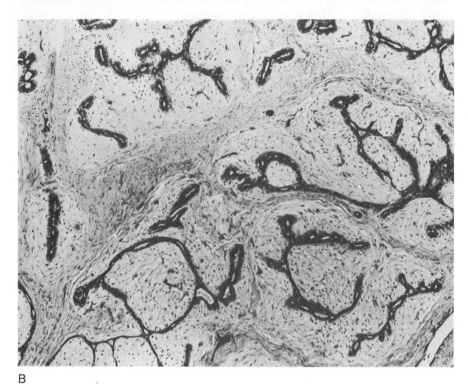

B

Figure 19-5. Fibroadenoma. (*A*) A well-circumscribed tumor can be easily enucleated from the surrounding breast. The septate and sometimes clefted gross appearance is caused by elongated epithelial duct structures (*B*). The predominant proliferation, however, is stromal.

large, lactiferous ducts. It is a solitary neoplasm, usually a few millimeters in diameter, and should be distinguished from papillomatosis, the form of duct epithelial hyperplasia that occurs as a component of fibrocystic disease. Intraductal papillomas occur most commonly in middle-aged and older women. Because they occur in the large, subareolar ducts, they may be associated with a serous or bloody nipple discharge. Although the solitary papilloma is not believed to be a premalignant lesion or to increase the risk of carcinoma in the breast, the lesion itself must be distinguished from well-differentiated papillary intraductal carcinoma.

CARCINOMA OF THE BREAST

EPIDEMIOLOGY

Carcinoma of the breast remains a leading cause of death from cancer in women. The incidence has remained relatively stable over the last 50 years. One in every 13 American women may be expected to develop breast cancer. Although breast cancer occasionally occurs in young women, it is uncommon before the age of 25.

Studies of the epidemiology of breast cancer have pinpointed several factors that are associated with increased risk (see Table 19-1). Among these is a **high socioeconomic and nutritional status.** Because improved overall health causes the age of menarche to occur earlier and menopause to occur later, the breast epithelium is mitotically active and vulnerable to carcinogenic influences for a longer period.

Women who have a full-term pregnancy at an early age display a decreased risk of cancer. Nulliparous women or those who become pregnant for the first time after age 35 are at a risk two to three times that of the general population.

The strongest association with an increased risk for breast cancer is a strong family history of breast cancer—specifically, breast cancer in first-degree relatives (mother, sister, daughter). Women who have previously had breast cancer themselves also have a markedly increased risk (four to five times that of the general population) of developing a second primary breast carcinoma.

Women with the diagnosis of fibrocystic disease have an increased risk of breast cancer if specific subsets of fibrocystic disease are identified histologically. The strongest association with increased risk appears to be in women with atypical ductal and lobular hyperplasia (four to five times that of the general popula-

tion). Women with both a first-degree family history of breast cancer and atypical hyperplasia have a tenfold increased risk of developing cancer.

MORPHOLOGY

Carcinomas of the breast are almost all adenocarcinomas; they are derived from the glandular epithelium of the terminal duct lobular unit.

CARCINOMA IN SITU

There are three major subtypes of noninvasive, or in situ, carcinoma, which correspond to the proliferative lesions described earlier. The most common is **intra ductal carcinoma.** A less common form is **lobular carcinoma in situ (lobular neoplasia).** The least common is **intraductal papillary carcinoma.** Both the ductal and lobular in situ forms arise in the terminal duct lobular unit, and there is frequent admixture of these two subtypes. Intraductal carcinoma exhibits a complex growth pattern, frequently showing cribriform, individual ductlike structures within the original duct (Fig. 19-6). Lobular carcinoma in situ, on the other hand, is composed of regular, small cells that grow in a solid pattern and fill the original ducts or lobules (Fig. 19-7).

It is the fibroblastic proliferation in the tissue surrounding the invading cancer cells that is responsible for the presence of a palpable hard mass. In situ carcinoma, which by definition is not at an invasive stage, may be an incidental finding in a biopsy specimen obtained because of the fibrosis and lumpiness associated with fibrocystic disease. An exception to this is the so-called **comedocarcinoma,** a form of intraductal carcinoma that may be associated with increased stromal fibrosis. A hallmark of this form of carcinoma is necrosis in the tumor cell aggregates, which plug the ducts. This expressible necrotic debris not uncommonly calcifies, resulting in multiple microscopic calcifications detectable radiographically.

Even when no invasive component is found on routine microscopic examination, up to 5% of women with intraductal carcinoma have metastatic carcinoma in axillary lymph nodes.

Papillary intraductal carcinoma is a more indolent neoplasm. If excised in its in situ state, it has a low risk of recurrence and metastasis.

INVASIVE CARCINOMA

Invasive, or infiltrating, ductal carcinoma is by far the most common form of breast cancer (Table 19-2). In this disease, the invasion by malignant epithelium

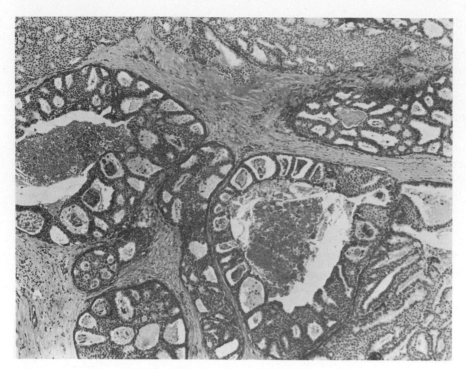

Figure 19-6. Intraductal carcinoma. Greatly distended terminal ducts with in situ carcinoma (intraductal carcinoma) are seen. The normal epithelium is replaced by malignant cells that commonly surround small spaces (giving a cribriform appearance). The cells are large, with prominent nuclei and abundant cytoplasm. Areas of necrosis are apparent in the lumina of the tumorous ducts.

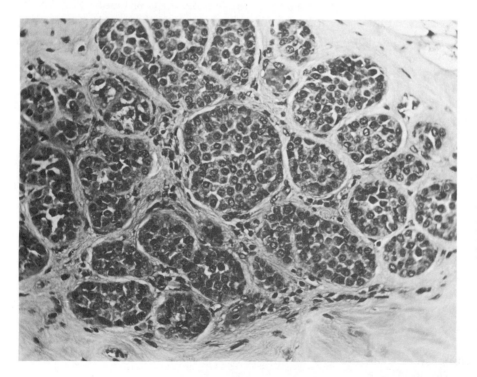

Figure 19-7. Lobular carcinoma in situ. In the lobular form of carcinoma in situ, the cells are smaller and have less cytoplasm than in the ductal type. Regular, round nuclei and small nucleoli are characteristic. The tumor cells usually completely obliterate the lumen without forming a cribriform pattern.

Table 19-2 Frequency of Histologic Subtypes of Invasive Breast Carcinoma

SUBTYPE	FREQUENCY (%)
Invasive ductal carcinoma	
Pure	
Mixed with others	52.6
(Mixed ductal and lobular 3.3)	28.0
Invasive lobular carcinoma (pure)	4.9
Medullary carcinoma (pure)	6.2
Mucinous carcinoma (pure)	2.4
Paget's disease	2.3
Other pure types	2.0
Other mixed types	1.6

incites a pronounced fibroblastic proliferation. Grossly, the tumors are firm and white, with irregular fingers extending into adjacent breast tissue (Fig. 19-8). These are the properties that result in a clinical impression of a hard, fixed mass. On cut section, the neoplasm commonly is flecked with yellow chalky streaks and has a gritty consistency. A frequently used descriptive term for this invasive tumor is **scirrhous carcinoma.**

The malignant epithelium of invasive ductal carcinoma appears as irregular nests and cords of cells (Fig. 19-9). The better-differentiated tumors may form glandular structures; the less-differentiated grow in solid sheets. Individually, the cells are similar to those of the in situ variety of ductal carcinoma.

Paget's disease of the nipple, although usually classified separately, is in fact an uncommon manifestation of ductal carcinoma. **Paget's disease is involvement of the epidermis of the nipple by the malignant ductal cells.**

The amount of fibrosis associated with **invasive lobular carcinoma** is much more variable than in invasive ductal carcinoma. Typically, the cells form single files, commonly termed "Indian filing," between the stromal fibers (Fig. 19-10).

MEDULLARY CARCINOMA

After ductal and lobular invasive carcinoma, medullary carcinoma is the most common type of breast cancer (see Table 19-2). Macroscopically, it is a well-circumscribed, fleshy, gray-white mass. Microscopically, it is composed of structureless sheets of cells, which are very pleomorphic and have a high mitotic index. **A sine qua non for the diagnosis of medullary carcinoma is a concomitant lymphoid infiltrate.** In spite of the highly malignant appearance of this neoplasm, it has a better prognosis than the ordinary infiltrating ductal carcinoma.

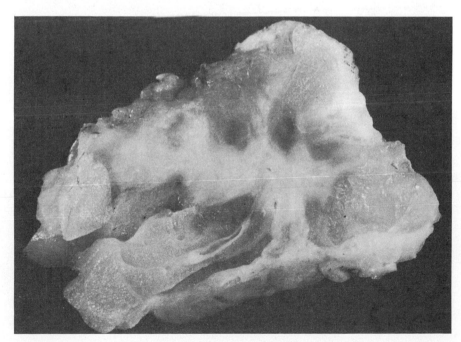

Figure 19-8. Scirrhous carcinoma. This gross appearance is most commonly associated with invasive ductal carcinoma. However, such tumors may also be produced by other subtypes of invasive carcinoma. The tumor mass is extremely firm and irregular, and tentacles from the main mass extend into the surrounding adipose tissue. The cut surface is gritty, owing to microcalcifications, which impart the characteristic appearance of breast cancer on mammography.

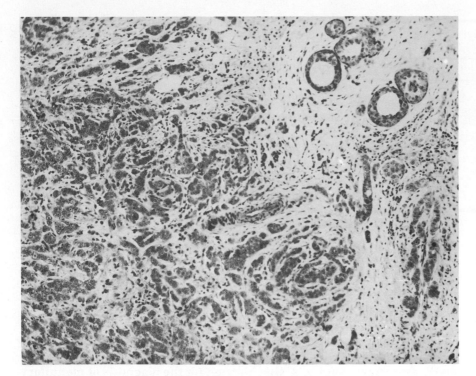

Figure 19-9. Infiltrating or invasive ductal carcinoma. The same cells that compose the intraductal component form irregular cords and nests of carcinoma invading the stroma. The cells may form ductlike structures. The invading epithelium is commonly accompanied by a marked fibrous tissue proliferation (desmoplasia). This latter characteristic is the cause of the clinically appreciated hard mass.

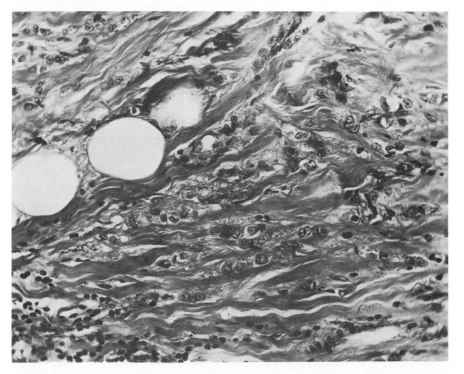

Figure 19-10. Invasive or infiltrating lobular carcinoma. The same cells seen in the in situ form of lobular carcinoma invade the stroma. In contrast to invasive ductal carcinoma, the "lobular" cells tend to form single strands of cells that line up in an Indian-file pattern between strands of collagen.

COLLOID CARCINOMA

A less common variant of breast carcinoma is the **mucinous** or **colloid carcinoma.** In its pure form this variant also has a better prognosis than the ordinary infiltrating ductal neoplasm. It tends to occur in older women. Grossly, the tumor has a glistening surface and mucoid consistency. Histologically, it is composed of small clusters of epithelial cells, occasionally forming glands, that float in a large amount of extracellular mucin.

MALE CANCER OF THE BREAST

Cancer in the male breast accounts for approximately one in every one hundred cases of breast cancer. As in women, by far the most common subtype is the infiltrating ductal variety. Although the normal man does not have development of the terminal duct lobular unit, rarely the lobular type of carcinoma is seen in men.

HISTOLOGIC PROGNOSTIC FEATURES

Breast tumors with poor histologic and cytologic differentiation display lack of gland formation, cellular pleomorphism, and a high mitotic index. **These histologic features correlate with a poor prognosis in invasive ductal carcinomas. A lack of circumscription and the presence of vascular and lymphatic invasion also indicate a worse prognosis. A particularly poor prognosis (less than 35% survival at 5 years) is associated with lymphatic invasion in the dermis of the overlying breast skin.** Dermal lymphatic invasion is the pathologic criterion for making the diagnosis of **"inflammatory"** carcinoma. This finding commonly correlates with clinical erythema and induration of the skin of the breast **(peau d'orange).**

STAGING OF CARCINOMA

The most common primary site for breast carcinoma is the upper outer quadrant. The second most common site is the central or subareolar area. The lower outer and inner quadrants are less commonly involved. The initial lymphatic spread is almost always to the axillary lymph nodes. Even in medially located lesions, the axillary nodes are as likely to be involved as the parasternal nodes.

Clinical staging of breast cancer is based on the size and extent of the primary tumor, regional lymph node status, and the presence of distant metastases. Clinical stage I refers to a primary tumor of less than 2 cm in diameter and uninvolved axillary lymph nodes. Stage II indicates metastases to axillary lymph nodes, or a primary tumor between 2 and 5 cm in diameter, with or without palpable axillary nodes. Stage III is characterized by a primary tumor greater than 5 cm in diameter and/or obvious axillary nodal involvement, with fixation of the nodes. Stage IV carcinoma refers to distant metastases or extensive local involvement, with **peau d'orange** of the breast skin.

The most common sites of metastasis from breast cancer are lung, bone, and liver. Brain, adrenal, and ovarian metastases are not uncommon.

OTHER NEOPLASMS

The phyllodes tumor may also be referred to as a **"cystosarcoma phyllodes."** It resembles the fibroadenoma in that it is composed of both stromal and ductal epithelial elements. The tumor is usually large, but the differentiation from fibroadenoma depends not on size but on the histologic and cytologic **characteristics of the stromal component.** A tumor that resembles a fibroadenoma may be given the designation of cystosarcoma solely on the basis of increased cellularity and mitotic activity of the stroma. In these cases, the term **"cellular fibroadenoma"** is preferred to "benign cystosarcoma." Such tumors are unlikely to metastasize, and are adequately treated by local excision. If incompletely excised, they may recur locally. A clearly malignant phyllodes tumor has an obviously sarcomatous stroma and usually is poorly circumscribed, with invasion into the surrounding breast tissue. The tumors may have various sarcomatous tissue types, such as malignant fibrous histiocytoma, chondrosarcoma, and osteosarcoma. Cystosarcomas preferentially metastasize to distant sites rather than the axillary lymph nodes.

20

THE BLOOD AND THE LYMPHOID ORGANS

HUGH BONNER

Disorders of Hemostasis

Anemia

Erythrocytosis (Polycythemia)

Benign Disorders of
   Polymorphonuclear
   Leukocytes

Proliferative Disorders
   of Mast Cells

Differentiated Histiocytoses

Benign Disorders
   of Lymphoid Cells

Disorders of the Spleen

Monoclonal Gammopathy of
   Unknown Significance

Chronic Myeloproliferative
   Syndromes

Acute Myeloproliferative
   Syndromes: The Acute
   Nonlymphocytic Leukemias

Malignant Disorders of the
   Mononuclear Phagocyte
   System

The Lymphocytic Leukemias

The Non-Hodgkin's Malignant
   Lymphomas

Plasma Cell Neoplasia

Hodgkin's Disease

Metastatic Tumors
   to the Bone Marrow

DISORDERS OF HEMOSTASIS

Congenital and acquired disorders of each of the three biologic systems involved in hemostasis, namely the blood vessels, platelets, and coagulation factors, predispose either to spontaneous bleeding or to excessive bleeding following trauma. Bleeding due to vascular disorders consists of petechiae and purpuric hemorrhages in the skin and in the gastrointestinal and genitourinary tracts. Bleeding due to platelet disorders is usually in the form of petechiae, from small vessels in the skin, mucous membranes, and the serosal surfaces of the body cavities. In platelet disorders bleeding usually occurs immediately following trauma or a surgical procedure. Bleeding due to coagulation factor deficiencies is seen as large areas of ecchymosis, as hematomas in sites such as the subcutaneous or muscle tissues, and as hemorrhage into the gastrointestinal system, genitourinary tract, and joint spaces (hemarthrosis). With coagulation factor deficiencies, the onset of bleeding may be delayed following trauma or a surgical procedure.

BLOOD VESSEL DISORDERS

Hereditary vascular disorders that are associated with bleeding include hereditary hemorrhagic telangiectasia (Osler-Weber-Rendu disease) and connective tissue disorders, such as Marfan's syndrome. **Acquired vascular defects** are an uncommon cause of clinical bleeding. In **vitamin C deficiency** (scurvy), collagen synthesis and deposition of intercellular cement are defective, and bleeding occurs in the subcutaneous tissues, skeletal muscle, gingiva, and skin around hair follicles. **Senile purpura** is caused by an age-related atrophy of the connective tissue supporting structures that predisposes to skin hemorrhage, particularly on sun-exposed areas. In **Cushing's syndrome** purpura is related to the catabolic effect of corticosteroids on the perivascular connective tissues. Purpura may also be due to **drug-induced vascular damage.** Serum paraproteins and cryoglobulins may also cause vascular damage and bleeding. **Allergic purpura** is a disorder generally discerned in children. It typically is preceded by an upper respiratory infection. Histopathologically, a vasculitis is characterized by perivascular neutrophils and eosinophils, and fibrinoid necrosis of vessel walls. Clinically, joint pain, gastrointestinal symptoms, and renal disease may be discerned.

DISORDERS OF PLATELETS

Thrombocytopenia is a decrease in the platelet count to less than the normal minimum of 150,000 platelets per microliter. A decrease in the platelet count to less than 50,000 per microliter increases the hazard of bleeding from trauma or surgical procedures. Spontaneous bleeding can occur with a platelet count below 20,000, and is especially likely to occur with a count below 5000 per microliter. Thrombocytopenia can result from decreased production of platelets, increased destruction of platelets, and splenic sequestration of platelets.

Decreased production of platelets is due either to a decreased number of megakaryocytes in the bone marrow or to ineffective thrombopoiesis (intramedullary destruction of megakaryocyte-platelets). A decreased megakaryocyte mass occurs in aplastic anemia, bone marrow infiltrative diseases (myelophthisis), and bone marrow hypoplasia caused by x-irradiation, myelotoxic agents, and viral infections.

Increased extramedullary destruction of platelets occurs both by immune and by nonimmune mechanisms and is accompanied by an increase in bone marrow megakaryocyte mass. Immune destruction of platelets is seen in idiopathic thrombocytopenic purpura, isoimmune neonatal purpura, posttransfusion purpura, drug-induced thrombocytopenic purpura, and secondary immunologic purpura.

Idiopathic thrombocytopenic purpura (ITP) generally occurs either as an acute disorder in children or as a chronic disorder in adults. **Acute ITP** usually follows an acute viral illness. There is a rapid decrease in the platelet count, frequently to less than 20,000 platelets per microliter. Petechiae or purpuric hemorrhages in the skin and mucous membranes are conspicuous. The mechanism of the thrombocytopenia may involve the binding of circulating antigen–antibody complexes to platelet Fc receptors. Such coated platelets are vulnerable to destruction by splenic macrophages. Eighty percent of the cases of acute ITP spontaneously remit in weeks or months. Recurrences are unusual.

Chronic ITP typically is a disorder of middle-aged women. IgG antiplatelet antibody is demonstrated in approximately 85% of the cases. Unlike acute ITP, chronic ITP is not generally precipitated by an infectious episode. Its course is usually punctuated by relapses and remissions. As with acute ITP, platelet destruction in chronic ITP occurs principally in the spleen. The pathologic hallmark in both acute and chronic ITP is an increase in young hyposegmented megakaryocytes in the bone marrow.

In **drug-induced thrombocytopenia,** an immunologic mechanism is also postulated. Platelets are destroyed, probably in the spleen, after being coated with drug–antibody complexes.

Disseminated intravascular coagulation (DIC) is a complex acquired disorder characterized by both widespread intravascular coagulation and diffuse hemorrhage. The pathophysiology of DIC (Fig. 20-1) relates

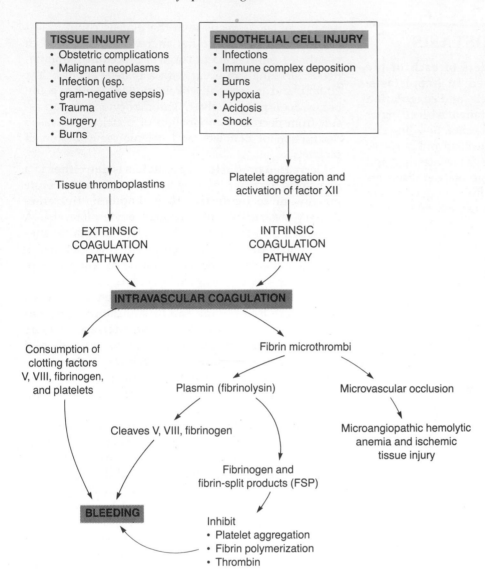

Figure 20-1. The pathophysiology of disseminated intravascular coagulation (DIC). The syndrome of DIC is precipitated either by tissue injury, with release of tissue thromboplastin and activation of the extrinsic coagulation pathway, or by endothelial cell injury, with activation of the intrinsic coagulation pathway. Intravascular coagulation is induced by either or, frequently, both mechanisms. Clinically, there is bleeding from multiple sites and microvascular occlusions or thromboses with secondary microangiopathic hemolytic anemia and ischemic tissue injury.

to an initial, widespread initiation of microvascular coagulation due to either tissue damage, with release of tissue procoagulants or thromboplastins into the peripheral circulation (extrinsic pathway), or extensive endothelial cell injury, with activation of factor XII and consequent initiation of platelet aggregation and release of platelet factor 3 (intrinsic pathway). Both mechanisms are commonly involved. **Widespread intravascular coagulation and fibrin deposition produces ischemia of severely affected organs.** In addition, red blood cells are fragmented in passage through the intravascular fibrin deposits **(microangiopathic hemolytic anemia).** Schistocytes (fragmented erythrocytes) are identified on the peripheral blood smear in 20% of the cases. **Fibrin–platelet microthrombi are**

seen in the microvasculature of essentially any organ. The most commonly involved sites, in decreasing order of frequency, are the brain, heart, lungs, kidneys, adrenal glands, spleen, and liver.

The hemorrhagic diathesis in DIC dominates the clinical picture. It results from the consumption of platelets, clotting factors V and VII, and prothrombin (consumption coagulopathy), as well as from the activation of plasminogen to plasmin (fibrinolysin). The presence of plasmin further depresses the blood levels of factors V and VIII and cleaves fibrinogen and fibrin to degradation products. These "split products" impair fibrin polymerization and platelet aggregation.

Disorders commonly associated with DIC include obstetric complications, certain malignancies, massive trauma, and infections, particularly those with accompanying sepsis. Laboratory findings include a low platelet count, low serum fibrinogen, prolonged prothrombin, partial thromboplastin and thrombin times, and elevated fibrinogen–fibrin split products.

Thrombotic thrombocytopenic purpura (TTP) is a rare, acute systemic disorder of the microvasculature. It occurs most commonly in young women. The pathogenesis appears to be related to immunologically mediated damage to small blood vessels. Fibrin–platelet microthrombi may be seen in the lumina of small arterioles and capillaries in essentially any organ or tissue. The clinical syndrome consists of the pentad of fever, thrombocytopenia, microangiopathic hemolytic anemia, renal failure, and fluctuating neurologic deficits.

Thrombocytopenia due to splenic sequestration reflects a redistribution of the peripheral blood platelet pool. A larger than normal proportion, over one-third, of the peripheral blood platelet pool is retained in the spleen. The platelet redistribution is roughly proportional to the size of the spleen. In massive splenomegaly as much as 90% of the peripheral blood platelet pool may be sequestered in the spleen.

DISORDERS OF COAGULATION FACTORS

Both quantitative and qualitative defects of all of the plasma protein clotting factors have been identified. These defects may be hereditary or acquired. Only **hemophilia A (factor VIII deficiency), von Willebrand's disease,** and **hemophilia B (factor IX deficiency),** are common.

Factor VIII is a complex composed of the factor VIII functional coagulant molecule (VIII:C), von Willebrand's factor (VIII R:WF), and the ristocetin cofactor (VIII R:RCo). **Hemophilia A,** or **classic hemophilia,** is a deficiency of factor VIII:C; it accounts for approximately 85% of the hereditary clotting factor disorders. An X-linked recessive trait, it is common only in males. One-quarter of the cases arise from a de novo mutation. Factor VIII levels vary widely. In severe hemophilia, a factor VIII level of approximately 1% of normal is usual. In moderate hemophilia a factor VIII level of 1% to 5% is characteristic, and in mild hemophilia levels vary from 5% to 10% of normal. **Severely affected persons manifest spontaneous bleeding into the weight-bearing joints (hemarthrosis).** Repeated hemarthroses eventually lead to joint deformities. Bleeding into the soft tissues and the viscera also occurs.

Von Willebrand's disease is due either to qualitative or to quantitative abnormalities of a factor (von Wille-brand's factor, factor VIII-related protein, VIII R:WF) that circulates as a complex with the factor VIII:C molecule.

Von Willebrand's factor is required for the normal adherence of platelets to subendothelial collagen. **In von Willebrand's disease, because of the intrinsic abnormality or deficiency of von Willebrand's factor, there is a lack of normal platelet adhesiveness.** Because of the **functional** platelet defect the bleeding time is prolonged. For poorly understood reasons a mild decrease in factor VIII coagulant activity is also usually observed.

In von Willebrand's disease there is also a decrease in or lack of the ristocetin cofactor. Because of this deficiency, upon the addition of the antibiotic ristocetin, aggregation of platelets either is decreased or does not occur. The demonstration of deficient or absent ristocetin-induced aggregation of platelets is a useful screening test for von Willebrand's disease.

The clinical severity of von Willebrand's disease varies. Generally, there is episodic mucosal bleeding, particularly from the gastrointestinal tract. Menorrhagia is also common. There is usually excessive bleeding following trauma. However, unlike hemophilia A, bleeding into the joint spaces is uncommon. The disorder tends to lessen in severity with age.

Hemophilia B is the result of factor IX deficiency. It is a less common disorder than either hemophilia A or von Willebrand's disease. Like hemophilia A, it is an X-linked recessive disorder. The clinical severity of the disorder is dependent on the level of factor IX. The disorder is severe when the factor IX level is 1% of normal, moderate when the factor IX level is 1% to 5% of normal, and mild when the factor IX level is at 5% to 10% of normal. The clinical syndrome is indistinguishable from that of hemophilia A. Recurrent hemarthroses may result in a crippling deformity of the joints.

ANEMIA

Anemia is a reduction below the normal range of the hemoglobin concentration in the peripheral blood. Disorders associated with anemia are classified according to either morphologic or pathophysiologic criteria (Table 20-1). The morphologic classification of anemia is based on a quantitative assessment of two of the erythrocyte indices: the mean corpuscular volume (MCV) and the mean corpuscular hemoglobin concentration (MCHC). An erythrocyte with a normal cell volume is said to be **normocytic.** An erythrocyte with a normal hemoglobin concentration is termed **normochromic.** On the basis of the erythrocyte indices,

Table 20-1   *Classification of Anemia*

PATHOPHYSIOLOGIC

Underproduction

Bone marrow failure
Deficiency of hematinic factors } ↓ **Reticulocyte count**
Bone marrow suppression

Increased Loss or Destruction

Hemorrhage } ↑ **Reticulocyte count**
Hemolysis

MORPHOLOGIC

	MCV	MCHC
Normocytic, normochromic	Normal	Normal
Macrocytic, normochromic	Increased	Normal
Microcytic, hypochromic	Decreased	Decreased
Normocytic, hyperchromic	Normal	Increased

(*MCV*, mean cell volume; *MCHC*, mean corpuscular hemoglobin concentration)

the anemias are morphologically classified as (1) normocytic, normochromic; (2) macrocytic, normochromic; (3) microcytic, hypochromic; and (4) normocytic, hyperchromic (see Table 20-10). **The pathophysiologic classification separates disorders associated with anemia into two major categories: those due to bone marrow failure, with underproduction of erythrocytes, and those caused by peripheral loss or destruction of erythrocytes.** Examination of the peripheral blood smear provides clues to the pathophysiology of the anemia (Fig. 20-2).

The pathophysiologic classification of the anemias is outlined in Table 20-2. This classification scheme is followed in the discussion of the specific anemias.

APLASTIC ANEMIA

Aplastic anemia (aplastic pancytopenia) is a common hematopoietic precursor cell disorder, characterized by a decrease in all peripheral blood cell types (pancytopenia) and a hypocellular marrow (Fig. 20-3). An apparent cause is identified in only half of the cases. Known causes include a variety of myelotoxic drugs and chemicals (e.g., chloramphenicol, benzene), ionizing radiation, certain viral infections (e.g., viral hepatitis), and immunologically mediated injury to the bone marrow precursor cells. The prognosis depends on the severity and duration of the bone marrow aplasia. Overall 5-year mortality for aplastic anemia is 70% in adults and 50% in children. Acute nonlymphocytic leukemia develops in 5% of the cases.

ANEMIA OF CHRONIC RENAL DISEASE

A mild normocytic, normochromic anemia is commonly observed in association with chronic renal disease. The severity of the anemia is proportional to the degree of the uremia. The causes of the anemia in chronic renal disease reflect both a decreased rate of erythrocyte production and an accelerated peripheral loss of erythrocytes. Decreased bone marrow production of erythrocytes results from **decreased production of erythropoietin** by the damaged kidneys and from the suppression of marrow erythroid precursors by unidentified factors in uremic serum. The administration of recombinant erythropoietin to anemic patients in renal failure has proved to be effective therapy. Blood loss due to gastrointestinal or gynecologic hemorrhage occurs in one-third to one-half of cases of chronic renal failure and may result in iron deficiency. The bleeding tendency is due to qualitative defects in platelet function or to abnormalities in vascular integrity that occur in uremia. The erythrocyte life span is also decreased, but the mechanism of hemolysis is incompletely understood. Finally, deficiencies in folic acid and iron may occur because of loss during hemodialysis. In chronic renal disease erythrocytes with regularly scalloped margins (burr cells) are characteristic.

MEGALOBLASTIC ANEMIAS

The megaloblastic anemias are due to a deficiency of either vitamin B_{12} or folic acid. Both types are characterized by abnormal DNA synthesis. In vitamin B_{12} deficiency the abnormal DNA synthesis is due to a coenzyme deficiency, with consequent impaired conversion of deoxyuridylate (dUMP) to deoxythymidylate (dTMP). This results in a delay in nuclear maturation and an abnormality in cell division. Cytoplasmic maturation, however, is normal. The mitotic abnormality is particularly expressed in such rapidly dividing cells as erythroid, granulocytic, and megakaryocytic precursor cells. Because of the delay in nuclear maturation, the nuclear chromatin is loose rather than condensed, an abnormality that persists even in the more mature precursor cells. **In vitamin B_{12} and folic acid deficiency, the abnormal and delayed cell division results in a population of unusually large precursor cells, a distinctive morphologic alteration called megaloblastosis** (Fig. 20-4). Because of the abnormal cell maturation and division, there is ineffective hematopoiesis,

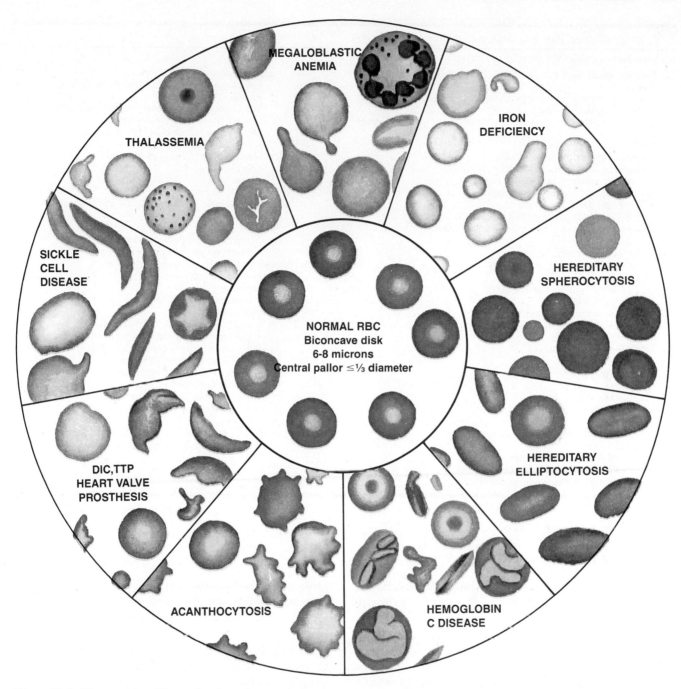

Figure 20-2. The anemias. The pathophysiology and characteristic morphologic features of the various anemias are shown. The morphology of normal erythrocytes is contrasted in the central circle.

Table 20-2   Anemia: Pathophysiologic Classification

Underproduction (Impaired Erythrocyte Production)

I. Hematopoietic stem cell proliferation and differentiation abnormality
   - Aplastic anemia (aplastic pancytopenia)
   - Myelodysplasia (dyshemopoiesis)
II. Erythroid-committed stem cell proliferation and differentiation abnormality
   - Pure red cell aplasia
   - Anemia of chronic renal disease
   - Anemia of endocrine disorders
   - Congenital dyserythropoietic anemias
III. Erythroblast proliferation and maturation abnormality
   A. Defective DNA synthesis
      - B_{12} deficiency or impaired utilization
      - Folate deficiency or impaired utilization
      - Inborn errors
   B. Defective hemoglobin synthesis
      1. Heme synthesis abnormality
         - Iron deficiency
      2. Globin synthesis abnormality
         - Thalassemias
IV. Unknown or multiple mechanisms
   - Anemia of chronic disease
   - Sideroblastic anemias
   - Myelophthisic anemias

Increased Loss or Destruction

I. Hemorrhage
   - Acute blood loss anemia
   - Chronic blood loss anemia
II. Hemolysis
   A. Intrinsic (intracorpuscular) abnormalities
      1. Hereditary
         (a). Membrane disorders
            - Hereditary spherocytosis
            - Hereditary elliptocytosis
            - Hereditary stomatocytosis
            - Acanthocytosis (abetalipoproteinemia)
         (b). Enzyme deficiency
            (i). Glycolytic (Embden-Myerhof) pathway
               - Pyruvate kinase deficiency
            (ii). Hexose monophosphate shunt pathway
               - G6PD deficiency
         (c). Structurally abnormal globin chain
            - Sickle cell anemia
            - Hemoglobin C disease
            - Unstable hemoglobins
            - Hemoglobins with abnormal oxygen affinity
            - Methemoglobinemia
      2. Acquired
         (a). Membrane complement sensitivity
            - Paroxysmal nocturnal hemoglobinuria
   B. Extrinsic (extracorpuscular) abnormalities
      1. Immune mediated
         (a). Isohemagglutinins
            - Erythroblastosis fetalis
         (b). Autoantibodies
            - Warm antibody-induced hemolysis
            - Cold antibody autoimmune hemolytic anemia
         (c). Drug-induced immunologic injury to erythrocytes
      2. Mechanical trauma to erythrocytes
         - Traumatic cardiac hemolytic anemia
         - March hemoglobinuria
         - Microangiopathic hemolytic anemia
      3. Hypersplenism (hyperactivity of mononuclear phagocyte system)
      4. Hemolytic anemia due to chemical or physical agents
      5. Hemolytic anemia due to infections

Multifactorial
   - Alcohol-induced anemia

---

with markedly increased intramedullary destruction of hematopoietic precursor cells. **Therefore, pancytopenia is characteristic of the megaloblastic anemias.**

VITAMIN B_{12} DEFICIENCY

In vitamin B_{12} deficiency the bone marrow is usually markedly hypercellular, and there is an increase in blast cells with dense, purple cytoplasm (megaloblasts). The maturing erythroid cells exhibit loose chromatin. In the granulocytic cell series, giant metamyelocytes and band neutrophils are observed. The megakaryocytes exhibit nuclear hypersegmentation, with widely separated, or "exploded," nuclear lobes.

In the peripheral blood, large erythrocytes with an oval shape, called oval macrocytes, are identified. There is prominent poikilocytosis. Teardrop-shaped erythrocytes are characteristic. Multilobed neutrophils, with five or more nuclear lobes, are seen. **This nuclear hypersegmentation of polymorphonuclear neutrophils is the first morphologic abnormality to appear in megaloblastic anemia and the last to disappear.** Characteristically, there is thrombocytopenia with large platelets (megathrombocytes).

Vitamin B_{12} is synthesized only by certain microorganisms. All animals depend ultimately on this microbiologic synthesis of the enzyme. Sources of vitamin B_{12} in the human diet include foods of animal origin, such as meat, seafood, liver, milk, and eggs.

The causes of B_{12} deficiency include dietary deficiency, defective absorption, increased requirements, and impaired utilization. Dietary deficiency is an exceedingly rare cause of B_{12} deficiency except in strict vegans—that is, persons who eat no food of animal origin. **Defective absorption in the gastrointestinal tract is the most common cause of B_{12} deficiency.** Absorption of vitamin B_{12} requires the initial complexing of B_{12} with intrinsic factor (IF), produced in the parietal cells of the gastric mucosa, and the presence of IF-B_{12} receptors in the mucosa of the terminal ileum

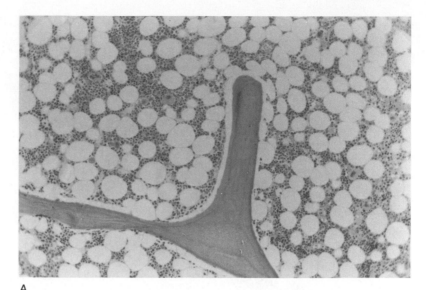

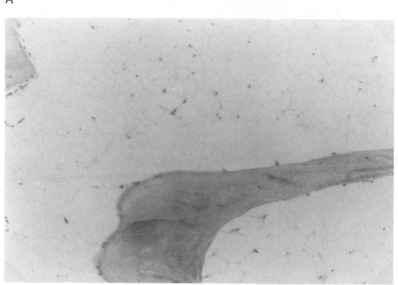

A

Figure 20-3. The bone marrow in aplastic ane-mia. (*A*) Normal bone marrow with a fat:cell ratio of 50:50. (*B*) Aplastic anemia. The marrow consists largely of fat cells and lacks normal he-matopoietic activity.

B

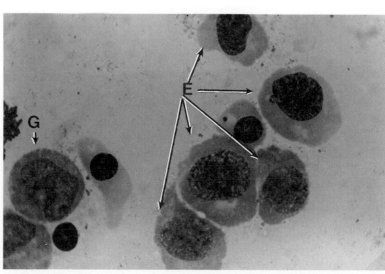

Figure 20-4. Bone marrow in megaloblastic anemia. Maturing erythroid (*E*) and granulo-cytic (*G*) precursor cells are large, and the chromatin is loose.

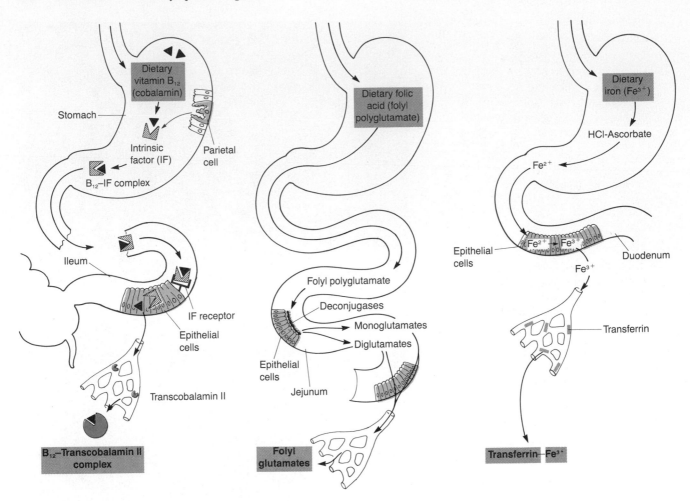

Figure 20-5. Absorption of vitamin B_{12}, folic acid, and iron. Absorption of vitamin B_{12} requires initial complexing with intrinsic factor (IF), which is produced by the parietal cells of the gastric mucosa. Absorption then occurs in the terminal ileum where there are receptors for the IF-B_{12} complex. Dietary folic acid is conjugated to polyglutamate. Absorption occurs in the jejunum following deconjugation in the intestinal lumen. Dietary ferric iron is reduced to ferrous iron in the stomach and absorbed principally in the duodenum.

(Fig. 20-5). **Defective absorption of vitamin B_{12} occurs in classic or pernicious anemia because IF is not produced by the gastric parietal cells** in this disorder. There is also a lack of secretion of gastric juice, gastric acid, and pepsin. This generalized deficiency of secretory function reflects an atrophy of the gastric mucosa, which is believed to be immunologically mediated. Antibodies to IF are found in half of cases of pernicious anemia. Because the daily requirement for vitamin B_{12} is only 1 μg and the total body stores are approximately 2 to 5 mg, it usually requires years for megaloblastic anemia to develop. Classic or pernicious anemia occurs most commonly in adults 40 to 80 years of age. Northern Europeans with a fair complexion are most commonly affected. A moderate to severe anemia is characteristic.

Combined system disease is a serious complication of B_{12} deficiency. Demyelination of the posterolateral columns of the spinal cord leads to peripheral neuropathy, spasticity, and ataxia. The pathogenesis of this demyelination is poorly understood. Personality changes, which may progress to "megaloblastic madness," may be observed.

FOLIC ACID DEFICIENCY

Folic acid deficiency is associated with a megaloblastic anemia that is similar to that caused by vitamin

B_{12} deficiency; however, the neurologic disorder of B_{12} deficiency, combined system disease, is not observed in folic acid deficiency.

Folic acid functions as a coenzyme in a variety of one-carbon transfer reactions, acting either as a donor or as an acceptor. The consequence of folic acid deficiency is abnormal DNA synthesis.

The principal sources of dietary folic acid are leafy vegetables, eggs, and meat products. The minimal daily requirement for folic acid is about 50 μg. Since total body stores are 2 to 5 mg, it takes 4 to 5 months for folic acid deficiency and megaloblastic anemia to develop. Folic acid deficiency occurs in: **alcoholism,** in which a poor nutritional status is common; impaired intestinal absorption, as in **nontropical or tropical sprue;** administration of certain anticonvulsant drugs, such as **dilantin,** which impair the intestinal deconjugation of polyglutamate forms of folic acid; conditions associated with increased requirements for folic acid, such as **pregnancy** or **chronic hemolysis;** and finally in conditions that impair utilization, such as treatment with **antineoplastic folic acid antagonists.**

IRON DEFICIENCY ANEMIA

Iron is utilized principally in the production of hemoglobin. It also functions as a cofactor with a variety of intracellular enzymes. An adequate dietary source provides approximately 20 mg of iron daily, of which 1 to 2 mg is absorbed, principally in the duodenum (see Fig. 20-5).

Iron deficiency is the most common medical disorder worldwide. The causes of iron deficiency include inadequate dietary sources of iron, impaired intestinal absorption of iron, loss of iron due to hemorrhage or intravascular hemolysis, and diversion of iron to the fetus during pregnancy and lactation. Dietary intake of iron is frequently inadequate in infants and young children on unsupplemented iron-poor milk diets. **Gastrointestinal hemorrhage is the most common cause of iron deficiency in the adult man and postmenopausal woman. In women of reproductive age, iron deficiency usually is caused by loss in the menses or during pregnancy.**

In iron-deficiency anemia, **bone marrow examination reveals a severe decrease in or absence of hemosiderin in macrophages and an absence of ferritin in developing normoblasts.** The normoblasts frequently have poorly hemoglobinized, or "ragged," cytoplasm. Hypochromic microcytic erythrocytes are seen on the peripheral blood smear. When the deficiency is severe, anisocytosis and poikilocytosis may be prominent. The common laboratory findings include a decreased serum iron level and an increased total iron binding capacity, the latter being a quantitative measure of the serum transferrin level. Iron saturation, the proportion of transferrin bound to iron, is generally less than 10%, the normal value being about 30%. The serum ferritin level, which reflects total body iron stores, is decreased.

THALASSEMIA SYNDROMES

The thalassemia syndromes are a heterogeneous group of genetic disorders that have in common a selective depression or absent synthesis of either the α- or the β-chains of the normal hemoglobin A tetramer ($\alpha_2\beta_2$). The specific thalassemia syndromes are defined by the globin chain affected. In the β-thalassemias, synthesis of the β-chain is defective, while in the α-thalassemias, there is an abnormal synthesis of the α-chain. **The pathophysiology of the thalassemias relates principally to the accumulation of excess globin chains, which precipitate and cause red cell membrane damage. Ineffective erythropoiesis and chronic hemolysis result.**

In the β-thalassemias, there may be either decreased (β^+) or absent (β°) synthesis of the β-chain. The genetic defects in β-thalassemia are heterogeneous but commonly relate to defective processing of messenger RNA. Heterozygous β-thalassemia (β-thalassemia minor) is the most common disorder. One β-globin gene is normal, but the second β-globin gene exhibits a variably impaired β-globin production. Hemoglobin A_1 ($\alpha_2\beta_2$) is slightly decreased, hemoglobin F ($\alpha_2\gamma_2$) is normal, and hemoglobin A_2 ($\alpha_2\delta_2$) is slightly increased (4% to 8%). In the peripheral blood, mild hypochromia, microcytosis, basophilic stippling of erythrocytes, and target cells are observed. The spleen is moderately enlarged. There is generally a mild anemia.

Homozygous β-thalassemia (Cooley's anemia) is caused by a severe reduction in or absence of β-chain production. Hemoglobin electrophoresis reveals principally fetal hemoglobin ($\alpha_2\gamma_2$). Hemoglobin A_2 ($\alpha_2\delta_2$) is normal to moderately elevated. Splenomegaly and hepatomegaly reflect the massive sequestration and destruction of the damaged erythrocytes. The peripheral blood erythrocytes are hypochromic and microcytic and show marked anisocytosis and poikilocytosis. The anemia is moderate to severe.

α-Thalassemias result from impaired α-chain synthesis. The defect appears to be a deletion of from one to all four α-globin genes found on chromosome 16. Excess γ- and β-chains precipitate as hemoglobin Barts (γ_4) in utero and during the neonatal period, and as hemoglobin H (β_4) in childhood and in adult life. A minor component of hemoglobin (δ_4) may be identified. The hemoglobin Barts, hemoglobin H, and δ-tetramers are more soluble and less toxic than the precipitated α-chains in the β-thalassemia syndromes. Red blood cell destruction is consequently generally less severe. However, the oxygen affinity of the tetramers is high, and the erythrocytes function poorly in the delivery of oxygen.

The clinical severity of the α-thalassemias reflects the number of α-genes deleted. In the silent carrier state, in which there is a deletion of one gene, the hematologic parameters are normal. In α-thalassemia trait, in which two genes are deleted, there is a mild hemolytic anemia. In hemoglobin H disease, in which three genes are deleted, there is a moderate hemolytic anemia with hypochromia and microcytosis of erythrocytes. If all four α-chains are deleted, death occurs either in utero or at the time of delivery. The predominance of the high-affinity hemoglobin Barts produces a severe impairment of oxygen delivery. There is massive hepatosplenomegaly as a result of compensatory extramedullary hematopoiesis. Generalized edema (hydrops fetalis) is a sequel of severe heart failure.

MYELOPHTHISIC ANEMIAS

The myelophthisic anemias are a consequence of bone marrow infiltrative disorders, most commonly metastatic carcinoma or malignant lymphoma. The pathogenesis involves damage to the normal hematopoietic microarchitecture. Because of disruption of the sinus endothelial cells, hematopoietic precursor cells are released prematurely. On the peripheral blood smear the erythrocytes display prominent anisocytosis and poikilocytosis. Teardrop-shaped erythrocytes are numerous. There may be leukoerythroblastosis, with circulating immature granulocytes, erythroid cells, and giant platelets. Commonly there is a mild to moderate normocytic normochromic anemia. The diagnosis is made by bone marrow biopsy. The course and prognosis are determined by the type of marrow infiltrative disorder.

ACUTE BLOOD LOSS ANEMIA

In acute hemorrhage, the clinical manifestations reflect both the rapidity and the volume of the blood loss. Following an acute hemorrhage, fluid shifts from the interstitial to the intravascular compartments in order to maintain the blood volume. This fluid shift accentuates the acute anemia due to hemorrhage because of the dilutional effect. The serum erythropoietin level rapidly increases and stimulates the pool of erythroid precursors. Since maturation and release of erythroid

cells requires 2 to 5 days, the fluid shift and subsequent dilution cause the hemoglobin level to reach a nadir in 2 to 3 days. Thereafter, depending on the adequacy of the total body iron stores, a gradual restoration of the red blood cell mass occurs. When bleeding occurs internally, such as into the body cavities, iron is recaptured and reutilized in the production of red blood cells.

CHRONIC BLOOD LOSS ANEMIA

Chronic blood loss anemia is caused by iron deficiency and occurs only after the total body iron stores are depleted. The old clinical dictum is still valid: occult blood loss in a man or a postmenopausal woman requires that the diagnosis of intestinal tumor be excluded.

HEREDITARY SPHEROCYTOSIS

Hereditary spherocytosis is an autosomal dominant disorder characterized by a distinctive spheroidal shape of the erythrocytes and hemolytic anemia. A defect in the cell membrane cytoskeleton leads to a low surface: volume ratio and dehydration of the red blood cells. The resulting spherocytes are incapable of the deformation required to traverse the splenic red pulp cords and are selectively destroyed by splenic macrophages. Macrophages and erythrocytes expand the red pulp cords, but the splenic sinusoids appear empty. Bone marrow examination reveals a marked compensatory erythroid hyperplasia. The common laboratory findings include a moderate normocytic hyperchromic anemia and a reticulocytosis. The erythrocyte osmotic fragility is increased.

Enlargement of the spleen is usual and splenectomy is curative.

SICKLE CELL DISEASE

In sickle cell disease, a single base mutation in DNA results in the substitution of valine for glutamic acid at the sixth position of the β-globin chain of hemoglobin. As a consequence of this point mutation, **aggregation and polymerization of globin chains occur under deoxygenated conditions, with the formation of rigid filamentous structures, or "tactoids."** These "tactoids" induce a characteristic deformity of the red blood cells, the sickled, or "hollyleaf," configuration. **Irreversibly sickled erythrocytes cannot traverse the red pulp cords of the spleen, and are destroyed by**

splenic macrophages. **Sickled erythrocytes can occlude small blood vessels in any visceral organ and produce multifocal ischemic infarctions.**

Approximately 10% of American blacks are heterozygous for the sickle cell gene. One β^S- and one β^A-chain are synthesized. Hemoglobin S constitutes 30% to 40% and hemoglobin A 60% to 70% of the total. **The associated disorder is called sickle cell trait.** In sickle cell trait the peripheral blood count and the red blood cell life span are normal. Generally, there are no symptoms. Rarely, sickling may occur in the renal medulla owing to low oxygen tension, low pH, and high osmolarity. There may be resultant ischemic infarction of the renal papillae. Sickling may occur in the lungs in conditions of low PO_2, such as pneumonia or atelectasis, or at high altitudes.

In homozygous sickle cell disease, only β^S-chains are synthesized. Hemoglobin S constitutes 80% to 95% of the total hemoglobin and hemoglobins F and A_2 constitute the residual minor components. The predominance of hemoglobin S leads to both **severe chronic hemolytic anemia and vaso-occlusive disease.** Vaso-occlusion of small vessels may cause painful infarctions in any visceral organ, the so-called **sickle cell crisis.** Ulceration of skin overlying the ankle malleoli due to occlusion of dermal and subcutaneous vessels is characteristic. Repeated splenic infarctions cause progressive fibrous scarring and eventual atrophy of the spleen (autosplenectomy). The lack of normal splenic function predisposes to infection, especially salmonella osteomyelitis and pneumococcal pneumonia.

GLUCOSE-6-PHOSPHATE DEHYDROGENASE DEFICIENCY

Glucose-6-phosphate dehydrogenase (G6PD), an enzyme of the hexose monophosphate shunt pathway, maintains glutathione in the reduced form. **When G6PD is deficient, the erythrocytes are more susceptible to oxidant stresses.** With exposure to oxidants, such as some of the antimalarial drugs, oxidized denatured hemoglobin precipitates as **Heinz bodies,** which adhere to the red cell membrane. The abnormal red cells are phagocytosed and removed in the spleen.

G6PD deficiency comprises a heterogeneous group of X-linked recessive disorders. Most G6PD-deficient males do not express clinical manifestations of their genetic trait. Fifteen percent of American blacks have the abnormal enzyme G6PD A, rather than the normal enzyme G6PD B. In this population hemolysis is generally mild, because G6PD levels are nearly normal in the reticulocytes. In the Mediterranean type of G6PD deficiency, a severe enzyme deficiency may lead to life-threatening hemolysis. Severe, occasionally lethal, reactions precipitated by ingestion of the fava bean may occur in this variant of G6PD deficiency.

PAROXYSMAL NOCTURNAL HEMOGLOBINURIA

Paroxysmal nocturnal hemoglobinuria (PNH) is an acquired disorder of the common hematopoietic precursor cell. In PNH the erythrocytes, granulocytes, and platelets demonstrate an inordinate sensitivity to complement-mediated lysis. The disorder probably results from a defect in the clearance of complement from the cell membrane, due to an absence of a decay-accelerating factor. The abnormal PNH cell clone frequently occurs in conjunction with a damaged bone marrow. The abnormality in the erythroid cell series is expressed either as intermittent episodes of acute hemolysis or as chronic hemolysis. The acute hemolytic episodes occur at night and are recognized by the passage of brown urine in the morning. Iron deficiency may result from the loss of hemoglobin. Because of complement-mediated platelet lysis, thrombocytopenia with secondary hemorrhages may occur. Venous thromboses, occasionally involving the hepatic veins (Budd-Chiari syndrome), are characteristic of PNH. This predisposition to thrombosis may reflect complement-mediated activation of platelets. Alternatively, adenosine diphosphate, which is released from damaged erythrocytes, may activate the circulating platelets.

Most individuals affected by PNH ultimately succumb to a complication of the disorder. Rarely, death is due to superimposed acute nonlymphocytic leukemia or to aplastic anemia.

AUTOIMMUNE HEMOLYTIC ANEMIA

Autoimmune hemolytic anemia is a heterogeneous group of disorders in which a shortened red cell survival is caused by an immune response against the autologous red blood cells. A positive Coombs' test confirms the presence of immunoglobulin on the erythrocyte cell membrane. Complement components are also identified on erythrocytes by the appropriate Coombs' reagents.

WARM-ANTIBODY TYPE

Warm-antibody autoimmune hemolytic anemia results from the production of antibodies, usually of the IgG class, that have maximum reactivity at 37°C

and that frequently exhibit specificity for Rh blood group determinants. **Warm antibodies cause 80% to 90% of cases of autoimmune hemolytic anemia.** Hemolysis occurs because of the coating of erythrocytes with anti-Rh antibody and complement components. Splenic macrophages have surface membrane receptors for the Fc portion of IgG and for the complement component C3b, and they therefore remove portions of the erythrocyte membrane. The result is the formation of spherocytes, which are ultimately destroyed by splenic macrophages.

Warm-antibody autoimmune hemolytic anemia occurs either as an idiopathic disease or as a secondary disorder in association with a variety of malignant or benign conditions. The lymphocytic lymphomas and chronic lymphocytic leukemia account for approximately half of all cases of secondary autoimmune hemolytic anemia. Secondary warm-antibody autoimmune hemolytic anemia may also occur in association with collagen vascular diseases, viral infections, some solid tumors, and certain inflammatory disorders. In warm-antibody autoimmune hemolytic anemia hemolysis is intermittent and the clinical course is unpredictable. The usual causes of death are thromboembolic episodes, infections, and severe anemia. The prognosis in secondary warm-antibody autoimmune hemolytic anemia reflects the course of the associated disorder.

COLD-ANTIBODY TYPE

Cold antibodies have maximal reactivity below 37°C and especially below 31°C. They usually are of the IgM class and generally have specificity for the I/i antigen complex. When blood is pooled in the extremities, IgM antibody fixes C3 to the erythrocyte membrane. Since IgM usually subsequently dissociates at 37°C, only complement components are identified on the erythrocyte surface membranes by the appropriate Coombs' reagents. These complement-coated red blood cells are removed principally by hepatic Kupffer cells. This extravascular hemolysis may be associated with a mild chronic anemia.

Cold antibodies cause 10% to 20% of cases of autoimmune hemolytic anemia. This type of hemolytic anemia may occur either as an idiopathic disorder in elderly individuals in whom a malignant lymphoma may subsequently be identified or as a secondary disorder in young persons who have acute infections, particularly mycoplasmal pneumonia or infectious mononucleosis.

DRUG-MEDIATED IMMUNOLOGIC INJURY OF ERYTHROCYTES

Many drugs have been implicated in the production of immunologic injury of erythrocytes. There are three principal mechanisms of drug-mediated immunologic injury of erythrocytes: (1) autoantibody induction, (2) immune complex formation, and (3) the hapten mechanism. In autoantibody induction a drug induces the formation of an autoantibody against a blood group determinant. The principal offender is the antihypertensive drug α-methyldopa. In 10% of those who take this medication the drug induces an IgG autoantibody directed against Rh blood group determinants, and in approximately 1% overt hemolytic anemia occurs. In the immune complex mechanism, a drug initially binds to a serum antibody, and the drug-antibody complex then reversibly binds to the erythrocyte. The erythrocyte is then destroyed by complement-mediated lysis. An example of this mechanism occurs with the anti-arrhythmic agent quinidine, which binds to an IgM antibody and forms quinidine-IgM complexes, which in turn bind to erythrocytes. In the hapten mechanism, a drug binds to an erythrocyte membrane protein, forming first a hapten. A serum antibody is then produced with specificity for this protein–drug complex. An example is the binding of penicillin to an erythrocyte membrane protein.

Drug-mediated immunologic destruction of erythrocytes is usually a benign process. In the hapten and autoantibody mechanisms of drug-mediated immunologic injury of erythrocytes, a mild to moderate hemolysis is usually observed. Severe hemolysis may occur in immune complex-mediated injury of erythrocytes.

TRAUMATIC CARDIAC HEMOLYTIC ANEMIA

Shear-stress forces on circulating erythrocytes due to cardiac prostheses are associated with traumatic rupture of the red blood cell membrane and hemolytic anemia. Plastic prosthetic aortic valves are most commonly implicated. **Schistocytes** are commonly identified on the peripheral blood smear.

MICROANGIOPATHIC HEMOLYTIC ANEMIA

A variety of disorders of the microvasculature are associated with intravascular fragmentation of erythrocytes, a condition termed **microangiopathic hemolytic anemia.** Disseminated intravascular coagulation plays a major role in the pathogenesis of most microvascular fragmentation syndromes.

HYPERSPLENISM

Hypersplenism is defined as an increased functional activity of the mononuclear phagocytes of the spleen

with increased sequestration and destruction of the peripheral elements of the blood. Variable anemia, leukopenia, and thrombocytopenia result. Although the increase in splenic phagocytic activity usually correlates directly with increasing size of the spleen, for poorly understood reasons hypersplenism is observed only in a minority of cases of splenomegaly.

ERYTHROCYTOSIS (POLYCYTHEMIA)

Relative erythrocytosis is defined as an increase in the hemoglobin level consequent upon a decrease in the plasma volume. The total red blood cell mass is normal. The decreased plasma volume generally reflects fluid loss from a variety of causes, such as water deprivation, diarrhea, diuresis, and extensive third-degree burns.

Secondary erythrocytosis (polycythemia) refers to a true increase in the red blood cell mass, due to either (1) appropriate increased production of erythropoietin due to tissue hypoxia or increased production of androgens or (2) inappropriate erythropoietin production in the absence of tissue hypoxia or increased androgens. In the first category (appropriate increased erythropoietin production) are included arterial hypoxemia related to high-altitude low PO_2, pulmonary disease with impaired gas exchange, and cardiac disease with right-to-left shunts, as well as a variety of abnormal hemoglobins with high oxygen affinity that

release oxygen poorly to the tissues. Tissue hypoxia stimulates erythropoietin production. Increased androgen production in Cushing's disease or in the adrenogenital syndrome may also cause increased erythropoietin production.

Inappropriate secondary erythrocytosis reflects secretion of erythropoietin in the absence of tissue hypoxia. Renal lesions such as cysts or hydronephrosis may produce localized renal hypoxia by a pressure effect and consequently cause enhanced erythropoietin production. Erythrocytosis may occur in association with a variety of tumors, probably because of aberrant production of erythropoietin by tumor cells. Such erythropoietin-producing tumors include renal cell carcinoma, cerebellar hemangioblastoma, uterine leiomyoma, primary hepatocellular carcinoma, and adrenal adenoma.

BENIGN DISORDERS OF POLYMORPHONUCLEAR LEUKOCYTES

NEUTROPHILIA

Neutrophilia is defined as an increase in the peripheral blood absolute neutrophil count to more than 7000 per microliter. Neutrophilia has many causes (Table 20-3). Kinetically, they relate to (1) increased neutrophil mobilization from the bone marrow storage pool or the peripheral blood marginal pool; (2) an increased bone marrow-effective granulocytopoiesis (i.e., a decreased destruction of maturing granulocyte precursor cells in the bone marrow); and (3) an increased neutrophil survival time in the peripheral blood, due either to immaturity of neutrophils because of premature release from the bone marrow or to diminished egress to the tissues.

A sustained neutrophilia is caused by the release of granulocytes from the bone marrow storage pool in the presence of an acute inflammatory disorder or acute infection. Chronic inflammation or infection, chronic blood loss, and malignant neoplasms increase effective granulocytopoiesis by augmenting the production of colony-stimulating factor neutrophil-monocyte (CSF-NM). In life-threatening infections there may be a pronounced neutrophilia, with circulating immature cells. This is termed a leukemoid reaction, since it may simulate leukemia.

NEUTROPENIA

Neutropenia is defined as a decrease in the absolute neutrophil cell count to less than 1800 neutrophils

Table 20-3 Principal Causes of Neutrophilic Leukocytosis

Infections (primarily bacterial)
Immunologic-inflammatory
  Rheumatoid arthritis
  Rheumatic fever
  Vasculitis
Tissue necrosis
  Infarction
  Trauma
  Burns
Neoplasia
Hemorrhage
Hemolysis
Metabolic disorders
  Acidosis
  Uremia
  Gout
Endocrinologic disorders
  Thyroid storm
  Glucocorticoids
Pregnancy
Toxins
Physical stimuli
  Cold
  Heat
  Stress
Emotional stress
Hereditary neutrophilia

per microliter. Neutropenia is due either to impaired bone marrow production of neutrophils or to their increased peripheral destruction of neutrophils. Causes of impaired bone marrow production of neutrophils include toxic bone marrow suppression by drugs, alcohol, and irradiation; idiosyncratic reactions to drugs; aplastic anemia; ineffective granulocytopoiesis; infection; and hereditary disorders, the prototype of which is Kostmann's disease (infantile genetic agranulocytosis). The causes of excessive peripheral destruction of neutrophils include (1) antibody-mediated destruction of neutrophils—idiopathic, related to drugs, or in association with immunologic disorders such as systemic lupus erythematosus or Felty's syndrome—and (2) hypersplenism.

Neutropenia is responsible for an increased susceptibility to infection, which is proportional to the severity of the neutropenia. Infection is particularly common when the absolute neutrophil count is less than 500 per microliter.

QUALITATIVE DISORDERS OF NEUTROPHILS

Bactericidal function in the neutrophil is mediated predominantly by hydrogen peroxide (H_2O_2) and by the enzyme myeloperoxidase, which is delivered to cytoplasmic phagosomes by the degranulation of lysosomes. In **chronic granulomatous disease,** there is a defect in oxygen metabolism, with consequent impaired production of bactericidal H_2O_2. As a result, bacteria multiply intracellularly. The common organisms involved in chronic granulomatous disease are *Staphylococcus aureus, Serratia marcescens,* and *Salmonella* species. Microscopically, both granulomatous inflammation and microabscesses, with necrosis and neutrophils, are observed.

The **Chediak-Higashi syndrome** is caused by a generalized defect in cell membrane formation. One consequence is impaired degranulation of neutrophils, with defective release of lysosomal enzymes into cytoplasmic phagosomes. Giant cytoplasmic inclusions represent abnormal lysosomes in all the circulating leukocytes. Poor function of both neutrophils and lymphocytes leads to an increased susceptibility to infection.

EOSINOPHILIA

Eosinophils respond to chemotactic substances produced by mast cells, including the eosinophil chemotactic factor of anaphylaxis and histamine. Because T-lymphocytes also produce eosinophilic chemotactic substances, eosinophils accumulate preferentially both in sites of mast cell degranulation and in sites of immune reactions. **Eosinophils function in the host immune defense against helminths and participate in some inflammatory reactions.** The causes of peripheral blood eosinophilia are outlined in Table 20-4.

Table 20-4   Principal Causes of Eosinophilia

Allergic disorders
Skin diseases
Parasitic infestations
Malignant neoplasms
   Lymphoma
   Leukemia
   Myeloproliferative syndromes
   Epithelial malignancy
Collagen vascular disorders
   Polyarteritis nodosa
   Dermatomyositis
Idiopathic
   Hypereosinophilic syndromes

PROLIFERATIVE DISORDERS OF MAST CELLS

Urticaria pigmentosa affects children and, less commonly, young adults. Multiple cutaneous reddish macules and papules contain mast cells. Histamine release from mast cells, induced by a variety of stimuli (e.g., friction, heat, cold), causes local skin wheals or systemic symptoms. The disorder is generally restricted to the skin and systemic involvement is unusual. In most cases urticaria pigmentosa resolves at the time of puberty. **Systemic mastocytosis** occurs at any age, the peak incidence being in the sixth and seventh decades. The male:female ratio is 2:1. Mast cell infiltration is seen in the skin, bone marrow, spleen, lymph nodes, and liver. Osseous lesions occur in approximately two-thirds of the cases. Mild hepatosplenomegaly and lymphadenopathy may be observed. **Mast cell leukemia** supervenes in 15% of cases of systemic mast cell disease, in which case the median survival is less than 2 years.

DIFFERENTIATED HISTIOCYTOSES

In the spectrum of disorders of the mononuclear phagocytes, the differentiated histiocytoses, a group of proliferative conditions of histiocytes, occupy a central position between the benign immunoreactive hyperplasias and the neoplastic malignant histiocytoses. These maladies are of unknown cause and pathogenesis. Three syndromes that reflect the age of presentation and the extent of tissue and organ involvement are recognized: **acute disseminated histiocytosis (Letterer-Siwe disease), chronic disseminated histiocytosis (Hand-Schüller-Christian disease),** and **eosinophilic granuloma.** In the differentiated histiocytoses the extent and clinical aggressiveness of the disease correlate inversely with the age of the patient; the younger the patient, the more serious the prognosis.

Despite their clinical heterogeneity, these disorders have common histopathologic features. Differentiated histiocytes are large cells with eccentric round or indented nuclei. They display a deep nuclear crease, a feature that is unusual for histiocytes and macrophages. The abundant cytoplasm is pink and may be vacuolated, reflecting an increased lipid content. **The cell surface markers, which include OKT-6 (common thymic antigen), are identical to those of the epidermal Langerhans cell, an antigen-processing and -presenting cell that is included in the mononuclear phagocyte system.** By electron microscopy a cytoplasmic inclusion, **the X-body, Birbeck granule, or Langerhans cell granule,** is occasionally identified in differentiated histiocytes. The Birbeck granule is rod-shaped or tubular with a dense core, a characteristic periodicity, and a bulbous end. **Because the Birbeck granule is found in epidermal Langerhans cells, it appears that the differentiated histiocytes may represent proliferative disorders of Langerhans cells;** the term **"Langerhans cell granulomatosis"** has therefore been applied to these disorders.

Acute disseminated histiocytosis (Letterer-Siwe disease) is an aggressive, frequently fatal, systemic disorder in children usually less than 3 years of age. Frequently the clinical features suggest a malignant disease. Fever, generalized lymphadenopathy, hepatosplenomegaly, and failure to thrive are usual. Involvement of the skin is common and is manifested by an eczematoid or seborrheic eruption, particularly of the scalp, face, and trunk. Interstitial pulmonary infiltration is frequently observed. Less commonly bone involvement with cystic lesions of the skull, pelvis, and long bones may be observed. Virtually any organ or tissue may be infiltrated by normal-appearing histiocytes or by histiocytes with nuclear atypia.

Chronic disseminated histiocytosis (Hand-Schüller-Christian disease) occurs in children usually under the age of 5 years. Although multifocal involvement of organs is frequent, the course is usually benign. Lytic bone involvement, particularly of the bones of the skull, is characteristic. Destruction of the orbital bones, with extension into the orbit, may result in proptosis. Involvement of the hypothalamus or of the pituitary stalk may induce diabetes insipidus. The Hand-Schüller-Christian triad of defects in membranous bones, diabetes insipidus, and exophthalmos is seen in less than 15% of cases. Seborrhea with involvement of the scalp and ear canals is common. Generally, there is mild lymphadenopathy and hepatosplenomegaly. Histologically, there is infiltration of differentiated histiocytes, usually admixed with numerous inflammatory cells, principally eosinophils.

Eosinophilic granuloma is most commonly observed in adolescent males or in young adults. There is single (monostotic) or multifocal (polyostotic) involvement of bone. The ribs, skull, and femur are most commonly affected. Occasionally extraskeletal involvement in sites such as the lymph nodes, skin, and the lungs occurs. Differentiated histiocytes, with numerous eosinophils, infiltrate the tissues. The course in eosinophilic granuloma is benign.

BENIGN DISORDERS OF LYMPHOID CELLS

LYMPHOCYTOSIS

Peripheral blood lymphocytosis is defined as an absolute increase in the number of circulating lymphocytes, that is, an absolute lymphocyte count that exceeds 4000 per microliter in adults, 7000 per microliter in children, and 9000 per microliter in infants. **The most frequent cause of lymphocytosis is an acute or chronic viral or other infection** (Table 20-5).

The morphologic hallmark of viral infections is the atypical lymphocyte, a term applied to a trans-

Table 20-5 Principal Causes of Absolute Lymphocytosis

Acute infections
Infectious mononucleosis
Cytomegalovirus
Bordetella pertussis
Acute infectious lymphocytosis
Toxoplasma gondii
Chronic infections
Tuberculosis
Brucellosis
Hematopoietic disorders
Chronic lymphocytic leukemia
Acute lymphocytic leukemia
Prolymphocytic leukemia
Hairy cell leukemia
Hypersensitivity reactions

formed lymphocyte in the blood. The atypical lymphocyte characteristically has a round to irregular nucleus with relatively coarsely clumped chromatin, one to several distinct nucleoli, and abundant blue cytoplasm. In infectious mononucleosis (Epstein-Barr virus infection), atypical lymphocytes usually constitute 20% or more of the peripheral blood nucleated cells. In cytomegalovirus and other viral infections, a moderate atypical lymphocytosis is observed.

REACTIVE HYPERPLASIA OF LYMPH NODES

A reactive hyperplasia of all or any combination of B cells, T cells, and mononuclear phagocytes of the lymph nodes occurs in many infectious, inflammatory, and neoplastic diseases (Fig. 20-6). **Hyperplasia of the follicles and plasmacytosis of the medullary cords indicate immunoreactivity of B cells. Lymphoid hyperplasia of the deep cortex or paracortex (interfollicular hyperplasia) reflects immunoreactivity of T cells.** In benign reactive hyperplasia of lymph nodes, more than one immunologic compartment is frequently involved, a feature termed a "mixed pattern of reactivity."

The site of enlarged lymph nodes often provides a clue as to the likely cause of benign reactive hyperplasia. For example, the posterior auricular lymph nodes are commonly prominent in rubella infection, the occipital lymph nodes in scalp infections, the posterior cervical lymph nodes in toxoplasmosis, the axillary lymph nodes in infections of the upper extremities, and the inguinal lymph nodes in venereal infections and infections of the lower extremities. A generalized enlargement of the lymph nodes occurs in systemic infections, hyperthyroidism, drug reactions, collagen vascular diseases, and malignant lymphoproliferative disorders. Enlargement of a supraclavicular lymph node occasionally heralds metastatic carcinoma from the lung or from a primary abdominal malignancy.

FOLLICULAR HYPERPLASIA

Nonspecific reactive follicular hyperplasia is characterized by prominent follicles in the lymph node cortex (Fig. 20-7). The follicles are enlarged and irregular and may be confluent. The activated follicular B-lymphocytes exhibit a spectrum of cell sizes and nuclear contours. A characteristic feature of benign follicles is the predominance of activated lymphoid cells toward one side of the follicle (the so-called polarized follicle.) In reactive follicles mitotic figures are numerous. Macrophages containing nuclear and cytoplasmic debris, so-called tingible bodies, are seen throughout such follicles (see Fig. 20-7). **The presence of tingible body macrophages is the hallmark of benign reactive follicular hyperplasia.** A perifollicular cuff of normal small lymphocytes is usually present and clearly demarcates the follicle from the surrounding interfollicular zone. A few immunoblasts and inflammatory cells may be located in the interfollicular zone, and an increase in medullary cord plasma cells is common. By definition, nonspecific reactive follicular hyperplasia is of unknown cause. Generally, a viral etiology is suspected. The course is typically benign, usually with rapid resolution of the lymphadenopathy.

Specific causes of follicular hyperplasia include rheumatoid arthritis, syphilis, toxoplasmosis, angiofollicular lymph node hyperplasia, and the acquired immunodeficiency syndrome (AIDS).

INTERFOLLICULAR HYPERPLASIA

In **nonspecific reactive interfollicular (paracortical) hyperplasia** low-power microscopy reveals a mottled

---

Figure 20-6. Lymph nodes—patterns of benign reactive hyperplasia. The patterns of benign reactive hyperplasia in lymph nodes are contrasted with the structure of a normal lymph node. Follicular hyperplasia with prominent enlarged and irregular benign follicles is characteristic of B-cell immunoreactivity. Interfollicular hyperplasia with expansion of the paracortex is characteristic of T-cell immunoreactivity. The sinusoidal pattern with expansion of sinuses by benign histiocyte-macrophages is characteristic of reactive proliferations of the mononuclear-phagocyte system. Mixed patterns of follicular, interfollicular, and sinusoidal hyperplasia are common in a variety of complex mixed immune reactions. In necrotizing lymphadenitis, variable necrosis of the lymph node architecture with residual cell debris is seen. In granulomatous inflammation, cohesive clusters of histiocytes with pink cytoplasm and occasional multinucleated giant cells are characteristic.

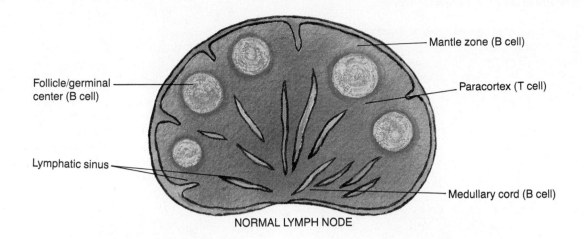

Follicle/germinal
center (B cell)

Lymphatic sinus

Mantle zone (B cell)

Paracortex (T cell)

Medullary cord (B cell)

NORMAL LYMPH NODE

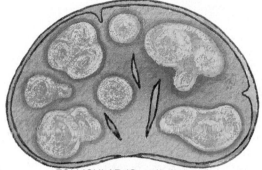

FOLLICULAR (Germinal center)

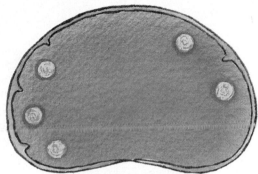

INTERFOLLICULAR

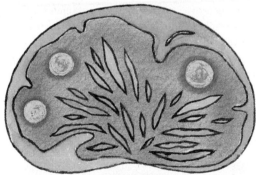

SINUSOIDAL

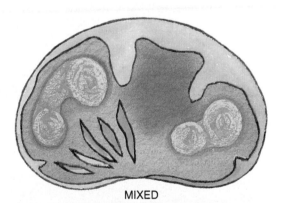

MIXED

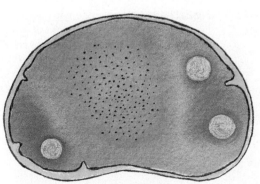

NECROTIZING

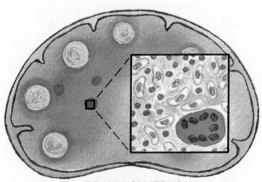

GRANULOMATOUS

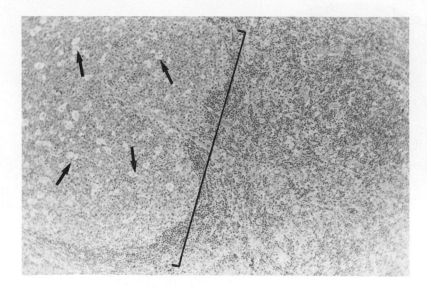

Figure 20-7. Lymph node with reactive follicular hyperplasia. A prominent follicle (*bracket*) containing pale cytoplasmic macrophages (*arrows*) is seen.

("salt and pepper") appearance of the lymph node paracortex. At high power an admixture of small lymphocytes, activated lymphocytes (including immunoblasts), and scattered histiocytes is seen (Fig. 20-8). Typically, the postcapillary venules are prominent and have conspicuous endothelial lining cells. This benign immunoblastic reaction may be florid and completely efface the normal lymph node architecture. Paracortical hyperplasia is seen in viral infections and in some immune reactions, but often no specific etiology is identified. However, there are occasionally histopathologic features that suggest a specific infectious agent.

In the lymphadenitis of **infectious mononucleosis** the immunoblastic reaction is usually severe and is ac-

companied by bizarre immunoblast variants, which may simulate or be indistinguishable from the Reed-Sternberg cells of Hodgkin's disease. A spectrum of noncohesive immunoblast variants may be observed "floating" in the lymph node sinuses.

In **varicella-herpes zoster lymphadenitis,** endothelial cells may exhibit intranuclear eosinophilic inclusions (Cowdry type A inclusions), which are surrounded by a clear nuclear halo. Such inclusion-containing endothelial cells are present in the typical cellular background of a viral lymphadenitis.

In **measles lymphadenitis,** multilobed or multinucleated cells with delicate nuclear chromatin called Warthin-Finbeldy giant cells (perikaryons or peri-

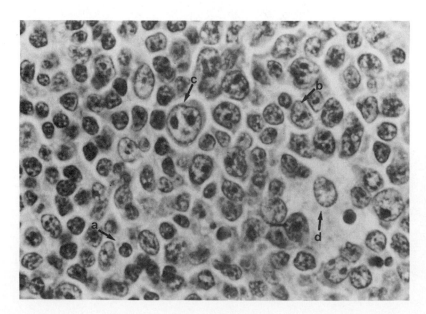

Figure 20-8. Lymph node with reactive interfollicular hyperplasia. A spectrum of lymphocytes undergoing transformation from a small lymphocyte (*a*) to a partially transformed lymphocyte (*b*) to a classic immunoblast (*c*) is seen in the T-dependent paracortex. One cytoplasmic histiocyte is seen (*d*).

karyocytes) are present in the prodromal phase of the infection.

In **cytomegalovirus lymphadenitis** the nuclei of endothelial cells may contain large eosinophilic, intranuclear inclusions, surrounded by a clear nuclear halo.

In **lymphadenopathy associated with systemic lupus erythematosus,** there is a diffuse or paracortical lymphoid hyperplasia with immunoblastic reaction, plasmacytosis, and extensive necrosis. The lymphoid follicles tend to be inconspicuous. Arteriolitis, with fibrinoid necrosis of vessel walls, is frequent. Extracellular, purple, amorphous deposits, which consist of altered DNA called "hematoxylin bodies," are diagnostic.

UNUSUAL FORMS OF LYMPHADENOPATHY

Angioimmunoblastic lymphadenopathy with dysproteinemia (AILD) comprises a spectrum of disorders that are characterized by generalized lymphadenopathy, hepatosplenomegaly, and a maculopapular rash. Middle-aged and elderly persons are most commonly affected. The common constitutional symptoms are fever, night sweats, and weight loss. Common laboratory findings include polyclonal hypergammaglobulinemia, peripheral blood eosinophilia, anemia, and a positive direct antiglobulin (Coombs') test. In approximately one-third of cases the disorder is precipitated by the administration of drugs. It has been speculated that AILD represents a hyperimmune disorder involving an altered or abnormal immunologic reactivity. **More recently there is evidence that many such disorders may in fact represent a subset of T cell lymphomas (AILD-like T cell lymphoma).**

In AILD the involved lymph nodes exhibit a diffuse effacement of the normal architecture, although a few "burnt-out," or depleted, follicles may persist. Typically, there is a polymorphous cell infiltrate consisting of a spectrum of activated lymphocytes with immunoblasts, plasmacytoid immunoblasts, plasma cells, histiocytes, neutrophils, and eosinophils. The lymph node vasculature is prominent and thick-walled (Fig. 20-9) and demonstrates an arborizing pattern. Deposition of an interstitial PAS-positive material, which represents either immunoglobulin secreted by B cells or the products of cell degeneration, is seen. A similar histologic picture is seen in involved skin, bone marrow, liver, and spleen. In one-third to one-half of cases, large transformed lymphoid cells appear in clusters and progressively obliterate the normal tissue architecture. The course and prognosis then are those of an aggressive large cell lymphoma. Even in the absence of malignant degeneration, the prognosis is poor because of progressive immune failure. Death usually is caused by superimposed infection.

DISORDERS OF THE SPLEEN

The spleen is an uncommon site of primary disease. However, enlargement (splenomegaly) is common because the spleen is involved in reactions to systemic infections, participates in systemic immunologic-inflammatory disorders, enlarges in storage diseases, and is involved in generalized hematopoietic and, less consistently, lymphopoietic disorders. The causes of splenomegaly are outlined in Table 20-6.

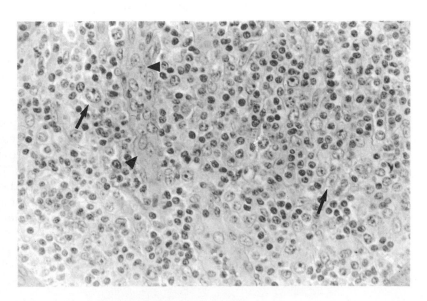

Figure 20-9. Angioimmunoblastic lymphadenopathy. A spectrum of lymphocytes undergoing transformation with scattered immunoblasts (*arrows*) is seen. Postcapillary venules are prominent and thick walled (*arrowheads*).

Table 20-6   Principal Causes of Splenomegaly

Infections
  Acute
  Subacute
  Chronic
Immunologic-inflammatory disorders
  Felty's syndrome
  Lupus erythematosus
  Sarcoidosis
  Amyloidosis
  Thyrotoxicosis
Hemolytic anemias
Pediatric immune thrombocytopenia
Splenic vein hypertension
  Cirrhosis
  Splenic and/or portal vein thrombosis or stenosis
  Right-sided cardiac failure
Primary or metastatic neoplasms
  Leukemia
  Lymphoma
  Hodgkin's disease
  Myeloproliferative syndromes
  Sarcoma
  Carcinoma
Storage diseases
  Gaucher's
  Niemann-Pick
  Mucopolysaccharidoses
Idiopathic
  Banti's disease

Splenomegaly is occasionally associated with the clinical syndrome of hypersplenism, a condition that reflects hyperplasia of splenic mononuclear phagocytes with macrophage-mediated destruction of sequestered elements of the blood. Any combination of anemia, leukopenia, and thrombocytopenia may result. Splenectomy is curative. The sporadic occurrence of hypersplenism in association with splenomegaly is poorly understood.

Immunoreactive hyperplasia of splenic lymphoid tissue ("activated spleen") may be observed in a number of chronic immunologic–inflammatory disorders. Follicles or germinal centers may be prominent. Hyperplasia of mononuclear phagocytes and increased immunoblasts, plasma cells, and eosinophils are seen in the red pulp. Features characteristic of specific disorders may be observed. For example, in **systemic lupus erythematosus** there may be fibrinoid necrosis of capsular and trabecular collagen and characteristic "onion-skin" thickening of penicilliary and central arterioles. In **infectious mononucleosis,** transformed lymphocytes (immunoblasts) prominently infiltrate the red pulp. Infiltration of the capsule, trabeculae, and blood vessels by activated lymphocytes, including immunoblasts, weakens the supporting structures of the spleen and accounts for the high incidence of splenic

rupture. **Typhoid fever** is characterized by lymphoid infiltrates of the red pulp and hyperplasia of macrophages, often accompanied by prominent erythrophagocytosis. **Chronic malarial infection** may result in massive splenomegaly with fibrous thickening of the capsule and trabeculae. Grossly, a slate-gray or black color reflects the presence of malarial pigment (hematin). Microscopically, myriads of macrophages contain malarial parasites and pigment.

Chronic passive congestion (fibrocongestive splenomegaly), is caused by prolonged elevation of pressure in the splenic vein. It is most commonly seen as a complication of hepatic cirrhosis, in which case it reflects portal hypertension. Other causes of portal hypertension, such as thrombosis of the portal or splenic veins secondary to pylephlebitis or tumors, may lead to chronic passive congestion of the spleen. An increase in splenic vein pressure may also result from right-sided heart failure, due either to cor pulmonale or to tricuspid or pulmonary valve disease.

With chronic passive congestion, the enlarged spleen (500 g to 1000 g) shows fibrosis of the capsule and red pulp. The sinusoids are dilated and empty. Foci of old hemorrhage persist as **Gamna-Gandy bodies,** fibrotic nodules containing iron and calcium salts encrusted on collagenous and elastic fibers. There is atrophy of the white pulp.

Infarctions of the spleen result from occlusion of the splenic artery or one of its tributaries. The vascular occlusion is frequently due to emboli from the left heart, originating in mural thrombi or in vegetations on mitral or aortic valves damaged by endocarditis. Splenic infarctions may also result from local thrombosis caused by disorders such as sickle cell disease, polyarteritis nodosa, and the chronic myeloproliferative syndromes. Infarcts are usually wedge-shaped, with their bases contiguous to the splenic capsule. After multiple infarcts, extensive fibrous scarring may result in atrophy of the spleen. Such "autosplenectomy" is especially characteristic of sickle cell disease.

Rupture of the spleen occurs most commonly as the result of blunt trauma. In the absence of trauma, an underlying predisposing disorder should be sought, since for practical purposes spontaneous rupture of a normal spleen does not occur. Diseases that predispose to rupture of the spleen include infectious mononucleosis, chronic malaria, typhoid fever, abscesses, and leukemia. Following rupture bits of splenic tissue may be seeded on the peritoneal surface, leading to the formation of splenic implants (splenosis).

In general, **the microenvironment of the spleen does not offer a favorable milieu for the implantation and growth of metastatic tumor cells.** Metastatic tumors to the spleen generally are observed only late in the course of most malignant neoplasms and are rare in the absence of extensive spread to other organ sites. The primary tumors that most commonly metastasize to the spleen include carcinomas of the lung, breast, stomach, colon, and prostate, and malignant melanoma.

MONOCLONAL GAMMOPATHY OF UNKNOWN SIGNIFICANCE

A detectable homogeneous immunoglobulin molecule, a portion of an immunoglobulin molecule, or a single predominant kappa or lambda light chain in the serum or urine is called a monoclonal gammopathy (M component). The abnormal protein is produced by a clone of B cells derived from a single aberrant B cell. Such a homogeneous protein is detected as a sharp peak, or "spike," in the serum or urine protein electrophoretic pattern (Fig. 20-10). By contrast, in benign or reactive processes a polyclonal immunoreactiv-

ity results in a polyclonal, or broad-based, increase in immunoglobulins.

In most persons in whom a monoclonal gammopathy is demonstrated, there is no evidence for an associated malignant tumor or other disorder. In the bone marrow, plasma cells are only slightly increased, and sheets of plasma cells, as seen in plasma cell neoplasia (multiple myeloma), are not observed. The incidence of monoclonal gammopathy of unknown significance increases from approximately 1% at age 25 years to 3% at age 70 years to 10% at age 80 years. Despite the alternative label of "benign monoclonal gammopathy," 10% of affected individuals subsequently develop either plasma cell neoplasia or a B-cell malignant lymphoma. A minority of persons with monoclonal gammopathy have an associated disorder, such as an epithelial malignancy or an infection. These associations are probably coincidental and may reflect an age-related increased incidence of all such disorders. **Monoclonal gammopathy of unknown significance is important because it is common and must be distinguished from plasma cell neoplasia.**

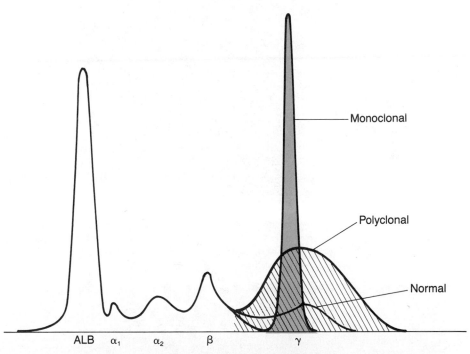

Figure 20-10. Serum protein electrophoretic patterns. Abnormal serum protein electrophoretic patterns are contrasted with a normal pattern. In polyclonal hypergammaglobulinemia, which is characteristic of benign reactive processes, there is a broad-based increase in immunoglobulins due to immunoglobulin secretion by a myriad of discrete reactive plasma cells. In monoclonal gammopathy, which is characteristic of monoclonal gammopathy of unknown significance or plasma cell neoplasia, there is a narrow peak, or spike, due to the homogeneity of the immunoglobulin molecules secreted by a single clone of aberrant plasma cells.

CHRONIC MYELOPROLIFERATIVE SYNDROMES

The chronic myeloproliferative syndromes are clonal disorders that arise from the neoplastic transformation of a single common hematopoietic precursor cell. Initially these cells retain their capacity for differentiation and maturation. **Thus, the bone marrow exhibits a trilineage hyperplasia (panhyperplasia), that is, a generalized increase in erythrocytic, granulocytic, and megakaryocytic cell lines. Cohesive clusters of atypical megakaryocytes with hyperchromatic nuclei are the morphologic hallmark of the chronic myeloproliferative syndromes** (Fig. 20-11).

Fibrosis of the bone marrow is common in the chronic myeloproliferative syndromes. Since the fibroblasts lack the restricted isoenzymes of G6PD and the marker chromosomes, identified in the neoplastic hematopoietic cells, the proliferation of fibroblasts appears to be a reactive phenomenon. The specific chronic myeloproliferative syndromes are defined by the predominant proliferating cell type. **Polycythemia vera** is characterized by predominant proliferation of erythroid precursor cells, **chronic granulocytic leukemia** by proliferation of cells of the granulocytic (myeloid) series, and **primary hemorrhagic thrombocythemia** by proliferation of megakaryocytes and megakaryocyte precursor cells. In **myelofibrosis with myeloid metaplasia,** all the hematopoietic cell lines are proliferative and reactive fibrosis is prominent.

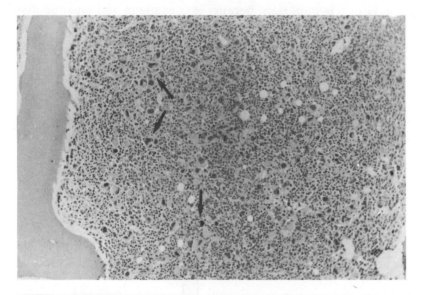

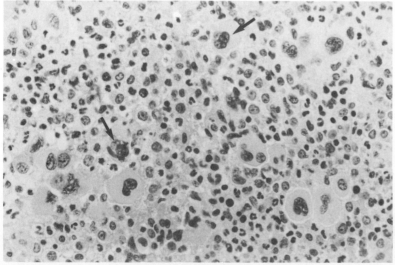

Figure 20-11. Bone marrow in chronic myeloproliferative syndrome. The marrow is cellular, with hyperplasia of all hematopoietic elements. Megakaryocytes (*arrows*) are atypical and show hyperchromatic nuclei.

Table 20-7   The Myeloproliferative Syndromes: Hematopathologic Features

	POLYCYTHEMIA VERA	CHRONIC MYELOGENOUS LEUKEMIA	MYELOFIBROSIS WITH MYELOID METAPLASIA
Bone Marrow			
Histopathology	Panhyperplasia (predominantly erythroid)	Panhyperplasia (predominantly granulocytic)	Panhyperplasia with fibrosis
M:E ratio	≤2:1	10:1 to 50:1	2:1 to 5:1
Marrow iron	↓ or absent	Normal or ↑	Normal or ↑
Marrow fibrosis	15–20%	<10%	90–100%
Liver, Spleen			
Extramedullary hematopoiesis (myeloid metaplasia)	Moderate (predominantly erythroid)	Moderate to marked (predominantly granulocytic)	Moderate to marked

POLYCYTHEMIA VERA

Polycythemia vera is a neoplastic disorder of the common hematopoietic precursor cell in which a pronounced increase in the production of erythroid cells is accompanied by a corresponding increase in the total red cell mass.

The principal hematopathologic features of polycythemia vera are presented in Table 20-7. In addition to hyperplasia of the erythroid series, all hematopoietic cell lines are increased. Clusters of atypical megakaryocytes, the morphologic hallmark of the chronic myeloproliferative syndromes, are often present. Bone marrow iron is depleted, owing both to diversion of storage iron to the developing erythroblasts and to blood loss from recurrent gastrointestinal hemorrhage. Bone marrow fibrosis may be observed even early in the course of the disease, and in one-fifth of the cases, severe fibrosis with depletion of hematopoietic cells is a late complication.

Generally, there is moderate enlargement of the spleen, reflecting expansion of the red pulp. (Fig. 20-12). The red pulp is congested and commonly exhibits myeloid metaplasia (neoplastic extramedullary hematopoiesis), that is, islands of erythroid normoblasts, scattered megakaryocytes, and immature granulocytic cells. The splenic white pulp is atrophic. Myeloid metaplasia of the liver is observed principally in the hepatic sinusoids.

The common laboratory findings are shown in Table 20-8. They include a hemoglobin concentration of greater than 20 g/dl, a hematocrit of 60% or more, and a red blood cell count of 6 million to 10 million per microliter. Arterial oxygen saturation is normal, thereby excluding a cardiopulmonary cause for the erythrocytosis. The peripheral blood erythrocytes usually appear morphologically normal. Hypochromia and microcytosis may be observed, with superimposed iron deficiency. With progression of the disease, the erythrocytes may exhibit marked anisocytosis and poikilocytosis. A leukocytosis of up to 25,000 per microliter occurs in two-thirds of the cases. The platelet count is moderately increased in half of the cases. The peripheral blood platelets are often abnormal, both morphologically (giant forms and abnormal granulation) and functionally. The leukocyte alkaline phosphatase (LAP) score is often high. Because levels of this enzyme activity vary in the different chronic myeloproliferative syndromes, the LAP score is useful in distinguishing these syndromes (see Table 20-8). In a quarter of the cases cytogenetic study reveals karyotypic abnormalities, such as aneuploidy or an extra C-group chromosome.

Polycythemia vera is most commonly a disorder of middle aged white men. The usual age at onset is 40 to 60 years. The clinical features are outlined in Table 20-9. The symptoms generally reflect the increased red blood cell mass, with secondary circulatory disturbances such as impaired blood flow, vascular stasis, and local tissue hypoxia. Any organ may be affected. Headache, dizziness, and visual disturbances result from impaired circulation in the central nervous system. Angina pectoris and intermittent claudication reflect poor circulation in the coronary and peripheral vascular systems, respectively. Hemorrhage and thrombosis occur in half of the cases and may involve the cerebral, coronary, and peripheral vascular systems.

The course of polycythemia vera is characterized by a protracted stable erythroid phase with polycythemia.

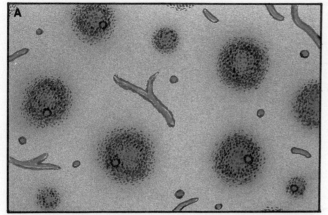

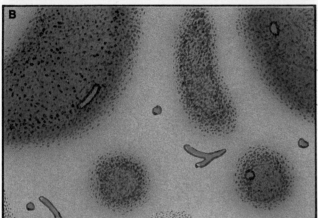

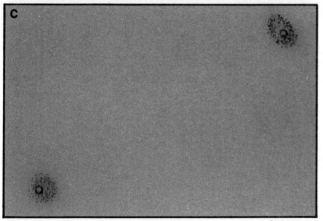

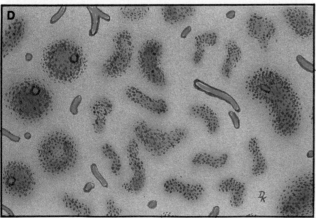

However, 20% of cases ultimately progress to a "spent" phase, typified by progressive anemia, an enlarging spleen with prominent myeloid metaplasia, a peripheral blood leukoerythroblastic picture, and marrow fibrosis with depletion of hematopoietic cells. The prognosis in the "spent" phase is poor. In untreated polycythemia vera the risk of acute nonlymphocytic leukemia is 2% to 4%, and this risk is further increased by treatment with ^{32}P or alkylating agents. With treatment the median survival is approximately 13 years. The most common cause of death is thrombosis.

CHRONIC MYELOGENOUS LEUKEMIA

Chronic myelogenous leukemia is a neoplastic disorder of the common hematopoietic precursor cell in which the granulocytic cell series is predominantly affected. Typically, there is an accompanying proliferation of erythroid cells and of megakaryocytes.

Ninety percent of individuals with chronic myelogenous leukemia have an acquired chromosomal abnormality, the Philadelphia chromosome (Ph[1]). This marker chromosome is identified in erythroid, granulocytic, and megakaryocytic cells and occasionally in lymphoid cells. **Translocation of half of the long arm of chromosome 22, usually to chromosome 9, is demonstrated. The critical event appears to be the loss of a portion of the long arm of chromosome 22.** An oncogene, c-abelson (c-abl), is present at the breakpoint of chromosome 9 and is reciprocally translocated to chromosome 22.

The hematopathologic features of chronic myelogenous leukemia are outlined in Table 20-7. **In the bone**

Figure 20-12. Hematopoietic malignancy—patterns of splenic involvement. The patterns of splenic involvement in hematopoietic malignancies are contrasted with the architectural structure of the normal spleen (*A*). (*B*) In malignancies that primarily involve the lymphoid white pulp (Hodgkin's disease and non-Hodgkin's lymphomas), there is variable expansion of the white pulp with encroachment on the red pulp. (*C*) In malignancies that primarily involve the red pulp (acute nonlymphatic leukemia, myeloproliferative syndromes, malignant histiocytosis, hairy cell leukemia, plasma cell neoplasia, and mast cell disease), there is expansion of the red pulp with encroachment on, and ultimately obliteration of, the white pulp. (*D*) Some malignant disorders both expand the white pulp and initially infiltrate the red pulp (prolymphocytic leukemia, mycosis fungoides, small lymphocytic lymphoma–leukemia, and small plasmacytoid lymphocytic lymphoma).

Table 20-8   The Myeloproliferative Syndromes: Laboratory Features

	POLYCYTHEMIA VERA	CHRONIC MYELOGENOUS LEUKEMIA	MYELOFIBROSIS WITH MYELOID METAPLASIA
Hemoglobin	>20 g/dl	Mild anemia	Mild anemia
RBC morphology	Slight aniso- and poikilocytosis	Slight aniso- and poikilocytosis	Immature erythrocytes and marked aniso- and poikilocytosis
Granulocytes	Normal to mildly increased, may be a few immature forms	Moderate to markedly increased with spectrum of maturation Basophilia	Normal to moderately increased with some immature WBC
Platelets	Normal to moderately increased	Normal to moderately increased	Increased to decreased
Leukocyte alkaline phosphatase (LAP)	Normal to increased	Decreased to absent	Variable
Cytogenetics	Aneuploid (25%)	Philadelphia chromosome (Ph^1) (90%)	Aneuploid (50%)

(*RBC*, red blood cells; *WBC*, white blood cells)

Table 20-9   The Myeloproliferative Syndromes: Clinical Features

	POLYCYTHEMIA VERA	CHRONIC MYELOGENOUS LEUKEMIA	MYELOFIBROSIS WITH MYELOID METAPLASIA
Male:female	1.2:1	3:2	1:1
Peak age range (years)	40–60	25 60	50–70
Clinical symptoms	Headache, dizziness, pruritus	Asymptomatic or LUQ discomfort, fatigability	Asymptomatic or LUQ discomfort, fatigability
Clinical signs	Bleeding, thrombosis	Easy bruising, bleeding	Weight loss, gouty arthritis
Splenomegaly	75%	90%	100%
Hepatomegaly	40%	50%	80%
Leukemia conversion	1–3%	70% (blast crisis)	15–20%
Median survival (years)	13	3–4	3–4

(*LUQ*, left upper quadrant)

marrow, there is trilineage hyperplasia with predominant proliferation of the granulocytic cell series. **The myeloid:erythroid ratio varies from 10:1 to 50:1 (normal, 2:1 to 4:5:1).** Megakaryocytes are numerous, but the clustering and atypia of megakaryocytes characteristic of the chronic myeloproliferative syndromes may be lacking. Significant marrow fibrosis is distinctly uncommon.

Splenomegaly, occasionally massive (>1000 g), is seen in 90% of cases. The cut surface of the spleen exhibits a homogeneous expansion of the red pulp (see Fig. 20-12). Microscopically, myeloid metaplasia of the sinuses, and less prominently of the cords, is identified.

Proliferation of immature granulocytic cells is predominant. Islands of erythroid normoblasts and variable numbers of megakaryocytes are also observed. Moderate hepatomegaly is common, with or without myeloid metaplasia in the hepatic sinusoids.

The common laboratory findings are shown in Table 20-8. **The peripheral blood white cell count is invariably elevated, typically exceeding 20,000 and often increased to up to 200,000 per microliter. The entire spectrum of maturing granulocytic cells, from myeloblast to neutrophil, is observed. Myelocytes and neutrophils constitute the most numerous cell types.** Myeloblasts and promyelocytes together account for less than 10% of the peripheral blood leukocytes. Frequently, circulating basophils and eosinophils are increased in number. Blood monocytes may also be increased. Initially there is a moderate thrombocytosis in one-third of the cases. **The leukocyte alkaline phosphatase (LAP) score is typically markedly decreased in chronic myelogenous leukemia.** This low LAP score is useful in distinguishing the leukemia from a leukemoid reaction caused by infection, in which case the LAP is typically increased. The LAP score increases when chronic myelogenous leukemia progresses to acute leukemia (blast crisis), an event that occurs in about 70% of cases.

In Western countries, chronic myelogenous leukemia constitutes 20% of all the leukemias. It is typically a disorder of middle-aged adults. The age at onset varies from 25 to 60 years, the median age being 45 years. A slight male predominance is observed. The clinical features are presented in Table 20-9. The symptoms relate either to a hypermetabolic state induced by the increased granulocytic cell turnover or to the prominent splenomegaly.

The course of the disease is usually characterized by an initial stable, chronic phase that persists for 2 to 8 years, with a mean of 3 years. Because only a subtle deficiency of granulocytic cell function is seen in the stable phase, with proper clinical management a normal life can be maintained.

In a minority of patients, an accelerated phase of the disease is heralded by an increasing or decreasing white blood cell count and frequently by a peripheral blood basophilia. Increasing splenomegaly and prominent symptoms of hypermetabolism are signs of disease progression. The accelerated phase is frequently a prelude to a terminal superimposed acute leukemia (blast crisis), the most common cause of death in chronic myelogenous leukemia. A loss of maturation capacity of the granulocytic cell series characterizes the blast crisis. Frequently, additional chromosomal abnormalities, including a second Ph[1] chromosome, are detected in this stage. The response to therapy in blast crisis is poor, with a median survival of 2 to 3 months. Although the blasts are usually of granulocytic origin, in one-quarter to one-third of the cases they originate from lymphoid elements. The median survival in lymphoid blast crisis is approximately 8 months.

MYELOFIBROSIS WITH MYELOID METAPLASIA

Myelofibrosis with myeloid metaplasia (MMM) is a neoplastic disorder of the common hematopoietic precursor cell. The bone marrow shows trilineage hyperplasia, with variable proliferative potential of the erythrocytic, granulocytic, and megakaryocytic cell lines. No single hematopoietic cell line is predominant. **A reactive marrow fibrosis (myelofibrosis) usually accompanies the neoplastic cell proliferation.**

In MMM there is prominent myeloid metaplasia in the sites of fetal extramedullary hematopoiesis. Myeloid metaplasia probably is the result of bone marrow precursor cells gaining access to the circulation and proliferating selectively in sites of fetal extramedullary hematopoiesis.

The hematopathologic features of MMM are listed in Table 20-7. **In the bone marrow, there is panhyperplasia of the hematopoietic cells, and clusters of atypical megakaryocytes with hyperchromatic nuclei are conspicuous.** Myelofibrosis involves particularly the central flat bones and the proximal long bones. Osteosclerosis (thickening of the bony trabeculae) may also be present. Early in the course of the disease, a cellular phase without accompanying myelofibrosis or osteosclerosis is common.

The spleen in MMM is customarily massively enlarged, weighing up to 4000 g. It is firm and homogeneously red-purple. The white pulp usually cannot be visualized (see Fig. 20-12). Microscopically, there is prominent myeloid metaplasia of the red pulp, especially of the sinusoids. Often the liver shows myeloid metaplasia of the hepatic sinusoids.

The common laboratory findings in MMM are listed in Table 20-8. In the peripheral blood typically a leukoerythroblastic picture is observed, with circulating immature erythroid and granulocytic cells and giant platelets. **Teardrop-shaped erythrocytes are characteristic of MMM and serve as a diagnostic feature because they are inconspicuous in chronic myelogenous leukemia and polycythemia vera.** A mild leukocytosis of up to 20,000 per microliter is common. Alternatively, there may be leukopenia. A blood basophilia or eosinophilia may be observed. The platelet count is usually normal to low. The LAP score is usually normal to increased, but in 20% of cases it is decreased. Chromosomal abnormalities, most commonly C-group trisomy, are found in half of the cases but are of no prognostic significance. **The Ph[1] chromosome is lacking, a finding which, together with the typically normal to high LAP score, is useful in distinguishing MMM from chronic myelogenous leukemia.**

The clinical features of MMM are presented in Table 20-9. The disorder occurs principally in middle-aged to elderly persons, with a median age of 60 years. There is no sex predominance. The course in MMM is usually characterized by progressive anemia, with gradually increasing transfusion requirements, and by progressive enlargement of the liver and spleen. The symptoms in MMM relate principally to the consequences of the anemia and to the splenomegaly. The median survival is 3 years. Infection, hemorrhage, and thromboses—due to leukopenia and conditions that reflect qualitative platelet abnormalities or thrombocytosis—are the usual causes of death. In 15% to 20% of cases death is due to a superimposed acute nonlymphocytic leukemia.

ACUTE MYELOPROLIFERATIVE SYNDROMES: THE ACUTE NONLYMPHOCYTIC LEUKEMIAS

The acute nonlymphocytic, or myelogenous, leukemias are a heterogeneous, but interrelated, group of neoplastic disorders of the hematopoietic precursor cells of the bone marrow. They are malignant proliferations that originate either from single multipotential precursor cells or from precursor cells with restricted lineage potential.

In the acute nonlymphocytic leukemias (ANLL), the pathophysiology involves a failure of maturation of the neoplastic cell clone. Because of this failure of maturation and the continued slow neoplastic cell proliferation, the bone marrow is gradually replaced by blast cells, with consequent encroachment upon and loss of normal hematopoiesis. **The most important complications in ANLL, therefore, are progressive anemia, leukopenia, and thrombocytopenia.**

The cause is unknown. The risk factors for the development of ANLL include myelotoxic agents, certain chromosomal abnormalities, and several predisposing hematologic disorders (Table 20-10).

On Wright-Giemsa-stained smears of blood or bone marrow aspirates, the neoplastic blast cells in ANLL

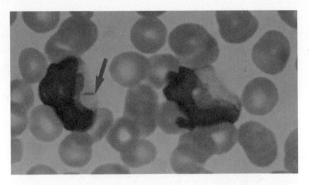

Figure 20-13. Acute nonlymphocytic leukemia. Two blast cells, one with a cytoplasmic Auer rod (*arrow*), are identified on a Wright-Giemsa-stained peripheral blood smear.

have delicate chromatin, frequently multiple nucleoli, and gray-blue cytoplasm. Pink-purple (azurophilic) cytoplasmic granules represent primary lysosomes. **Auer rods, an aberrant morphologic expression of the primary lysosomes, are azurophilic, rod-shaped, cytoplasmic structures that are noted in up to 40% of cases** (Fig. 20-13). The morphologic variants of ANLL, described by the French–American–British (FAB) task force on acute leukemia, are shown in Figure 20-14. In general, the FAB morphologic variants exhibit a similar clinical course. In acute promyelocytic leukemia (FAB M3) the neoplastic blast cells have abundant azurophilic granules and Auer rods, both of which have tissue thromboplastin-like activity. Release of the granules, especially with therapy-associated cell lysis, may trigger the syndrome of disseminated intravascular coagulation. Acute monocytic leukemia, (FAB M5), an aggressive variant of ANLL, is characterized by prominent infiltration of the skin, gums, and perirectal soft tissues; a high white blood cell count; and a poor response to therapy. Acute megakaryoblastic leukemia, a recently described variant now included as FAB M7 in the French–American–British classification, presents either as a usual variant of ANLL or as a rare disorder known as acute myelofibrosis. The clinical syndrome of acute myelofibrosis includes pancytopenia, hyperplasia of all marrow elements, conspicuous fibrosis, and a rapid progression to acute leukemia. Typically, the spleen is not enlarged.

The significance of the FAB classification lies in its precise identification of variants of the acute nonlymphocytic and, as will be discussed, the lymphoblastic leukemias, thus aiding in their distinction. The differentiation of acute nonlymphocytic from acute lymphoblastic leukemia is important because of markedly different prognoses and appropriate therapies. In addition to precise morphologic subclassification as defined by the FAB criteria, cyto-

Table 20-10   Factors Predisposing to Acute Nonlymphocytic Leukemia

Genetic influences
  Sibling with leukemia
Down's syndrome
Syndromes with chromosome instability
  Bloom's syndrome
  Fanconi's anemia
  Ataxia telangiectasia
  Kostman's syndrome
Chemical exposure
  Benzene
Alkylating agent chemotherapy
Ionizing radiation
Myelodysplastic syndromes
Chronic myeloproliferative syndromes
Aplastic anemia
Paroxysmal nocturnal hemoglobinuria

MORPHOLOGY	CLASSIFICATION	NUCLEUS	NUCLEOLUS	CHROMATIN	CYTOPLASM
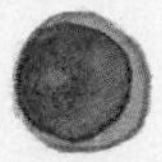	L1 ACUTE LYMPHOBLASTIC (principally pediatric)	Uniformly round, small	Single, indistinct	Slightly reticulated with perinucleolar clumping	Scant, blue
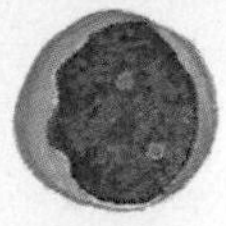	L2 LYMPHOBLASTIC (principally adult)	Irregular	Single to several, indistinct	Fine	Moderate, pale
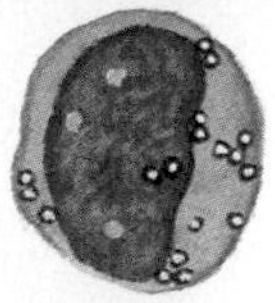	L3 BURKITT'S	Round to oval	Two to five	Coarse with clear parachromatin	Moderate, blue, vacuolated
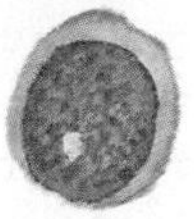	M1 MYELOBLASTIC (without maturation)	Round to oval	Single to multiple, distinct	Fine	Scant, nongranulated
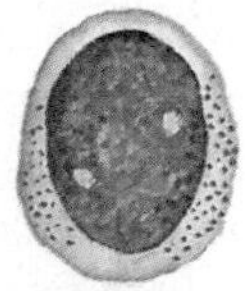	M2 MYELOBLASTIC (with maturation)	Round to oval	Single to multiple, distinct	Fine	Moderate azurophilic granules with or without Auer rods
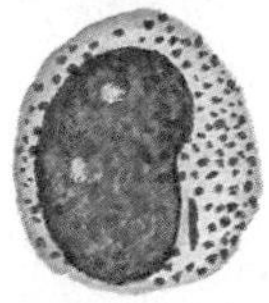	M3 PROMYELOCYTIC	Round to indented to lobed	Single to multiple (granules obscure)	Fine	Prominent azurophilic granules and/or Auer rods
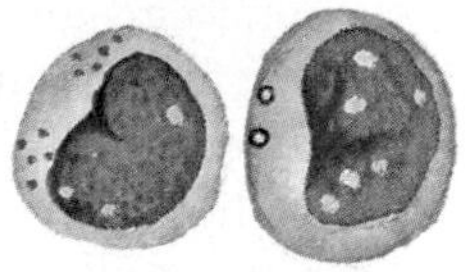	M4 MYELOMONOCYTIC (biphasic M1 and M5)	Round to indented, folded	Single to multiple, distinct	Fine	Moderate, blue to gray, may be granulated
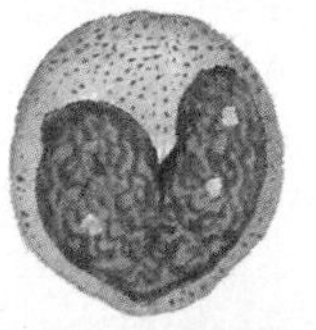	M5 MONOCYTIC	Round to indented, folded	Single to multiple, distinct	Variable, lacy or ropy	Scant to moderate, gray-blue, dustlike lavender granules
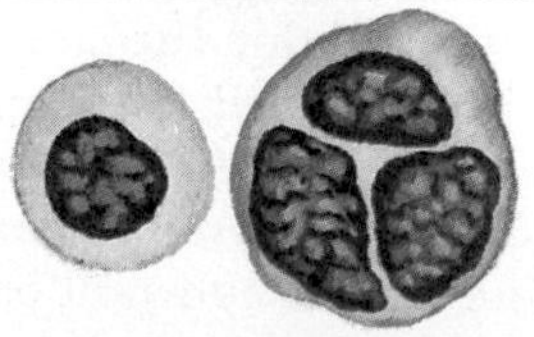	M6 ERYTHROLEUKEMIA	Single to bizarre multinucleated, multilobed	Single to multiple, distinct	Open "megaloblastoid"	Abundant, red to blue

Figure 20-14. Acute leukemia—French–American–British classification.

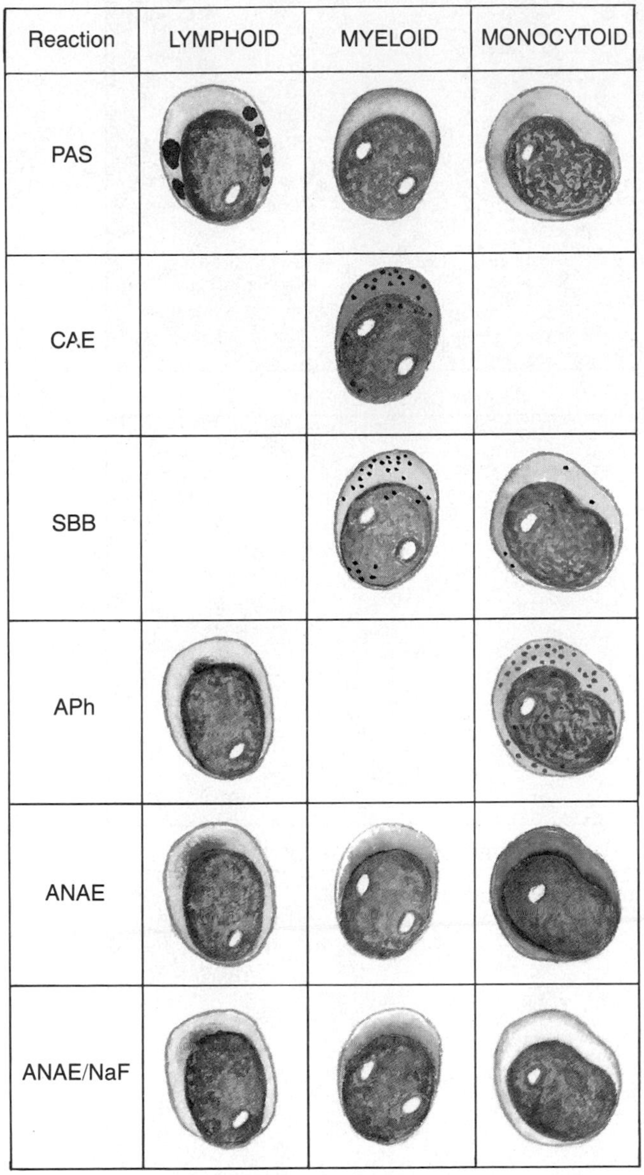

Reaction	LYMPHOID	MYELOID	MONOCYTOID
PAS			
CAE			
SBB			
APh			
ANAE			
ANAE/NaF			

Figure 20-15. Acute leukemia-cytochemistry.

Table 20-11   Terminal Deoxynucleotidyl Transferase (Tdt) in Hematologic Disease

DISEASE	PERCENT POSITIVE
Acute lymphoblastic leukemia	80–90
Lymphoblastic lymphoma	90
Chronic granulocytic leukemia in blast crisis	30
Acute undifferentiated leukemia	60
Acute nonlymphocytic leukemia	2–5

Variable bone marrow replacement by blast cells is found in ANLL (Fig. 20-16). Although initially the leukemic blast cells are interspersed among the normal hematopoietic cells, with time progression to complete bone marrow replacement usually occurs (Fig. 20-17). Morphologic abnormalities of the residual maturing erythroid and granulocytic precursor cells, an abnormality termed "dyspoiesis," are often present. Dyspoiesis is distinctly uncommon in the acute lymphoblastic leukemias. **A characteristic abnormality is an increase in small, single-lobed megakaryocytes.** Myelofibrosis may occur in any variant of ANLL.

Clinically, variable splenomegaly, hepatomegaly, and lymphadenopathy are observed. The initial leukemic cell infiltration involves the red pulp of the spleen (see Fig. 20-12), the sinusoids of the liver, and the paracortex of the lymph nodes (Fig. 20-18). Occasionally, in bone and in the soft tissues, there are discrete tumor masses composed of variable proportions of myeloblasts and promyelocytes. These tumors, termed **granulocytic sarcomas** or **chloromas,** commonly are located in the bones and the adjacent soft tissues of the orbit, the facial bones, the lymph nodes, and other soft tissue sites. Histologically, granulocytic sarcomas are difficult to distinguish from the large cell lymphomas or undifferentiated carcinomas. A positive chloroacetate esterase stain, the demonstration of lysozyme by the immunoperoxidase technique, and the presence of azurophilic granules confirm the diagnosis of granulocytic sarcoma (Fig. 20-19).

The common laboratory findings in ANLL reflect the depletion of normal hematopoietic cell elements and the presence of blast cells. The total white blood cell count may be decreased, normal, or increased up to 200,000 per microliter. Blast cells are generally predominant, particularly when the white blood cell count is increased. A moderate normocytic, normochromic anemia is common. Basophilic stippling, circulating normoblasts, and other features of erythroid dyspoiesis may be observed. Thrombocytopenia is a common finding, although generally not as marked as in acute lymphoblastic leukemia. Serum and urinary lysozyme

chemical studies are frequently required to distinguish acute nonlymphocytic from acute lymphoblastic leukemia (Fig. 20-15). In general, demonstration of the nuclear DNA-polymerizing enzyme terminal deoxynucleotidyl transferase (Tdt) identifies the acute leukemia as having a lymphoid rather than a nonlymphocytic phenotype; however, Tdt activity is also demonstrated in 2% to 5% of otherwise typical cases of ANLL (Table 20-11), so results must be interpreted cautiously.

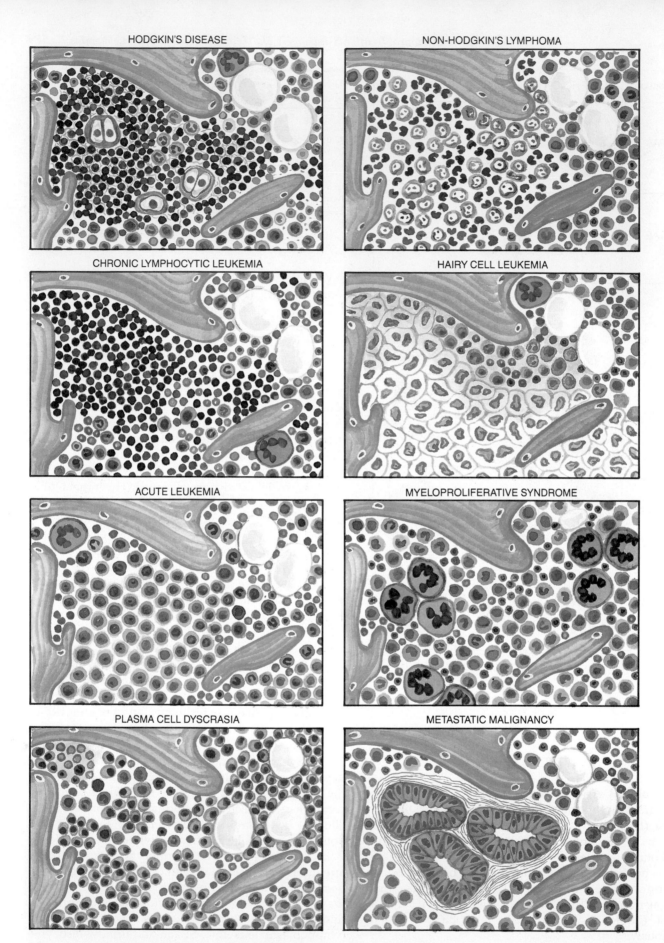

HODGKIN'S DISEASE

NON-HODGKIN'S LYMPHOMA

CHRONIC LYMPHOCYTIC LEUKEMIA

HAIRY CELL LEUKEMIA

ACUTE LEUKEMIA

MYELOPROLIFERATIVE SYNDROME

PLASMA CELL DYSCRASIA

METASTATIC MALIGNANCY

Figure 20-16. Bone marrow biopsy in hematologic disease.

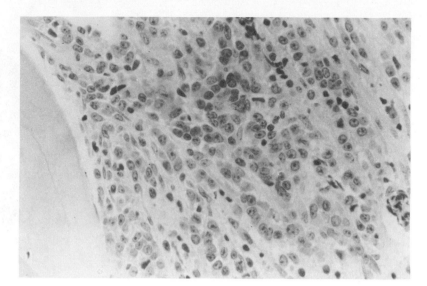

Figure 20-17. Acute nonlymphocytic leukemia. The bone marrow is diffusely hypercellular and consists largely of myeloblasts.

levels are elevated, particularly in acute monocytic leukemia, because monocyte cytoplasmic lysosomes contain abundant lysozyme. In acute promyelocytic leukemia (FAB M3) cytogenetic study reveals a characteristic translocation in approximately half of the cases (t15q+:17q−). Acute myeloid leukemia with maturation (FAB M2) frequently exhibits a characteristic translocation (t8q−:21q+).

ANLL constitutes 20% of all the leukemias, 85% of the acute leukemias in adults, and 15% to 20% of the acute leukemias in children. The clinical manifestations include fatigue due to anemia, infection following granulocytopenia, and bleeding secondary to thrombocytopenia. The risk of infection correlates directly with the severity and duration of the granulocytopenia. Leukostasis, i.e., the occlusion of small blood vessels by blast cells, occurs when the white blood cell count exceeds 100,000 per microliter. The complication of leukostasis is most common in the central nervous system and in the lungs. Blast cell infiltration of the leptomeninges produces the syndrome of leukemic meningitis. Arthralgias and bone pain are caused by expansion of the bone marrow spaces and by periosteal infiltration by leukemic blast cells. Hyperuricemia due to leukemic blast cell turnover predisposes to the complications of uric acid nephropathy and kidney stones.

The most common cause of death in ANLL is infection. Hemorrhage is a less frequent cause of death than in the past because of the efficacy of platelet transfusions. Leukostasis in patients with high blast cell counts may cause fatal brain hemorrhage.

MALIGNANT DISORDERS OF THE MONONUCLEAR PHAGOCYTE SYSTEM

MALIGNANT HISTIOCYTOSIS

Malignant histiocytosis is an aggressive and rapidly fatal systemic neoplasm of the mononuclear phagocytes. Malignant transformation of fixed tissue histiocytes and macrophages affects any organ in which the mononuclear phagocytes are normally found.

The cause is unknown. The pathophysiology relates to the systemic proliferation of functioning malignant histiocytes and nonfunctioning precursor cells of histiocytes. Typically, pancytopenia is caused by (1) phagocytosis by malignant histiocytes, with destruction of erythrocytes, leukocytes, and platelets, and (2) replacement of the normal bone marrow hematopoietic tissues by the tumor cells. The physical findings include splenomegaly, hepatomegaly, mild lymphadenopathy, and papulonodular skin lesions.

Cytologically, the malignant histiocytes exhibit bizarre and atypical morphologic features. The nuclei are single or multiple, are often eccentrically situated, and may be multilobed. The heterochromatin is irregularly clumped in a background of clear parachromatin, and the nucleoli are prominent. The pale to pink cytoplasm is abundant, particularly in the more mature histio-

(Text continues on p. 584)

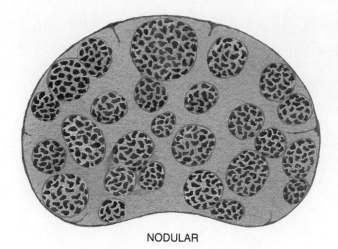

NODULAR

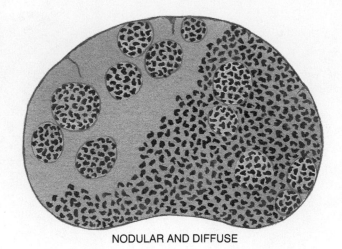

NODULAR AND DIFFUSE

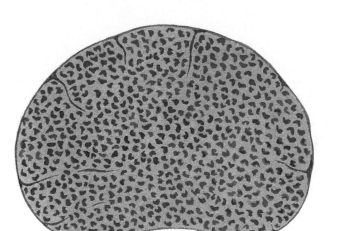

DIFFUSE

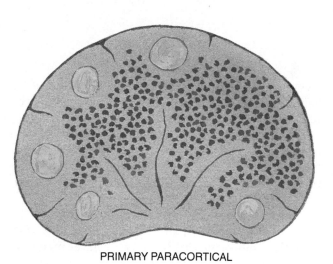

PRIMARY PARACORTICAL

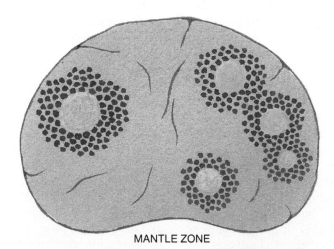

MANTLE ZONE

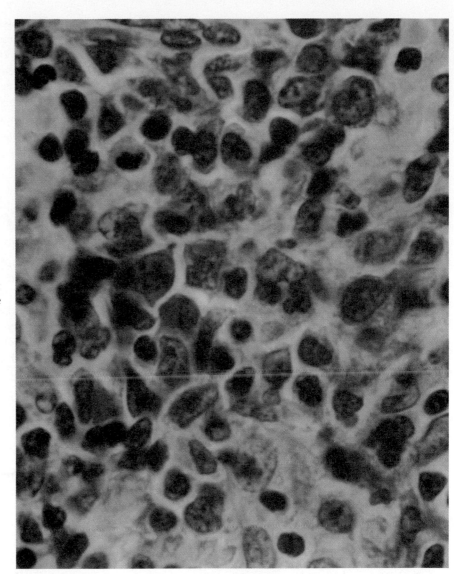

Figure 20-19. Granulocytic sarcoma (chloroma). A diffuse soft tissue infiltrate of the orbit contains primitive blast cells with round to lobulated nuclei. The napthol-AS-D chloroacetate esterase stain is focally positive (*red*).

Figure 20-18. The lymph node—patterns of involvement in leukemia and lymphoma. In the follicular lymphomas, there is replacement of the normal lymph node architecture by uniform nodular aggregates of neoplastic B-lymphocytes. In the follicular and diffuse lymphomas, there is variable replacement of the node architecture by neoplastic B-lymphocytes in both follicular and diffuse architectural patterns. In the diffuse lymphomas, there is partial to (frequently) total obliteration of the normal nodal architecture by neoplastic B- or T-lymphocytes. The architectural pattern is diffuse without proclivity to form follicles. With primary paracortical involvement, there is initial neoplastic cell infiltration of the T-cell–dependent paracortex. Involvement may progress to total effacement of the lymph node architecture. In mantle zone lymphomas, there is initial variable expansion of the B-cell cuff that surrounds normal germinal centers. Ultimately, there may be progression to total obliteration of the normal lymph node architecture.

cytes. The mitotic rate is high and abnormal configurations, such as tripolar or quadripolar forms may be observed. **Striking phagocytosis of erythrocytes, leukocytes, platelets, and nuclear and cytoplasmic debris is seen, particularly in the more differentiated histiocytes** (Fig. 20-20). Detection of elevated lysozyme levels in serum or urine, produced by the malignant histiocytes, suggests the diagnosis of malignant histiocytosis.

Prominent sites of neoplastic histiocytic cell infiltration include the spleen, liver, lymph nodes, bone marrow, and skin. In the spleen the neoplastic histiocytic cells principally infiltrate the cords and sinusoids of the red pulp and eventually obliterate the white pulp (see Fig. 20-12). Erythrophagocytosis by the malignant histiocytes is best appreciated in the spleen. In the liver atypical neoplastic Kupffer cells are observed in the hepatic sinusoids. The subcapsular and radiating sinuses represent the sites of initial involvement of the lymph nodes (see Fig. 20-20). Infiltration of the lymph node stroma by malignant histiocytes may occur secondarily, and the nodal architecture may ultimately be effaced.

"Malignant histiocytosis" has traditionally been defined as an aggressive and generally rapidly fatal systemic neoplasm of mononuclear phagocytes. More recently, many cases previously termed "malignant histiocytosis" have been identified as T cell lymphomas with possible secondary lymphokine activation of benign macrophages. Therefore the incidence of true neoplasms of fixed tissue histiocytes is unknown and probably exceedingly rare.

"TRUE" HISTIOCYTIC LYMPHOMA

In approximately 1–2% of malignant neoplasms with the histologic appearance of a large cell lymphoma, neoplastic cell markers characteristic of mononuclear phagocytes are identified. Malignant tumors with these phenotypic markers are therefore not lymphomas or neoplasms of lymphoid cells, but rather true neoplasms of the mononuclear phagocyte system. Cytologically and clinically, **they are indistinguishable from some lymphomas of the large cell type** (see Fig. 20-20).

MALIGNANT HISTIOCYTOSIS

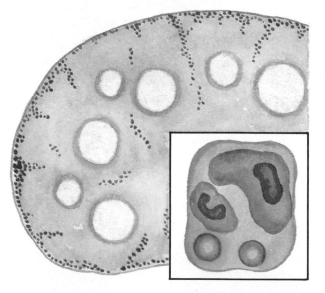

"TRUE" HISTIOCYTIC LYMPHOMA

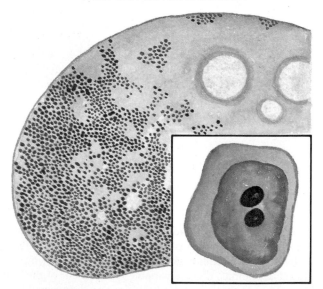

Figure 20-20. Malignant histiocytosis and "true" histiocytic lymphomas. The patterns of lymph node involvement in malignant disorders of the mononuclear phagocyte system are shown. In malignant histiocytosis there is initial involvement of the nodal sinuses, which are expanded by morphologically atypical malignant histiocytes. Neoplastic cell phagocytosis of erythrocytes and other formed elements of the blood may be observed. Ultimately, there may be progression to complete obliteration of the lymph node architecture. In "true" histiocytic lymphoma there is partial to total obliteration of the lymph node architecture by large, transformed cells that are morphologically indistinguishable from those of the large cell lymphomas.

THE LYMPHOCYTIC LEUKEMIAS

CHRONIC LYMPHOCYTIC LEUKEMIA

Chronic lymphocytic leukemia is a malignant, clonal disorder, commonly of B-lymphocytes. The neoplastic cell is a hypoproliferative, immunologically incompetent small lymphocyte. The disease distribution in chronic lymphocytic leukemia is leukemic, with primary involvement of the bone marrow and secondary release to the peripheral blood. The recirculating lymphocytes selectively infiltrate the lymph nodes, the spleen, and the liver. Therefore, with disease progression, lymphadenopathy, splenomegaly, and hepatomegaly develop.

The cause is unknown. Genetic influences may be important. **Of all the leukemias, chronic lymphocytic leukemia most conclusively demonstrates familial case clustering.** The disease is rare in Japan and other Asian countries, **whereas in Western countries it is the most common type of leukemia** (Fig. 20-21).

Male predominance is more accentuated in this disorder than in the other leukemias, with a male:female ratio of 2:1. The disease is observed most frequently in the elderly, the mean age at diagnosis being 60 years.

The pathophysiology is traced to the progressive accumulation of malignant lymphocytes in the bone marrow and in extramedullary tissue sites and to the secondary immunologic deficiency with hypogammaglobulinemia. Localized or generalized lymphadenopathy may be observed. The spleen is frequently moderately enlarged and on cut surface exhibits a generalized enlargement of the white pulp with occasional prominent tumor nodules (Fig. 20-22). The liver may also be mildly to moderately enlarged. The respiratory and gastrointestinal tracts may be infiltrated. Cutaneous involvement appears as papulonodular lesions or as a more diffuse dermatitis.

In the bone marrow three distinctive microscopic patterns of lymphocytic infiltration are recognized: interstitial, nodular, and diffuse (see Fig. 20-16). The initial pattern of lymphocytic cell infiltration is often interstitial, with an increased population of lymphocytes irregularly distributed among normally maturing hematopoietic cells. The lymphocytes often cluster into cohesive nodular aggregates separated by normal hematopoietic stroma. Both the interstitial and the nodular patterns of tumor cell infiltration are associated with a favorable prognosis. Progression to a diffuse pattern of involvement, with obliteration of normal hematopoietic elements and fat cells, is associated with a poor prognosis.

In tissue sections the neoplastic cells of chronic lymphocytic leukemia generally resemble normal small lymphocytes. The nuclei are round, the chromatin compact, the nucleoli inconspicuous, and the cytoplasm scant. Mitotic figures are rare. Clusters of partially transformed lymphoid cells or prolymphocytes, with round vesicular nuclei and more abundant cytoplasm, are common. These clusters are called proliferation centers. Rarely, the transformed cells in these proliferation centers are pleomorphic and may simulate the Reed-Sternberg cells of Hodgkin's disease.

In the blood the absolute lymphocyte count is elevated, exceeding 15,000 and occasionally 100,000 per microliter. The predominant circulating cell is a normal small lymphocyte, but often there is a variable size range, with admixed medium-sized lymphocytes (Fig. 20-23). Some tumor cells display large central nucleoli, in which case they are termed "prolymphocytes." Occasionally primitive lymphoblastlike cells are noted. The neoplastic lymphocytes are fragile and rupture easily on preparation of the blood smear. The resultant amorphous, dark-blue nuclear remnants, called "smudge cells," are characteristic of chronic lymphocytic leukemia.

The neoplastic B cells express limited surface membrane monoclonal immunoglobulin, usually IgM kappa. If the absolute peripheral blood lymphocyte count is only modestly increased and the diagnosis of chronic lymphocytic leukemia is in doubt, the demonstration of monoclonality or light-chain restriction is accepted as evidence of B-cell neoplasia. Hypogammaglobulinemia is detected in half of the cases. In 5% of cases a monoclonal serum immunoglobulin (paraprotein), usually IgM kappa, is detected. Trisomy of chromosome 12 has been reported in up to one-third of patients. A specific chromosomal translocation, t(11;14), may be identified.

The natural history of chronic lymphocytic leukemia is highly variable. The Rai clinical staging system (Table 20-12), which is based on the extent of soft tissue involvement and the degree of compromise of bone marrow function at the time of diagnosis, has clinical utility in assessing prognosis. As the disease progresses, anemia may be caused by hypersplenism, bone marrow replacement, or autoimmune hemolytic anemia. Bleeding may result from thrombocytopenia due to hypersplenism, marrow replacement, and to immunologic destruction of platelets. Bacterial pneumonia and other infections are common, reflecting both hypogammaglobulinemia and neutropenia induced by the disease or by therapy. Occasionally there may be complicating viral infections, such as herpes zoster. The median survival in chronic lymphocytic leukemia is 6 years. Infection is the leading cause of death.

T-cell chronic lymphocytic leukemia is uncommon, constituting less than 5% of cases of chronic lymphocytic leukemia. It is characterized by a high periph-

(Text continues on p. 589)

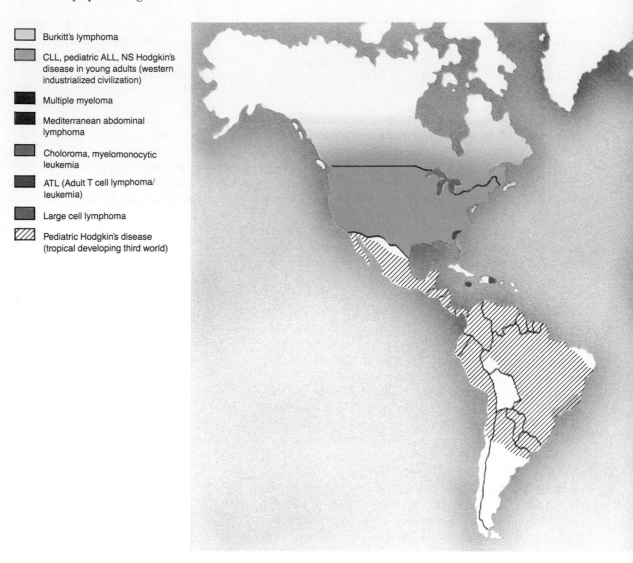

◻ Burkitt's lymphoma

▨ CLL, pediatric ALL, NS Hodgkin's disease in young adults (western industrialized civilization)

▮ Multiple myeloma

▮ Mediterranean abdominal lymphoma

▮ Choloroma, myelomonocytic leukemia

▮ ATL (Adult T cell lymphoma/ leukemia)

▮ Large cell lymphoma

▨ Pediatric Hodgkin's disease (tropical developing third world)

Figure 20-21. Global epidemiology of lymphoma and leukemia. Burkitt's lymphoma is prominent in tropical equatorial Africa and in parts of New Guinea. In Western industrialized countries, including the United States and Western Europe, chronic lymphocytic leukemia, pediatric acute lymphoblastic leukemia, and nodular sclerosing Hodgkin's disease in young adults are common. Multiple myeloma is common in South Africa. Mediterranean abdominal lymphoma occurs commonly in the Eastern Mediterranean basin. Adult-type T-cell leukemia-lymphoma is common in the Southwestern islands of Japan, in certain Caribbean islands, and in the southeastern United States. Acute myelomonocytic leukemia with chloromas is common in parts of Turkey. Large cell lymphomas are common in Japan, China, and Egypt. In tropical Third World countries, aggressive Hodgkin's disease is common in children.

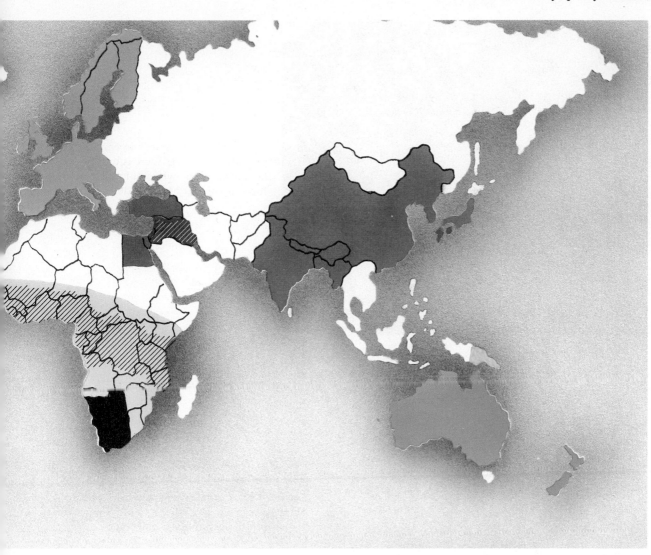

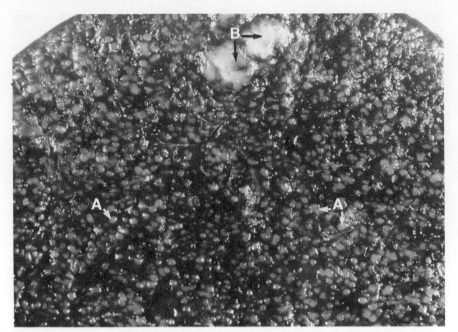

Figure 20-22. The spleen in chronic lymphocytic leukemia. There is diffuse enlargement of the white pulp (*A*), with focal prominent tumor nodules (*B*).

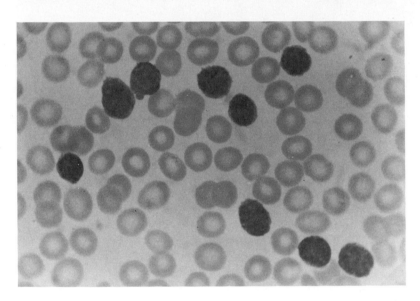

Figure 20-23. Chronic lymphocytic leukemia. Numerous small- to medium-sized lymphocytes are seen in the peripheral blood smear.

Table 20-12   Chronic Lymphocytic Leukemia: Rai Clinical Staging System

STAGE	ABSOLUTE LYMPHOCYTOSIS (≥15,000/μl)	ENLARGED NODES	HEPATOMEGALY/ SPLENOMEGALY	ANEMIA	THROMBOCYTOPENIA
0	+	−	−	−	−
I	+	+	−	−	−
II	+	±	+	−	−
III	+	±	±	+	−
IV	+	±	±	±	+

eral blood white cell count, skin involvement, and prominent splenomegaly, without lymphadenopathy. The cells are medium-sized and have round or irregular nuclei, generally a single nucleolus, and moderate blue cytoplasm, with azurophilic granules. The disease is generally aggressive, with a median survival of 6 months.

PROLYMPHOCYTIC LEUKEMIA

Prolymphocytic leukemia is an aggressive variant of chronic lymphocytic leukemia. The neoplastic cell, the prolymphocyte, is distinctive. It is medium-sized, with a round nucleus in which the chromatin is reticulated. The most characteristic morphologic feature is the large central nucleolus. About 60% of cases are of B-cell origin, although T-cell (and, less commonly, null cell) prolymphocytic leukemias have been described.

Prolymphocytic leukemia is most common in middle-aged to elderly men, the male:female ratio being 2:1 to 3:1. Patients present with massive splenomegaly, a high white blood cell count, and a low platelet count. Lymph nodes are often only modestly enlarged. Regardless of cell type, the prognosis is poor, and the median survival is less than 2 years.

HAIRY CELL LEUKEMIA

Hairy cell leukemia is a distinctive variant of chronic leukemia. The clinicopathologic features include circulating neoplastic cells with prominent cytoplasmic membrane filamentous processes, or "hairs"; splenomegaly; pancytopenia; a marrow that is difficult to aspirate; and an indolent clinical course. Hairy cell leukemia, also called leukemic reticuloendotheliosis, constitutes only 2% of all the leukemias. The cell of origin is usually a B-lymphocyte with aberrant morphologic and functional properties. The pathophysiology relates to (1) tumor cell infiltration of the spleen, with resulting splenomegaly and secondary hypersplenism, and (2) marrow infiltration, with replacement of normal hematopoietic elements.

The principal clinicopathologic finding is marked enlargement of the spleen, which occurs in 85% of cases. The splenic parenchyma is a homogeneous dark red color, reflecting expansion of the red pulp and obliteration of white pulp (see Fig. 20-12). Mild hepatomegaly occurs in half of the cases. Histologically, the spleen exhibits a diffuse infiltration of the red pulp cords and sinusoids by bland medium-sized lymphoid cells with round to indented nuclei and poorly visualized cytoplasm. Mitotic figures are rare. In the liver,

mild infiltration, primarily in the portal areas, is seen. Circulating hairy cells may also be observed in their traverse through the hepatic sinusoids. The lymph nodes reveal patchy involvement of the paracortex, cortex, and sinuses; eventually, the normal lymph node architecture is obliterated.

There is patchy to diffuse infiltration by hairy cells in the bone marrow. Biopsy sections of marrow show a distinctive mosaiclike histologic pattern with bland, round to indented lymphoid nuclei surrounded by a clear zone, or halo, representing the moderate cytoplasm and well-defined cytoplasmic margins (see Fig. 20-16). Mild, diffuse marrow fibrosis, with reticular fibers surrounding individual neoplastic cells, is common.

In smears of blood or marrow aspirates stained by the Wright-Giemsa method, hairy cells are 10 to 15 μm in diameter and show eccentric round, indented, or occasionally lobed nuclei; moderately delicate chromatin; indistinct nucleoli; and scant to moderate gray-blue cytoplasm. **The filamentous cytoplasmic membrane projections, for which this disorder is named, are usually well visualized on smears** (Fig. 20-21).

In 90% of cases, a specific isoenzyme of acid phosphatase, number 5, is identified in the cytoplasm of the neoplastic cells. When the cytochemical stain for acid phosphatase is performed in the presence of inhibitory tartaric acid, there is little loss of activity. Such cells are said to have tartrate-resistant acid phosphatase (TRAP) activity. With rare exceptions, other lymphoproliferative disorders are TRAP-negative. Therefore, a positive TRAP stain in the appropriate clinicopathologic setting confirms the diagnosis of hairy cell leukemia.

Usually the hairy cells express B-cell markers. However, immunologic and cytochemical markers indicative of monocyte differentiation may also be identified. Rare T-cell variants have been described. Thus, **hairy cell leukemia may constitute a neoplastic disorder of a pluripotential precursor cell that is principally committed to B-cell differentiation but that remains capable of expressing heterogeneous cell markers.**

The principal laboratory finding is pancytopenia, reflecting hypersplenism and neoplastic cell replacement of bone marrow. In 10% of cases, leukocytosis, with circulating hairy cells, occurs late in the clinical course.

Hairy cell leukemia most commonly occurs in middle-aged to elderly men. The male:female ratio is 4:1. The onset is insidious, and the clinical course is generally indolent. In 10% to 15% of cases, a more aggressive clinical course characterized by progressive enlargement of visceral organs and peripheral blood cytopenias is observed. The median survival in hairy cell leukemia is 4 years, but a prolonged survival of

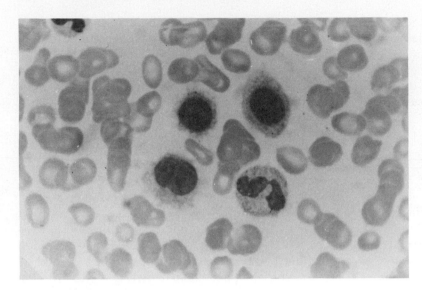

Figure 20-24. Hairy cell leukemia. Three typical hairy cells with fibrillar cytoplasmic margins are seen in the peripheral blood smear.

over 10 years is not unusual. The most common cause of death is infection.

ACUTE LYMPHOBLASTIC LEUKEMIA

Acute lymphoblastic leukemia is a malignant, clonal disorder of bone marrow lymphopoietic precursor cells. The cause is unknown. Certain observations suggest a genetic predisposition, at least in some cases. The incidence of leukemia, usually acute lymphoblastic leukemia, is increased 15-fold in Down's syndrome (trisomy 21), and if one identical twin develops acute lymphoblastic leukemia before the age of 6 years, there is a 20% chance that the other twin will also develop it.

The pathogenesis in acute lymphoblastic leukemia involves a progressive medullary and extramedullary accumulation of lymphoblasts that lack the potential for differentiation and maturation. **An important clinical feature is inhibition by the expanding leukemic cell mass of the development of normal hematopoietic cell elements. Therefore, the clinical presentation is dominated by the untoward effects of progressive weakness and fatigue due to anemia, infection due to leukopenia, and bleeding due to thrombocytopenia.** There may be prominent extramedullary soft tissue infiltration, frequently with generalized lymphadenopathy. Mild to moderate hepatosplenomegaly is also common. Before the era of modern therapy, involvement of the brain, particularly of the leptomeninges (leukemic meningitis), was common even early in the course of the disease. The complication of leukemic meningitis is now usually prevented by initial prophylactic treatment of the

craniospinal axis, although, late relapse may still occur. Bone pain is common, owing both to leukemic cell expansion of medullary spaces and to infiltration of the subperiosteum. There may be infiltration of the joint synovia with polyarthralgias that mimic rheumatic fever.

Acute lymphoblastic leukemia cells are morphologically and immunologically heterogeneous. The FAB morphologic classification distinguishes three cell variants (see Fig. 20-15). L1 cells are small and have fine chromatin, commonly a single indistinct nucleolus, and scant blue cytoplasm. **L1 cells are predominant in 85% of cases of childhood acute lymphoblastic leukemia and in approximately 35% of cases in adults.** L2 cells are moderate to large in size and exhibit finely reticulated chromatin, frequently irregular or cleaved nuclei, one to several nucleoli, and moderately abundant gray-blue cytoplasm. **L2 cells predominate in 65% of cases of adult acute lymphoblastic leukemia and in 10% of cases in children.** L3 cells are uniform and moderate in size, with round to oval nuclei, 2 to 5 small distinct nucleoli, coarsely reticulated chromatin, and a moderate deeply basophilic and vacuolated cytoplasm. **L3 cells represent the leukemic or circulatory phase of Burkitt's lymphoma.** They are seen in less than 5% of cases of acute lymphoblastic leukemia, predominantly in children.

The immunologic classification recognizes B-cell, B-precursor, and T-cell variants of acute lymphoblastic leukemia. It is based on the recognition of specific B- and T-cell markers as well as of a common acute lymphoblastic leukemia antigen (CALLA) (Table 20-13). The B-cell origin of most L3 cells (B acute lymphoblastic leukemia) is demonstrated by the presence

Table 20-13   *Acute Lymphoblastic Leukemia (ALL): Immunologic Phenotypes*

SUBTYPES	CALLA	TdT	IA	PAN-T	PAN-B	C-μ	SIG	IG GENE REARRANGEMENT
T ALL	−	+	−	+	−	−	−	−
B ALL	±	−	+	−	+	−	+	+
B Precursor ALL								
Pre-B	+	+	+	−	+	+	−	+
Non-Pre-B	+	+	+	−	+	−	−	+
Unclassified ALL	−	+	+	−	−	−	−	−

of monoclonal surface membrane IgM. **In 80% of cases of acute lymphoblastic leukemia, an origin of neoplastic blast cells from early B-cell precursors is suggested by immunologic marker studies and by the demonstration of gene rearrangements of the immunoglobulin heavy and light chains. Fifteen percent to 20% of cases of acute lymphoblastic leukemia are of T-cell origin, as demonstrated by reactivity with monoclonal anti-T-cell antibodies and by rearrangement of the gene for the beta chain of the T-cell receptor.** T-cell acute lymphoblastic leukemia is morphologically classified in the FAB classification as either L1 or, more commonly, as L2 acute lymphoblastic leukemia. A small minority of leukemias lack any distinguishing immunologic or other cell markers and are labelled null, or unclassified, leukemias.

A characteristic cytochemical finding in B-precursor and T-cell acute lymphoblastic leukemia is coarse cytoplasmic staining with the periodic acid-Schiff reaction in over half of all cases. Focal cytoplasmic staining with acid phosphatase and alpha-naphthyl acetate esterase is observed in a majority of cases of T-cell acute lymphoblastic leukemia (see Fig. 20-16). **Ninety percent of T- and B-precursor cell acute lymphoblastic leukemias contain the nuclear DNA-polymerizing enzyme Tdt.** This marker is lacking only in the morphologically distinctive FAB L3 variant. Tdt is useful in distinguishing lymphoblastic from primitive nonlymphocytic or myelogenous leukemias, which are positive for Tdt only 2% to 5% of the time (see Table 20-11). **Demonstration of Tdt has important therapeutic and prognostic implications, because acute lymphoblastic leukemia has a much better prognosis than acute nonlymphocytic leukemia and responds to a less intensive chemotherapeutic regimen.**

The leukemic cells in most cases of acute lymphoblastic leukemia have an abnormal karyotype. Aneuploidy, usually hyperdiploidy, and marker chromosomes, commonly involving the C and G groups, are the most frequent cytogenetic findings. The finding of hyperdiploidy is a favorable prognostic sign in acute lymphoblastic leukemia. The blast cells of 25% of adults and 5% of children with acute lymphoblastic leukemia have the Ph[1] chromosome. Ph[1]-positive acute lymphoblastic leukemia usually is an aggressive disorder with a poor prognosis. L3 (Burkitt's) leukemia is characterized by a translocation, involving the oncogene c-myc between chromosomes 2 and 8, 14 and 8, or 22 and 8. The specific translocation determines whether the neoplastic cells express surface membrane kappa or lambda light chains with the IgM heavy chain.

Acute lymphoblastic leukemia is predominantly a disease of childhood, 85% of all cases occurring in the pediatric age group. In children the incidence peaks between 3 and 6 years of age. In this age group, most acute lymphoblastic leukemia is morphologically L1 and immunologically CALLA- and Tdt-positive **(B-precursor cell acute lymphoblastic leukemia).** White males are most commonly affected. L3 (Burkitt's) leukemia occurs in a slightly older age group, with a peak age range of 6 to 11 years.

The prognosis in the 3- to 6-year-old age group with acute lymphoblastic leukemia has improved dramatically, and cure can be anticipated in over half of the cases. The prognosis in adult acute lymphoblastic leukemia is much less favorable. In acute lymphoblastic leukemia adverse risk factors include FAB L3 and T-cell subtypes of leukemia, the presence of the Ph[1] chromosome, a high peripheral blood blast cell count, the presence of a mediastinal mass, central nervous system involvement, and onset of disease either in infancy or in adulthood.

THE NON-HODGKIN'S MALIGNANT LYMPHOMAS

The non-Hodgkin's malignant lymphomas are a clinically and pathologically diverse group of neo-

Table 20-14   Hodgkin's Disease Versus Non-Hodgkin's Malignant Lymphoma—Clinical Features

CLINICAL FEATURE	HODGKIN'S DISEASE	NON-HODGKIN'S MALIGNANT LYMPHOMA
Age range	Bimodal (15–34, >50) (Western or type III)	Increases with age (median, 50)
Sex incidence	Male:female, 1.5:1 (nodular sclerosis: male:female, 1:1)	Male:female, 1.5:1 (Mediterranean abdominal lymphoma: male:female, 1:1)
Pathologic stage at presentation	Frequently stage I or II (localized)	Generally stage III or IV (<20% localized)
Constitutional symptoms at presentation	40%	15%
Pattern of spread	Predictable (to contiguous nodal groups)	Random
Leukemic conversion	Never	Variable (cell-type dependent)

plastic disorders of lymphoid cells. **The heterogeneity of the lymphomas reflects the potential for malignant transformation at any stage of B- or T-lymphocyte differentiation.** The malignant lymphomas commonly first involve the lymph nodes or other lymphopoietic tissues. They have traditionally been called the non-Hodgkin's malignant lymphomas to distinguish them from Hodgkin's disease. This distinction may on occasion be difficult because of overlapping clinical and pathologic features. Clinical features helpful in distinguishing non-Hodgkin's lymphoma from Hodgkin's disease are shown in Table 20-14. Differences in preferential sites of initial involvement are outlined in Table 20-15.

The malignant lymphomas are characterized by the following: homogeneous neoplastic cell populations; a histologic pattern of tumor cell growth, either as cohesive cellular aggregates (called the follicular, or nodular, pattern,) or as diffuse infiltration; a prognosis determined principally by the histopathologic subtype; unpredictable spread of disease; frequent presentation as widespread or systemic disease; and pronounced clinical and pathologic differences between the malignant lymphomas of children and those of adults. In addition to characteristic morphologic patterns, e.g., all follicular lymphomas are of B cell origin, the demonstration of light-chain restriction, with the expression of only kappa or only lambda light chains, is confirmatory of monoclonality and hence of B-cell neoplasia (Fig. 20-25). The diagnosis of a T-cell lymphoma requires the demonstration of a homogeneous population of cytologically atypical lymphoid cells that express T-cell markers or rearrangement of the gene for the beta chain of the T-cell receptor.

ETIOLOGY

The cause of most non-Hodgkin's malignant lymphomas is unknown, but variations in global epidemiologic patterns provide clues (Table 20-16). Two uncommon clinicopathologic subtypes are associated with specific viruses. **There is a strong correlation between infection with the Epstein-Barr virus and endemic**

Table 20-15   Hodgkin's Disease Versus Non-Hodgkin's Malignant Lymphoma—Preferential Sites of Involvement

SITE	HODGKIN'S DISEASE	NON-HODGKIN'S MALIGNANT LYMPHOMA
Initial involvement	Nodal (>95%), extranodal (rare)	Nodal (80%), extranodal (20%)
Epitrochlear nodes	Rare	Occasional
Mesenteric nodes	Rare	Common
Mediastinal or hilar nodes	50%	20%
Pharyngeal lymphoid tissue (Waldeyer's ring)	Rare	Common
Spleen	Common	Common
Bone marrow	<10%	Cell-type dependent: Small cleaved (50–70%) Large cell (5–10%)
Gastrointestinal tract	Rare	Diffuse (20%), follicular (<10%)
Testicle	Rare	Common with lymphoblastic and large cell lymphoma
Central nervous system	Rare	Cell-type dependent: lymphoblastic (common), large cell (common after marrow involvement)
Skin	Rare	Common
Liver	Uncommon	Small cleaved (common), large cell (uncommon)

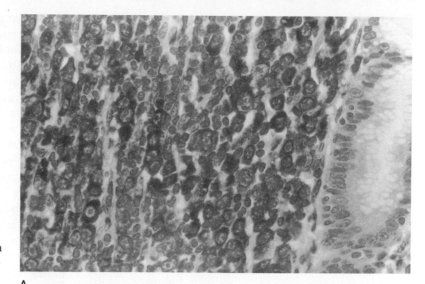

A

Figure 20-25. Plasmacytoid large cell lymphoma in the large bowel. (*A*) A positive immunohistochemical (peroxidase–antiperoxidase) stain for cytoplasmic kappa light chains. (*B*) A negative immunohistochemical stain for cytoplasmic lambda light chains.

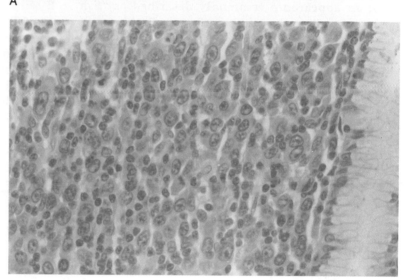

B

Table 20-16 Geographic Pathology of Lymphomas: Global Epidemiologic Patterns

Type I	Tropical countries with high prevalence of Burkitt's lymphoma
Type II	Tropical countries where Burkitt's lymphoma not prevalent but where there is high incidence of aggressive Hodgkin's disease in children
Type III	Tropical and subtropical countries with high incidence of aggressive Hodgkin's disease in children and high incidence of nodular sclerosing Hodgkin's disease in young adults
Type IV	Industrialized countries with low incidence of Hodgkin's disease in children and high incidence of nodular sclerosing Hodgkin's disease in young adults
Type V	Asian countries with low incidence of Hodgkin's disease and high incidence of large cell lymphoma

Burkitt's lymphoma in central equatorial Africa (see Fig. 20-21). A specific C-type retrovirus, the human T-cell leukemia/lymphoma virus (HTLV-I), is commonly associated with the adult T-cell leukemia/lymphoma that occurs in several geographically restricted areas of the world (see Fig. 20-21).

A number of disorders are associated with an increased risk for the development of B-cell large cell immunoblastic lymphomas (Table 20-17).

GENERAL FEATURES

In the non-Hodgkin's malignant lymphomas, the involved lymph nodes are enlarged, soft, and pale

Table 20-17   Disorders Associated With Significantly Increased Risk of Secondary Malignant Lymphoma

Sjögren's syndrome
Renal and cardiac transplant
Acquired immunodeficiency syndrome (AIDS)
Congenital immune deficiency syndromes
   Chediak-Higashi
   Wiskott-Aldrich
   Ataxia telangiectasia
   IgA deficiency
   Severe combined immune deficiency
Alpha heavy-chain disease
Celiac disease
Hodgkin's disease posttreatment
X-linked lymphoproliferative disorder

gray, an appearance commonly described as "fish flesh." However, they may be firm or "rubbery" if there is an associated fibrosis.

In non-Hodgkin's lymphomas involving the spleen, there is primary involvement of the white pulp (see Fig. 20-12). Initially, the follicular centers are involved in B-cell lymphomas and the periarteriolar lymphoid sheath in T-cell lymphomas. There may be generalized expansion of the white pulp or discrete tumor masses. The liver may be grossly normal or variably enlarged, with accentuation of the normal lobular pattern. Uncommonly, tumor masses may be evident. Microscopically, the portal areas are first involved. In the bone marrow initial involvement is usually focal and paratrabecular in distribution (see Fig. 20-16), but multifocal or diffuse involvement with marrow re-

placement may be observed. Radiologically, osteolytic or, less commonly, osteoblastic, lesions are identified.

Histologic examination reveals a monotonous cell population that infiltrates and obliterates the normal lymph nodal or other tissue architecture. Characteristically, the neoplastic cells exhibit uniformly atypical cytologic features. A spectrum of neoplastic cell size may be seen, but careful histologic examination usually reveals cytologic atypia of all of the infiltrating lymphoid cells. Only in small or well-differentiated lymphocytic lymphoma is cellular atypia generally lacking.

Microscopically, in 40% of the malignant lymphomas in adults, the initial tumor cell pattern is one of uniform discrete aggregates of neoplastic cells, referred to as follicles or nodules (Fig. 20-26). All malignancies that exhibit a follicular pattern are of B-cell origin. A specific chromosomal translocation t(14;18) is present in 85% of the follicular lymphomas. Follicular lymphomas are generally indolent disorders and typically follow a chronic course. However, relapses are common, and cure is exceptional. Follicular lymphomas progressively infiltrate the normal interfollicular tissues to become both follicular and diffuse. The final growth pattern is frequently diffuse. Follicular lymphomas are most common in middle-aged to elderly adults, are uncommon under the age of 30 years, and are exceedingly rare in children. The vast majority of malignant lymphomas in the pediatric age group are diffuse neoplasms that exhibit an aggressive clinical course and frequent leukemic distribution e.g., with circulating cells in the peripheral blood (Table 20-18). Follicular lymphomas must be

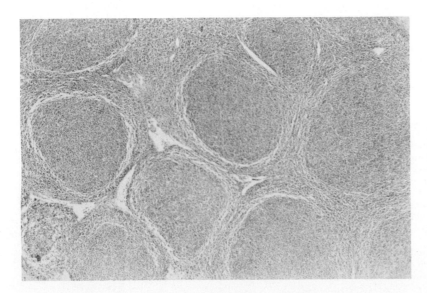

Figure 20-26. The lymph node in follicular lymphoma. The normal nodal architecture is replaced by homogeneous nodular aggregates of neoplastic B-lymphocytes.

Table 20-18   Non-Hodgkin's Malignant Lymphoma: Pediatric Versus Adult

	PEDIATRIC	ADULT
Sites of initial involvement	Commonly extranodal	Predominantly nodal
Histopathologic subtypes	Aggressive high-grade	Indolent to high-grade
Pattern of tumor cell growth	Diffuse, rarely follicular	Diffuse (60%), follicular (40%)
Leukemic conversion	Common	Occasional, cell-type dependent
Initial central nervous system involvement	Common	Common only with lymphoblastic lymphoma
Monoclonal gammopathy	Rare	Infrequent, cell-type dependent
Late relapse after 2 years	Rare	Common with follicular lymphomas

distinguished from the benign or reactive follicular hyperplasias (Table 20-19).

In 60% of the malignant lymphomas in adults, the tumor is initially diffusely infiltrative, without a proclivity to form follicles or nodules. These diffuse lymphomas are of B- or T-cell origin. **With the exception of small lymphocytic lymphoma, diffuse lymphomas exhibit a more aggressive clinical course than the follicular lymphomas.** However, a clinical cure can now be anticipated in many of these more aggressive diffuse (large cell) lymphomas. The patterns of neoplastic involvement of the lymph nodes by the non-Hodgkin's malignant lymphomas are shown in Figure 20-18.

CLASSIFICATION

Because the malignant lymphomas are pathologically diverse, a number of classification systems have been proposed to identify subtypes that have therapeutic and prognostic relevance. All require the identification of tumor cell types and tumor growth patterns. Three such classification systems (Table 20-20) are relevant to a current understanding of the malignant lymphomas: Rappaport, Lukes-Collins, and the International Working Formulation.

The Rappaport classification (1966) is based on morphologic evaluation of tumor cell size and cytologic appearance, and was formulated before the application of modern immunologic concepts to the study of the malignant lymphomas. Nevertheless, this classification is clinically relevant and prognostically significant and has been widely employed in clinical therapeutic trials.

The Lukes-Collins classification (1974) is based on a combined morphologic and functional or immunologic identification of B- and T-cell malignant lymphomas and tumors of true histiocytes. The Lukes-Collins classification applies immunologic concepts to the understanding of the malignant lymphomas, but its therapeutic and prognostic relevance has not been fully assessed.

The International Working Formulation (1982) is based on an international pathologic review and clinical correlation of almost 1200 cases of malignant lymphoma. The Working Formulation compared six major lymphoma classifications and found that each defined three major subgroups: lymphomas with a

Table 20-19   Lymph Nodes—Reactive Follicular Hyperplasia Versus Follicular Lymphoma

REACTIVE FOLLICULAR HYPERPLASIA	FOLLICULAR LYMPHOMA
Follicles composed of spectrum of activated normal lymphoid cells	"Follicles" composed of uniformly atypical or spectrum atypical neoplastic cells
Follicles with "starry sky" pattern due to presence of intrafollicular phagocytic macrophages and dendritic reticular cells	"Follicles" without "starry sky" pattern due to absence of phagocytic macrophages and dendritic reticular cells
Marked variation in size and shape of follicles	Minor variation in size and shape of follicles
Follicles sharply demarcated from surrounding lymph node tissue by cuff of normal lymphocytes	"Fading follicles" poorly demarcated from surrounding lymph node tissue
Follicles predominantly in cortex	"Follicles" closely apposed and evenly distributed in cortex and medulla
Preservation of normal lymph node architecture	Partial to complete effacement of normal lymph node architecture
Absent to moderate capsular and perinodal soft tissue infiltration in predominantly perivascular distribution	Frequent extensive capsular and perinodal soft tissue infiltration not selectively perivascular in distribution
Polyclonal B-cell population	Monoclonal B-cell population

Table 20-20 *Comparative Classification of Non-Hodgkin's Lymphoma*

1982 NCI INTERNATIONAL WORKING FORMULATION (SURVIVAL)	1974 (MODIFIED 1979) LUKES-COLLINS (MORPHOLOGIC-IMMUNOLOGIC)	1966 (MODIFIED 1976) RAPPAPORT (MORPHOLOGIC-CELL SIZE)
Low-Grade		
Small lymphocytic		
Consistent with chronic lymphocytic leukemia	Diffuse small lymphocytic	Diffuse well-differentiated lymphocytic
Plasmacytoid	Plasmacytoid lymphocytic	Well-differentiated lymphocytic with plasmacytoid differentiation
Follicular, predominantly small cleaved cell	Follicular small cleaved	Nodular poorly differentiated lymphocytic
Diffuse areas, sclerosis	Follicular and diffuse small cleaved	Nodular and diffuse poorly differentiated lymphocytic
Follicular, mixed small cleaved and large cell	Follicular small cleaved and large cell	Nodular mixed lymphocytic-histiocytic
Diffuse areas, sclerosis	Follicular and diffuse small cleaved and large cell	Nodular and diffuse, mixed lymphocytic-histiocytic
Intermediate-Grade		
Follicular, predominantly large cell	Follicular, large cell	Nodular histiocytic
Diffuse areas sclerosis	Follicular and diffuse large cell	Nodular and diffuse histiocytic
Diffuse small cleaved cell	Diffuse small cleaved	Diffuse poorly differentiated lymphocytic
Diffuse mixed small and large cell	Diffuse mixed small cleaved and large cell	Diffuse poorly differentiated lymphocytic-histiocytic
sclerosis, epithelioid component		
Diffuse large cell		
Cleaved cell	Diffuse large cleaved	Diffuse mixed lymphocytic-histiocytic or histiocytic
Noncleaved sclerosis	Diffuse large noncleaved	Diffuse histiocytic
High-Grade		
Large cell immunoblastic	Immunoblastic sarcoma	Diffuse histiocytic
Plasmacytoid	B-cell type	
Clear cell	T-cell type	
Polymorphous	B- or T-cell type	
Epithelioid cell component	T-cell type	
Lymphoblastic	Lymphoblastic, diffuse	Diffuse lymphoblastic
Convoluted	Convoluted	
Nonconvoluted		
Small noncleaved cell	Small noncleaved	Diffuse undifferentiated
Burkitt's	Burkitt's	Burkitt's
Follicular areas (same as Burkitt's)	Burkitt's-like	non-Burkitt's

low-grade (indolent) clinical course, an intermediate-grade clinical course, and a high-grade (aggressive) clinical course. The schema of the Working Formulation is employed in the following discussion of the salient features of subtypes of the malignant lymphomas; corresponding terminology in the Rappaport and Lukes-Collins classifications is shown in Table 20-20. The cytologic features of each of the neoplastic cell subtypes, following the order of the Working Formulation, are illustrated in Figure 20-27. The preferential sites of involvement of the specific non-Hodgkin's malignant lymphomas and, for comparison, Hodgkin's disease are presented in Figure 20-28.

LOW-GRADE NON-HODGKIN'S MALIGNANT LYMPHOMAS

In the Working Formulation low-grade non-Hodgkin's lymphomas are classified as **small lymphocytic, small lymphocytic plasmacytoid, follicular small cleaved,** and **follicular small cleaved and large cell.**

SMALL LYMPHOCYTIC LYMPHOMA

Small lymphocytic lymphoma is a diffuse lymphoma of morphologically normal but immunologi-

SMALL LYMPHOCYTIC
Nucleus: round
Chromatin: dense
Nucleolus: indistinct
Cytoplasm: scant, blue

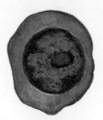

IMMUNOBLASTIC, B
Nucleus: round to oval
Chromatin: vesicular
Nucleolus: prominent
Cytoplasm: moderate, dense, blue

SMALL LYMPHOCYTIC, PLASMACYTOID
Nucleus: round, eccentric
Chromatin: dense
Nucleolus: variable
Cytoplasm: moderate, blue

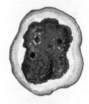

IMMUNOBLASTIC, T
Nucleus: round to irregular
Chromatin: variable
Nucleoli: variable
Cytoplasm: clear

SMALL CLEAVED
Nucleus: indented
Chromatin: coarse
Nucleolus: small
Cytoplasm: scant

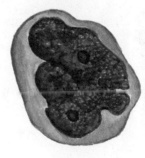

IMMUNOBLASTIC, POLYMORPHOUS
Nucleus: pleomorphic
Chromatin: variable
Nucleoli: variable
Cytoplasm: moderate

SMALL NONCLEAVED (BURKITT'S)
Nucleus: round to oval
Chromatin: coarsely reticulated
Nucleoli: small, 2-5
Cytoplasm: blue, vacuolated

LYMPHOBLASTIC, CONVOLUTED
Nucleus: irregular
Chromatin: delicate
Nucleolus: variable
Cytoplasm: blue, scant

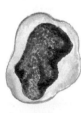

LARGE CLEAVED
Nucleus: irregular, indented
Chromatin: delicate
Nucleoli: indistinct
Cytoplasm: scant, pale

LYMPHOBLASTIC, NONCONVOLUTED
Nucleus: round to oval
Chromatin: delicate
Nucleolus: variable
Cytoplasm: scant, blue

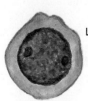

LARGE NONCLEAVED
Nucleus: round to oval
Chromatin: vesicular
Nucleoli: contiguous to membrane
Cytoplasm: moderate

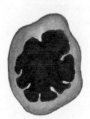

MYCOSIS FUNGOIDES
Nucleus: irregular, convoluted
Chromatin: dense
Nucleolus: indistinct
Cytoplasm: scant

Figure 20-27. Non-Hodgkin's malignant lymphomas—neoplastic cells.

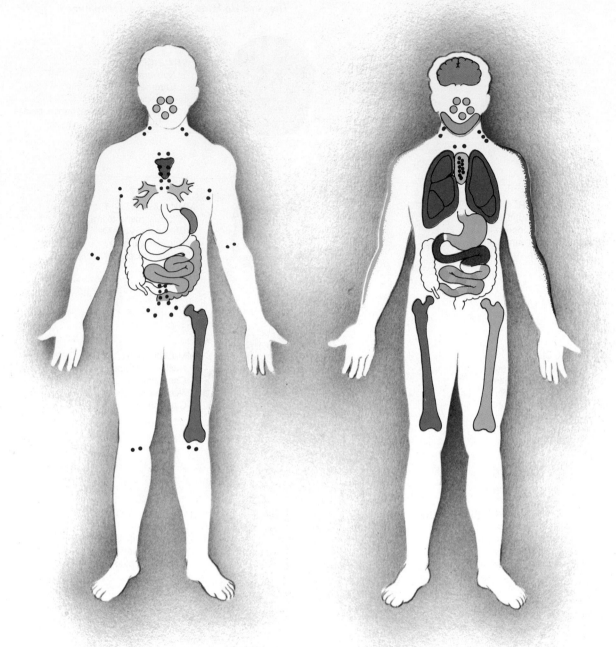

LYMPH NODES

SPLEEN (white pulp)

BONE MARROW

THYMUS

WALDEYER'S RING (lymphoid tissue of oronasopharynx)

GALT (gut-associated lymphoid tissue)

BALT (bronchial-associated lymphoid tissue)

HODGKIN'S DISEASE—lymph nodes
  Lymphocyte predominant—high cervical
  Mixed cellularity—left cervical
  Nodular sclerosis—mediastinal and supraclavicular

SMALL LYMPHOCYTIC LYMPHOMA/LEUKEMIA—bone marrow

MEDITERRANEAN ABDOMINAL LYMPHOMA—proximal small bowel

BURKITT'S LYMPHOMA—maxilla, mandible, terminal ileum

EXTRANODAL LARGE CELL LYMPHOMA—stomach, terminal ileum, bone, skin, Waldeyer's ring

POST-TRANSPLANT IMMUNOBLASTIC SARCOMA (B cell)—central nervous system

T CELL LYMPHOMA—skin, pleura, lungs, nodes

LYMPHOBLASTIC LYMPHOMA—mediastinum

Figure 20-28. (*Left*) Normal immune system. (*Right*) Sites of preferential tumor involvement.

cally incompetent small B lymphocytes. Most often it represents the tissue phase of chronic lymphocytic leukemia. **Histologically, the normal architecture of the lymph node is replaced by a monotonous population of morphologically normal small lymphoid cells with round hyperchromatic nuclei** (Fig. 20-29). Scattered pale clusters of larger, partially transformed round lymphoid cells, called pseudoreaction or proliferation centers, are characteristic. Mitotic figures are typically rare, and an increased mitotic rate (> 30 per 20 high-power fields) predicts a more aggressive clinical course. In the spleen the white pulp is uniformly expanded and spills over into the red pulp. In the liver the portal areas are first affected. The bone marrow shows involvement similar to that in chronic lymphocytic leukemia.

The **tumor cell immunologic markers of small lymphocytic lymphomas are comparable to those of chronic lymphocytic leukemia.** These include weakly expressed monoclonal surface membrane immunoglobulin, usually IgM kappa, and pan B-cell antigens. A specific chromosomal translocation t(11;14) is found in some cases of small lymphocytic lymphoma.

The clinical features of small lymphocytic lymphoma are similar to those of chronic lymphocytic leukemia. Generalized lymphadenopathy and hepatosplenomegaly are usual. The disease tends to be indolent. Middle-aged to elderly men are most commonly affected. Less than 5% of small lymphocytic lymphomas are of T-cell origin, and these are frequently characterized by an aggressive clinical course, with frequent leukemic distribution and extensive soft tissue involvement.

SMALL LYMPHOCYTIC PLASMACYTOID LYMPHOMA

Small lymphocytic plasmacytoid lymphoma is a diffuse B-cell lymphoma of small lymphoid cells that exhibits variable plasmacytoid differentiation. The neoplastic cells usually secrete monoclonal IgM macroglobulin. Small lymphocytic plasmacytoid lymphoma usually represents the clinical entity termed **Waldenström's macroglobulinemia.**

Generalized lymphadenopathy and hepatosplenomegaly are characteristic, and involvement of the bone marrow is common. A leukemic phase with circulating tumor cells occurs in 10% to 15% of cases. The neoplastic cell population is heterogeneous, being composed of small lymphoid cells and plasmacytoid lymphoid cells that display eccentric lymphoid nuclei and abundant dark blue plasmacytoid cytoplasm. Histologic evidence for immunoglobulin production includes refractile eosinophilic globules of immunoglobulin in the nuclei (Dutcher bodies) and cytoplasm (Russell bodies).

The clinical symptoms frequently are due to an increased serum viscosity secondary to the circulat-

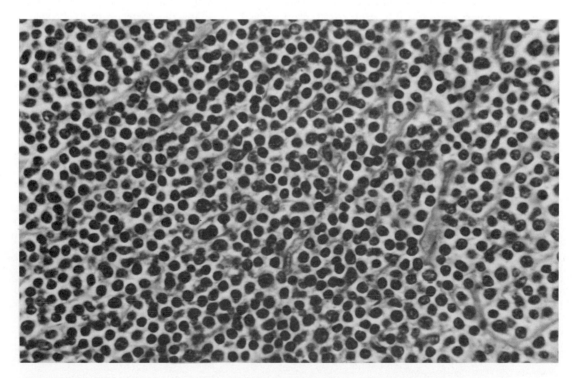

Figure 20-29. The lymph node in small lymphocytic lymphoma. Normal nodal architecture is replaced by a diffuse infiltration of normal-appearing small lymphocytes.

ing IgM paraprotein of high molecular weight. When the serum viscosity exceeds 4.0 (normal, 1.4 to 1.8), circulatory disturbances, with symptoms referable particularly to the central or peripheral nervous systems, may be observed. These include headache, dizziness, deafness, paresis, coma, and peripheral neuropathy. Small lymphocytic plasmacytoid lymphoma has an average survival of 3 to 4 years. Occasionally, a superimposed large cell immunoblastic lymphoma, with the same surface membrane immunoglobulin (idiotype), may usher in the terminal phase.

Rare B-cell tumors are associated with the secretion of an immunoglobulin heavy-chain molecule or portion of heavy-chain molecule. **Heavy-chain diseases** include IgA, IgG, and IgM heavy-chain diseases. Each is associated with a distinctive clinicopathologic picture.

FOLLICULAR SMALL CLEAVED CELL LYMPHOMA

Follicular small cleaved cell lymphoma, the most common variant of follicular lymphoma, is characterized by cohesive aggregates of small cleaved or notched and clefted lymphocytes. These cells, 10 to 15 μm in diameter, have small, hyperchromatic angulated nuclei, indistinct nucleoli, and scant or indistinguishable cytoplasm. Few mitoses are seen. The common finding that up to 20% of the cells are large or transformed lymphoid cells suggests an incomplete block to transformation of follicular center cells.

Small cleaved cells exhibit prominent monoclonal surface membrane immunoglobulin, most commonly IgM kappa, complement receptors, and Fc receptors.

Pan B-cell antigens are expressed, and in a minority of cases, the tumor cells also express common acute lymphoblastic leukemia antigen (CALLA).

Follicular small cleaved cell lymphoma is typically a disorder of middle and old age, the mean age at diagnosis being 50 years. Men and women are equally affected. Initially, lymphadenopathy and, frequently, splenomegaly are observed. Early in the clinical course there is usually widespread dissemination of disease, with hepatic and bone marrow involvement in at least 50% of cases. Frank leukemic dissemination occurs late in the course of the disease in 10% to 15% of cases. **The natural history of follicular small cleaved cell lymphoma is often characterized by progression to a follicular and diffuse, and finally to a diffuse, lymphoma, frequently of the large cell type.** Late relapses are frequent, and cure is exceptional. The median survival is 9 to 11 years.

FOLLICULAR SMALL CLEAVED AND LARGE CELL LYMPHOMA

Follicular small cleaved and large cell lymphoma is similar clinically and pathologically to follicular small cleaved cell lymphoma, but the proportion of large lymphoid cells exceeds 20%, (with 5 to 15 large cells per high power field). Histologically, a spectrum of neoplastic cell size is observed, with admixed small cleaved and transformed large lymphoid cells (Fig. 20-30). The median survival is similar to that associated with follicular small cleaved cell lymphoma, but early relapse is more common. Progression to a diffuse small cleaved and large cell lymphoma or to a diffuse large cell lymphoma may be observed.

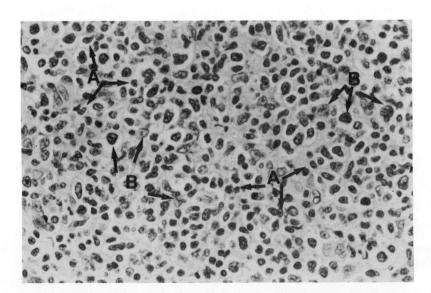

Figure 20-30. The lymph node in mixed small-cleaved and large cell lymphoma. There is a variety in cell size, from small (*A*) to large (*B*) lymphocytes.

INTERMEDIATE-GRADE NON-HODGKIN'S MALIGNANT LYMPHOMAS

Intermediate-grade malignant lymphomas are classified as: **follicular large cell, diffuse small cleaved cell, diffuse mixed small cleaved and large cell,** and **diffuse large cell, cleaved and non-cleaved.**

FOLLICULAR LARGE CELL LYMPHOMA

Follicular large cell lymphoma is a distinctly uncommon subtype of follicular lymphoma. The malignant follicles are composed predominantly of large neoplastic lymphoid cells, which may be cleaved or non-cleaved. **Follicular large cell lymphoma is the only follicular lymphoma characterized by an aggressive clinical course.** In follicular large cell lymphoma the neoplastic follicles are usually eventually obliterated and the disease progresses to a diffuse large cell lymphoma. Indeed, in a follicular large cell lymphoma, the identification of accompanying diffuse areas suggests a biologic behavior similar to that of the diffuse large cell lymphomas.

DIFFUSE SMALL CLEAVED CELL LYMPHOMA

Diffuse small cleaved cell lymphoma is typically a B-cell lymphoma of follicular center cell origin in which there is a diffuse infiltration of small cleaved lymphocytes. The age range of persons affected is similar to that of adults with follicular lymphomas; however, the clinical course is more aggressive.

DIFFUSE MIXED SMALL AND LARGE CELL LYMPHOMA

Diffuse mixed small and large cell lymphomas are of B- or T-cell type. In mixed small cleaved and large cell B-cell lymphomas, the neoplastic cells are of follicular center cell origin. Cytologically, they are identical to the malignant cells observed in follicular mixed small cleaved and large cell lymphomas. Tumor cells may be compartmentalized into small clusters of aggregates outlined by a delicate reticular fibrosis. The disorder is usually widespread at the time of diagnosis, with involvement of the lymph nodes, bone marrow, liver, and other tissues. In mixed small and large cell lymphomas of T-cell type, a spectrum of neoplastic cell size is also observed. **The contour of the tumor cell nuclear membranes is commonly irregular or cerebriform but may be round.** The cytoplasm is typically pale and clear. Tumor cells may be compartmentalized by reticular fibrosis. Postcapillary venules are frequently prominent. Admixed inflammatory cells and histiocytes are not unusual.

Immunologic studies may be required to establish that a particular tumor is of T-cell origin. Findings consistent with T-cell malignancy include marked predominance of helper or suppressor cell populations, loss of mature or postthymic T-cell markers, and demonstration of gene rearrangement of the beta chain of the T-cell receptor.

Mixed small and large cell lymphomas of T-cell type are aggressive neoplasms manifested by generalized lymphadenopathy, particularly involving the retroperitoneal lymph node groups. Commonly, there is neoplastic involvement of such sites as the skin, lungs, pleura, palatine tonsils, bone marrow, and spleen.

DIFFUSE LARGE CLEAVED CELL LYMPHOMA AND LARGE NONCLEAVED CELL LYMPHOMA

Diffuse large cleaved cell lymphoma and diffuse large noncleaved cell lymphoma occur in persons of any age and may be manifested by either local or widespread systemic disease. The most common sites of origin are the lymph nodes or other lymphopoietic sites, but in 25% to 40% of cases an extranodal site of origin, such as the gastrointestinal tract (especially the stomach and distal small bowel), thyroid gland, bone, or skin, is identified.

Histologically, there is diffuse infiltration by large transformed lymphoid cells with vesicular nuclei. The nuclear membrane contours may be either irregular (cleaved) or round (noncleaved) (Fig. 20-31). One to several nucleoli are noted. The tumor cell cytoplasm is scant to moderately abundant and pale to eosinophilic. Numerous mitoses are the rule.

More than half of all diffuse large cell lymphomas are of B-cell origin. The remainder are largely of T-cell origin, although in a minority of cases no identifying cell markers are observed. Surface membrane immunoglobulin is frequently lacking in B-cell diffuse large cell lymphomas, in which case B-cell origin is confirmed by the demonstration of specific B-cell antigens or by the rearrangement of an immunoglobulin light chain gene.

Diffuse large cell lymphoma, cleaved or non-cleaved, is an aggressive neoplasm. Large cleaved cell lymphoma generally follows a more indolent clinical course than does large noncleaved cell lymphoma. The clinical course in B-cell, T-cell, and null cell large cell lymphomas is generally similar. Clinical cure can be anticipated in approximately 40% to 50% of such neoplasms.

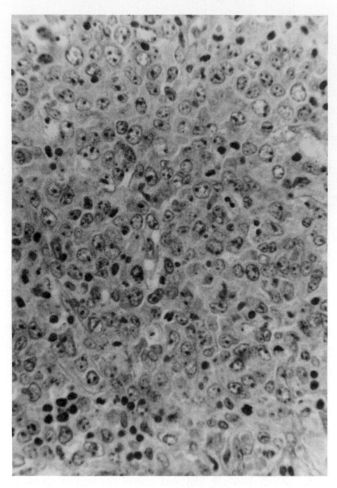

Figure 20-31. The lymph node in large noncleaved cell lymphoma. The normal nodal architecture is replaced by a diffuse infiltration of transformed lymphoid cells with round vesicular nuclei.

HIGH-GRADE NON-HODGKIN'S MALIGNANT LYMPHOMAS

High-grade malignant lymphomas are classified as: **large cell immunoblastic, lymphoblastic,** and **small noncleaved cell (Burkitt's** and **Burkitt's-like lymphoma).**

LARGE CELL IMMUNOBLASTIC LYMPHOMA

Large cell immunoblastic lymphoma is the most aggressive subtype of the large cell lymphomas. Variants of the immunoblastic lymphomas are described in the Working Formulation as plasmacytoid, clear cell, polymorphous, and epithelioid cell component.

The plasmacytoid variant is typically a B-cell neoplasm and is commonly termed **B immunoblastic lymphoma.** The neoplastic cells exhibit nuclei with vesicular chromatin, a large central, eosinophilic nucleolus, and a moderate amount of dark blue plasmacytoid cytoplasm. **B immunoblastic lymphomas arise commonly in disordered immune states;** they include the lymphomas that arise in the central nervous system in renal allograft recipients, the lymphomas that complicate chronic lymphocytic thyroiditis and the lymphoepithelial lesions of the salivary glands, the lymphomas that arise in one-third to one-half of the cases of immunoblastic lymphadenopathy, and the Mediterranean abdominal lymphoma, which may be superimposed on alpha heavy-chain disease of the proximal small bowel.

Variants of immunoblastic lymphoma defined as clear cell, polymorphous, and epithelioid cell component are generally of T-cell origin. **Clear cytoplasm is particularly characteristic of the T-cell malignant lymphomas.** Occasionally T-cell lymphomas exhibit bizarre or polymorphous cytologic features. Pleomorphic tumor cells, which morphologically simulate the Reed-Sternberg cells of Hodgkin's disease, may be identified. B-cell immunoblastic lymphomas may also exhibit such pleomorphic cytologic features. The distinction between non-Hodgkin's malignant lymphoma and Hodgkin's disease is based on the abnormal or neoplastic cytologic features of the background small lymphoid cells in T-cell (or polymorphous B-cell) lymphomas, as opposed to the background of normal small lymphocytes in Hodgkin's disease. Additionally, immunohistochemical staining for the granulocyte antigen Leu-M1 may be helpful in this distinction. Leu-M1 is commonly positive in Hodgkin's disease in a focal paranuclear and plasma membrane distribution. In T-cell lymphomas, staining for Leu-M1 is generally negative, although a minority of cases may exhibit positive staining frequently indistinguishable from that seen in Hodgkin's disease. The presence of benign epithelioid cell histiocytes, which may be sufficiently numerous to partially obscure the underlying neoplastic lymphoid cell population, is a histologic feature that suggests a T-cell lymphoma.

Common clinical features of T-cell immunoblastic lymphomas include widespread (stage III-IV) disease, an aggressive clinical course, and frequent involvement of such anatomic sites as the skin, retroperitoneal lymph nodes, lungs, and pleura.

A distinctive T-cell malignancy, **the adult T-cell leukemia/lymphoma** (ATL), has recently been described. It is associated with a C-type retrovirus, HTLV-1. **The disease is endemic in the islands of Southwestern Japan and in certain Caribbean islands** (see Fig. 20-21). There is also an increased incidence of this disorder in the southeastern United States. Morphologically, the neoplastic T cells display conspicuous nuclear membrane convolutions, which are best appreciated on peripheral blood smears. Both leukemic and lymphomatous distributions are seen, with involvement of the bone marrow, blood, lymph nodes, liver, spleen, and skin. Hypercalcemia secondary to bone lysis may be a complication. The bone destruction may reflect tumor cell secretion of an osteoclast-activating factor. **ATL is aggressive and is associated with a median survival of less than 1 year.**

LYMPHOBLASTIC LYMPHOMA

Lymphoblastic lymphoma is a diffuse malignant lymphoma, usually of mid-thymic or late thymic T-cell origin, that is closely related to the acute lymphoblastic leukemias. The neoplastic cell is a lymphoblast, 10 to 15 μm in diameter, that contains a round or convoluted nucleus. The chromatin is delicate, and one to several inconspicuous nucleoli are present. The cytoplasm is usually scant. The mitotic rate is extremely high. In 90% of cases the neoplastic cells express the nuclear DNA-polymerizing enzyme Tdt.

Lymphoblastic lymphoma is an aggressive malignancy most commonly observed in adolescent and young adult males. In half of the cases a mediastinal mass is identified. Supradiaphragmatic lymphadenopathy is also common. The disease usually spreads rapidly to the bone marrow with a subsequent leukemic phase in which the white blood cell count is high, frequently greater than 100,000 per microliter. Commonly, there is involvement of the central nervous system, with secondary leukemic meningitis.

SMALL NONCLEAVED CELL LYMPHOMA

Small noncleaved cell lymphomas include **Burkitt's lymphoma** and similar clinicopathologic disorders that lack the distinctive uniform morphologic features of Burkitt's lymphoma (Burkitt's-like lymphoma). **Initially described as a common malignant tumor of the jaw in young African children, Burkitt's lymphoma is endemic in tropical equatorial Africa and in certain areas of New Guinea** (see Fig. 20-21); it also occurs sporadically in other geographic locations. In endemic areas there is a high frequency of association with the Epstein-Barr (EB) virus. **Burkitt's lymphoma is an aggressive neoplasm of children that rarely occurs in adults.** In Africa the median age of onset is 7 years, and commonly the bones of the maxilla and mandible are initially involved; in Western countries the median age of onset is 9 to 11 years, and abdominal sites, including the terminal ileum, ovaries, and kidneys, are frequently initially affected. The lymph nodes tend to be spared. In the preterminal stage there may be leukemic distribution (FAB L3 or Burkitt's leukemia),

with secondary involvement of the central nervous system.

Burkitt's lymphoma has a distinctive histologic and cytologic appearance; it is a diffuse lymphoma. Tumor cells in tissue sections are uniform and have round to oval nuclei, with coarsely reticulated chromatin, 2 to 5 small nucleoli, and a modest rim of dense cytoplasm. The cytoplasm is deep blue with clear cytoplasmic vacuoles. **Mitotic figures are numerous, reflecting the fact that Burkitt's lymphoma is one of the most rapidly dividing human neoplasms. Phagocytic macrophages containing nuclear and cytoplasmic debris impart the "starry sky" pattern. Burkitt's lymphoma is a B-cell tumor, and monoclonal surface membrane IgM usually is demonstrated.**

MISCELLANEOUS LYMPHOMAS

In the Working Formulation, several distinctive neoplastic disorders are included in a miscellaneous category.

Mycosis fungoides is a cutaneous malignant disorder of mature or postthymic T-helper lymphocytes. The evolution of mycosis fungoides is typically indolent, and the disorder is initially manifested by a localized or generalized chronic erythematous or eczematous rash. In the early eczematous phase the histologic appearance is not diagnostic; focal perivascular and periadnexal lymphoid cell, and occasionally mixed inflammatory cell infiltrates in the superficial dermis are characteristic. **Over the course of months to years, the lesions progress to raised, flattened, indurated plaquelike papules and subsequently to fungating tumor nodules.** Both in the plaque and in the tumor stages a bandlike dermal infiltrate lies contiguous to the epidermis. The infiltrate is composed of a spectrum of atypical lymphoid cells. Medium to large lymphoid cells with hyperchromatic cerebriform nuclei are termed "mycosis cells." Admixed inflammatory cells, including eosinophils and plasma cells, may be observed, particularly early in the course of the disease. Aggregates of atypical lymphoid cells in the epidermis, called **Pautrier's microabscesses, are characteristic but not diagnostic of mycosis fungoides.** Draining lymph nodes show dermatopathic lymphadenopathy and subsequently neoplastic cell infiltration. Tumor infiltration is first observed in the T-dependent paracortex (see Fig. 20-18). Subsequent involvement of such sites as the lungs, spleen, and liver is common.

The Sézary syndrome represents the leukemic phase of mycosis fungoides. A high white blood cell count reflects the presence of circulating neoplastic lymphoid cells with bizarre cerebriform nuclei (Fig.

20-32). Frequently a ring of perinuclear PAS-positive cytoplasmic vacuoles is demonstrated. Skin involvement is prominent in the Sézary syndrome, with diffuse eczema or erythroderma.

PLASMA CELL NEOPLASIA

Plasma cell neoplasia is a malignant, clonal disorder of the terminally differentiated B cell, namely the plasma cell. It is characterized by neoplastic plasma cell infiltration of the bone marrow and, less frequently, of the soft tissues. In most cases there is secretion either of a monoclonal immunoglobulin molecule or of a light chain. A serum or urine paraprotein is therefore generally detected.

There are three well-defined clinical presentations, of which only one is common. Most plasma cell neoplasia occurs as multifocal disease of the bone marrow (**multiple myeloma**). Uncommonly, a single destructive lesion of bone, **solitary myeloma,** is identified. With time, solitary myeloma usually progresses to multiple myeloma. Localized plasma cell tumors of the soft tissues, called **extramedullary plasmacytomas**, are rare. They are located in the upper respiratory tract in 75% of cases (Fig. 20-33). Less commonly involved locations include the lower respiratory tract and other soft tissue sites. Extramedullary plasmacytomas usually do not progress to multiple myeloma.

The cause of multiple myeloma is unknown. A genetic predisposition is suggested by an increased incidence of multiple myeloma and monoclonal gammopathy of unknown significance in family members of patients with myeloma, an increased frequency of the 4c complex of the HLA system in myeloma patients, and an increased incidence of multiple myeloma in blacks.

The pathophysiology in multiple myeloma relates to both progressive infiltration and destruction of bone by malignant plasma cells and to the secondary effects of the serum or urine paraprotein.

In histologic sections of bone marrow, **clusters or diffuse sheets of plasma cells are identified** (see Fig. 20-16). **Unlike reactive processes, neoplastic plasma cell infiltration is not selectively perivascular.** Ultimately both normal hematopoietic tissues and fat cells are replaced. Although neoplastic plasma cells may be indistinguishable from normal plasma cells, they are more commonly immature and display atypical morphologic features. These include the presence of nucleoli, irregular chromatin distribution, binucleation or multinucleation, and a primitive blastlike appearance. Marrow osteoclast activity is frequently increased, with

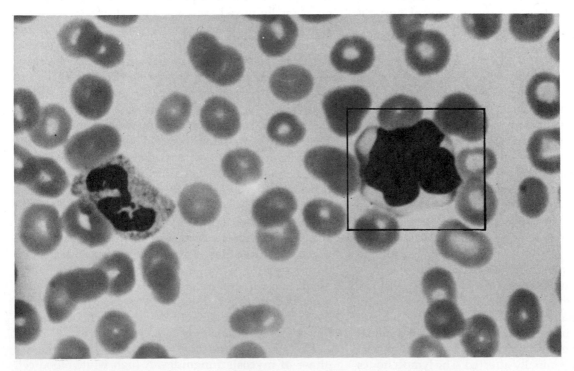

Figure 20-32. Sézary syndrome. A circulating neoplastic T-helper cell with prominent nuclear convolutions (*inset*).

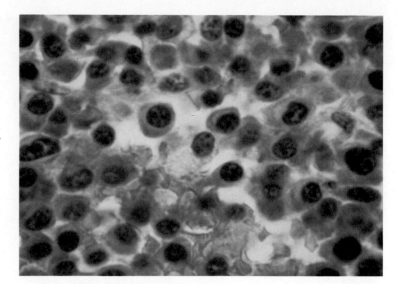

Figure 20-33. Extramedullary plasmacytoma. Infiltration of the larynx by neoplastic plasma cells, with eccentric hyperchromatic nuclei and abundant purple cytoplasm.

numerous osteoclasts located in resorption lacunae along the margins of bony trabeculae. This osteoclast proliferation may represent a response to the secretion of osteoclast-activating factor by the neoplastic plasma cells. The bone resorption induced by the increased osteoclast activity may be responsible, at least in part, for the hypercalcemia that is a common complication of multiple myeloma.

In the spleen the red pulp is principally involved, with plasma cell infiltration of both the cords and the sinuses (see Fig. 20-12). The liver may show infiltration of the portal areas or, in the case of a leukemic phase, of the sinusoids. In the lymph nodes there may be initial patchy involvement of the medullary cords, which rarely progresses to extensive infiltration and obliteration of the normal nodal architecture.

Renal involvement (myeloma kidney) occurs in up to 80% of cases. The kidneys may be normal in size, slightly enlarged, or contracted owing to the multiple damaging effects of hypercalciuria, hyperuricosuria, and acute and/or chronic pyelonephritis. Plasma cell infiltration of the kidneys, usually focal and interstitial, is common, but even extensive involvement may not affect renal function. Light chains are toxic to the renal tubular epithelium and are important in the genesis of the renal failure that is common in multiple myeloma. Frequently proteinaceous casts containing light chains and other proteins are found in the distal convoluted and collecting tubules. Such casts may induce destruction of the renal tubules, occasionally with an accompanying giant cell reaction or with proliferation of the tubular epithelium.

The diagnosis of multiple myeloma is made only after careful consideration of both the clinical and the pathologic findings. **The diagnosis requires the findings of sheets of plasma cells or a significant population of atypical plasma cells in the bone marrow, the presence (in the vast majority of cases) of a monoclonal paraprotein, and the radiologic demonstration (in the majority of cases) of lytic bone lesions** (Fig. 20-34) **or of diffuse osteoporosis.** Lytic bone lesions of the skull and other flat bones are a characteristic but not diagnostic radiologic finding in multiple myeloma.

The distribution of the serum and urine immunoglobulin abnormalities in multiple myeloma is shown in Table 20-21. In the majority of cases levels of the normal circulating immunoglobulins are depressed. A small serum or urine monoclonal protein can be identified in up to one-third of cases of solitary myeloma or of extramedullary plasmacytoma. These generally disappear following treatment of the isolated tumor.

Common laboratory findings include a mild normocytic, normochromic anemia and a mild neutropenia. Circulating plasma cells may be seen on the blood smear. Because of the increased serum immunoglobulin levels due to the paraprotein, there is typically a high erythrocyte sedimentation rate. Occasionally the peripheral blood smear exhibits rouleaux formation, described as a stacked coin appearance of erythrocytes. Serum calcium and uric acid levels are frequently elevated. Normal alkaline phosphatase levels attest to an absence of increased bone marrow osteoblast activity.

Multiple myeloma is usually a disease of the older age groups, the average age at diagnosis being 60 years. However, the disease may occur in middle-aged and young adults and has even been seen in teenagers. There is a slight male predominance. **The most common symptom is bone pain. Lower back pain occurs**

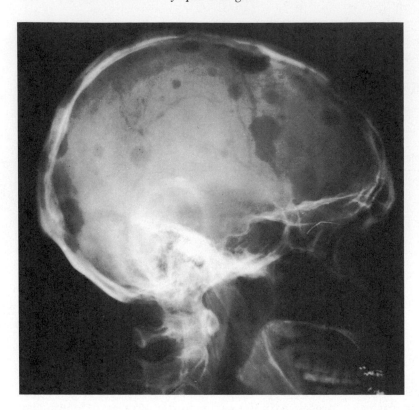

Figure 20-34. Multiple myeloma. A radiograph of the skull shows numerous "punched-out" radiolucent areas.

in 70%, rib pain in 20%, and leg pain in 10% of the cases. The bone pain may be intermittent and chronic, owing to slowly progressive plasma cell infiltration, or acute and severe, as in the case of pathologic fractures. Pathologic fractures most commonly involve the vertebrae, ribs, and long bones. Weakness and fatigue due to the normocytic, normochromic anemia are also frequently encountered. Less commonly, there may be neurologic symptoms due either to spinal cord com-

pression or to infiltration of nerve trunks by neoplastic plasma cells. Nerve root symptoms may also be due to amyloid deposition. **Amyloidosis occurs in 10% to 15% of cases of multiple myeloma.**

Complicating acute infections are common and often involve the lungs and genitourinary tract. The increased incidence of infection is caused by decreased levels of normal serum immunoglobulins and by therapy-induced neutropenia. The hyperviscosity syndrome, which reflects the high serum levels or unusual physicochemical properties of the paraprotein, is observed in 7% of cases.

The clinical course of multiple myeloma is frequently biphasic, with an initial chronic stable phase followed by an accelerated preterminal phase. The median survival in multiple myeloma is 30 months. The prognosis is worse if there is a large tumor cell burden, indicated by a hemoglobin level of less than 8.5 g/dl, a serum calcium level greater than 12 mg/dl, marked elevation of serum or urine paraproteins, and extensive lytic bone lesions.

A poor prognosis is associated with the presence of a lambda light-chain paraprotein, since lambda light chains are particularly toxic to the renal tubular epithelium. A poor prognosis is also associated with those

Table 20-21   Multiple Myeloma: Distribution of Immunoglobulin Abnormalities

Immunoglobulin Abnormality	Percent
Serum monoclonal gammopathy	75
IgG	55–60
IgA	15–20
IgD	<1
IgE	Rare
IgM	Very rare
Urine light chain only (Bence-Jones protein)	20–25
Combined serum monoclonal gammopathy and urine light chain	70
Two or more serum monoclonal immunoglobulins	0.5
Nonsecretory	1

cases in which there is secretion of IgD heavy chain. This form of myeloma is aggressive and frequently involves prominently the extramedullary soft tissues. The common causes of death in multiple myeloma are infection and renal failure. A small minority of patients succumb to superimposed acute nonlymphocytic leukemia, usually following chemotherapy with alkylating agents.

HODGKIN'S DISEASE

Hodgkin's disease is a unique malignant disorder that commonly first involves the lymph nodes. Hodgkin's disease has traditionally been classified with the malignant lymphomas, but a number of unusual clinical and pathologic features distinguish Hodgkin's disease from the non-Hodgkin's malignant lymphomas and other malignant neoplasms. First, the clinicopathologic presentation frequently simulates an infectious process. Second, a significant proportion of tumor tissue commonly consists of benign host immune and inflammatory cells. Third, the classification of histopathologic subtypes is based on the type of host immune response rather than on the architectural or cytologic features of the neoplastic cells. Fourth, the origin of the neoplastic cell, the Reed-Sternberg cell, is controversial. Finally, Hodgkin's disease usually spreads predictably from involved nodes to adjacent nodal groups.

ETIOLOGY AND PATHOGENESIS

The cause of Hodgkin's disease is unknown. **The pathogenesis appears to involve a gradual malignant transformation of indigenous cells in lymph nodes or, less commonly, other tissues.** The process of transformation seems to follow an orderly progression from normal to disordered cellular proliferation to overt neoplasia.

GROSS PATHOLOGY

Grossly, lymph nodes and other tissues involved by Hodgkin's disease are usually soft and pale gray, producing the so-called "fish flesh" appearance. Less commonly, firm, or "rubbery," tumor tissue reflects a variable degree of fibrosis. The lymph nodes may be matted together if tumor extends beyond the nodal capsules.

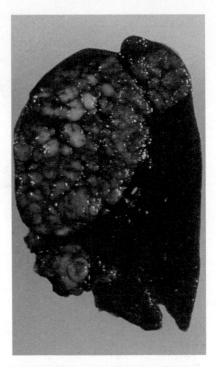

Figure 20-35. Hodgkin's disease involving the spleen. Several multinodular tumor masses partially replace the normal splenic parenchyma.

The spleen in Hodgkin's disease exhibits variable enlargement of the white pulp or a few dominant tumor nodules (Fig. 20-35). With early involvement (first in the T-dependent periarteriolar lymphoid sheath), there may be slight enlargement of one or several areas of the white pulp. In the liver the portal areas are first involved. Tumor nodules may be identified in the liver, usually late in the course of the disease. Focal, multifocal, or diffuse infiltration of the bone marrow may be observed (see Fig. 20-16). Osteolytic or osteoblastic bone lesions are demonstrated radiographically.

HISTOPATHOLOGY

Histopathologically, Hodgkin's disease exhibits a considerable heterogeneity of cell types, including classic Reed-Sternberg cells, variants of Reed-Sternberg cells that are characteristic of subtypes but not fully diagnostic of Hodgkin's disease, normal lymphocytes, and a spectrum of inflammatory cells. There may be delicate or dense fibrosis. **The diagnosis of Hodgkin's disease requires the demonstration of the Reed-**

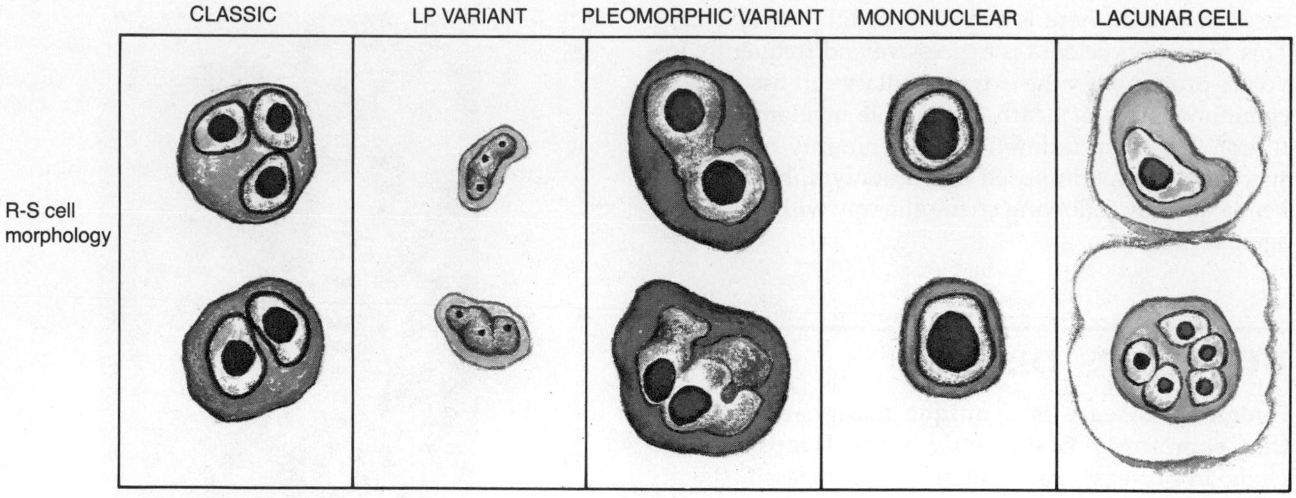

	CLASSIC	LP VARIANT	PLEOMORPHIC VARIANT	MONONUCLEAR	LACUNAR CELL
R-S cell morphology					

	CLASSIC	LP VARIANT	PLEOMORPHIC VARIANT	MONONUCLEAR	LACUNAR CELL
Nuclear Configuration	Binucleated to multinucleated to multilobulated	Single to multilobed	Single to multinucleated or multilobed	Single	Single to multilobed
Nucleoli	large (≥1/3 diameter of nucleus), eosinophilic	Small, punctate	Variable, prominent	large (≥1/3 diameter of nucleus), eosinophilic	Variable (generally <1/3 diameter of nucleus), eosinophilic
Chromatin	Clear parachromatin	Delicate	Variable, clear parachromatin to hyperchromatic	Abundant, clear parachromatin	delicate to clear parachromatin
Cytoplasm	Moderate to abundant, pale to pink	Scant, pale	Moderate to abundant, eosinophilic	Moderate, pale to pink	Abundant, pale[†]
Associated histologic subtype	Diagnostic in lymphocyte predominant, mixed cellularity, may be seen (diagnostic) in lymphocyte depleted, nodular sclerosis	Lymphocyte predominant (suggestive, not diagnostic)	Lymphocyte depleted[‡]	May be seen in any subtype	Nodular sclerosis[§]

[*] Mononuclear R-S cell variants are not diagnostic of Hodgkin's disease. However, these cells, in the appropriate environment, indicate involvement either in the staging work-up or in relapse

[†] Formalin fixation artifact: the cytoplasm of these cells may retract and the cell appears to lie in a clear space (lacuna or lake).

[‡] Pleomorphic large cell lymphoma of T-cell type must be ruled out

[§] Similar cells may occasionally be seen in mixed cellularity

Figure 20-36. Hodgkin's disease—Reed-Sternberg cells. Morphology of the classic Reed-Sternberg cell of Hodgkin's disease and variants of the Reed-Sternberg cell that are characteristic of Hodgkin's disease subtypes. Criteria for the identification of each cell type are shown in the accompanying table.

Sternberg cell, a distinctive tumor giant cell, in an environment of normal small lymphocytes or a heterogeneous population of benign inflammatory cells.

The classic Reed-Sternberg cell (Fig. 20-36) is binucleated and has large eosinophilic nucleoli centrally located in nuclei which exhibit abundant clear parachromatin. Delicate threads of heterochromatin frequently extend from the nucleoli to a marginal rim of dense heterochromatin that accentuates the nuclear membranes. The cytoplasm is a pale pink. Multinucleated cells or cells with multilobed nuclei may be seen and are also considered diagnostic Reed-Sternberg cells. The identification of necrobiotic (mummified) Reed-Sternberg cells is characteristic of Hodgkin's disease.

Cells with single nuclei and similar nuclear features are called mononuclear variants, or Hodgkin's cells (see Fig. 20-36). They may be seen in any subtype but are not diagnostic. Mononuclear variants may be difficult to distinguish from atypical reactive immunoblasts. Three additional Reed-Sternberg cell variants, the lymphocyte predominant, the pleomorphic, and the lacunar variants, are characteristic of several subtypes but are not diagnostic of Hodgkin's disease (see Fig. 20-36).

Four histopathologic subtypes of Hodgkin's disease are recognized, on the basis of specific cellular and stromal fibroblastic components of the host immune response (Fig. 20-37): lymphocyte predominant (LP), mixed cellularity (MC), lymphocyte depleted (LD), and nodular sclerosis (NS). The subdivisions LP, MC, and LD are based on the ratio of normal lymphocytes to neoplastic Reed-Sternberg cells. The progression from lymphocyte predominant to mixed cellularity to lymphocyte depleted is characterized by decreasing numbers of normal small lymphocytes and by increasing numbers of Reed-Sternberg cells. Before the era of modern therapy, the histopathologic subtype represented an important prognostic indicator (LP>MC>LD). With current therapy, the prognostic differences due to histopathologic subtype have largely evaporated.

Nodular sclerosis is a distinctive subtype of Hodgkin's disease characterized by dense, bandlike fibrosis and by a specific Reed-Sternberg cell variant, the lacunar cell. This cell has abundant pale cytoplasm and a lobulated nucleus, with eosinophilic nucleoli that are generally intermediate in size. The lacunar cell is so named because, in formalin-fixed tissue, the cytoplasm artifactually retracts toward the nucleus and the cell appears to lie in a lacuna, or lake. Classic binucleated Reed-Sternberg cells may be diffi-

cult to identify among the clearly predominant lacunar cell variants. In nodular sclerosis, the fibrosis or sclerosis is prominent and initially involves the lymph node capsule. Subsequently, bandlike fibrosis extends into the nodal parenchyma to circumscribe nodules of lymphoid tissue. Characteristic lacunar cells are identified singly or in clusters in these lymphoid nodules.

CLINICAL FEATURES

Clinically, Hodgkin's disease generally presents as a nontender enlarged lymph node or group of lymph nodes. Central, or axial, lymph nodes are most commonly involved, particularly cervical (60% to 80% of cases) and mediastinal (50% to 60% of cases) (Fig. 20-38). Preferential sites of involvement are outlined in Table 20-15.

The spread of Hodgkin's disease appears to be by direct contiguity; that is, by direct spread between adjacent lymph node groups.

In Western countries, nodular sclerosis accounts for 50% to 60% of cases of Hodgkin's disease, mixed cellularity for 30%, lymphocyte predominant for 5% to 10%, and lymphocyte depleted for 5% to 10%. The nodular sclerosis subtype commonly involves the lower cervical, supraclavicular, and mediastinal lymph nodes, particularly in young women. A mediastinal mass is common. Clinically, nodular sclerosing Hodgkin's disease is an indolent disorder, but late relapse is not uncommon. The mixed cellularity subtype involves any lymph node group, but the left cervical lymph nodes are most commonly affected. Although any age group may be afflicted, but the disease is most common in middle-aged and elderly men. The lymphocyte-predominant subtype commonly involves the high cervical and, less frequently, the inguinal lymph nodes in men under the age of 35 years. It follows an indolent course and, before the era of modern therapy, was the only subtype associated with a good prognosis, even in the presence of widespread or systemic disease. Recent evidence indicates that at least some disorders with the histopatholic features of lymphocyte-predominant Hodgkin's disease, unlike other subtypes, may express B cell immunologic markers and lack cell markers usually associated with Hodgkin's disease. Therefore lymphocyte-predominant Hodgkin's disease may represent an unusual subtype of B cell lymphoma. Lymphocyte depleted is the most aggressive subtype of Hodgkin's disease. Visceral involvement, especially of the liver and bone marrow, is common at the time of

(Text continues on p. 612)

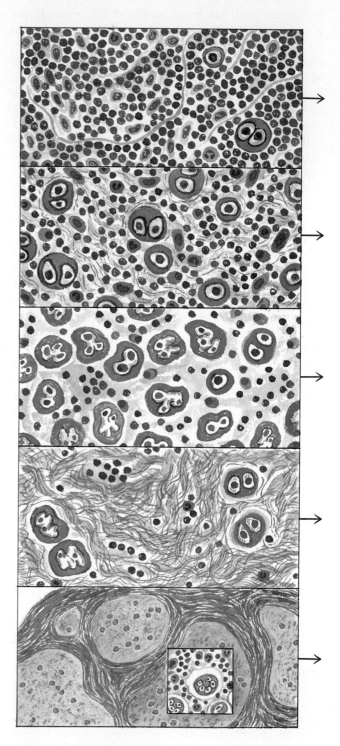

Figure 20-37. Histopathologic subtypes of Hodgkin's disease. The characteristic histopathologic appearance of each of the principal subtypes of Hodgkin's disease is shown. The sequence from lymphocyte-predominant Hodgkin's disease to lymphocyte-depleted Hodgkin's disease is characterized by progressively fewer normal lymphocytes and by increasing numbers of Reed-Sternberg cells. The subtype of lymphocyte-depleted diffuse fibrosis is characterized by few lymphocytes, few Reed-Sternberg cells, and abundant loose fibrosis. The subtype nodular sclerosing Hodgkin's disease is distinctive because of dense, bandlike, collagenous fibrosis, which envelops cellular aggregates that contain lymphoid and inflammatory cells and the specific lacunar cell variants of the Reed-Sternberg cell. The specific criteria that define each of the Hodgkin's disease subtypes are outlined in the accompanying table.

SUBTYPE	LYMPHOCYTE/REED-STERNBERG (R-S) CELL RELATIONSHIP			BACKGROUND ENVIRONMENT			LYMPH NODE INVOLVEMENT	
	NORMAL SMALL LYMPHOCYTES	REED-STERNBERG (R-S) CELL		MIXED INFLAMMATION (eosinophils, plasma cells, polys, histiocytes)	FIBROSIS	NECROSIS	PATTERN	EXTENT
		CLASSIC	VARIANT					
Lymphocyte predominant	Predominant*	Rare	Variable LP variants	Rare	Rare	Rare	Diffuse or vaguely nodular	Complete effacement
Mixed cellularity	Moderate	Variable (easily identified)	Mononuclear, lacunar, pleomorphic variants may be seen	Variable	Delicate	May be seen	Diffuse	Focal paracortical to complete effacement
Lymphocyte depleted, reticular	Scant	May be seen	Pleomorphic variant may be predominant	Scant	Delicate	May be seen	Diffuse	Complete effacement
Lymphocyte depleted, diffuse fibrosis	Scant	Rare	Rare pleomorphic variant	Scant	Abundant loose mesh-like	May be seen	Diffuse	Complete effacement
Nodular sclerosis	Predominant to scant	Rare to absent	Variable lacunar variant	Variable	Dense band-like	May be seen	Nodular (defined by collagenous fibrosis)**	Focal paracortical to complete effacement

*Benign histiocytes may constitute predominant population (histiocytic variant of lymphocyte-predominant Hodgkin's Disease).

**Vaguely nodular pattern without collagenous fibrosis (cellular phase nodular sclerosis) may be seen rarely.

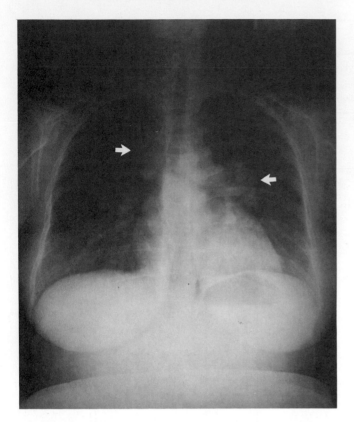

Figure 20-38. Hodgkin's disease—nodular sclerosis subtype. A radiograph of the chest shows enlarged hilar lymph nodes (*arrows*).

diagnosis. Bulky lymphadenopathy may or may not be observed but is most common in the reticular subtype. In Western countries, lymphocyte depleted Hodgkin's disease is most common in middle-aged and elderly men.

The salient clinical features of Hodgkin's disease are listed in Table 20-14. Fever, night sweats, and weight loss of 10% or more of baseline body weight within the 6 months before diagnosis are observed in 40% of cases. Patients with these symptoms are in the B group and have a worse prognosis than A-group patients, who lack these symptoms. Other distinctive symptoms include localized or generalized pruritus and alcohol-induced pain in involved sites.

All ages are affected in Hodgkin's disease. There is a distinctive bimodal age peak, with an increased incidence between ages 15 and 34 years and over 50 years. The younger age peak principally reflects the increased incidence of nodular sclerosing Hodgkin's disease in

young women. Overall there is a slight male predominance because of the higher incidence of Hodgkin's disease in middle-aged and elderly men.

The prognosis in Hodgkin's disease is principally dependent on the age of the patient and the extent of the disease or stage. In general, younger patients do better than older patients. **A more favorable prognosis is also associated with a lower clinical stage (localized disease).**

The therapy of Hodgkin's disease is increasingly effective, and in a majority of cases, clinical cure can be anticipated.

The complications of Hodgkin's disease include compromise of vital organs by progressive tumor growth, infections due to defects in delayed-type hypersensitivity or to the immunosuppressive effects of therapy, direct toxicity of therapy, and second malignancies, due probably to the immunosuppressive and mutagenic effects of therapy (acute nonlymphocytic leukemia in less than 5% of cases and large cell malignant lymphoma in less than 1% of cases).

METASTATIC TUMORS TO THE BONE MARROW

The bone marrow is a common site of metastatic malignancy. The incidence of metastatic tumors exceeds that of primary bone tumors. In adults, carcinomas that arise in glandular or ductular epithelium are the most common cancers that metastasize to the bone marrow. **Carcinomas of the breast, lung, and prostate account for over 80% of the tumors that metastasize to the bone marrow.** In children, neuroblastomas and Ewing's tumor are the types of tumor that most commonly metastasize to the bone marrow.

The axial skeleton, including the cranium, vertebrae, ribs, and sacrum, is involved in 70% of cases of metastatic malignancy to bone. Secondary neurologic symptoms are common, resulting from encroachment on and damage to the brain, spinal cord, and nerve roots. In 30% of cases of metastatic tumor, the appendicular skeleton, particularly the metaphyses of the proximal long bones, is first involved. Metastasis to the distal long bones below the elbows and knees is distinctly uncommon.

Most metastatic tumors to the bone marrow cause osteolysis (destruction of underlying bone). Such osteolytic metastases are particularly characteristic of metastatic thyroid, renal, and breast carcinomas. Some tumors induce new bone formation. These osteoblastic metastases are characteristic of metastatic prostatic carcinoma, carcinoid tumors, and some breast carcinomas. Frequently, mixed osteolytic and osteoblastic metastases are observed. A reactive fibrosis is especially characteristic of metastatic gastric and breast carcinomas.

Laboratory findings include an elevated serum acid phosphatase in metastatic carcinoma of the prostate gland and an elevated alkaline phosphatase in any osteoblastic bone metastasis. The increased serum alkaline phosphatase is due to hyperplasia of marrow osteoblasts involved in laying down new bone.

The principal clinical symptom in metastatic tumor to the bone marrow is the gradual onset of bone pain. The pain is usually localized and generally worse at night. There may be pathologic fractures in sites of metastasis, usually involving the weight-bearing bones. The clinical syndrome is characterized by the sudden onset of severe pain in the site of the fracture.

21

THE ENDOCRINE SYSTEM

VICTOR E. GOULD AND SHELDON C. SOMMERS

Endocrine function refers to the transmission of a biologic message by a chemical substance synthesized *in vivo* and acting on specific receptors. Chemical messengers that qualify as endocrine include amines, polypeptides, organic acids, and steroids. Other substances of varying chemical compositions are also regarded as having endocrine functions. These include the widely distributed prostaglandins; thymus-produced thymosin and related materials; erythropoietin, mostly produced by the kidney and playing an important role in red blood cell maturation; kinins and related vasoactive substances; factors produced by B lymphocytes; nerve and epithelial growth factors; and a host of chemical messengers produced by mast cells, platelets, certain macrophages, and other cells.

It is now generally accepted that closely related, or even identical, transmitter substances, including certain amino acids, amines, and peptides ("common peptides"), are produced in the following:

- Neurons of the central nervous system
- Peripheral nerves
- "Traditional" endocrine glands such as the pituitary
- Less clearly defined aggregates of endocrine cells, such as pancreatic islets and pulmonary neuroepithelial bodies
- A system of widely distributed cells located in numerous organs and tissues, including the gastrointestinal tract, the bronchopulmonary tree, and the skin

Cells that produce, store, and secrete endocrine substances were originally classified together because of their capability to take up and decarboxylate relatively simple amine precursor substances. Such cells were designated by the acronym, **APUD cells,** and as a whole they were said to constitute the APUD system. These cells are now collectively designated as neuroendocrine (NE), and the complex array of organs and tissues composed of or containing such cells is currently designated as the **dispersed neuroendocrine system (DNS).**

Neuroendocrine cells are readily characterized immunohistochemically by the demonstration of **neuron specific enolase,** a glycolytic enzyme common to all of these cells. Other significant markers are **chromogranin,** a protein of the secretory granule matrix, and **synaptophysin,** a membrane protein of neuronal presynaptic vesicles. Peptide hormones can also be shown immunohistochemically. By electron microscopy, neuroendocrine cells contain characteristic granules that consist of an electron-dense core, surrounded by a single membrane.

PITUITARY GLAND

Anterior pituitary lobe cells are of four histologic types and six ultrastructural–immunohistochemical types. They produce seven important peptide hormones:

Growth hormone (somatotropic hormone) is produced by classic acidophilic cells.

Prolactin (mammotropic hormone) is also produced by acidophils.

Follicle stimulating hormone (FSH) is produced by classic basophilic cells.

Luteinizing hormone (luteotropic hormone, LH) is produced by the same type of basophils as FSH; together these cells are called gonadotropic basophils or gonadotropes.

Adrenocorticotropic hormone (corticotropin, ACTH), is secreted by a subset of basophils.

Thyroid-stimulating hormone (thyrotropin, TSH) is produced by pale basophilic or amphophilic cells.

Melanocyte-stimulating hormone (melanotropin, MSH), part of the molecule of ACTH prohormone, increases skin pigmentation.

The posterior pituitary lobe (or neurohypophysis) is a downward projection of the central nervous system ectoderm, and is normally joined to the anterior lobe. There are two posterior lobe hormones: vasopressin and oxytocin. **Arginine vasopressin** (antidiuretic hormone, ADH), has the key function of promoting water resorption from the distal renal tubular fluid, thus conserving it for the body. Should any process sufficiently damage the posterior pituitary lobe or stalk, notable chronic water diuresis results, a disorder called **diabetes insipidus** (Fig. 21-1). **Oxytocin** is important in stimulating vigorous uterine muscle contractions during and after childbirth.

HYPOTHALAMIC–PITUITARY AXIS

The hypothalamus, pituitary stalk, and pituitary gland constitute an integrated "neuroendocrine system," both anatomically and functionally. Neuron groups in the hypothalamus secrete at least five factors that stimulate the anterior pituitary lobe:

Growth hormone releasing factor (GRF)
Gonadotropin releasing hormone (GnRH)
Thyrotropin releasing hormone (TRH)
Corticotropin releasing factor (CRF)
Melanotropin releasing hormone

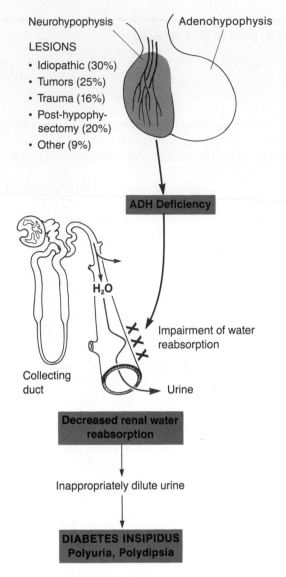

Figure 21-1. The mechanism of diabetes insipidus.

There are three hypothalamic inhibitory hormones:

Prolactin inhibiting factor (PIF)
Growth hormone inhibitory factor (GHIF)
Melanotropin inhibitory factor

These hypothalamic hormones are polypeptides, some of which have been synthesized. They are stored in and released from neuronal endocrine granules.

HYPOPITUITARISM

In adults, severe panhypopituitarism may be caused by any process that destroys pituitary tissue, such as isch-

emia, infarction, or metastatic tumor. The disorder presents clinically as **Simmonds' disease** or "pituitary cachexia," most commonly caused by infarction of the pituitary. The patient undergoes massive weight loss, and appears "skeletal," as if reduced to skin and bones. A psychiatric condition, anorexia nervosa, may simulate Simmonds' disease, but is not caused by a hypothalamic or pituitary lesion.

Sheehan's syndrome, a subcategory of Simmonds' disease, is caused by shock-induced infarction of the pituitary in women who suffer considerable blood loss as a result of a traumatic abortion or delivery. Thereafter, they become amenorrheic and lack energy, muscle strength, and normal drive (Fig. 21-2). All normal anterior lobe trophic functions are reduced.

PITUITARY TUMORS

CRANIOPHARYNGIOMA

The anterior lobe (or adenohypophysis) is ectodermally derived, developing from Rathke's duct, which in embryos extends upward from the palatal region. "Rathke" rests are considered the source of **craniopharyngioma**, a locally invasive solid and cystic neoplasm that closely resembles the tooth germ tumor called ameloblastoma.

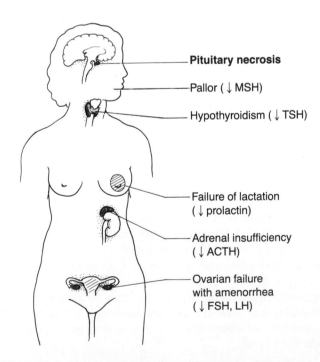

Figure 21-2. The major clinical manifestations of Sheehan's syndrome.

ADENOMAS

Pituitary adenomas are benign neoplasms of the anterior lobe. In the familial disorder known as multiple endocrine neoplasia (MEN) syndrome type I, pituitary adenoma and adenomas of the thyroid gland, adrenal cortex, parathyroid gland, and sometimes the pancreatic islets, coexist. Pituitary adenomas most commonly present as enlarging, space-occupying masses, without overt endocrine effects. They have classically been subdivided histologically according to the tinctorial properties of the neoplastic cells with conventional stains. Thus, pituitary tumors were classified as acidophil, basophil, or chromophobe. However, histochemical studies have demonstrated a lack of correlation between these properties and the type of hormone secreted

Chromophobe Adenomas

These tumors generally are over 1 cm in diameter, and consist of soft, pale tissue. Microscopically, there is a monotonous growth of small, regular cells with poorly stained cytoplasm (Fig. 21-3). **The majority of chromophobe adenomas contain prolactin.** The remainder include null cell and stem cell adenomas, which lack identifiable hormones or secretory granules.

Somatotropic Adenomas

Pituitary adenomas that secrete growth hormone produce dramatic bodily changes. If a somatotropic adenoma develops before adult growth is achieved, the individual becomes a **giant.** Most true giants, defined as over seven feet tall, have been found at autopsy to have had an acidophil pituitary adenoma. Sometimes a somatotropic adenoma so damages gonadotropic pituitary function that the individual eventually develops a eunuchoid habitus. The eunuchoid person is tall, exhibits elongated arms and legs, and suffers from deficient genital and secondary sex characteristics.

Should the somatotropic pituitary adenoma first develop after the long bone epiphyses have fused and the full adult height has been achieved, only the bones of the hands, feet, mandible, and maxilla respond to excess growth hormone. The afflicted person develops coarse facial features, with (1) overgrowth of the mandible, (2) mandibular and maxillary prognathism, with spaces between the upper incisor teeth, (3) a thickened nose, and (4) enlarged, broad "spade-shaped" hands and feet. These abnormalities are encompassed under the term **acromegaly** (Greek *acron*, extremities; *megalē*, great) (Fig. 21-4). The viscera are also hypertrophied.

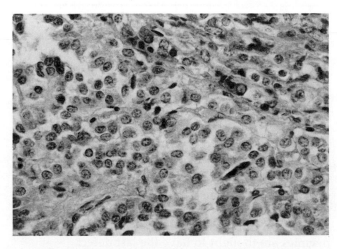

Figure 21-3. Chromophobe adenoma of the anterior pituitary. Compressed normal cells are evident at the upper right. The patient had no endocrine syndrome, but prolactin was shown by immunohistochemistry.

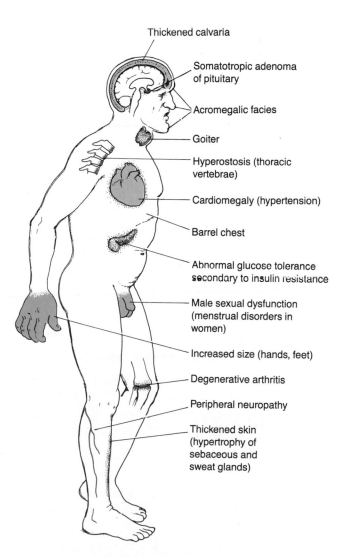

Thickened calvaria

Somatotropic adenoma of pituitary

Acromegalic facies

Goiter

Hyperostosis (thoracic vertebrae)

Cardiomegaly (hypertension)

Barrel chest

Abnormal glucose tolerance secondary to insulin resistance

Male sexual dysfunction (menstrual disorders in women)

Increased size (hands, feet)

Degenerative arthritis

Peripheral neuropathy

Thickened skin (hypertrophy of sebaceous and sweat glands)

Figure 21-4. The clinical manifestations of acromegaly.

Although these persons are deformed to a greater or lesser degree, they are not necessarily handicapped.

The somatotropic pituitary adenoma is composed of sheets of acidophilic (pink) cells; thus, the old name "acidophil pituitary adenoma." Since prolactin cells are also acidophilic, there are adenomas that secrete both growth hormone and prolactin.

Among the various chromophobe and acidophil pituitary adenomas described, the most important are microadenomas, defined as tumors smaller than 1 cm. Such lesions are usually prolactinomas. The **microprolactinoma** is a frequent cause of irregular menses, anovulation, and consequent infertility.

Oncocytomas

Oncocytoma is another acidophilic pituitary adenoma, but, from the hormonal viewpoint, it is nonfunctional.

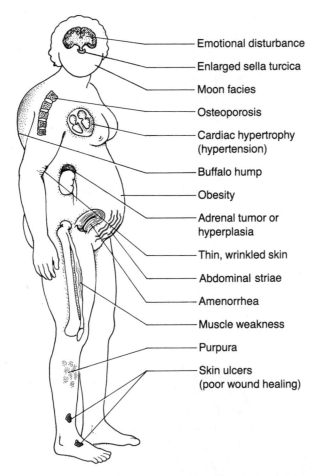

— Emotional disturbance

— Enlarged sella turcica

— Moon facies

— Osteoporosis

— Cardiac hypertrophy (hypertension)

— Buffalo hump

— Obesity

— Adrenal tumor or hyperplasia

— Thin, wrinkled skin

— Abdominal striae

— Amenorrhea

— Muscle weakness

— Purpura

— Skin ulcers (poor wound healing)

Figure 21-5. The major clinical aspects of Cushing's syndrome.

Basophil Adenomas

Basophil pituitary adenoma is the classic cause of Cushing's disease. Excessive ACTH secretion induces adrenocortical hypersecretion of cortisol/cortisone. The hypercortisolemia in turn brings on the panoply of typical somatic, biochemical, and metabolic changes seen in Cushing's syndrome (Fig. 21-5). (See Adrenocortical Hyperfunction, under Adrenal Cortex, this chapter). The pituitary tumor is often small, and its removal is curative.

ANTERIOR PITUITARY SYNDROMES

Most dwarfs and midgets suffer from defects of constitutional origin. However, a few true pituitary dwarfs lack anterior lobe somatotropic cells that secrete growth hormone. African pygmies have normal growth hormone secretion, but their target tissues are relatively unresponsive.

Corticotropic basophils in humans who are exposed to elevated levels of corticosteroids, whether administered therapeutically or endogenously produced by adrenocortical hyperfunction, undergo a cobweb vacuolar degeneration and loss of their basophilic cytoplasmic granules. These glassy-appearing cells containing whorled intermediate filaments, called **hyaline basophils** or **Crooke's cells,** are a marker for hypercortisolemia and Cushing's syndrome.

HYPOTHALAMUS

HYPOTHALAMIC SYNDROMES
GROWTH DISORDERS

Dwarfism in children that is idiopathic or follows psychosocial deprivation is thought to reflect neurotransmitter dysfunction in the central nervous system. Other children, adolescents, and young adults with growth hormone (GH) deficiency may have (1) hypothalamic dysfunction, with impaired synthesis or secretion of GH releasing hormone, (2) isolated GH deficiency, (3) absent or low pituitary GH activity as a result of abnormal GH molecules or polymeric GH ("pituitary dwarfism, type I"), or (4) unresponsiveness of the target organ to GH ("pituitary dwarfism, type II"). African pygmies are thought to have the last defect.

HYPOTHALAMIC CAUSES OF GONADAL DYSFUNCTION

Precocious Puberty

Sexual precocity is usually, but not invariably, constitutional rather than pathologic. A midline hypothalamic hamartoma is the classic neoplastic cause of precocious puberty. Its neurons contain luteinizing hormone releasing hormone. Suprasellar cysts and hypothalamic gliomas also may cause precocious puberty.

Amenorrhea and Related Disorders

Primary amenorrhea has many possible causes, among which hypothalamic dysfunction or lesions are infrequent. Isolated pituitary gonadotropin deficiency, a cause of primary amenorrhea, may be identified by the failure of the plasma prolactin level to rise after the injection of thyrotropin releasing hormone, a potent stimulator of prolactin secretion.

Secondary amenorrhea is often caused by increased circulating levels of prolactin. About one-third of cases are associated with a pituitary adenoma that secretes prolactin. In another third, patients are thought to have a functional disorder of the hypothalamic-pituitary axis.

Hyperprolactinemia has many causes besides hypothalamic disease, including hypothyroidism, chronic renal failure, and the administration of various therapeutic drugs and hormones.

Menstrual Cycle and Fertility

In some young postpubertal women, ovulation is irregular, because the maturing hypothalamic-pituitary axis does not provide a luteinizing hormone spike essential to ovulation every month. Consequently, the average fertility of women 13 to 15 years of age is less than that of older women.

Hypopituitarism in either sex prevents ovulation or spermatogenesis. Ordinarily, neither hypothalamic lesions nor functional disturbances are identified.

Beyond 47 years of age most women cease to ovulate, and the menses stop, an event termed the menopause. The primordial ova disappear, and the ovaries become incapable of cyclic function and undergo atrophy. Since pituitary gonadotropins are released in menopausal women, and the feedback effects of ovarian estrogens and progestogens on the hypothalamus cease, a hypothalamic-pituitary basis for hot flashes is suspected.

ANOREXIA NERVOSA

Anorexia nervosa is currently regarded as a predominantly psychiatric condition of adolescent girls who refuse to eat. Young women on diets, sometimes models, ballerinas, or schizophrenic women, and possibly male "obligatory runners," also may be afflicted. Amenorrhea and several endocrine dysfunctions are typical. Although gonadal dysfunctions predominate, other abnormalities occur, such as impaired thermoregulation and diabetes insipidus, with subnormal or erratic vasopressin secretion. **These changes are regarded as adaptive mechanisms in chronic starvation.**

OBESITY

The obverse of anorexia nervosa, namely obesity, also has cultural, psychosocial, and psychosomatic aspects. The relative unresponsiveness of obese individuals to internal cues of satiety could be of hypothalamic or higher origin, but the cause is unknown.

THYROID GLAND

METABOLIC AND INFLAMMATORY DISEASES

GOITER

Goiter, or struma, means thyroid enlargement; a deficiency of iodine in the diet is its major cause. Goiters are—or used to be—common in the Great Lakes area, Switzerland, south Austria (Styria), central Africa, and the Himalayas.

Endemic goiter due to iodine deficiency has various clinical and pathologic names, of which **nodular goiter** is the simplest. Other, synonymous terms are multinodular goiter, nontoxic nodular goiter, and adenomatous goiter. The normal adult thyroid weighs about 20 to 35 g, whereas a nodular goiter may weigh 100 g or even 1000 g. It forms a palpable and often visible mass in the lower anterior neck. On removal the thyroid is grossly and microscopically nodular, and shows translucent gelatinous regions and foci of hemorrhage, fibrosis, and calcification (Fig. 21-6). **Congenital goiter** most often reflects severe maternal iodine deficiency.

Sporadic cretinism is associated with thyroid agenesis, an anomaly due to intrauterine exposure to maternal antithyroid antibodies. **Endemic cretinism** occurs in remote, usually mountainous districts. Chil-

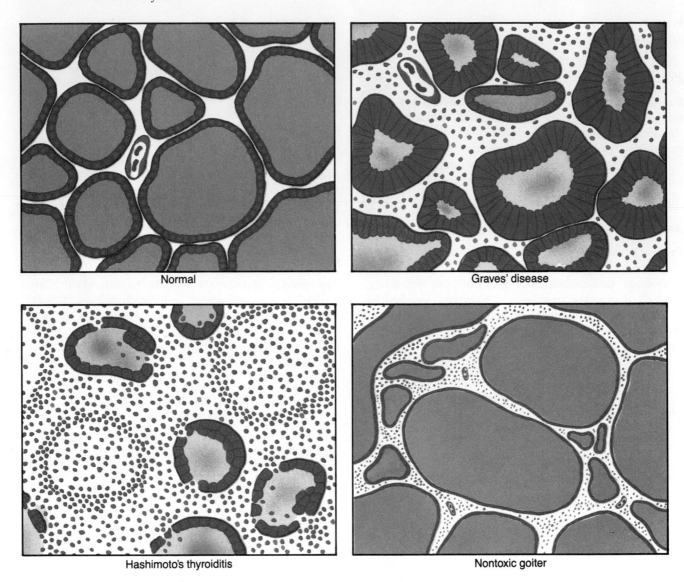

Normal

Graves' disease

Hashimoto's thyroiditis

Nontoxic goiter

Figure 21-6. Thyroid gland histology. Note the differences in size, architectural organization, and tinctorial affinities of the cells. (*A*) Normal. (*B*) Graves' disease. (*C*) Hashimoto's disease. Lymphoid infiltrates are evident. (*D*) Nontoxic goiter.

dren with this disorder, with or without goiter, suffer from the prenatal metabolic and developmental effects of **nearly total maternal thyroid iodine insufficiency.** They have large tongues, defective nervous system development, mental deficiency, neuromuscular abnormalities, and short stature. **Irreversible neurologic damage is their most serious handicap.**

Increased thyroid stimulating hormone levels indicate an inadequate feedback control by thyroid T_3 and T_4. **If the diagnosis of neonatal hypothyroidism is missed and replacement thyroid hormone is not given promptly, by age six months the infant will**

have irreversible mental deficiency. Most American states and all Canadian provinces have established mandatory testing programs to prevent neonatal hypothyroidism.

Adults with unrecognized and neglected recurrent hyperthyroidism eventually develop a nodular goiter. Foci of reddish thyroid hyperplasia may be evident on section of the enlarged gland. **Goitrogenic foods or medications cause a few nodular goiters.** "Cabbage goiter" designates one food fad.

About half of adults over the age of 40 years have one or two thyroid nodules, either palpable or impalpable. These nodules, like those in nodular goiters, are not neoplasms. They are foci of excessive colloid storage, with or without fibrosis. Since the thyroid gland containing such isolated nodules is of normal weight, it is not a goiter. Over 90% of solitary "cold" thyroid masses surgically removed because they may represent benign or malignant tumors prove to be simply the dominant nodule of a nodular thyroid.

HYPERTHYROIDISM

Graves' disease is the classic **primary hyperthyroidism.** The disorder is also termed **diffuse toxic goiter** and **primary thyroid hyperplasia.** In florid cases, Graves' disease is an arresting condition. The patient's eyes bulge, a condition called **exophthalmos,** and there is a symmetrical goiter. Heat intolerance and hypomenorrhea or amenorrhea are the rule. Tachycardia, palpitations, and cardiomegaly are evident (Fig. 21-7). Older patients may present with a clinical picture of congestive heart failure. Women are especially affected, and, as in most thyroid diseases, predominate over men by approximately 6:1.

Excessive thyroid hormonal activity is responsible for the hypermetabolic effects, with the probable exception of the exophthalmos. If there is a sudden,

excessive thyroid hormonal discharge, a potentially lethal **"thyroid storm"** may develop, comprising a crisis of fever, abdominal pain, cardiorespiratory insufficiency, and shock. At another extreme, elderly people develop **apathetic hyperthyroidism,** in which there are no dramatic symptoms or signs.

The thyroid in Graves' disease is symmetrically enlarged, usually weighing 35 to 40 g, and has a thin translucent capsule covering firm, dark red, glandular parenchyma. The tan translucence of the normal cut surface of the thyroid, attributable to stored colloid, is notably absent. Microscopically, colloid within the follicles is depleted or absent. If colloid remains, it is typically scalloped around the edges, as a result of reabsorption into the epithelium prior to hormone secretion. The follicular thyroid epithelium is normally regular and cuboidal, but in hyperthyroid states it becomes tall, cuboidal, or columnar (Fig. 21-8). Typically, intrafollicular folds or pleats of crowded thyroid epithelium are formed.

Less common causes of primary hyperthyroidism are hyperfunctioning thyroid adenoma and carcinoma. The rare hyperplastic or genuine toxic adenoma presents as a clinically "hot" nodule that concentrates a test dose of radioactive technetium and proves to be a benign follicular neoplasm. Similarly, a follicular adenocarcinoma may on occasion be hyperfunctional.

Secondary hyperthyroidism affects some individuals with nodular goiter, a disorder termed **toxic multinodular goiter.** Usually the patient is elderly, the obvious goiter is longstanding, and the clinical presentation is less dramatic than in full-blown Graves' disease.

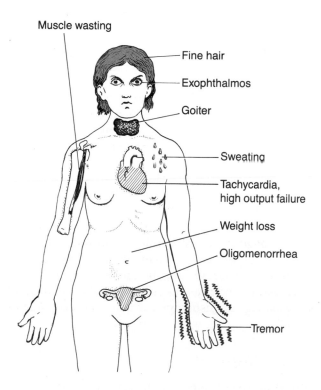

Figure 21-7. The major clinical manifestations of Graves' disease.

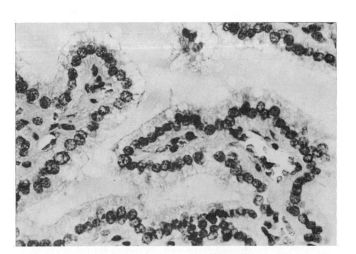

Figure 21-8. Graves' disease. Note the abnormal follicular architecture and the tall epithelial cells with vacuolated cytoplasm. Scalloping of pale-staining colloid is evident (compare with Fig. 21-11*B*).

THYROIDITIS

Thyroiditis may be acute or chronic. **Hashimoto's disease, struma lymphomatosa,** and **lymphadenoid goiter** are mellifluous names for the best known and clinically significant type of chronic thyroiditis. Characteristically, Hashimoto's disease develops in perimenopausal women; the patients present with an enlarged, hard thyroid gland, clinically believed to represent thyroid carcinoma. Grossly, the thyroid gland in Hashimoto's struma is diffusely and uniformly enlarged. The capsule is thin, smooth, and intact, an unlikely feature if the lesion were a thyroid carcinoma or lymphoma of this size. Microscopic scrutiny reveals small, degenerated follicles containing minute droplets of colloid and scattered epithelial remnants of destroyed follicles. The tissue is overrun by sheets of lymphocytes, with many lymph follicles that contain germinal centers. Few plasma cells are present. The remaining thyroid epithelium characteristically has an eosinophilic, often granular, cytoplasm, and is arranged in cords, nests, and follicles. This metaplasia is often called "Hürthle cell" metaplasia (Fig. 21-9).

The pathogenesis of Hashimoto's disease, like that of Graves' disease, is thought to be based on autoimmune phenomena. The most frequently demonstrated antibodies in patients with Hashimoto's disease are those against thyroid stimulating hormone receptors and against thyroid microsomal fractions. Other antithyroid antibodies include those against thyroglobulin, against the nonthyroglobulin protein of the colloid material, and against the membrane of follicular cells.

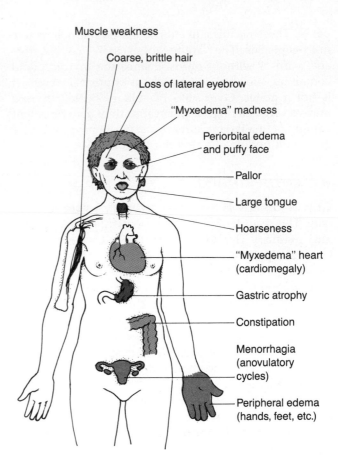

Figure 21-10. The dominant clinical manifestations of hypothyroidism.

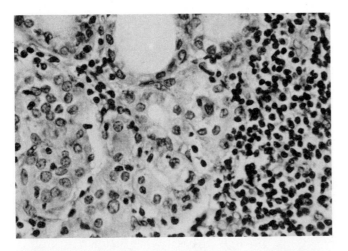

Figure 21-9. Hashimoto's disease. A dense lymphocytic infiltrate is evident on the right, and thyroid follicles can be recognized in the upper portion. The remaining epithelial cells are larger than normal and compactly arranged; their cytoplasm is granular and intensely pink (compare with Fig. 21-6C).

Subacute thyroiditis is also called **granulomatous, pseudotuberculous,** or **de Quervain's thyroiditis.** It typically presents in a woman as a tender, enlarged, firm thyroid gland. Microscopically, many thyroid follicles are disrupted. There are nonspecific epithelioid cell granulomas and usually a prominent giant cell reaction to released colloid. This pattern should not be confused with that of tuberculosis, which sometimes affects the thyroid.

Riedel's struma is a rare form of chronic thyroiditis. It is also called ligneous thyroiditis, meaning "hard as wood." At surgery a dense white scar involves part of the gland, the thyroid capsule, and the adjacent connective tissues and muscles. The original thyroid gland may be difficult to distinguish grossly, and even microscopically.

HYPOTHYROIDISM

Hypothyroidism refers to a decrease in thyroid function. Degeneration of the gland, often following chronic thyroiditis, is a common cause. The most extreme forms of thyroid atrophy and degeneration lead to **myxedema,** a term that refers to hard edema of subcutaneous tissue. Patients who suffer from myxedema are sluggish, irritable, and display dry skin, loss of lateral eyebrow hairs, pasty swollen faces, an enlarged tongue, intolerance to cold, and excessive (anovulatory) menstrual bleeding in premenopausal women (Fig. 21-10).

The thyroid gland in myxedema may weigh as little as 6 g and may consist largely of connective tissue and blood vessels. Microscopically, only isolated minute thyroid follicles with colloid droplets remain in a fibrofatty stroma. Pituitary insufficiency may cause secondary hypothyroidism. Following the radioiodine treatment of Graves' disease, not surprisingly, hypothyroidism is noted in half or more of the patients.

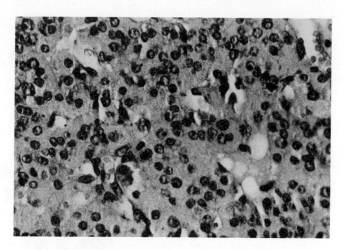

Figure 21-12. Hürthle cell adenoma of the thyroid. Note the solid architecture; no follicles are recognized. The cytoplasm is granular and intensely pink.

THYROID TUMORS

THYROID ADENOMA

Follicular Adenoma

Follicular adenoma is the prototypical endocrine adenoma. Recall that only 10% or less of clinical solitary thyroid nodules prove to be genuine adenomas. The distinction is made because a true adenoma is a benign clonal neoplasm, with small but clear cancerous potential, while a thyroid nodule is not neoplastic.

The typical follicular adenoma ordinarily presents as a solitary "cold" thyroid nodule—that is, one that does not take up radioiodine. When removed it is entirely encapsulated, and on transection the compressed tissue everts. The adenoma is tan, usually 2 to 3 cm in diameter and may have a central scar or degenerative cysts. The follicles are small and uniform, and show limited colloid storage (Fig. 21-11). Less commonly one sees solid cords of embryonal-type epithelium, admixed with follicles of small or ordinary size; an adenoma may also comprise variable proportions of oncocytes or Hürthle cells—a Hürthle cell adenoma (Fig. 21-12). Current classifications lump all these varieties under the designation of follicular thyroid adenoma.

Papillary Adenoma

Papillary thyroid adenoma is morphologically unusual as well as uncommon. There is a fibrous shell around a cystic tumor, which is filled with dark red fluid. The cyst lining has small, granular, gray, papillary projections covered by uniform, cuboidal, follicular-type epithelium, with fibrovascular cores. **Complete encapsulation is the exception, and hence most or all papillary adenomas may in fact be papillary carcinomas.** Removal, nonetheless, is curative.

Atypical Adenoma

Atypical adenoma refers to a solid encapsulated growth of closely packed, uniform spindle cells, which are unlike ordinary thyroid follicular epithelium. It is not precancerous.

THYROID CARCINOMA

Papillary Carcinoma

Papillary carcinoma is the most common thyroid cancer, and is not unusual in the young. It may form a visible and palpable thyroid nodule, or first become

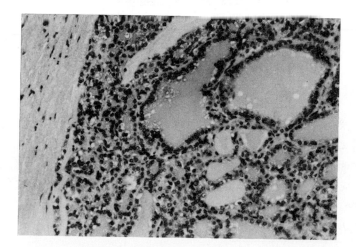

Figure 21-11. Follicular adenoma of the thyroid. A dense capsule is evident on the left. The size and shape of the follicles and solid areas are notably irregular.

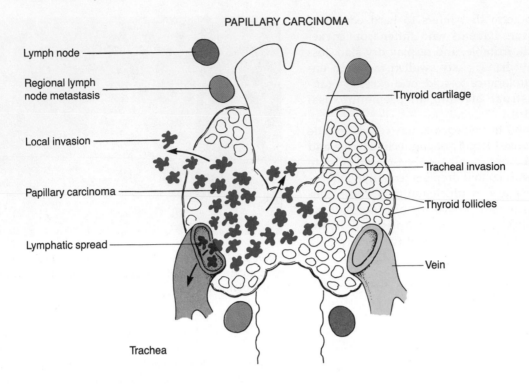

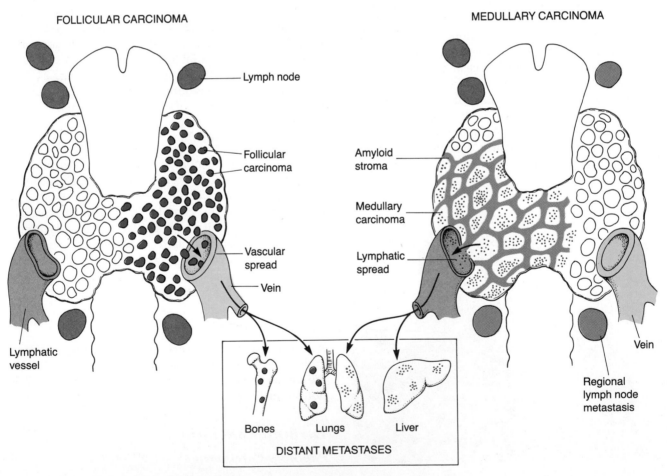

Figure 21-13. Principal gross characteristics and patterns of growth and metastases of papillary, follicular, and medullary carcinomas of the thyroid gland.

evident as a lymph node metastasis in the lateral neck (Fig. 21-13). **If a papillary tumor is incompletely encapsulated and has spread into the adjacent thyroid tissue, or if it is multifocal without a dominant mass, it is almost certainly carcinoma.** Papillary thyroid carcinoma is recognized by (1) epithelium piled up on the surfaces of papillae, (2) empty, ground glass, "Orphan Annie eye" nuclei, and (3) laminated masses of calcareous material (so-called "psammoma bodies") in half of the cases (Fig. 21-14).

Papillary thyroid carcinoma typically invades lymphatics and spreads to the regional cervical lymph nodes. Sometimes the primary carcinoma is small, about 2 mm, and the involved lymph nodes are large. In these different clinical presentations, papillary thyroid carcinoma ordinarily grows sluggishly. With local surgical excision alone, the 5-year survival is now over 90%, and the 10-year survival rate is over 85%.

Therapeutic irradiation to the face, neck, and upper chest regions was given several decades ago, often to infants and children, for various benign conditions. These patients subsequently displayed a higher than usual incidence of papillary thyroid carcinomas.

Follicular Carcinoma

Follicular thyroid carcinoma is the prototype of the moderately differentiated, grossly identifiable carcinoma. It forms a hard thyroid mass that, on section, appears as a granular, pale gray-white, stellate invasive tissue, resembling many other visceral carcinomas. The neoplastic follicles are formed by cells with abnormally enlarged, crowded, and misshapen nuclei. These follicles closely abut, with scanty intervening stroma; the

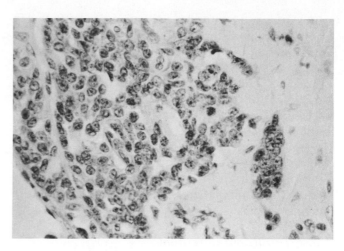

Figure 21-15. Medullary thyroid carcinoma. A solid arrangement of rather small cells (compare with Fig. 21-14, at identical magnification) is surrounded by solid stroma containing abundant amyloid.

tumor invades the adjacent thyroid tissue, the thyroid gland capsule, and blood vessels.

Follicular thyroid carcinoma typically spreads via the bloodstream and metastasizes to the lungs and bones (see Fig. 21-13). The prognosis is less favorable than that for papillary carcinoma. After the extirpation of follicular carcinoma about 40% have a five-year survival without disease.

Medullary Carcinoma

Medullary thyroid carcinoma is different from all other thyroid carcinomas because of its cellular differentiation, its endocrine activities, and its morphologic appearance. The tumor forms bulky, soft, gray masses, sometimes bilaterally. Despite its ominous gross and microscopic appearance, it ordinarily grows slowly. The 5-year survival rate, usually with residual tumor present, is about 40%. It readily metastasizes via lymphatic channels to regional lymph nodes, but may also invade blood vessels and metastasize to the liver, lungs, and bones (see Fig. 21-13).

Medullary carcinoma does not resemble normal thyroid tissue, for it is composed of pale, cuboidal, and often spindle-shaped cells. In sections stained with hematoxylin and eosin the compact masses of tumor cells are surrounded by abundant, uniformly pink or violet stroma that represents amyloid (Fig. 21-15). Because of the characteristic stromal change, the diagnostic term often employed is "medullary carcinoma with amyloid stroma."

Immunohistochemical studies of medullary carcinoma show not only calcitonin, but also serotonin, so-

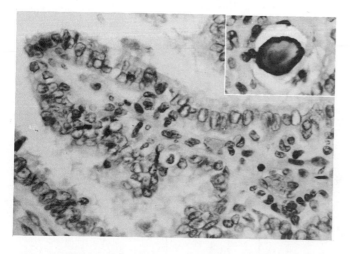

Figure 21-14. Papillary carcinoma of the thyroid. A papilla projects toward the upper left, and vesicular "Orphan Annie" nuclei are evident. (*Inset*) Typical psammoma body.

matostatin, and bombesin, a situation similar to that in normal C-cells. Ectopic hormones such as ACTH are sometimes present. Hence medullary thyroid carcinoma may cause the carcinoid syndrome or Cushing's syndrome. **These characteristics mark C-cells as a component of the dispersed neuroendocrine system, and medullary thyroid carcinoma as a neuroendocrine tumor.**

Familial medullary thyroid carcinoma is part of a genetic condition associated with pheochromocytoma, often bilateral, and parathyroid hyperplasia or adenoma. This combination is designated as multiple endocrine neoplasia (MEN) type IIa.

Undifferentiated Carcinoma

Undifferentiated thyroid carcinomas are usually clinically obvious and rapidly lethal. The fast growing, hard neck mass is composed of dense, granular grayish tissue. These aggressive cancers typically occur in older women; they often develop in a preexistent goiter, with or without associated, better-differentiated carcinomas.

Microscopically, the best known pattern is a bizarre cellular proliferation of spindle and giant cells, with polyploid nuclei, many mitoses, tumor necrosis, and stromal fibrosis. Such lesions are termed spindle and giant cell thyroid carcinomas. Less common types of undifferentiated thyroid carcinoma are small cell anaplastic carcinoma, which vaguely resembles a breast carcinoma, and small cell diffuse carcinoma.

As mentioned above, some cases of undifferentiated thyroid carcinoma have a long history, beginning with goiters in youth. Others have preceding papillary or follicular carcinoma, and terminate 20 or more years later with a spindle and giant cell thyroid carcinoma.

THYROID LYMPHOMA

Malignant lymphomas of the thyroid, though uncommon, appear to be increasing in frequency. They usually are of the large cell or mixed large cell and lymphocytic types.

PARATHYROID GLANDS

The parathyroid glands are not under anterior pituitary control, but are most directly influenced by circulating ionized calcium and magnesium concentrations.

HYPOPARATHYROIDISM

Hypoparathyroidism most often occurs after thyroidectomy, when three or four glands are either removed or have their vasculature damaged. The result is a prompt fall in the blood calcium level, with clinical tetany. Hypoparathyroidism less commonly is an infantile condition, due either to gland agenesis or congenital hypoplasia, and is characterized by tetany or convulsions and a failure to thrive.

Pseudohypoparathyroidism designates a group of conditions that exhibit target organ resistance or insensitivity to parathyroid hormone (PTH). The blood calcium level is low; phosphate levels and alkaline phosphatase activity are high. Some patients display short metacarpals or metatarsals, short stature, cataracts, subcutaneous calcifications, or mental deficiency—the so-called **Albright hereditary osteodystrophy somatotype.** Type I pseudohypoparathyroidism patients are resistant not only to PTH, but also to thyrotropin (TSH), glucagon, and the gonadotropins, follicle stimulating hormone and luteinizing hormone. In type II pseudohypoparathyroidism, after PTH is given the serum calcium does not rise, and renal phosphate reabsorption remains excessive.

HYPERPARATHYROIDISM

Hyperparathyroidism (i.e., parathyroid hyperfunction) most often is due to a parathyroid adenoma that secretes PTH. In its originally recognized, most florid state, hyperparathyroidism is clinically characterized by rubbery, deformed long bones, attributable to excessive calcium reabsorption. The bone lesions are called either brown tumors, because the fibrous tissue

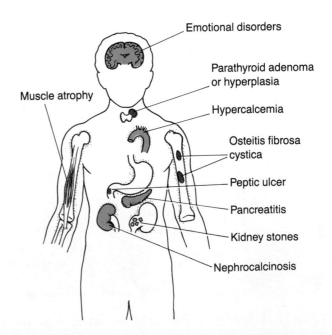

Figure 21-16. The major clinical features of hyperparathyroidism.

is pigmented by hemosiderin, or osteitis fibrosa cystica, a term that describes the radiologic appearance. The blood calcium level is elevated, because calcium is mobilized from bones. Deposition of calcium in the kidneys can result in kidney stones, secondary renal infections, and even renal failure.(Fig. 21-16).

PARATHYROID ADENOMA

Primary hyperparathyroidism is due to a single parathyroid adenoma in about 80% of cases, two adenomas in 5%, and diffuse parathyroid hyperplasia in 15%. Functioning parathyroid carcinoma may account for 1% or 2%. The size and weight of the responsible parathyroid adenoma are correlated with the severity of the hypercalcemia.

Hyperparathyroid crisis is a life-threatening emergency caused by an unrecognized or neglected, usually rather large, parathyroid adenoma. Palpation of the neck may set off the crisis. The blood calcium level rises above 15 mg/dl, renal failure follows, and about 60% of the patients die.

Surgical neck exploration, with removal of the abnormal parathyroid(s), is the curative procedure for primary hyperparathyroidism. An elongated, typically mustard-colored, thinly encapsulated soft mass is removed. Microscopic examination reveals a solid parathyroid cell growth, partly surrounded by a rim of unaltered parathyroid gland, half of which is adipose tissue. The most common diagnosis is parathyroid chief cell adenoma (Fig. 21-17).

PARATHYROID HYPERPLASIA

Primary parathyroid hyperplasia, as already noted, is a less common cause of primary hyperparathyroidism. Because of claims that parathyroid adenomas represent the dominant nodule of a general parathyroid hyperplasia, some surgeons, after removing an adenoma, will biopsy one additional parathyroid gland to prove it is histologically normal. Primary parathyroid hyperplasia involves all four glands. The glands are grossly enlarged and tan, and are composed of nearly solid chief cell parenchyma, with little residual adipose tissue.

Secondary parathyroid hyperplasia is commonplace at autopsy. It is encountered in patients with renal insufficiency. The inadequate renal conservation of calcium lowers blood calcium levels and causes the parathyroids to increase their PTH secretion, a sequence that results in increasing calcium resorption from bones.

The hyperplastic parathyroids are enlarged two-fold or more, and parathyroid cells replace part or most of the adipose tissue normally present. Chief, transitional, or water-clear cells may predominate, the hypersecretion of PTH increasing in that order.

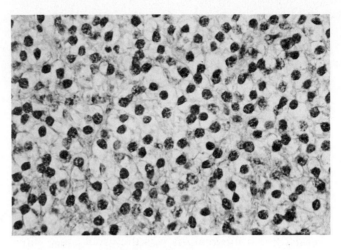

Figure 21-17. Parathyroid adenoma. Solidly arranged epithelial cells with pale cytoplasm are evident.

A diagrammatic outline of the various forms of primary and secondary hyperparathyroidism is presented in Figure 21-18.

PARATHYROID CARCINOMA

Parathyroid carcinoma is very uncommon. Some cases are nonfunctional. A neck mass that is difficult to distinguish from a clear cell or small cell thyroid carcinoma possesses ultrastructural features of parathyroid cells. In parathyroid carcinoma, with or without previous surgery, multiple metastases in the lungs, soft tissues, and bones may accompany the clinical onset or a recurrence of hyperparathyroidism.

Microscopically, some parathyroid carcinomas are cytologically overtly malignant neoplasms, with lymphatic and blood vessel invasion. Others have a bland growth pattern and monotonous cellularity. The prognosis is generally poor.

ADRENAL CORTEX

CONGENITAL ANOMALIES

Congenital adrenal hyperplasia comprises important inborn functional deficiencies of adrenocortical steroidogenesis. One of five enzymes required for the formation of intermediate steroids from cholesterol is lacking or defective.

The absence of 21-hydroxylase is the most common. No step in cortisol synthesis beyond 17-α-hydroxyprogesterone is completed. **The affected infants or children are susceptible to lethal shock after trivial trauma or respiratory infections.** Excessive androgenic steroid synthesis is characteristic. At birth affected females have external genitalia that resemble a penis and scrotum, owing to clitoral and labial hypertrophy. Congenital adrenal hyperplasia is the most common cause of female pseudohermaphroditism, in which a genetic female appears male at birth, and may be so reared.

ADRENOCORTICAL INSUFFICIENCY

Chronic adrenocortical insufficiency has the classical name **Addison's disease.** In times past, destructive bilateral adrenal tuberculosis was the usual cause. Now autoimmune destruction of the adrenal cortex is the most common cause, infiltrates of lymphocytes and macrophages populating the residual connective tissue. Patients with Addison's disease experience muscle weakness, asthenia, low blood pressure, low serum sodium, and a tendency to suffer shock after minor infections or injuries. Their skin and mucous membranes are pigmented brown.

Systemic viral infections, especially herpesvirus or cytomegalovirus, tend to damage the adrenals, and

their viral inclusion bodies are evident in cortical cell nuclei. Numerous other infections and toxic states produce foci of adrenocortical necrosis. Such conditions rarely result in adrenocortical insufficiency.

Adrenocortical atrophy is a result of long continued therapy with adrenocortical steroids. The adrenal glands shrink from the normal weight of 6 g each to 3 g or less. Should the corticosteroid therapy be abruptly discontinued, a temporary addisonian state may develop.

In children and some adults the most **acute adrenocortical destruction** is known as the **Waterhouse-Friderichsen syndrome.** This often lethal condition is characterized by sudden shock, associated with massive bilateral adrenal hemorrhage and necrosis. Most commonly, meningococcal septicemia is responsible, but gram-positive cocci may be found. It probably is a form of endotoxic shock reaction analogous to the Shwartzman phenomenon.

In chronic illness the steroids are secreted as fast as they are formed, and there is little intracellular lipid storage. Hence, bright-yellow, lipid-rich adrenocortical tissue is an indicator of sudden death without preexisting chronic disease. Conversely, autopsies performed on chronically ill patients yield adrenal glands that are

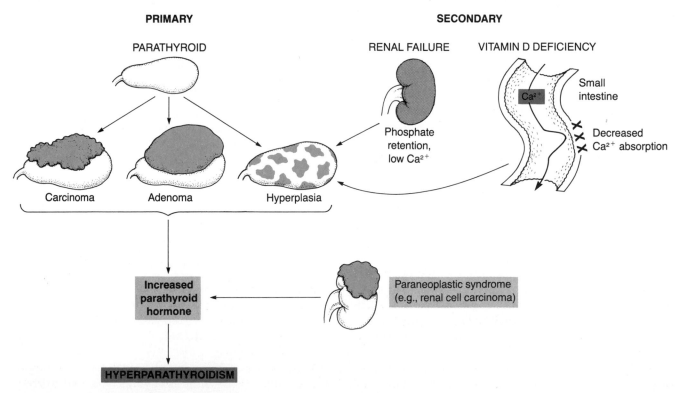

Figure 21-18. Major pathogenetic pathways leading to clinical primary and secondary hyperparathyroidism.

less yellow than their normal counterparts; these glands are said to be "lipid depleted."

ADRENOCORTICAL HYPERFUNCTION

Hyperfunction, hypertrophy, and hyperplasia of the adrenal cortex follow appropriate stimulation. The zona glomerulosa, site of aldosterone synthesis, is normally discontinuous in humans. If chronically stimulated, as by the salt and water imbalance associated with liver cirrhosis and ascites, the cells form a continuous subcapsular zone. This is designated as **adrenocortical hyperplasia of secondary hyperaldosteronism.**

Hypertrophy and hyperplasia of the zona fasciculata constitute the major adrenal reactions to chronic illness. The zona fasciculata, which contains the cells that secrete cortisol, comprises about 75% of the gland mass, so that its changes are often evident both grossly and microscopically. The glands reach weights of 10 to 12 g each, compared to the normal 6 g.

Cells of the zona reticularis, which produce sex steroids, are enlarged and their numbers increased in **adrenal virilism.** This uncommon condition affects some perimenopausal women, who develop male hair patterns in the facial, limb, chest, and pubic areas.

Specific adrenocortical hyperfunctional states also may involve any one or two of the three cortical zones. The most important of these hyperfunctional states is **Cushing's syndrome.** These patients, unlike those with Cushing's disease, do not have a definable pituitary adenoma. However, many have irregular aggregates of corticotropin-producing cells called pituitary microadenomas. "Pituitary Cushing's syndrome" accounts for two-thirds of the cases.

When excess ACTH is produced by an extra-pituitary neoplasm, the condition is termed **ectopic Cushing's, or ectopic ACTH syndrome.** The tumors most frequently implicated are neuroendocrine carcinomas of the lung, thymus, and pancreatic islets. The direct hormonal effects of Cushing's syndrome are due to hypercortisolism; thus Cushing's syndrome can also be based on functional adenomas, carcinomas, or unilateral hyperplasia of the adrenal cortex (Fig. 21-19).

Patients with Cushing's syndrome typically present with a rounded, moon-shaped face, obesity around the shoulder girdle (called a buffalo-hump), thin skin that may stretch and show red striae over the abdomen, osteoporosis, plethoric features reflecting erythrocythemia, a diabetic type of glucose tolerance test, and psychological disturbances (see Fig. 21-5). These changes are common side effects of prolonged treatment with large doses of corticosteroids. Indeed, **iatro-genic Cushing's syndrome is, by far, the most common variety seen today.**

Typically, the adrenal glands in spontaneous Cushing's syndrome are both enlarged to 8 to 12 g and display hyperplasia of the zona fasciculata. Three-quarters of cases of spontaneous Cushing's syndrome are due to this type of bilateral adrenocortical hyperplasia, which in turn, may be either primary or secondary to pituitary lesions.

Some patients with Cushing's syndrome are partly virilized women or, rarely, feminized men. The bilateral adrenocortical hyperplasia in such individuals involves the zona reticularis as well as the fasciculata.

NEOPLASMS

ADRENOCORTICAL ADENOMAS

Adrenocortical adenoma is a frequent incidental finding at autopsy. The adenoma is a bright yellow, spheroidal mass of some 2 cm in diameter, compressing the adjacent uninvolved adrenal gland and sometimes possessing a partial fibrous capsule. Microscopically, the enlarged adenoma cells, which have a lipid-rich cytoplasm, are arranged in nodules and cords (Fig. 21-20). Since there is no overt endocrine disease, the adenoma is considered nonfunctional.

Cushing's syndrome due to adrenal adenoma is clinically indistinguishable from that due to bilateral hyperplasia of the zona fasciculata. Pathologically, the nontumorous adrenal cortices are narrowed, and their cells are atrophic, because the adenoma overproduces cortisol-type steroids, which in turn, inhibit pituitary ACTH secretion.

Aldosteronoma is functionally the most notable type of adrenocortical adenoma. It is usually small, 0.9 to 2.0 cm in size. The sectioned aldosteronoma is orange and histologically resembles other adrenocortical adenomas. **Conn's syndrome,** characterized by **hypertension, low plasma potassium, high sodium, alkalosis, and edema,** is relieved by the removal of an aldosteronoma. Curiously, typical primary hyperaldosteronism in Conn's syndrome is closely imitated by pseudoprimary aldosteronism, a condition in which no adrenal adenoma is found.

ADRENAL CARCINOMA

Adrenal carcinomas are usually first recognized as upper abdominal masses. **At least half are clinically nonfunctional.** The diagnostic criteria of adrenocortical carcinoma include large tumor size, capsular and vascular tumor invasion, hemorrhage and necrosis within the mass, and occasional local or distant metas-

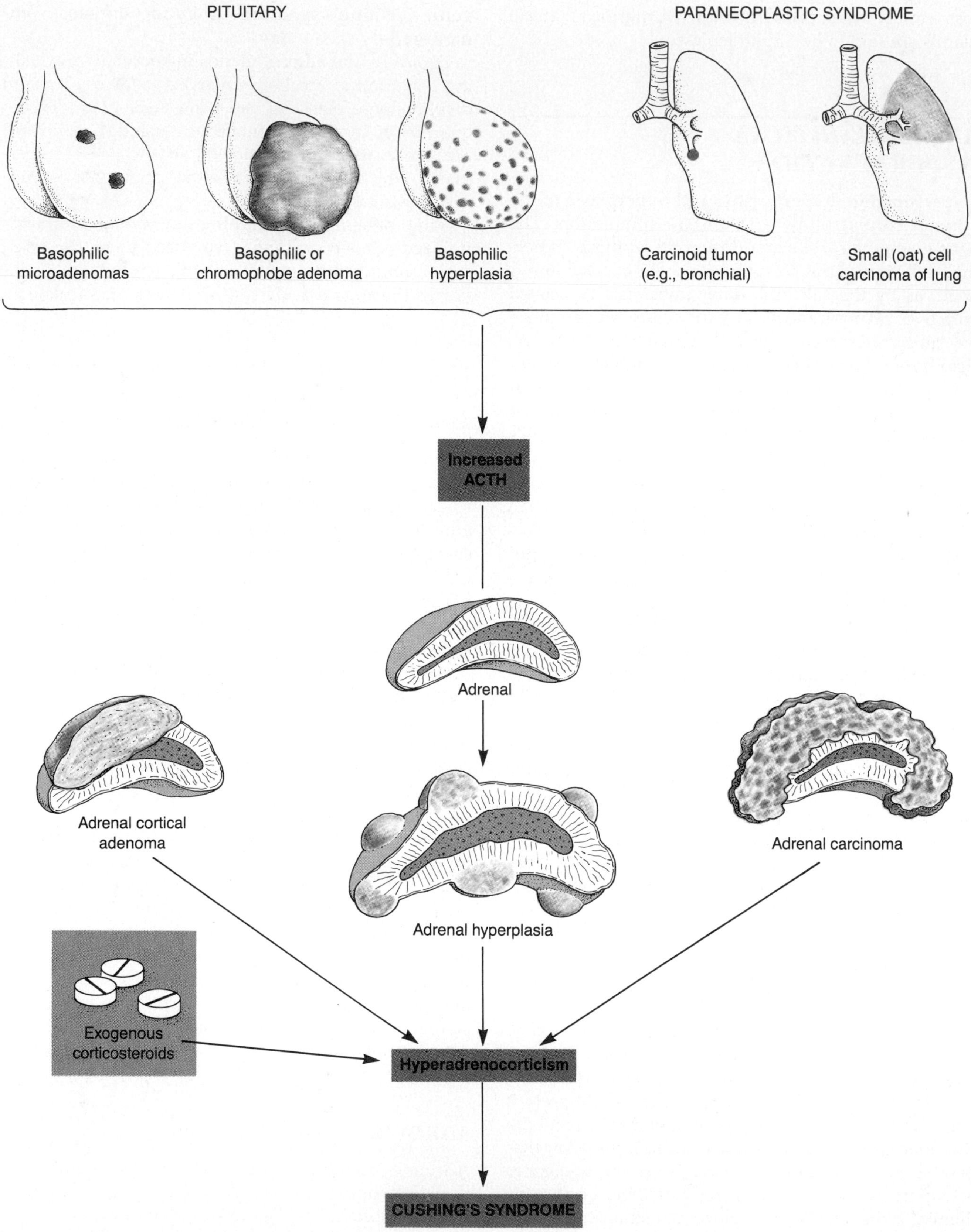

Figure 21-19. The pathogenetic pathways of Cushing's syndrome.

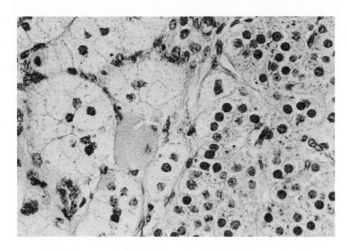

Figure 21-20. Adrenal cortical adenoma without clinical manifestations. Small, normal cortical cells are evident on the right, and notably larger adenoma cells can be seen on the left.

tases. Microscopically, cytologic atypicality and abundant mitoses are common.

In the case of functional tumors, Cushing's syndrome, virilization, feminization, and hyperaldosteronism occur in decreasing order of frequency.

METASTATIC CANCER

Metastatic cancer to the adrenal glands commonly originates from carcinomas of the lung or breast or from malignant melanoma. The glands may be unilaterally or bilaterally massively enlarged and largely replaced by carcinoma.

ADRENAL MEDULLA AND PARAGANGLIA

NEOPLASMS

PHEOCHROMOCYTOMA

Pheochromocytoma, also referred to as a type of chromaffin paraganglioma, is the most important neoplasm of the adrenal medulla in adults and older children. "Chromaffin" refers to the dark brown color that typically develops when fresh pheochromocytoma tissue is dipped in chromate solutions. The majority of pheochromocytomas produce norepinephrine as well as epinephrine.

Clinical presentations of pheochromocytoma are of four types:

1. Episodic hypertension
2. Persistent hypertension
3. Multiple endocrine neoplasia, types IIa and IIb
4. Silent asymptomatic pheochromocytoma

Multiple endocrine neoplasia (MEN) type IIa is a familial syndrome, with unilateral or bilateral adrenal tumors, thyroid medullary carcinoma, and parathyroid hyperplasia or adenoma (Fig. 21-21). In MEN type IIb, there are mucosal neuromas, particularly affecting the lips and tongue.

A pheochromocytoma may be silent and then first manifest as extreme or lethal hypertension during an unrelated surgical procedure. A sudden massive infusion of epinephrine and norepinephrine is responsible. Pheochromocytoma is diagnosed by finding increased urinary levels of catecholamine metabolites, particularly vanillyl-mandelic acid (VMA).

Most pheochromocytomas are encapsulated, spongy, reddish masses, with prominent central scars and enlarged vascular spaces. The tumor cells are of variable size and shape, forming twisted cords or rounded clusters, with cytoplasmic basophilic granules. The nuclei are large and irregular (Fig. 21-22). **Only a few pheochromocytomas are malignant,** as defined by the development of metastases. In this neoplasm **histologic atypicality is not an accurate indicator of biologic behavior.**

The cytoplasmic granules represent, for the most part, packaged catecholamines. Pheochromocytomas may also produce and store other peptide hormones, including calcitonin, bombesin, vasoactive intestinal peptide (VIP) and ACTH, which occasionally are associated with clinical syndromes.

NEUROBLASTOMA

Neuroblastoma is principally a neoplasm of children. Approximately two-thirds of neuroblastomas are found in children under 5 years of age, but they may be encountered in young adults. They may occasionally be congenital. The overwhelming majority of neuroblastomas occur sporadically. There have been a few reports of increased incidence of neuroblastomas in families.

The adrenal medulla is the most frequent site of origin of neuroblastomas. However, they may develop anywhere in the retroperitoneal space, the posterior mediastinum, and the neck, and within or around the brain.

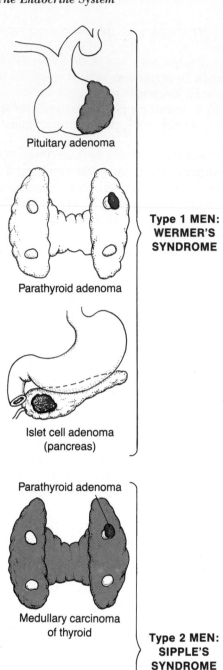

Pituitary adenoma

Parathyroid adenoma

Type 1 MEN: WERMER'S SYNDROME

Islet cell adenoma (pancreas)

Parathyroid adenoma

Medullary carcinoma of thyroid

Type 2 MEN: SIPPLE'S SYNDROME

Pheochromocytoma

Figure 21-21. The major forms of multiple endocrine neoplasia (MEN) syndromes.

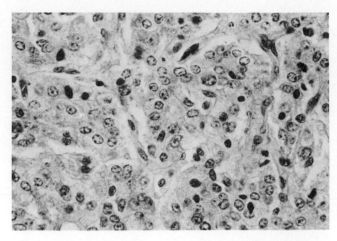

Figure 21-22. Adrenal pheochromocytoma with the classic syndrome of paroxysmal hypertension. The tumor cells are arranged in solid clusters, and mild pleomorphism is evident.

Neuroblastomas range from minute, barely discernible nodules to masses readily palpable through the abdominal wall. They are round, irregularly lobulated, soft, friable masses that may weigh 150 g or more. The cut surface ranges from gray to dark red and hemorrhagic.

The cells are small, but slightly larger than lymphocytes. Neuroblastoma cells range from round to fusiform; their nuclei are very dark and the cytoplasm is scanty. Mitoses are frequent. The neoplastic cells are arranged in ill-defined sheets that show areas of necrosis. The classic microscopic rosettes are defined by a rim of dark tumor cells in a circumferential arrangement around a central pale circle (Fig. 21-23).

Neuroblastomas infiltrate surrounding structures and metastasize to regional lymph nodes, liver, lungs, bones, and other sites. Occasionally metastases may be found earlier than the primary tumor.

Neuroblastomas secrete variable amounts of dopamine and catecholamines. **The overwhelming majority of patients with neuroblastoma excrete catecholamines and some of their metabolites in the urine.** Among the latter VMA and homovanillic acid are significant aids in the diagnosis and in monitoring the response to therapy. Rare but well-documented cases of total spontaneous regression of neuroblastomas occur. Maturation of neuroblastomas to ganglioneuroma has been reported "spontaneously" and also following various forms of therapy.

The majority of neuroblastomas discovered over the age of 1 year already have demonstrable metastases at the time of the initial diagnosis. Combined forms of therapy have dramatically improved the prognosis.

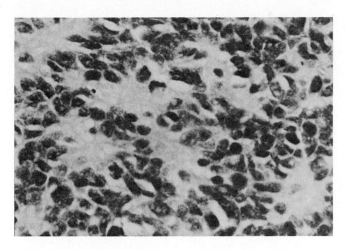

Figure 21-23. Neuroblastoma of the adrenal gland. Round to slightly spindle-shaped cells define irregular, round spaces with faintly fibrillar contents (rosettes).

GANGLIONEUROMAS

Ganglioneuromas appear grossly as well-encapsulated tumors, with myxoid, glistening, cut surfaces. Microscopically, they show differentiated, mature ganglion cells, associated with scanty spindle cells in abundant stroma. The cytoplasmic processes of the ganglion cells contain neurosecretory granules.

There are close embryogenetic, structural, and functional relationships among the group of neoplasms comprising neuroblastomas, ganglioneuromas, pheochromocytomas, and paragangliomas of all sites. All are regarded as neural crest neoplasms, with close anatomic relations to blood vessels.

THYMUS

AGENESIS AND HYPOPLASIA

Agenesis or congenital hypoplasia of the thymus may be found in the newborn or in young infants, and is associated with combined immunodeficiency disorders, telangiectatic ataxia, reticular dysgenesis, Nezelof's syndrome, or DiGeorge's syndrome, in which the thymus disorder is accompanied by parathyroid agenesis. In all these instances the thymus may be "represented" by scattered groups of lymphocytes in fibrous tissue. **With advancing age, the thymus normally atrophies and is progressively replaced by fibroadipose tissue.**

HYPERPLASIA

The most reliable criterion of thymic hyperplasia is the presence of lymphoid follicular structures. Thymic follicular hyperplasia may be found in association with a spectrum of chronic inflammatory and immunologic disorders, with myasthenia gravis, and in numerous other diseases in which autoimmunity plays a role.

TUMORS

The term **thymoma** is currently applied to tumors of the thymus in which the thymic epithelial cells are neoplastic. Whether scarce or prominent, the lymphocytic elements are not considered neoplastic.

The vast majority of thymomas (80% to 95%) are clinically benign. Benign thymomas are irregularly shaped masses that range from a few centimeters to 15 cm or more in major diameter. They are encapsulated, firm, and gray to yellow. Fibrous tissue septa divide the tumors into lobules. The epithelial cells of thymomas may be obvious or may be obscured by the dominating non-neoplastic lymphocytes. In such cases, ultrastructural or immunohistochemical studies for cytokeratin or other epithelial markers will uncover the epithelial cells (Fig. 21-24). The most characteristic microscopic pattern is one of irregular sheets of epithelial cells. Squamous features are frequent. The dominant lym-

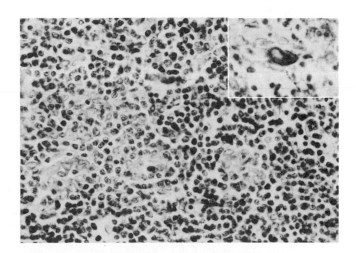

Figure 21-24. Thymoma. The picture is dominated by small, dark-staining lymphocytes. However, larger and paler epithelial cells represent the neoplasm. The inset (*upper right*) shows one of these epithelial cells immunostained with antibody against keratin.

phoid component of occasional thymomas may result in an erroneous diagnosis of lymphoma.

Malignant thymomas are carcinomas of the thymus. They are diagnosed by marked cellular and nuclear atypism and a brisk mitotic activity of the neoplastic epithelial cells. More often than not, however, the diagnosis is based on macroscopic criteria, particularly invasion of the surrounding structure, including the lung, pericardium, and large vessels. Microscopic penetration of the capsule, and lymphatic and vascular invasion, is important.

Neuroendocrine tumors of the thymus may be carcinoids (benign) or carcinomas (malignant). Thymic carcinoids are morphologically similar to those occurring in the bronchi and other sites, showing well-defined cellular cords, nests, and ribbons separated by delicate fibrovascular septa. Neurosecretory granules are common. Neuroendocrine carcinomas of the thymus are composed of intermediate-sized or small oat cells.

Miscellaneous tumors in the thymus or anterior mediastinum include seminomas or dysgerminomas, choriocarcinomas, and teratomas. Primary thymic lymphomas occur, as does Hodgkin's disease, which is often of the nodular sclerosing type.

PINEAL GLAND

NEOPLASMS

Tumors of the pineal gland are rare, and represent less than 1% of brain tumors. The most frequent neoplasms are apparently not derived from pineal parenchymal cells or their precursors, but from germ cells. Germinomas, or dysgerminomas, account for about 60% of pineal tumors. They are thought to be equivalent to testicular seminomas, ovarian dysgerminomas, and their counterparts in other sites.

Pinealomas presumably arise from the pinealocyte. These rare tumors are of two types, pineoblastomas and pineocytomas. **Pineoblastomas** occur in the young. **Pineocytomas** represent the better-differentiated counterpart of the pineoblastomas. They tend to be clinically less aggressive; they impinge upon surrounding tissues but do not invade them. Pineocytomas often show a dual neuronal and glial differentiation, somewhat reminiscent of primitive neural neoplasms in other sites.

Destruction of the pineal, neoplastic or otherwise, in children is frequently associated with precocious puberty.

ECTOPIC HORMONES

Occasional neoplasms developing in "nonendocrine" organs are associated with significant endocrine syndromes. According to the traditional concept, a carcinoma of the lung that produced ACTH and was associated with Cushing's syndrome was regarded as a typical example of ectopic hormone production, because the tumor developed in an organ presumed to be nonendocrine. The development of the concept of a dispersed neuroendocrine system has seriously challenged older notions. We now know that the bronchi include a significant population of solitary neuroendocrine cells and aggregates, termed neuroepithelial bodies. Cells that produce serotonin, bombesin, calcitonin, and leucine enkephalin are found in normal bronchial epithelium. Therefore, the demonstration of elevated levels of calcitonin in association with a neuroendocrine carcinoma of the lung may no longer be regarded as an "ectopic" marker. On the other hand, we may still regard ACTH production by a small cell neuroendocrine lung carcinoma as ectopic. Whereas the lung may be rightly viewed as an endocrine organ, ACTH production is currently not regarded as indigenous to the normal lung. The same may be said when islet cell neoplasms produce hormonal material such as gastrin or vasoactive intestinal peptide (VIP).

22

DIABETES

JOHN E. CRAIGHEAD

Type I Diabetes Mellitus

Type II Diabetes Mellitus

Complications of Diabetes

Diabetes has been defined as "a **genetically determined** disorder of carbohydrate metabolism...with **specific microvascular complications** and **accelerated atherogenesis.**" Functionally it has been termed "a **complex metabolic derangement,** characterized by either **relative** or **absolute insulin deficiency.**"

The two most common types of diabetes are referred to simply as type I and type II diabetes. Although type I diabetes generally occurs in children and teenagers, it occasionally develops in adults. Type II also is sometimes seen in the young, but most cases appear during the later decades of life. Type I diabetes is uncommon compared to type II; the latter affects 5 to 10 million Americans (Fig. 22-1). There are also rare clinical syndromes that cause either frank hyperglycemia or abnormal glucose metabolism.

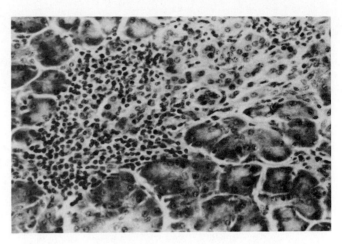

Figure 22-2. Type I diabetes. Mononuclear inflammatory cells infiltrate in and around an islet of Langerhans. Such inflammation is found in the pancreas of many type I diabetics at the time of diagnosis.

TYPE I DIABETES MELLITUS

Before insulin became commercially available, type I diabetes usually was fatal. **In this form of the disease, the islets of Langerhans contain few if any functional beta cells, and insulin secretion is either substantially reduced or nonexistent.** As a result, body fat is metabolized as a source of energy, and ketone bodies (acetoacetic acid and β-hydroxybutyric acid) are released into the blood. Systemic metabolic acidosis

develops as a result. Hyperglycemia and glucosuria produce fluid and electrolyte imbalances that can ultimately lead to coma and death. Patients with type I diabetes usually experience an increase in urine output (polyuria) caused by glucosuria and the resulting thirst (polydipsia). Many patients have an insatiable appetite (polyphagia), but nonetheless lose weight because of defective carbohydrate metabolism and wasted calories. Often the appearance of diabetes coincides with the metabolic stresses of an acute illness, such as an infection.

Fewer than 20% of type I diabetics have a parent or sibling with the disease. Many investigators argue that inheritance of this form of diabetes is autosomal recessive with variable penetrance, but this claim is not universally accepted. It now appears that the gene or genes influencing the development of diabetes are located close to the DR locus. **Environmental factors seem to contribute to the causation of the disease, possibly superimposed on a heritable predisposition.**

The concept of an **autoimmune pathogenesis** is appealing, because type I diabetics who die shortly after the onset of disease display an infiltrate of mononuclear cells in and around the islets of Langerhans (Fig. 22-2). This possibility is supported by the observation that serum antibodies to islet cells are present in almost all newly diagnosed diabetics. Many of these patients develop islet cell antibodies.

Although these serum antibodies might play a role in the causation of diabetes, other immune mechanisms could be involved. Considerable evidence now points to cellular immunity, perhaps resulting from the action of cytolytic T cells on the beta cells.

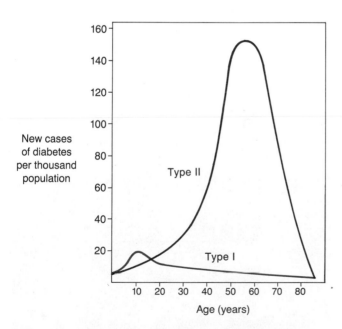

Figure 22-1. Age of onset of new cases of types I and II diabetes in a large clinic population. Note the relative proportions of cases of the two types of diabetes.

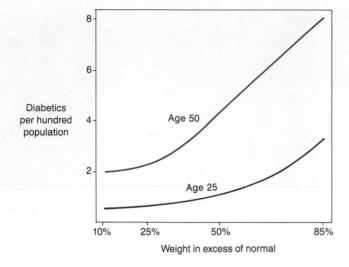

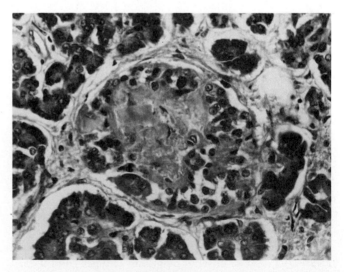

Figure 22-3. Occurrence of diabetes in relation to body weight in younger and older adults of both sexes.

TYPE II DIABETES MELLITUS

Type II diabetes usually develops in the adult, and its prevalence increases with advancing age. Indeed, almost 10% of persons over 65 years of age are affected. Four out of every five patients with type II diabetes are overweight (Fig. 22-3).

The pathogenesis of types I and II diabetes differ in most respects. **Genetic influences are a key factor in the occurrence of type II diabetes;** about 60% of patients have either a parent or a sibling with this type of diabetes. **Constitutional factors, such as obesity and exercise, influence the expression of the condition** and thus confuse genetic analyses.

Two pathogenetic factors appear to be critical to the development of type II diabetes. First, in many but not all hyperglycemic patients **insulin release by the beta cells is impaired.** Second, **tissue sensitivity to insulin is reduced in major organs,** with the exception of the brain. There also appear to be changes in the function of intracellular mediators of insulin action. Thus, uptake and metabolism of glucose are altered. A variety of microscopic lesions are found in the islets of Langerhans of many, but not all, patients with type II diabetes. In the islets of some patients, fibrous tissue accumulates, sometimes with sufficient prominence to obliterate the islets. In other patients, one may see a hyaline material that has many of the properties of amyloid (Fig. 22-4).

Type II diabetics have either normal or only slightly reduced amounts of insulin in the pancreas. The islet lesions appear to develop late in the course of the disease and generally are found in older patients.

Metabolic studies provide further insight into the pathogenesis of type II diabetes. **Deficient insulin release occurs during the early response of the beta cell to glucose stimulation, a defect most prominent in those with severe hyperglycemia.** Although recognition of glucose by the beta cell is impaired, the blood insulin concentration of many type II diabetics is actually increased. This paradoxical finding is now attributed to a reduction in the number of functional insulin receptors in the plasma membranes of cells that utilize insulin. Thus, **patients with type II diabetes are hy-**

Figure 22-4. Type II diabetes. Hyalinization and fibrosis of a pancreatic islet in an elderly patient are prominent.

perglycemic, but their cells are relatively deficient in insulin receptors, and so they metabolize glucose inefficiently despite normal or elevated levels of insulin in the blood** (Fig. 22-5).

OBESITY

There is a high incidence of obesity among type II diabetics. Although it is difficult to distinguish genetic factors from environmental influences, the importance of heredity in predisposing to obesity is becoming clear. Of greater relevance are the apparent polygenic influ-

ences on metabolism, which often seem to translate into familial tendencies to obesity. **Studies of monozygotic twins who have lived apart since birth have demonstrated the prevailing influence of heredity on physique and body weight.**

Some overweight people accumulate fat on the upper trunk, shoulders, and arms, whereas others exhibit pelvic girdle obesity. The former usually can reduce these body fat deposits by diet, whereas those in the latter group seem to retain their obese configuration despite rigorous control of food consumption. Curiously, those with upper-body obesity develop type II diabetes more often than persons of equal weight whose fat accumulates around the pelvic girdle.

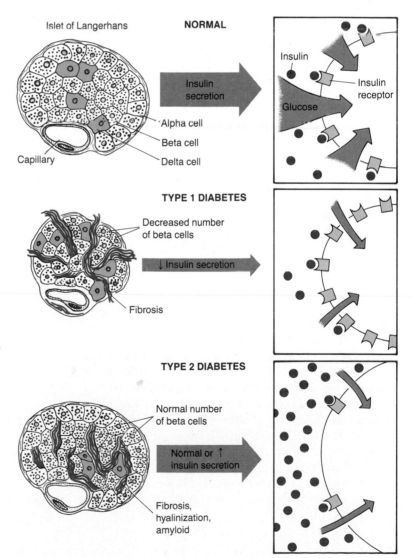

Figure 22-5. Pathogenesis of diabetes. In normal persons, insulin secreted by the beta cells binds to receptors on the effector cells (represented here by an adipocyte), thereby enhancing the entry of glucose. In type I diabetes the islets are atrophied and insulin production is reduced. This results in an absolute deficiency in the supply of insulin to tissues. In type II diabetes the output of insulin is variable but the cells prove "resistant" to the metabolic effects of insulin. Thus, there is a relative deficiency of insulin even when the concentration of insulin in the blood is increased.

COMPLICATIONS OF DIABETES

Virtually every tissue and organ is biochemically and structurally altered as a consequence of the hyperglycemia of diabetes. The development of secondary lesions has been claimed to relate largely to the severity and chronicity of hyperglycemia.

Two biochemical mechanisms appear to be involved in the development of many complications. In the first, glucose reversibly binds to a wide variety of body proteins, roughly in proportion to the degree of hyperglycemia. This is a nonenzymatic event that can occur with any free amino group, and one that can cause structural and functional abnormalities of the involved proteins.

The second biochemical mechanism operates in the aorta, lens of the eye, kidney, and peripheral nerves. These tissues are endowed with an enzyme, aldose reductase, that facilitates the accumulation of sorbitol and fructose in cells of the hyperglycemic patient. As a result of the intracellular accumulation of sorbitol and fructose, an osmotic gradient is established, and excessive amounts of water enter the cells from the extracellular compartment. Presumably the cells then swell and are damaged. Another consequence of the high intracellular concentration of sorbitol is the failure of myoinositol, a key to polyol energy metabolism, to enter cells. Many investigators believe that an intracellular deficiency of myoinositol plays a causative role in the long term complications of diabetes.

DISEASE OF LARGE AND MEDIUM-SIZED BLOOD VESSELS

The extent and severity of atherosclerosis is increased by diabetes. Significant atherosclerosis is rarely found in healthy premenopausal women, but diabetes predisposes them to its early appearance. Thrombotic occlusions of atherosclerotic large and medium-sized vessels are increased severalfold in diabetics. Thus, **myocardial and cerebral infarcts are extremely common complications of diabetes.** Indeed, atherosclerotic coronary heart disease is the major cause of death among adults with diabetes. The vasculature of the lower extremities is also compromised in many diabetics, a complication that results in pain in the legs because of inadequate circulation during exercise (intermittent claudication). Ulcers and gangrene of the toes and feet commonly develop, ultimately leading to amputation.

DISEASE OF ARTERIOLES AND CAPILLARIES

Arteriolosclerosis and capillary basement membrane thickening are characteristic changes in the vasculature of diabetics. The effects of disease in small vessels on tissue perfusion and wound healing are profound. For example, microvascular disease is believed to reduce blood flow to a heart already compromised by coronary atherosclerosis. It also plays a role in the susceptibility of the diabetic to chronic ulcers following trauma and infection of the feet.

DISEASE OF THE KIDNEYS

About 30% to 40% of those with type I diabetes develop renal failure (Fig. 22-6); a somewhat smaller proportion of patients with the type II form of the disease are similarly affected. It is not known why only some diabetics have kidney disease, but poor metabolic control may be an important consideration, since the prevalence increases with the severity and duration of

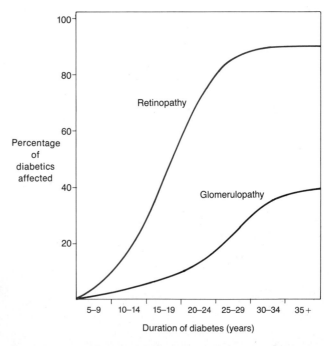

Figure 22-6. Frequency of clinically evident retinopathy and glomerulopathy in type I diabetes.

the disease. Hypertension and cigarette smoking appear to be additional contributory factors.

The glomeruli in the kidney of the diabetic exhibit a unique form of sclerosis, a lesion frequently referred to as **diabetic glomerulosclerosis** or **Kimmelstiel-Wilson disease.** Two microscopic patterns are seen. In the more common pattern, spherical masses of basement-membranelike material accumulate in the lobules of the glomeruli (Fig. 22-7). The second form is characterized by a more diffuse deposition of this material throughout the glomerulus. The second pattern must be differentiated from membranous glomerulonephritis.

DISEASE OF THE EYES

Lesions of small blood vessels commonly develop in the retina of the diabetic. The prevalence of retinopathy relates to the duration and control of diabetes (see Fig. 22-6). Although glaucoma, cataracts, and corneal disease occur with increased frequency in people with diabetes, **progressive retinopathy is the most devas-**

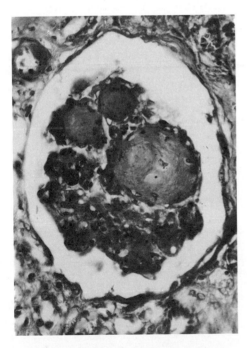

Figure 22-7. Diabetic glomerulosclerosis. This lesion, characteristically found in the kidneys of diabetics, is also referred to as Kimmelstiel-Wilson disease.

tating complication, and about 10% of those with type I diabetes of 30 years duration are legally blind.

DISEASE OF PERIPHERAL AND AUTONOMIC NERVES

Peripheral sensory and autonomic nerve dysfunction is one of the most common and distressing complications of diabetes. The lesions of the nerves are complex, and abnormalities of axons, myelin sheath, and Schwann cells have all been found. In addition, lesions of the small blood vessels of the nerves contribute to the disorder. Peripheral neuropathy is a major factor in the initiation of ulcers of the toes and feet, which are so common with severe diabetes, as well as in the painless, destructive joint disease that occasionally develops.

INFECTION

Bacterial and mycotic infections complicate the life of the diabetic whose metabolic disease is poorly regulated. Urinary tract infections pose a particular problem, in part because the dystonic bladder retains urine. Pyelonephritis is a threat to the diabetic. **Necrotizing papillitis,** a unique and devastating manifestation of infection, complicates vascular disease of the kidney, and kidney failure follows.

DIABETES AND PREGNANCY

Evidence of diabetes develops in about 1% to 2% of seemingly healthy women during pregnancy, and it continues after parturition in a small proportion of these patients. The metabolic basis for this syndrome, termed **gestational diabetes,** is uncertain.

Perinatal complications occur with unusual frequency in the diabetic. About 5% to 10% of infants of diabetic mothers are born with major developmental abnormalities. A variety of lesions of the heart and great vessels are found, and many of these prove fatal during the early days of life. Neural tube defects, such as anencephaly and spina bifida, also occur with increased frequency.

Diabetic mothers tend to give birth to large babies, so that obstetric complications are common.

23

AMYLOIDOSIS

ROBERT KISILEVSKY

General Features of Amyloid
  Deposits

Types of Amyloid Deposits

Mechanisms Involved in
  Amyloid Deposition

Clinical Features
  of Amyloidosis

Amyloid, a generic term that refers to a group of diverse extracellular protein deposits, is associated with many different diseases. Amyloid deposits have common morphologic properties, stain with specific dyes, and have a characteristic appearance under polarized light. Though varying in amino acid sequence, all amyloid proteins are folded in such a way as to share common ultrastructural and physical properties.

Amyloid deposits are composed of at least three constituents:

1. A fibrillary protein, the nature of which varies with the underlying disease. The tertiary structure of this protein and the manner in which it interacts with fellow molecules are responsible for the morphologic, structural, and some staining characteristics of amyloid. Furthermore, it is the particular nature of this fibrillary protein that is now the determining factor in the classification of amyloid.
2. Stacks of a pentagonal, doughnut-shaped protein, called the amyloid P, or AP, component. All types of amyloid, with only one exception, possess the AP component. AP is identical to, and is derived from, a normal circulating serum protein termed serum amyloid P, or SAP, component.
3. A complex carbohydrate (a glycosaminoglycan—in most cases, heparan sulfate). This molecule is probably responsible for the iodine-staining properties of amyloid.

It is important to emphasize that not all amyloids are the same. The protein responsible for the fibrillary characteristics varies significantly. In amyloid associated with multiple myeloma, the fibrillary component is a product of immunoglobulin light chains produced by the myeloma cells. In amyloid associated with inflammatory diseases, the fibrillary component is derived from the amino-terminal two-thirds of an acute phase protein. This protein is produced by the liver and is unrelated to immunoglobulins. Amyloid in medullary carcinoma of the thyroid is restricted to the tumor deposits, and its fibrillary component is derived from a polypeptide hormone.

GENERAL FEATURES OF AMYLOID DEPOSITS

STAINING PROPERTIES

The staining properties and general appearance of amyloid are governed primarily by its protein nature.

All amyloids stain red with Congo red dye (Fig. 23-1A). When the sections stained with Congo red are viewed under polarized light, the deposits exhibit a red-green birefringence (Fig. 23-1B). The fibrillary deposits organized in one plane have one color and those organized perpendicularly to the first have the other color.

The presence of glycosaminoglycans in virtually all amyloid deposits is demonstrated with a variety of alcian blue stains, which cause the glycosaminoglycans to appear blue.

The recent success in isolating various amyloid proteins has led to the preparation of both polyclonal and monoclonal antibodies directed against the different proteins. In turn, immunohistochemical techniques have been devised to demonstrate the presence of the AP component, as well as the specific protein present in each type of amyloid.

DEFINITION OF AMYLOID

The staining and structural properties allow a general definition of amyloid, based primarily on its morphologic characteristics. **All amyloid stains positively with Congo red and shows red-green birefringence when viewed under polarized light.** Ultrastructurally, all amyloids consist of **interlacing bundles of parallel arrays of fibrils,** which have a diameter of 70Å to 100Å. When examined by x-ray diffraction **the adjacent fibrils are organized in a crossed β-pleated sheet pattern.**

TYPES OF AMYLOID DEPOSITS

CLINICAL CLASSIFICATION

The classification used most commonly is one based on the clinical presentation of the patient (Table 23-1). On this basis, amyloidosis is categorized as either primary, secondary, familial, or isolated.

PRIMARY AMYLOIDOSIS

Amyloid appearing de novo—that is, without any preceding disease—has been called primary amyloidosis. In 25% to 40% of these cases, primary amyloidosis is the harbinger of frank plasma cell neoplasia, such as multiple myeloma or other B cell lymphomas. Regardless of whether amyloidosis or multiple myeloma presents first, the type of amyloid protein is the same.

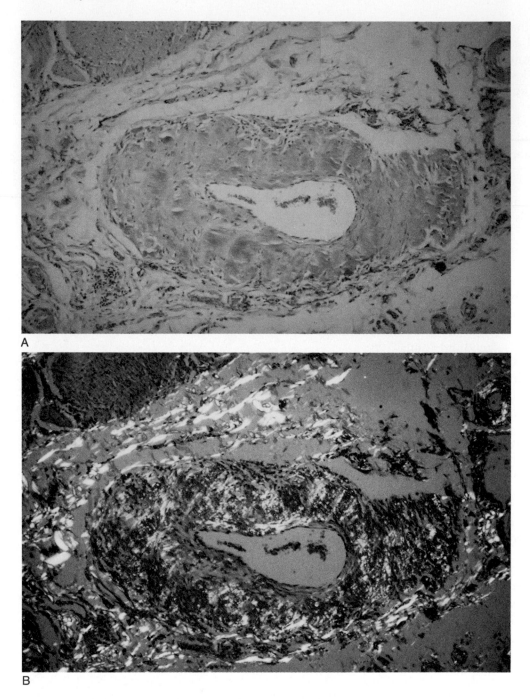

Figure 23-1. AL amyloid involving the wall of an artery, stained with Congo red. The appearance under ordinary light (*A*) and polarized light (*B*) is shown. Note the red-green birefringence of the amyloid. Collagen has a silvery appearance.

Table 23–1   *Classification of Amyloidosis*

CLASSIFICATION BY PROTEIN TYPE	RELATED OR PRECURSOR PROTEIN	ASSOCIATED DISEASES	CLINICAL CLASSIFICATION
AA	SAA	Recurrent inflammation 　Arthritis 　Tuberculosis 　Skin and lung abscesses	Secondary
		Cancer 　Kidney 　Hodgkin's disease 　Nonlymphomatous tumors	Secondary
		Familial 　Mediterranean fever	Familial
AL	λ or κ light chains	Multiple myeloma	Primary and secondary
		Immunoblastic lymphomas	Secondary
		Nodular pulmonary amyloidosis	Isolated
A prealbumin	Serum prealbumin	Familial amyloidotic polyneuropathy	Familial
		Cardiac amyloidosis	Isolated
		Amyloidosis of senescence	Senile
A-4	Membrane protein	Alzheimer's disease	Isolated
AE	Procalcitonin	Medullary carcinoma of thyroid	Endocrine
	Peptide related to calcitonin	Insulinomas	Endocrine
AP	SAP	Component of all forms of amyloid	

SECONDARY AMYLOIDOSIS

Secondary amyloidosis is the form of disease that appears as a complication of a previously existing disorder. While 10% to 15% of patients with multiple myeloma eventually develop amyloidosis, most patients with secondary amyloidosis have a preexisting chronic inflammatory disorder, which may or may not have an immunologic basis. Patients with rheumatoid arthritis, ankylosing spondylitis, and occasionally those with systemic lupus erythematosus can develop secondary amyloidosis. Most other patients with secondary amyloidosis have long-standing inflammation—for example, lung abscesses, tuberculosis, or osteomyelitis.

FAMILIAL AMYLOIDOSIS

Several geographic populations display genetically inherited forms of amyloidosis. One group, those with familial Mediterranean fever, is found in Israel, predominantly among Sephardic Jews. This disorder is characterized by polymorphonuclear leukocyte dysfunction and recurrent episodes of serositis, including peritonitis. Since there is recurrent inflammation, the type of amyloid protein deposited is identical to that seen in amyloidosis secondary to acquired inflammatory disorders.

A second grouping, familial amyloidotic polyneuropathy, has been described in at least three nationalities: Swedish, Portuguese, and Japanese. This type exhibits a predilection for peripheral and autonomic nerves. The nature of the protein deposited is quite different from that found in familial Mediterranean fever. All three national groups have the same basic genetic disorder—a single amino acid substitution in one particular protein.

ISOLATED AMYLOIDOSIS

The isolated forms of amyloidosis tend to involve a single organ system. Isolated amyloidosis has been described in the lung, heart, and various joints, and in association with endocrine tumors that secrete polypeptide hormones. In endocrine tumors the amyloid usually is a part of a hormone or prohormone product.

By far the most common organ-specific amyloid is found in Alzheimer's disease. In this disorder, the amyloid is restricted to the brain and its vessels. In most instances it occurs as a sporadic case within a family, but it can also be found in a familial form. The deposited protein is a 4-kd peptide (A-4) whose gene has been localized to chromosome 21.

CLASSIFICATION BY TYPE OF PROTEIN

Amyloidosis is not one disease, but a grouping of diseases, all of which have tissue protein deposits with similar morphologic, structural, and staining properties, despite fundamentally different amino

acid sequences. A grouping of the amyloids and the diseases with which they are associated can be made according to the type of protein (see Table 23-1).

AL AMYLOID

The first amyloid protein to be isolated and sequenced was AL amyloid from patients who had primary amyloidosis or multiple myeloma. **This amyloid usually consists of the variable region of immunoglobulin light chains,** and it can be derived from either the κ or λ moieties.

The AL protein is common to primary amyloidosis and amyloidosis secondary to either multiple myeloma or B cell lymphomas. Since many of the patients who first present with "primary" amyloidosis subsequently develop plasma cell abnormalities or frank myeloma, one can appreciate that "primary" amyloidosis, multiple myeloma, and immunoblastic lymphomas form part of the spectrum of a single disorder.

AA AMYLOID

AA amyloid is common to a host of seemingly unrelated disorders. **Clinically, it can be a complication of long-standing inflammation, familial disorders, and various forms of cancer.** The serum protein has been called SAA. SAA is an acute phase protein, the serum concentration of which rapidly increases (500- to 1000-fold) during any inflammatory process. **In contrast to the AL protein, the amino acid sequence of the AA protein is identical in all patients,** regardless of the underlying nature of the inflammatory disturbance.

A PREALBUMIN (TRANSTHYRETIN)

Prealbumin, or transthyretin, serves as a serum carrier of thyroid hormones and vitamin A. **A variant of this protein is deposited in all forms of familial amyloidotic polyneuropathy. A normal prealbumin molecule is deposited in the isolated form of cardiac amyloidosis and in a systemic form of amyloidosis associated with aging.**

AE–ENDOCRINE FORMS OF AMYLOID

Several forms of isolated amyloid associated with endocrine tumors have been described. Medullary carcinoma of the thyroid originates from the C-type cells of the thyroid, which normally secret calcitonin. The amyloid in this tumor is a fragment of procalcitonin. Similarly, in insulin-secreting tumors of the pancreas, the amyloid seems to be a peptide related to but distinct from calcitonin.

MECHANISMS INVOLVED IN AMYLOID DEPOSITION

For many years it was widely held that a disturbance in immunologic mechanisms underlies virtually all forms of amyloid deposition. We now appreciate that different clinical forms of amyloidosis exhibit proteins that are not uniform and need not be related to immunoglobulins. Present data suggest that common mechanisms are involved when there is a common amyloid protein, and that different mechanisms are invoked for the genesis of different amyloid proteins.

DEPOSITION OF AL AMYLOID

In most instances AL amyloid deposition is associated with disturbances in B cell function, resulting in excessive immunoglobulin production, usually in the form of a monoclonal gammopathy (Fig 23-2).

AL amyloid is a fragment of a larger protein molecule and is derived from its proteolysis. The close anatomic association between AL amyloid deposits and phagocytic cells suggests that the proteolytic process resides in these cells. It appears that large quantities of substrate (κ or λ chains), in association with cells possessing proteolytic enzymes, can lead to AL amyloid deposits.

DEPOSITION OF AA AMYLOID AND INFLAMMATION

AA amyloid is associated with inflammatory diseases, viral infections, a variety of cancers, and familial Mediterranean fever. This is the type of amyloid induced in the standard experimental models of amyloidosis. AA amyloid is clearly related to the SAA protein. Recently, direct conversion of SAA into AA has been demonstrated.

SAA has the characteristics of an apoprotein of high-density lipoprotein, yet it is present in significant quantities only during inflammation. When the lipoprotein is denatured, it releases a 12,000- to 14,000-molecular-weight subunit (apo-SAA) that has all the immunologic cross-reactivity found between the SAA and AA protein. Apo-SAA is synthesized primarily in the liver and binds to a high-density lipoprotein upon entering the circulation. Hepatic apo-SAA synthesis is induced by a cytokine, interleukin-1, which is released from activated inflammatory cells. Thus, part of the pathogenetic pathway involved in AA deposition involves the natural reaction of the body to acute inflammatory stimuli (Fig. 23-3).

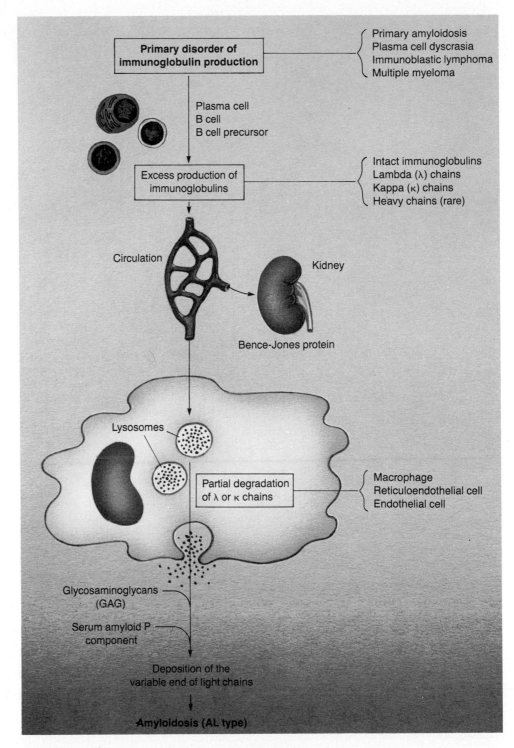

Figure 23-2. The mechanism of AL amyloid deposition.

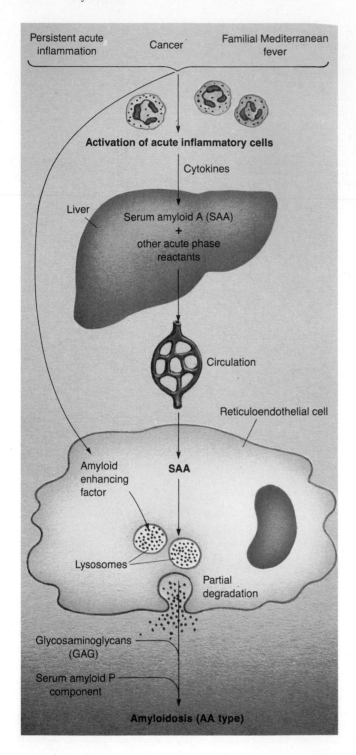

Figure 23-3. The mechanism of AA amyloid deposition. A variety of diseases are associated with the activation of polymorphonuclear leukocytes, which in turn leads to the release of acute phase reactants, including SAA, by the liver. These disorders also are accompanied by the appearance of amyloid enhancing factor. SAA, in the presence of amyloid enhancing factor, is partially degraded by reticuloendothelial cells, and the released product complexed with GAG and SAP is deposited as AA amyloid.

Whereas only a small percentage of patients with high levels of SAA actually develop amyloidosis, there are experimental models in which all animals deposit amyloid within a matter of days. It has been shown that persistent acute inflammation in such animals induces not only the synthesis of the amyloid precursor, SAA, but also the appearance of a protein that has been termed **amyloid enhancing factor (AEF.)** AEF is a naturally occurring glycoprotein, the concentration of which increases markedly during inflammation, that alters the metabolic processing of SAA. **Thus, during inflammation at least two coincident processes are apparently necessary for AA amyloid deposition. The first is the generation of amyloid precursor; the second is the generation of AEF.**

In both AA and AL amyloid deposition, partial degradation of a protein by a phagocytic cell occurs. It is the distribution of phagocytic cells that seems to determine the anatomic distribution of the AL and AA forms of amyloid.

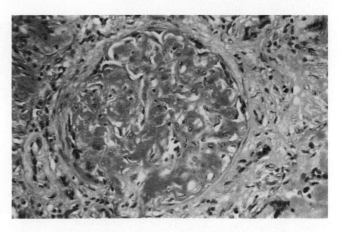

Figure 23-4. The microscopic appearance of AA amyloid from glomeruli. Note the lobular pattern of the deposit and the involvement of the afferent arteriole.

DEPOSITION OF AMYLOIDS ASSOCIATED WITH PREALBUMIN

Familial amyloidotic polyneuropathy is inherited in an autosomal dominant fashion. Apparently the entire molecule of A prealbumin is deposited, rather than a fragment. **In contrast to the AL and AA amyloids, a proteolytic mechanism is not involved in the pathogenesis of familial amyloidotic polyneuropathy.**

FEATURES OF AMYLOID DEPOSITS IN DIFFERENT TISSUES

While amyloid deposits share common structural features, they also exhibit features related to the tissues in which they are laid down. **Because amyloid is deposited along stromal networks, the deposits take on the architectural framework of the organs involved.** For example, in the medulla of the kidney, amyloid is laid down in a longitudinal fashion, parallel to the tubules and vasa recta. In the glomerulus (Fig. 23-4), amyloid is deposited in a pattern determined by the lobular architecture of the glomerulus itself.

Amyloid adds interstitial material to sites of deposition, a process that increases the size of affected organs. This increase may be counterbalanced by the deposition of amyloid in vessels, an effect that may impair circulation and lead to organ atrophy. Affected organs may, therefore, increase or decrease in size. The compact protein deposits are essentially avascular, a property that makes organs paler and adds a firmness to their consistency.

The fibrils are usually in close association with subendothelial basement membranes when they are first deposited (Fig. 23-5). **Regardless of whether amyloid is laid down in a systemic or local fashion, the deposits tend to occur between parenchymal cells and their blood supply. Extension of these deposits eventually entraps the parenchymal cells, interferes with their nutrition, and leads to their strangulation and atrophy** (Fig. 23-6).

CLINICAL FEATURES OF AMYLOIDOSIS

The symptomatology of amyloidosis is governed by both the underlying disease and the type of protein deposited. **No single set of symptoms points unequivocally to amyloidosis as a diagnosis.** In fact, amyloidosis may be found as a completely unexpected disorder, with no clinical manifestations. Renal and cardiac complications are common in several varieties of amyloidosis.

Amyloid involvement of the myocardium should be suspected in systemic forms of amyloidosis, in which congestive failure or cardiomegaly is associated with low voltage on the electrocardiogram. Entrapment of the conduction system may lead to arrhythmias, which in turn can result in sudden death. Sufficient amyloid

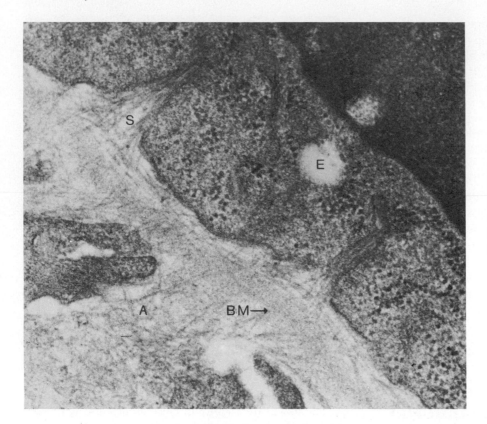

Figure 23-5. Electron micrograph of glomerular amyloid (*A*) illustrating its location relative to the basement membrane (*BM*). Amyloid spicules (*S*) extend into the cytoplasm of the glomerular epithelial cells (*E*).

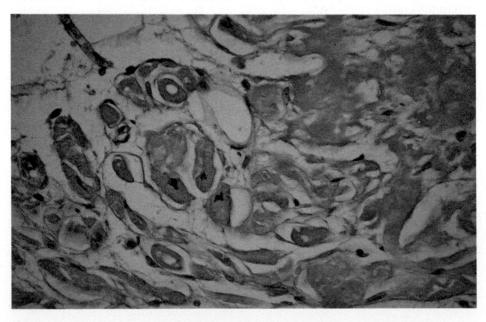

Figure 23-6. Myocardial amyloid (AL type), showing the encroachment upon and strangulation of individual myocardial fibers.

deposition within the myocardium also impairs ventricular distensibility and filling, an effect that appears clinically as a restrictive form of cardiomyopathy.

Gastrointestinal ganglia, smooth muscle vasculature, and submucosa all may be involved by amyloid. Deposits in these locations alter gastrointestinal motility and absorption. Enlargement of the tongue and interference with its motor function may be of sufficient degree to affect speech and swallowing.

For the most part, amyloid is a stable, static protein deposit. However, successful treatment of the underlying condition, may on rare occasion lead to the resorp-tion and resolution of these deposits. **In all systemic forms of amyloidosis, the patient's course is usually unremitting and ultimately fatal.**

DIAGNOSIS OF AMYLOIDOSIS

Even when one suspects amyloidosis, the diagnosis ultimately rests on its histologic demonstration in biopsy specimens. Amyloid is readily demonstrated in gingival and rectal biopsy specimens and in abdominal subcutaneous fat.

24

THE SKIN

WALLACE H. CLARK, JR.

DISEASES PRIMARILY AFFECTING THE EPIDERMIS

HERITABLE DISORDERS ASSOCIATED WITH EXCESSIVE CORNIFICATION

PSORIASIS

Definition and Clinical Features

Psoriasis is an epidermal–dermal disease characterized by persistent epidermal hyperplasia. It is chronic, frequently familial, and worldwide, affecting 1% to 2% of the population. **In its classical form it is characterized by large, erythematous, scaly plaques commonly observed on the extensor–dorsal cutaneous surfaces.** The severity of the disease varies from annoying scaly lesions over the elbows to a serious debilitating disorder, involving most of the skin, that at times may be associated with arthritis. A single lesion of psoriasis may be a small focus of scaly erythema or an enormous confluent plaque covering much of the trunk. A typical plaque is 4 to 5 cm in diameter, is sharply demarcated at its margin, and has a surface of silvery scales. When the scales are detached, pinpoint foci of bleeding dot the underlying glossy erythematous surface.

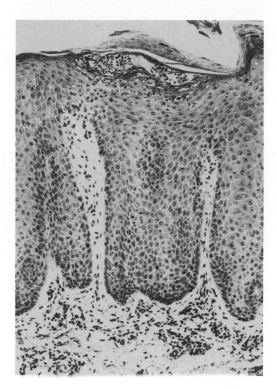

Figure 24-2. Intraepidermal neutrophils are a manifestation of the transepidermal migration of these cells in psoriasis. They emerge from the venulized capillaries at the tips of the dermal papillae and migrate to the location illustrated here. In time, they extend into the stratum corneum, which commonly is parakeratotic, as shown in this micrograph.

Pathology

The most distinctive pathologic changes in psoriasis are seen at the periphery of a classical psoriatic plaque. **The epidermis is thickened and shows both hyperkeratosis (thickened stratum corneum) and parakeratosis (persistence of nuclei into the stratum corneum).** The nucleated layers of the epidermis are thickened several-fold in the rete, and frequently are thinner over the dermal papillae (Fig. 24-1). The papillae, in turn, are elongated and appear as sections of cones, with their apices toward the dermis. In chronic lesions, the papillae may appear as bulbous clubs with short handles. The rete ridges of the epidermis have a profile reciprocal to that of the dermal papillae, and the skin shows interlocked mesenchymal and epithelial clubs with alternating reversed polarity. The capillaries of the papillae are dilated and tortuous. Electron micrographs show the capillaries to be venulelike; neutrophils may emerge at their tips and migrate into the epidermis above the apices of the papillae. The acute inflammatory cells may become localized in the epidermal spinous layer or in small collections in the stratum corneum, and may be associated with circumscribed areas of parakeratosis (Fig. 24-2).

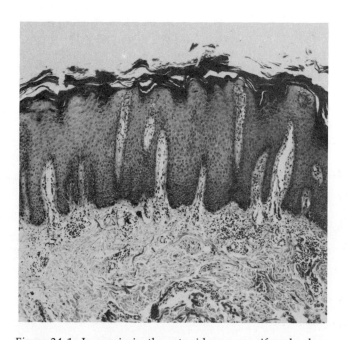

Figure 24-1. In psoriasis, the rete ridges are uniformly elongated. The dermal papillae are elongated, and some present prominent, elongated venules.

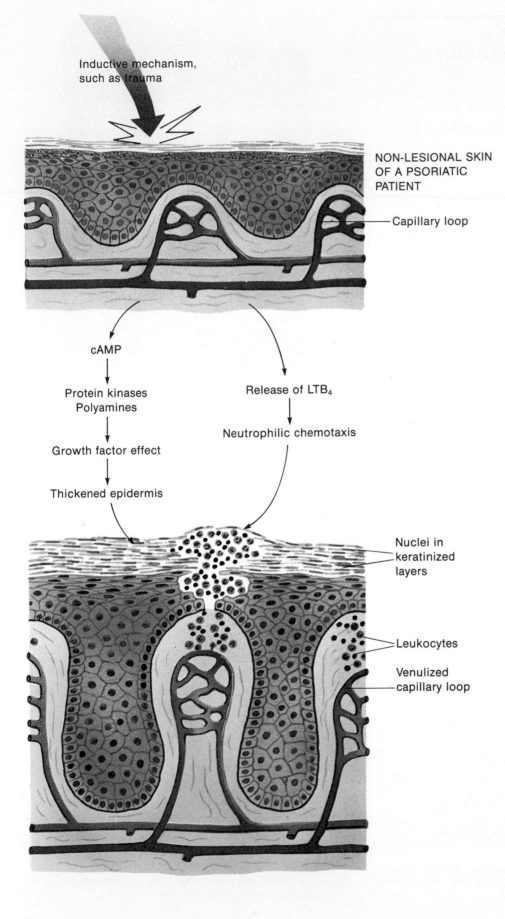

Inductive mechanism,
such as trauma

NON-LESIONAL SKIN
OF A PSORIATIC
PATIENT

Capillary loop

cAMP

Protein kinases
Polyamines

Release of LTB$_4$

Growth factor effect

Neutrophilic chemotaxis

Thickened epidermis

Nuclei in
keratinized
layers

Leukocytes

Venulized
capillary loop

Figure 24-3. Pathogenetic mechanisms in psoriasis. The drawing depicts the deregulation of epidermal growth, venulization of the capillary loop, and a unique form of neutrophilic inflammation. The altered epidermal growth is thought to be caused by defective epidermal cell surface receptors. This results in a decrease in cAMP, together with the effects indicated. The decrease in cAMP is also likely to be related to the increased production of arachidic acid which, in turn, leads to activation of LTB-4. This potent neutrophilic chemotactic agent acts on a venulized capillary loop. Neutrophils then emerge from the tips of the capillary loop at the apex of the dermal papilla, rather than from the postcapillary venule, as is the rule in most inflammatory skin diseases.

Etiology and Pathogenesis

In psoriasis, the entire skin—both that with lesions and that without—is abnormal. About one-third of affected patients have a family history of the disease. The pathogenesis of the psoriatic plaques may be appreciated by contrasting the effect of chronic cutaneous trauma in persons with and without psoriasis. Chronic trauma (for instance, that caused by rubbing) of the skin of a normal person produces a tough, scaly, cutaneous plaque that is psoriasiform both clinically and histologically. However, with cessation of the trauma the lesion disappears. In the psoriatic patient, even less severe trauma produces a distinctive psoriatic plaque that may persist for years after the initial injury. Although there is no universally accepted explanation for this unique response to injury, evidence suggests that a **deregulation of epidermal proliferation and an abnormality in the microcirculation of the dermis are responsible** (Fig. 24-3).

DYSHESIVE DISORDERS

PEMPHIGUS

Definition and Clinical Features

The term pemphigus, derived from the Greek *pemphix*, meaning bubble, defines a blistering disease. All blistering diseases were once classified as pemphigus. **Pemphigus vulgaris is but one of a group of diseases**

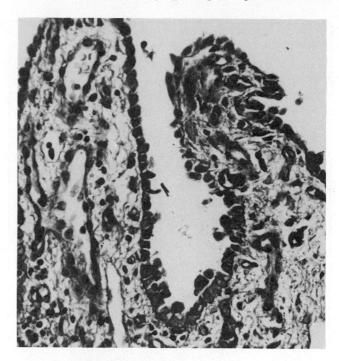

Figure 24-5. Higher power magnification of the suprabasal dyshesion in pemphigus vulgaris. The crisply delineated basal cells, slightly separated from each other and completely separated from the stratum spinosum, are still firmly attached to the basement membrane zone.

characterized by blister formation secondary to diminished cohesiveness (dyshesion) of epidermal cells. This dyshesion is related to the reaction of autoantibodies to surface antigens on the cells of stratified squamous epithelia. Pemphigus vulgaris, a severe dyshesive disorder that is usually fatal without corticosteroid therapy, is the prototype for this group of blistering diseases. The characteristic lesion of pemphigus vulgaris is a large, easily ruptured blister that leaves extensive denuded or crusted areas. The lesions are most common on the scalp and mucous membranes, and in the periumbilical and intertriginous areas. Without treatment, the disease is progressive, and much of the epidermis may become denuded.

Pathology

The blister in pemphigus vulgaris forms because of the separation of the stratum spinosum and outer epidermal layers from the basal layer. This suprabasal dyshesion results in a blister that has the intact basal layer as a floor and the remaining epidermis as a roof (Figs. 24-4 and 24-5). The vesicle contains a moderate number of lymphocytes, macrophages, eosinophils, neutrophils, and distinctive, rounded keratinocytes that shed into the vesicle during the process of dyshesion. These keratinocytes are called **acantholytic cells,**

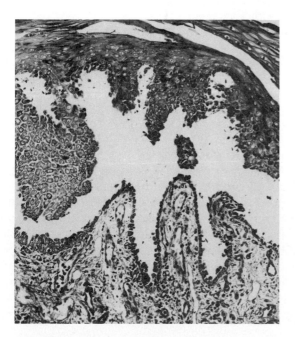

Figure 24-4. Suprabasal dyshesion in pemphigus vulgaris. A classic suprabasal vesicle is evident.

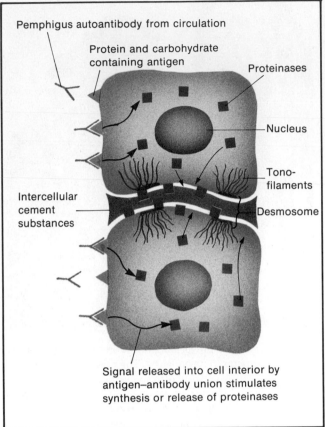

Pemphigus autoantibody from circulation

Protein and carbohydrate containing antigen

Proteinases

Nucleus

Tono-filaments

Desmosome

Intercellular cement substances

Signal released into cell interior by antigen–antibody union stimulates synthesis or release of proteinases

1. Antigen–antibody union activates intracellular proteinases.

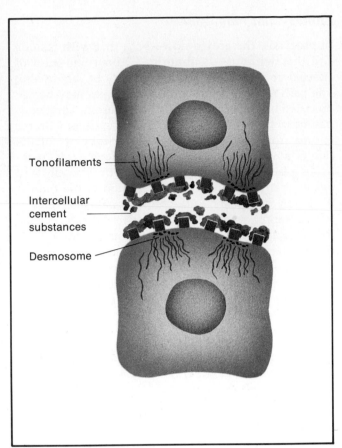

Tonofilaments

Intercellular cement substances

Desmosome

2. Proteinases interact with intercellular cement, initiating cellular dyshesion (acantholysis).

Figure 24-6. The pathogenetic mechanisms of suprabasal dyshesion in pemphigus vulgaris. A circulating autoantibody of unknown origin reacts with an antigen on the outer leaflet of the plasma membrane of epidermal cells, especially in the basilar regions. (*1*) Antigen–antibody union results in release of a proteinase (plasmin). (*2*) The proteinase interacts with intercellular cement, initiating dyshesion. (*3*) Desmosomes deteriorate, tonofilaments clump about the nucleus, the cells round up, and separation is complete. (*4*) A vesicle, which is usually suprabasal, forms.

a term that implies "lysis of a spine." The flawed cohesiveness of the epidermal cells that is characteristic of this disorder is due to the action of proteases on many of the epidermal cohesive forces. Consequently, the term dyshesion aptly describes the "flawed sticking" of the epidermal cells in this disease. The dyshesion may extend along the adnexa, and is not always strictly suprabasal. The subjacent dermis shows a moderate infiltrate of lymphocytes, macrophages, eosinophils, and neutrophils, predominantly about the capillary venular bed. Occasionally, eosinophils are numerous.

Etiology and Pathogenesis

There are specific circulating autoantibodies in pemphigus, as well as in vivo-bound IgG in the intercellular substance of the epidermis and other stratified squamous epithelia. Electron microscopy suggests that the antibody reacts with a component of the outer layer of the epidermal plasma membrane. The circulating antibodies in patients with pemphigus vulgaris react with an epidermal surface antigen that is not species-specific, and is found in other mammals and birds. Pem-

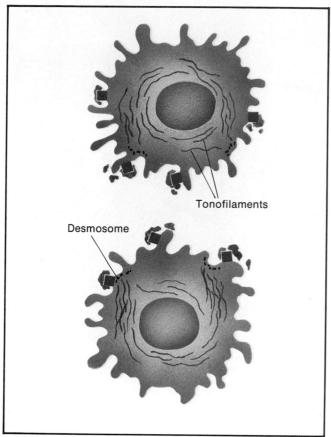

3. Complete dyshesion (acantholysis). Acantholytic cells separate, round up, and form micropapillary projections on the cell surface. Desmosomes deteriorate and tonofilaments clump about nucleus.

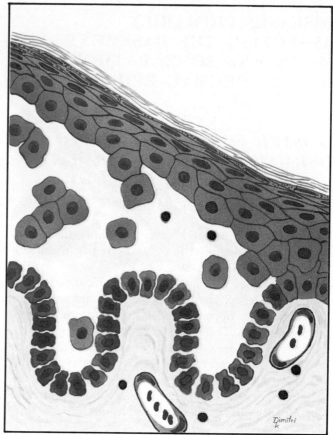

4. Intraepidermal bulla

phigus may be associated with other autoimmune diseases, such as myasthenia gravis and lupus erythematous, and may also be seen with benign thymomas. The clinical activity of the disease correlates with the titer of pemphigus autoantibodies. The autoantibodies are related to the dyshesion, and the purified antibodies can induce dyshesion in animal skin. Moreover, antibodies produced in rabbits in response to the administration of purified antigen cause lesions similar to pemphigus in the skin of the newborn mouse.

Present evidence suggests that the binding of antibody to antigen causes an increase in synthesis of plasminogen activator and, hence, activation of plasmin. This proteolytic enzyme acts on the intercellular substance and is probably the dominant factor in dyshesion. Cytopathologic processes within the cell may also contribute to dyshesion. Internalization of the antigen–antibody complex, disappearance of attachment plaques, and perinuclear tonofilament retraction all may act in concert with proteinases to cause dyshesion and vesiculation (Fig. 24-6).

DISEASES PRIMARILY AFFECTING THE BASEMENT MEMBRANE ZONE: PATHOLOGY OF THE DERMAL–EPIDERMAL INTERFACE

BLISTER FORMATION DUE TO DERMAL–EPIDERMAL SEPARATION

BULLOUS PEMPHIGOID

Definition and Clinical Features

Bullous pemphigoid is a blistering disease with clinical similarities to pemphigus vulgaris, hence the name "pemphigoid." The disease has a predilection for the later decades of life, but has no significant racial or sexual prevalence. The blisters are large and tense, and may appear on normal-appearing skin or on an erythematous base. The medial thighs and flexor aspects of the forearms are commonly affected, but the groin, axilla, and other cutaneous sites may also develop blisters. The disease is self-limited but chronic, and the patient's general health is usually unaffected. The course of the disease is greatly shortened by systemic steroids.

Pathology

The blisters of pemphigoid are subepidermal, with the roof of the blister being formed by an intact epidermis, and the base by the lamina densa of the basement membrane zone (Fig. 24-7 and 24-8). The blister contains fibrin, lymphocytes, neutrophils, and eosinophils,

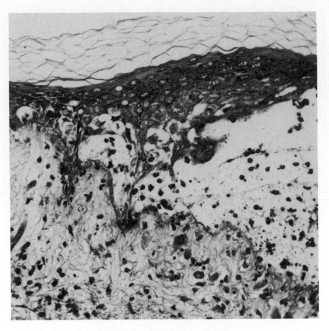

Figure 24-8. The subepidermal vesicle is above the lamina densa (*arrows*) in bullous pemphigoid.

with the last usually appearing as the dominant cell form. Even before becoming erythematous, the normal skin around the lesions of pemphigoid shows mast cell migration from the venule toward the epidermis. With the onset of erythema, eosinophils appear in the upper dermis and are occasionally arranged in a linear array at the basement membrane zone. By electron microscopy, the first site of dermal–epidermal separation is in the lamina lucida, and is associated with disruption of anchoring filaments.

Etiology and Pathogenesis

Bullous pemphigoid is thought to be an autoimmune disease, characterized by circulating IgG antibodies to a normal glycoprotein of the lamina lucida in or near the basal keratinocyte hemidesmosome. This glycoprotein, known as BP-antigen, together with laminin and anchoring filaments, contributes to dermal–epidermal adherence. Most cases of pemphigoid display a linear deposit of IgG and C3 in the lamina lucida of the basement membrane zone. The BP-antigen-antibody complex in the lamina lucida may injure the basal cell plasma membrane through the formation of C5b-C9 membrane attack complex, and this damage might interfere with the elaboration of adherence factors by basal cells. Of greater importance is the production of the anaphylatoxins C3a and C5a following activation of complement. In turn, these anaphylatoxins cause

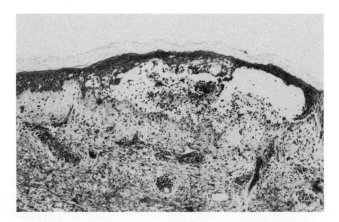

Figure 24-7. Subepidermal vesicle in bullous pemphigoid. Inflammatory cells are prominent in the vesicle and in the dermis.

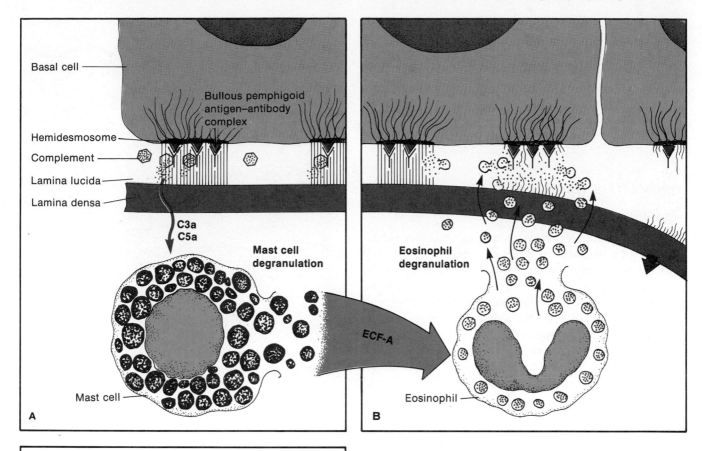

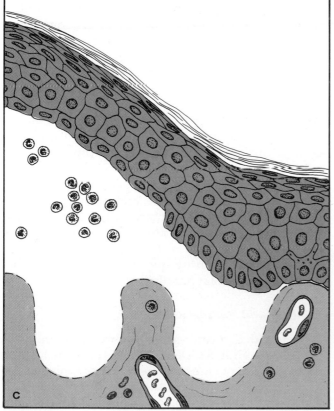

Figure 24-9. Pathogenetic mechanisms of blister formation in bullous pemphigoid. A circulating antibody to an apparently normal glycoprotein—BP antigen—in the lamina lucida precipitates the pathogenetic events in bullous pemphigoid. (*A*) Antigen–antibody union activates complement, and the anaphylatoxins C3a and C5a are produced. These degranulate mast cells, resulting in release of eosinophilic chemotactic factor. (*B* and *C*) The tissue-damaging substances of eosinophilic granules cause vesicle formation at the lamina lucida, with some breakdown of the lamina densa. (ECF-A = eosinophil chemotactic factor-A)

degranulation of mast cells and the release of factors that are chemotactic for eosinophils, neutrophils, and lymphocytes. The eosinophilic granules contain tissue-damaging substances, including eosinophil peroxidase and major basic protein. These, together with proteases of neutrophilic and mast cell origin, cause dermal–epidermal separation, primarily within the lamina lucida (Fig. 24-9).

DERMATITIS HERPETIFORMIS

Definition and Clinical Features

Dermatitis herpetiformis is an intriguing disease characterized by urticarialike plaques, which may develop small vesicles, over the extensor surfaces of the body. The lesions are especially prominent over the elbows, knees, and buttocks. The intensely pruritic vesicles may become grouped in a fashion similar to herpes. Because they are so pruritic, emerging vesicles may be rubbed until broken, and a patient may first present with crusted lesions only, and no intact vesicles. Although the disease is of varying severity and is characterized by remissions, it is disturbingly chronic. The healing lesions often leave scars. **The ailment is related to gluten sensitivity in patients of the HLA-B8/DRW3 haplotype; most of these patients also have a gluten sensitivity enteropathy.** The cutaneous lesions are related to deposits of granular IgA at the dermal–epidermal interface, mainly at the tips of the dermal papillae.

Pathology

The pathologic changes associated with dermatitis herpetiformis are best appreciated by studying sequential biopsies over a 72-hour period after cessation of therapy. Dapsone or sulfapyridine completely control the signs and symptoms of the disease, probably by inhibiting the inflammatory cascade and neutrophilic lysosomal functions. Twenty-four hours after cessation of therapy, however, patients develop erythematous, urticarial plaques about the elbows and knees. In these lesions, concomitant with the emergence of a delicate perivenular lymphocytic infiltrate, a row of neutrophils appears immediately deep to the lamina densa. Within 36 hours, **the neutrophils aggregate in clusters of 10 to 25 at the tips of the dermal papillae to create a highly distinctive, essentially diagnostic histologic picture.** There are two related mechanisms of dermal–epidermal separation. In one, associated with the sheetlike spread of a layer or two of neutrophils at the dermal–epidermal interface, the entire epidermis detaches from the papillary dermis, carrying the base-

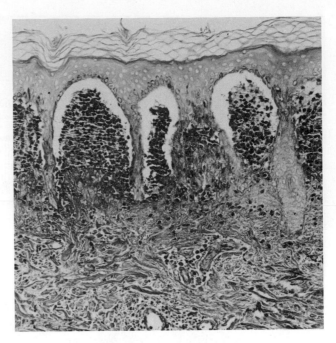

Figure 24-10. Dermal papillary abscesses with early dermal–epidermal separation at that site are essentially unique to dermatitis herpetiformis.

ment membrane zone with it (Fig. 24-10). The roof of such a vesicle contains the intact lamina densa, whereas the floor is made up of papillary dermis with a prominent neutrophilic infiltrate. In striking contrast to bullous pemphigoid, eosinophils are uncommon early in the course of dermatitis herpetiformis. When an increased number of neutrophils rapidly accumulate at the tips of dermal papillae, the release of large amounts of neutrophilic lysosomal enzymes in the outer portion of the dermal papillae results in **the uncoupling of the epidermis from the dermis at the tips of dermal papillae, disruption of the basement membrane zone in the outer part of the papillae, and tearing of the epidermis across the adjacent rete ridges. In the resulting vesicle, the roof has alternating tears across its epidermal covering, whereas the floor shows residual epidermal covering, pegs alternating with the basal half of dermal papillae.**

Etiology and Pathogenesis

Patients with dermatitis herpetiformis are, for the most part, of the HLA-B8/DRW3 haplotype. This locus is physically close to the immune response gene that determines gluten sensitivity, and most patients develop a gluten sensitivity enteropathy, although it may be only minimally expressed. There is a receptor for gluten—a protein found in wheat, barley, rye, and oats—in the dermal papillae of human skin. Granular deposits of IgA immune complexes are present at the tips of dermal papillae, and are greater in perilesional skin than in nonlesional skin. Importantly, a gluten-free diet controls the disease, whereas reintroduction of dietary gluten provokes new lesions.

It has been suggested that patients of the B8/DRW3 haplotype express two genes. One is responsible for gluten sensitivity enteropathy, while the other controls dimeric IgA antibody formation in response to partially digested forms of gluten and other dietary proteins. These proteins pass through a defective mucosal epithelial barrier that has been damaged by gluten sensitivity. The resultant IgA immune complexes are deposited in the skin at gluten receptor sites, where they accumulate at locations, such as the elbow, that frequently sustain trauma.

IgA immune complexes are inefficient in complement activation, and only a few neutrophils are attracted to the site. However, the neutrophils elaborate the leukotrienes, which attract more neutrophils. Through their lysosomal enzymes, the epidermis is cleaved from the dermis. The immune complexes are deposited deep to the lamina densa in intimate relation to the collagen rootlets (microfibrils) which, along with anchoring fibrils, are important in the attachment of the lamina densa to the subjacent papillary dermis (Fig. 24-11).

BASAL KERATINOCYTIC INJURY, EXCESSIVE SYNTHESIS OF LAMINA DENSA, AND IMMUNE REACTANTS AT THE BASEMENT MEMBRANE ZONE

LUPUS ERYTHEMATOSUS

Definition and Clinical Features

The various forms of cutaneous lupus erythematosus have been classified as chronic (discoid), subacute, or acute. Chronic cutaneous lupus erythematosus is usually a disease of the skin alone. Subacute cutaneous lupus may be accompanied by involvement of the musculoskeletal system, but severe disease of other organs is uncommon. By contrast, acute cutaneous lupus is associated with serious involvement of a variety of organ systems, especially progressive renal disease (systemic lupus erythematosus).

The lesions of chronic cutaneous lupus erythematosus are generally above the neck—on the face, scalp, and ears. The lesions begin as slightly elevated, violaceous papules that have a rough scale of keratin on the surface. As they enlarge, the lesions assume a disclike appearance, with a hyperkeratotic margin and a depigmented center. This form of the disease is not associated with involvement of other organs. These cutaneous lesions may culminate in disfiguring scars.

Subacute cutaneous lupus erythematosus, a disease of young and middle-aged Caucasian women, differs from chronic cutaneous lupus erythematosus in a number of ways. The lesions are seen in the "V" areas of the upper chest and upper back, and extensor surfaces of the arms, a distribution that suggests that light may have a role in the pathogenesis of this form of the disease. Indeed, photosensitivity is common. The early lesions are scaly erythematous papules, but they enlarge into psoriasiform or annular lesions which, in turn, may fuse. Significant scarring does not occur.

The most serious form of lupus—namely, acute systemic lupus erythematosus—may be associated with inconspicuous and transient acute cutaneous lesions. Frequently, the only manifestation is the **classic butterfly rash**—a delicate erythema of the malar area of the face that may pass in a few hours or a few days. Occasionally, the upper chest or extremities may be involved.

Pathology

There is an inverse relationship between the prominence of skin pathology and the extent of systemic pathology in lupus erythematosus. Chronic cutaneous lupus erythematosus (discoid lupus erythematosus) presents distinctive and diagnostic histologic changes, but is rarely associated with systemic pathology. The nucleated epidermal layers are modestly thickened or somewhat thin, but hyperkeratosis and plugging of hair follicles are prominent. The rete papillary pattern of the dermal epidermal interface is partially effaced (Fig. 24-12). Unique changes are seen in the basal cells and the basement membrane zone. The basal cells are vacuolated, and fibrillary bodies, which provide evidence of the death of keratinocytes (see the discussion of lichen planus that follows), are noted. The lamina densa is greatly thickened and reduplicated. On periodic acid-Schiff staining, multiple layers of lamina densa are found to extend into the subjacent dermis. The excessive quantity of lamina densa, a product of the basal cells, reflects a response of basal cells to damage. **The vacuolated basal cells, the fibrillary bodies,**

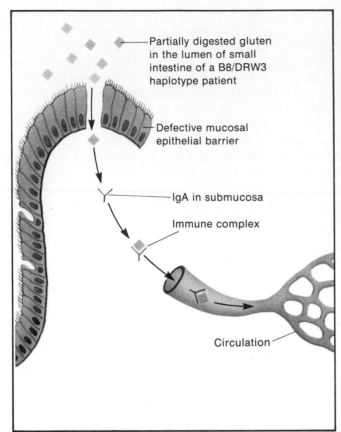

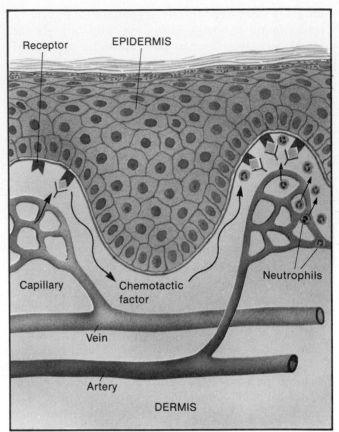

1. Formation of immune complexes in submucosa of small intestine. Passage of immune complexes into circulation.

2. Receptor–immune complex union releases neutrophil chemotactic factor. Neutrophils migrate to the tips of the papillae.

Figure 24-11. The pathogenesis of the cutaneous lesions in dermatitis herpetiformis. The disease is initiated in the small intestine and is expressed in the skin because of a gluten receptor immediately deep to the lamina densa.

and the alterations of the lamina densa all indicate **one essential pathogenetic characteristic of lupus-induced skin disease—namely, injury to basal keratinocytes** (Figs. 24-13 and 24-14). A variety of immune complexes are present in the basement membrane zone. These are located predominantly deep to the lamina densa, but are also seen on the lamina densa and within the lamina lucida; a haphazard array is to be expected in a disease involving numerous, diverse antigens.

Etiology and Pathogenesis

The mechanisms underlying the pathology of the skin lesions of lupus are complex. First, epidermal injury seems to be caused by exogenous agents, such as ultra-violet light, and by cell-mediated immune reactions similar to those in graft-versus-host disease. The manifestations of epidermal injury include vacuolization of basal cells with some diminution in epidermal thickness and hyperkeratosis, release of DNA and other nuclear and cytoplasmic antigens into the circulation, and deposition of DNA and other antigens in the basement membrane zone (lamina densa and immediately subjacent dermis) (Fig. 24-15). The deposition of circulating immune complexes in the kidney and skin is accompanied by the local formation of immune complexes in the basal laminae of the two organs (see Fig. 24-15). **Thus, epidermal injury, local immune complex formation, and deposition of circulating complexes all seem to act in concert in the pathogenesis of cutaneous lupus.**

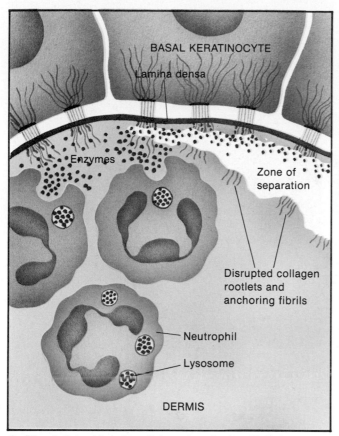

3. Dissolution of basal rootlets and anchoring fibrils by enzymes released by neutrophils. Early dermo-epidermal separation.

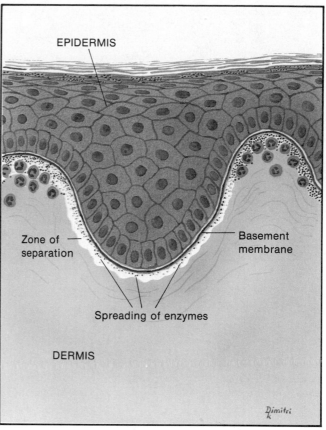

4. Concentration of neutrophils at the tips of the papillae. Spreading of enzymes along basement membrane. Lifting away of lamina densa.

BASAL KERATINOCYTIC INJURY WITH A LYMPHOCYTIC INFILTRATE OBSCURING THE DERMAL–EPIDERMAL INTERFACE —LICHENOID TISSUE REACTIONS AND DISEASES

LICHEN PLANUS

Definition and Clinical Features

Disorders involving lichenoid tissue reactions are so named because of a fancied or actual resemblance to certain lichens that form a scaly growth on rocks or tree trunks. Microscopically, lichen planus is distinguished by a **dense, bandlike infiltrate of lymphocytes and macrophages at the dermal–epidermal interface,** which is frequently obscured by the infiltrate. This infiltrate is so characteristic that the term **lichenoid** is used to describe other diseases that have a similar histologic appearance. Lichen planus is characterized by violaceous, flat-topped papules that usually appear on the flexor surface of the wrists. White patches or streaks may also be present on the oral mucous membranes. The lesions may be pruritic and chronic, lasting one or more years.

Pathology

The prototypic disorder of the group is lichen planus itself. The lesions of this disease present with compact hyperkeratosis, with little or no parakeratosis. The

(Text continues on p. 666)

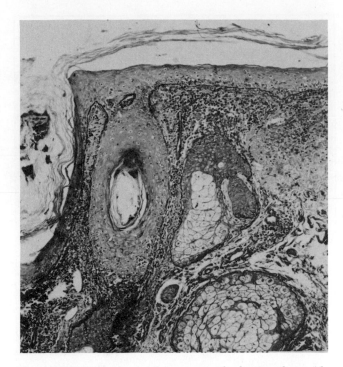

Figure 24-12. In lupus erythematosus, the lamina densa (the dark line separating the epidermis from the dermis) is thickened, and there is plugging of the hair follicle with keratin.

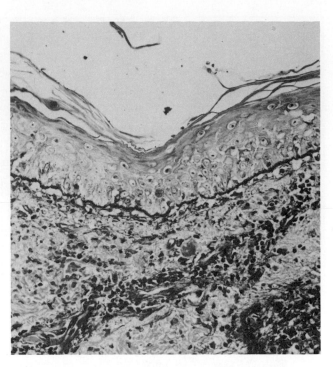

Figure 24-13. In this case of lupus erythematosus, the prominently thickened lamina densa with sublaminar vacuolization is evident.

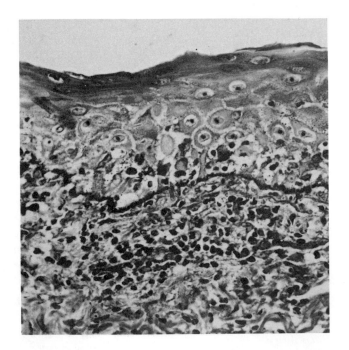

Figure 24-14. In this case of lupus erythematosus, the basal lamina is again prominently thickened. In this instance, the basal cells are vacuolated and poorly preserved, which is evidence of damage to these cells.

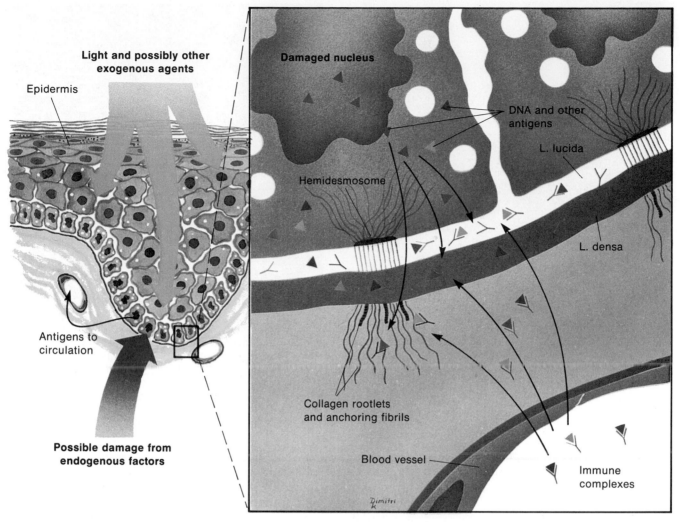

Figure 24-15. In lupus erythematosus, there is epidermal generation of a variety of autoantibodies, as well as deposition of diverse immune complexes in and about the basement membrane zone. The epidermis is damaged by light, other exogenous agents, and endogenous mechanisms, especially cell-mediated immune reactions. Such injury releases a large number of antigens into the circulation, some of which return as immune complexes. Immune complexes are also formed in the skin, and the complexes are deposited throughout the basement membrane zone.

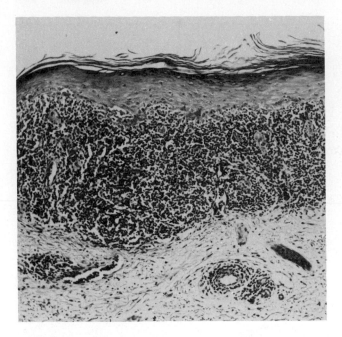

Figure 24-16. In lichen planus, there is a prominent band-like lymphocytic infiltrate.

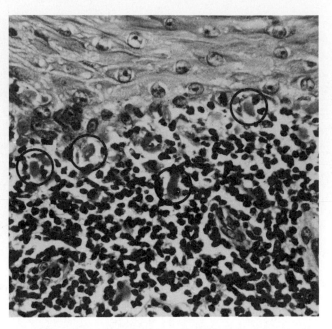

Figure 24-17. Lichen planus is often associated with a thickened granular layer, fibrillary bodies, and lymphocytic infiltrate. The pale grey, irregular bodies (*circled*) at the dermal–epidermal interface are fibrillary bodies.

stratum granulosum is thickened, frequently in a distinctive, focal, wedge-shaped pattern. The base of the wedge abuts against the stratum corneum. The stratum spinosum is variably thickened. **The distinctive pathology is at the dermal–epidermal interface.** The basal layer is no longer a distinctive row of cuboidal cells, but is replaced by flattened or polygonal keratinocytes. The normal, gently undulating, interface, which passes from the dermal papilla to the rounded profile of the rete ridge, is replaced by papillae that are densely infiltrated with lymphocytes and macrophages and separated by sharply pointed (saw-toothed), inwardly projecting wedges of keratinocytes. The entire interface is obscured by the infiltrate of lymphocytes, macrophages, and melanophages (Fig. 24-16). Commonly admixed with the infiltrate (in the epidermis or dermis) are circular, fibrillary, eosinophilic bodies that

are 15 to 20 μm in diameter (Fig. 24-17). These structures, which are variously termed colloid, Civatte, Sabouraud, or fibrillary bodies, are, in all likelihood, a manifestation of the focal death of keratinocytes. The fibrils within the bodies are similar to keratin filaments when studied by electron microscopy and with monoclonal antibodies.

Etiology and Pathogenesis

The etiology of classic lichen planus is unknown. It has been suggested that idiopathic lichen planus is similar in pathogenesis to graft-versus-host disease. An unknown agent injures the epidermal cells, thereby altering their antigenic structure (Fig. 24-18). The altered antigen is then presented by epidermal and dermal Langerhans cells to T-cells which, in turn, stimulate

Figure 24-18. Pathogenetic mechanisms in lichen planus. Lichen planus is apparently initiated by epidermal damage. This damage causes some epidermal cells to be treated as "foreign." The antigens of such cells are processed by Langerhans cells. The processed antigen induces lymphocytic proliferation and macrophage activation. The macrophages, along with T-cytotoxic lymphocytes, injure the epidermal basal cells, resulting in a reactive epidermal proliferation and the formation of fibrillary bodies.

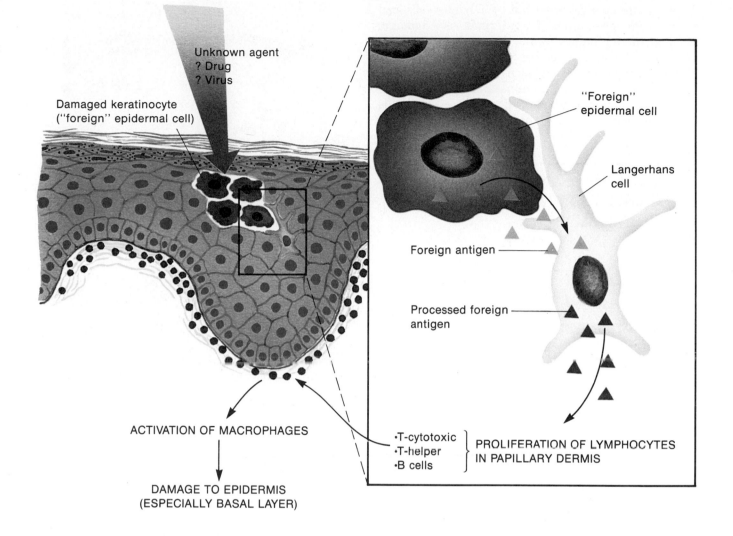

Unknown agent
? Drug
? Virus

Damaged keratinocyte
("foreign" epidermal cell)

"Foreign" epidermal cell

Langerhans cell

Foreign antigen

Processed foreign antigen

ACTIVATION OF MACROPHAGES

•T-cytotoxic
•T-helper
•B cells

PROLIFERATION OF LYMPHOCYTES IN PAPILLARY DERMIS

DAMAGE TO EPIDERMIS
(ESPECIALLY BASAL LAYER)

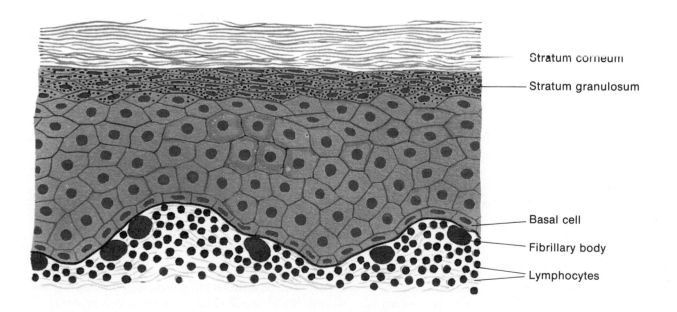

Stratum corneum

Stratum granulosum

Basal cell

Fibrillary body

Lymphocytes

B-cells. Lymphokines produced by T-helper cells lead to macrophage-mediated epidermal cell damage, whereas the antibodies formed by the B-cells are deposited in the skin, especially within the eosinophilic fibrillary bodies. Excessive reactive proliferation of the epidermis in response to immune-mediated damage is manifested by a brisk lymphocytic response and results in the distinctive pathology of lichen planus.

DISORDERS MANIFESTED PRIMARILY BY ALTERATIONS OF THE DERMAL CONNECTIVE TISSUE

SCLEROSIS OF THE RETICULAR DERMIS

PROGRESSIVE SYSTEMIC SCLEROSIS: SCLERODERMA

Definition and Clinical Features

Scleroderma is defined by progressive sclerosis and tightening of the skin. Its initial manifestation is frequently on the distal portion of the upper extremities and on the face about the mouth. Progression of the disease results in widespread thickening of the skin, with dense fibrosis and a striking decrease in cutaneous motility. A similar disease that involves only patchy circumscribed areas of the skin is designated **morphea.** Scleroderma is characterized by varying structural and functional involvement of internal organs, including the kidneys, lungs, heart, esophagus, and small intestine.

Pathology

The initial manifestations of scleroderma are in the lower reticular dermis, but eventually the entire reticular dermis and even the papillary dermis become involved. There is a diminution of interbundle space in the reticular dermis and a tendency for the collagen bundles to be ill-defined and parallel to each other. A patchy lymphocytic infiltrate with a few plasma cells is common, and may also be present in the underlying subcutaneous tissue. Sweat ducts are entrapped in the thickened fibrous tissue, and hair follicles are completely lost (Fig. 24-19).

Etiology and Pathogenesis

The cause of progressive systemic sclerosis is unknown. The presence of a variety of autoantibodies, which is

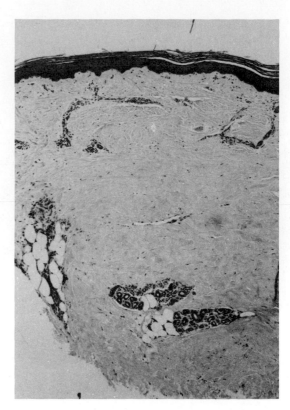

Figure 24-19. In scleroderma, the dermis is sclerotic and displays entrapped eccrine ducts.

somewhat reminiscent of the multiple autoantibodies of lupus erythematosus, suggests that some form of autoimmunity is involved in the pathogenesis of scleroderma. In this regard, chronic graft-versus-host disease is characterized by diffuse sclerosis that simulates scleroderma, at least in its cutaneous manifestations. There is some evidence that the patient with scleroderma forms antibodies to the centromere, as well as a distinctive antibody, referred to as SCL-70 antibody.

INFLAMMATORY DISORDERS OF THE PANNICULUS

PREDOMINANTLY SEPTAL PANNICULITIS

ERYTHEMA NODOSUM

A number of ailments are manifested by inflammation, of one sort or another, in subcutaneous tissue. These disorders are classified according to involvement of the subcutaneous septa, the lobule, or the subcutaneous blood vessels. One of the most common of these disorders—erythema nodosum—is seen in patients who have some other systemic disease, commonly one characterized by granulomatous inflammation. Erythema nodosum may also be an abnormal immune response to a drug.

Definition and Clinical Features

Erythema nodosum classically presents acutely on the anterior portion of the lower limbs of women as **dome-shaped, exquisitely tender, elevated, erythematous nodules.** These lesions come to resemble bruises and, finally, less tender, firm nodules that may disappear in time, only to be followed by other evolving nodose lesions. Many affected patients prove to have sarcoidosis, tuberculosis, or deep fungus infections, such as histoplasmosis.

Pathology

Early in the course of the malady, the lesions are in the fibrous septa of the subcutaneous tissue, where a neutrophilic inflammation associated with the extravasation of erythrocytes is seen. In chronic lesions, the septa are widened and show focal giant cell inflammation about small areas of altered collagen, as well as an ill-defined lymphocytic infiltrate (Fig. 24-20). At the

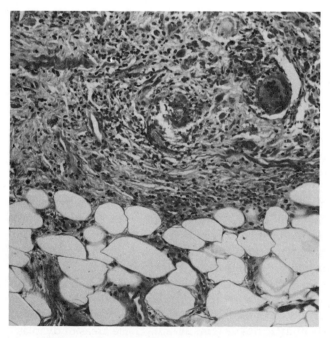

Figure 24-20. Erythema nodosum. A septal panniculitis with foreign body giant cells is evident.

interface between the septum and the surrounding fat lobule, giant cells and inflammation extend into the lobule.

Etiology and Pathogenesis

Erythema nodosum occurs so commonly in association with a variety of infectious diseases that it may be accepted as an altered immune response. However, the precise mechanisms underlying its development have not been elucidated.

PRIMARY NEOPLASMS OF THE SKIN

COMMON ACQUIRED MELANOCYTIC NEVI (MOLES)

Most people, regardless of their native skin color, who are exposed to a significant amount of light in the first 15 years of life, develop 10 to 50 moles on their skin. The moles do not ordinarily develop in areas protected from light, such as the breasts of women. Melanocytic nevi begin to appear between the first and second year of life and continue to emerge for the first two decades of life. The advent of significant numbers of moles beyond the twentieth year is regarded as abnormal. A mole is first recognized as a small tan dot that does not exceed 0.1 to 0.2 cm in diameter. Over a period of 3 to 4 years, the dot enlarges as a uniformly colored, tan to brown area. During this period of enlargement, the outline of the melanocytic nevus is regular and either circular or oval. When the nevus is 4 to 5 mm in diameter, it is flat or slightly elevated and stops enlarging at the periphery. When peripheral enlargement ceases, the uniformly colored, rich brown mole becomes sharply demarcated from the surrounding normal skin. Over the next 10 years, the lesion begins to elevate and the color is slightly diminished. Gradually, the mole becomes a tan skin tag. For one to two decades, it gradually flattens and the skin may return to a normal appearance. Most people experience a gradual decrease in the number of moles through the years.

HISTOLOGIC CHANGES

At the very beginning, an increased number of melanocytes in the basal epidermal layer is associated with hyperpigmentation. Subsequently, the melanocytes form nests at the tips of rete ridges, and melanocytes migrate into the dermis, where they form a cellular lesion. These small cells are circular and bear a superfi-

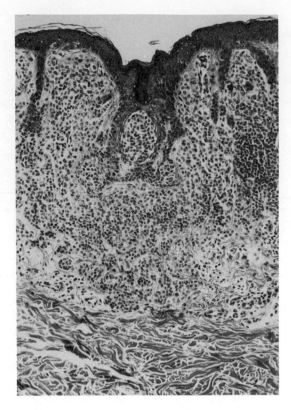

Figure 24-21. The melanocytes that form a compound nevus are within the epidermis and dermis.

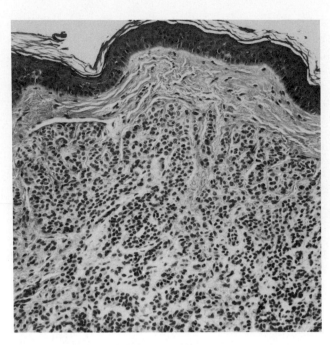

Figure 24-22. The cells of the dermal nevus are entirely confined to the dermis.

cial resemblance to a lymphocyte. With further passage of time, as the lesion becomes clearly elevated, the dermal component differentiates, and the cells evolve along the lines of Schwann cells, forming small structures similar to nerve endings. Gradually, this differentiation encompasses the entire dermal component of the lesion, and the core of a 20-year-old nevus may be composed of a delicate neuromesenchyme. This stage is followed by fibrosis, flattening, and eventual disappearance of the revus.

CLASSIFICATION

When the cells are limited to the basal layer of the epidermis, the lesion is called **lentigo.** At the stage of nest formation by melanocytes in the epidermis, the term **junctional nevus** is used. When nests of melanocytes are seen in both the epidermis and dermis, the lesion is labeled a **compound nevus** (Fig. 24-21). After intraepidermal melanocytic growth has ceased, the lesion is identified as a **dermal nevus** (Fig. 24-22).

DYSPLASTIC NEVI

Occasionally, common acquired nevi do not follow the normal pattern of growth, differentiation, and disappearance described above. Their evolution is flawed, and their differentiation aberrant. One or several moles in a patient with dysplastic nevi show focal areas of eccentric melanocytic growth, and become larger and more irregular. The peripheral irregular area is flat (macular) and extends asymmetrically from the parent mole. Initially, in these areas, the growth of melanocytes in the basal region of the epidermis appears no different from that which occurs at the beginning of the development of a common mole. It is abnormal in pattern, not in cytologic features. With the passage of time, melanocytes with large atypical nuclei that have some similarities to cancer cells appear. The combination of an abnormal growth pattern and cytologic abnormality of melanocytes (melanocytic nuclear atypia) defines a **dysplastic nevus** (Fig. 24-23). These areas of dysplasia are usually associated with a subjacent lymphocytic

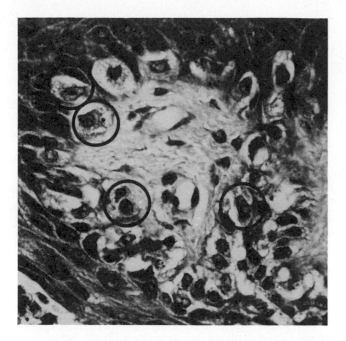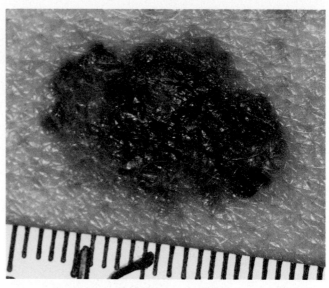

Figure 24-23. The large, epithelioid melanocytes with atypia that are characteristic of a compound nevus with melanocytic dysplasia are shown (*circled*).

Figure 24-24. The clinical appearance of the radial growth phase in malignant melanoma of the superficial spreading type. The larger diameter is 1.8 cm.

infiltrate. More than half of the malignant melanomas of the superficial spreading type have a mole precursor, the majority of which show melanocytic dysplasia, or have dysplastic nevi away from the site of the primary melanoma.

MALIGNANT MELANOMAS

MALIGNANT MELANOMA OF THE SUPERFICIAL SPREADING TYPE

The incidence of malignant melanoma of the superficial spreading type is increasing at a rate greater than that of any other form of human cancer. It is estimated that 1% of children born today will develop malignant melanoma.

Radial Growth Phase

Initially, the lesions of superficial spreading melanoma usually have a diameter of 10 mm or more and have a

slightly elevated and palpable border. The neoplasm is variably and haphazardly colored. Some parts are unusually black or dark brown, while lighter brown shades are mingled with pink and light blue tints. On the other hand, the entire lesion may be uniformly dark brown (Fig. 24-24).

On microscopic examination, large, epithelioid melanocytes are dispersed in nests and as individual cells throughout the entire thickness of the epidermis (Fig. 24-25). They invade the dermis, but are confined to the papillary zone. Here, the disposition of the cells is highly characteristic of the radial growth phase. The cells are arranged in small nests or as individual cells. No nest of cells has a growth preference over the surrounding cells (see Fig. 24-25). As a rule, the cells of the radial growth phase are associated with a brisk lymphocytic response. The cells of the radial growth phase grow in all directions: upward in the epidermis, peripherally in the epidermis, downward from the epidermis into the dermis, and peripherally in the papillary dermis. The net clinical enlargement of these lesions is

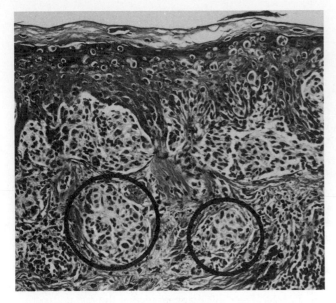

Figure 24-25. The histology of the radial growth phase in malignant melanoma of the superficial spreading type. Tumor cells grow at all levels of the epidermis, including the granular layer. Tumor cells are present in the papillary dermis (*circled*) but no nest has preferential growth over any other nest.

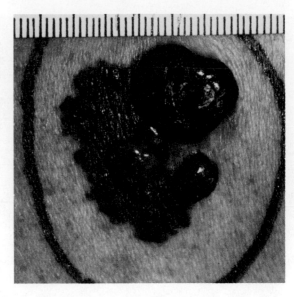

Figure 24-26. Clinically, the radial growth phase in malignant melanoma of the superficial spreading type is represented by the relatively flat, dark, brown-black portion of the tumor. There are three areas in this lesion that are characteristic of the vertical growth phase. All are nodular in configuration; two have a pink coloration, and the largest is a rich, ebony black.

at the periphery, along the radii of an imperfect circle —thus the name radial growth phase. It is critical that this phase be recognized by clinicians and pathologists because **tumors having the characteristics of the radial growth phase have not been observed to metastasize.**

Vertical Growth Phase

After a variable time (usually 1 to 2 years), the character of the growth of cells in the dermis changes focally. Foci of new cells appear in the dermis and the primary tumor possesses metastatic potential. The cells grow as spheroidal nodules (in a manner similar to the growth of metastatic nodules), expanding more rapidly than the rest of the tumor in the surrounding papillary dermis (Fig. 24-26). The net direction of growth tends to be perpendicular to that of the radial growth phase —hence, the term **vertical growth phase** (Fig. 24-27).

Although malignant melanoma was once regarded as a particularly malignant tumor, its reputation is no longer deserved. The prognosis is excellent if the lesion is recognized before it enters the vertical growth phase. **When the vertical growth phase produces a lesion that is more than 4 mm in thickness, however, 75% to 80% of affected patients will die of metastatic dis-**

ease, a figure to be contrasted with the negligible mortality in the radial growth phase. With proper awareness on the part of physicians and the general public, the mortality from melanoma should be less than 5%.

Metastatic Melanoma

Metastatic melanoma, the final stage in tumor progression, arises from the cells of the vertical growth phase. Initial metastases in malignant melanoma usually involve the regional lymph nodes, but metastases via the bloodstream are also common. When bloodstream metastases do occur, they are unusually widespread in comparison with other neoplasms; virtually every organ system may be involved.

MALIGNANT MELANOMA OF THE NODULAR TYPE

Even though a cancer generally acquires its properties in a stepwise fashion, occasional cancers may arise that have all of their characteristics expressed in the initial lesion. Nodular malignant melanoma illustrates this form of tumor progression. These lesions, which fortunately are the rarest form of melanoma in man, appear as circumscribed, elevated nodules that tend to be

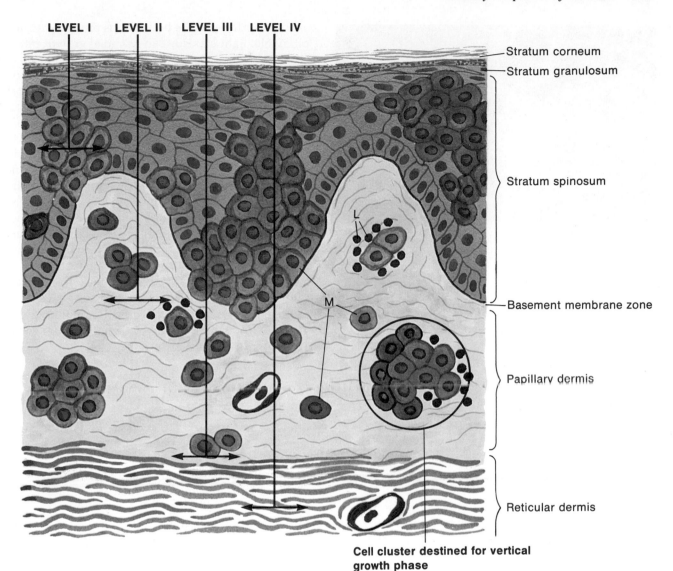

LEVEL I LEVEL II LEVEL III LEVEL IV

Stratum corneum
Stratum granulosum
Stratum spinosum
Basement membrane zone
Papillary dermis
Reticular dermis

Cell cluster destined for vertical growth phase

Figure 24-27. Schematic depiction of the radial growth phase in malignant melanoma of the superficial spreading type. In the **radial growth phase,** cells grow in the epidermis and are present in the dermis. They grow in all directions: outward, peripherally, and downward. However, the net direction of growth is peripheral—along the radii of an imperfect circle. Growth, as manifested by mitotic activity, is largely in the epidermis. No cells in the dermis seem to have a growth preference over others. The nest depicted here then evolves into a **vertical growth phase.** The anatomic landmarks of the levels of invasion are shown. Level III is not simply the occasional impingement of a tumor cell against the reticular dermis, but indicates a collection of cells that fills and widens the papillary dermis and broadly abuts the reticular dermis. Level III invasion is usually a manifestation of the vertical growth phase. Level IV invasion should be designated only when tumor cells clearly permeate between otherwise unaltered collagen bundles of the reticular dermis.

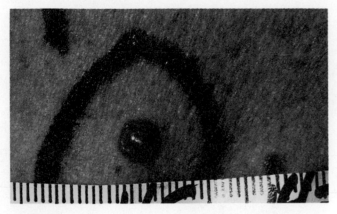

Figure 24-28. In malignant melanoma of the nodular type, the primary focus of growth of this 0.5-cm lesion is in the dermis.

exposed surfaces of the body and is probably related to ultraviolet light exposure. In its radial growth phase, it is a flat, irregular, brown to black lesion that may cover a large part of the face or back of the hand prior to the onset of the vertical growth phase (Fig. 24-29). The cells of the radial growth phase are seen predominantly in the basal layer, occasionally forming small nests that "hang down" into the papillary dermis. Invasion is not as prominent or as extensive in the radial growth phase of lentigo maligna melanoma as it is in superficial spreading melanoma. Cells of the radial growth phase, especially those disposed in nests, are of variable size. The subjacent dermis shows a modest lymphocytic infiltrate and, almost invariably, advanced solar degeneration of the elastic tissue. In the vertical growth phase, the cells tend to be spindle-shaped. Occasionally, cells of this phase synthesize connective tissue and form a firm plaque; this condition is called **desmoplastic melanoma.** Cells of the vertical growth phase may also grow along small nerves, forming a **neurotropic vertical growth phase.**

spheroidal initially—that is, they do not develop through a radial growth phase (Fig. 24-28). Histologically, the tumor is composed of one or more nodules of cells that clearly grow in an expansile (balloonlike) fashion in the dermis. The tumor is in the vertical growth phase from the outset. The prognosis is dependent, in part, upon the thickness of the spheroidal nodule when the tumor is removed.

LENTIGO MALIGNA MELANOMA

Lentigo maligna melanoma, which occurs almost exclusively in fair, usually elderly Caucasians, affects the

ACRAL LENTIGINOUS MELANOMA

Acral lentiginous melanoma is the most common form of melanoma in dark-skinned people. The tumor is essentially limited to the palms of the hands, soles of the feet, and subungual regions. Although rare, a similar tumor affects the mucous membranes, and is termed **mucosal lentiginous melanoma.** In the radial growth phase, acral lentiginous melanoma forms an irregular, brown to black, flat area that covers a large part of the palm or sole or arises under a nail, usually the large toe or thumb (Fig. 24-30). Microscopically, the cells are, for the most part, confined to the basal layer, and maintain

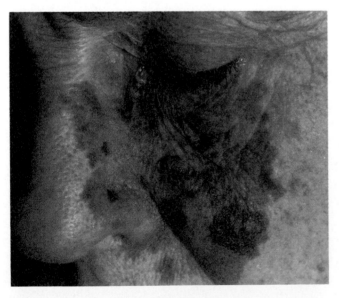

Figure 24-29. The radial growth phase in malignant melanoma of the lentigo maligna type.

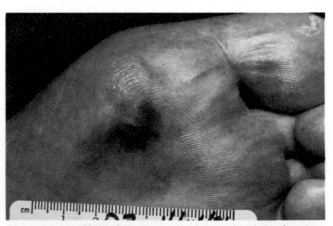

Figure 24-30. Clinical appearance of the sole of the foot in a patient with malignant melanoma of the acral lentiginous type (radial growth phase).

long dendrites. Frequently, a brisk lichenoid lymphocytic response is present. As the vertical growth phase approaches, cells may grow upward in the epidermis and become more epithelioid. The vertical growth phase is similar to that of lentigo maligna melanoma, and spindle cells are common. Neurotropism is also occasionally seen.

KERATINOCYTIC NEOPLASMS

BENIGN KERATINOCYTIC NEOPLASMS (INCLUDING THOSE OF VIRAL ETIOLOGY)

Seborrheic Keratosis

Although seborrheic keratosis is one of the most common keratoses of man, its etiology is unknown. It generally presents in the later years of life, and tends to be familial. The lesion is a scaly, frequently pigmented, elevated lesion, the scales of which are easily rubbed off by hand. Microscopically, the lesions seem to be tacked onto the skin, and are composed of broad anastomosing cords of mature, stratified, squamous epithelium, associated with small cysts of keratin called **horn cysts.** These lesions are innocuous, but represent a cosmetic nuisance.

Verruca Vulgaris

A number of interesting papillary hyperplasias of the epidermis are induced by viruses. Some of these are venereally transmitted (for example, condyloma acuminatum), whereas others are apparently spontaneous in origin. **An example of a viral papilloma is the common wart, termed verruca vulgaris.** It is characterized by pale, delicate, pointed spines that represent a circumscribed area of epidermal hyperplasia. Microscopically, there is marked hyperkeratosis and hyperplasia of mature stratified squamous epithelium. Early lesions show distinct, eosinophilic, intranuclear, and intracytoplasmic inclusions that are diagnostic of the viral infection.

Actinic Keratosis

Actinic keratosis ("from the sun's rays") is an atypical hyperplasia of keratinocytes. It presents in **solar-damaged skin** as a circumscribed area of hyperkeratosis, commonly on the backs of the hands or on the face. Microscopically, the stratum corneum is no longer loose and basket-weaved, but is replaced by a dense parakeratotic material (a result of the retention of nuclei in the stratum corneum). The underlying basal cells show significant atypia (Fig. 24-31). With passage of time, **these lesions may evolve into squamous cell carcinoma in situ, and finally into invasive squa-**

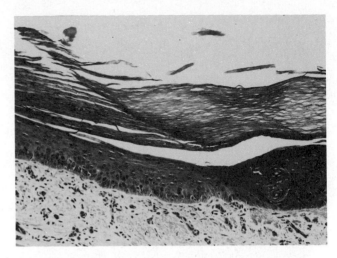

Figure 24-31. Actinic keratosis is shown on the left. Parakeratosis and loss of polarity are evident. The lesion is separated from the relatively normal epidermis by a diagonal line, which is a common histologic appearance.

mous cell carcinoma. The lesions are generally stable or may even regress.

MALIGNANT KERATINOCYTIC NEOPLASMS

Squamous Cell Carcinoma

The end stage of keratinocytic tumor progression, except for metastasis, is squamous cell carcinoma. These lesions characteristically arise on the backs of the hands or on the face. An area of localized hyperkeratosis, which is usually actinic, produces increasing amounts of keratin. Microscopic examination reveals atypical keratinocytic hyperplasia involving all of the epidermal layers (Fig. 24-32). However, of far greater importance is the extension of atypical keratinocytes into the underlying connective tissue as an invasive squamous cell carcinoma. These tumors have only a limited potential for metastasis, which is expressed more prominently in lesions of the lip.

Basal Cell Carcinoma

Basal cell carcinoma, probably the most common malignant tumor affecting humans, characteristically occurs in the same light-exposed areas as does squamous cell carcinoma. However, there are important exceptions, for basal cell carcinomas are associated with several unusual heritable syndromes, in which case they may occur in dark-skinned persons. Classically, basal cell carcinomas present as circumscribed, pearly papules, but they may also be associated with overlying hyperkeratosis and appear flat. Microscopi-

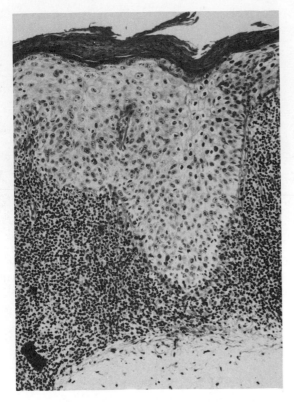

Figure 24-32. In this case of squamous cell carcinoma in situ, the entire epidermis is replaced by atypical keratinocytes. A brisk lymphocytic response is evident.

cally, buds of deeply basophilic cells protrude from the epidermis or extend into the dermis, forming large nests. These nests are separated from the surrounding mesenchyme by a delicate cap of connective tissue containing mucin (Fig. 24-33). It is unusual for lymphocytes to traverse this zone of mucin-containing connective tissue. Basal cell carcinomas have an interesting and favorable aspect in that they do not metastasize, except with exquisite rarity.

VASCULAR NEOPLASMS

ANGIOMA

Beginning in the middle years of life, scattered, small, cherrylike dots appear over the trunk and face; these angiomas are more prominent on the trunk than on the face. Microscopically, these tumors are composed of large, dilated, vascular spaces immediately deep to the epidermis. The small angioma is of no clinical consequence. Other forms of angiomas, such as cavernous hemangiomas, may be present at birth, and are responsible for disfiguring vascular birthmarks.

KAPOSI'S SARCOMA AND ACQUIRED IMMUNODEFICIENCY SYNDROME (AIDS)

Kaposi's sarcoma was once regarded as an esoteric, rare, cutaneous neoplasm, with genetic predominance

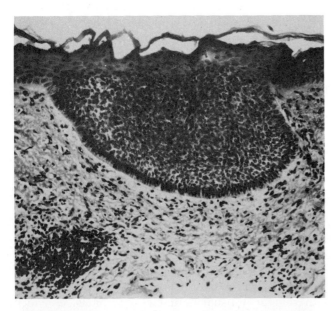

Figure 24-33. The tumor cells of basal cell carcinoma bud down from the epidermis, but are still attached to it. The peripheral, palisaded layer of cells is common in these lesions.

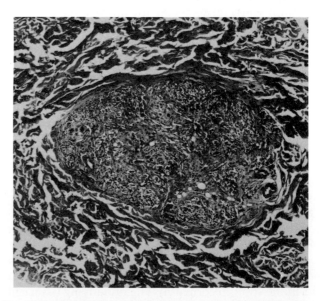

Figure 24-34. Nodular proliferative lesion in Kaposi's sarcoma. The blood vessels and spindle cells are growing as a tumor nodule.

in Africans, Ashkenazi Jews, and possibly, Italians. The disease usually occurred in the elderly male and had a distinctive clinical and histologic appearance. It is important to be able to recognize the classical form of Kaposi's sarcoma, for a similar neoplasm is one of the important manifestations of the acquired immunodeficiency syndrome (AIDS).

The classical form of the tumor generally presents on the lower extremities, often as a firm, brownish, circumscribed area. Microscopic study shows only **vascular proliferation throughout the entire thickness of the skin.** This proliferating vascular tissue, which may not be atypical, is associated with fibroplasia, patchy infiltrates of lymphocytes and plasma cells, and hemosiderin deposition. With the passage of time, these lesions undergo tumor progression. The plaques become firmer and present as elevated nodules. **Tumor progression is reflected by proliferation of fibroblast-like spindle cells,** which have the form of perithelial fibroblasts, immediately outside the proliferating vascular spaces. The cells gradually grow to confluence, forming a distinctive nodule (Figs. 24-34 and 24-35). The elongated spindle cells are tightly compacted and are associated with small columns of erythrocytes that are not apparently enclosed by an endothelial lining. The periphery of the neoplastic nodules exhibits patches of lymphocytes, true vascular proliferation, fibroplasia, and a scattering of plasma cells.

A similar neoplasm occurs in some patients with AIDS. These lesions are not necessarily present on the lower extremities, but may affect all areas of the body. Kaposi's sarcoma associated with AIDS may also be seen at sites of sexual contact. The vascular proliferation is typically more prominent than the typical spindle cell proliferation of classical Kaposi's sarcoma. However, with the passage of time, the lesions of Kaposi's sarcoma in AIDS may completely overlap classical Kaposi's sarcoma. Kaposi's sarcoma, when associated with AIDS, may result in widespread systemic lesions.

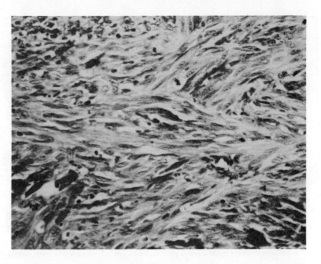

Figure 24-35. A higher magnification of the nodular proliferative lesion in Kaposi's sarcoma. In this last stage of tumor progression, the lesion is composed almost entirely of large spindle cells. These cells are sometimes separated from each other by erythrocytes in a single-file, linear array.

PRIMARY CUTANEOUS T-HELPER CELL LYMPHOMA (MYCOSIS FUNGOIDES)

Mycosis fungoides (cutaneous T-helper cell lymphoma) is a primary lymphoreticular neoplasm that originates in the skin. In its late stages, the disease may disseminate systemically, and is frequently manifested by the presence of circulating atypical lymphoid cells in the blood. This late stage of the disease is referred to as the **Sézary syndrome.** Early stages of mycosis fungoides are distinguished by the proliferation of lymphoreticular cells that do not have cytologic characteristics that permit a diagnosis of cancer. Occasional late stages have histologic features that are characteristic of malignant lymphoma.

25

THE HEAD AND NECK

KÁROLY BALOGH

Oral Cavity

Salivary Glands

Nose and Paranasal Sinuses

Nasopharynx

Ear

ORAL CAVITY

DEVELOPMENTAL ANOMALIES

LINGUAL THYROID NODULE

During its normal development, the thyroid gland descends from the base of the tongue to its final position in the neck. Heterotopic functioning thyroid tissue or a developmental cyst **(thyroglossal duct cyst)** may occur anywhere along the path of descent. The most common location is at the foramen cecum of the tongue.

BRANCHIAL CLEFT CYST

Branchial cleft cysts are thought to originate from remnants of the branchial arches (Fig. 25-1). Branchial cleft cyst occurs on the lateral anterior aspect of the neck or in the parotid gland, mostly in young adults. It contains

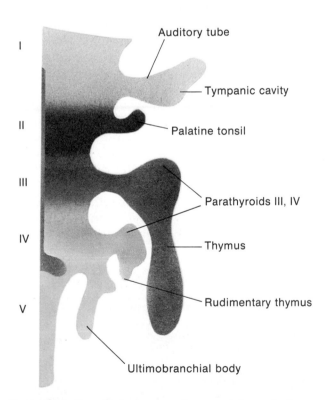

Figure 25-1. Branchial apparatus in man. Schematic diagram of the pharyngeal pouches (left half, ventral view) in a human embryo of six weeks. Five pairs of pouches give rise to many important structures of the head, neck, and chest. A wide spectrum of congenital malformations results from abnormalities of the branchial apparatus.

thin watery fluid, mucoid, or gelatinous material and is usually lined by squamous epithelium, although foci of ciliated respiratory or pseudostratified columnar epithelium are also seen.

INFECTIONS

The bacteria, spirochetes, viruses, fungi, and parasites found in the normal oral cavity are usually harmless. If the mucosa is injured or the defense mechanisms are impaired, for instance by immunosuppression, the organisms can cause disease, as in fusospirochetal gingivitis. Healthy persons may be carriers for pathogens such as *Corynebacterium diphtheriae* or meningococcus.

Inflammation of the lips is termed **cheilitis;** of the gum, **gingivitis;** of the tongue, **glossitis;** and of the oral mucosa, **stomatitis.**

BACTERIAL INFECTIONS

Aphthous Stomatitis (Aphthae, Canker Sores)

Aphthous stomatitis is a common disease characterized by painful, recurrent, solitary or multiple ulcers of the oral mucosa. The causative agent is a pleomorphic, transitional L-form of an α-hemolytic organism, *Streptococcus sanguis*. The disease is thought to be a hypersensitivity reaction to the bacterium. Microscopically, a nonspecific superficial ulcer shows marked inflammation and a covering fibrinopurulent membrane. The lesions heal without scar formation.

Acute Necrotizing Ulcerative Gingivitis (Vincent's Infection)

Acute necrotizing ulcerative gingivitis is caused by fusospirochetosis, that is, infection with two symbiotic organisms, one a fusiform bacillus and the other the spirochete *Borrelia vincentii*. The most important predisposing factor appears to be decreased resistance to infection associated with poor nutrition or poor oral hygiene. The disorder is characterized by punched-out erosions of the interdental papillae. The ulceration tends to spread and eventually involve all gingival margins, which become covered by a necrotic pseudomembrane. Severe fusospirochetal infection in persons who are malnourished, debilitated from infections, or weakened by blood dyscrasias, causes a rapidly spreading gangrene of the oral and facial tissues, termed **noma.** Large masses of tissue slough and leave the bones exposed (Fig. 25-2). This extreme complication of fusospirochetosis is more common in children.

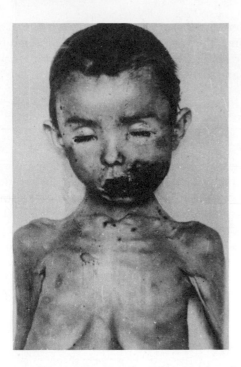

Figure 25-2. Noma. This 10-year-old boy had undergone starvation and contracted typhoid fever during World War II in Europe. The debilitated child developed an oral fuso-spirochetal infection with massive gangrene of the oral and facial tissues.

Syphilis

The lips or oral mucosa may be the portal for *Treponema pallidum* (primary stage). The secondary stage is characterized by diffuse mucocutaneous eruptions also involving the oral mucosa. The tertiary stage is characterized by necrotizing granulomas (gummas), which may occur in any organ, including the palate and tongue. (See Syphilis in Chapter 9.)

Systemic bacterial infections may manifest changes in the oral mucosa, e.g. in scarlet fever (see Chapter 9). Other bacterial infections that may specifically affect the oral cavity are diphtheria, gonorrhea, tularemia, anthrax, and leprosy.

FUNGAL INFECTIONS

Candidiasis (thrush, moniliasis) is caused by a yeast-like fungus, *Candida albicans*. To cause disease the fungus must penetrate the tissues, albeit superficially. The oral lesions appear as white, slightly elevated soft patches that consist mainly of fungal hyphae. Oral candidiasis is the most common fungal infection of the oral mucosa. It also is frequently seen in the mouths of diabetics and immunocompromised persons.

Other fungal infections of the oral cavity are rare in the United States, and include histoplasmosis, actinomycosis, coccidioidomycosis, cryptococcosis, sporotrichosis, North American blastomycosis, South American blastomycosis, and rhinosporidiosis.

VIRAL INFECTIONS

Herpetic stomatitis (also known as herpes labialis, cold sores, or fever blisters) is caused by herpes simplex. It is one of the most common viral infections of the oral mucosa in both children and young adults. The disease starts with painful inflammation of the affected mucosa, followed shortly by formation of vesicles. These rupture and form shallow, painful ulcers, ranging from punctate lesions to a centimeter in diameter. The ulcers heal spontaneously without scar formation. Transmission occurs by droplet infection, and the virus can be recovered from the saliva of infected persons. Microscopically, the herpetic vesicle forms as a result of "ballooning degeneration" of the epithelial cells. Some epithelial cells show intranuclear inclusion bodies.

Once the herpes simplex virus has been introduced into the body, it appears to survive in a dormant state and can be reactivated in diverse ways, including trauma, allergy, menstruation, pregnancy, exposure to ultraviolet light, and other viral infections. This is known as **recurrent herpetic stomatitis.** The recurrent vesicles almost invariably develop on a mucosa that is tightly bound to the periosteum, for example the hard palate.

Other viral infections that involve the oral mucosa are herpangina (caused by various strains of Coxsackie virus), measles, rubella, chickenpox, and herpes zoster.

TUMORS AND TUMORLIKE CONDITIONS OF THE ORAL SOFT TISSUES

BENIGN TUMORS

Papilloma

Papilloma is a common benign tumor that is often found on the tongue, buccal mucosa, gingiva, and palate, particularly adjacent to the uvula. The exophytic growth consists of numerous, small, fingerlike projections, which are covered by stratified squamous epithelium. Mitoses, particularly in irritated papillomas, may be frequent, but malignant transformation is exceptional.

Fibroma

Fibroma is the most common benign mesenchymal tumor of the oral cavity. It is seen at any age, but is most common in young adults. Fibromas are elevated lesions of varying size, and are sessile or pedunculated. They occur at any site of the mouth, but by far the most common location is the gingiva.

A condition microscopically similar to fibroma is known as **inflammatory hyperplasia of the gum.** This lesion, which can be focal or diffuse, is due to chronic low-grade irritation.

Peripheral Giant Cell Granuloma

Peripheral giant cell granuloma is a common lesion that has been known under a variety of names, such as epulis, giant cell reparative granuloma, giant cell tumor of gum, and osteoclastoma. The adjective "peripheral" denotes the superficial, extraosseous location of the lesion, as opposed to the "central" giant cell granulomas that occur within bones.

The prevailing view is that peripheral giant cell granuloma is not a neoplasm but an unusual proliferative reaction to local injury. In a few cases it is caused by hyperparathyroidism, in which case it can be regarded as a brown tumor of soft tissues. Although the growth has a variable clinical appearance, it always occurs on the gingiva or the alveolar process and seems to originate from the deeper soft tissues.

Histologic examination reveals a nonencapsulated lesion, with a striking and characteristic appearance. Numerous multinucleated giant cells are embedded in a fibrous stroma that also contains ovoid or spindle-shaped mesenchymal cells (Fig. 25-3). The lesion is vascular and shows foci of old hemorrhage, with hemosiderin-laden macrophages and chronic inflammation. The origin of the multinucleated giant cells remains unclear.

Hemangioma

Hemangioma, a common tumor of vascular tissue, is probably a hamartoma and not a true neoplasm, usually being present at birth or appearing shortly thereafter. Hemangiomas in the soft tissues of the mouth are similar to those of the skin, and may also be associated with a number of syndromes, such as **hered-**

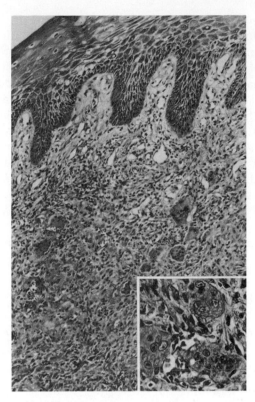

Figure 25-3. Peripheral giant cell granuloma. A protruding gingival mass contains multinucleated giant cells and spindle-shaped stromal cells. (*Inset*) Foreign body giant cells.

itary hemorrhagic telangiectasia (Rendu-Osler-Weber syndrome) and Sturge-Weber syndrome.

Lymphangioma

Most cases of lymphangioma are congenital, and almost all develop before adulthood. They are often seen in the head and neck area, particularly on the tongue, lips, cheek, and palate. Usually the lesion forms a diffuse, poorly delineated, soft and compressible pink mass without any gross or microscopic boundaries.

MALIGNANT TUMORS

Leukoplakia

Leukoplakia designates a white patch on the surface of a mucous membrane. A variety of diseases present clinically as leukoplakia, including various keratoses, hyperkeratosis, and intraepidermal (in situ) carcinoma. Thus, leukoplakia is not a histologic diagnosis, but rather **a descriptive clinical term.**

The etiology of leukoplakia is diverse, the most common incriminated factors being **tobacco, alcoholism,** and **local irritation.** The same factors are also important in the etiology of oral carcinoma. Leukoplakia may occur anywhere in the oral cavity, but the buccal mucosa, tongue, and floor of the mouth are the most frequently involved sites. The white plaques, which may be solitary or multiple, vary from small lesions to large diffuse patches of considerable size.

Biopsies of patients with oral leukoplakia have revealed dysplasia or carcinoma in situ in 7% to 12% of the cases and invasive carcinoma in 3% to 8% of the cases.

Carcinoma in Situ (Intraepithelial Carcinoma)

The biologic and morphological characteristics of this lesion in the oral mucosa are essentially the same as in other body sites.

Squamous Cell (Epidermoid) Carcinoma

Squamous cell carcinoma is the most common malignant tumor of the oral mucosa and may occur at any site. It most frequently involves the tongue, followed in descending order by the floor of the mouth, alveolar mucosa, palate, and buccal mucosa. The male to female ratio is 2:1.

Environmental etiologic factors in the pathogenesis of oral cancer include tobacco, alcoholism, syphilis, nutritional deficiencies (Plummer-Vinson syndrome), physical and chemical irritants, chewing of betel nut, ultraviolet light on the lips, and poor oral hygiene (craggy teeth and ill-fitting dentures).

Lymphatic metastases from oral carcinoma occur mainly in the submandibular, superficial, and deep cervical lymph nodes. Lymph node involvement at the time of diagnosis carries a poor prognosis. More than half of patients who die of squamous cell carcinoma of the head and neck have distant, blood-borne metastases, most commonly in the lungs, liver, and bones.

DISEASES OF THE TONGUE
MACROGLOSSIA

The tongue may be involved by various localized or systemic diseases, some of which can lead to its enlargement (**macroglossia.**) If present at birth, macroglossia is usually due to diffuse lymphangioma or hemangioma. Secondary or acquired macroglossia is due to amyloidosis, acromegaly, and infiltration or lymphatic obstruction by tumors.

GLOSSITIS

Inflammation of the tongue is caused by various microorganisms, physical effects, or chemical agents. Some forms of glossitis are associated with systemic diseases or vitamin deficiencies, such as pernicious anemia, riboflavin (vitamin B_2) deficiency, pellagra, and pyridoxine (vitamin B_6) deficiency.

DISEASES OF THE TEETH AND PERIODONTAL TISSUES
DENTAL CARIES

One of the most prevalent chronic diseases is dental caries. It affects persons of both sexes and every age group throughout the world, and its incidence has increased with modern civilization.

The cause of dental caries is complex; the main factors are microorganisms, host, and environment, with numerous interrelations among them. The colonies of several species coalesce to form a soft, nonmineralized mass known as **dental plaque.** The essential characteristics of cariogenic microorganisms (including *Streptococcus mutans* as well as other streptococci, lactobacilli, and actinomyces) in the dental plaque are their ability to (1) colonize and proliferate on tooth surfaces, (2) metabolize carbohydrates, and (3) produce acid, which demineralizes enamel.

One of the most important factors in the development of caries is a high carbohydrate intake. Raw and unrefined foods contain roughage that cleanses the teeth and necessitates more mastication, which further contributes to the cleansing of the teeth. By contrast, soft and refined foods tend to stick to the teeth and also require less chewing.

The presence of fluoride in drinking water protects against dental caries. Fluoride is incorporated into the crystal lattice structure of enamel, where it forms fluoroapatite, a less acid-soluble compound than the apatite of enamel. The fluoridation of drinking water in many communities has been followed by a dramatic reduction in the incidence of dental caries in children, whose teeth are formed while they drink fluoride-containing water.

Microscopically, caries begins with the disintegration of the enamel prisms after decalcification of the interprismatic substance, events that lead to the accumulation of debris and microorganisms (Figs. 25-4, 25-5). When the process reaches the dentinoenamel junction, it spreads laterally and also penetrates the dentin along

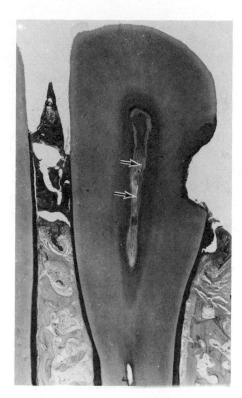

Figure 25-4. Dental caries. A large cavity close to the gingival margin is illustrated. *Arrows* point to the band of secondary dentin that lines the pulp chamber. This newly formed dentin is opposite the area of tooth destruction and was produced by the stimulated odontoblasts.

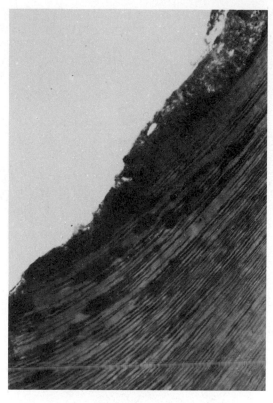

Figure 25-5. Dental caries. A deposit of debris covers the surface. Bacterial colonies (*black*) have extended into dentinal canals.

the dentinal tubules. Decalcification of dentin usually continues and leads to a focal coalescence of the destroyed dentinal tubules. Damage to dentin stimulates the odontoblasts that line the wall of the pulp chamber to form secondary dentin. Unfortunately, this reparative process usually does not prevent the microorganisms of the oral flora from reaching the dental pulp and causing pulpitis.

PULPITIS

Inflammation of the dental pulp, known as **pulpitis,** is a complication of dental caries, usually due to invasion by oral bacteria. In **acute pulpitis,** pain is caused by the increase in pressure of the pulp chamber by edema and exudate. Acute pulpitis may be accompanied by the formation of a small pulp abscess, and several small abscesses may lead to necrosis of the entire pulp. **Chronic pulpitis** may be the outcome of a subsiding

acute inflammation, or may be a chronic inflammation from its onset.

The most common sequel of pulpitis is the formation of chronically inflamed periapical granulation tissue, termed **periapical granuloma** (Fig. 25-6). Histologic examination of periapical granulomas reveals the presence of stratified squamous epithelium, which may be derived from a periodontal pocket, or from oral epithelium lining a fistula. Since this epithelium proliferates, a cavity lined by stratified squamous epithelium forms in this inflammatory tissue, and is labelled an **apical periodontal cyst.** A **periapical abscess** develops as a result of pulpitis, either directly or after the formation of periapical granulomas and cysts. This abscess, if not contained, rapidly extends to the adjacent bone, where it produces osteomyelitis. Bacteriologic cultures in all stages of pulpitis and periapical infection grow *Staphylococcus aureus, Staphylococcus albus,* various streptococci, or mixed organisms.

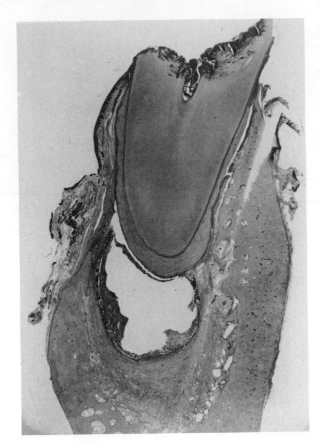

Figure 25-6. Advanced caries with periapical granuloma. The crown of the tooth has been destroyed by caries. Chronic infection of the pulp has led to chronic inflammation and the development of periapical granulation tissue.

DISEASES OF THE PERIODONTAL TISSUES

Scurvy, due to vitamin C deficiency, frequently affects the marginal and interdental gingiva, which becomes swollen and bright red and readily bleeds and ulcerates. Hemorrhage into the periodontal membrane causes loosening and loss of teeth.

A number of hematologic disorders affect the oral tissues, but some strike the gums with particular frequency. **Agranulocytosis** causes necrotizing ulcers anywhere in the oral and pharyngeal mucosa, but involvement of the gingiva is particularly common. **Infectious mononucleosis** is frequently accompanied by acute gingivitis and stomatitis, with exudate and ulceration.

Acute and chronic **leukemias** of all types cause oral lesions, including gingivitis, gingival hyperplasia, petechiae, hemorrhage, and ulceration.

Chronic **gingivitis** is one of the most widespread disorders of the periodontal tissues. Local factors that cause gingivitis include microorganisms, calculus, food impaction, tooth malposition or defects, irritating restorations or prostheses, topical drugs, and chemicals. The most important and most frequent causes of chronic gingivitis are microorganisms, alone or in combination with physical or chemical irritants.

Often the inflammation starts as a marginal gingivitis and, if untreated, progresses to severe chronic **periodontitis.** This disease occurs particularly in individuals with poor oral hygiene. Chronic inflammation weakens and destroys the periodontium, causing loosening and eventual loss of teeth. **Chronic periodontitis causes loss of more teeth in the adult than does any other disease, including caries.**

ODONTOGENIC CYSTS AND TUMORS

The mandible and maxilla, similar to other bones, are affected by both generalized and localized forms of skeletal diseases.

Odontogenic cysts have been classified according to the stage of odontogenesis during which they originate. The most common is the **radicular, or apical periodontal, cyst,** which involves the apex of an erupted tooth, usually following an infection of the dental pulp. The cyst is lined by stratified squamous epithelium.

Dentigerous cysts are associated with the crown of an impacted, embedded, or unerupted tooth, most often with the mandibular and maxillary third molars. The cyst forms after the crown of the tooth has completely developed, and fluid accumulates between the crown and the overlying enamel epithelium (Fig. 25-7). Dentigerous cysts are usually unilocular and are lined by a thin layer of stratified squamous epithelium. Among the potential complications of a dentigerous cyst are recurrence after incomplete removal, development of an ameloblastoma from the cyst lining or from epithelial rests of Malassez, and the development of squamous cell carcinoma.

Ameloblastoma is a tumor of the jaws, although rare cases have been reported in other sites (long bones, sella turcica). The origin of the tumor is not clear, but it clearly derives from odontogenic epithelium, most likely from cell rests of the enamel organ.

The large majority of ameloblastomas arise in the mandible, although they can also involve the maxillary antrum or floor of the nasal cavity. Radiographs, particularly of advanced tumors, show a multilocular cystlike appearance, with a smooth periphery, expansion of the bone, and thinning of the cortex. Microscopically, the ameloblastoma resembles the enamel organ in its various stages of differentiation; a single tumor may show various histologic patterns. Accordingly, the tumor cells resemble ameloblasts at the periphery of the epithelial nests or cords, where columnar cells are

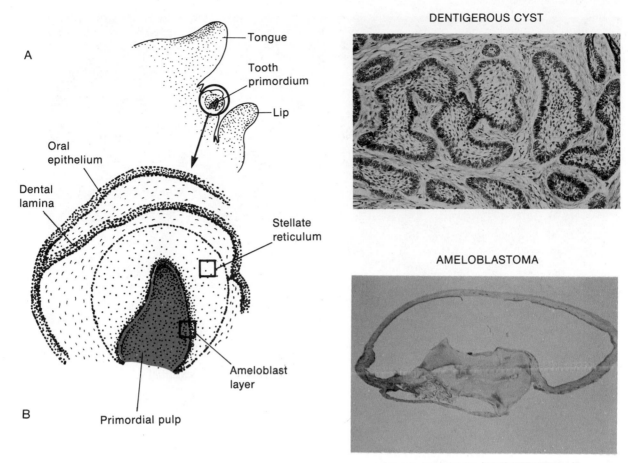

Figure 25-7. Development of dental and odontogenic tumors. Diagrammatic representation of the normal development of a tooth and the mode of formation of a dentigerous cyst and ameloblastoma. (*A*) Sagittal section of the lower jaw of a human embryo at 14 weeks, through the primordium of the lower central incisor. (*B*) Higher power representation of the circled area in *A*. The enamel organ at this stage is a double-walled sac, composed of an outer convex wall and an inner concave wall. Between the two are looser ectodermal cells (stellate reticulum). The stellate reticulum gives rise to dentigerous cysts, while the ameloblasts may form an ameloblastoma.

oriented perpendicularly to the basement membrane (Fig. 25-8). The centers of these cell nests consist of loosely arranged, larger polyhedral cells that resemble the stellate reticulum of the developing tooth. Frequently the complete breakdown of these looser areas results in the formation of microcysts.

The prognosis of ameloblastomas is favorable. Incompletely excised tumors recur, but malignant transformation is exceedingly rare.

SALIVARY GLANDS

INFLAMMATION

Acute suppurative parotitis is caused by the ascent of bacteria (usually *Staphylococcus aureus*) from the oral cavity when the salivary flow is reduced. It is most frequently seen in debilitated or postoperative patients.

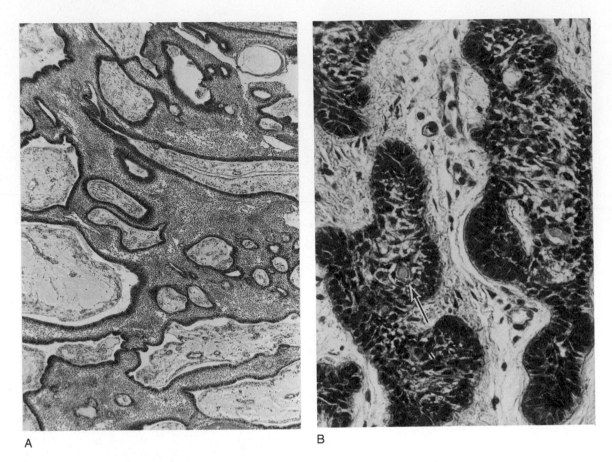

A   B

Figure 25-8. Ameloblastoma. (*A*) A common histologic pattern is characterized by
confluent islands of epithelium. The peripheral cells form a band that separates the
tumor from the stroma. (*B*) A higher magnification of *A* shows tumor nests with central areas of stellate cells and squamous cells. The arrow indicates focal keratinization.
The peripheral layer of cuboidal cells rests on a basement membrane.

Acute and chronic inflammation of the major salivary glands is often associated with stricture or obstruction of the ducts by calculi (sialoliths). The stagnant secretions serve as a medium for retrograde bacterial invasion.

Epidemic parotitis (mumps) is an acute viral disease of the parotid glands that spreads with infected saliva. The submandibular and sublingual salivary glands may also be involved (See Mumps, Chapter 9).

Sjögren's syndrome is a chronic inflammatory disease that is probably of autoimmune etiology. It is characterized by a set of inflammatory changes consisting of keratoconjunctivitis sicca (dry eyes), pharyngolaryngitis sicca, rhinitis sicca, rheumatoid arthritis, enlargement of the parotid gland (and sometimes, submandibular salivary gland), and xerostomia. Sjögren's syndrome may be accompanied by other presumably autoimmune disorders, such as primary biliary cirrhosis, chronic active (lupoid) hepatitis, dermatomyositis, systemic lupus erythematosus, scleroderma, polyarteritis nodosa, Waldenström's macroglobulinemia, and Hashimoto's thyroiditis. The overwhelming majority of the patients are postmenopausal women.

The involved salivary glands are, unilaterally or bilaterally, enlarged. Histologically, an initial periductal round cell infiltrate gradually extends to the acini until the glands are completely replaced by a sea of lymphocytes, immunoblasts, germinal centers, and plasma cells. Proliferating myoepithelial cells surround remnants of the damaged ducts and form so-called "epimyoepithelial islands" (Fig. 25-9). The irreversible destruction of the glandular acini causes marked dryness of the mucous membranes, and the rate of flow of saliva is below normal. Similar changes can be seen in the lacrimal glands and in the minor salivary glands (Fig. 25-10). (See Sjögren's Disease, Chapter 4.)

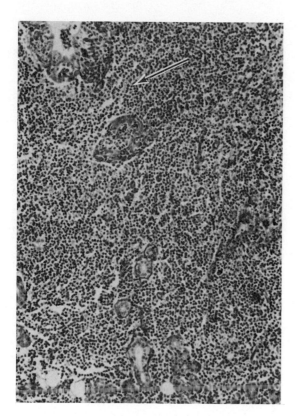

Figure 25-9. Sjögren's syndrome. A massive lymphoid infiltrate (*arrow*) and epimyoepithelial islands in the parotid gland are shown. Marked acinar atrophy caused xerostomia.

TUMORS OF MAJOR AND MINOR SALIVARY GLANDS

PLEOMORPHIC ADENOMA (MIXED TUMOR)

Pleomorphic adenoma is the most common tumor of the salivary glands, and is considered of epithelial origin. The tumor is about nine times more frequent in the parotid than in the submandibular salivary gland. It occurs most frequently in middle-aged persons and shows a female preponderance. Pleomorphic adenoma usually presents as a slow-growing, painless, movable, firm mass with a smooth surface.

Pleomorphic adenomas are characterized microscopically by a mixture of epithelial tissue intermingled with myxoid, mucoid, or chondroid areas (Fig. 25-11). The epithelial component consists of two cell types, ductal and myoepithelial. The cells lining the ducts form tubules or small cystic structures and contain clear fluid or eosinophilic, PAS-positive material. Around the duct epithelial cells are the smaller myoepithelial cells, which form well-defined sheaths, cords, or nests. Often the myoepithelial cells are separated by acellular matrix that resembles cartilaginous, myxoid, or mucoid material.

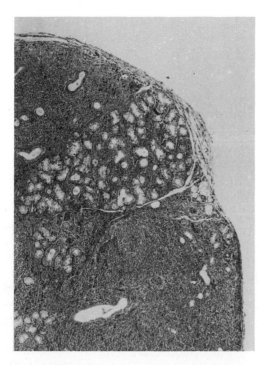

Figure 25-10. Sjögren's syndrome. A lip biopsy shows lobules of mucous glands infiltrated by lymphocytes and plasma cells. Slightly dilated ducts without acini indicate glandular atrophy.

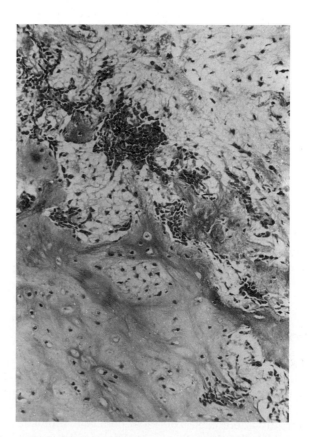

Figure 25-11. Pleomorphic adenoma of the parotid gland. Myoepithelial cells spread out into myxoid (*top*) and chondroid (*bottom*) areas.

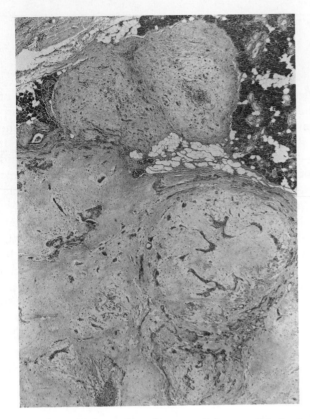

Figure 25-12. Pleomorphic adenoma of the parotid gland. The tumor contains characteristic myxoid and chondroid portions. The tumor is partly encapsulated, but a nodule protruding into the parotid gland lacks a capsule. If such nodules are not included in the resection, the tumor will recur.

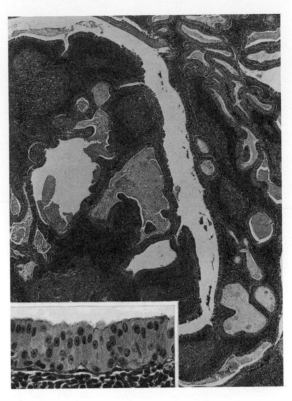

Figure 25-13. Adenolymphoma (Warthin's tumor) of the parotid gland. A compact portion of the tumor shows a papillary adenomatous arrangement in follicular lymphoid tissue. The cystic spaces and ductlike structures are lined by oncocytes. (*Inset*) Oncocytes have finely granular cytoplasm.

If the tumor is not carefully dissected at surgery so as to leave an intact capsule and an adequate margin of surrounding glandular parenchyma, tumor cells implanted during surgery or unresected tumor nodules continue to grow as recurrences in the scar tissue of the previous operation (Fig. 25-12). It is important to remember that recurrence of the tumor represents local growth and does not reflect metastatic disease.

MONOMORPHIC ADENOMA

About 5% to 10% of benign epithelial tumors of the salivary glands consist of epithelium arranged in a regular, usually glandular, pattern without a mesenchymal component. Such lesions are designated as monomorphic adenomas. The most common tumor in this group is **adenolymphoma,** or **Warthin's tumor,** which occurs almost exclusively in the parotid gland.

Adenolymphomas generally arise after age 50 years. The tumors are composed of glandular spaces, which tend to become cystic and show papillary projections. The cysts are lined by characteristic eosinophilic epithelial cells (oncocytes) and are embedded in lymphoid tissue with germinal centers (Fig. 25-13). The histogenesis of this peculiar tumor has been much debated. Lymph nodes, which are normally found in the parotid gland and in its immediate vicinity, usually contain a few ducts or small islands of salivary gland tissue. It has been suggested that adenolymphomas arise from the proliferation of these salivary gland inclusions.

Oncocytes are benign epithelial cells that are swollen with mitochondria, which impart a granular appearance to the cytoplasm. These cells may form **oncocytomas** (oxyphilic adenomas), solid tumors composed of nests or cords of benign oncocytes (Fig. 25-14). Most of these rare tumors occur in the parotid glands of elderly persons.

MUCOEPIDERMOID CARCINOMA

Mucoepidermoid carcinomas are composed of malignant squamous cells, mucus-secreting cells, and cells of an intermediate type. These tumors probably originate from ductal epithelium, which has a considerable potential for metaplasia. They account for 5% to 10% of major salivary gland tumors, mostly in the parotid gland, and 10% of those in the minor salivary glands. Mucoepidermoid carcinomas grow slowly and present as a firm painless mass. Microscopically, well-differentiated mucoepidermoid carcinomas form irregular ductlike and cystic spaces that are lined by squamous or mucus-secreting cells (Fig. 25-15). Even well-differentiated tumors can metastasize, but the 5-year survival is better than 90%, regardless of the primary site. On the other hand, poorly differentiated mucoepidermoid tumors have a much lower survival rate (20% to 40%).

ADENOID CYSTIC CARCINOMA (CYLINDROMA)

Adenoid cystic carcinomas constitute about 5% of all tumors of the major salivary glands and about 20% of all tumors of the minor salivary glands. Of all adenoid cystic carcinomas, a third arise in the major salivary glands and two-thirds in the minor ones. These tumors occur not only in the oral cavity, but also develop in the lacrimal glands, nasopharynx, nasal cavity, paranasal sinuses, and lower respiratory tract. They are most common between 40 and 60 years of age. The tumor grows slowly, but invades adjacent tissues. It is notorious for its predilection to infiltrate the perineural spaces and is, therefore, frequently painful.

Histologically, adenoid cystic carcinomas present varying patterns of cellular arrangement. The tumor cells are small, have scant cytoplasm, and grow in solid sheets or as small groups, strands, or columns. Within

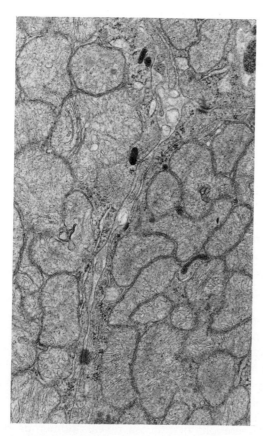

Figure 25-14. Oncocytoma of the parotid gland. An electron micrograph of oncocytes shows cytoplasm packed with mitochondria.

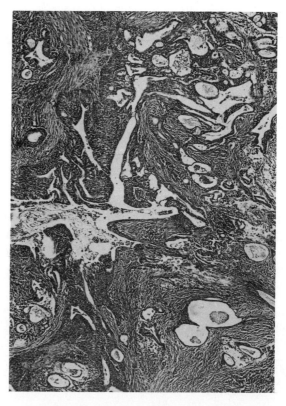

Figure 25-15. Mucoepidermoid carcinoma of a minor salivary gland. This tumor invades the fibrous stroma and forms irregular ductlike and cystic spaces. The cysts, lined by squamous and mucus-secreting cells, contain mucus.

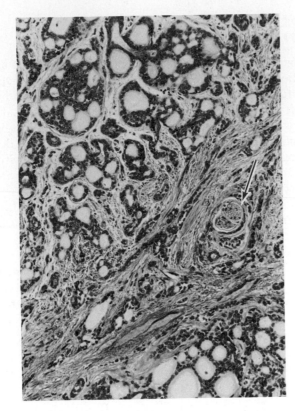

Figure 25-16. Adenoid cystic carcinoma. Groups and strands of small tumor cells surround round or oval spaces. The homogeneous material (hyaline cylinders) in the center of the cell groups is a product of myoepithelial cells, which have secreted it in contact with the stroma of the tumor. Perineural spread (*arrow*) is also a common feature.

these structures, the tumor cells interconnect to enclose cystic spaces, resulting in a cribriform (sievelike) arrangement. The tumors probably originate from the intercalated ducts. The myoepithelial cells produce the homogeneous material that is deposited around the cell groups and that gives them the characteristic cylindromatous appearance (Fig. 25-16). **Although adenoid cystic carcinomas grow slowly and do not metastasize for many years, their long-term prognosis is poor, because of local recurrence.**

NOSE AND PARANASAL SINUSES

DISEASES OF THE EXTERNAL NOSE AND NASAL VESTIBULE

Virtually all diseases of the skin can occur on the external nose, including lesions due to solar damage (for example, actinic keratosis, basal cell carcinoma, and epidermoid carcinoma). Marked hyperplasia of the sebaceous glands and chronic inflammation of the skin in **acne rosacea** are reflected in a protuberant bulbous mass on the nose, called **rhinophyma.**

The nasal vestibule is affected by various diseases of the skin, the most important being inflammatory or neoplastic. **Pyogenic granuloma** is an inflammatory lesion on the anterior nasal septum that appears clinically to be an ulcerated capillary hemangioma, but in some instances is produced by trauma.

DISEASES OF THE NASAL CAVITY AND PARANASAL SINUSES

INFLAMMATORY PROCESSES

Rhinitis

Rhinitis is defined as inflammation of the mucous membranes of the nasal cavity and sinuses. Causes range from the common cold to diphtheria, anthrax, and glanders.

The most common causes of **acute rhinitis** are viral infections and allergic reactions. One of the most frequent viral infections is the common cold (acute coryza). In viral rhinitis the virus replicates in the epithelial cells, after which the degenerating epithelial cells are shed. The mucosa is edematous and engorged, and infiltrated by neutrophils and round cells. Viral rhinitis is usually followed within a few days by secondary bacterial infections; the organisms are mostly normal inhabitants of the nasal and pharyngeal mucosa. Viral rhinitis causes abundant serous discharge that becomes mucopurulent after the bacterial infection and is accompanied by shedding of the surface epithelium. After the inflammation subsides, the epithelial cells regenerate rapidly.

Repeated bouts of acute rhinitis may lead to the development of **chronic rhinitis.** This disorder is characterized by thickening of the nasal mucosa because of persistent hyperemia, hyperplasia of the mucous glands, and infiltration by lymphocytes and plasma cells.

A large number of allergens is constantly present in our environment, and sensitivity to any one of them can cause **allergic rhinitis.** Often called **hay fever,** allergic rhinitis may be acute and seasonal, or chronic and perennial. The typical clinical and microscopic finding is **edema of the nasal mucosa,** especially of the inferior turbinates. Microscopic examination of the nasal secretions or mucosa reveals numerous eosinophils.

Polyps

If an allergic reaction is recurrent, fluid accumulates in the mucosa of the nose and paranasal sinuses, causing chronic mucosal swelling and enlargement of the turbinates. Eventually, mucosal edema may lead to localized bulging that grows to form polyps. **Allergic polyps** are usually multiple and appear as smooth, pale, movable, rounded tumors. They may be sessile or pedunculated, although the stalk is often not well seen. Polyps protrude into the airway and cause symptoms of nasal obstruction or, in the case of the paranasal sinuses, changes that are visible radiographically.

Nonallergic polyps arise in cases of chronic rhinitis and chronic sinusitis and are not related to allergic diseases of the nose.

Sinusitis

Acute sinusitis is caused predominantly by the extension of inflammation from the nasal mucosa. **Chronic sinusitis** is a sequel of acute inflammation, either as a result of incomplete resolution of the infection or because of recurrent acute complications. Any condition (inflammation, neoplasm, foreign body) that interferes with drainage or aeration of a sinus renders it liable to infection.

The accumulation of mucous secretions in a nasal sinus leads to the formation of a **mucocele;** a collection of purulent exudate results in **empyema.** Mucoceles occur most often in the anterior compartments ("cells") of the ethmoid sinus and in the frontal sinus. They develop slowly and by pressure cause resorption of bone (pressure atrophy). Mucoceles of the anterior ethmoid or frontal sinuses may be large enough to displace the contents of the orbit. Infection of a mucocele results in a **pyocele,** a sinus filled with mucopurulent exudate. Suppurative inflammation of the frontal sinus may extend to bone and cause **osteomyelitis.** The infection may also penetrate the bone and spread to the frontal and diploic venous system, thereby producing **septic thrombophlebitis.**

A life-threatening complication of sinusitis is the **spread of septic (or aseptic) thrombophlebitis to the cavernous venous sinus** via the superior ophthalmic veins.

Syphilis

The mucosal lesions of secondary syphilis are commonly observed in the nose and nasopharynx. In tertiary syphilis the inflammatory process may involve large portions of the nasal mucosa, the underlying cartilage, and bone. The gumma, a necrotizing granuloma, is usually perichondrial or periosteal, and therefore destroys nasal cartilage and bone. The nasal bridge collapses and the so-called **saddle nose** of syphilis develops.

Leprosy

Since *Mycobacterium leprae* multiplies more readily at a lower body temperature, it frequently infects cooler body sites, such as the nares and anterior nasal mucosa. Indeed, **nasal involvement is commonly the first manifestation of leprosy.** The skin around the nares and the anterior nasal mucosa shows nodules, ulceration, or perforations. The diagnosis is made by demonstrating the intracellular bacilli.

Scleroma

Originally named **rhinoscleroma,** this chronic inflammatory process usually begins in the nose and remains localized to this region, although it may extend slowly into the nasopharynx, larynx, and trachea. Scleroma is endemic in some Mediterranean countries, and in parts of Asia, Africa, and Latin America. Although the gram-negative diplobacillus, *Klebsiella rhinoscleromatis,* was identified more than a century ago, Koch's postulates were only fulfilled in the 1970s. The organisms, also known as **von Frisch's bacilli,** are present in the throats of many healthy persons, but the mode of transmission is unknown. The disease is successfully treated with various antibiotics.

The infected tissues appear firm, greatly thickened, irregularly nodular, and often ulcerated. Microscopically, the granulation tissue is strikingly rich in plasma cells, lymphocytes, and foamy histiocytes (Fig. 25-17). The characteristic histiocytes, referred to as **Mikulicz's cells,** are large macrophages that contain the phagocytosed bacilli.

NECROTIZING GRANULOMAS OF UNKNOWN ETIOLOGY

Wegener's Granulomatosis

Wegener's granulomatosis is a rare disease characterized by necrotizing tuberculoid granulomas that affect the upper airways. In its fully developed form it involves the lungs, kidneys, and small arteries throughout the body. The disease usually first presents as a mucosal thickening and granulations in the nose. In about half of the cases, the disease progresses to the classical triad of Wegener's granulomatosis, namely **involvement of (1) the nasal or sinus mucosa, (2) the lungs, and (3) the kidneys.** Microscopically the lesions reveal **necrotizing granulomas** with multinucleated

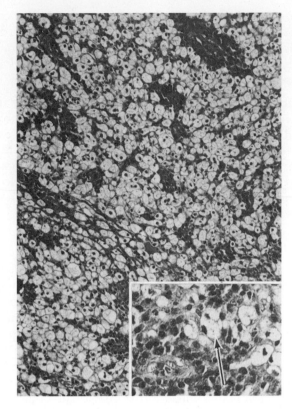

Figure 25-17. Scleroma. Granulation tissue contains numerous foamy histiocytes (Mikulicz's cells) and plasma cells. (*Inset*) Bacilli in the cytoplasm of foam cells appear as small granules (*arrow*).

- It is characterized by necrotizing, ulcerating mucosal lesions of the upper respiratory tract.
- If untreated, it is invariably fatal.

The clinical course is characterized by an insidious onset, with symptoms of nonspecific rhinitis or sinusitis. Gradually the nasal mucosa becomes focally swollen and indurated, and eventually ulcerated. The ulcers are covered by a black crust, under which the lesions progress to erode and destroy cartilage and bone. This destruction causes defects of the nasal septum and hard palate, with serious functional consequences.

There is now an increasing body of evidence that **lethal midline granuloma is probably a peripheral T cell lymphoma.** Similar infiltrates can also occur in the upper airways, lungs, and alimentary tract, but any organ may be involved, including the skin, lymph nodes, spleen, bone marrow, liver, kidneys, and central nervous system. Death is due to secondary bacterial infection, aspiration pneumonia, or hemorrhage from

giant cells (Fig. 25-18). Necrotizing arteritis and corresponding infarcts occur in such disparate sites as skeletal muscle and the spleen, and are often *not* associated with necrotizing granulomas. Focal necrotizing glomerulitis, as well as renal arteritis, may occur.

The etiology of Wegener's granulomatosis is unknown. Circulating immune complexes can be found during the initial phase of the disease and during relapses associated with infections.

The natural history of Wegener's granulomatosis is dismal. Untreated patients usually succumb within a year of the onset of symptoms, often in renal failure. However, immunosuppressive therapy (azathioprine) achieves prolonged remissions.

Lethal Midline Granuloma

Lethal midline granuloma, also known as midline lethal reticulosis of the face, shares two major features with Wegener's granulomatosis:

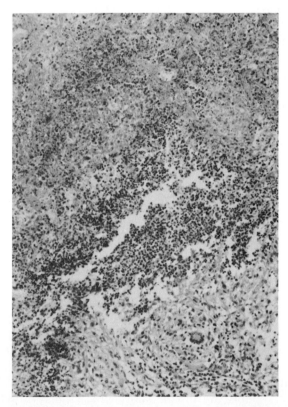

Figure 25-18. Wegener's granulomatosis. A necrotizing granuloma contains Langhans' giant cells. Extensive necrosis and acute inflammatory cells are seen in the upper half of the picture.

an eroded large blood vessel. The infiltrates are, at least initially, radiosensitive, and remission with cytotoxic agents has been reported.

INTRANASAL NEOPLASMS

Benign Neoplasms

Inverted papillomas involve the lateral nasal wall and may spread into the paranasal sinuses. They occur mainly in middle-aged persons. As the name implies, these papillomas show characteristic inversions of the surface epithelium into the underlying stroma (Fig. 25-19). Inverted papillomas recur frequently, unless surgical resection extends beyond the boundaries of the grossly visible lesion. Although inverted papillomas are benign, in about 5% of the cases they give rise to epidermoid carcinomas.

Malignant Neoplasms

Most cancers of the nasal cavity and paranasal sinuses are epidermoid carcinomas; about 15% are adenocarcinomas, transitional cell carcinomas, or anaplastic carcinomas. More than half of carcinomas of the nasal cavity and paranasal sinuses originate in the antrum (maxillary sinus); one-third originate in the nasal cavity, 10% in the ethmoid, and 1% in the sphenoid and frontal sinuses.

Several industrial chemicals have been implicated in the causation of cancer of the nose and sinuses, including nickel, chromium, and aromatic hydrocarbons. Occupational settings that carry an increased risk for cancer of the nose and sinuses (but for which a specific chemical agent has not been identified) are woodworking in the furniture industry, the use of cutting oils, and employment in the shoe and textile industries.

NASOPHARYNX

INFLAMMATION

TONSILS

Tonsillitis

Tonsillar enlargement is due to inflammation and hyperplasia of lymphoid tissue. **Acute tonsillitis is usually due to bacterial infection, most often with** *Streptococcus pyogenes.* **Follicular tonsillitis** refers to pinpoint exudates that can be extruded from the crypts. In **pseudomembranous tonsillitis** the necrotic mucosa is covered by a coat of exudate, for instance in diphtheria or in Vincent's angina.

Adenoids

Adenoids represent chronic inflammatory hyperplasia of the pharyngeal lymphoid tissue, which is often accompanied by chronic tonsillitis or rhinitis (almost always in children). Enlarged adenoids may cause partial or complete blockage of the eustachian tube, leading to serous or suppurative otitis media.

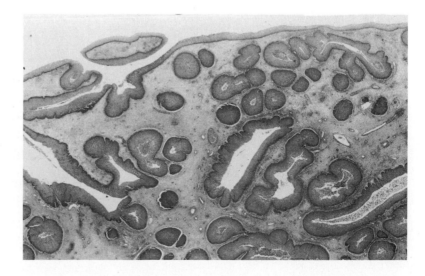

Figure 25-19. Inverted papilloma. Stratified nonkeratinizing squamous epithelium covers the surface and inverts into the underlying stroma.

Peritonsillar Abscess

A **peritonsillar abscess (quinsy),** usually the sequel of inappropriately treated acute tonsillitis, is an important local complication of tonsillitis.

NEOPLASMS

BENIGN TUMORS

Juvenile Nasopharyngeal Angiofibroma

Juvenile angiofibroma is a rare, highly vascular, non-encapsulated tumor of the nasopharynx that is histologically benign but locally aggressive. It occurs almost exclusively in adolescent males. Angiofibroma may grow into the fissures and foramina of the skull, or may destroy bone and thus spread into adjacent structures,

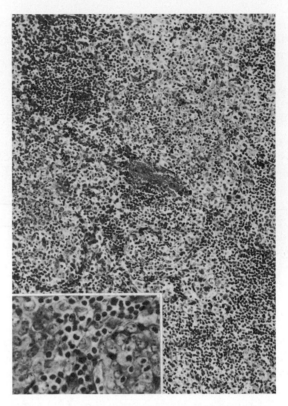

Figure 25-21. Anaplastic carcinoma of the nasopharynx. The cellular tumor is heavily infiltrated by lymphocytes. (*Inset*) Higher magnification reveals clusters of tumor cells with large nuclei and scant cytoplasm. The intermingled lymphocytes have smaller, dark, round nuclei.

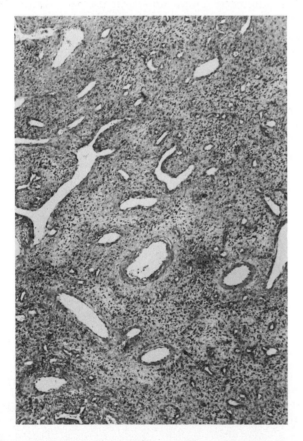

Figure 25-20. Juvenile angiofibroma. The tumor contains dense cellular fibrous tissue with numerous interspersed vascular channels of different caliber. The blood vessels have a varying configuration and a smooth muscle wall, which is often incomplete.

such as the nasal cavity, paranasal sinuses, orbit, middle cranial fossa, or pterygomaxillary fossa. Histologically, the tumor has two components, vascular and stromal (Fig. 25-20). Although surgery has been the treatment of choice, equally good results are obtained with radiation therapy.

MALIGNANT TUMORS

Epidermoid Carcinoma

Squamous carcinoma of the oropharynx often metastasizes because of the rich lymphatic network in this region. The primary lymphatics drain into the superior deep jugular and submandibular lymph nodes.

Anaplastic Carcinoma of the Nasopharynx (Nasopharyngeal Carcinoma)

By far the most common of all cancers of the nasopharynx, anaplastic carcinoma is the most frequent of all malignant tumors in the Chinese. In Hong Kong, nasopharyngeal carcinoma represents 18% of all cancers.

The Epstein-Barr virus (EBV) is present in the tumor cells and B lymphocytes of patients with nasopharyngeal carcinoma. Although a direct cause and effect relationship between EBV and nasopharyngeal carcinoma remains to be proved, the presence of EBV is a useful tumor marker, and serologic studies can help monitor the tumor burden or response to treatment in patients with known nasopharyngeal carcinoma.

Anaplastic carcinoma of the nasopharynx is a squamous cell carcinoma, with the passive participation of the nasopharyngeal lymphoid tissue. It displays clusters of poorly delimited cells with large oval nuclei and scant eosinophilic cytoplasm. The tumor is infiltrated by numerous lymphocytes (Fig. 25-21).

Because of their location, most nasopharyngeal carcinomas remain asymptomatic for a long time. Palpable cervical lymph node metastases are the first sign of disease in about half of the cases, and even then many patients have no complaints referable to the nasopharynx. The tumor does not form a large space-occupying mass or extend into contiguous cavities. Rather, it infiltrates neighboring regions, such as the parapharyngeal space, orbit, and cranial cavity.

Nasopharyngeal carcinomas are radiosensitive, and more than half of the patients with no tumor outside the nasopharynx survive 5 or more years. Metastasis to the cervical lymph nodes considerably lowers the survival rate, and cranial nerve involvement or distant metastases carry a dismal prognosis.

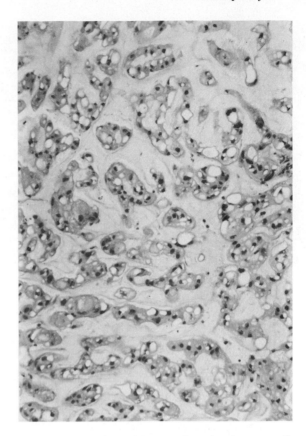

Figure 25-22. Chordoma. Nests and cords of tumor cells are surrounded by abundant acellular ground substance. The tumor cells have a characteristic vacuolated, bubbly cytoplasm (physaliferous cells).

Malignant Lymphomas of Waldeyer's Ring

Enlargement of a single tonsil in any age group or bilateral painless tonsillar enlargement in adults suggests the possibility of a lymphoma. The palatine tonsils are the most common primary site of malignant lymphoma, followed by tonsils of the nasopharynx and the base of the tongue. In these cases the cervical lymph nodes are most often involved by metastases. Histologically, 90% of nasopharyngeal lymphomas are diffuse, and more than half have been classified as large cell lymphomas. Virtually all malignant lymphomas of Waldeyer's ring are of B-cell origin.

Chordoma

About one-third of chordomas, tumors that arise from the vestigial remnants of the embryonic notochord,

occur at the base of the skull and extend to the nasopharynx. In the cranial region, chordomas originate from the region of the spheno-occipital synchondrosis. Histologically, these tumors show a variable appearance, but they characteristically have **large vacuolated (physaliferous) cells surrounded by abundant intercellular matrix** (Fig. 25-22). Chordomas usually grow slowly, but they infiltrate bone and are ordinarily not accessible to complete surgical removal. Few patients survive longer than 5 years.

Other Malignant Tumors

Other malignant tumors of the nasopharynx are rare. They may arise from various components of the mucosa or adjacent supportive soft tissues and skeleton. **Embryonal rhabdomyosarcomas** (Fig. 25-23) arise in the pharyngeal tissues of young children.

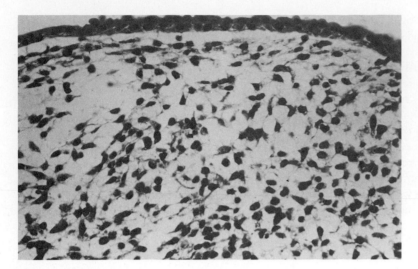

Figure 25-23. Embryonal rhabdomyosarcoma from the middle ear of a 3-year-old girl. This highly malignant tumor arose in the parapharyngeal space and invaded the adjacent structures. The oval or tadpole-shaped tumor cells under the middle ear epithelium have hyperchromatic, eccentric nuclei. The cells have immunohistochemical and ultrastructural features of rhabdomyoblasts.

EAR

EXTERNAL EAR

RELAPSING POLYCHONDRITIS

Relapsing polychondritis is a rare, chronic disorder of unknown etiology that may involve hyaline cartilage, elastic cartilage, or fibrocartilage. Relapsing polychondritis occurs alone or in association with one of the connective tissue diseases. The disease is characterized by intermittent inflammation that destroys the cartilaginous structures in the ears, nose, larynx, tracheobronchial tree, ribs, and joints. Noncartilaginous tissues, such as the sclera and cardiac valves, may also be affected. Aortitis can cause fatal rupture of the aorta.

Microscopically, the perichondrium is infiltrated with lymphocytes, plasma cells, and neutrophils, which also extend into the adjacent cartilage (Fig. 25-24). The chondrocytes die, and the cartilaginous matrix degenerates and fragments. Ultimately, the cartilage is destroyed and replaced by granulation tissue and fibrosis. The cause of the cell damage is obscure, although immune mechanisms are suspected.

AURAL POLYPS

Aural polyps are benign lesions that arise from within the external ear canal or extrude into the canal from the

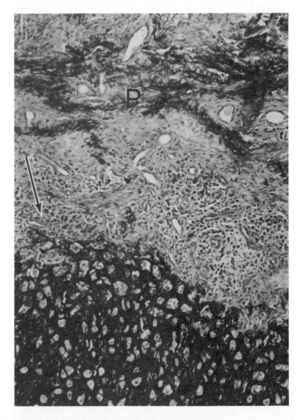

Figure 25-24. Relapsing polychondritis of the external ear. The perichondrium (*P*) is disrupted, and the underlying elastic cartilage is partly replaced by an ingrowth of vascular and chronically inflamed granulation tissue. The inflammation has extended into the cartilage (*arrow*). Elastic fibers are black (Verhoeff's elastin stain).

middle ear. The polyps are composed of ulcerated and inflamed granulation tissue, which readily bleeds. Polyps arising in the middle ear are secondary to chronic otitis media and can cause hearing loss.

MIDDLE EAR

OTITIS MEDIA

Inflammation of the middle ear cleft is usually the result of an upper respiratory infection that extends from the nasopharynx. The inflammation of the middle ear almost invariably extends through the mastoid antrum into the mastoid cells. In the presence of an infection in the nasopharynx, microorganisms may reach the middle ear by passing through the lumen of the eustachian tube or by spreading in the lamina propria of the mucosa as an extending cellulitis or thrombophlebitis. Acute otitis media may be due to viral or bacterial infections or to obstruction of the eustachian tube without microorganisms. Viral otitis media may resolve without suppuration, or the middle ear may be secondarily invaded by suppurative bacteria.

Dysfunction or obstruction of the eustachian tube plays an important role in the production of middle ear effusion. When the pharyngeal end of the eustachian tube is swollen, air cannot enter the tube. If the tube is blocked, the mucosa absorbs gases in the middle ear, and negative pressure develops. Over a period of time, this negative pressure causes transudation of plasma and, occasionally, bleeding in the middle ear. Acute otitis media is commonly classified as serous, secretory, hemorrhagic, or suppurative.

Chronic Serous Otitis Media

In chronic serous otitis media, the mucosal lining of the middle ear cleft undergoes changes that render it secretory, and mucus-producing goblet cells become preponderant. If an episode of obstruction occurs acutely, for example in the mastoid cells, there may be accompanying hemorrhage. Extravasation of blood and the degradation of red blood cells liberate cholesterol. Crystals of cholesterol stimulate a foreign body reaction, with the formation of granulation tissue, referred to as a **cholesterol granuloma.** Large cholesterol granulomas may destroy tissue in the mastoid or antrum. If the cholesterol granuloma is allowed to persist for many months, the granulation tissue may become fibrotic, a process that eventually results in complete obliteration of the middle ear and mastoid by fibrous tissue.

Acute Suppurative Otitis Media

One of the most common infections of childhood, **acute suppurative otitis media, is caused by virulent pyogenic bacteria that invade the middle ear.** Infection of the nasopharynx may lead to the passage of bacteria up the eustachian tube. When tubal obstruction is partially relieved, reflux of mucus-containing microorganisms may infect the middle ear. *Streptococcus pneumoniae* is the most common causative agent in all age groups (30% to 40%). *Haemophilus influenzae* causes about 20% of cases and is less frequent with increasing age. In about a quarter of cases, no bacteria can be cultured.

If the pressure of the purulent exudate in the middle ear sufficiently increases, the eardrum spontaneously ruptures, and the pus is then discharged. In most cases the infection is self-limited, and even without therapy tends to heal. A few untreated patients continue to have suppuration and develop chronic otitis media.

Chronic Suppurative Otitis Media and Mastoiditis

Neglected or recurrent infection of the middle ear and mastoid process may eventually produce a chronic inflammation of the mucosa or destruction of the periosteum covering the ossicles. Chronic otitis media is much more common in persons who had ear disease in early childhood.

Chronic otitis media can be active, quiescent, or inactive. Usually the process is insidious, persistent, and destructive. By definition, the eardrum is always perforated; consequently, painless discharge (otorrhea) and varying degrees of hearing loss are constant symptoms of chronic otitis media. If the granulation tissue becomes exuberant, it may form polyps, which can extend through the perforated ear drum into the external ear canal.

Perforation of the eardrum may allow squamous epithelium from the external ear canal to grow into the middle ear, where it continues to produce keratin. The resultant mass, composed of accumulated keratin, is known as a **cholesteatoma.** Microscopically, cholesteatomas are identical to epidermal inclusion cysts, and are surrounded by granulation tissue and fibrosis. They frequently become infected, and the keratin mass harbors bacteria that are inaccessible to antibiotic therapy. The principal dangers of cholesteatoma arise from erosion of bone, a process that may lead to the destruction of important contiguous structures (auditory ossicles, facial nerve, labyrinth).

Many different bacteria are associated with chronic suppurative otitis media. Some are obvious or probable pathogens, while others are common saprophytes. Most organisms are aerobes; *Streptococcus pneumoniae, Haemophilus influenzae,* staphylococci, gram-negative bacilli, and diphtheroids are common.

Complications of Acute and Chronic Otitis Media

As a result of antibiotic treatment, complications of otitis media are now rare. However, a potential for serious, and even fatal, complications still exists with any suppurative inflammation of the middle ear cleft. Factors influencing the spread of infection beyond the middle ear space include the type and virulence of pathogenic organisms, the adequacy of treatment, and host resistance (for instance diabetes, leukemia, immunosuppressive therapy).

Infection can extend from the middle ear cleft to other contiguous structures. The following cranial and intracranial complications may develop:

- Destruction of the facial nerve (chorda tympani)
- Deep cervical or subperiosteal abscess, when the cortical bone of the mastoid process is eroded
- Petrositis, when the infection spreads to the petrous portion of the temporal bone via the chain of air cells
- Suppurative labyrinthitis, when the infection extends to the internal ear
- Epidural, subdural, or cerebral abscess, after extension of the infection through the inner table of the mastoid bone

- Meningitis, when the infection extends to the meninges
- Thrombophlebitis of the sigmoid sinus, which occurs when the infection spreads through the dura to the posterior cranial fossa

INTERNAL (OR INNER) EAR

OTOSCLEROSIS

Otosclerosis is defined as a new formation of spongy bone about the stapes and the oval window that results in progressive deafness. The disorder, a hereditary defect of unknown etiology, is the most common cause of conductive hearing loss in young adults and middle-aged people in the United States. An autosomal dominant gene, with variable penetrance, transmits this trait. About 10% of white and 1% of black adult Americans have some degree of otosclerosis, although 90% of cases are asymptomatic. The female to male ratio is 2:1, and both ears are usually affected.

Though any part of the petrous bone may be affected, otosclerotic bone tends to form at particular points. The most frequent site is immediately anterior to the oval window (80% to 90% of all cases). The focus of sclerotic bone extends posteriorly and may infiltrate and replace the stapes. This process progressively immobilizes the footplate of the stapes, and the developing bony ankylosis (Fig. 25-25) is functionally

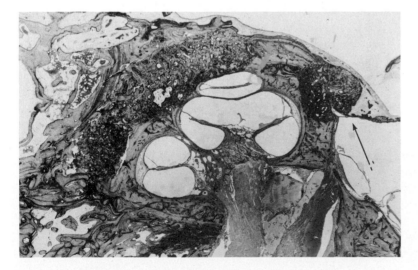

Figure 25-25. Otosclerosis. Otosclerotic foci appear as dark areas in the bony labyrinth. The arrow points to the anterior margin of the oval window, where otosclerosis has involved the footplate of the stapes and has caused bony ankylosis.

manifested by a slowly progressive conductive hearing loss.

MENIERE'S DISEASE

This common disorder is characterized by episodes of vertigo, sensorineural hearing loss, and usually tinnitus. A wide variety of etiologic factors has been incriminated, but the cause of Meniere's disease remains uncertain. Its pathologic correlate is **hydropic distention of the endolymphatic system,** which is bilateral in about 15% of patients. It is believed that the symptoms of Meniere's disease occur when the endolymphatic hydrops causes ruptures, and the endolymph escapes into the perilymph.

LABYRINTHINE TOXICITY

Drug-induced damage to the inner ear, usually dose-related, is the most frequent and serious cause of labyrinthine toxicity. The best-known drugs that manifest ototoxic side effects are the aminoglycoside antibiotics, which cause irreversible damage to the vestibular or cochlear sensory cells. Other antibiotics, diuretics, antimalarial drugs, nitrogen mustard, and salicylates may also cause transient or permanent sensorineural hearing loss. The labyrinth of the embryo is especially sensitive to some drugs (congenital deafness due to thalidomide, quinine, chloroquine).

VIRAL LABYRINTHITIS

Viral infections are becoming increasingly recognized as the cause of several inner ear disorders, particularly **deafness.** Most cases represent a hematogenous invasion of the labyrinth by the virus. The best-known prenatal viral infections that cause congenital deafness through maternal-to-fetal transmission include **cytomegalovirus** and **rubella** syndromes. Among the postnatal viral infections, **mumps** is the most common cause of deafness.

ACOUSTIC TRAUMA

Noise-induced hearing loss is a significant health problem in industrialized countries. The earliest changes occur in the external hair cells of the organ of Corti. The loss of sensory hairs is followed by deformation, swelling, and disintegration of the hair cells.

NEOPLASMS

Schwannomas

Nearly all of the schwannomas in the internal auditory canal originate from the **vestibular nerves.** Vestibular schwannomas, which account for about 10% of all intracranial tumors, are generally slow-growing and encapsulated. Larger tumors protrude from the internal auditory meatus into the cerebellopontine angle and may deform the brain stem and adjacent cerebellum. The tumor causes vestibular and auditory symptoms that are usually slowly progressive.

Von Recklinghausen's disease is characterized by a high incidence of bilateral vestibular schwannomas. Histologically, these tumors are indistinguishable from other vestibular schwannomas.

Meningiomas

Meningiomas of the cerebellopontine angle originate from the meningothelial cells in the arachnoid villi. The favored sites for these tumors are the sphenoid ridge and the petrous pyramid. Meningiomas may extend into the adjacent temporal bone or dural sinuses.

26

BONES AND JOINTS

ALAN L. SCHILLER

BONES

DISORDERS OF GROWTH AND MATURATION OF THE SKELETON

DELAYED OR DISORGANIZED CARTILAGE MATURATION

CRETINISM

Cretinism, which results from maternal iodine deficiency, has profound effects on the skeleton, including severe dwarfism and delayed appearance of the deciduous teeth. The fontanels of the skull do not close, and there is a delay in closure of the epiphyses, as well as radiologic stippling of the epiphyses. **The histopathology is related to a defect in cartilage maturation.** Endochondral ossification does not proceed appropriately, and metaphyseal transverse bars of bone seal off the epiphyseal plate from further capillary invasion. The failure of endochondral ossification produces severe dwarfism.

DISORDERS OF THE EPIPHYSEAL PLATE

ACHONDROPLASIA

Achondroplasia, a genetic disease characterized by dwarfism with short extremities and a normal trunk for which the specific defect is unknown, is one of the most common types of dwarfism. The epiphyseal plate is greatly thinned, and the zone of proliferative cartilage is either absent or extensively attenuated. The zone of provisional calcification, if present, undergoes endochondral ossification, but at a greatly reduced rate. A transverse bar of bone often seals off the epiphyseal plate, thus preventing extensive bone formation and causing dwarfism.

OSTEOCHONDROMA

An osteochondroma is frequently classified as a neoplasm, but it is actually an abnormality that arises from a defect at the ring of Ranvier of the epiphyseal plate. If the ring of Ranvier is absent or defective, epiphyseal cartilage grows laterally into the soft tissue. Vessels originating in the marrow cavity of the bone extend into this cartilage mass. If this process continues, a cartilage-capped, bony, stalked osteochondroma results,

which is in direct continuity with the marrow cavity of the parent bone (Fig. 26-1).

There are two forms of this disease. The most common is a **solitary osteochondroma,** which may have to be removed if it is cosmetically displeasing or presses on an artery or nerve. A second form of the disease, termed **hereditary multiple osteochondromatosis,** is inherited as an autosomal dominant disorder, and is characterized by multiple osteochondromas.

MODELING ABNORMALITIES

OSTEOPETROSIS

Osteopetrosis, or marble bone disease of Albers-Schönberg, is a rare disorder characterized by abnormally dense bone. The autosomal recessive form is a severe, sometimes fatal disease affecting infants and children. The death of infants with this severe variant is attributable to marked anemia, cranial nerve entrapment, hydrocephalus, and infections. A more benign form, which is transmitted as an autosomal dominant trait and presents in adulthood or adolescence, is associated with mild anemia or no symptoms at all. The defect involves defective bone remodeling and, more specifically, the function of osteoclasts. Hypofunction of the osteoclasts results in the retention of the primary spongiosum with its cartilage cores, lack of funnelization of the metaphysis, and a thickened cortex. The result is short, blocklike, radiodense bones—hence, the term marble bone disease (Fig. 26-2).

DELAYED BONE MATURATION

OSTEOGENESIS IMPERFECTA

Osteogenesis imperfecta refers to a group of heritable disorders of the connective tissues, which tend to affect the skeleton, joints, ears, ligaments, teeth, sclerae, and skin. The basic disorder is the defective synthesis of collagen. There are at least four types of osteogenesis imperfecta, each with a different mode of inheritance and clinical features.

Osteogenesis Imperfecta Type I

Type I osteogenesis imperfecta, inherited as an autosomal dominant disorder, is a common form of the disease. It is characterized by multiple fractures after birth, blue sclerae, and hearing abnormalities. The initial fractures usually occur after the infant begins to sit and walk. There may be hundreds of fractures a year initiated by minor movement or trauma. On radiologic ex-

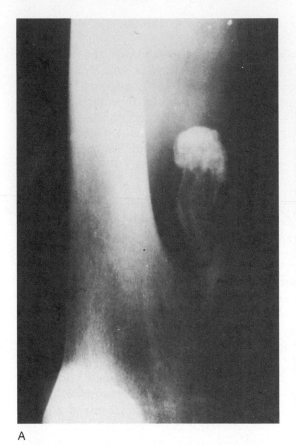

A

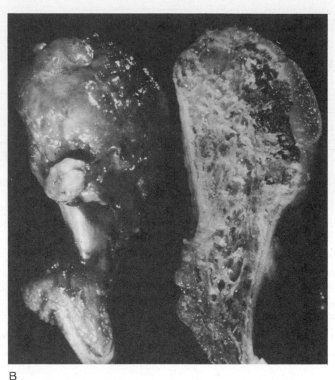

B

Figure 26-1. Osteochondroma. (*A*) A radiograph of an osteochondroma growing at the distal end of the femur shows a lesion that is directly contiguous with the marrow space. The osteochondroma grows away from the joint and is capped by radiodense, calcified cartilage. (*B*) The gross specimen of the resected osteochondroma shows the cap of calcified cartilage, the coarse cancellous bone, and the communication with the medullary cavity of the femur.

amination, the bones are extremely thin, delicate, and abnormally curved (Fig. 26-3).

Osteogenesis Imperfecta Type II

Type II osteogenesis imperfecta is a lethal, perinatal disease. In some families, it is inherited as an autosomal recessive disorder, although it also occurs sporadically. Those affected are stillborn or die within a few days. These infants are, in a sense, crushed to death. Almost all of the bones sustain fractures during delivery or during uterine contractions in labor. As in type I, the sclerae are blue.

Osteogenesis Imperfecta Type III

Type III osteogenesis imperfecta, the progressive, deforming type of this disease, is characterized by many bone fractures, growth retardation, and severe skeletal deformities. It seems to be inherited as an autosomal recessive disorder. The fractures are present at birth,

but the bones seem to be less fragile than in the type II form. These patients may eventually develop severe shortening of their stature because of progressive bone fractures and severe kyphoscoliosis.

Osteogenesis Imperfecta Type IV

Type IV osteogenesis imperfecta, which is inherited as an autosomal dominant disorder, is similar to type I, except that the sclerae are normal.

ENCHONDROMATOSIS (OLLIER'S DISEASE)

Although enchondromatosis is not specifically a disease of delayed maturation of bone, it is a condition in which residual hyaline cartilage, anlage cartilage, or cartilage from the epiphyseal plate does not undergo endochondral ossification and remains in the bones. As a consequence, the bones show multiple, tumorlike masses of abnormally arranged hyaline cartilage, with

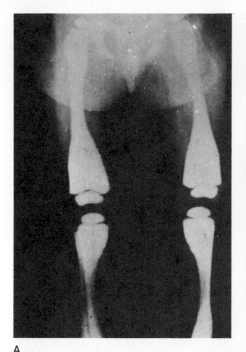
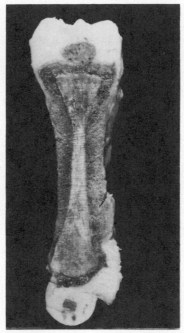
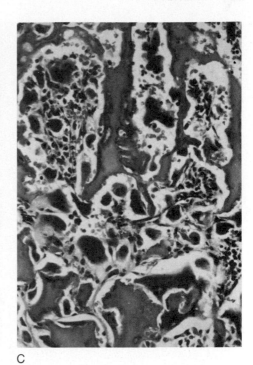

A B C

Figure 26-2. Osteopetrosis. (*A*) A radiograph of a child shows markedly dense bones of the lower extremities secondary to the preservation and retention of primary trabeculae, along with their calcified cores of cartilage. This increased density gives rise to the term "marble bone disease." The bones are also misshapen. (*B*) A gross specimen of the femur shows the original femur in the center, with virtually no marrow space remaining. The new bone deposited on the surface of the original femur accommodates the marrow space, which has been crowded out by osteopetrosis. The developing secondary centers of ossification at both ends of the specimen are also deficient in normal marrow elements. (*C*) A photomicrograph illustrates the preservation of the primary trabeculae, together with their cores of calcified cartilage and osteoclasts. Although the osteoclasts are more numerous than normal, they do not function appropriately.

zones of proliferative and hypertrophied cartilage (Fig. 26-4). These cartilage masses are all called **enchondromas,** and to some investigators they represent true neoplasms. These cartilage nodules exhibit a strong tendency to undergo malignant change into chondrosarcomas in adult life.

FRACTURE

The most common bone lesion is a fracture, which is essentially defined as a discontinuity of the bone.

FRACTURE HEALING

In the repair of a bone fracture, **anything other than the formation of bone tissue at the fracture site represents incomplete healing.** The healing of a fracture

is divided into three phases: the inflammatory phase, the reparative phase, and the remodeling phase (Fig. 26-5).

INFLAMMATORY PHASE

In the first 1 to 2 days after a fracture, there is extensive tearing of the periosteum. The resultant rupture of blood vessels in the periosteum and adjacent soft tissue leads to extensive hemorrhage. There is extensive necrosis of bone at the fracture site because of the disruption of large vessels in the bone and the interruption of the cortical vessels (i.e., the Volkmann and haversian canals). **The hallmark of dead bone is the absence of osteocytes and empty bone lacunae.**

In about 2 to 5 days, the hemorrhage forms a large clot, with formation of fibrin. This is a relatively avascular area that must be resorbed so that the fracture can heal. Peripheral to this blood clot, neovascularization

(Text continues on p. 706)

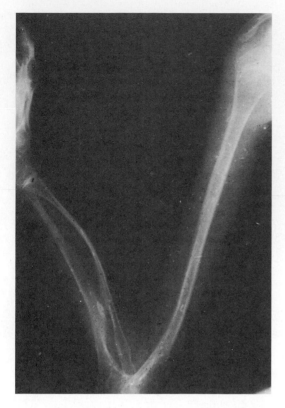

Figure 26-3. Osteogenesis imperfecta. A radiograph illustrates the markedly thin and attenuated humerus and bones of the forearm. There is a fracture callus in the proximal ulna.

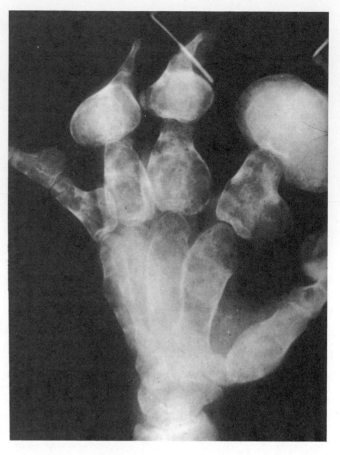

Figure 26-4. Multiple enchondromatosis (Ollier's disease). A radiograph of the hand shows bulbous swellings that represent cartilage masses composed of hyaline cartilage, which is sometimes admixed with more primitive myxoid cartilage.

Figure 26-5. Healing of a fracture. (*A*) Soon after a fracture is sustained, an extensive blood clot forms in the subperiosteal and soft tissue, as well as in the marrow cavity. The bone at the fracture site is jagged. (*B*) The inflammatory phase of fracture healing is characterized by neovascularization and beginning organization of the blood clot. Because the osteocytes in the fracture site are dead, the lacunae are empty. The osteocytes of the cortex are necrotic well beyond the fracture site, owing to the traumatic interruption of the perforating arteries from the periosteum. (*C*) The reparative phase of fracture healing is characterized by the formation of a callus of cartilage and woven bone near the fracture site. The jagged edges of the original cortex have been remodeled and eroded by osteoclasts. The marrow space has been revascularized and contains reactive woven bone, as does the periosteal area. (*D*) In the remodeling phase, during which the cortex is revitalized, the reactive bone may be lamellar or woven. The new bone is organized along stress lines and mechanical forces. Extensive osteoclastic and osteoblastic cellular activity is maintained.

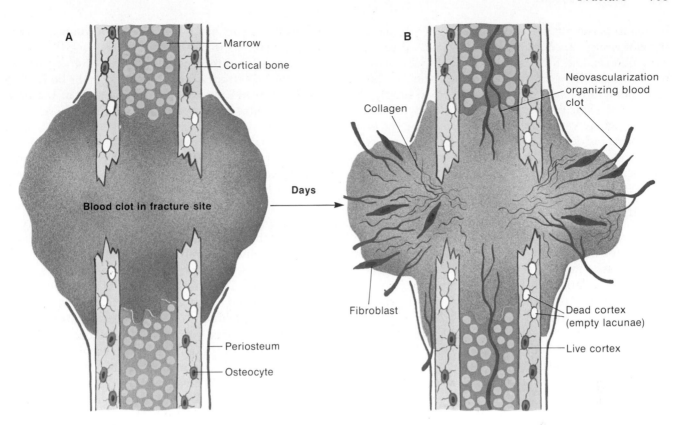

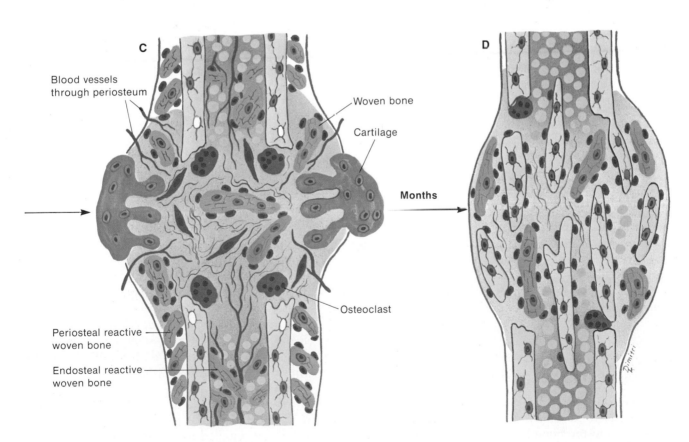

begins to occur. By the end of the first week, most of the clot is organized by invasion of blood vessels and early fibrosis, and the earliest bone (invariably woven) has formed. This corresponds to the "scar" of bone. Since bone formation requires a good blood supply, the woven bone spicules begin to form at the periphery of the clot, where vascularization is greatest. Woven bone also forms inside the marrow cavity at the periphery of the blood clot because vascular tissue is also present in this location.

REPARATIVE PHASE

The reparative phase begins after the first week and extends for months. By this time, the acute inflammatory cells seen in the first week have dissipated. Extensive neovascularization introduces mononuclear cells that form osteoclasts. The repair process proceeds from the most peripheral portion toward the fracture site, and accomplishes two objectives: (1) it organizes and resorbs the blood clot, and more importantly, (2) it furnishes neovascularization for the construction of granulation tissue (callus) that will eventually bridge the fracture site.

REMODELING PHASE

After the bone ends have been sealed by ingrowth of callus (generally, several weeks after the fracture occurs), remodeling begins. In the remodeling phase, the bone is reorganized so that the original cortex is restored.

INFECTION

OSTEOMYELITIS

Osteomyelitis is an inflammation of bone caused by a pyogenic organism. Despite the common use of antibiotics, osteomyelitis is still a major diagnostic and therapeutic problem. The most common pathogens are Staphylococcus species, but other organisms, such as *Escherichia coli, Neisseria gonorrhea, Haemophilus influenzae,* and *Salmonella* species, are also seen.

PATHOGENESIS AND CLINICAL PRESENTATION

The organisms are introduced either through the **hematogenous** route or by **direct introduction** of the organisms into the bone by penetrating wounds, fractures, or surgery. **Infection by direct penetration or extension of bacteria is now the most common cause of osteomyelitis in the United States.**

In **hematogenous osteomyelitis,** the organisms reach the bone from a focus elsewhere in the body. **The most common sites affected are the ends of the long bones, such as the knee, ankle, and hip.** Hematogenous osteomyelitis principally affects boys 5 to 15 years of age, usually in the metaphyseal area (Fig. 26-6).

Once the bacteria have penetrated the bone they proliferate in the marrow and extend into the cortex. Pus may form underneath the periosteum, shearing off the perforating arteries of the periosteum and further devitalizing the cortex. Pus flows between the periosteum and the cortex, isolating more bone from its blood supply, and may even invade the joint. Eventually, the pus penetrates the periosteum and the skin to form a draining sinus. The hole formed in the bone during this process is termed a **cloaca.** A fragment of necrotic bone, called a **sequestrum,** is often embedded in the pus.

The bone generally has several options for repair. Marrow cells may modulate into osteoblasts and osteoclasts in an attempt to wall off the infection. Alternatively, a **Brodie's abscess** may form, consisting of reactive bone from the periosteum and the endosteum that contained the infection. The third option occurs when periosteal new bone formation is extensive. In such cases the reactive new bone forms a sheath around the necrotic sequestrum, giving rise to an **involucrum.**

COMPLICATIONS

The complications of osteomyelitis include the following:

- Septicemia may occur in infants secondary to bone infection.
- Acute bacterial arthritis may arise as a result of osteomyelitis. Direct digestion of cartilage by inflammatory cells destroys the articular cartilage and leads to osteoarthritis.
- Pathologic fractures may occur as a result of osteomyelitis. These fractures heal poorly because of the infected tissue, and may require surgical drainage.
- Squamous cell carcinoma develops in the bone or in the sinus tract of long-standing chronic osteomyelitis, often years after the initial infection. Squamous tissue arises from the epithelialization of the sinus tract.
- Amyloidosis was a common complication of chronic osteomyelitis in the preantibiotic era, and patients often died from cardiac and renal disease. Currently, it is rare in industrialized countries.

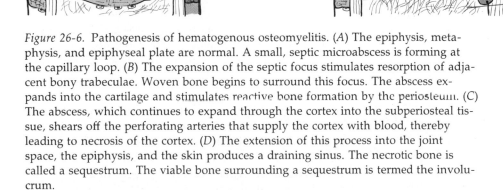

Figure 26-6. Pathogenesis of hematogenous osteomyelitis. (*A*) The epiphysis, metaphysis, and epiphyseal plate are normal. A small, septic microabscess is forming at the capillary loop. (*B*) The expansion of the septic focus stimulates resorption of adjacent bony trabeculae. Woven bone begins to surround this focus. The abscess expands into the cartilage and stimulates reactive bone formation by the periosteum. (*C*) The abscess, which continues to expand through the cortex into the subperiosteal tissue, shears off the perforating arteries that supply the cortex with blood, thereby leading to necrosis of the cortex. (*D*) The extension of this process into the joint space, the epiphysis, and the skin produces a draining sinus. The necrotic bone is called a sequestrum. The viable bone surrounding a sequestrum is termed the involucrum.

- Chronic osteomyelitis, especially that involving the entire bone, is incurable because antibiotic therapy does not eradicate all the organisms.

TUBERCULOSIS

Tuberculosis of bone is invariably secondary to a primary focus elsewhere in the body—the lungs or lymph nodes in the human type, or the gut or tonsils in the rare bovine type. The mycobacteria spread to the bone hematogenously; only rarely is there direct spread into the rib, spine, or sternum from a lung or lymph node.

TUBERCULOUS SPONDYLITIS (POTT'S DISEASE)

Tuberculous spondylitis, inflammation of the spine, is a feared complication of childhood tuberculosis. It affects the vertebral bodies, sparing the lamina and spines and adjacent vertebrae. With antibiotic treatment, Pott's disease is rare. The thoracic vertebrae are usually affected, especially T11, with the lumbar and cervical vertebrae being less commonly involved.

The pathologic process is similar to that in other sites. The tuberculous granulomas first produce caseous necrosis of the bone marrow, an effect that leads to slow resorption of bony trabeculae, and occasionally, to cystic spaces in the bone. Because there is little or no reactive bone, **collapse of the affected vertebra is usual,** after which kyphosis and scoliosis ensue.

ARTHRITIS

In tuberculous arthritis, the focus of tuberculosis, reflecting hematogenous spread, begins in the joint capsule, synovium, or intracapsular portion of the bone. Tuberculosis induces proliferation of granulomas in synovial tissue. This tissue then becomes edematous and papillary, and may fill the entire joint space. There is also massive destruction of the articular cartilage from undermining granulation tissue in the bone. The destroyed joint is replaced by osseous tissue, the result being bony ankylosis.

OSTEOMYELITIS OF THE LONG BONES

Osteomyelitis of the long bones is the least common bone manifestation of tuberculosis. Tuberculous osteomyelitis in a long bone occurs near the joint, and produces a simultaneous arthritis.

METABOLIC BONE DISEASE

The term "metabolic disease" refers to a number of generalized skeletal disorders; these disorders involve **all** of the bones of the skeleton. **In metabolic bone disease, there are no normal areas of bone tissue in the skeleton.** A disease such as Paget's disease, which is discussed in a later section, is not considered a metabolic bone disease because, although it may be widespread, foci of normal bone tissue are also present.

OSTEOPOROSIS

Osteoporosis refers to a **group of diseases** of many etiologies (Table 26-1) that have as their **common denominator a reduction in the bone mass to a level below that required for normal bone support.** Although reduced in mass, the bones are normal with respect to mineralization. Histologically, there is a decrease in the thickness of the cortex and the number and size of trabeculae of the coarse cancellous bone. By contrast, the osteoid seams are of normal width (Fig. 26-7). The major problem in this disease is that the **rate of bone resorption exceeds that of bone formation.**

In general, after the age of 40 or 50 years, the skeletal mass begins to decrease at a faster rate in women than in men, and at different rates in various parts of the skeleton. The degree of bone loss may be striking, amounting to as much as a 30% to 50% reduction in skeletal mass, compared to that at age 30 to 40 years. In elderly patients, the rate of resorption is high, whereas the rate of bone formation remains in the normal range. The cause for this age-associated decrease in bone mass and increase in osteoclastic resorption is unknown. The disease is not as common in American blacks as in whites.

In Cushing's syndrome, either the spontaneous form or that caused by the administration of corticosteroids, there may be deficient bone production as well as an increased rate of bone resorption. An increased rate of bone resorption seems also to be the mechanism for osteoporosis in hyperthyroidism, even though the rate is only slightly higher than normal. Thus, **the combination of decreased osteoblastic activity and increased osteoclastic activity is responsible for the striking changes seen in osteoporosis.**

EPIDEMIOLOGY

Osteoporosis is the most common metabolic bone disease in the United States. Fifteen percent of white

Table 26-1 *Classification of Osteoporosis*

Primary

Postmenopausal osteoporosis
Involutional osteoporosis
Idiopathic osteoporosis (juvenile, adult)

Secondary

Primary biliary cirrhosis
Rheumatoid arthritis
Chronic pulmonary disease
Endocrine causes
    Hyperthyroidism
    Cushing's syndrome (endogenous or exogenous)
    Diabetes
    Lactation and pregnancy
    Hypogonadism
    Hyperparathyroidism
Nutritional causes
    Intestinal malabsorption
    Protein malnutrition
    Scurvy
    Calcium deficiency (?)
Immobilization
Drugs
    Anticonvulsants
    Heparin
Heritable disorders of the connective tissue
    Osteogenesis imperfecta
    Menkes' syndrome
    Homocystinuria
    Adult hypophosphatasia
Neoplasms
    Multiple myeloma
    Myelomonocytic leukemia
    Systemic mastocytosis
    Waldenström's macroglobulinemia

women older than 65 years of age have significant osteoporosis. Thirty percent of those women 75 years of age or older have suffered fractures secondary to osteoporosis. **These fractures usually occur in the proximal humerus, lower forearm, hip, spine, and pelvis.** A typical patient with osteoporosis is a thin, sedentary, postmenopausal, white woman of Northern European descent who smokes and has breastfed several children. Her diet is usually deficient in calcium and vitamin D, and she has little sun exposure.

DIAGNOSIS

The diagnosis of osteoporosis is primarily made on the basis of the radiologic finding of thin cortices, a condition labelled **osteopenia** (meaning "little bone"). Radiologists use this term because they are unable to distinguish between loss of bone with normal mineralization (osteoporosis), and osteoid with incomplete mineralization (osteomalacia) (Fig. 26-8). The laboratory findings, including serum calcium and phosphorus levels, are basically normal.

OSTEOMALACIA

Osteomalacia ("soft bones") refers to a group of diseases in which there is a failure to form the normal inorganic calcium phosphate phase in relation to the organic matrix of bone. This defective mineralization results in exaggeration of the osteoid seams, both in the thickness and in the proportion of trabecular surface covered (see Fig. 26-7). The term **rickets** means osteomalacia of the growing skeleton, a disorder that involves not only bone but also cartilage. The mechanisms underlying osteomalacia are related to the type of disease producing it. Causes include **deficiency of dietary or endogenous vitamin D** (see Chapter 8), **intestinal malabsorption, and acquired or hereditary renal disorders.**

Osteomalacia is a cause of the **osteopenic** x-ray pattern. The only findings may be compression fractures and a decrease in bone thickness, as seen in osteoporosis.

RICKETS

Clinical Presentation

Children with rickets are short and exhibit characteristic changes of bone and teeth. Flattening of the skull, prominent frontal bones ("frontal bossing"), and prominent suture lines are typical. The teeth show delayed dentition, with severe dental caries and enamel defects. The chest has the classic rachitic "rosary" appearance, which is produced by the enlargement of the costal cartilages and indentations of the lower ribs at the insertion of the diaphragm. The sternum is marked by pectus carinatum, or "pigeon breast," which is an outward curvature. The limbs are shortened and deformed, with severe bowing of the arms and forearm, and frequent fractures.

Radiologic and Histologic Findings

Because rickets affects children, there are extensive changes at the epiphyseal plate. The epiphyseal plate is not adequately mineralized, and the calcified cartilage and the zones of hypertrophy and proliferative cartilage continue to grow, because osteoclastic activity does not resorb the cartilage growth plate. As a consequence, the epiphyseal plate is conspicuously thickened, irregular, and lobulated. Endochondral ossifica-

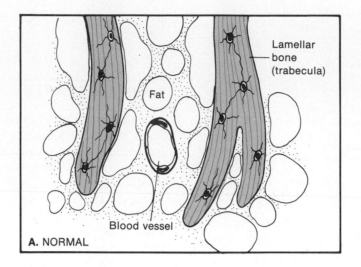

A. NORMAL

Lamellar bone (trabecula)

Fat

Blood vessel

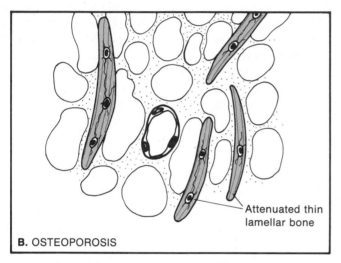

B. OSTEOPOROSIS

Attenuated thin lamellar bone

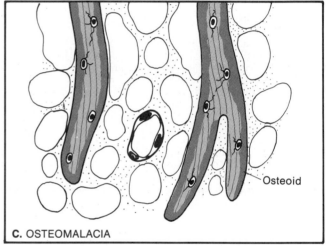

C. OSTEOMALACIA

Osteoid

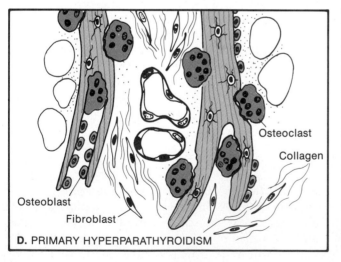

D. PRIMARY HYPERPARATHYROIDISM

Osteoclast

Collagen

Osteoblast

Fibroblast

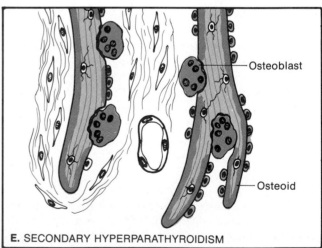

E. SECONDARY HYPERPARATHYROIDISM

Osteoblast

Osteoid

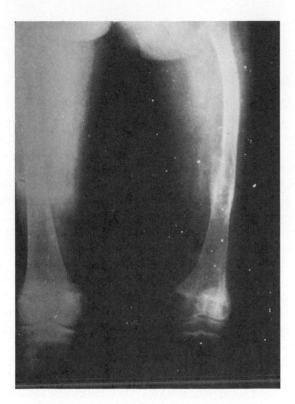

Figure 26-8. Disuse osteoporosis. A radiograph shows thin cortices, attenuated trabeculae, and associated soft tissue atrophy in a previously fractured left femur.

tion proceeds very slowly and preferentially at the peripheral portions of the metaphysis. The net result is a flared and cup-shaped epiphysis. The largest part of the primary spongiosum is composed of lamellar or woven bone, which is unmineralized.

Pathogenesis

Rickets is rare in the United States, but it is sometimes encountered in children who have abnormal diets as a result of food fads, in premature infants, and in patients hospitalized in mental institutions. In the industrialized countries, osteomalacia is more often caused by diseases associated with intestinal malabsorption than by poor nutrition. For instance, in obstructive jaundice, the lack of bile salts in the intestine precludes adequate absorption of lipids and lipid-soluble substances, among which is the fat-soluble vitamin D. Calcium absorption from the gut is also impaired. Furthermore, with sufficient liver damage, the hydroxylation of vitamin D is reduced. The absorption of vitamin D and calcium is also decreased in gluten-sensitive enteropathy, Crohn's disease, sarcoidosis, and intestinal tuberculosis. In dietary vitamin D deficiency, the serum levels of calcium and phosphorus are both low owing to decreased intestinal absorption, particularly of calcium. **A low serum calcium level stimulates the parathyroid glands, thus producing secondary hyperparathyroidism.**

RENAL OSTEODYSTROPHY

A distinct syndrome in which bone is directly affected by renal failure is termed **renal osteodystrophy.** The pathogenesis of renal osteodystrophy is essentially similar to that of osteomalacia, with **secondary hyperparathyroidism exerting its influence by way of osteoclastic resorption on the bone** (see Fig. 26-7). The pathophysiology of renal osteodystrophy may be summarized as follows:

Figure 26-7. Metabolic bone diseases. (*A*) Normal trabecular bone and fatty marrow. The trabecular bone is lamellar and contains evenly distributed osteocytes. (*B*) Osteoporosis. The lamellar bone exhibits discontinuous, thin trabeculae. (*C*) Osteomalacia. The trabeculae of the lamellar bone have abnormal amounts of nonmineralized bone (osteoid). These osteoid seams are thickened, and cover a larger than normal area of the trabecular bone surface. (*D*) Primary hyperparathyroidism. The lamellar bone trabeculae are actively resorbed by numerous osteoclasts that bore into each trabecula. The appearance of osteoclasts dissecting into the trabeculae, a process termed dissecting osteitis, is diagnostic of hyperparathyroidism. Osteoblastic activity is also pronounced. The marrow is replaced by fibrous tissue adjacent to the trabeculae. (*E*) Secondary hyperparathyroidism. The morphologic appearance is similar to that of primary hyperparathyroidism, except that prominent osteoid covers the trabeculae. Osteoclasts do not resorb osteoid, and wherever an osteoid seam is lacking, osteoclasts bore into the trabeculae. Osteoblastic activity, in association with osteoclasts, is again prominent.

1. Damage to the glomerulus causes retention of phosphate, thereby producing hyperphosphatemia.
2. Tubular injury leads to a reduction in 1,25-dihydroxyvitamin D.
3. Intestinal calcium absorption is, in turn, decreased, leading to profound hypocalcemia.
4. Hypocalcemia stimulates the elaboration of parathyroid hormone and, within a short time, there is marked secondary hyperparathyroidism, with clear cell hyperplasia of all four glands.
5. This increased amount of parathyroid hormone does not effectively promote intestinal calcium absorption or renal tubular resorption of calcium because of the absence of vitamin D and the increased level of phosphate. Therefore, the principal action of parathyroid hormone is resorption of skeletal calcium.

The four components of renal osteodystrophy are osteomalacia, secondary hyperparathyroidism, osteosclerosis (new bone), and ectopic calcification or ossification. Acidosis and hypoalbuminemia are accompanied by low serum calcium and elevated inorganic phosphate levels. The alkaline phosphatase and parathyroid hormone levels are increased, but the concentrations of 1,25-dihydroxy vitamin D are also decreased. The urinary calcium level is low, whereas fecal calcium is increased.

PRIMARY HYPERPARATHYROIDISM

Primary hyperparathyroidism, the oversecretion of parathyroid hormone, is prominently associated with bone disease. The disorder may be caused by one or more parathyroid adenomas (90% of cases), hyperplasia of all four glands (10% of cases), or more rarely, by parathyroid carcinoma. Since parathyroid hormone promotes excretion of phosphate in the urine, low serum phosphate and high serum calcium levels are characteristic.

CLINICAL PRESENTATION

The symptoms related to this abnormality of calcium ion homeostasis have been summarized as "stones, bones, moans, and groans." The "stones" refer to kidney stones, and the "bones" to the usual skeletal changes. The "moans" relate to psychiatric depression and other abnormalities associated with hypercalcemia, while the "groans" characterize the gastrointestinal irregularities associated with a high serum calcium level.

RADIOGRAPHIC APPEARANCE

The skeletal disease of hyperparathyroidism is also called **von Recklinghausen's disease.** On radiologic examination, there is a generalized decalcification of the entire skeleton, and the weakened bones are associated with deformities such as platybasia, biconcave vertebrae, and bowing of the long bones, and with fractures. Similar deformities are also seen in osteomalacia and, less frequently, in osteoporosis. A distinctive radiologic peculiarity, referred to as **subperiosteal bone resorption,** is seen in the subperiosteal outer surface of the cortex.

In addition to the generalized osteopenia seen on radiography, there are multiple, localized, lytic lesions that represent hemorrhagic cysts or masses of fibrous tissue, called **brown tumors** (Fig. 26-9). These eccentric and well-demarcated lesions are separated from the soft tissue by a periosteal shell of bone. The lesions may be multiple or solitary. **It is important to remember that these focal, tumorlike, lytic lesions always occur in the context of an abnormal skeleton produced by hyperparathyroidism.**

HISTOPATHOLOGIC CHANGES

The histopathology of primary hyperparathyroidism that culminates in **osteitis fibrosa cystica** may be classified into three stages.

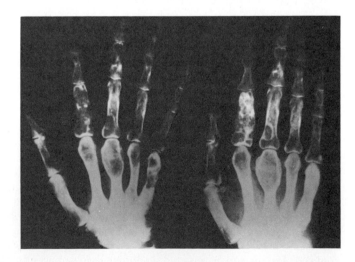

Figure 26-9. Primary hyperparathyroidism. A radiograph of the hands reveals bulbous swellings ("brown tumors") and numerous cavities, both representing bone resorption.

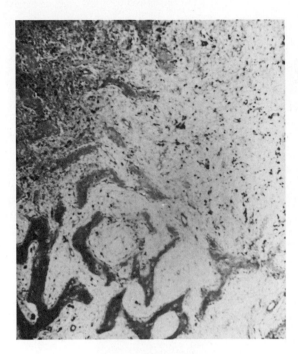

Figure 26-10. Primary hyperparathyroidism. A photomicrograph of a "brown tumor" shows reactive woven bone, numerous macrophages filled with hemosiderin, fibrosis, and foci of hemorrhage.

In the early stage of the disease, osteoclasts are stimulated by the elevated parathyroid hormone levels to resorb bone. The pattern of osteoclasts boring into the trabecular bone is termed **dissecting osteitis** (see Fig. 26-7) because each trabeculum is continually hollowed out by osteoclastic activity. At the same time, the endosteal marrow modulates into fibrous tissue and additional osteoclasts that also penetrate bone.

In the second stage of hyperparathyroidism, the trabecular bone is ultimately resorbed, and the marrow is replaced by loose fibrosis, hemosiderin-laden macrophages, areas of hemorrhage from microfractures, and reactive woven bone. This combination of features constitutes the **osteitis fibrosa** portion of the complex.

As the disease progresses and hemorrhage progressively increases, cystic degeneration ultimately occurs, leading to **osteitis fibrosa cystica,** the third and final stage of the disease. The areas of fibrosis with reactive woven bone and hemosiderin-laden macrophages often display many giant cells of the foreign body type, as well as osteoclasts, an appearance that has been termed a **brown tumor** (Fig. 26-10). This is not a true tumor, but rather a repair reaction as an end stage of hyperparathyroidism.

PAGET'S DISEASE OF BONE

Paget's disease, a generalized disorder of the skeleton characterized by both thickening and weakening of the bones, is common, and some manifestation of the disorder is found in 3% to 4% of all autopsies in elderly individuals. On radiographic examination, about 4% of aged persons exhibit some changes that are characteristic of Paget's disease. The disease is seen in both sexes, and generally affects persons older than 60 years of age.

In Paget's disease, there is an uncoupling of osteoblastic and osteoclastic activities. The disease is triphasic, having a "hot" or osteoclastic resorptive stage, a mixed stage of osteoblastic and osteoclastic activity, and a "cold" or burnt-out stage characterized by little cellular activity. The disease need not progress through all three stages, and in polyostotic disease, different foci may be in different stages.

The radiologic appearance of the disease correlates with the histopathologic stage of the disease (Fig. 26-11). For example, if the disease is in the lytic, or "hot," phase, the bone shows a characteristic, sharply defined, **flame-shaped** or **wedged-shaped lysis of the cortex,** which often mimics a tumor. In the mixed stage, the bones are generally larger than normal; in fact, Paget's disease is one of two diseases that produces **larger than normal bones,** the other being fibrous dysplasia (discussed later). The cortex in the mixed phase is thickened, and the accentuation of the coarse cancellous bone makes the bone look heavy and enlarged.

The bones involved in this disease tend to be those of the axial skeleton, including the spine, skull, pelvis, proximal femur, tibia, and humerus. Solitary Paget's disease rarely involves the humerus, but in polyostotic disease, lesions involving this bone are common.

CLINICAL FEATURES

The most common symptom of Paget's disease is pain, although its cause is not clear. The skull may exhibit localized lysis, generally in the frontal and parietal bones, which is termed **osteoporosis circumscripta.** Alternatively, there may be thickening of the outer and inner tables, which is most pronounced in the frontal and occipital bones. The skull becomes very heavy and may collapse over the C1 vertebra, thereby producing **platybasia,** with compression of the neurologic structures in the posterior fossa and spinal cord. Hearing loss is caused by involvement of the ossicles and bony impingement on the eighth cranial nerve at the fora-

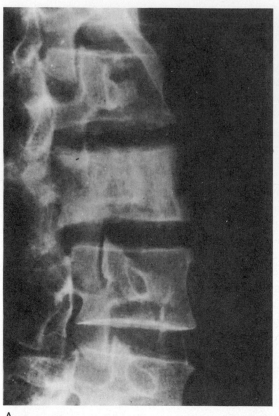

A

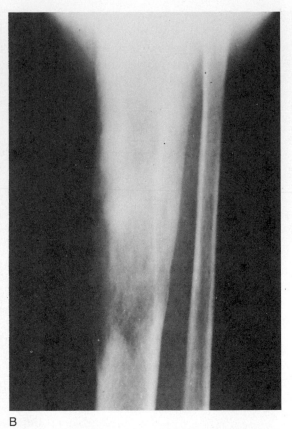

C

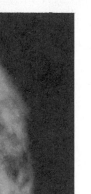

B

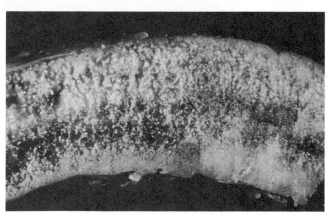

D

men. Occasionally patients feel light-headed, a symptom thought to be due to so-called **pagetic steal,** in which blood is shunted from the internal carotid system to the bone, rather than to the brain. The jaws may be grossly affected and misshapen, and the teeth may fall out. Often, the facial bones increase in size, producing the so-called **leontiasis ossea,** the "lion-like" face. Fractures in Paget's disease are common, the bones snapping transversely like a piece of chalk. Sarcomatous change in a focus of Paget's disease occurs in less than 1% of all cases.

HISTOLOGIC FEATURES

The diagnostic feature of Paget's disease is the abnormal arrangement of lamellar bone, in which islands of irregular bone formation resembling pieces of a jigsaw puzzle are separated by prominent "cement lines" (Fig. 26-12). The result is a **mosaic pattern** in the bone, which can be seen particularly well under polarized light. Although the changes in lamellar bone are diagnostic, it is not uncommon to see woven bone as part of the pathologic process.

The osteoclast of Paget's disease is characteristic, and to some, diagnostic. The osteoclast is very large, possessing more than 12 nuclei, each of which is hyperchromatic. The osteoclast thus appears as a large cell with dark, smeared nuclei.

NEOPLASMS OF BONE

Bone tumors are uncommon, but are nevertheless important neoplasms, particularly in young people. A primary bone tumor may arise from any one of the cellular elements of bone. Most neoplasms of bone occur near the metaphyseal area, and more than 80% of primary tumors occur in either the distal femur or the proximal tibia (Fig. 26-13). In the growing child these areas are characterized by conspicuous growth activity and are, therefore, more likely to develop a tumor.

BENIGN TUMORS

SOLITARY BONE CYST

The solitary bone cyst is a benign, fluid-filled, usually unilocular lesion found in children and adolescents. There is a male predilection of 3:1 over females. About 65% to 75% of all solitary bone cysts occur in the upper humerus or femur, often in the metaphysis adjacent to the epiphyseal plate. The lesion seems to be not a true neoplasm but rather a disturbance of bone growth with superimposed trauma.

The cyst is lined by fibrous tissue, a few giant cells, hemosiderin-laden macrophages, chronic inflammatory cells, and reactive bone. Osteoclasts, seen in the advancing front of the cyst, enable the expansion of the lesion. Curettage and the deposition of bone chips are curative.

OSTEOID OSTEOMA

Osteoid osteoma, a small, painful lesion that is often about 1 cm in diameter, occurs in persons ranging in age from 5 to 24 years. It occurs more commonly in males than in females, with a ratio of 3:1. The pain is diaphyseal and intracortical, and principally affects the lower extremity, including the small bones of the foot. The severity of the pain is out of proportion to the size of the lesion.

Osteoid osteoma is characterized by a dense, vascular center of woven bone and osteoid (Fig. 26-14), which may be partially mineralized and is seen radiographically as a radiolucent nidus surrounded by very dense, reactive bone. If the nidus is calcified, the lesion resembles a target on radiography, having a dense center, a thin, peripheral, radiolucent zone, and a very dense outer zone of bone. Surgical excision is usually curative.

Figure 26-11. Paget's disease of bone. (*A*) A radiograph of the spine demonstrates a sclerotic and enlarged vertebral body (*arrow*) in which the trabeculae and the cortex are coarsened and thickened. Paget's disease is one of the few diseases that can enlarge a bone. (*B*) The lytic phase of Paget's disease is illustrated in this radiograph. A sharply defined, lucent lesion has thinned the cortex. (*C*) A radiograph of the skull shows the thickening and distortion of the bone by osteoblastic and osteolytic foci. (*D*) A gross specimen of bone from the skull demonstrates marked thickening of the outer and inner tables, which narrows the diploë (hematopoietic marrow).

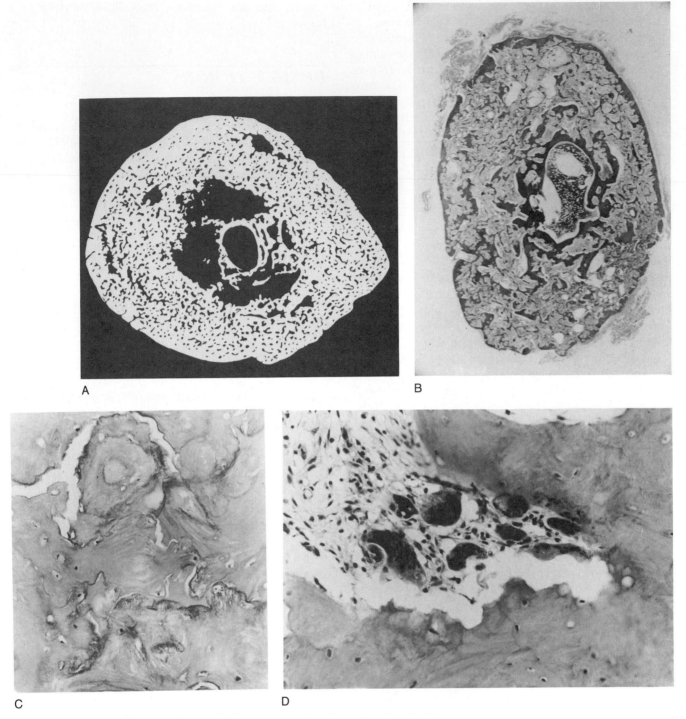

Figure 26-12. Paget's disease of bone. (*A*) Cross-sectional radiograph of a rib. The cortex is markedly thickened, and the marrow space is narrowed. (*B*) A histologic section of the specimen in *A*. (*C*) The characteristic mosaic pattern of lamellar bone units fastened together in a random fashion is evident. The mosaic pattern is produced by the interfaces of the units of lamellar bone, termed cement lines. Artifactual cracks along the cement lines separate the units of lamellar bone. (*D*) The osteoclasts in Paget's disease have numerous hyperchromatic nuclei.

BENIGN TUMORS

EPIPHYSIS

Chondroblastoma,.
Giant cell tumor

METAPHYSIS

Osteoblastoma
Osteochondroma
Non-ossifying fibroma
Osteoid osteoma
Chondromyxoid fibroma
Giant cell tumor

DIAPHYSIS

Enchondroma
Fibrous dysplasia

MALIGNANT TUMORS

DIAPHYSIS

Ewing's sarcoma
Chondrosarcoma

METAPHYSIS

Osteosarcoma
Juxtacortical osteosarcoma

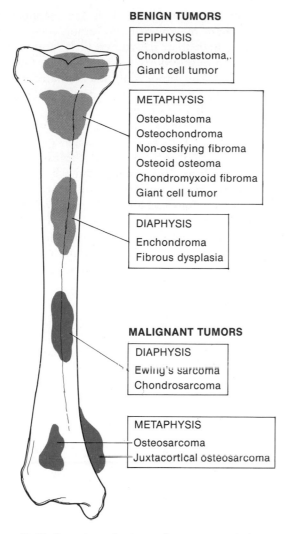

Figure 26-13. Location of primary bone tumors in long tubular bones.

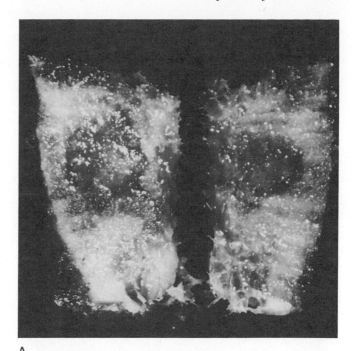

A

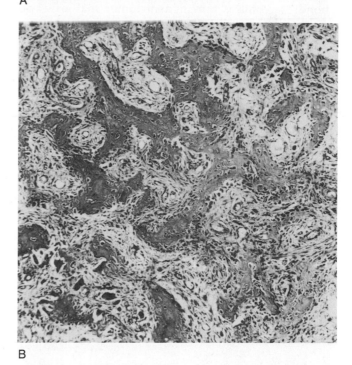

B

Figure 26-14. (*A*) A gross specimen of an osteoid osteoma shows the nidus, which is less than 1 cm in diameter, as a small hemorrhagic area. (*B*) A photomicrograph of the nidus reveals irregular trabeculae of woven bone surrounded by osteoblasts, osteoclasts, and fibrovascular marrow.

MALIGNANT TUMORS

OSTEOSARCOMA (OSTEOGENIC SARCOMA)

Osteosarcoma is the most common primary malignant bone tumor, representing one-fifth of all malignant bone tumors. It is a highly malignant lesion that often requires amputation for treatment, and is associated with a poor prognosis (the 5-year survival rate ranges from 10% to 60%). The tumor most commonly occurs in persons between the ages of 10 and 20 years, and it affects males more often than females. It is often found around the knee—that is, the lower femur, upper tibia, or fibula—but any metaphyseal area of a long bone may be affected. Radiologic evidence of bone destruction and bone formation is characteristic, with the latter representing tumor bone. Often, the periosteum is elevated by reactive bone adjacent to the tumor, a pattern that appears on radiographic studies as a triangular area between the cortex and the periosteal bone (Codman's triangle).

Histologic examination reveals malignant mesenchymal cells that modulate into malignant osteoblasts, producing osteoid and tumor bone (Fig. 26-15). This almost wholly woven bone is laid down haphazardly, and is not aligned along stress lines. Thus, it is the tumor bone that gives the radiologic "sunburst" appearance. Often, foci of malignant cartilage cells or malignant giant cells are intermixed with the stromal tumor. In areas of lysis, osteoclasts are found at the advancing front of the tumor. The tumor spreads via the bloodstream to the lungs (more than 90% of patients who die from this disease have lung metastases) and, less commonly, to other bones (14%).

CHONDROSARCOMA

Chondrosarcoma is a malignant tumor that arises de novo in a pre-existing cartilaginous rest or in a benign chondroma. It usually presents within the bone rather than as a juxtacortical lesion. It is the second most common primary malignant bone tumor, occurs more commonly in men than in women (2:1), and is most frequently seen in the fourth to sixth decades (average age of 45 years). The tumor is often a lobulated mass in the pelvic bones, but may be seen in the long bones, ribs, spine, scapula and sacrum.

Histologically, chondrosarcomas are composed of malignant cartilage cells in various stages of maturity. Occasionally, a well-differentiated chondrosarcoma would be difficult to differentiate from a benign cartilaginous tumor were it not for its large size. Zones of calcification are often conspicuous, and are seen on radiography as splotches or bulky masses (Fig. 26-16). Most tumors grow slowly, but hematogenous metastases to the lungs are common. Amputation is often necessary, and the 5-year survival rates vary between 45% and 75%.

GIANT CELL TUMOR

Giant cell tumors are locally aggressive bone lesions with the capacity to metastasize, especially if manipulated surgically. They are thought to arise from primi-

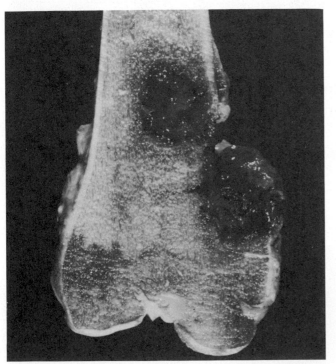

A

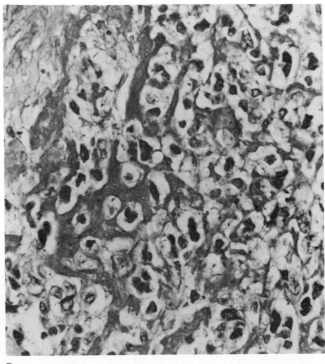

B

Figure 26-15. Osteosarcoma. (*A*) The distal femur contains a tumor composed of hemorrhagic tissue. The dense white tissue that fills the metaphyseal marrow represents new bone formation. (*B*) A photomicrograph of the tumor in *A* shows malignant osteocytes and woven bone matrix.

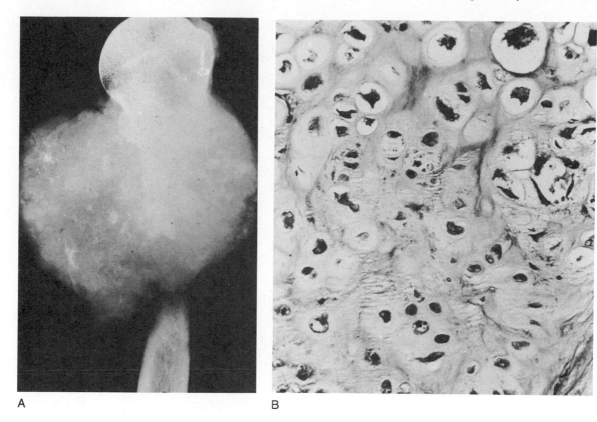

A   B

Figure 26-16. Chondrosarcoma. (*A*) A radiograph of the resected proximal humerus reveals a bulky, destructive, mineralized lesion in the diaphysis. There is extensive bone destruction and extension of the tumor into the soft tissue. (*B*) A photomicrograph of *A* reveals a hypercellular tumor composed of malignant chondrocytes embedded in a sparse matrix.

tive stromal cells that have the capacity to modulate into osteoclasts. Indeed, the giant cell tumor is often a lytic lesion that grows slowly enough to allow a periosteal reaction. Thus, the tumor is usually surrounded by a thin, bony shell and expands the bone (Fig. 26-17). The tumor usually occurs in the third and fourth decades, predominantly in women. In the long bones, it invariably involves the metaphysis after the epiphysis is closed, but it often extends into the epiphysis. It may also be found in the pelvis and sacrum. The mononuclear "stromal" cells are plump and oval, with large nuclei and scanty cytoplasm. Large osteoclastic giant cells, some with more than 100 nuclei, are scattered throughout the richly vascularized tumor. Amputation may be necessary for treatment if an en bloc excision cannot be performed.

EWING'S SARCOMA

Ewing's sarcoma is an uncommon lesion, representing only about 4% to 5% of all bone tumors. It is primarily a tumor of the long bones, especially the humerus, tibia, and femur, where it occurs as a midshaft or metaphyseal lesion. However, it may occur in any bone of the body, including those in the hands and feet. It is a tumor of childhood and adolescence, with two-thirds of the cases occurring in patients younger than 20 years of age. Males are affected more often than females (2:1). The onion-skin pattern that is seen on radiologic examination represents a circumferential layer of reactive periosteal bone that is associated with a lytic lesion of the medulla and endosteal surface of the cortex. The tumor cells are found in sheets that permeate all the bony interstices, including the haversian canals. The malignant cells extend along the shaft in both directions.

On histologic examination, the cells resemble primitive lymphocytes, and are visualized as small, closely packed cells with little cytoplasm; they are two to three times larger than a lymphocyte (Fig. 26-18). There is little or no interstitial stroma, and mitoses occur infrequently. Ewing's sarcoma metastasizes to many organs, including the lungs and brain. Other bones, especially

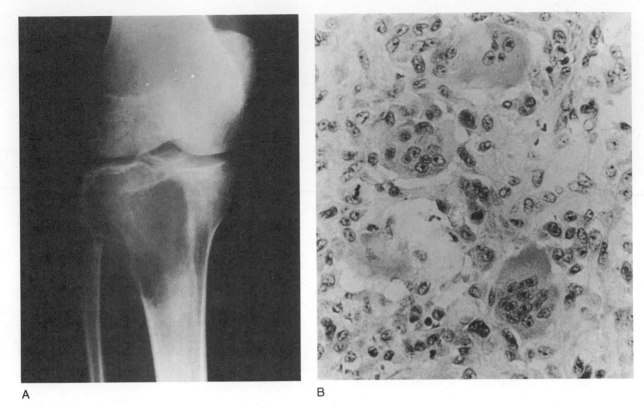

A   B

Figure 26-17. Giant cell tumor of bone. (*A*) A radiograph of the proximal tibia shows
an eccentric lytic lesion, with virtually no new bone formation. The tumor extends to
the subchondral bone plate and breaks through cortex into the soft tissue. (*B*) A photomicrograph shows osteoclast-type giant cells and plump, oval, mononuclear cells.
The nuclei of both types of cells are identical.

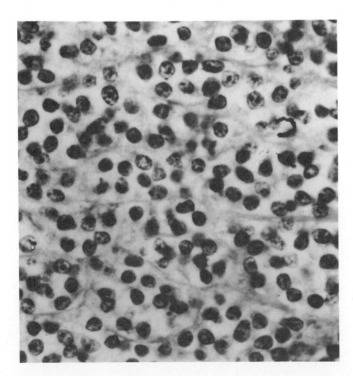

Figure 26-18. Ewing's sarcoma. Small, round cells, with
glycogen-filled clear cytoplasm, are uniformly distributed.

the skull, are common sites for metastases (45% to 75% of cases). With irradiation and chemotherapy, the 5-year survival rate is approximately 50%.

METASTATIC TUMORS

The most common malignant tumor of bone is metastatic cancer, with carcinomas comprising the vast majority of lesions. Specifically, tumors of the breast, prostate, lung, thyroid, and kidney frequently spread to bone. Tumor cells usually arrive in the bone via the bloodstream; in the case of spinal metastases, they are transported particularly by the vertebral veins. It is estimated that skeletal metastases are found in at least 85% of cancer cases that have run their full clinical course. The vertebral column is, by far, the most commonly affected bony structure. Some tumors (cancers of the thyroid, gastrointestinal tract, kidney, and neuroblastoma) produce mostly lytic lesions by stimulating osteoclasts. A few tumors (prostate, breast, lung, and stomach cancers) stimulate osteoblastic components to make bone; these appear on radiographic studies as

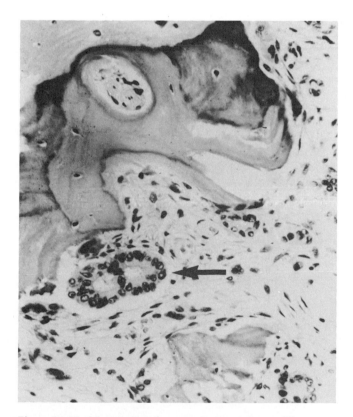

Figure 26-19. Metastatic adenocarcinoma to bone. The neoplastic glands (*arrow*) have stimulated new woven bone formation. The marrow has been replaced by loose fibrosis. This focus is an osteoblastic metastasis.

dense, bony foci (Fig. 26-19). However, most foci of metastatic cancer have mixtures of both lytic and blastic elements. It is important to remember that the cancer itself does not resorb or make bone, but instead stimulates, by unknown mechanisms, the mesenchymal elements of the marrow.

FIBROUS DYSPLASIA

Fibrous dysplasia is a condition characterized by a disorganized mixture of fibrous and osseous elements in the interior of affected bones. The disorder probably represents a peculiar developmental abnormality of the skeleton rather than a neoplasm, although it is neither familial nor hereditary. It occurs in children or adults, and may involve a single bone (monostotic) or many bones (polyostotic). The skeletal lesions may be associated with skin pigmentation and endocrine dysfunction, in which case the term "Albright's syndrome" is applied.

Monostotic fibrous dysplasia is the most common form of the disease and is most often seen in the second and third decades. The bones that are commonly involved are the proximal femur, tibia, ribs, and facial bones, but any bone may be involved. The disease may be asymptomatic, or it may lead to a pathologic fracture.

In **polyostotic fibrous dysplasia** (osteitis fibrosa disseminata) more than one bone is involved; 25% of patients exhibit disease in more than half of the skeleton, including the facial bones. Symptoms usually present in childhood, and almost all patients suffer from pathologic fractures, limb deformities, or limb length discrepancies. Polyostotic fibrous dysplasia is more common in females.

The endocrine dysfunctions of **Albright's syndrome** may include acromegaly, Cushing's syndrome, hyperthyroidism, and vitamin-D–resistant rickets. However, the most common endocrine abnormality is precocious puberty in females (males rarely have Albright's syndrome). The most frequent extraskeletal manifestations of this form of fibrous dysplasia are the characteristic skin lesions. These are pigmented macules (café au lait spots) which are usually located on the buttocks (Fig. 26-20A), back, and over the sacrum.

The radiographic features of fibrous dysplasia are distinctive. The bone lesion has a lucent ground-glass appearance with well-marginated borders and a thin cortex. The bone may be ballooned, deformed, or enlarged, and involvement may be focal, or it may encompass the entire bone (Fig. 26-20B).

All the forms of fibrous dysplasia have an identical histologic pattern—benign fibroblastic tissue arranged

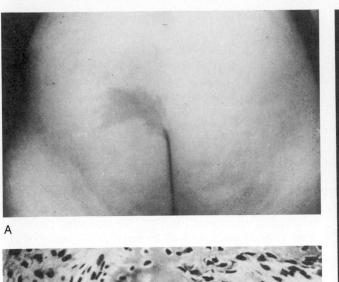

A

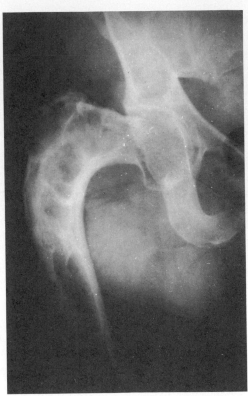

B

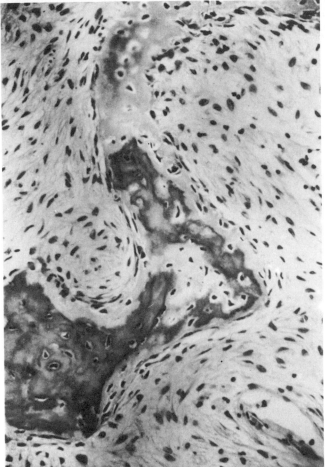

C

Figure 26-20. Fibrous dysplasia. (*A*) A café au lait spot on the skin involves the gluteal crease. The spot has an irregular ("coast of Maine") border and does not cross the midline. (*B*) A radiograph of the proximal femur shows a "shepherd's crook" deformity, caused by fractures sustained over the years. There are irregular, marginated, ground-glass lucencies, which are surrounded by reactive bone. The shaft has an appearance that has been likened to a soap bubble. (*C*) A photomicrograph reveals loose, fibrous marrow in which a fragment of partially mineralized woven bone is embedded. The lack of osteoblastic palisading is characteristic of fibrous dysplasia.

in a loose, whorled pattern. Irregularly arranged, purposeless, woven bone spicules that lack osteoblastic rimming are embedded in the fibrous tissue (Fig 26-20C). Treatment consists of curettage, repair of fractures, and prevention of deformities.

JOINTS

OSTEOARTHRITIS

Osteoarthritis, the most common form of joint disease in the United States, **is a slowly progressive degeneration of the articular cartilage that generally is manifested in the weight-bearing joints and fingers of elderly individuals.** The prevalence and severity of this disease increase with age, so that people 18 to 24 years of age have incidence rates of 4%, whereas those who are 75 to 79 years of age have an 85% rate. Before the age of 45 years, the disease predominantly affects men; after the age of 55 years, however, osteoarthritis is more common in women. The disease is not a single nosologic entity, but rather a group of disorders that have in common the mechanical destruction of a joint. Osteoarthritis has variously been called "wear and tear" arthritis and "degenerative joint disease" because of the progressive degradation of articular cartilage that leads to joint narrowing, subchondral bone thickening, and eventually, a nonfunctioning, painful joint. Although it is not primarily an inflammatory process, a mild inflammatory reaction may occur within the synovium.

Radiologically, osteoarthritis is characterized by (1) narrowing of the joint space, which represents the loss of articular cartilage; (2) increased thickness of the subchondral bone; (3) subchondral bone cysts; and (4) large peripheral nodules of bone, called **osteophytes,** which represent the bone's attempt to grow a new articular surface. **Chondromalacia,** a term applied to a subcategory of osteoarthritis that affects the patellar surface of the femoral condyles of young people, produces pain and stiffness of the knee.

ETIOLOGY

The factors that play a major role in the etiology of osteoarthritis include an increased unit load on the chondrocyte, decreased resilience of the subchondral coarse cancellous bone, and increased stiffness of the coarse cancellous bone of the epiphysis. These three factors may lead to increased degradation of articular cartilage, with accompanying focally increased synthesis of cartilage matrix, and even increased replication of chondrocytes. Both of these effects represent an attempt to heal the articular cartilage. However, the degree of synthesis and cell replication is not enough to keep pace with the continuing stress, and eventually **the articular cartilage is degraded and disappears.**

PATHOLOGY

The earliest histologic changes of osteoarthritis involve the loss of proteoglycans from the surface of the articular cartilage, manifested as a decrease in metachromatic staining. At the same time, empty lacunae in the articular cartilage indicate the death of chondrocytes (Fig. 26-21). The viable chondrocytes become large, aggregate into groups or **clones,** and are surrounded by basophilic-staining matrix, called the **territorial matrix.** The disease may arrest at this stage for many years before it proceeds to the next stage, which is characterized by **fibrillation,** the development of surface cracks parallel to the long axis of the articular surface. These fibrillations also may persist for many years before further progression occurs. As these cracks propagate, synovial fluid begins to flow into the defects. Eventually, pieces of articular cartilage break off and lodge in the synovium, there inducing mild inflammation and a foreign body giant cell reaction. The result is a hyperemic and hypertrophied synovium.

As a crack extends downward neovascularization from the epiphysis and subchondral bone extend into the area of the crack, inducing subchondral osteoclastic bone resorption. Adjacent osteoblastic activity also occurs, and the net result is a thickening of the subchondral bone plate in the area of the crack. As neovascularization progressively extends into the area of the crack, mesenchymal cells invade, and fibrocartilage forms as a poor substitute for the articular hyaline cartilage. These fibrocartilaginous plugs may persist, or they may be swept into the joint. The subchondral bone becomes exposed and burnished as it grinds against the opposite joint surface, which is undergoing the same process. These thick, shiny, and smooth areas of subchondral bone are referred to as **eburnated** ("ivorylike") bone (Figs. 26-22 and 26-23). In some areas, the eburnated bone eventually cracks, allowing synovial fluid to extend from the joint surface into the subchondral bone marrow, where it eventually leads to a **subchondral bone cyst.**

An **osteophyte** may be formed (usually, in the lateral portions of the joint) when the mesenchymal tissue of the synovium modulates into osteoblasts and chondroblasts, cells that form a mass of cartilage and bone. On gross examination, these osteophytes are pearly, grayish-bone nodules appearing on the peripheral

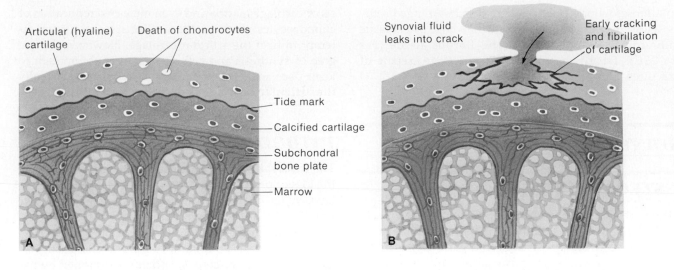

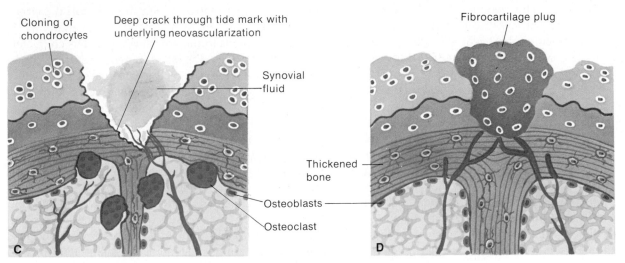

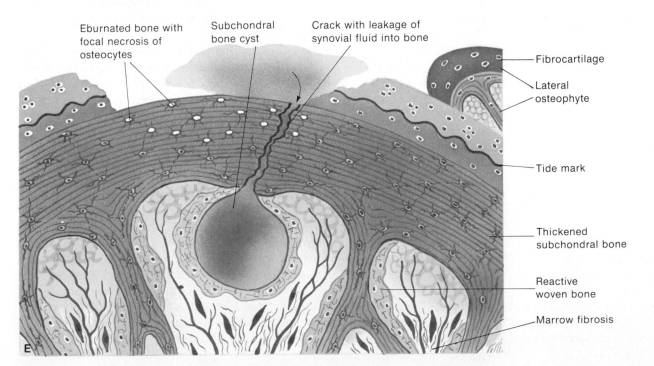

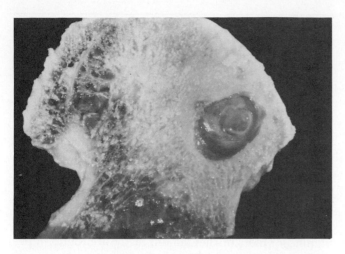

Figure 26-22. Osteoarthritis. The femoral head is flattened, with loss of articular cartilage and an eburnated subchondral bone plate. A subchondral bone cyst, surrounded by new bone, is evident.

portion of the joint surface. These osteophytes, or bony spurs, also occur at the lateral portions of the intervertebral discs, extending from the adjacent vertebral bodies and producing the "lipping" pattern seen on radiologic studies as osteoarthritis of the spine. In the fingers, osteophytes at the distal interphalangeal joints are termed **Heberden's nodes.**

RHEUMATOID ARTHRITIS

Rheumatoid arthritis is a systemic, chronic, inflammatory disease that involves the joints. Its onset usually occurs in the third or fourth decade, but it may occur at any age. The joints that are commonly affected are those of the extremities, which are usually afflicted at the same time and often in a symmetrical pattern. The

Figure 26-23. Osteoarthritis. The articular cartilage has been lost (*right*). Remnants of the articular cartilage are evident on the left. The thickened subchondral bone corresponds to the eburnated bone seen on gross inspection.

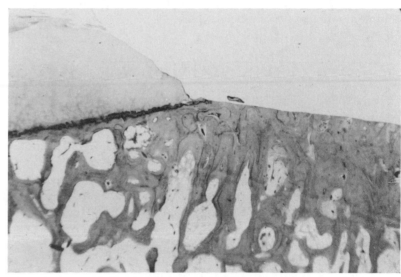

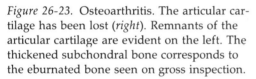

Figure 26-21. Histogenesis of osteoarthritis. The death of chondrocytes leads to a crack in the articular cartilage that is followed by an influx of synovial fluid and further loss and degeneration of cartilage. As a result of this process, cartilage is gradually worn away. Below the tide mark, new vessels grow in from the epiphysis, and fibrocartilage is deposited. The fibrocartilage plug is not mechanically sufficient and may be worn away, thereby exposing the subchondral bone plate, which becomes thickened and eburnated. If there is a crack in this region, synovial fluid leaks into the marrow space and produces a subchondral bone cyst. Focal regrowth of the articular surface leads to the formation of osteophytes.

course of the disease is variable, and is often punctuated with remissions and exacerbations. The broad spectrum of clinical manifestations ranges from barely discernible and mild forms to severe, destructive, and mutilating disease.

The diagnosis is based primarily on the clinical course, rather than the histopathology, because there is no one specific finding that is diagnostic of rheumatoid arthritis. Rheumatoid factor is usually present in the serum, but some patients are persistently seronegative. Furthermore, rheumatoid factor is not specific for rheumatoid arthritis. It is now thought that classic rheumatoid arthritis probably comprises a heterogeneous group of disorders; patients who are persistently seronegative for rheumatoid factor may have disease of a different etiology than do those who are seropositive. While in the classic form of rheumatoid arthritis joint manifestations are predominant, rheumatoidlike diseases exist; they are associated with underlying maladies such as inflammatory bowel disease and cirrhosis.

Rheumatoid arthritis and its variants are characterized histologically by a progressive proliferation of the synovium, which eventually destroys the articular cartilage and leads to severe osteoarthritis as the final common pathway of joint destruction.

CLASSIFICATION AND INCIDENCE

Clinically rheumatoid arthritis is considered to be a disease without a specific biologic marker. The diagnosis is based primarily on a number of criteria, and the incidence varies depending upon which criteria are employed. Rheumatoid arthritis affects less than 1% of the adult population; its incidence is greater in women than in men (with a ratio of 3:1). A genetic origin for the disease in white patients is suggested by the association of the haplotype HLA-DW4 and a related B-cell alloantigen, HLA-DRW4, with severe seropositive rheumatoid arthritis.

PATHOGENESIS

The cause of rheumatoid arthritis is unknown. It is thought that immunologic mechanisms play an important role in the pathogenesis of the disease. Lymphocytes and plasma cells, which are increased in number in the synovium, produce immunoglobulins, mainly of the IgG class. Deposits of immunoglobulins and complement components are present in the articular cartilage and the synovium.

Rheumatoid factor actually represents multiple antibodies, principally IgM, directed against the Fc fragment of IgG. **Up to 80% of patients with classic rheumatoid arthritis are positive for rheumatoid factor.** Significant titers of rheumatoid factor are found in patients with related diseases, such as systemic lupus erythematosus, progressive systemic sclerosis, and dermatomyositis. Rheumatoid factor also may occur in a wide variety of nonrheumatic disorders, including pulmonary fibrosis, cirrhosis, sarcoidosis, Waldenström's macroglobulinemia, tuberculosis, kala-azar, lepromatous leprosy, and viral hepatitis. Healthy elderly people, particularly women, may also test positive for rheumatoid factor. Interestingly, although patients with classic rheumatoid arthritis may be seronegative, the presence of high titer rheumatoid factor is frequently associated with severe and unremitting disease, many systemic complications, and a grave prognosis. In addition to IgM, rheumatoid factors may also be IgG and IgA. The presence of IgG may be associated with the development of systemic complications, such as necrotizing vasculitis. In addition, IgG immune complexes may be found in the synovial fluid.

PATHOLOGY

The early synovial changes of rheumatoid arthritis are edema and the accumulation of plasma cells, lymphocytes, and macrophages (Fig. 26-24). There is a con-

Figure 26-24. Histogenesis of rheumatoid arthritis. A virus or an unknown stress stimulates the synovial cells to proliferate. The influx of lymphocytes, plasma cells, and mast cells, together with neovascularization and edema, leads to hypertrophy and hyperplasia of the synovium. Lymphoid nodules are prominent. The proliferating synovium extends into the joint space, burrows into the bone beneath the articular cartilage, and covers the cartilage as a pannus. The articular cartilage is eventually destroyed by direct resorption or by deprivation of its nutrient synovial fluid. The synovial tissue continues to proliferate in the subchondral region, as well as in the joint. Eventually, the joint is destroyed and becomes fused, a condition termed ankylosis.

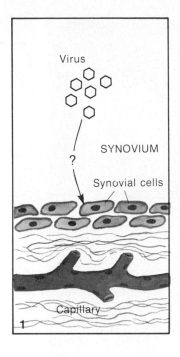

Virus

SYNOVIUM

Synovial cells

Capillary

1

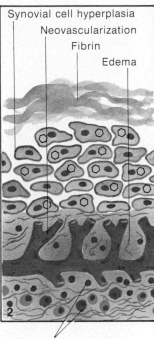

Synovial cell hyperplasia
Neovascularization
Fibrin
Edema

2

Lymphocytes and plasma
cells and mast cells

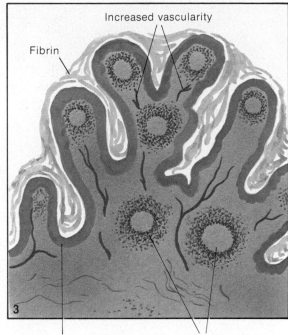

Increased vascularity

Fibrin

3

Papillary synovium with
synovial cell hyperplasia

Nodules of lymphocytes
and plasma cells

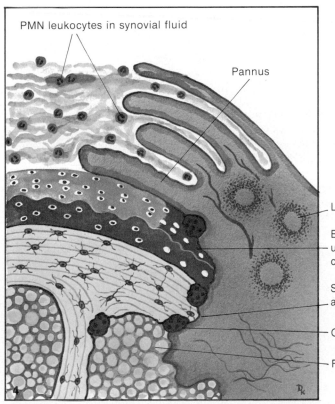

PMN leukocytes in synovial fluid

Pannus

Lymphoid follicle

Erosion of cartilage and
underlying dead
chondrocytes

Subchondral pannus
and bone erosion

Osteoclast

Fatty marrow

4

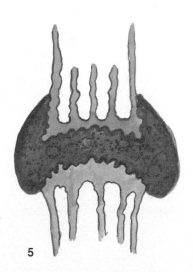

5

Destruction of joint by fibrosis and
loss of articular cartilage, with
periarticular bone loss

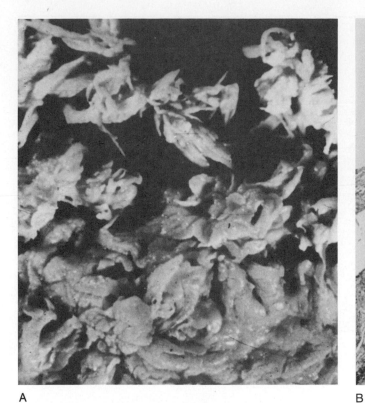

A

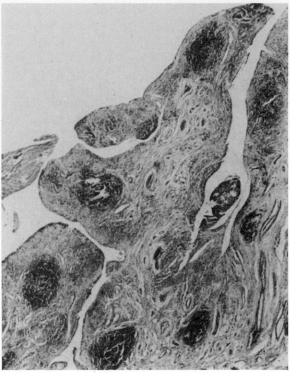

B

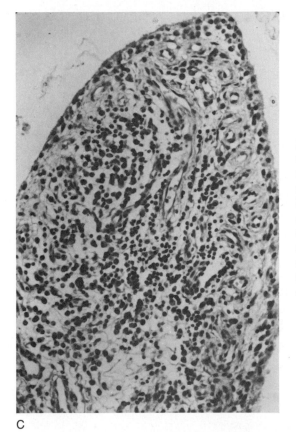

C

Figure 26-25. Rheumatoid arthritis. (*A*) On gross examination, the synovium shows numerous papillary folds, swelling, and thickening of the synovial membrane. (*B*) A microscopic view reveals prominent lymphoid follicles (Allison-Ghormley bodies), synovial hyperplasia and hypertrophy, villous folds, and thickening of the synovial membrane by fibrosis and inflammation. (*C*) A higher-power view of a single villus demonstrates the synovial cell hyperplasia. More than two or three cell layers of synovial cells are present. The subsynovial tissue is filled with lymphocytes, plasma cells, and scattered mast cells. The capillaries are congested.

comitant increase in vascularity, and exudation of fibrin in the joint space. Conspicuous fibrin deposition may result in small fibrin nodules that float in the joint, termed **rice bodies.** The synovial lining cells, which are normally one to three layers thick, undergo hyperplasia and form layers 8 to 10 cells thick. Multinucleated giant cells are often found among the synovial cells. **The net result is a synovial lining thrown into the numerous villi and frondlike folds that fill the peripheral recesses of the joint.** As the synovium undergoes hyperplasia and hypertrophy, it creeps over the surface of the articular cartilage and adjacent structures. This inflammatory synovium, now containing mast cells, is termed a **pannus** ("cloak"). The pannus proceeds to cover the articular cartilage and isolate it from its nutritional synovial fluid. **The pannus erodes the articular cartilage and the adjacent bone, probably through the action of collagenase produced by the pannus.** Lymphocytes aggregate into masses and eventually develop a follicular center, an appearance termed an **Allison-Ghormley body** (Fig. 26-25).

The **synovial fluid** contains abundant polymorphonuclear leukocytes, although they are rarely present in the **synovial tissue.** As the disease waxes and wanes over the years, the degree of acute inflammation also correlates with the varying activity of the rheumatoid process. The pannus may burrow deep to the subchondral bone plate, where it erodes the bone as well as the cartilage. It may also extend through the joint capsule into adjacent tissues. The tendon sheaths, which are lined by synovial tissue, may undergo the same rheumatoid change; this occasionally produces rupture of the affected tendons.

The characteristic bone loss of rheumatoid arthritis is juxta-articular; that is, it is immediately adjacent to both sides of the joint. Since the remaining bone is normal, juxta-articular bone loss is probably related to a factor elaborated locally by the rheumatoid synovium. The pannus invades the joint and subchondral bones as if it were a neoplasm. Eventually, the joint is destroyed and undergoes fibrous fusion, or ankylosis (Fig. 26-26). Longstanding disease leads to a fused joint with bony bridging, called **bony ankylosis** of a joint.

RHEUMATOID NODULES

Rheumatoid arthritis is a systemic disease that also involves tissues other than the joints and tendons. A characteristic lesion, termed the **rheumatoid nodule,** is found in other systemic locations. The rheumatoid nodule resembles a granulomatous reaction to a centrally located core of so-called "fibrinoid necrosis," which is a mixture of fibrin and other proteins, such as degraded collagen (Fig. 26-27). A surrounding rim of histiocytes is arranged in a radial, or palisading, fashion. Peripheral to the histiocytes is an outer circle of lymphocytes, plasma cells, and other mononuclear cells. Such nodules may also be seen in lupus erythematosus and rheumatic fever. Rheumatoid nodules, which are usually found in areas of pressure (for example, the skin of the elbow and legs), are movable, firm, rubbery, and not painful, although they may be tender. Rheumatoid arthritis is occasionally accompanied by acute necrotizing vasculitis affecting virtually any organ. Vasculitis may produce a myocardial infarction, cerebrovascular occlusion, renal failure, mesenteric infarction, or gangrene of a digit.

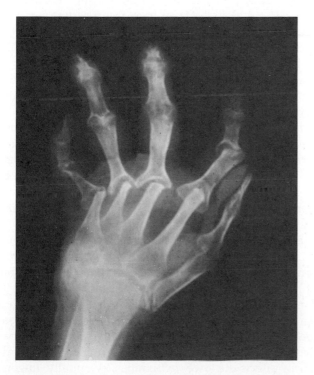

Figure 26-26. Rheumatoid arthritis. A radiograph of the hand reveals joint destruction, particularly of the proximal interphalangeal and metacarpalphalangeal joints. Periarticular loss of bone (osteoporosis) is confined to the joint areas. The metacarpal heads are destroyed.

URATE GOUT

Gout represents a heterogeneous group of diseases in which the common denominator is an increased serum uric acid level. Recurrent attacks of acute arthritis are associated with the deposition of urate crystals in and about the joints of the extremities.

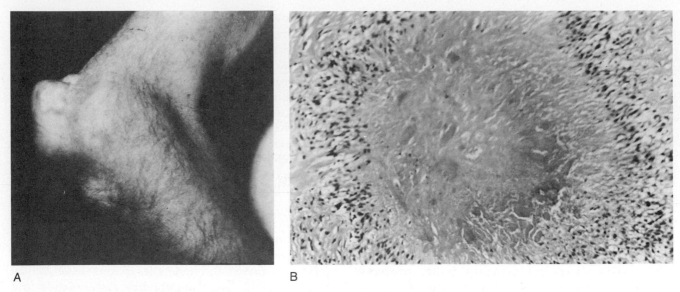

A　　　　　　　　　　　　　B

Figure 26-27. Rheumatoid nodule. (*A*) A patient with rheumatoid arthritis has a mass on the extensor surface of the elbow. (*B*) A central area of fibrinoid necrosis is surrounded by palisaded histiocytes.

CLASSIFICATION

Primary gout, a diagnosis made when no other intercurrent disease is present, may be caused by increased urate production (termed primary metabolic gout), decreased renal excretion of urate (primary renal gout), or a combination of the two. **Secondary gout** refers to hyperuricemia caused by another disease in which there is both an increased urate production secondary to cell lysis and release of nucleic acids (secondary metabolic gout), as well as decreased renal excretion (secondary renal gout).

EPIDEMIOLOGY AND ETIOLOGY

The serum uric acid level in gout is elevated beyond 7 mg/dl, a value that exceeds the limit of solubility of monosodium urate in the blood, although the prevalence of gout is less than that of hyperuricemia. **Gout is a disease that primarily affects adult men; indeed, only about 5% of cases occur in women.** The peak incidence is in the fifth decade. A family history is elicited in up to 75% of patients.

There are two enzymatic causes of primary gout—namely, a deficiency of hypoxanthine guanine phosphoribosyl transferase, and overactivity of 5-phosphoribosyl-l—pyrophosphate (PRPP) synthetase. Both enzymes are X-linked. Some studies indicate that autosomal dominant inheritance may be a factor in the development of gout.

CLINICAL FEATURES

Classic gout presents with characteristic clinical features. These include (1) an increase in serum uric acid concentration; (2) recurrent attacks of acute arthritis, with sodium urate crystals demonstrable in the synovial fluid leukocytes; (3) the presence of aggregates of urate crystals, termed tophi, in or around joints of the extremities (Fig. 26-28); (4) renal disease; and (5) urate nephrolithiasis.

The clinical features of gout may be divided into four stages: asymptomatic hyperuricemia, acute gouty arthritis, intercritical gout, and chronic tophaceous gout. Renal stones may occur in any stage except the first. In most cases, symptomatic gout appears before the renal stones, which usually require 20 to 30 years of sustained hyperuricemia.

Acute gouty arthritis is a painful condition that usually involves one joint and is unaccompanied by constitutional symptoms. However, later in the course of the disease, polyarticular involvement with fever is common. At least 50% of patients first present with a painful and red first metatarsophalangeal joint (great toe), designated **podagra.** Eventually, 90% of all patients experience podagra. Although the disease primarily affects the lower extremities, eventually, fingers, elbows, and wrists also become involved. Classically, a gouty attack is triggered by consuming a large meal or drinking alcoholic beverages, but other specific events, such as trauma, certain drugs, and surgery, may also be responsible.

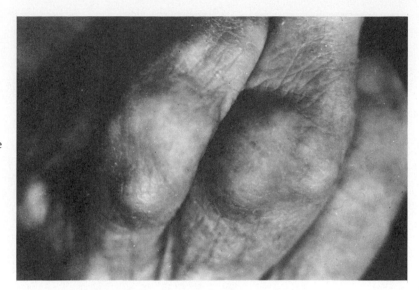

Figure 26-28. Gout. Tophi project from the fingers as rubbery nodules.

The **intercritical period** is the asymptomatic phase that represents the interval between the initial acute attack and subsequent attacks. These periods may last up to 10 years, but later attacks may be increasingly severe and prolonged, polyarticular, and febrile.

In the untreated patient **tophaceous gout** eventually appears in the form of tophi in the cartilage, synovial membranes, tendons, and soft tissues. **A tophus** is a chalky, cheesy, yellow-white, pasty deposit of monosodium urate crystals. A classic location of a tophus is in the external ear. Tophi also occur along pressure points of the body, in the olecranon bursa, and in the Achilles tendon. In patients treated with antihyperuricemic drugs, tophi are rarely seen.

Renal dysfunction, manifested as albuminuria, occurs in up to 90% of patients with gouty arthritis and, when left untreated, may progress to renal failure. **Renal damage occurs as a result of crystal deposition in the renal interstitial tissue and obstruction of the collecting tubules by the uric acid crystals** (see Chapter 16).

PATHOLOGY

The presence of long, needle-shaped crystals that are negatively birefringent under polarized light is diagnostic of gout (Fig. 26-29). Extracellular soft tissue deposits of these crystals in tophi are surrounded by foreign body giant cells and an associated inflammatory response of mononuclear cells. These granulomalike areas are found in cartilage, in any of the soft tissues around joints, and even in the subchondral bone marrow adjacent to joints. Grossly, any chalky, white deposit on the surfaces of intra-articular structures (Fig.

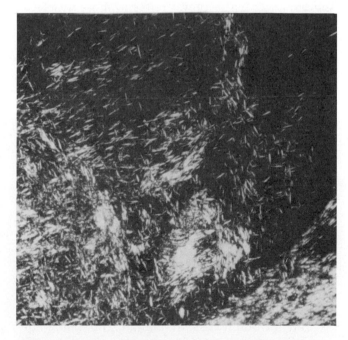

Figure 26-29. Gout crystals. Needle-shaped, elongated, highly refractile crystals are seen on exposure to polarized light.

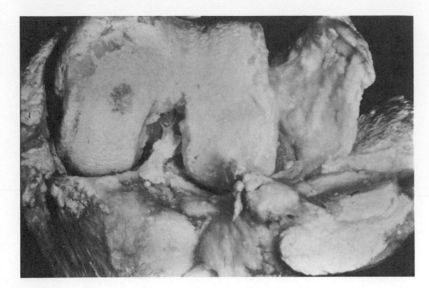

Figure 26-30. Gouty arthritis. A gross specimen of a knee shows crystals covering the articular surface of the distal femur. The patella (*lower right*) and the synovial membrane display chalky, white deposits.

26-30), including articular cartilage, is suspicious for gout.

SOFT TISSUE TUMORS

The term **soft tissue tumor** refers to those neoplastic conditions that arise in extraskeletal tissues of the body, excluding epithelia, visceral organs and their connective tissue framework, the reticuloendothelial system, meninges, and glia. Thus, tumors arising in the skeletal muscle, fat, fibrous tissue, blood and lymphatic vessels, and peripheral nerves are considered to be soft tissue tumors.

Soft tissues tumors are rare, and benign neoplasms are 100 times more common than malignant ones. Soft tissue sarcomas comprise less than 1% of all cancers in the United States, and only 5,000 are reported yearly.

A few important general principles relate to soft tissue tumors:
- The more superficial the location of the tumor, the more likely it is to be benign.
- The larger the tumor, the more likely it is to be malignant.
- A rapidly growing tumor is more likely to be malignant than one that develops slowly.
- Calcification exists in benign and malignant tumors.
- Deep lesions tend to be malignant.

- Benign tumors are relatively avascular, whereas most malignant ones are hypervascular, as documented on angiography.

TUMORS OF FIBROUS ORIGIN

NODULAR FASCIITIS

Nodular fasciitis is actually a benign lesion, not a neoplasm (Fig. 26-31). It is a reactive phenomenon, probably secondary to trauma, that occurs in young boys and most commonly affects the forearm, trunk, and back. Usually, the rapid growth of this lesion prompts the adolescent to seek medical attention. Histologically, nodular fasciitis may be mistaken for a sarcoma because it is hypercellular and has abundant mitoses and numerous, pleomorphic, spindle-shaped cells. Its true nature is defined when it is recognized that the entire "mass" is the counterpart of granulation tissue in response to trauma. The lesion is self-limited and is cured by surgical excision.

FIBROSARCOMA

Fibrosarcoma is a malignant tumor of fibroblasts that is most commonly found in the thigh, particularly around the knee. It is characterized histologically by pleomorphic fibroblasts that form densely interlacing bundles

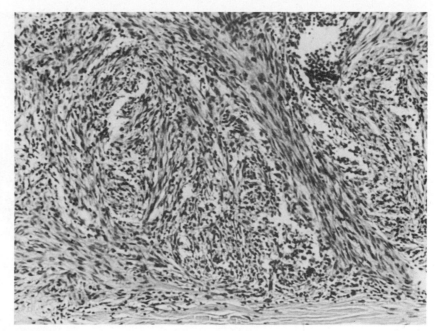

Figure 26-31. Nodular fasciitis. Swirls of tightly woven spindle cells and collagen are admixed with lymphocytes and plasma cells. Although the abundance of spindle cells is suggestive of a neoplastic process, the presence of an inflammatory component indicates the non-neoplastic nature of the lesion.

and fascicles, producing a so-called "herringbone" pattern (Fig. 26-32). Poorly differentiated fibrosarcomas have a poor prognosis, whereas the well-differentiated forms have a 5-year survival rate of 60% or more.

MALIGNANT FIBROUS HISTIOCYTOMA

Some malignant soft tissue tumors contain foci of histiocytic differentiation, in which case they are called malignant fibrous histiocytomas. Regardless of the name, the prognosis depends on the degree of cytologic atypia. The recurrence rate is high if the tumor is incompletely removed and, depending upon the grade of tumor, at least 50% metastasize to the lungs.

TUMORS OF FAT (ADIPOSE TUMORS)

The most common soft tissue mass is a benign, well-defined proliferation of adipocytes termed a **lipoma.** Histologically, a lipoma is often indistinguishable from normal adipose tissue. Lipomas are generally seen in

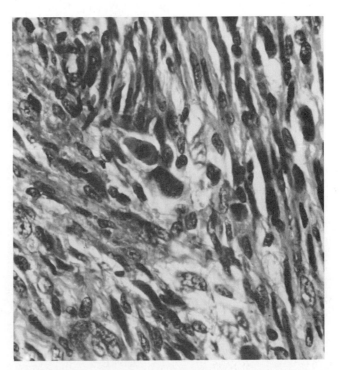

Figure 26-32. Fibrosarcoma. The tumor exhibits bizarre spindle cells. A mitosis is seen in the center of the field.

middle-aged individuals and may occur at any site in the body.

Liposarcomas are the most common sarcomas in adults, comprising 20% of all soft tissue sarcomas. They generally appear in persons 50 years of age or older, and are found in the deep thigh and retroperitoneal regions. They tend to grow slowly but may become extremely large. Liposarcomas with extensive pleomorphism have a poor prognosis (Fig. 26-33). Recurrence rates following surgery are high, depending on the location of the tumor.

VASCULAR TUMORS

Tumors arising from endothelial cells may be either benign or malignant. Benign vascular tumors are called **hemangiomas,** and are the most common benign neoplasms of childhood. These lesions are characterized by blood-filled spaces lined by benign endothelial cells. A tumor with large endothelial spaces is labeled a **cavernous hemangioma,** whereas one with small endothelial spaces is designated a **capillary hemangioma** (Fig. 26-34). **Arteriovenous malformations** are composed of large, tortuous arteries and misshapen, veinlike structures.

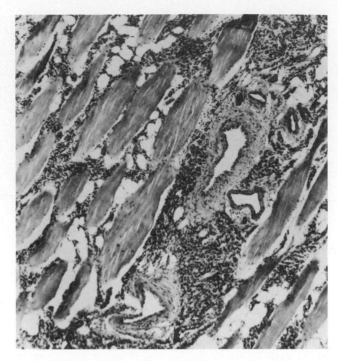

Figure 26-34. Capillary hemangioma. Benign vascular spaces, lined by flat endothelial cells, infiltrate between muscle fibers.

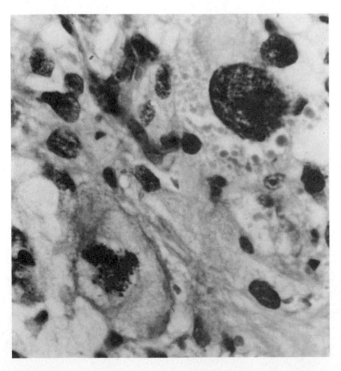

Figure 26-33. Liposarcoma. Large pleomorphic cells with vacuolated cytoplasm and atypical mitoses are evident.

Angiosarcoma, a malignant vascular tumor, usually occurs in subcutaneous tissues, especially those of the face and scalp, and is highly invasive. Histologically, the endothelial cells pile up, proliferate into vascular spaces, and display numerous mitotic figures.

RHABDOMYOSARCOMA

Rhabdomyosarcoma is a malignant tumor that displays features of striated muscle differentiation. The histogenesis of rhabdomyosarcoma is controversial, but it is probable that most of these tumors derive from primitive mesenchyme that retains the capacity for skeletal muscle differentiation. Alternatively, rhabdomyosarcoma may arise from embryonal muscle tissue that is displaced into the soft tissues during embryogenesis.

Rhabdomyosarcoma is an uncommon tumor in adults, but is the most frequent soft tissue sarcoma of children and young adults. Most cases can be classified according to four histologic categories: embryonal, botryoid embryonal, alveolar, and pleomorphic.

Embryonal rhabdomyosarcoma is most common in children 15 years of age or younger, and most frequently involves the head and neck (see Chapter 25), genitourinary tract, and retroperitoneum. The morphologic appearance varies from that of a highly differentiated tumor, containing rhabdomyoblasts with a large eosinophilic cytoplasm and cross striations, to that of a poorly differentiated neoplasm that is difficult to classify.

The botryoid variant of embryonal rhabdomyosarcoma is distinguished by the formation of polypoid, grapelike tumor masses. Microscopically, there are only a few malignant cells, scattered in an abundant myxoid stroma. Botryoid foci may occur in any type of embryonal rhabdomyosarcoma, but they are most common in tumors of the visceral organs, including the vagina (see Chapter 18) and the bladder.

Alveolar rhabdomyosarcoma occurs less frequently than the embryonal type, and principally affects persons between the ages of 10 and 25 years. It is most common in the upper and lower extremities, but it can also be distributed in the same sites as the embryonal type. Typically, club-shaped tumor cells are arranged in clumps that are outlined by fibrous septa. The loose arrangement of the cells in the center of the clusters leads to the ''alveolar'' pattern. Malignant rhabdomyoblasts, identifiable by their cross striations, occur less commonly in the alveolar variant than in embryonal rhabdomyosarcoma, being present in only 25% of cases.

Pleomorphic rhabdomyosarcoma, the least common form of rhabdomyosarcoma, is found in the skeletal muscles of older persons. This tumor differs from the other types of rhabdomyosarcoma in the pleomorphism of its irregularly arranged cells. Large, granular, and eosinophilic rhabdomyoblasts are common, although cross striations are virtually nonexistent.

The previously dismal prognosis associated with most rhabdomyosarcomas has improved in the last 20 years as a result of the introduction of combined therapeutic modalities, including surgery, radiotherapy, and chemotherapy. Today, more than 80% of patients with localized or regional disease are cured.

KAPOSI'S SARCOMA

A lesion worthy of special attention is Kaposi's sarcoma, a skin tumor of endothelial cell origin that is typified by irregular bundles of spindle-shaped cells with vascular, slitlike spaces. These spaces are lined by atypical endothelial cells, and contain extravasated erythrocytes. Hemosiderin-laden macrophages are scattered throughout the tumor.

The disease was first described in the 19th century, and was seen in two forms. One occurred among elderly, white people, many of whom had another disease that impaired the immune system. This neoplasm was indolent, but was often followed by another malignant disease, usually a lymphoproliferative disorder. A more aggressive variant of Kaposi's sarcoma commonly occurred in African blacks. There is a high incidence of this tumor in patients with acquired immunodeficiency syndrome (AIDS).

SYNOVIAL SARCOMA

Synovial sarcoma should be considered a soft tissue tumor. The lesion is classically described as having a **biphasic pattern** that forms microscopic spaces in a sarcomatous spindle cell background (Fig. 26-35). These slitlike spaces are filled with fluid similar to hyaluronic acid. If these spaces are not present, a diagnosis of **monophasic sarcoma** may be established, but it is difficult to differentiate such a tumor from fibrosarcoma. The recurrence rate of this tumor after resection is high, and metastases occur in over 60% of cases. The 5-year survival rate is about 50%, and those who die have extensive lung metastases.

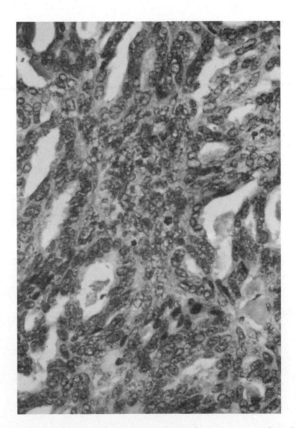

Figure 26-35. Synovial sarcoma. Irregular spaces are lined by plump, synovial-like, neoplastic cells. The intervening tissue contains neoplastic cells with similar nuclei. There are no basement membranes separating the joint-like spaces from the more spindle-shaped interstitial tumor cells. This pattern is typical of a biphasic synovial sarcoma.

27

SKELETAL MUSCLE

VERNON W. ARMBRUSTMACHER

Noninflammatory Myopathies

Inflammatory Myopathies

Metabolic Diseases

Denervation

NONINFLAMMATORY MYOPATHIES

MUSCULAR DYSTROPHY

The term muscular dystrophy was developed to describe a primary degeneration of muscles, which was frequently hereditary, or at least familial, and relentlessly progressive. Morphologic study showed degeneration of muscle fibers, with regenerative activity, progressive fibrosis, and infiltration of the muscle with fatty tissue (Fig. 27-1). No inflammation was recognized. In subsequent years many variants of this type of muscle disease were described, and a classification of hereditary, progressive, noninflammatory degenerative conditions of muscle has been developed.

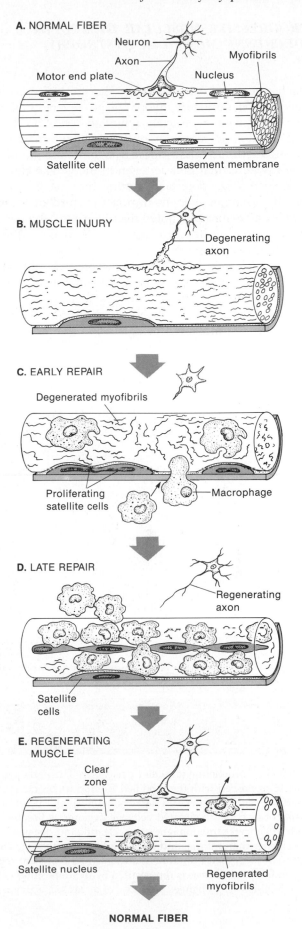

Figure 27-1. Degeneration/regeneration.
(*A*) A normal muscle fiber communicates with the lower motor neuron via the motor endplate. It contains subsarcolemmal nuclei, is packed with myofibrils, and is covered by a basement membrane. Scattered satellite cells are situated on the surface of the sarcolemma, but inside the basement membrane. These are dormant myoblasts, capable of proliferating and differentiating into muscle fibers. They constitute 3% to 5% of the nuclei seen in a cross section of skeletal muscle.
(*B*) In types of injury to the muscle fiber that preserve the integrity of the basement membrane (such as alcoholic rhabdomyolysis, Duchenne muscular dystrophy, or polymyositis) the sarcoplasmic structures begin to disintegrate and the terminus of the motor endplate breaks down.
(*C*) The damaged fiber attracts circulating macrophages, which penetrate the basement membrane and begin to digest and engulf the sarcoplasmic contents (myophagocytosis). In the meantime, regenerative processes begin with the activation and proliferation of the satellite cells, which, in contrast to the macrophages, are confined by the intact cylinder of basement membrane.
(*D*) At a later stage, myophagocytosis is prominent, satellite cells have proliferated and are beginning to fuse, protein synthesis has begun, and the damaged axon terminus is beginning to regenerate.
(*E*) Regeneration is prominent. The nuclei of the regenerating fiber are immature (large, vesicular with nucleoli) and centrally located. Myofibrils are developing, mostly at the periphery, and the ribosome-rich sarcoplasm appears basophilic with a hematoxylin and eosin stain. The motor endplate has reformed at its original site. This fiber will process to complete maturity, reconstituted as in *A*.

PROGRESSIVE MUSCULAR DYSTROPHY (DUCHENNE MUSCULAR DYSTROPHY)

Duchenne muscular dystrophy, the most clearly defined noninflammatory myopathy, is a severe, progressive, sex-linked, recessively inherited condition. Boys with Duchenne muscular dystrophy have markedly elevated serum creatine kinase from birth and morphologically abnormal muscle, even in utero. The clinical weakness is not detectable during the first year and usually becomes evident during the third or fourth year. The weakness is noted mainly around the pelvic and shoulder girdles (proximal muscle weakness) and is relentlessly progressive.

The weak muscles eventually become atrophic and are replaced by fibrofatty tissue. Eventually, a "pseudohypertrophy" of the calf muscles develops. The patients are usually wheelchair-bound by the age of 10 years and bedridden by the age of 15. The most common causes of death are complications of respiratory insufficiency caused by the muscular weakness, or cardiac arrhythmia due to myocardial involvement.

The earliest pathologic changes in the muscle tissue consist of scattered foci of degenerating and regenerating muscle fibers, together with scattered, large, hyalinized dark fibers, which are overly contracted and in an early stage of degeneration (Fig. 27-2). Breakdown of the sarcolemma, which probably accounts for the early striking elevation of serum creatine kinase in these patients, is one of the earliest ultrastructural changes noted. Myophagocytosis, the infiltration of histiocytes into degenerating muscle fibers, is almost invariable but does not reflect an inflammatory process. There is a brisk regenerative response to the degeneration. These regenerating fibers, which are alkaline phosphatase positive, have more basophilic sarcoplasm, as seen with the hematoxylin and eosin stain, and have large vesicular nuclei with prominent nucleoli (see Fig. 27-2).

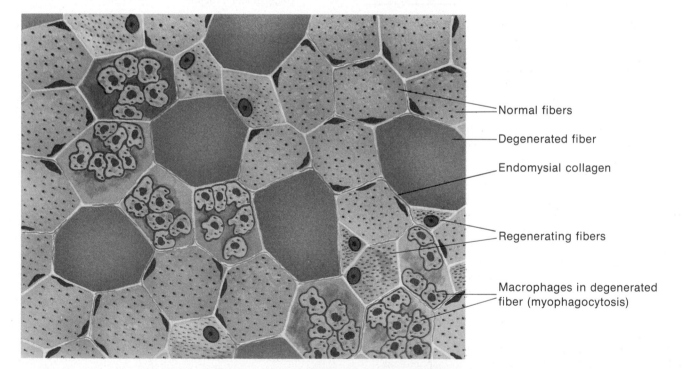

Normal fibers

Degenerated fiber

Endomysial collagen

Regenerating fibers

Macrophages in degenerated fiber (myophagocytosis)

Figure 27-2. Duchenne muscular dystrophy. The pathologic changes seen in skeletal muscle as stained with the modified Gomori trichrome stain are illustrated. Some fibers are slightly larger and darker than normal. These represent overcontracted segments of sarcoplasm situated between degenerated segments. Some fibers are packed with phagocytes (myophagocytosis) clearing out degenerated sarcoplasm. Some fibers are smaller than normal and have granular sarcoplasm. These fibers have enlarged, vesicular nuclei with prominent nucleoli, and represent regenerating fibers. Developing endomysial fibrosis is represented by the deposition of collagen around individual muscle fibers. The changes are those of a chronic, active noninflammatory myopathy.

Another typical change of Duchenne dystrophy is endomysial fibrosis, which develops early and becomes prominent with time. The process consists of constant focal degeneration of muscle fibers, with a prolonged effort at repair and regeneration, together with progressive fibrosis. The degenerative process eventually outstrips the regenerative capacity of the muscle. As a consequence there is a progressively decreasing number of muscle fibers and increasing amounts of fibrofatty connective tissue. The end stage is characterized by an almost complete loss of skeletal muscle fibers, but an interesting sparing of the muscle spindle fibers. The muscle spindle is surrounded by a capsule that creates a blood-spindle barrier similar to the blood-brain barrier.

Enzyme histochemical studies of skeletal muscle demonstrate that skeletal muscle fibers and muscle spindle fibers are equally affected, and there is no excess staining of the endomysial connective tissue with the alkaline phosphatase reaction, such as is seen in primary inflammatory myopathies. Although the pathogenesis of Duchenne's muscular dystrophy remains enigmatic, it may be related to an inability of the abnormal muscle to produce a protein termed dystrophin.

CONGENITAL MYOPATHIES

Occasionally a newborn infant manifests generalized hypotonia, with decreased deep tendon reflexes and muscle bulk. Some of these infants suffer from neurologic or metabolic disorders, which are often fatal. Other hypotonic patients have a "benign" course. Although the hypotonia persists throughout their lives, it is not progressive and they become ambulatory and live a normal life span; however, they continue to experience secondary skeletal complications of the hypotonia. It is the latter group of patients that is subsumed in the category of "congenital myopathies."

Morphologic study of the muscle of patients with congenital myopathy reveals three distinct groups of conditions, although variations in presentation often make the exact diagnosis difficult. The three groups are central core disease, nemaline (rod) myopathy, and central nuclear myopathy (Fig. 27-3).

Some generalizations can be made about these three conditions. In addition to presenting with congenital hypotonia, decreased deep tendon reflexes, decreased muscle bulk, and delayed motor milestones, the morphologic abnormality expressed in the muscle biopsy in all three conditions is confined to the type I (red) fibers. Furthermore, these patients have an abnormal predominance of type I fibers or, perhaps more accurately, a failure of type II (white) fibers to develop. The skele-

tal muscle does not show signs of active degeneration, and the patients do not ordinarily have elevated levels of serum creatine kinase.

CENTRAL CORE DISEASE

Central core disease can be sporadic, autosomal recessive, or autosomal dominant. It is characterized by congenital hypotonia, with proximal muscle weakness, decreased deep tendon reflexes, and delayed motor development. A typical patient does become ambulatory, although muscle strength never develops to a normal level.

Muscle biopsy typically reveals a striking predominance of type I fibers. In many or all of the type I fibers there is a central zone of degeneration that is best seen with the NADH tetrazolium reductase reaction. This is referred to as a central core abnormality and is characterized by loss of membranous organelles, with or without disorganization of the myofibrillar architecture. This central core runs the entire length of the fiber. It is difficult to see with the hematoxylin and eosin stain, but can often be demonstrated with a periodic acid-Schiff reaction (see Fig. 27-3B). Electron microscope study reveals that membranous organelles are absent in the central portion of the core but condense around its margin. The ultrastructure of the fiber is otherwise unremarkable. The myofibrils may show considerable disorganization or may be intact.

ROD (NEMALINE) MYOPATHY

This myopathy was initially named "nemaline" myopathy because the inclusions within the muscle fiber were interpreted as a tangled, threadlike mass. Since then it has been determined that the inclusions are clusters of rod-shaped inclusions, and the term rod myopathy has become established.

This entity probably includes a heterogeneous group of diseases that have in common the accumulation of rodlike inclusions within the sarcoplasm of skeletal muscle. The classic congenital form is characterized by congenital hypotonia and a clinical course of delayed motor milestones of variable clinical severity, with associated secondary skeletal changes, such as kyphoscoliosis. Later-onset (childhood and adult) forms have been noted, and these tend to be associated with some muscle degeneration, elevations of serum creatine kinase levels, and a slowly progressive course.

The pathologic findings on muscle biopsy consist of a variable predominance of type I fibers and the accumulation of rod-shaped structures within the sarcoplasm of the skeletal muscle. These inclusions, found mostly in the type I fibers, are brilliant red when

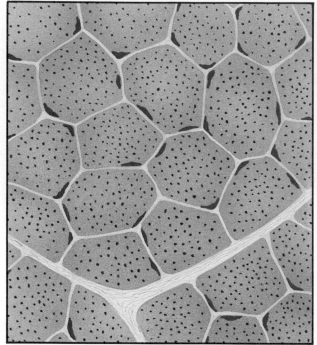

A. NORMAL

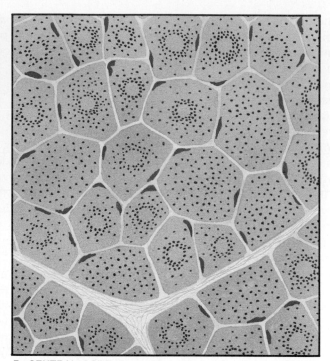

B. CENTRAL CORE DISEASE

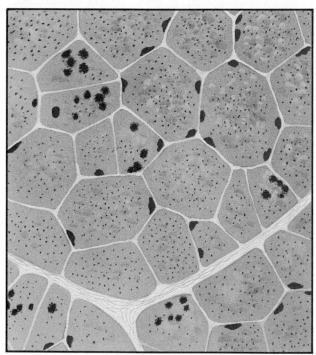

C. ROD MYOPATHY

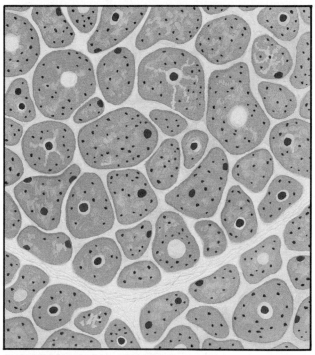

D. CENTRONUCLEAR MYOPATHY

stained with the modified Gomori trichrome stain (Fig. 27-3C) and may or may not be visible with a standard hematoxylin and eosin stain. Ultrastructural studies demonstrate that the inclusions are indeed rod-shaped and can be seen to arise from the Z-band, which they resemble ultrastructurally. The etiology of the condition is unknown.

CENTRAL NUCLEAR MYOPATHY (MYOTUBULAR MYOPATHY)

Central nuclear myopathy has been recognized as an autosomal recessive, autosomal dominant, and X-linked recessive condition. In the X-linked recessively inherited condition the newborn infant is strikingly weak and hypotonic and may die of respiratory insufficiency during the neonatal period. The autosomal dominant form tends to be of later onset and is associated with modestly elevated serum creatine kinase levels.

Biopsy specimens from patients with central nuclear myopathy are characterized by type I predominance; many of the type I fibers are small and round, with a single central nucleus (see Fig. 27-3D). The later onset forms of central nuclear myopathy are characterized morphologically by more mature muscle fibers (i.e., the fibers are larger and have more numerous myofibrils). The single central nucleus also appears more mature.

INFLAMMATORY MYOPATHIES

Inflammatory myopathies are easily recognized, the hallmark being an unequivocal inflammatory infiltrate within the skeletal muscle. In this category we do not include conditions caused by known infectious agents, but rather those in which the muscle tissue itself is the primary target of the inflammatory reaction. This targeting may be highly specific, as in polymyositis, or generalized, as in some of the diffuse collagen vascular diseases.

POLYMYOSITIS/DERMATOMYOSITIS

Polymyositis, an inflammatory myopathy of unknown etiology, is characterized by an inflammatory reaction of mononuclear cells (lymphocytes and histiocytes) confined to the striated muscle. Cardiac muscle is not involved. The onset of the disease is usually subacute and often follows a "viral syndrome" by several days or weeks. Untreated, the disease is characterized by exacerbations and remissions, with progressive weakness and, ultimately, a high mortality rate. The patients present with muscular pain and proximal muscle weakness, often accompanied by difficulty in swallowing. Most often seen in young adult women, the

Figure 27-3. Congenital myopathies.
(A) **Normal.** A microscopic field of a frozen section of normal skeletal muscle stained with the modified Gomori trichrome (MGT) stain is depicted. The nuclei are purple, the membranous organelles (mitochondria and sarcoplasmic reticulum) are red, myofibrils are light green, and perifascicular collagen is light green. The fibers are of uniform size and somewhat polygonal.
(B) **Central core myopathy** (MGT stain). Many fibers are slightly smaller than normal and contain a round central core that is devoid of membranous organelles, which form a condensed ring around the core. Staining for ATPase identifies the fibers with cores as type I. The cores run the length of the muscle fiber. "Core fibers" resemble target fibers, although, as yet, no neuropathic process has been demonstrated in central core disease.
(C) **Rod myopathy** (MGT stain). Many fibers are slightly smaller than normal and contain brilliant red granules. The abnormal fibers are identified as type I with an ATPase stain. Electron microscopy reveals the granules to be clusters of electron-dense, rod-shaped structures that arise from the Z-band.
(D) **Central nuclear myopathy** (MGT stain). Many fibers are smaller and rounder than normal. Some contain a round central pale zone, while others contain a single, central nucleus. Again, ATPase staining identifies the abnormal fibers as type I. These fibers resemble the myotube stage of the embryogenesis of skeletal muscle.

disease also occurs in young children and older patients.

In addition to the skeletal muscle symptoms and signs, some develop an erythematous skin rash, in which case the disease is designated dermatomyositis. Whether or not there is skin involvement, the disease typically responds to corticosteroid therapy. When dermatomyositis or polymyositis occurs in a middle-aged man, there is an associated increased risk of an epithelial cancer, most commonly carcinoma of the lung.

Biopsy of skeletal muscle in patients with polymyositis ordinarily demonstrates the inflammatory nature of the myopathy (Fig. 27-4). Scattered degenerating and regenerating muscle fibers are surrounded by a focal or diffuse mononuclear infiltrate that occurs in the endomysium and the interstitium, as well as around blood vessels. Another morphologic feature that reveals the inflammatory nature of polymyositis is a pattern recognized as "perifascicular atrophy." In these biopsy specimens the periphery of a fascicle or group of fascicles shows degeneration and regenera-

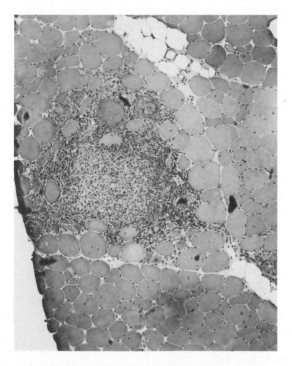

Figure 27-4. Polymyositis. With hematoxylin and eosin staining a cross section of skeletal muscle shows a focus of mononuclear inflammation within a muscle fascicle. At the perimeter of the inflammatory focus there is a zone of degenerating and regenerating fibers. A biopsy could easily miss the focus of inflammation but would probably show the scattered degenerating and regenerating fibers.

tion. Even in the absence of an inflammatory infiltrate, this pattern strongly suggests polymyositis.

METABOLIC DISEASES

Skeletal muscle tissue is dramatically affected by a variety of generalized diseases, such as Cushing's disease, Addison's disease, hypothyroidism, hyperthyroidism, and conditions associated with hepatic or renal failure. In the following disorders, however, a primary abnormality in the metabolism of skeletal muscle results in its abnormal function.

GLYCOGEN STORAGE DISEASES (GLYCOGENOSES)

TYPE II GLYCOGENOSIS

Various genetic mutations affect the acid maltase activity of muscle and lead to distinctly different clinical syndromes. The first acid maltase deficiency to be recognized, described by Pompe, is the most severe form and occurs in the neonatal or early infantile stage. It is known by various names: type II glycogenosis, acid maltase deficiency, alpha-1,4- glucosidase deficiency, and Pompe's disease. These patients have severe hypotonia and areflexia. Sometimes the patients have an enlarged tongue and cardiomegaly. In fact, cardiac failure is a common cause of death, usually within the first year or two of life. Many tissues are affected, but the most significant involvement is in skeletal and cardiac muscle, the central nervous system, and the liver.

Pompe's disease displays massive accumulation of membrane-bound glycogen and apparent lysis of the myofilaments and other sarcoplasmic organelles. Surprisingly, there is very little regeneration, and apparently inactive satellite cells are seen on the surface of muscle fibers that have been almost completely destroyed by the disease process.

TYPE V GLYCOGENOSIS

Type V glycogenosis, also known as McArdle's disease or myophosphorylase deficiency, is usually not progressive or severely debilitating. The absence of myophosphorylase causes muscle cramps with exercise. If the patients avoid strenuous exercise, the disease does not seriously interfere with their lives. However, persistence in exercise may lead to massive rhabdomyolysis and severe metabolic consequences. The absence of myophosphorylase activity renders the skeletal muscle

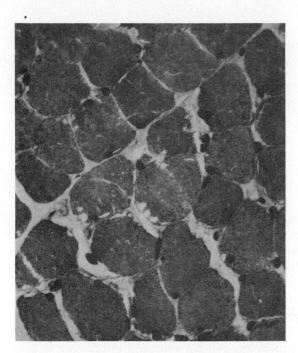

Figure 27-5. McArdle's disease (myophosphorylase deficiency). A cross section of skeletal muscle treated with hematoxylin and eosin shows that some fibers have subsarcolemmal vacuoles that appear empty. Electron microscopy, however, demonstrates that they consist of masses of glycogen granules, nonmembrane-bound, in the sarcoplasm.

glycogen inaccessible for energy production during periods of physical exertion.

The patients are unable to produce lactate during ischemic exercise, a defect that is the basis of a metabolic test for the condition. The muscle biopsy may appear completely normal, except for the complete absence of phosphorylase activity. However, there is usually some evidence of abnormal accumulation of glycogen granules within the sarcoplasm, predominantly within the subsarcolemmal area (Fig. 27-5). The diagnosis can be specifically made histochemically or biochemically by the absence of myophosphorylase activity.

LIPID MYOPATHIES

Occasionally, the muscle biopsy specimen from patients with exercise intolerance or muscle weakness exhibits an accumulation of neutral lipid vacuoles. When the number of mitochondria is also increased, the cases are referred to as mitochondrial myopathies. Such conditions are probably caused by a variety of metabolic conditions affecting lipid metabolism.

CARNITINE PALMITOYL TRANSFERASE DEFICIENCY

Patients with carnitine palmitoyl transferase deficiency are unable to metabolize long-chain fatty acids because of an inability to transport these lipids into the mitochondria for beta oxidation. After prolonged exercise, these individuals characteristically have muscular pain, which may progress to severe rhabdomyolysis. Prolonged fasting can produce the same symptoms. Biopsy specimens show no microscopic abnormalities. The diagnosis depends on the biochemical assay for carnitine palmitoyl transferase activity.

CARNITINE DEFICIENCY

Carnitine, which is synthesized in the liver and is present in large quantities in skeletal muscle, is necessary for the transport of long-chain fatty acids into the mitochondria. Patients with muscle carnitine deficiency have progressive proximal muscle weakness and atrophy and often show signs of denervation and peripheral neuropathy.

The absence of carnitine leads to massive accumulation of lipids outside the mitochondria. The activity of carnitine palmitoyl transferase activity is normal, but carnitine levels are diminished. Sometimes oral carnitine therapy, with or without associated corticosteroid therapy, may alleviate the symptoms.

RHABDOMYOLYSIS

Rhabdomyolysis refers to a diffuse destruction or lysis of skeletal muscle fibers. It is analogous to hemolytic anemia and has many causes, only some of which are known. Rhabdomyolysis may be acute, subacute, or chronic. When acute, the sarcoplasmic contents are poured into the circulation, an event that may result in myoglobinuria and acute renal failure. During acute rhabdomyolysis the muscles are swollen and tender, and there is profound weakness. Occasionally, an episode may complicate or follow an episode of "flu".

Some patients develop rhabdomyolysis with apparently mild exercise and probably have some form of ill-defined metabolic myopathy. After recovery a subsequent biopsy may reveal muscle that is morphologically normal.

Rhabdomyolysis may also complicate heat stroke and malignant hyperthermia after the administration of a triggering anesthetic agent, such as halothane. Alcohol intoxication is occasionally associated with either acute or chronic rhabdomyolysis.

The pathologic changes are classified as a noninflammatory myopathy, with varying degrees of degeneration and regeneration of muscle fibers. Clusters of macrophages are seen in and around muscle fibers, but these are not accompanied by lymphocytes or other inflammatory cells (see Fig. 27-1).

PERIODIC PARALYSIS

Periodic paralysis, a disease characterized by abrupt onsets of complete paralysis, is associated with abnormalities in potassium metabolism. Although there are three clinically and genetically distinct syndromes, the pathologic changes and the therapy (carbonic anhydrase inhibitors) for all three are similar. The three conditions are hyperkalemic, hypokalemic, and normokalemic periodic paralysis.

Biopsy specimens from patients with periodic paralysis appear completely normal between attacks, although occasionally, large, central vacuoles containing periodic acid-Schiff–positive material are seen. Electron microscopic examination reveals that these vacuoles are composed of markedly dilated sarcoplasmic reticulum.

DENERVATION

The pathology of denervation reflects lesions of the lower motor neuron. Lesions of the upper motor neuron, as seen in multiple sclerosis or cerebral vascular stroke, result in paralysis and atrophy. In lesions of the upper motor neuron the lower motor neuron is intact and the pathologic changes are those of a nonspecific diffuse atrophy rather than of denervation atrophy.

When a skeletal muscle fiber becomes separated from contact with its lower motor neuron, it invariably becomes progressively more atrophic, owing to progressive loss of myofibrils and myofilaments. On cross section the atrophic fiber has a characteristic angular atrophic configuration, being compressed by surrounding normal muscle fibers. If the fiber is not reinnervated, the atrophy progresses to complete loss of myofibrils and myofilaments, and the nuclei condense into aggregates. In longitudinal section, the end-stage of atrophy consists of an aggregate of nuclei connected by a thin strand of sarcoplasm to another aggregate of nuclei. On cross section these nuclei are seen as pyknotic nuclear clumps. A section between clusters of nuclei may fail to demonstrate that a muscle fiber was even present.

Angular atrophic fibers that are denervated are excessively dark when stained with the nonspecific esterase and the NADH tetrazolium reductase reactions, in contrast to a case involving nonspecific atrophy due to disuse or wasting. With the adenosinetriphosphatase (ATPase) reaction, the clusters of angular atrophic fibers that are excessively dark-stained are found to be a mixture of type I and type II fibers.

With every episode of of denervation there is an effort at reinnervation. In a slowly progressive denervating process reinnervation may actually keep pace with denervation. New sprouting nerve endings make synaptic contact with muscle fiber at the site of the previous motor endplate. There is a tendency for a given lower motor neuron to take over the innervation of a given field of fibers, and a group of fibers of one type is seen adjacent to fibers of another type. **This pattern is designated type grouping and is pathognomonic of denervation followed by reinnervation.**

Patients with striking type grouping often have symptoms of muscle cramping in addition to progressive muscular weakness. After a single episode of denervation, such as occurs with poliomyelitis, there is often a remarkable recovery of strength, due to reinnervation.

Occasionally a biopsy specimen reveals an abnormal prominence of one fiber type over the other. This situation is designated **type predominance** and may involve either type I or type II fibers. The explanation for this is often not clear, but frequently there is also evidence of denervation.

TYPE II ATROPHY

A commonly misinterpreted pathologic pattern in muscle biopsy specimens is atrophy due to disuse, wasting, upper motor neuron disease, and corticosteroid toxicity. This diffuse, nonspecific atrophy is manifested histologically by a selective angular atrophy of type II fibers. Using the routine hematoxylin and eosin stain, it is sometimes impossible to distinguish this pattern of atrophy from that of denervation (Fig. 27-6). However, with the ATPase reaction all of the angular atrophic fibers are type II, and virtually all of the type II fibers are angular and atrophic (Fig. 27-7). Furthermore, these angular atrophic fibers do not stain excessively with the nonspecific esterase reaction or the NADH tetrazolium reductase reaction. Type II atrophy is a common condition that is often an epiphenomenon associated with a more chronic problem.

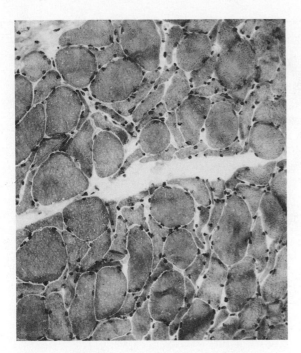

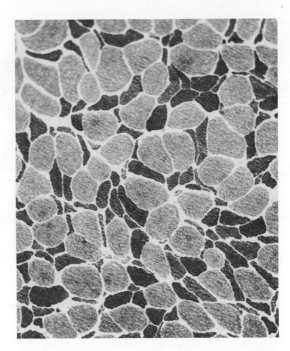

Figure 27-6. Type II fiber atrophy. This cross section of striated muscle treated with a modified Gomori stain is from a man who had suffered an unexplained 30-pound weight loss and proximal muscle weakness. He was found to have a malignant tumor. The numerous angular atrophic fibers suggest denervation.

Figure 27-7. Type II fiber atrophy. The angular atrophic fibers here stained for ATPase were not excessively stained with the esterase stain and are virtually all type II fibers. Denervating conditions do not involve only type II fibers. Selective atrophy of type II fibers is associated with wasting, chronic inactivity (disuse atrophy), and corticosteroid toxicity and is often mistaken for denervation atrophy.

28

THE NERVOUS SYSTEM

F. STEPHEN VOGEL AND THOMAS W. BOULDIN

THE CENTRAL NERVOUS SYSTEM

F. STEPHEN VOGEL

TRAUMA

EPIDURAL HEMATOMA

The anatomical features relevant to epidural hematoma are the following: The two middle meningeal arteries that occupy the theoretical space between the dura and the calvarium are grooved into the inner table of the bone and are fixed securely by the underlying dura. Branches of the middle meningeal artery splay across the temporoparietal area, generally as three major tributaries. The temporal bone is the thinnest bone of the skull, with the exception of the orbital surfaces of the frontal bone.

The classic epidural hematoma results from a fracture of the temporoparietal bone, with severance of a branch of the middle meningeal artery (Figs. 28-1 and 28-2). A regional skull fracture frequently causes transection of one or several of the branches of the middle meningeal artery. Skull fractures may also traverse a dural sinus, initiating less forceful venous bleeding into the epidural space.

Transection of one or several branches of the middle meningeal artery permits the escape of blood under arterial pressure and slowly deflects the dura from the calvarium. The firm adhesiveness of the dura to the calvarium is slowly but progressively overcome by this relentless arterial force, which eventually creates a true epidural compartment engorged with blood.

During the first 4 to 8 hours post-trauma the intracranial events characteristically are asymptomatic. After the hematoma has attained a volume of 30 to 50 ml, it acts as a space-occupying lesion. When the increased intracranial pressure exceeds the intravenous pressure, the veins (represented principally by large venous sinuses) are compressed. This collapse of the venous conduits impedes arterial flow and creates circulatory stagnation, thereby causing cerebral ischemia and hypoxia.

The hematoma attains a volume of approximately 60 ml within 6 to 10 hours, and the brain shifts laterally away from the side of the lesion. The medial aspect of the temporal lobe on the same side as the hematoma is compressed against the midbrain and displaced downward through the horseshoe-shaped opening of the tentorium. This important phenomenon, termed **trans-**

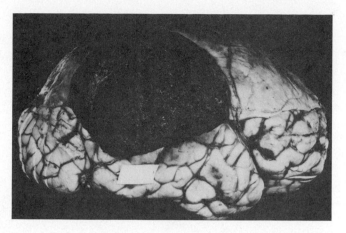

Figure 28-1. Epidural hematoma. A fracture of the temporparietal bone transected the right middle meningeal artery, permitting blood (under arterial pressure) to create a discoid hematoma between the skull and the dura. The patient died of transtentorial herniation.

tentorial herniation, compresses the tissues of the uncus of the hippocampus against the midbrain and contiguous structures. The herniated uncus compresses the vasculature of the midbrain—most importantly, the mesencephalic veins (great veins of Rosenthal). This creates venous stagnation in the midbrain. Stagnation and hypoxia impair neuronal function, notably that of the reticular formation; this is expressed clinically as a decline in the level of consciousness. Shortly thereafter, stagnation causes hemorrhage and necrosis, after which the regional injury to the reticular formation becomes irreversible. Death of the injured patient is then imminent or, if supratentorial pressure is relieved, unconsciousness is permanent. Epidural hematomas are invariably progressive; when not recognized and evacuated, they are lethal, usually within 24 to 48 hours (Fig. 28-3).

SUBDURAL HEMATOMA

The cerebral hemispheres are displaced in an anteroposterior direction when the frontal or occipital portion of the moving head strikes a fixed object. Alternatively, the forehead or posterior portion of the stationary head may be struck by a blunt object. **Subdural hematomas occur most frequently when the moving head strikes a fixed object** (Fig. 28-4). The abrupt arrest of movement of the skull forcefully brings the moving cerebral hemispheres against the inner aspect of the occipital or frontal bone. Since the dura is adherent to the skull and the arachnoid is attached to the cerebrum, the interface between these two disparately moving membranes lo-

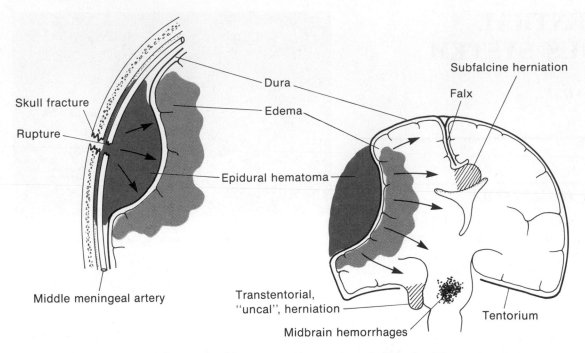

Skull fracture

Rupture

Middle meningeal artery

Dura

Edema

Epidural hematoma

Subfalcine herniation

Falx

Transtentorial, "uncal", herniation

Midbrain hemorrhages

Tentorium

Figure 28-2. Development of an epidural hematoma. Transection of a branch of the middle meningeal artery by the sharp edge of a fracture initiates bleeding under arterial pressure. This bleeding slowly dissects the dura from the calvarium and produces an expanding hematoma. After an asymptomatic interval of several hours, transtentorial herniation becomes life-threatening.

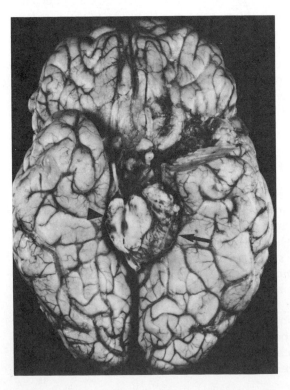

Figure 28-3. Transentorial herniation. An expanding lesion above the tentorium in the left cerebral hemisphere caused a left-to-right shift of midline structures, notably of the midbrain, and initiated downward displacement of a ridge of neural tissue, the uncus of the hippocampus, through the aperture of the tentorium (*arrow*). Compression of the venous drainage from the midbrain resulted in secondary midbrain hemorrhages. As a terminal event, the shift of the brain stem brought the right cerebral peduncle into forceful contact with the edge of the tentorium, causing laceration of the posterior aspect of the right cerebral peduncles, a lesion referred to as Kernohan's notch (*arrowhead*).

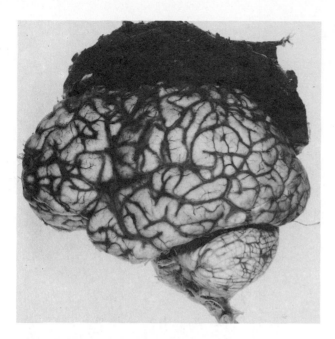

Figure 28-4. Subdural hematoma. A recent subdural hematoma is exposed by upward deflection of the dura. Note the absence of blood in the subarachnoid space. The patient died of transtentorial herniation.

calizes a shearing phenomenon to the subdural space. **This motion cleaves the cortical veins as they pass through the theoretical subdural compartment.** Thus, with rare exceptions, the bleeding is venous in origin. The liberated blood enters a compartment that is readily expansile, unlike the restricted epidural space. Fortunately, because the bleeding is venous in origin, in most instances it stops spontaneously after an accumulation of 25 to 50 ml. The hematoma compresses the severed veins and initiates thrombosis. As brain structures are bilateral and symmetric, and the force is usually directed sagittally, it is not surprising that **subdural hematomas are frequently bilateral.**

The surface of contact between the hematoma and the inferior aspect of the dura becomes the site of granulation tissue formation. This layer of granulation tissue, which is rich in capillaries and fibroblasts, is referred to as the "outer membrane." From it, migratory fibroblasts enter the subjacent hematoma and knit a fibrous membrane across the deep, or inner, aspect of the blood clot. Approximately 2 weeks pass before this "inner membrane" is grossly visible.

The hematoma, which is static in size and generally asymptomatic, has three potential routes of evolution: **reabsorption, maintenance of the status quo,** or **enlargement.** Expansion of the hematoma and the onset of symptoms is most often the result of rebleeding from the outer membrane. The granulation tissue is vulnerable to minor trauma, even the mild pressure exerted by shaking the head. Rebleeding creates a new hematoma that lies subjacent to the outer membrane. With time, it becomes compartmentalized from the original hematoma by the development of a second inner membrane. Such episodes of sporadic rebleeding may expand the lesion periodically and at unpredictable time intervals.

The symptoms of a subdural hematoma are protean. Stretching of the meninges may cause headaches. Pressure on the motor cortex may produce contralateral weakness. Irritation of the cortex may initiate seizures. Diffuse, often bilateral, subdural hematomas may impair cognitive function, an effect that may be manifested as dementia and that is often misinterpreted as senility. One or several rebleeds may enlarge the mass sufficiently to cause transtentorial herniation and death (Fig. 28-5).

CEREBRAL CONTUSION

Cerebral contusions, like subdural hematomas, are generally the result of energetic anteroposterior displacement when the moving head strikes a fixed object. When the contusion occurs immediately internal to the point of surface impact, the lesion is referred to as a coup contusion. When the occipital area strikes the ground in a backward fall, the resultant abrasions are situated on the opposite sides of the brain in the frontal or temporal cortex, and the lesion is designated a contrecoup contusion (Figs. 28-6 and 28-7).

If the force is minimal, the contusion is limited to the gray cortex and is restricted to the apex of one or several gyri. Greater forces destroy larger expanses of the cortex, creating deeper cavitary lesions that extend into the white matter, or that lacerate the cortex and initiate cortical or subcortical hemorrhages. Large lesions are associated with considerable edema which, together with hemorrhage, forms a mass lesion that threatens life by transtentorial herniation.

Contusions are permanent. Bruised, necrotic tissue is promptly phagocytized by macrophages and is transported into the blood stream. Mild, regional, astrocytic proliferation forms a regional scar, and the lesions persists as a telltale crater.

The presence of blood in the cerebrospinal fluid of a patient who has sustained head trauma usually denotes a cerebral contusion or laceration that has torn the pia, permitting blood from the contused cortex to gain entry into the cerebrospinal fluid.

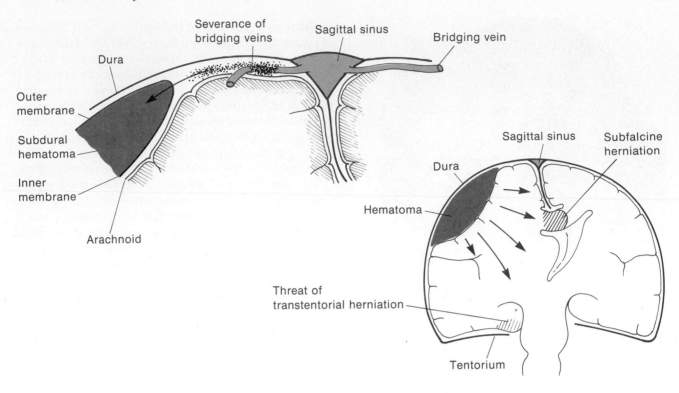

Figure 28-5. Development of a subdural hematoma. With head trauma, the dura moves with the skull and the arachnoid moves with the cerebrum. As a result, the bridging veins are sheared as they cross between the dura and the arachnoid. Venous bleeding creates a hematoma in the expansile/subdural space. Subsequent transtentorial herniation is life-threatening.

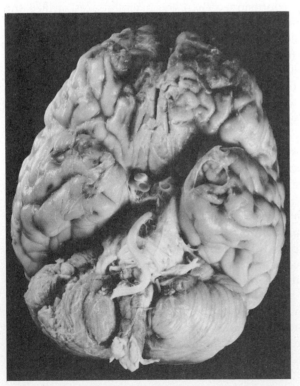

Figure 28-6. Cerebral contusion. The orbital surfaces of both frontal lobes and the tips of both temporal lobes are the sites of superficial lesions caused by the forceful impact of the soft cortical tissues against the rough surfaces of the base of the skull. The initial hemorrhage and edema have regressed, and the injured cortical tissue has been removed by the action of macrophages.

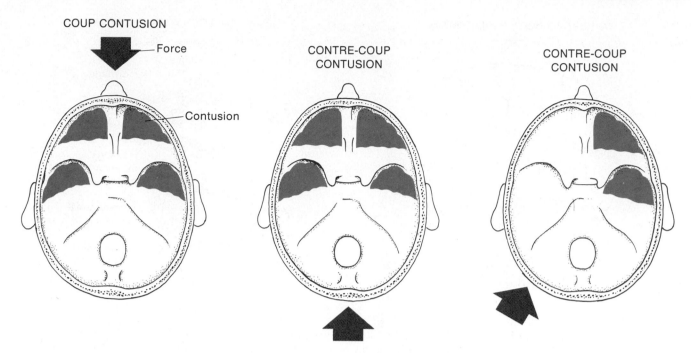

COUP CONTUSION

Force

Contusion

CONTRE-COUP
CONTUSION

CONTRE-COUP
CONTUSION

Figure 28-7. Mechanisms of cerebral contusion. The cerebral hemispheres float in the cerebrospinal fluid. Rapid deceleration or, less commonly, acceleration of the skull causes the cortex to impact forcefully into the anterior and middle fossa. The position of a contusion is determined by the direction of the force and the intracranial anatomy.

PENETRATING HEAD WOUNDS

Objects such as bullets and knives may enter the cranium and traverse the brain at variable velocities. In the absence of direct injury to the vital medullary centers, the immediate threat to life is hemorrhage (Fig. 28-8). Bleeding creates a space-occupying mass which, when present in or about the cerebrum, may lead to transtentorial herniation. When the hemorrhage occurs in the cerebellum, the immediate threat is herniation of the cerebellar tonsils into the foramen magnum and compression of the medulla.

Velocity contributes a blast effect to a projectile. Thus, a high-caliber bullet, as it traverses the brain, disrupts tissues not only by its own mass but also by a centrifugal blast that enlarges the diameter of the cylinder of disruption. A high-velocity military bullet can cause immediate death through an explosive increase in intracranial pressure. This pressure forcefully herniates the cerebellar tonsils into the foramen magnum and compresses the medulla, thereby causing immediate cardiac or respiratory paralysis (Fig. 28-9).

When **hemorrhage** has been less than lethal, or when it is controlled by surgery, a second complication arises from the introduction of microorganisms by the projectile. **Infection** is usually anticipated clinically, and is generally controlled by antibiotics. The onset of

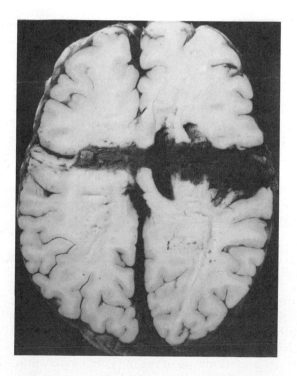

Figure 28-8. Penetrating head wound. A 22-caliber bullet entered the cranial compartment on the right. Its course through the cerebral hemispheres was attended by considerable hemorrhage. Note the petechiae in the area of the shock wave beyond the point of penetration of the bullet.

A. HIGH VELOCITY BULLET WOUND

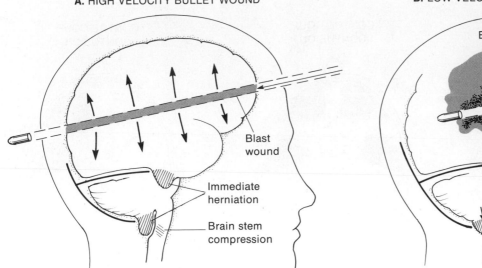

B. LOW VELOCITY BULLET WOUND

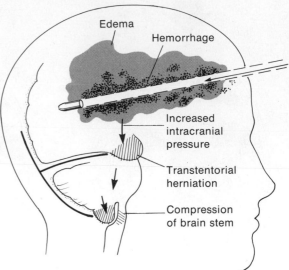

Figure 28-9. Consequences of high- and low-velocity bullet wounds. (*A*) The "blast effect" of a high-velocity projectile causes an immediate elevation in supratentorial pressure and results in death because of impaction of the cerebellum and medulla into the foramen magnum. (*B*) A low-velocity projectile elevates the pressure at a more gradual rate through hemorrhage and edema.

seizures is a tertiary manifestation that may appear 6 to 12 months after sustaining a penetrating wound. Seizures are caused by the displacement of collagen into the brain from the scalp or dura and the subsequent fibroblastic proliferation that forms a dense scar. The collagen scar causes distortion of neurons, which causes seizures.

SPINAL CORD INJURIES

The angulation of the bony vertebral column brings the spinal cord forcefully into contact with bone or, alternatively, interferes with the regional circulation. Thus, a **hyperextension injury** occurs when the forehead is driven posteriorly, as in the impact of a dive into shallow water. This posterior displacement tears the anterior spinal ligament and permits a sharp, posterior angulation of the spinal canal. At the point of angulation, the posterior aspect of the spinal cord is brought into forceful contact with the posterior process of the sta-

tionary vertebral body—that is, the vertebra that lies immediately caudal to the angulation (Fig. 28-10).

Hyperflexion injuries result when the head or shoulders are struck from behind by an object of considerable weight, or when the falling body strikes the ground in a flexed position. The head is driven forcefully forward and caudal. The force causes one vertebral body to impact on the underlying one. This frequently causes a fracture of a lip of the underlying vertebral body, with forward slippage of the underlying one and downward displacement. This disfigurement of the spinal canal results in sharp angulation of the spinal cord. The ventral surface of the angulated cord forcefully contacts the posterosuperior edge of the stable, underlying vertebral body.

A consequence of spinal injury is hemorrhage into the central core of the cord, a condition termed **hematomyelia.** Intramedullary hemorrhage is invariably accompanied by edema and softening, a combination designated **myelomalacia.** Severe trauma may cause transection of the spinal cord.

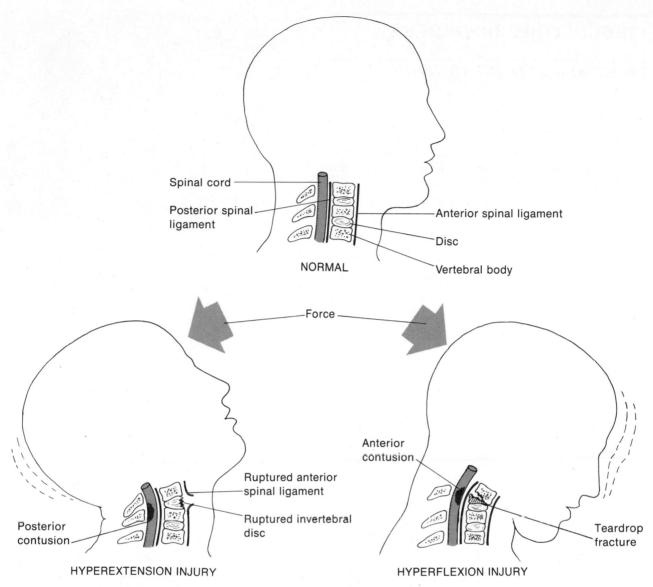

Figure 28-10. Spinal injury. Numerous angles of force can be applied to the highly vulnerable cervical spine. Posterior (hyperextension) and anterior (hyperflexion) injuries are the most common. Hyperextension injury causes rupture of the anterior spinal ligament and permits excessive posterior angulation. Hyperflexion injury causes compression, frequently associated with a "teardrop" fracture of a vertebral body, and produces excessive forward angulation of the cord.

CIRCULATORY DISORDERS

ISCHEMIA AND INFARCTION

LARGE EXTRACRANIAL AND INTRACRANIAL VESSELS

The progressive character of atherosclerosis dictates that, in the course of time, the circulation to the brain will become compromised and the incidence of lesions, such as infarcts and hemorrhages, will increase. A recent infarct of the brain transforms the cerebral tissue into puttylike material, and the necrotic tissue is ultimately phagocytized by macrophages (Figs. 28-11 and 28-12).

Unlike infarcts of the heart and kidneys, **cerebral infarcts are not repaired by fibroblasts.** In accord with the size of the lesion, but generally within a period of months, the necrotic area is excavated by phagocytosis, and the lesion becomes a **permanent cyst** (Fig.

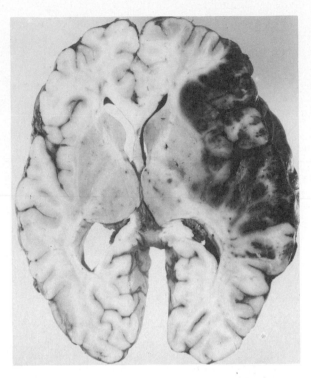

Figure 28-12. Hemorrhagic cerebral infarct. The trifurcation of the left middle cerebral artery was occluded by an embolus of thrombotic material from a mural thrombus in the heart. The hemorrhage and edema in the left hemisphere caused left-to-right displacement of the ventricular system. Death resulted from transtentorial herniation.

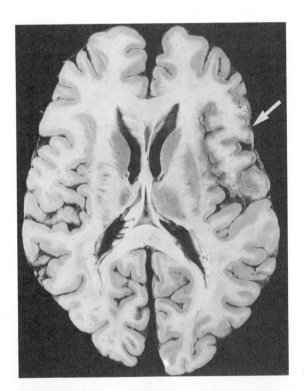

Figure 28-11. Ischemic cerebral infarct. A horizontal section of the cerebral hemisphere shows an area of ischemic necrosis (*arrow*) of about 5 days duration in the distribution of the left middle cerebral artery distal to the trifurcation. Note the preservation of the lenticulate nuclei, structures supplied by the striate branches from the middle cerebral artery. The occlusion resulted from thrombosis in situ initiated by severe atherosclerosis.

28-13). Because the cyst is filled with fluid, cerebral infarcts have been referred to as examples of liquefactive necrosis. However, the fluid is derived from seepage, and is not the end product of necrosis. Thus, it is more accurate to speak of cerebral infarctions as examples of coagulative, rather than liquefactive, necrosis.

Cerebral infarcts are either hemorrhagic or bland. In general, **infarcts that are caused by embolization are the sites of varying degrees of hemorrhage, whereas those initiated by thrombotic occlusion in situ are largely ischemic and, therefore, bland.** An embolus occludes vascular flow abruptly, after which the ischemic region undergoes necrosis. The collateral blood vessels that traverse the area of infarction also become necrotic and leak blood into the area of infarction. Occlusion by thrombosis in situ progresses more slowly, and the collateral vessels also thrombose, thus guarding against secondary hemorrhage.

Frequent sites of atherosclerosis are the large vessels in the neck, most notably the common carotid artery at its bifurcation—that is, the point of origin of the external and internal branches. Occlusion or severe stenosis of the internal carotid artery affects the ipsilateral hemisphere proportional to the degree of collateral

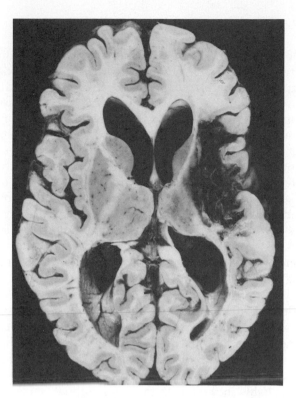

Figure 28-13. Remote cerebral infarct. An occlusion of the left middle cerebral artery at the trifurcation caused infarction in the left hemisphere in the region supplied by the distal branches of this major vessel. Note that the left caudate nucleus is preserved, as it is supplied predominantly by the anterior cerebral artery. The thalamus, which receives its circulation principally from the posterior cerebral artery, also remains intact. Over a period of months, macrophages removed the necrotic tissue and established a permanent cystic lesion.

PARENCHYMAL ARTERIES AND ARTERIOLES

The parenchymal arteries and arterioles are of small caliber and are not disposed to atheromatous deposition. However, they are often affected by hypertension, and become stenotic because of fibromuscular hyperplasia. The integrity of their walls is further compromised by the deposition of lipid and hyalin material, a transformation that is spoken of as lipohyalinosis. **The weakening of the wall leads to the formation of Charcot-Bouchard aneurysms.** These small, fusiform aneurysms, which are located on the trunk of a vessel rather than at a bifurcation, are disposed to rupture and hemorrhage. Alternatively, as a result of hypertension, fibromuscular proliferation impinges on the caliber of these arteries and leads to microinfarction. The microinfarcts, like the hemorrhages, are small. They are conventionally referred to as **lacunar infarcts.** When multiple, these minute infarcts impair cognition and create the entity referred to as **multiple infarct dementia.**

CEREBRAL CAPILLARIES

The capillary bed is the site of occlusion by small emboli, notably those of fat and air. Droplets of fat are carried downstream through the cerebral vessels until the caliber of the embolus exceeds that of the tributaries beyond a bifurcation. When they lodge, their semifluid consistency creates a major, but not absolute, barrier to blood flow. The distant capillary endothelium becomes hypoxic and permeable, and petechiae develop. Typically, these petechiae are restricted to the white matter (Fig. 28-14). Similarly, the introduction of air into the vascular system liberates a multitude of bubbles. Upon lodgment, a bubble of air acts in a manner comparable to that of a droplet of fat.

circulation through the anterior and posterior communicating arteries. **Most often, it initiates infarction in the distribution of the middle cerebral artery,** with a less intense insult to the ipsilateral frontal lobe. The latter area is partially spared because of circulation through the anterior communicating artery.

CIRCLE OF WILLIS AND ITS BRANCHES

Among the immediate branches of the circle of Willis, the middle cerebral artery is most often occluded by emboli, as well as by atherosclerosis and thromboses. Because the trifurcation represents a major step-down in vascular caliber, it is the predominant site of occlusion by embolized thrombotic material derived from a mural thrombus in the heart.

CEREBRAL VEINS

Venous sinus thrombosis is a serious complication of (1) **systemic dehydration,** as occurs in the adult with chronic alcoholism or in the infant with gastrointestinal fluid loss; (2) **phlebitis,** as might result from regional mastoiditis or from bacteremia; (3) **obstruction by a neoplasm,** notably a meningioma; and (4) **red blood cell sickling** in a sickle cell disease. Abrupt thrombosis of the sagittal sinus frequently results in bilateral hemorrhagic infarctions of the frontal regions of the cerebral hemispheres. A more indolent mechanism of occlusion, such as occurs with invasion by a meningioma, permits the recruitment of collateral circulation through the inferior sagittal sinus.

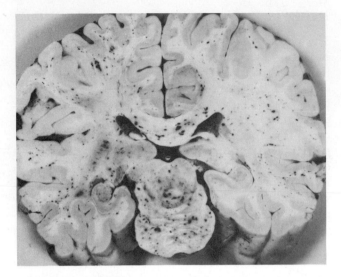

Figure 28-14. Fat embolization. Droplets of fat liberated from the bone marrow at the site of a fracture of the femoral bone passed through the pulmonary vascular bed and lodged in the cerebral capillaries. The white matter is more vulnerable to the ischemia of partial occlusion by a fat droplet because the white matter contains fewer capillaries than does the gray matter. Diapedesis of red cells and petechiae result when the endothelial integrity is compromised. Thus, petechiae are restricted to the white matter, although fat droplets are also present in the capillaries of the gray matter.

GLOBAL ISCHEMIA

Global ischemia or hypoxia, as results from cardiac arrest (ischemia) or from near-drowning (hypoxia), imparts a generalized, or global, insult to the brain. The topography of the cerebral vasculature is primarily responsible for two lesions: **watershed infarcts** and **laminar necrosis.** The major cerebral vessels—notably the anterior, middle, and posterior cerebral arteries—provide overlapping collateral circulation where they interface with the distribution of a contiguous vessel. A precipitous decline in circulatory flow, as occurs during cardiac arrest, abruptly diminishes the circulation in the terminal branches of both the anterior and middle cerebral arteries, and thus inflicts a dual insult to the zones of collateral circulation, or "watershed" areas (Fig. 28-15).

Similarly, laminar necrosis is an injury whose pattern reflects the topography of the normal cerebral vasculature. The cerebral gray matter receives its major blood supply through the "short penetrators" that originate at right angles from larger vessels in the pia and construct a rich plexus of capillaries deep in the gray matter, notably in the fourth to sixth neuronal cell layers. An abrupt loss of circulatory pressure selectively diminishes flow through this terminal capillary plexus. The necrotic zone is laminar in configuration, parallel

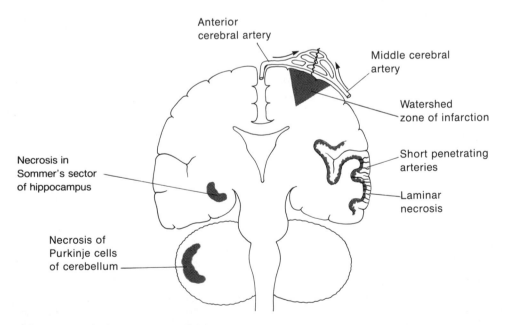

Figure 28-15. Consequences of global ischemia. A global insult induces lesions that reflect the vascular architecture (watershed infarcts, laminar necrosis) and the sensitivity of individual neuronal systems (pyramidal cells of Sommer's sector, Purkinje cells).

to the surface of the cortex, and the necrosis is understandably most severe in the deep layers of the gray cortex.

Selective neuronal sensitivity to hypoxia is expressed most dramatically by necrosis of the Purkinje cells of the cerebellum and the pyramidal neurons of Sommer's sector in the hippocampus.

ANEURYSMS

Fluid under pressure exploits weaknesses of the arterial wall and may produce focal dilatations, or aneurysms. Such weaknesses may be the result of developmental defects, which give rise to (1) berry (saccular or medial defect) aneurysms; (2) atherosclerosis; (3) hypertensive lipohyalinosis, the harbinger of Charcot-Bouchard aneurysms; (4) bacterial inflammation, the forerunner of mycotic aneurysms; or (5) trauma, which is rarely the instigator of a dissecting aneurysm.

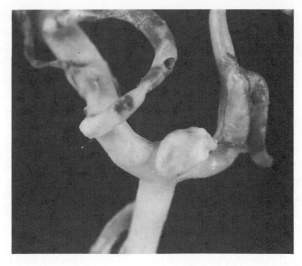

Figure 28-17. Saccular aneurysm. A small spherical outpouching occurred at the bifurcation of the middle cerebral artery in the crotch of two branches. This is the point of impact of the circulatory stream. The apical wall of the aneurysm consists only of adventitial fibrous tissue; it lacks a muscularis, and the internal elastic membrane has disintegrated.

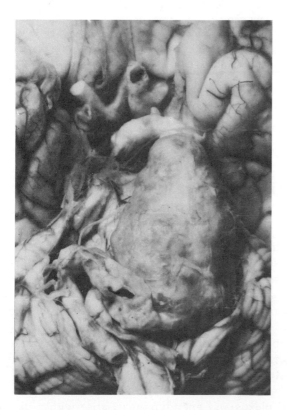

Figure 28-16. Atherosclerotic aneurysm. Atherosclerosis weakens the wall of the major cerebral vessels—notably, the basilar and carotid arteries—and aneurysms may result. In this photograph, the basilar artery is greatly dilated. A redundancy in length permitted the mass lesion to shift from the midline into the left cerebellopontine angle.

Intracranially, atherosclerosis preferentially localizes in the major vessels—namely, the vertebral, basilar, and internal carotid arteries. Characteristically, atherosclerotic aneurysms are fusiform. As an aneurysm acquires girth, the vessel also becomes elongated. Thus, an atherosclerotic aneurysm of the basilar artery moves laterally into the cerebellar pontine angle, where it constitutes a mass that compresses cranial nerves and produces neurologic deficits. The major clinical complication of a cerebral atherosclerotic aneurysm is thrombosis, not rupture. Thus, pontine infarctions are the anticipated sequelae of atherosclerotic aneurysms of the basilar artery (Fig. 28-16).

The terms saccular and berry aneurysm are synonymous with medial defect aneurysm. A point of congenital muscular weakness is bridged only by endothelium, internal elastic membrane, and a slender coating of adventitia. The point of the angle is also the site of impact of the bloodstream from the parent vessel. Time and trauma exploit the weakness. When the internal elastic membrane degenerates or fragments, the endothelium yields. A saccular aneurysm evolves, with its apical portion precariously formed only by adventitia. Rupture of a berry aneurysm causes life-threatening subarachnoid hemorrhage, associated with a 35% mortality during the initial bleed (Fig. 28-17). For reasons not understood, **more than 90% of saccular aneurysms occur at branch points in the carotid system.**

Mycotic aneurysms result from the embolization of thrombotic material, usually from an infected cardiac valve, which contains microorganisms.

VASCULAR MALFORMATIONS

There are four major categories of vascular anomalies: **arteriovenous malformations, cavernous angiomas, telangiectasia,** and **venous angiomas.** The arteriovenous malformation is the most common, and it has the greatest clinical significance. The lesion evolves during embryonic development from disordered angiogenesis. The resultant conglomeration of abnormal vessels usually involves a region of the cerebral cortex and the contiguous underlying white matter. Symptoms usually appear in the second or third decades and include seizure disorders and cerebral hemorrhages.

HEMORRHAGES

Hemorrhages that occur in the brain independent of trauma are referred to as spontaneous, but most are secondary to a vascular anomaly or are the consequence of long-standing hypertension. **The common sites of hypertensive hemorrhage are the basal ganglia-thalamus (65%), the pons (15%), and the cerebellum (8%).**

Long-standing hypertension is associated with the occurrence of Charcot-Bouchard aneurysms, which are fusiform, segmental dilatations along the course of small arteries and arterioles. The aneurysmal site is marked by lipohyalinosis, i.e., lipid deposition within the media and hyaline replacement of the muscularis.

Most hypertensive cerebral hemorrhages begin in the region of the external capsule—that is, peripheral to the basal ganglia and thalamus. The onset of symptoms is abrupt, and is dominated by weakness. When hemorrhage is progressive (and it usually is), the time span during the appearance of symptoms is a period of hours or several days. During this interval, the hematoma may attain a size that is sufficient to cause death by transtentorial herniation or rupture into a lateral ventricle. The latter event initiates massive intraventricular hemorrhage (Fig. 28-18). **Intraventricular hemorrhage** rapidly distends the entire ventricular system with blood and causes death by distention of the fourth ventricle, with compression of the vital centers in the medulla.

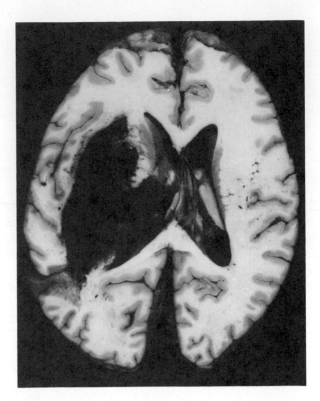

Figure 28-18. Cerebral hemorrhage. The basal ganglia–thalamus is the most frequent site of hypertensive hemorrhage. Note the contouring of the hematoma on the left by the external capsule. Blood has dissected through the thalamus into the left lateral ventricle.

HYDROCEPHALUS

Obstruction to the flow of cerebrospinal fluid results in hydrocephalus. When the obstruction is within the ventricular chambers, the hydrocephalus is designated as **noncommunicating.** By contrast, an impediment in the subarachnoid space creates **communicating** hydrocephalus (Fig. 28-19).

Flow through a ventricular chamber or a foramen may be obstructed by a congenital malformation, a neoplasm, inflammation, or hemorrhage. **The aqueduct of Sylvius is the most common location of an obstructive congenital malformation.** Some neoplasms, notably papillomas or carcinomas of the choroid plexus and ependymomas, arise within the ventricular chambers. Obstruction with hydrocephalus and increased intracranial pressure predominate in the production of the clinical symptomatology. Interest-

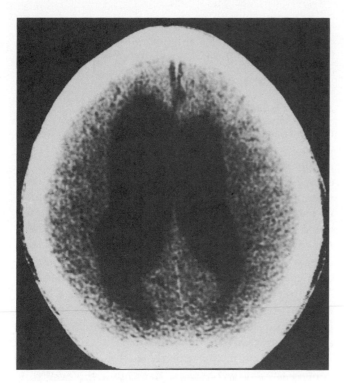

Figure 28-19. Hydrocephalus. In this computed tomography (CT) scan of the brain, the ventricular system is remarkably dilated, even though the brain is contained within the limiting confines of the cranial compartment.

ingly, in addition to physical obstruction, neoplasms of the choroid plexus form excessive volumes of spinal fluid. Tumors of the parenchyma, notably gliomas, compress the aqueduct or a ventricular chamber, causing hydrocephalus behind the point of obstruction. The ependyma is sensitive to viral infections, particularly during embryonic development; thus, ependymitis is possibly a cause of congenital aqueductal stenosis. Inflammation of the meninges produces fibrosis and may obstruct cerebrospinal fluid flow, thereby inducing communicating hydrocephalus.

INFLAMMATORY DISEASES

MENINGITIS

The term **leptomeningitis** denotes an inflammatory process that is localized on the interfacing surfaces of the pia and arachnoid, the encasement for the cerebrospinal fluid.

Pachymeningitis is inflammation of the dura. It is usually the consequence of focal, contiguous inflammation, such as chronic sinusitis or mastoiditis. The dura is a substantial barrier, and the inflammation is usually restricted to its outer surface.

With few exceptions, all forms of meningitis are initiated by microorganisms, with bacteria being the principal offender. **Because most organisms initiate a purulent or suppurative response, the presence of polymorphonuclear leukocytes in the spinal fluid is the most definitive index of meningitis.** However, lymphocytes are the hallmark of tuberculosis, the viral meningitides, and chronic infections, such as those attributable to *Cryptococcus neoformans.*

Gross examination of the brain in meningitis discloses an exudate of leukocytes and fibrin that imparts opacity to the arachnoid. (When extreme, this membrane appears creamy.) Since the intracranial and intraspinal subarachnoid spaces are in continuity, the exudate passes freely between these conjoined compartments.

BACTERIAL MENINGITIS

Many organisms are capable of initiating acute, purulent inflammation in the meninges or the brain. The list is headed by *E. coli* and *H. influenzae* in the neonate and child, and by pneumococcus, meningococcus, staphylococcus, and streptococcus at older ages.

The cross-placental transfer of maternal IgG imparts protection to the neonate against many bacteria. However, IgM, which is required to neutralize *E. coli* and similar gram-negative organisms, is not normally transported across the placental barrier. Meningitis induced by gram-negative organisms quickly produces a dense, purulent exudate, and is often lethal in infancy.

H. influenzae is also a gram-negative organism. However, environmental exposure is somewhat delayed, and the incidence of meningitis is maximal between 3 months and 3 years.

The meningococcus frequents the human nasopharynx. Its airborne transmission in crowded environments causes epidemic meningitis, a serious problem in military barracks.

TUBERCULOUS MENINGITIS AND TUBERCULOMAS

The granulomatous expression of tuberculosis in the meninges is analogous to that in visceral sites. Individ-

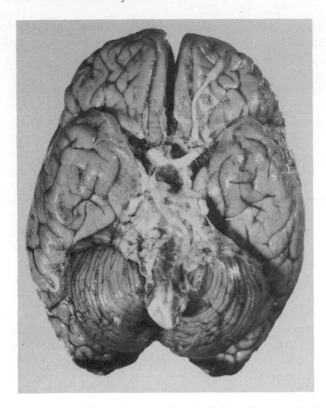

Figure 28-20. Tuberculous meningitis. Tuberculous meningitis involves the base of the brain. Granulomatous lesions are scattered in the leptomeninges of the pons, in the interpeduncular fossa, and in the Sylvian fissure.

ual tubercles, with epithelioid cells, Langerhans giant cells, and lymphocytes, are arranged about areas of caseous necrosis. Inadequately treated tuberculous meningitis expresses two further attributes—namely, a propensity for scar formation and a tendency to involve blood vessels. Meningeal fibrosis is responsible for the sequel of communicating hydrocephalus, whereas involvement of vessels leads to parenchymal infarcts. These infarcts are most often found in the distribution of the striate arteries, as tuberculosis has a strong predilection for the base of the brain, and particularly for the Sylvian fissure. Untreated tuberculous meningitis is uniformly fatal within 2 to 4 weeks (Fig. 28-20).

Parenchymal involvement by tuberculosis produces a solitary mass which, typically, is a spherical lesion with a central area of caseous necrosis surrounded by granulomatous tissue. In the early era of neurosurgery, these tuberculomas accounted for 10% or more of intracranial "tumors" (Fig. 28-21).

Tuberculosis of the spinal column (Pott's disease) produces an epidural mass of granulomatous tissue. Frequently, it causes destruction and angulation of the spine, and carries the risk of spinal cord compression. Classically, the typical "hunchback" was often a victim of Pott's disease.

CRYPTOCOCCAL MENINGITIS

Cryptococcal meningitis is an indolent form of infection wherein the virulence of the causative agent marginally exceeds the resistance of the host. In most instances the organism acts opportunistically, producing meningitis in an immunosuppressed host. It customarily enters the human host by the inhalation of contaminated particulates. Birds are a major reservoir for *Cryptococcus neoformans*, and their excreta is a vehicle of disease transmittal to humans. The organisms are encapsulated spheres that are 5 to 15 μm in diameter. They have an external gelatinous capsule and reproduce by budding. The inhaled organisms initiate a pneumonitis, after which they enter the bloodstream and the intracranial compartment. Although the organisms may abound, particularly in the Virchow-Robin spaces, the tissue response is meager. It features an occasional multinucleated giant cell, sometimes with phagocytized organisms, accompanied by scant epithelioid cells and a scattering of lymphocytes.

SYPHILITIC MENINGITIS AND RELATED LESIONS

Syphilis attests to the potential chronicity of intracranial infections. The spirochete *Treponema pallidum*

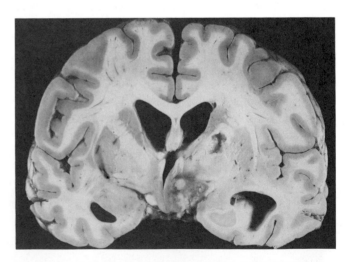

Figure 28-21. Tuberculoma. A tuberculoma in the right hypothalamus produced a mass lesion that disfigures the third ventricle. It impaired circulation through the striate arteries and caused an infarct in the right internal capsule.

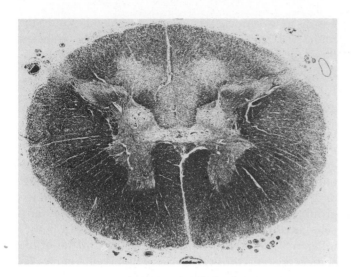

Figure 28-22. Tabes dorsalis. A myelin preparation shows the loss of axonal cylinders in the posterior column. The lesion is an expression of wallerian degeneration that results from constriction of the dorsal spinal roots proximal to the dorsal root ganglia. Axons that do not synapse in the spinal cord degenerate in a cephalad direction in the posterior fasciculus.

enters the bloodstream from a primary lesion, the chancre. The onset of secondary syphilis is indicated externally by the appearance of a maculopapular rash on the skin and mucous membranes, and internally by a few lymphocytes and plasma cells and an elevated protein level in the spinal fluid. This is also the period when the blood-borne spirochetes come to reside, at least transiently, in the meninges. Spirochetes can also infect the cerebral tissues during this interval. The organisms do not survive for long in the meninges. Nevertheless, on occasion, the transitory presence of the spirochete initiates a fibroblastic response in the meninges that is accompanied by a **proliferative, obliterative endarteritis** of the subjacent cortical arterioles. **Plasma cells are the hallmarks of syphilis.** They are the inflammatory cells that prominently cuff the cortical arterioles in meningovascular syphilis. Obliterative endarteritis induces multiple, small, cortical infarcts.

The initial lesion of tabes dorsalis is a variant of chronic luetic meningitis. The dorsal nerve roots that approach the spinal cord proximal to the dorsal root ganglia are met by a conical sleeve of arachnoid. This sleeve is filled with cerebrospinal fluid, and may be the site of chronic luetic inflammation. With time, the inflammatory response generates fibrous tissue that con-

stricts the nerve root and causes wallerian degeneration, which, in turn, extends directly into the posterior fasciculi. This is the most readily visualized morphologic lesion of tabes dorsalis (Fig. 28-22).

The spirochetes that lodge in the cerebral parenchyma may be clinically latent for one or several decades. They induce (1) a focal loss of cortical neurons; (2) a disfigurement in the topography of the residual nerve cells, producing a "wind-blown appearance;" (3) a marked astrogliosis; (4) a conversion of the microglia into elongated forms encrusted with iron, termed rod cells; and (5) a nodular ependymitis. These morphologic alterations are accompanied by marked decrements in cognitive function, referred to as **dementia paralytica.**

ABSCESS FORMATION

Microorganisms carried by the bloodstream lodge preferentially in the cerebral gray matter and the immediately subjacent white matter, which are vascularized by a rich plexus of branching capillaries. In the cortex, they replicate and generate a colony that stimulates inflammation. As a result, the vascular bed becomes permeable, and the escape of fluid produces regional edema, which is soon permeated by leukocytes. Within several days, the leukocytic component intensifies, and lytic enzymes produce **liquefactive necrosis.** The lesion then becomes an abscess.

An abscess threatens life, either by **transtentorial herniation** or by **rupture into a ventricle.** Although astrocytes are usually the designated cell for cerebral repair, in this unique situation, they yield the role of containment to fibroblasts. The fibroblasts knit a capsule about regions of liquefactive necrosis. Frequently, a secondary abscess forms subjacent to the primary lesion. Through the evolution of one or several generations of contiguous abscesses, the inflammatory process is carried inward, to threaten intraventricular rupture. This event is promptly fatal, presumably because of the absorption of toxic products. Alternatively, the expansion of an abscess may threaten life through transtentorial herniation (Fig. 28-23).

VIRAL INFECTIONS

Viral infections are prone to localize in specific areas of the nervous system. Thus, poliomyelitis selects the motor neurons of the spinal cord and bulbar area. Rabies assails the brain stem. Herpes simplex targets the temporal lobes. von Economo's encephalitis ac-

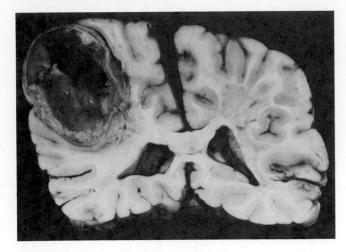

Figure 28-23. Cerebral abscess. An abscess of the left cerebral hemisphere is encapsulated by dense fibrous tissue. The center of the abscess is liquid; the wall is coated with a purulent exudate, fibrin, and necrotic tissue debris. The patient died of transtentorial herniation.

quired the synonym "sleeping sickness" because the inflammation localizes in the midbrain and hypothalamus. In this region, it also produces post-encephalitic parkinsonism through its destruction of the substantia nigra. Subacute sclerosing panencephalitis and progressive multifocal leukoencephalopathy afflict the cerebral hemispheres.

Perivascular cuffs of lymphocytes, principally in small arteries and arterioles, are the classic, but not universal, hallmark of viral infections of the central nervous system. A more precise diagnostic feature is the formation of inclusion bodies. Inclusion bodies are not present in some classic infections, such as poliomyelitis, nor are they features of atypical infections, such as Creutzfeldt-Jakob disease. The inclusions of **herpes simples** and **herpes zoster** are small, intranuclear, and eosinophilic, but their morphologic appearance does not distinguish one from the other. By contrast, the cytoplasmic **Negri body** is unequivocal evidence of **rabies encephalitis.** The inclusions of **progressive multifocal leukoencephalopathy,** caused by a papovavirus ("JC virus"), are intranuclear, distinctively within oligodendroglial cells, are typically associated with mild nucleomegaly, and exhibit a "ground glass" appearance. The inclusions of **subacute sclerosing panencephalitis** are intranuclear, frequently basophilic, and characteristically discrete, with a prominent halo. The inclusions of an infection by the **cytomegalovirus** are present both in the nucleus and cytoplasm, but are most conspicuous in the nucleus, where they are discrete, associated with nucleomegaly, and surrounded by a halo. Thus, inclusions add significant direction and security to a diagnosis but are rarely pathognomonic.

POLIOMYELITIS (INFANTILE PARALYSIS)

Generically, **the term poliomyelitis refers to inflammation of the gray matter of the spinal cord.** However, in common usage, it implies an inflammation by one of three strains of poliovirus (Brunhilde, Lancing, or Leon). The organism belongs to the enterovirus group, which also contains the coxsackievirus and echovirus. On occasion, the latter two viruses induce inflammation, predominantly in the gray matter of the spinal cord, and thus can mimic poliomyelitis clinically.

The polio virus binds to receptor sites on motor neurons, enters these cells, and produces injury and death of the cells. An influx of fluid into the cytoplasmic compartment of an infected cell disperses the Nissl substance (rough endoplasmic reticulum) and displaces the nucleus peripherally. These structural events are collectively termed **chromatolysis.** Thereafter, the dead neuron appears contracted, and is phagocytosed by macrophages. This process is referred to as **neuronophagia.** These events produce inflammation that transiently features polymorphonuclear leukocytes; however, these cells soon yield to lymphocytes. The inflammation is centered in the anterior horns of the spinal cord and in the medulla. Inflammatory cells surround parenchymal blood vessels and involve the meninges to a lesser degree. The motor cortex usually does not exhibit frank inflammation, but may contain **glial nodules.** These are focal collections of small, round cells that are thought to represent microglia or lymphocytes.

RABIES

Rabies has been recognized throughout recorded time. In humans it is a lethal encephalitis. Carnivores, such as the dog, wolf, fox, and skunk, are the principal reservoirs, but the infection extends to bats and to some domesticated animals, such as cattle, goats, and swine. The infectious agent is transmitted to humans through contaminated saliva introduced into the wound of a bite. The virus enters a peripheral nerve and is transported by centripetal axoplasmic flow to the spinal cord and brain. The latent interval varies from days to months.

Although it is not understood why the virus seeks out the brain stem, this pattern of localization initiates the classic symptoms of difficulty in swallowing and the painful spasms of the throat that justify the term **hydrophobia.** The clinical symptoms—namely, irritability, agitation, seizures, and delirium—also reflect a **general encephalopathy.** The spinal fluid is altered in accord with the "typical viral response:" a modest pleocytosis by lymphocytes, a moderate elevation of protein content (50 to 100 mg/ml), and an unaltered glucose level and spinal fluid pressure. The illness progresses to death within one to several weeks.

Lymphocytes aggregate about the small arteries and veins in the brain stem. Scattered neurons show chromatolysis and neuronophagia. Glial nodules attest to the infectious nature of the process. The geographic distribution of the inflammation, centered in the brain stem with spillage into the cerebellum and hypothalamus, strongly suggests rabies. The presence of **Negri bodies** validates the diagnosis. Negri bodies are discrete, intracytoplasmic, deeply eosinophilic inclusions that measure several micrometers in diameter. They occur in neurons of the brain stem, particularly those in the hippocampus, and in the Purkinje cells of the cerebellum.

HERPES SIMPLEX ENCEPHALITIS AND RELATED INFECTIONS

An important genus of pathogenic viruses includes herpes simplex (types I and II), the varicella-zoster virus, cytomegalovirus, Epstein-Barr virus, and the simian B virus.

Type I herpesvirus is largely responsible for the "cold sore." This vesicular cutaneous lesion is connected anatomically with the gasserian ganglion through its man-

dibular nerve trunk. The virus resides latently within the gasserian ganglion, where it proliferates during periods of stress, and is transmitted centrifugally through the nerve trunk to the lip. Similarly, type II herpesvirus initiates a vesicular lesion on the genital labia of women and is coupled with a latent infection in the pelvic ganglia.

At the present time, herpes encephalitis constitutes the most important viral infection of the human nervous system. In adults, the encephalitis is caused principally by the type I virus, and curiously is localized predominantly in one or both temporal lobes.

The temporal lobes become swollen, hemorrhagic, and necrotic. The exudate is predominantly lymphocytic and perithelial, an appearance consistent with inflammation initiated by a virus (Fig. 28-24). However, because the small arteries and arterioles characteristically become necrotic and filled with fibrin thrombi, the parenchyma becomes hemorrhagic and edematous. Intranuclear inclusions occur predominantly in neurons, but also involve astrocytes and oligodendrocytes (Fig. 28-25). They are weakly eosinophilic, occupy less than half the volume of a nucleus, and are usually surrounded by an inconspicuous halo. The detection of viral proteins by immunohistochemical techniques is diagnostic.

In neonates, encephalitis is induced predominantly by type II herpesvirus, as an acquired infection from the birth canal. At this age, the neural tissues are extremely vulnerable, and the infection promptly causes extensive necrosis in the cerebrum and cerebellum.

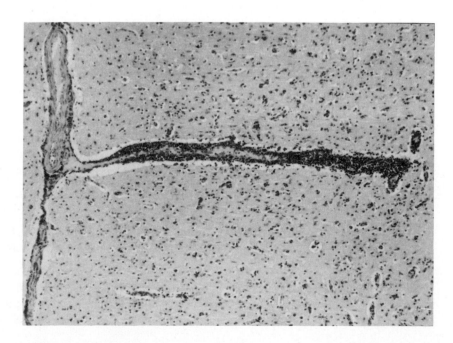

Figure 28-24. Herpes simplex encephalitis. A photomicrograph illustrates perivascular lymphocytic cuffing, a feature shared by most viral encephalitides.

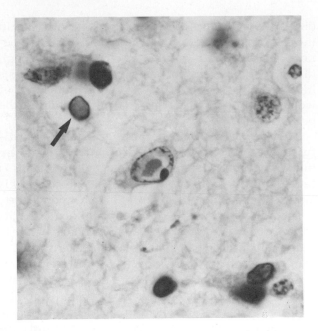

Figure 28-25. Herpes simplex encephalitis. A photomicrograph shows the inclusion bodies of herpes simplex encephalitis. They are intranuclear and may be discrete, with a halo, as depicted in the neuron in the center of the field, or they may occupy the entire nucleus, as is shown in an astrocyte (*arrow*).

The pattern of **herpes zoster-varicella viral infection** is anatomically analogous to the gasserian ganglion cold sore complex of herpes simplex. **The vesicular cutaneous eruption of "shingles" occurs in the distribution of a dermatome, the dorsal root ganglion of which harbors the virus.** Rarely does this infection spread to the central nervous system.

Cytomegalovirus induces encephalitis in utero as a crossplacental infection and also initiates encephalitis lesions in the brain of adult immunocompromised hosts. Characteristically, the lesions in the embryonic nervous system predominantly occur in the periventricular areas, and are characterized by necrosis and calcification. Because of their proximity to the third ventricle and the aqueduct, they are prone to induce hydrocephalus.

ENCEPHALITIS LETHARGICA (VON ECONOMO'S ENCEPHALITIS)

Unlike the lengthy histories of poliomyelitis and rabies, the agent of encephalitis lethargica induced a single, severe epidemic which began in the winter of 1916,

lasted for about 5 years, and was concurrent with the influenza epidemic. Although the infectious agent was neither isolated nor identified, the characteristics of the inflammation testified unequivocally to its viral nature. It featured perivascular cuffs of lymphocytes in the region of the midbrain and hypothalamus. As the name implies, the dominant symptom was somnolence which, on occasion, persisted for weeks. In a few patients, the period of lethargy was followed by the onset of parkinsonism, a symptom complex of hyperkinesia, involuntary movements, athetosis, and tremors. These symptoms reflected injury to the substantia nigra. Other patients developed parkinsonism (postencephalitic parkinsonism) a decade or so later. This occurrence gave rise to the theory that subclinical injury to the substantia nigra during an acute encephalitis episode may compromise the longevity of the neurons.

SUBACUTE SCLEROSING PANENCEPHALITIS

Subacute sclerosing panencephalitis primarily affects children, but also occurs in adults. Its course is characteristically protracted, but may be as brief as several months. The inflammation centers in the cerebral gray matter, but may also involve the white matter.

The classic, protracted disease insidiously disturbs cognitive function, alters personality and behavior, produces motor sensory deficits, and ultimately leads to stupor and death over a period of several years. The spinal fluid is minimally altered, but typically displays an elevated titer against the measles virus. The inflammation is highlighted by the presence of (1) prominent, haloed, intranuclear inclusions within neurons; (2) a marked astrogliosis; (3) a patchy loss of myelin; and (4) the customary perivascular cuffs of lymphocytes and macrophages.

An agent having the general properties of the measles virus proliferates in cells maintained in co-culture with infected tissues of the host. The protracted course of subacute sclerosing panencephalitis is thought to result from a defect in the cycle of measles virus replication and release in the infected neuron. As a consequence, the virus is not released from the cell, and viral products accumulate intracellularly, creating inclusions and causing neuronal dysfunction and cell death.

PROGRESSIVE MULTIFOCAL LEUKOENCEPHALOPATHY

Progressive multifocal leukoencephalopathy exemplifies many fundamental characteristics of neurotropic viruses, including (1) opportunism; (2) selectivity for an individual cell species—in this instance, for oligoden-

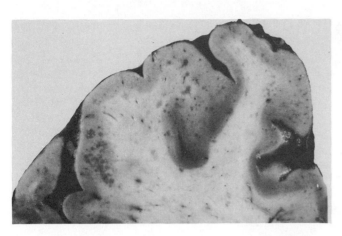

Figure 28-26. Progressive multifocal leukoencephalopathy. Focal demyelinating lesions are widespread in the cerebral hemispheres, with a preference for the gray-white junction.

drocytes; (3) the capacity to induce demyelination through interference in the normal functional relationship of oligodendrocytes to the metabolism of myelin; and (4) oncogenicity.

The causative agent of progressive multifocal leukoencephalopathy is a papovavirus bearing the name **JC virus.** The human nervous system becomes vulnerable through immunosuppression. Thus, with few exceptions, the encephalitis is a terminal complication in patients with cancer or lupus erythematosus, in recipients of organ transplants, and particularly, in patients with acquired immunodeficiency syndrome (AIDS).

Characteristically, the lesions appear as discrete foci of demyelination near the gray-white junction in the cerebral hemispheres (Fig. 28-26). Nevertheless, in most instances, they are also widely disseminated through the cerebrum and brain stem. A typical lesion (1) is spherical, measuring several millimeters in diameter; (2) exhibits a central area that is largely devoid of myelin but contains axons; (3) is sparsely populated by oligodendrocytes; (4) displays no necrosis, although it is infiltrated by macrophages; and (5) is distinguished by the presence of pleomorphic astrocytes, which appear to be anaplastic. The diagnosis is established on the basis of a peripheral area of demyelination in the presence of enlarged oligodendrocytes, which are homogeneously dense and hyperchromatic, and which contain intranuclear inclusions that lack a halo and have a ground-glass appearance. The nuclei of the pleomorphic astrocytes are often multiple and irregular, and possess dense chromatin material. This anaplastic morphologic appearance is occasionally associated with the development of astrocytomas.

SLOW VIRAL INFECTIONS

The category of infectious disease caused by "slow viruses" and its relationship to certain degenerative disorders of the human central nervous system remain enigmatic. An awareness of this possible relationship dates from 1956, when a medical officer in New Guinea provided an account of individuals in an isolated tribe whose illness was characterized by trembling. The disease, known as **kuru,** takes its name from the word "trembling" in the Fore language of this tribe.

The morphologic lesions of kuru, and the more widespread Creutzfeld–Jacob disease, are limited to the central nervous system and are descriptively represented by the term **spongiform degeneration.** Their morphologic appearance is analogous to that of scrapie, a disease of sheep that had been studied extensively, principally in England and Iceland, and that had been shown to be transmissible by the inoculation of infected tissue. Curiously, such inoculation was followed by a prolonged latent period of a year or more. Subsequently, infected tissues from patients with kuru were inoculated into chimpanzees, and the disease was successfully transmitted.

As the term spongiform degeneration connotes, the cardinal feature of Creutzfeldt-Jakob disease and kuru is the presence of small aggregates of microcysts (Fig. 28-27). These are most prevalent in the cortical gray matter, but also involve the deeper nuclei of the basal ganglia and hypothalamus and, importantly, the cerebellum. The involvement of the cerebellum adds ataxia to the predominant symptom of dementia and distinguishes Creutzfeldt-Jakob disease clinically from Alzheimer's disease. Within the areas of spongiform degeneration, neurons disappear, and astrogliosis becomes prominent. The corticospinal pathways degenerate. Of singular interest is the absence of inflammatory cells, a factor that accounts for the fact that Creutzfeldt-Jakob disease was mistakenly classified as a degenerative disorder for many years.

ACQUIRED IMMUNODEFICIENCY SYNDROME (AIDS)

Approximately 50% of patients with AIDS manifest an encephalopathy. Of these patients, half were found at postmortem examination to exhibit a recognizable infection of the central nervous system (such as toxoplasmosis, cytomegalovirus, progressive multifocal leukoencephalopathy, or herpes simplex encephalitis) or a neoplasm (e.g., primary lymphoma or Kaposi's sarcoma).

Recent evidence indicates that the AIDS virus possesses neurotropic properties. Particularly in

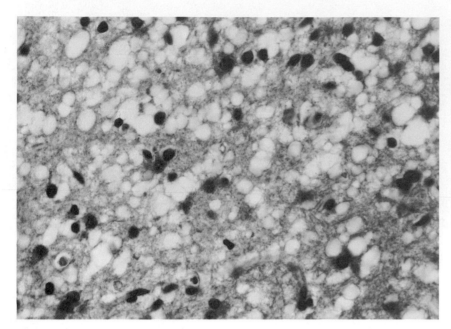

Figure 28-27. Creutzfeldt-Jakob disease. A photomicrograph shows spongiform degeneration, with the characteristic moth-eaten appearance that results from multiple small microcysts. As is typical of this lesion, neurons have undergone degeneration, and there is a marked astrocytic proliferation.

childhood cases of AIDS, scattered perivascular cuffs of lymphocytes and distinctive, solitary, multinucleated glia attest to a response to infection by the virus.

CONGENITAL MALFORMATIONS

ANENCEPHALY

Anencephaly is characterized by an absence of the cranial vault; the cerebral hemispheres are represented by a discoid mass of highly vascularized, poorly differentiated, neural tissue, the so-called **cerebrovasculosa** (Fig. 28-28). This diminutive mass lies upon the flattened base of the skull, behind two well-formed and normally positioned eyes. Most often, the entire brain stem and cerebellum are rudimentary. The upper spinal cord is generally hypoplastic and deformed. A **rachischisis** may involve the cervical area, appearing as a dysraphic bony defect of the posterior spinal column.

Typically, the discoid mass, which represents a residuum of the underdeveloped cerebral hemispheres, contains discrete islands of immature neural and glial tissue. It also contains cavities that are partially lined by ependyma and that occasionally contain choroid plexus. However, the discoid mass is composed predominantly of variably sized vascular channels that are lined by endothelium, but that are largely devoid of muscularis. Beneath this discoid mass, but sharing a common origin with the brain, are cranial nerves and intraosseous ganglia.

The incidence of anencephaly is second only to that of spina bifida with meningomyelocele among lethal malformations of the nervous system. Anencephalic fetuses are either stillborn or die within the first few days of life.

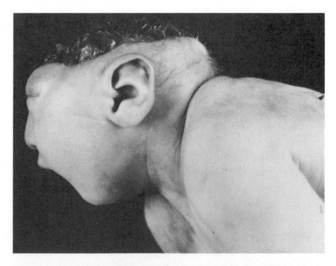

Figure 28-28. Anencephaly. The absence of a calvarium has exposed a discoid mass of highly vascularized tissue, in which there are rudimentary neuroectodermal structures. Characteristically, the lesion of anencephaly involves the cerebral hemispheres; thus, it is usually bounded anteriorly by normally formed eyes and posteriorly by the brain stem.

SPINA BIFIDA

A dysraphic state refers to a defective closure in the dorsal aspects of the vertebral column. Spina bifida is a dysraphic state that occurs most commonly in the lumbosacral region. When the defect is restricted to the vertebral arches, the entity is termed **spina bifida occulta.** Generally, this condition is asymptomatic, although its presence is frequently marked by a dimple or small tuft of hair. A more extensive bony and soft tissue defect, known as a **meningocele,** permits protrusion of the meninges as a fluid-filled sac. The lateral aspects of the sac are characteristically covered by skin, whereas the apex is usually ulcerated. More extensive defects expose the spinal canal and cause the nerve roots, particularly those of the cauda equina, to be entrapped in subcutaneous scar tissue. Characteristically, the spinal

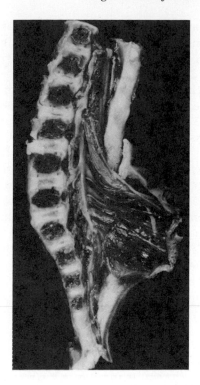

Figure 28-30. Spina bifida with meningomyelocele. A sagittal section of the spine reveals displaced nerve roots of the cauda equina entering the meningomyelocele.

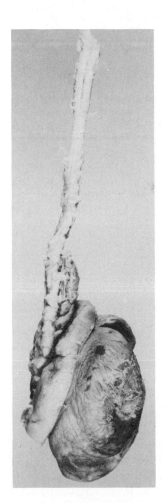

Figure 28-29. Spina bifida with meningomyelocele. The illustration shows a cystic lesion that protrudes above a discoid mass of skin and subcutaneous tissue in which the underlying lumbosacral segment of the spinal cord is enmeshed.

cord appears as a flattened, ribbonlike structure, suggesting lack of closure of the neural tube. The term **meningomyelocele** is applied to this entity (Figs. 28-29 and 28-30.). The extreme defect converts the spinal column into a gaping canal, often without a recognizable spinal cord. This lesion is termed a **rachischisis.**

The spectrum of neurologic deficits is similarly scaled, ranging from an absence of symptoms in spina bifida occulta to lower limb paresis or paralysis, sensory loss, and rectal and vesical incontinence with meningomyelocele. Importantly, the appearance of such a lesion implies the possibility of other malformations. In the case of meningomyelocele, Arnold-Chiari malformation, hydrocephalus, polymicrogyria, and hydromyelia may also be present.

ARNOLD-CHIARI MALFORMATION

The Arnold-Chiari malformation is usually associated with a lumbosacral meningomyelocele and involves structures in the posterior fossa and the upper cervical cord. The brain stem and cerebellum are compacted into a shallow, bowl-shaped, posterior fossa, with a low-positioned tentorium. A cardinal sign of the deformity is herniation of the caudal aspect of the cerebellar vermis through an enlarged foramen magnum (Figs. 28-31 and 28-32).

This cerebellar tissue protrudes as a tongue upon the dorsal aspect of the cervical cord, often reaching the level of C3-C5. The herniated tissue shows pressure atrophy. As viewed from a lateral aspect, the lower medulla is sharply angulated in its midsegment, thereby creating a dorsal protrusion. The foramina of Magendie and Luschka are compressed by the bony ridge of the foramen magnum. The cerebellum is typically flattened and resembles a clam; it has discoid, rather than an ovoid, contour. Frequently, the quadrigeminal plate is also deformed by a beak-shaped, dorsal protrusion of the inferior colliculus.

Consideration of the Arnold-Chiari malformation is important in the clinical management of a patient with meningomyelocele. It is also a cause of hydrocephalus,

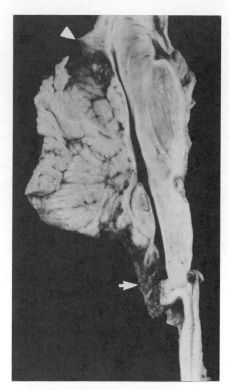

Figure 28-32. Arnold-Chiari malformation. A sagittal section of the brain stem illustrates the features enumerated in Figure 28-31. A tongue of tonsillar tissue extends downward over the dorsum of the cervical cord (*arrow*). Note the sharp beak of the posterior colliculus (*arrowhead*).

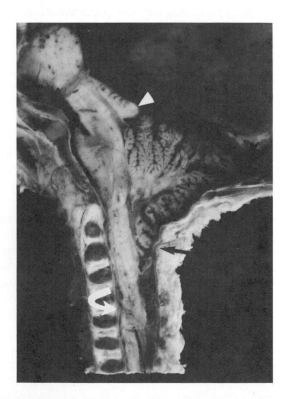

Figure 28-31. Arnold-Chiari malformation. The cerebellar tonsils are herniated below the level of the foramen magnum (*arrow*). The excessive downward displacement of the dorsal portion of the cord causes the obex of the fourth ventricle to occupy a position below the foramen magnum. The beaking of the inferior colliculus of the quadrigeminal plate (*arrowhead*) and the S-shaped angulation of the upper cervical cord (*curved arrow*) are seen.

through obstruction of the foramina of Magendie and Luschka.

CONGENITAL HYDROCEPHALUS

The excessive accumulation of cerebrospinal fluid intracranially is termed hydrocephalus. The entity is classified as **noncommunicating** when the blockage is situated within the ventricular system, and is considered to be **communicating** when the obstruction is positioned distal to the foramina of Magendie and Luschka.

The most frequent solitary malformation responsible for congenital hydrocephalus is an obstruction in the continuity of the aqueduct. Histologic examination usually reveals multiple, small, ependymal-lined canals that lack directional orientation, caliber, and continuity. In some instances, the single aqueduct or the clustered, aborted canals are surrounded by astrogliosis, in which case the condition is thought to represent an inflammatory ependymitis, probably attributable to an intrauterine viral infection.

POLYMICROGYRIA

A significant number of infants with meningomyelocele and the Arnold-Chiari malformation not only develop hydrocephalus, but also show abnormalities in gyral topography. Abnormalities of the cerebral gyri cause numerous deviations from normal and are regularly associated with mental retardation. These deviations include a spectrum of entities, such as **polymicrogyria,** a term descriptive of the presence of small and excessive gyri (Fig. 28-33); **pachygyria,** a condition in which the gyri are too few and too broad; and **lissencephaly,** a disorder in which the cortical surface is smooth or only lightly furrowed.

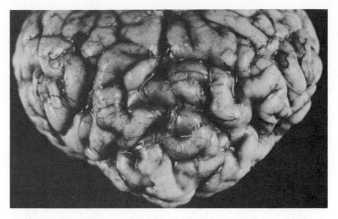

Figure 28-34. Holoprosencephaly. A view from the frontal aspect of the brain shows horizontally positioned gyri without the cleavage of the interhemispheric fissure. This malformation is commonly associated with trisomy 13.

CONGENITAL DEFECTS ASSOCIATED WITH CHROMOSOMAL ABNORMALITIES

Derangements of the larger autosomes (1 through 12) are incompatible with sustained intrauterine life, and affected fetuses are spontaneously aborted. Structural and functional abnormalities attributable to gross chromosomal derangements are best exemplified by the trisomies of groups 13-15 and 21.

Trisomy 13-15 results in deformities that involve the brain, facial features, and extremities. Holoprosencephaly, arhinencephaly, microphthalmia, cyclopia, low-set ears, harelip, and cleft palate dominate the complex.

Holoprosencephaly refers to a microcephalic brain that features an absence of the interhemispheric fissure (Fig. 28-34). The noncleaved cerebral hemispheres are horseshoe-shaped with an uncleaved frontal pole, across which the gyri have an irregular, horizontal orientation. Behind this lens-shaped cortex, there is a common ventricular chamber created by the lateral displacement of the posterior portions of the cerebral hemispheres. Holoprosencephaly is rarely compatible with life beyond a few weeks or months. The absence of the olfactory tracts and bulbs, either associated with holoprosencephaly or as a solitary malformation, is designated **arhinencephaly.**

The corpus callosum is regularly absent in holoprosencephaly, but its absence can also be a solitary lesion. The **absence of the corpus callosum** is a remarkably latent maldevelopment, usually without significant impairment of interhemispheric functional coordination.

Down's syndrome is an expression of several chromosomal abnormalities, each of which involves chromosome 21, and is predominantly associated with duplication and the formation of a trisomy. The weight of the brain is moderately reduced, and the organ is shortened in its anteroposterior dimension. There is a simple gyral pattern, with disproportionately slender superior temporal gyri. Of interest is the predisposition of patients to the **precocious development of the histologic features of Alzheimer's disease** before the middle of the fourth decade of life.

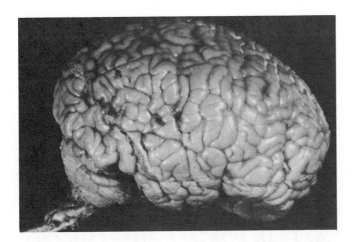

Figure 28-33. Polymicrogyria with Arnold-Chiari malformation. The surface of the brain exhibits an excessive number of small, irregularly sized and randomly distributed gyral folds.

DEMYELINATING DISEASES

THE LEUKODYSTROPHIES

Metachromatic leukodystrophy is the most common and also the best understood disorder among a group of entities that include Krabbe's disease, Alexander's disease, and **adrenoleukodystrophy.** The disease is an autosomal recessive disorder of the central and peripheral myelin. Metachromatic leukodystrophy occurs predominantly in infancy, but also has a rare juvenile or adult form. The course is progressive and the disease is always fatal, usually within several years. Postmortem examination discloses a diffuse, confluent loss of myelin that is most advanced in the cerebrum. The degradation of myelin is attributed to an inborn error of metabolism in which the enzyme arylsulfatase-A, although present, is enzymatically inactive. The functional inadequacy of this enzyme leads to the breakdown of myelin and the accumulation of sulfatide-rich lipids, which exhibit a metachromatic reaction to staining with toluidine blue.

Krabbe's disease also appears in the early months of life, and progresses to death within a year or two. The symptomatology reflects a diffuse involvement of the nervous system, with severe motor, sensory, and cognitive impairments. The disorder, an autosomal recessive trait caused by a deficiency of galactocerebroside, β-galactosidase, is expressed histologically by the presence of perivascular aggregates of globoid cells. These cells have an epithelial quality and are often multinucleated, so that they mimic a foreign body reaction. The loss of myelin is diffuse, and marbled areas of partial and total demyelination are present. Both central and peripheral myelin are involved. Astrogliosis is typically severe.

The degradation of myelin into lipid products was the basis for the identification of a childhood condition that was initially referred to as sudanophilic leukodystrophy or **Schilder's disease.** It is now appreciated that most of these cases represent an X-linked recessive entity, termed **adrenoleukodystrophy,** which conjoins an inborn metabolic error of lipids in the adrenals and a disturbance in the preservation of myelin. Again, the clinical signs, which are variably motor, sensory, or cognitive, develop in the first decade of life and progress insidiously for about a year. The central nervous system and, to a lesser degree, the peripheral nervous system, are depleted of myelin. The adrenals are characteristically atrophic, and electron microscopy reveals pathognomonic, cytoplasmic, membrane-bound, curvilinear inclusions, or clefts, in the cortical cells of the adrenal.

Alexander's disease is characterized by a lack of formation of myelin, suggesting an inborn error of metabolism. The histologic appearance of the central nervous system is strikingly abnormal because of the presence of innumerable **Rosenthal fibers.** These irregular, beaded formations of lipoproteins, which stain like myelin, are deposited in the subpial mantle of the cerebrum, in the molecular cortex of the cerebellum, in the periphery of the spinal cord, and in the outer margins of the optic and olfactory nerves. The content of myelin in the white matter is strikingly deficient.

MULTIPLE SCLEROSIS

Classically, multiple sclerosis has its clinical onset during the third or fourth decades of life. The disease is marked thereafter by indolent periods, punctuated by abrupt and brief episodes of clinical progression. The disease has a protracted course of 5 to 20 years or more. Each exacerbation is the expression of additional focal plaques of demyelination. The visual system is particularly vulnerable, whereas the peripheral nerves are uniformly spared.

The plaque is the hallmark of multiple sclerosis. Characteristically, plaques of variable size, rarely more than 2 cm in diameter, accumulate in great numbers, usually in the white matter. The lesions exhibit a preference for the optic nerves and chiasm, and almost always localize in the periventricular white matter of the corona radiata. Otherwise, their distribution is highly random, and they indiscriminately involve the cerebrum, cerebellum, brain stem, and spinal cord.

The evolving plaque is marked by a selective loss of myelin in a region of axonal preservation, a few lymphocytes that cluster about small veins and arteries, an influx of macrophages, and considerable edema. As the lesion ages, the plaque becomes more discrete and edema regresses. The aging plaque acquires astrocytes and, with time, the tissue becomes dense with glial processes that presumably impair the structural integrity of the axons. Oligodendroglia are lost without evidence of abortive attempts of remyelination.

There have been many theories about the etiology and pathogenesis of multiple sclerosis, but none are proved. At the moment, a viral etiology is particularly popular.

CENTRAL PONTINE MYELINOLYSIS

Discrete areas of selective demyelination occur as solitary lesions in the pons of chronic alcoholics who enter the hospital with severe electrolyte disturbances. **The**

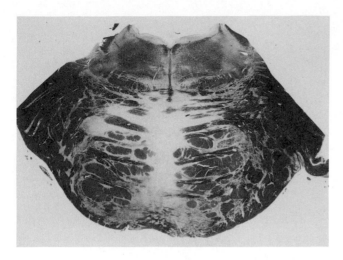

Figure 28-35. Central pontine myelinolysis. The crossed fibers of the pons have lost myelin in the region of the central raphe. As this early lesion progresses, it will widen laterally.

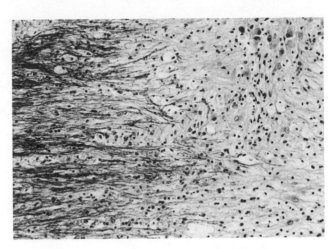

Figure 28-36. Central pontine myelinolysis. A photomicrograph shows a myelinated tract as it approaches the zone of demyelination (*right*). The neurons within the area of demyelination are preserved, emphasizing the selectivity of the injury for myelin.

electrolyte abnormality is of primary significance, and chronic alcoholism is merely the setting for its occurrence. It is thought that the rapid correction of hyponatremia is instrumental in the initiation of the selective demyelination that characterizes central pontine myelinolysis (Figs. 28-35 through 28-37).

NEOPLASIA

DERIVATION AND BEHAVIOR

Neoplastic lesions in the cranial cavity can be classified according to five fundamental origins: (1) the neuroectoderm (principally, gliomas), (2) mesenchymal structures (notably, meningiomas and schwannomas), (3) tissues and cells that have been ectopically displaced intracranially during embryonic development (craniopharyngiomas, dermoid and epidermoid cysts, lipomas, and dysgerminomas), (4) retained embryonal structures, and (5) metastases. Primary intracranial tumors constitute approximately 2% of "malignant" neoplasms, but their frequent occurrence in childhood weighs heavily upon their clinical importance. About 60% of primary intracranial neoplasms are gliomas, slightly less than 20% are meningiomas, and all others account for the remainder (Fig. 28-38).

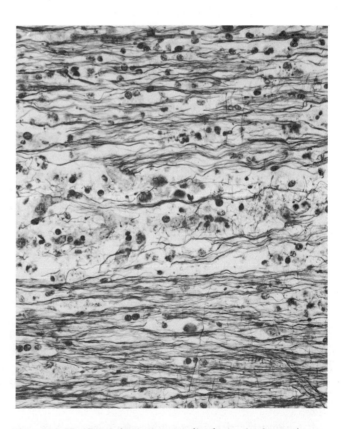

Figure 28-37. Central pontine myelinolysis. A photomicrograph demonstrates that the zone of demyelination retains axons that are splayed by an influx of macrophages.

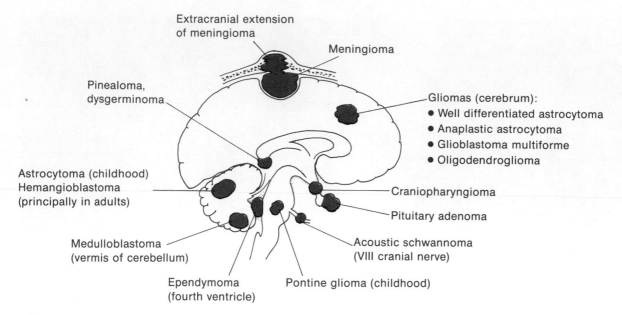

Figure 28-38. The distribution of common intracranial tumors.

Tumors of neuroectodermal origin are predominantly glial. They are derived from astrocytes, oligodendroglia, or ependyma, and are designated accordingly as **astrocytomas, oligodendrogliomas,** and **ependymomas.** Within each of these three cell species, there is a spectrum or gradient of anaplasia. Thus, the astrocytic gliomas are conventionally subclassified in a three-tiered fashion as astrocytoma, anaplastic astrocytomas, and glioblastoma multiforme, in increasing degrees of anaplasia. In accord with the degree of anaplasia, tumors of oligodendrogliomas and ependymal origins are conventionally designated as oligodendrogliomas or anaplastic oligodendrogliomas and, by analogy, either ependymomas or anaplastic ependymomas.

The descriptive terms "benign" and "malignant" require qualification when these intracranial tumors, particularly the gliomas, are contrasted with tumors in other body sites. For example, even the cytologically well-differentiated astrocytoma infiltrates freely through the surrounding brain tissue and has a poorly defined margin. The term "benign" is frequently applied to this lesion because its growth is indolent, despite the fact that its expansion and infiltration ultimately cause death in 5 to 10 years. Conventionally, anaplastic astrocytoma and glioblastoma multiforme are designated as malignant neoplasms. These lesions grow rapidly, infiltrate without restraint, and are rapidly fatal. **Yet, unlike malignant tumors elsewhere in the body, these anaplastic gliomas rarely metastasize.**

Infrequently, the neuroectoderm gives rise to a neoplasm of neuronal heritage. These neoplasms occur most often in childhood, and the cellular composition is usually primitive. An important example is the medulloblastoma that arises in the cerebellum, generally in the first decade of life. This tumor is usually situated in the vermis; its growth is rapid, and regional infiltration is extensive. It has been emphasized that the neuroectodermal tumors, even though highly anaplastic, rarely metastasize outside the cranial cavity. However, certain tumors—notably, the medulloblastoma and less commonly, the ependymoma and pinealoma—have a propensity to disseminate or "seed" by way of the spinal fluid. The implants involve the subarachnoid compartment over the spinal cord and cauda equina. Because neuronal replication occurs in infancy and childhood, medulloblastomas and the better-differentiated ganglionic tumors typically present in children. Many originate during embryonic development.

SYMPTOMS

The many symptoms of an intracranial tumor stem from its location and biologic behavior. Plainly, an infiltrative neoplasm that destroys functional neural tissue will cause a neurologic deficit. Alternatively, a neoplasm that "irritates" a functional area may initiate an involuntary release of neuronal activity, and its presence may then be manifested clinically as a seizure.

As a third mechanism for the production of symptoms, the mass of a neoplasm, combined with edema or the presence of hydrocephalus, causes increased intracranial pressure, which typically causes headaches and a predilection for vomiting. A mass effect, if progressive, ultimately causes herniation of neural tissue in the following manner: (1) the cingulate gyrus herniates beneath the falx (subfalcine herniation); (2) the medial aspect of the hippocampus (uncus) herniates into the aperture of the tentorium (transtentorial herniation); and (3) the cerebellar tonsils herniate into the foramen magnum. The latter two events are rapidly fatal.

TUMORS OF NEUROECTODERMAL ORIGIN

Astrocytoma is defined as a glioma composed of well-differentiated astrocytes. Fibrillary, pilocytic, and gemistocytic varieties are identified. This tumor constitutes approximately 20% of primary intracranial neoplasms. It frequents the cerebral hemispheres in adults; the optic nerve, walls of the third ventricle, midbrain, pons (Fig. 28-39), and cerebellum in the first two decades of life; and the spinal cord, predominantly the thoracic and cervical segments, in young adults. Astrocytomas of the cerebellum in childhood predominantly involve the hemispheres, where they are frequently cystic.

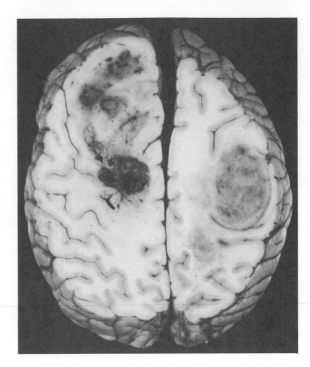

Figure 28-40. Glioblastoma multiforme. This extremely anaplastic tumor of the astrocytic series is represented by a necrotic, hemorrhagic lesion that has crossed the corpus callosum and has spread throughout both hemispheres.

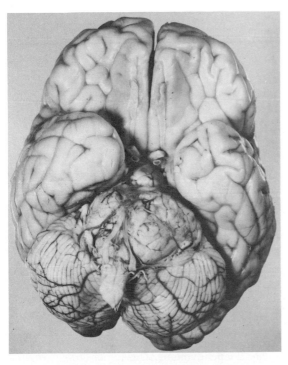

Figure 28-39. Astrocytoma of the brain stem. The expansile nature of an astrocytoma is shown by the enlargement of the pons, particularly laterally, but also ventrally, where it encircles the basilar artery. Pontine gliomas involve the cranial nerve nuclei and interfere with the long tracts that pass through the pons. The tumor may also obstruct the flow of cerebrospinal fluid, producing hydrocephalus.

On gross examination, the tumor is poorly defined, and infiltrates the brain. Microscopically, astrocytomas are variably cellular, and are distinguished by a matrix of slender, glial, cytoplasmic processes. Most astrocytic neoplasms, particularly those in the cerebral hemispheres of adults, have moderately dense glial processes and are called **fibrillary astrocytomas.**

The life expectancy of affected patients is widely variable, but generally approximates 5 years. In approximately 10% of cases, the tumor becomes more anaplastic. An **anaplastic astrocytoma is distinguished from the usual astrocytoma by a greater degree of cellularity, by cellular pleomorphism, and by the features of anaplasia. Its growth is accelerated, and life expectancy is reduced to about 3 years.**

Glioblastoma multiforme, the extreme expression of anaplasia among the glial neoplasms, accounts for 40% of all primary intracranial tumors. Most glioblastomas have constituent cells with recognizable astrocytic properties, but they generally display marked cellular pleomorphism, frequent mitoses, regional zones of necrosis, and endothelial proliferation.

Characteristically, the glioblastoma infiltrates across the corpus callosum and produces a bilateral lesion, likened to a butterfly in its gross configuration and mottled red and yellow color (Fig. 28-40). These colors

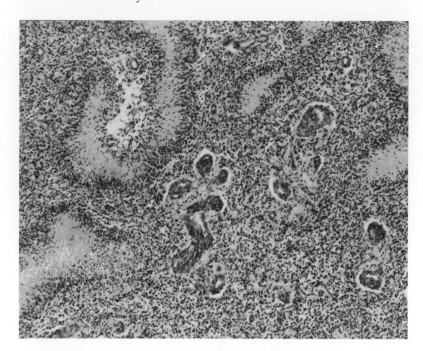

Figure 28-41. Glioblastoma multiforme. The characteristic microscopic features of this anaplastic tumor include prominent cellularity, areas of necrosis around which nuclei are palisaded, and the presence of numerous blood vessels that show endothelial proliferation.

are imparted by multiple areas of recent (red) and remote (yellow) hemorrhage and necrosis. The cardinal histologic features of a glioblastoma multiforme are (1) dense cellularity, with variable degrees of cellular pleomorphism, often accompanied by multinucleation; (2) serpentine areas of necrosis surrounded by zones of increased tumor cell density ("palisading"); and (3) endothelial cell proliferation that creates clusters of small vessels (Fig. 28-41).

The clinical course of this neoplasm rarely exceeds a year and a half. Glioblastoma multiforme predominates in the latter decades of life, and has a frequency twice that of the astrocytomas.

Oligodendroglioma, in accord with the cell of origin, arises in the white matter, predominantly in the cerebral hemispheres of adults. Although the lesion is infiltrative, its slow growth permits survival for 5 to 10 years. Seizures are often the first symptom.

Ependymoma, a lesion that occurs most commonly in the fourth ventricle, is accompanied by symptoms that are predominantly caused by obstruction and hydrocephalus (Fig. 28-42). Together with astrocytomas, the ependymoma is the second most common intramedullary tumor of the spinal cord. It arises from

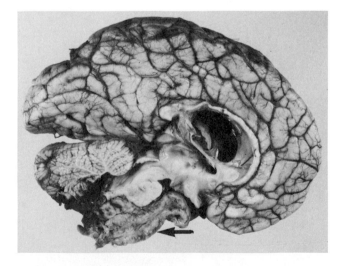

Figure 28-42. Ependymoma. This tumor (*arrow*) originated in the fourth ventricle and spread outward over the base of the brain. The obstruction to the flow of cerebrospinal fluid caused dilatation of the aqueduct of Sylvius, enlargement of the third ventricle, dilatation of the foramen of Monro, and a marked expansion of the lateral ventricles. The symptomatology associated with ependymoma of the fourth ventricle often reflects increased intracranial pressure.

the central canal or the filum terminale, and generally presents at the lumbosacral level. This differs from the preference of astrocytomas for the cervicothoracic level of the spinal cord. The tumor generally grows slowly, but it can seed the subarachnoid space.

Medulloblastoma, the most common intracranial neuroblastic tumor, arises exclusively in the cerebellum and has its highest frequency in the first decade of life. The progenitor cell is of neuronal origin and is derived from the transient, external, granular cell layer of the cerebellum. The lesion infiltrates aggressively and frequently disseminates throughout the spinal fluid. The neuroblastic quality of the cells is occasionally expressed in a rosette formation, a distinctive feature of embryonic and neoplastic neuroblasts. The tumor, in accord with embryonic neuroblasts, is highly sensitive to ionizing radiation.

TUMORS OF MESENCHYMAL ORIGIN

Meningiomas account for almost 20% of all primary intracranial neoplasms, having a maximum frequency in the fourth to fifth decades, but with a significant incidence in young adults, as well. They originate in the arachnoid villi and produce a globoid or discoid ("meningioma en plaque") mass. The superficial position of meningiomas in relation to the brain and spinal cord, coupled with neural displacement rather than infiltration, permits total surgical excision (Fig. 28-43). However, particularly with lesions at the base of the brain, invasion of the bone may limit complete resection, and recurrence is common. The histologic hallmark of meningiomas is the whorled pattern of "meningothelial" cells in association with psammoma bodies (Fig. 28-44). The latter are small, laminated calcospherites.

The indolent growth of meningiomas creates a symptomatic interval that often spans years. Because the lesion displaces rather than infiltrates the brain, seizures, rather than neurologic deficits, frequently characterize the clinical presentation. In some locations, meningiomas compress functional structures. For instance, those in the olfactory groove produce anosmia, those in the suprasellar region cause visual deficits, those in the cerebellopontine angle are associated with cranial nerve palsies, and those in the spinal column produce spinal nerve root and cord dysfunctions.

Schwannoma (neurilemoma, perineural fibroblastoma, neurinoma) is derived from Schwann cells, a cell species that produces collagen as well as myelin. Histologically, schwannomas feature spindle cells in fascicles and occasionally in parallel, picketed, and regimented patterns termed Verocay bodies. Malignant transformation is a rare event among Schwann cell tumors.

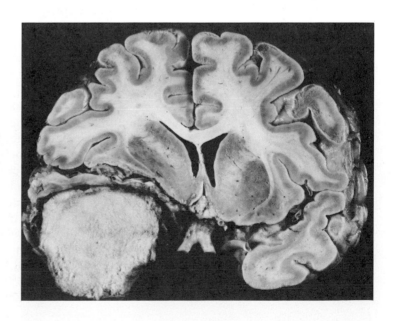

Figure 28-43. Meningioma. This globoid tumor, which underlies the temporal lobe, compresses but does not infiltrate this portion of the brain. The presence of the meningioma "irritated" the cortex, initiating a seizure disorder.

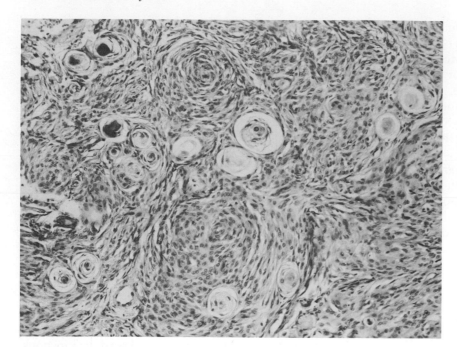

Figure 28-44. Meningioma. A photomicrograph shows the classic features of a meningioma. Whorls of uniform, round nuclei are interspersed with dark psamoma bodies. The general absence of mitotic activity and necrosis attests to the slow growth of this neoplasm.

Intracranial schwannomas are largely restricted to the eighth nerve, and are often referred to as acoustic neurinomas. The lesion not only initiates tinnitus and deafness, but also expands the bony meatus. Growth causes the lesion to protrude into the cerebellopontine angle, where compression initiates cranial nerve palsies. Schwannomas also arise on spinal nerve roots. Together with meningiomas, Schwann-cell tumors constitute the greatest proportion of intradural-extramedullary neoplasms. Tumors of Schwann cell origin also occur on peripheral nerves as schwannomas or neurofibromas.

TUMORS DERIVED FROM ECTOPIC TISSUES

Craniopharyngiomas arise from epithelium derived from Rathke's pouch, a derivative of the embryonic nasopharynx that migrates cephalad and gives origin to the anterior lobe of the pituitary. It is thought that remnants of this epithelium are positioned above the sella turcica, where they may generate cystic and solid lesions, termed craniopharyngiomas (Fig. 28-45). These tumors generally become symptomatic in the first two decades of life, creating visual deficits and causing headaches.

Dermoid and epidermoid cysts represent cutaneous structures that may be displaced into the bone of the skull and occasionally into the intracranial compartment. These displaced squamous cells proliferate and develop into a cyst whose inwardly oriented epithelium desquamates keratotic debris.

Lipomas arise from rudiments of adipose tissue that have been carried inward as the brain infolded embryologically. Not surprisingly, therefore, lipomas are positioned either along the superior aspect of the corpus callosum, across the dorsum of the quadrigeminal plate, or down the dorsal sagittal plane of the spinal cord to the level of the cauda equina. They enlarge slowly, if at all.

Dysgerminomas comprise a spectrum of lesions derived from displaced germ cells. Tumors derived therefrom show a strong preference for the pineal area or the region of the infundibulum above the sella turcica. Subsequent neoplastic growth permits a number of phenotypic morphologic expressions that parallel gonadal neoplasms—namely, seminomas, choriocarcinomas, embryonal carcinomas, endodermal sinus tumors, and teratoid tumors. As a family, these lesions greatly exceed the incidence of true neoplasms of the pineal gland, or **pinealomas.**

Hemangioblastomas originate principally in the cerebellum, without a well-defined cell of origin. These tumors are highly vascularized and feature endothelial-lined canals interspersed with plump cells. In about 20% of cases, these cells secrete erythropoietin and induce polycythemia.

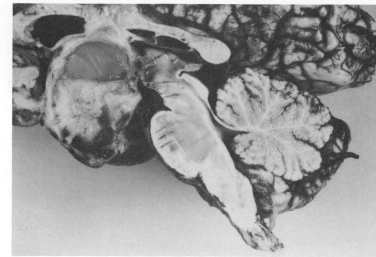

Figure 28-45. Craniopharyngioma. This cystic tumor, which originates from rudiments of Rathke's pouch in the suprasellar area, has a fibrous capsule that adheres to the undersurface of the corpus callosum. The lower portion of the cyst contains cellular debris; a coagulum of protein-rich fluid occupies the upper part of the cyst. Obstruction of the third ventricle is reflected in the dilatation of the lateral ventricles.

METASTATIC TUMORS

Metastatic tumors are the most common neoplasms of the central nervous system, reaching the intracranial compartment through the bloodstream. It is not clear why tumors of different organs or different cell types exhibit differences in the incidence of intracranial metastases. In this respect, a patient with disseminated malignant melanoma has a greater than a 50% likelihood of acquiring intracranial metastases, whereas the incidence of cerebral metastases in patients with carcinoma of the breast and lung is about 35%, and that in carcinoma of the kidney or bowel is 5%. Sarcomas and certain carcinomas, such as those of the prostate, liver, and adrenals, rarely metastasize to the brain.

TUMORS DERIVED FROM EMBRYONIC STRUCTURES

Colloid cysts (paraphyseal cyst, third ventricular cyst) are distinctive for their anterior, midline location in the segmental portion of the third ventricle. The colloid cyst is lined by cuboidal epithelium. The lesion enlarges slowly, usually over decades, because of the accumulation of desquamated and secretory products. The origin of the colloid cyst remains in doubt, but it is conjectured that it arises from the paraphysis, a sense organ of lower vertebrates that may remain as a vestigial structure in man.

GENETIC CONTRIBUTIONS TO INTRACRANIAL NEOPLASMS

Three genetically expressed entities deserve consideration. They include von Recklinghausen's disease, tuberous sclerosis, and Lindau's disease.

von Recklinghausen's disease (neurofibromatosis) is inherited as an autosomal dominant disorder, with a high degree of penetrance. In addition, a high mutation rate accounts for cases without a familial history. There is a high incidence of neurofibromas and schwannomas of the peripheral nerves. In addition, there is a high incidence of meningiomas, acoustic and spinal schwannomas, and gliomas (Fig. 28-46).

Tuberous sclerosis (Bourneville's disease) is transmitted as a mendelian dominant disorder. In this entity, disordered migration and arrested maturation of the neuroectoderm result in "tubers" of the cerebral cortex and the appearance of subependymal astrocytic nodules. The "tubers" are discrete, firm, cortical areas composed of bizarre cells that possess both neuronal and glial features. The subependymal nodules have been likened to candle drippings, and provide the substrate for the highly characteristic gemistocytic astrocytomas

A. CENTRAL NERVOUS SYSTEM

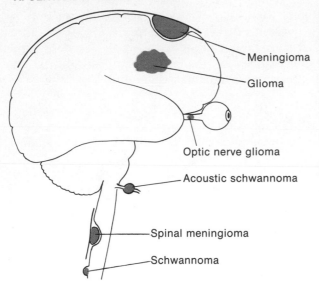

Meningioma

Glioma

Optic nerve glioma

Acoustic schwannoma

Spinal meningioma

Schwannoma

B. PERIPHERAL NERVOUS SYSTEM

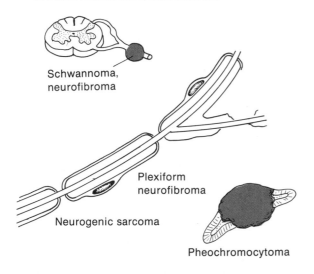

Schwannoma, neurofibroma

Plexiform neurofibroma

Neurogenic sarcoma

Pheochromocytoma

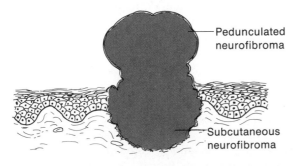

Pedunculated neurofibroma

Subcutaneous neurofibroma

Figure 28-46. Tumors associated with von Recklinghausen's disease.

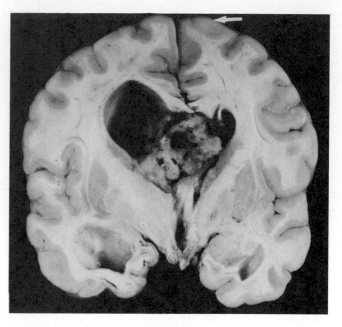

Figure 28-47. Tuberous sclerosis with secondary neoplasia. A neoplasm occupies the midline between the two cerebral hemispheres, creating a bosselated mass that histologically is composed of large, gemistocytic astrocytes. This neoplasm originated from subependymal "candle drippings," a stigma of tuberous sclerosis. A cortical tuber (*arrow*) is present in the right parasagittal region of the gray cortex, where the definition of the gray mantle is obscured.

(Fig. 28-47). In addition to the intracranial neuroectodermal lesions, the syndrome includes angiofibromas of the face (adenoma sebaceum) rhabdomyomas of the heart, and mixed mesenchymal tumors of the kidney (angiomyolipomas).

Some hemangioblastomas of the cerebellum display a hereditary pattern (**Lindau's** syndrome). An identical tumor may occur in the retina (**von Hippel-Lindau** syndrome).

METABOLIC DISORDERS

NEURONAL STORAGE DISEASES

Tay-Sachs disease (amaurotic familial idiocy) is the morphologic and functional expression of an autosomal recessive genetic disorder. A deficiency of hexosaminidase A permits the accumulation of a ganglioside within the neurons of the central and peripheral nervous systems. Retinal involvement increases the transparency of the macula, resulting in a cherry-red spot (see Chapter 29). The infant appears normal at birth, but shows a delay in motor development by the age of 6 months. Thereafter, the child deteriorates to a state of flaccid weakness, blindness, mental inactivity, and ultimately death, generally by the end of the second year. The brain becomes heavier, and on histologic examination, shows the universal presence of lipid droplets within the cytoplasm of distended nerve cells, both in the central and peripheral nervous systems.

Hurler's syndrome reflects a hereditary disturbance in glycosaminoglycan metabolism that results in the intraneuronal accumulation of mucopolysaccharides. Typically, Hurler's syndrome is expressed in infancy or early childhood by dwarfism, corneal opacities, skeletal deformities, and hepatosplenomegaly. The intraneuronal storage distends the cytoplasmic compartment.

Gaucher's disease results from an autosomal recessive genetic disorder involving a deficiency of glucocerebroside β-glucosidase. As a result, glucocerebroside accumulates, principally in the reticuloendothelial system. The central nervous system is most severely involved in the infantile type (type II) of Gaucher's disease, in which intraneuronal storage is not as conspicuous as neuronal loss, which is accompanied by severe, diffuse astrogliosis. These infants fail to thrive, and die at an early age.

Niemann-Pick disease is an autosomal recessive disorder characterized by intraneuronal storage of sphingomyelin that results from a deficiency of sphingomyelinase. The clinical symptoms occur early, and the disease is marked by failure of the infant to develop and thrive. The reticuloendothelial system is targeted for storage, but symptoms may predominantly affect the nervous system during infancy. The brain becomes atrophic and shows marked astrogliosis. Retinal degeneration may produce a cherry-spot similar to that which occurs in Tay-Sachs disease.

IMPAIRED NEURONAL METABOLISM

Phenylketonuria is an autosomal recessive disorder that is clinically manifested in homozygotes as an enzymatic deficiency in phenylalanine hydroxylase (see Chapter 6). This abnormality results in the excessive accumulation of phenylalanine in the blood and tissues because of a block in the conversion of phenylalanine to tyrosine. Symptoms of the disease include mental retardation, seizures, and retarded physical development, and generally become apparent in the early months of life. This entity exemplifies an inborn metabolic error that seriously impairs cognitive function without consistent alterations of neuronal cytoarchitecture.

Cretinism is a consequence of maternal iodine deficiency, with a resulting lack of thyroxin (see Chapter 21). Severe hypothyroidism in infancy alters the functional capacity of the central nervous system.

Wilson's disease is an autosomal recessive disorder of copper metabolism (see Chapter 14). Copper accumulates in toxic amounts in the liver and the brain, especially the putamen—hence, the term **hepatolenticular degeneration.** The cerebral intoxication is generally manifested in the second decade by athetoid movements. Before, during, or after the appearance of neurologic symptoms, an insidiously developing cirrhosis of the liver may present as hepatic failure. The deposition of copper in the limbus of the cornea produces a visible golden-brown band, the Kayser-Fleischer ring.

DEFICIENCIES OF DIETARY INTAKE AND NUTRIENT UTILIZATION

Wernicke's syndrome results from a deficiency of thiamine (vitamin B_1) (see Chapter 8). **In the industrialized world, the disease is most commonly associated with chronic alcoholism.** Typically, the onset of symptoms is precipitous. Lesions in the hypothalamus and mamillary bodies, in the periaqueductal regions of the midbrain, and in the tegmentum of the pons are manifested clinically by a disturbance in thermal regulation, altered consciousness, ophthalmoplegia, and nystagmus. The condition may progress rapidly to death, but is promptly reversible with the administration of thiamine. The acute tissue response features petechiae about small capillaries (Fig. 28-48). The mamillary bodies become atrophic.

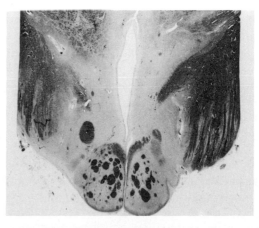

Figure 28-48. Wernicke's encephalopathy. A coronal section through the hypothalamus, the third ventricle, and mamillary bodies discloses clusters of "ring hemorrhages" in the mamillary bodies.

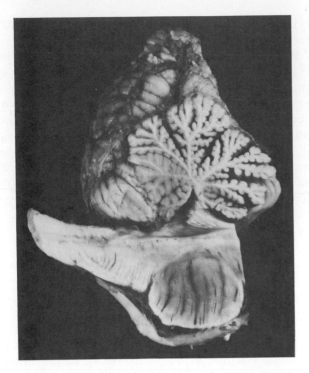

Figure 28-49. Alcoholic cerebellar atrophy. The cerebellum shows atrophy of the superior portion of the vermis. The open, fernlike appearance is indicative of a loss of parenchyma, which accentuates the individual folia.

DEGENERATIVE DISEASES

PARKINSONISM

Parkinsonism (paralysis agitans) is a neuronal disorder that primarily involves the substantia nigra. Neurons of the substantia nigra exert their action principally by secreting dopamine. The clinical expression of tremors at rest, muscular rigidity, and emotional lability are usually evidenced in the sixth to eighth decade of life.

Gross examination of the brain typically reveals a loss of pigment in the substantia nigra and locus ceruleus (Fig. 28-50). Microscopic examination reveals a depletion of pigmented neurons in these areas. Some residual nerve cells are atrophic, and a few contain spherical, eosinophilic, cytoplasmic inclusions termed **Lewy bodies.**

HUNTINGTON'S DISEASE

Huntington's disease is an autosomal dominant, hereditary disorder in which the expression of an abnormal gene alters the metabolism of a specific neuronal cell species and initiates a progressive functional deficiency

Alcoholism creates a complex problem that embraces both nutrition and intoxication (see Chapter 8). Four cerebral conditions are associated with alcoholism: cortical atrophy, atrophy of the superior aspect of the vermis of the cerebellum, Wernicke's syndrome, and central pontine myelinolysis. Atrophy of the Purkinje and granular cells of the cerebellum (Fig. 28-49) is, perhaps, the most common corollary of the chronic alcoholism, and is ostensibly the cause of the truncal ataxia that persists during periods of sobriety. As noted previously, central pontine myelinolysis is presumably an iatrogenic complication related to the rapid correction of hyponatremia.

Subacute combined degeneration (posterolateral combined degeneration) results precipitously from a deficiency of vitamin B_{12}, most often in association with pernicious anemia treated only with folic acid. The lesion begins as a symmetric loss of myelin and axons in the midthoracic or lower thoracic level of the spinal cord, and extends caudally and cephalad, producing an edematous, spongiform appearance in the posterolateral areas.

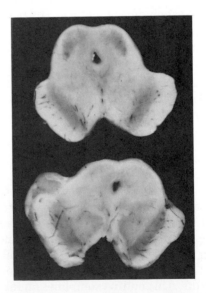

Figure 28-50. Parkinsonism. Transverse sections of the midbrain show a marked loss of melanin pigmentation in the substantia nigra, reflecting a loss of neurons in that area.

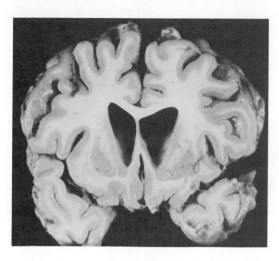

Figure 28-51. Huntington's chorea. Selective degeneration of the caudate nuclei bilaterally has straightened the normal concave contour of the lateral walls of the lateral ventricles, and has brought the ependyma in close proximity to the internal capsules. There is a moderate degree of cortical atrophy.

SPINOCEREBELLAR DEGENERATION

Spinocerebellar degeneration represents a category of disease that contains numerous heterogeneous entities. However, they are unified by three features: a broad but system-based geographic topography, a genetic influence, and a precocious loss of neurons and tracts in the cerebellum, brain stem, and spinal cord. The symptomatology reflects the topography of the lesions. Thus, patients display ataxia and intention tremor with involvement of the cerebellum, rigidity and tremor with degeneration of the brain stem; and loss of deep tendon reflexes, vibratory sense, and pain sensation with involvement of the spinal cord (Fig. 28-52).

Friedreich's ataxia is an autosomal dominant disorder that involves the spinal cord (Fig. 28-53). The symptoms of this disorder first appear during the first and second decades of life, and the course is insidiously progressive for 10 years or more. The classic lesion features degeneration of the posterior columns, the corticospinal pathways, and the spinocerebellar tracts.

that terminates in cell death. The abnormal gene resides on the short arm of chromosome 4. The patients remain asymptomatic through the first three to five decades of life. The primary disorder concerns the extrapyramidal system, and initial symptoms usually include an athetoid movement disorder. Subsequent involvement of the cortex leads to a loss of cognitive function, often accompanied by paranoia and delusions. Death occurs a decade or so later, and postmortem examination shows marked, symmetrical atrophy of the caudate nuclei, with lesser involvement of the putamen (Fig. 28-51).

AMYOTROPHIC LATERAL SCLEROSIS

Amyotrophic lateral sclerosis is a disease that relates specifically to motor neurons—that is, the anterior horn cells of the spinal cord; the motor nuclei of the brain stem, particularly the hypoglossal nuclei; and the upper motor neurons of the cerebral cortex. Initially, the lateral columns degenerate at the lumbosacral level. Thereafter, the degeneration progresses retrograde or cephalad. With time, the cell body itself undergoes atrophy and disappears.

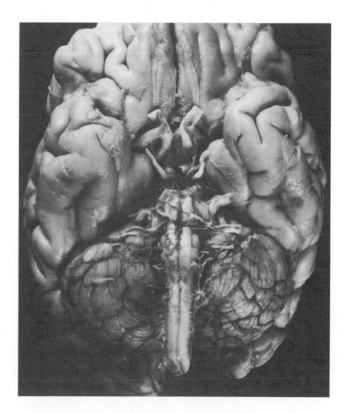

Figure 28-52. Spinocerebellar degeneration. Degeneration of the pons is conspicuous in this case of olivopontocerebellar degeneration.

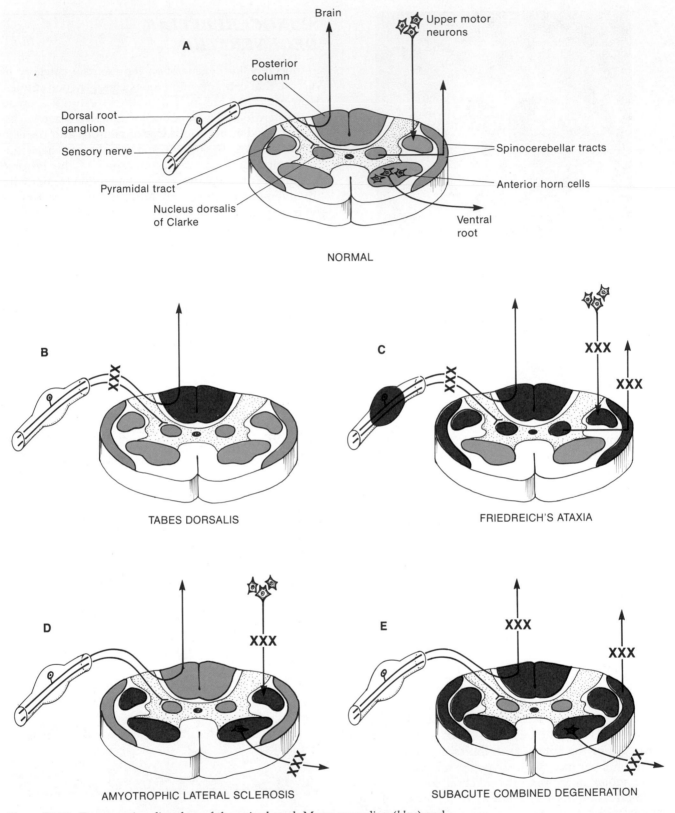

Figure 28-53. Degenerative disorders of the spinal cord. Many ascending (*blue*) and descending (*green*) pathways traverse the spinal cord. The four diseases illustrated produce differing patterns of disruption (*red*) of these pathways depending on the location of the primary pathologic process.

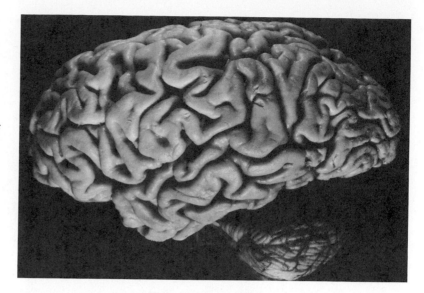

Figure 28-54. Alzheimer's disease. The cortex of the frontal, temporal, and parietal areas of the brain is atrophic.

Interestingly, but for reasons not understood, a chronic, interstitial cardiomyopathy develops. Cardiac hypertrophy and fibrosis may lead to heart failure.

Alzheimer's disease is characterized by the formation of senile (neuritic) plaques, neurofibrillary tangles, and granulovacuolar degeneration. These structural changes are most likely responsible for the **dementia** that affects about two-thirds of persons who are institutionalized because of impaired cognitive function.

During the course of Alzheimer's disease, neurons and neuritic processes are lost, the gyri narrow, the sulci widen, and cortical atrophy becomes apparent. The brain weight is reduced by about 200 g in an interval of 3 to 8 years. The atrophy is bilateral and symmetric and principally involves the cortex of the frontal lobes and hippocampus (Fig. 28-54). The most conspicuous histologic lesion, the **senile or neuritic plaque,** is a focal, discrete area that is several hundred micrometers in diameter. The maturing neuritic plaque is argentophilic and contains abundant glial processes and deposits that stain positively for amyloid.

The second member of the morphologic triad, **neurofibrillary tangles,** comprises helical filaments within neurons, which are formed in such abundance as to engorge the perikaryon (Fig. 28-55). These filaments have the same protein composition and diameter (10

nm) as normal neurofilaments and neurotubules. However, they are present in great excess and are abnormally paired into helical complexes. The third constituent of the morphologic triad is **granulovacuolar degeneration,** which is largely restricted to the pyramidal cells of the hippocampus. The term is used to describe multiple, small, cytoplasmic vacuoles, each of which contains one or several dark granules (Fig. 28-56). There is a predictable and precocious development of neuritic plaques, neurofibrillary tangles, and granulovacuolar degeneration in persons with Down's syndrome.

Pick's disease (lobar sclerosis) is expressed clinically as **dementia that is essentially indistinguishable from that of Alzheimer's disease.** The brain in Pick's disease is atrophic, but unlike Alzheimer's disease, the atrophy is typically localized in a frontal or a temporal lobe, and it may attain extreme proportions (Fig. 28-57). Histologically, the involved cortex is markedly depleted of neurons, and their absence is accentuated by a marked astrogliosis (Fig. 28-58). Many residual neurons have a "ballooned" cytoplasm, and in some, there are one or several faintly eosinophilic inclusions, termed **Pick bodies,** whose presence is validated by their intense argentophilia (Fig. 28-59). These bodies are formed of densely aggregated neurofilaments.

(Text continues on p. 786)

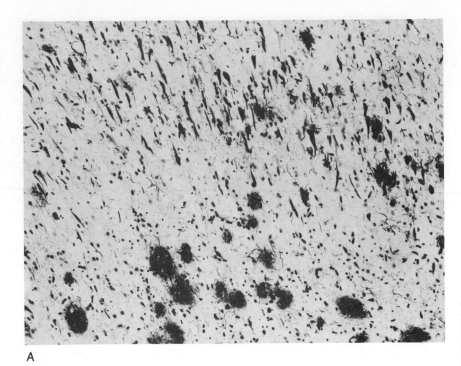

A

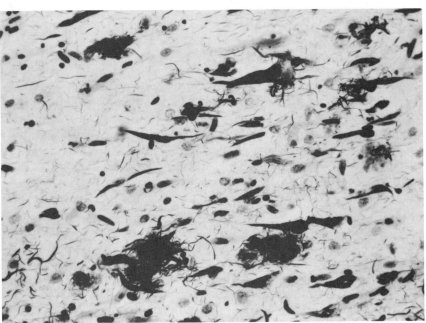

B

Figure 28-55. Alzheimer's disease. (*A*) A photomicrograph of the hippocampal cortex demonstrates extensive neurofibrillary degeneration of many neurons. There are numerous senile plaques, the presence of which is made apparent by their argentophilia. (*B*) High-power view of *A*.

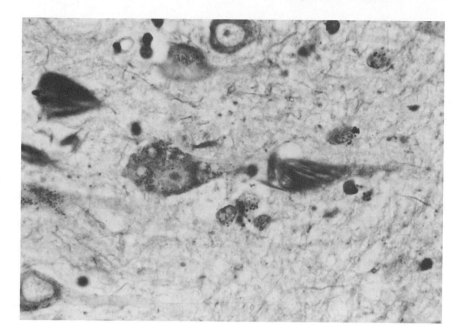

Figure 28-56. Alzheimer's disease. The neurofibrillary tangles are also argentophilic. Note that the neuron with granulovacuolar degeneration (*center*) does not show neurofibrillary degeneration.

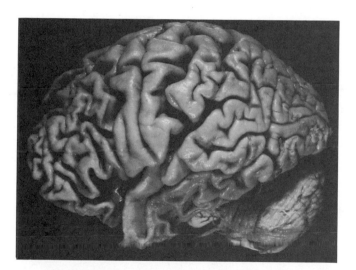

Figure 28-57. Pick's disease. Atrophy is extreme in the temporal lobe, pronounced in the frontal region, and moderate in the parietal area.

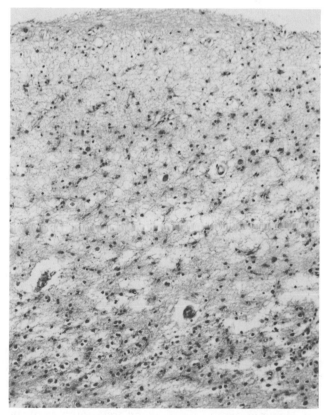

Figure 28-58. Pick's disease. A photomicrograph shows advanced neuronal depopulation and marked astrogliosis.

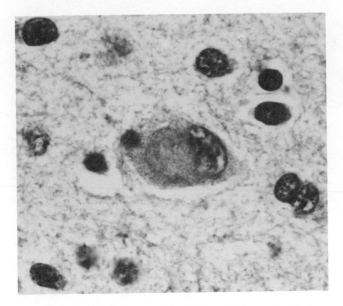

Figure 28-59. Pick's disease. The Pick body is a spherical accumulation of neurofibrillary material that displaces the nucleus.

THE PERIPHERAL NERVOUS SYSTEM

THOMAS W. BOULDIN

GENERAL PATHOLOGY

AXONAL DEGENERATION

Degeneration (necrosis) of the axon occurs in many neuropathies and reflects significant injury of the neuronal cell body or its axon. Axonal degeneration is quickly followed by breakdown of the myelin sheath and Schwann cell proliferation. The myelin debris is cleared by Schwann cells and macrophages. In many neuropathies, axonal degeneration is initially restricted to the distal ends of the larger, longer fibers (Fig. 28-60). Peripheral neuropathies exhibiting this selective degeneration of distal axons are known as **dying-back neuropathies (distal axonopathies)** and typically present as distal ("glove-and-stocking") neuropathies. Axonal degeneration may also be secondary to degen-

eration of the neuronal cell body, as occurs in poliomyelitis.

Neuropathies characterized by selective degeneration of the neuronal soma are referred to as **neuronopathies,** and are much less common than distal axonopathies. The axonal degeneration that occurs in a nerve distal to a transection or crush of the nerve is termed **wallerian degeneration.**

SEGMENTAL DEMYELINATION

The loss of myelin from one or more internodes (segments) along a myelinated fiber is common in many neuropathies and reflects Schwann cell dysfunction (see Fig. 28-60). Schwann cell dysfunction may be caused by direct injury of the Schwann cell/myelin

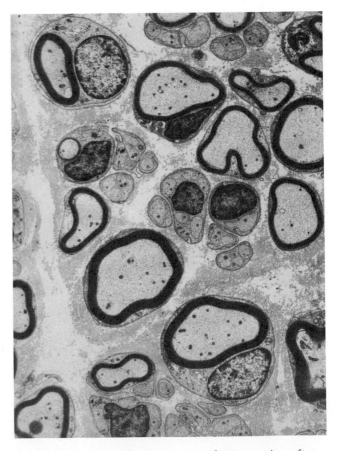

Figure 28-60. Axonal degeneration and regeneration after peripheral nerve injury.

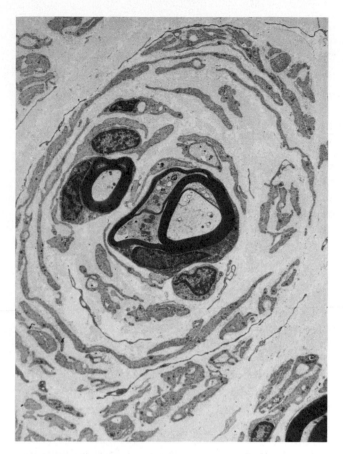

Figure 28-61. Onion bulb formation in peripheral nerve. An electron micrograph shows multiple layers of flattened Schwann cell processes encircling two myelinated axons. Onion bulb formations are common in certain hereditary neuropathies and in chronic inflammatory demyelinating neuropathy.

PERIPHERAL NEUROPATHIES

The major clinical manifestations of peripheral neuropathy are muscle weakness, muscle atrophy, alterations of sensation, and autonomic dysfunction. Motor, sensory, and autonomic functions may be equally or preferentially affected. The clinical manifestations may have an acute (within days), subacute (within weeks), or chronic (within months or years) evolution. They may be localized to one nerve (mononeuropathy) or several individual nerves (mononeuropathy multiplex), or they may be diffuse and symmetric (polyneuropathy). On pathologic examination, a neuropathy may show mainly axonal degeneration (axonal neuropathy), mainly segmental demyelination (demyelinating neuropathy), or a mixture of axonal degeneration and segmental demyelination. The etiologic classification of peripheral neuropathies is presented in Table 28-1.

sheath, or it may be secondary to underlying axonal abnormalities **(secondary demyelination).** The myelin debris is cleared by Schwann cells and macrophages. Degeneration of the internodal myelin sheath is followed sequentially by Schwann cell proliferation, remyelination of the demyelinated segments, and recovery of function. Repeated episodes of segmental demyelination and remyelination of peripheral nerves, as occurs in chronic demyelinating neuropathies, lead to the accumulation of supernumerary Schwann cells around axons **(onion bulb formation)** and nerve enlargement (hypertrophy) (Fig. 28-61). Neuropathies characterized by conspicuous onion bulb formation and nerve hypertrophy are known as **hypertrophic neuropathies.**

INFLAMMATORY DEMYELINATING NEUROPATHY

Acquired inflammatory demyelinating neuropathy usually presents as an acutely evolving, predominantly motor, polyneuropathy **(Landry-Guillain-Barré syndrome).** Occasional patients have a chronic course characterized by multiple relapses or a slow, continuous progression **(chronic inflammatory polyneuropathy).** Resolution of the neuropathy commences 2 to 4 weeks after onset, and most patients make a good recovery. The pathogenesis of the demyelination is unknown, but current evidence suggests that it may be immunologically mediated. The neuropathy may be sporadic; may follow immunization, surgery, or viral and mycoplasmal infections; or it may complicate cancer.

The neuropathy may involve all levels of the peripheral nervous system, including spinal roots, ganglia, craniospinal nerves, and autonomic nerves, with the distribution of the lesions varying from case to case. The involved regions show endoneurial infiltrates of lymphocytes and macrophages, segmental demyelination, and relative sparing of axons. The chronic form of the disease may show numerous onion bulb formations, owing to the recurring episodes of demyelination and remyelination. Lumbar puncture characteristically reveals an increase in the protein level of the cerebrospinal fluid, but only slight pleiocytosis.

Table 28–1   Etiologic Classification of Neuropathies

Autoimmune
Inflammatory demyelinating neuropathy

Metabolic
Diabetic polyneuropathy
Uremic neuropathy
Hypothyroid neuropathy
Hepatic neuropathy
Porphyric neuropathy

Nutritional
Alcoholic neuropathy
Beriberi neuropathy
Neuropathy related to vitamin B_{12} deficiency
Neuropathy related to vitamin E deficiency
Neuropathy related to the postgastrectomy state
Neuropathy related to celiac disease

Ischemic
Vasculitic neuropathy
Neuropathy of peripheral vascular disease
Some diabetic mononeuropathies

Toxic (see Table 28-2)

Paraneoplastic

Amyloid

Paraproteinemic

Inherited (See Table 28-3)

Infectious
Herpes zoster
Leprosy
Diphtheria (toxin)
Acquired immunodeficiency syndrome (AIDS)

Sarcoid

Radiation-induced

Cryptogenic

DIABETIC NEUROPATHY

Diabetes mellitus, a major cause of neuropathy, is associated with distal sensory or sensorimotor polyneuropathy, autonomic neuropathy, mononeuropathy, or mononeuropathy multiplex. Symmetric polyneuropathy is characterized by a mixture of segmental demyelination and axonal degeneration.

ALCOHOLIC NEUROPATHY

The distal sensorimotor polyneuropathy associated with alcohol abuse is generally attributed to concomi-

tant nutritional deficiencies, rather than to a direct toxic effect of alcohol on the peripheral nerves. Peripheral nerves show loss of nerve fibers secondary to axonal degeneration of the dying-back type.

TOXIC NEUROPATHIES

Many drugs and toxic agents produce peripheral neuropathy (Table 28-2). Most toxic neuropathies are characterized by axonal degeneration, usually of the dying-back type. Buckthorn and diptheria toxins are notable for producing demyelinating neuropathies.

PARANEOPLASTIC NEUROPATHIES

The remote effects of cancer on the nervous system include (1) encephalomyelitis, (2) necrotizing myelopathy, (3) cerebellar degeneration, (4) several types of peripheral neuropathy, and (5) the Eaton-Lambert syndrome. The paraneoplastic neuropathies are of several clinicopathologic types: (1) a distal sensorimotor polyneuropathy showing axonal degeneration and a variable amount of segmental demyelination, (2) a subacute sensory polyneuropathy secondary to dorsal root ganglionitis, (3) a subacute motor polyneuropathy caused by the loss of anterior horn cells, and (4) an acute or chronic inflammatory demyelinating polyneuropathy of the Landry-Guillain-Barré type.

Table 28–2   Agents Associated with Toxic Neuropathy

DRUGS	ENVIRONMENTAL AGENTS
Amiodarone	Acrylamide
Amytriptyline	Arsenic
Chloramphenicol	Buckthorn toxin
Dapsone	Carbon disulfide
Disulfiram	Chlordecane
Glutethimide	2,4-Dichlorophenoxyacetic
Gold	acid (2,4-D)
Hydralazine	Dimethylaminopropionitrile
Isoniazid	Diphtheria toxin
Lithium	*n*-Hexane
Metronidazole	Methyl-*n*-butyl ketone
Misonidazole	Lead
Nitrofurantoin	Methyl bromide
Perhexiline	Organophosphates
Platinum	Polybrominated biphenyls
Pyridoxine (Vitamin B_6)	Thallium
Vincristine	Trichloroethylene

AMYLOID NEUROPATHY

A distal sensorimotor polyneuropathy, often with prominent autonomic dysfunction, complicates hereditary systemic amyloidosis or the acquired form of systemic amyloidosis that is associated with plasma cell dyscrasias (primary amyloidosis, multiple myeloma, Waldenström's macroglobulinemia). The neuropathy is characterized pathologically by the deposition of amyloid in peripheral nerves, dorsal root ganglia, and autonomic ganglia.

The chronic entrapment neuropathy of the median nerve at the wrist **(carpal tunnel syndrome)** is a complication of systemic amyloidosis. The nerve entrapment is secondary to amyloid infiltration of the flexor retinaculum.

HEREDITARY NEUROPATHIES

Peripheral neuropathy is a manifestation of a number of inherited diseases. Among these inherited diseases are several in which peripheral neuropathy is the major clinical manifestation. The biochemical abnormalities for most of these hereditary neuropathies are unknown; thus, current classifications are based on the mode of inheritance, clinical presentation, and pathologic features (Table 28-3).

NERVE TRAUMA

TRAUMATIC NEUROMA

Shortly after the transection of a peripheral nerve, regenerating axonal sprouts arise from the distal ends of the intact axons in the proximal nerve stump. If the severed ends of the proximal and distal nerve stumps are closely approximated, the regenerating axonal sprouts may find and reinnervate the distal stump. In many instances, however, the severed ends of the nerve are not closely approximated, and there is considerable scar tissue between the proximal and distal stumps. This scar tissue and the wide gap between the proximal and distal stumps prevent the regenerating sprouts from successfully reinnervating the distal stump. In this situation, the axonal sprouts ensheathed by Schwann cells grow haphazardly into the scar tissue

Table 28-3 Hereditary Neuropathies

DISEASE	INHERITANCE	CLINICAL PRESENTATION	PATHOLOGY
HMSN type I (Peroneal muscular atrophy; Charcot-Marie-Tooth disease)	AD	Distal sensorimotor neuropathy; onset after first decade; slow progression; palpably enlarged nerves, severe slowing of nerve conduction	Extensive demyelination with numerous onion bulbs and nerve hypertrophy; distal axonal degeneration
HMSN type II (Peroneal muscular atrophy; Charcot-Marie-Tooth disease)	AD	Similar to HMSN type I except no nerve hypertrophy and less slowing of nerve conduction	Distal axonal degeneration
HMSN type III (Dejerine-Sottas disease)	AR	Distal sensorimotor neuropathy; onset in infancy; palpably enlarged nerves; severe slowing of nerve conduction	Extensive demyelination with numerous onion bulbs and nerve hypertrophy; distal axonal degeneration
HMSN type IV (Refsum's disease)	AR	Distal sensorimotor neuropathy; pigmentary retinopathy; enlarged nerves; accumulation of phytanic acid in serum	Extensive demyelination with onion bulbs and nerve hypertrophy; distal axonal degeneration
HSN type I	AD	Distal sensory neuropathy; onset in adolescence; sensory loss leads to mutilation of feet	Axonal degeneration
HSN type II	AR	Similar to HSN type I except earlier onset and mutilation of hands and feet	Axonal degeneration
Werdnig-Hoffman disease (acute infantile spinal muscular atrophy)	AR	Motor neuropathy; onset in infancy; proximal muscle weakness; progressive and fatal	Axonal degeneration with chromatolysis and loss of lower motor neurons

HMSN, hereditary motor and sensory neuropathy; HSN, hereditary sensory neuropathy; AD, autosomal dominant; AR, autosomal recessive.

at the end of the proximal stump to form a painful swelling known as a traumatic or amputation neuroma.

PLANTAR NEUROMA (MORTON'S NEUROMA)

Plantar neuroma, a painful, sausage-shaped swelling of the plantar digital nerve between the second and third or third and fourth metatarsal bones, is probably caused by repeated nerve compression. The swelling is not a true neuroma, as it is secondary to endoneurial, perineural, and epineural fibrosis, rather than a mass of regenerating axons.

TUMORS

SCHWANNOMA (NEURILEMOMA)

Schwannoma, a benign, slowly growing neoplasm of Schwann cells, may arise in any nerve. The tumor is oval and well demarcated, and varies in diameter from a few millimeters to several centimeters. The cut surface of the schwannoma is firm and tan to gray, and often shows foci of hemorrhage, necrosis, xanthomatous change, and cystic degeneration. Microscopically, the proliferating Schwann cells form two distinctive histologic patterns (Fig. 28-62). One pattern, termed **Antoni type A,** is characterized by interwoven fascicles of spindle cells with elongated nuclei, eosinophilic cytoplasm, and indistinct cytoplasmic borders. The nuclei may palisade in areas to form structures known as **Verocay bodies.** The second histologic pattern, termed **Antoni type B,** is characterized by spindle or oval cells with indistinct cytoplasm in a loose, vacuolated background.

Schwannomas may arise from cranial nerves, spinal roots, or peripheral nerves, and most often present in adults. Intracranial schwannomas are most common, accounting for 8% of all intracranial tumors. With rare exceptions, the intracranial schwannomas arise from the eighth cranial nerve **(acoustic schwannoma)** within the internal auditory canal or at the meatus, and cause unilateral hearing loss and tinnitus.

Intraspinal schwannomas usually arise from the dorsal (sensory) spinal roots. They typically present as intradural, extramedullary tumors producing radicular (root) pain and spinal cord compression.

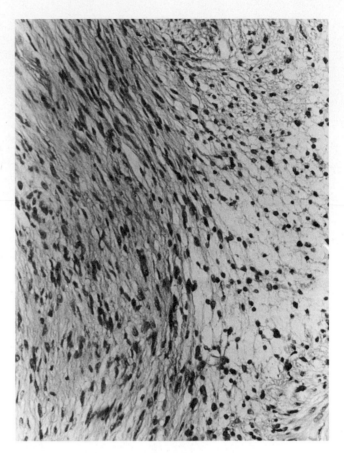

Figure 28-62. Schwannoma. A photomicrograph shows the characteristically abrupt transition between the compact Antoni type A cellular pattern (*left*) and the spongy Antoni type B cellular pattern (*right*).

NEUROFIBROMA

The Schwann cell is the principal constituent of neurofibroma, which may be more hamartomatous than neoplastic. A distinction between neurofibroma and schwannoma is warranted because of the close association of neurofibroma with von Recklinghausen's neurofibromatosis and its potential for sarcomatous degeneration. On gross examination, the neurofibroma involves the large nerves, appearing as a poorly circumscribed, fusiform enlargement of the nerve. The diffuse, intrafascicular growth of the tumor within multiple nerve fascicles may so enlarge the nerve's fascicles that they appear grossly as the cords of a nerve plexus (plexiform neurofibroma). Cutaneous neurofibromas arise from dermal nerves and present as soft, nodular, or pedunculated skin tumors.

The cut surface of a neurofibroma is soft and light gray, and the enlarged nerve fascicles of the plexiform neurofibroma may be prominent. Microscopically, the neurofibroma arising in large nerves is characterized by an endoneurial proliferation of spindle cells with elongated nuclei, eosinophilic cytoplasm, and indistinct cell borders. Interspersed among the spindle cells are wavy bands of collagen, an extracellular myxoid matrix, and residual nerve fibers. A small but clinically significant proportion of neurofibromas exhibits sarcomatous transformation.

Neurofibromas are solitary or multiple, arise on any nerve, and are found in children or adults. Most commonly, they involve the skin, major nerve plexuses, large deep nerve trunks, retroperitoneum, and gastrointestinal tract. Most **solitary cutaneous neurofibromas** occur outside the context of neurofibromatosis, and these tumors do not have the potential for sarcomatous degeneration of their deeper counterparts. **The presence of multiple neurofibromas is diagnostic of neurofibromatosis.**

MALIGNANT SCHWANNOMA (NEUROFIBROSARCOMA)

The histogenesis of malignant schwannoma, a poorly differentiated, spindle cell sarcoma of the peripheral nerve, is uncertain. The tumor may arise de novo or from malignant transformation of a neurofibroma. The malignant schwannoma rarely arises from malignant transformation of a schwannoma. **About half of these sarcomas are found in patients with neurofibromatosis.** The tumor is prone to local recurrence and blood-borne metastases, and has a worse prognosis in the context of neurofibromatosis.

29

THE EYE

GORDON K. KLINTWORTH

Largely because of its superficial location, the eye is exposed to a myriad of microorganisms, antigens, and toxic chemicals, as well as to solar radiation and adverse climatic conditions. The unprotected position of the eye also makes it vulnerable to a host of injuries. Disorders of the eye are common and many of its afflictions result in loss of sight.

INFECTIONS, INFLAMMATION, AND IMMUNOLOGIC DISORDERS

CONJUNCTIVA

CONJUNCTIVITIS

Conjunctivitis, the most common eye disease, is characterized by hyperemic conjunctival blood vessels ("pink eye"). The conjunctival discharge may be purulent, fibrinous, serous, or hemorrhagic, and contains inflammatory cells that vary with the etiologic agent.

TRACHOMA AND RELATED INFECTIONS

About 500 million people are afflicted by trachoma, an acute, infectious, cicatrizing keratoconjunctivitis due to *Chlamydia trachomatis* and other associated bacteria. **This is the most common cause of blindness in the world and is especially prevalent in the Asia, the Middle East, and parts of Africa. In the United States it is almost restricted to the American Indian population in the southwestern region of the country.** Trachoma is not very contagious, but overcrowding and poor hygienic conditions favor its transmission by fingers, fomites, and flies. Spontaneous healing is common in children, but in adults the disease progresses more rapidly and rarely heals in the absence of treatment.

Trachoma is virtually always bilateral and involves the upper half of the conjunctiva more extensively than the lower. The cellular infiltrate is predominantly lymphocytic, and conjunctival lymph follicles with necrotic germinal centers are characteristic. Eventually lymphocytes and blood vessels invade the superior portion of the cornea between its epithelium and Bowman's zone (trachomatous pannus), and scarring of the conjunctiva and eyelids distorts the lids. On microscopic examination the desquamated conjunctival epithelium exhibits glycogen-rich intracytoplasmic inclusion bodies and large macrophages containing nuclear fragments (Leber cells).

Chlamydia is responsible for a purulent conjunctivitis that develops in the newborn. The infection is also acquired by swimming in nonchlorinated pools or exposure to discharges of lesions of the conjunctiva, urethra, or cervix uteri. In adults and older children, chlamydia causes a chronic follicular conjunctivitis with intracytoplasmic inclusion bodies indistinguishable from those of trachoma. In contrast to trachoma, however, the lower tarsal conjunctiva is involved, scarring and necrosis do not develop, and keratitis is rare and mild.

OPHTHALMIA NEONATORUM

Neisseria gonorrhoeae causes a severe, acute conjunctivitis with a copious purulent discharge, especially in the newborn. The infection, a common cause of blindness in some parts of the world, is complicated by corneal ulceration, perforation and scarring, and panophthalmitis. The infant usually becomes infected while passing through the birth canal of an infected mother. Aside from gonorrhea, ophthalmia neonatorum has other causes, including other pyogenic bacteria, *C. trachomatis,* and even the silver nitrate administered to the conjunctiva of newborns to prevent gonococcal conjunctivitis.

CORNEA

HERPES SIMPLEX

Herpesvirus has a predilection for the corneal epithelium, but it can invade the corneal stroma and occasionally other ocular tissues. Primary infection by herpes simplex type I usually causes subclinical or undiagnosed localized ocular lesions in childhood, these often being accompanied by regional lymphadenopathy, systemic infection, and fever. Herpes simplex type II can produce widespread infection of the cornea and retina, especially in the neonate who becomes infected during natural birth when the mother harbors genital herpes.

A high rate of recurrence at one site characterizes secondary herpes infection (reactivation disease). The herpes simplex virus commonly causes multiple, minute, discrete, intraepithelial ulcers. While some of these lesions heal, others enlarge and eventually coalesce to form linear or branching fissures called dendritic ulcers; (from Greek *dendron,* a tree). The epithelium between the fissures desquamates, causing sharply demarcated, irregular geographic ulcers.

ONCHOCERCIASIS

The nematode *Onchocerca volvulus,* which is transmitted by bites of infected black flies (*Simulium* species) is by far the most important helminthic infection of the eye. This parasite is estimated to account for blindness in at least half a million individuals in endemic regions of Africa and Latin America. Five to six years after the appearance of subcutaneous nodules (cercomas), the living microfilaria that are released from fertilized adult female onchocerca migrate into the superficial cornea, bulbar conjunctiva, aqueous humor, and other ocular tissues. Following the demise of intracorneal microfilaria, an inflammatory response causes corneal opacification and visual impairment ("river blindness").

UVEA

Inflammation of the iris and ciliary body, termed uveitis typically causes a red eye, sensitivity to bright light (photophobia), moderate pain, blurred vision, a pericorneal halo, dilated deep ciliary vessels (ciliary flush), and slight constriction of the pupil (miosis). As a sequel to iritis, adhesions develop between the iris and the lens (posterior synechiae) or between the peripheral iris and the anterior chamber angle (peripheral anterior synechiae), thereby causing glaucoma.

SYMPATHETIC OPHTHALMIA

An important complication of a perforating ocular injury and prolapse of uveal tissue is a progressive, bilateral, diffuse, granulomatous inflammation of the uvea. This uveitis, which also rarely follows evisceration and intraocular melanomas, develops in the originally injured eye ("exciting eye") after a latent period of at least 10 days (usually 4 to 8 weeks, sometimes many years). The uninjured eye ("sympathizing eye") becomes affected at the same time or shortly thereafter. Nodules containing reactive retinal pigment epithelium, epithelioid cells, and macrophages commonly appear between Bruch's membrane and the retinal pigment epithelium (Dalen-Fuchs nodules). It is widely believed that the condition is an autoimmune reaction to sensitization by uveal isoantigens.

EYELIDS

Inflammation of the eyelids (blepharitis) is common and sometimes presents as an acute, red, tender inflammatory mass in the eyelid called a sty or hordeolum. Acute inflammation of the meibomian glands (internal hordeolum) and acute folliculitis of the glands of Zeis (external hordeolum) are common. Chronic, foreign-body, granulomatous inflammation centered around the meibomian or Zeis glands produces a painless swelling in the eyelid known as a chalazion.

NEOPLASMS

The eye and the structures around it contain a wide variety of cell types and, as one might expect, benign and malignant neoplasms arise from them. However, the frequency with which the different cell types become neoplastic varies immensely. **Intraocular neoplasms arise mostly from immature retinal neurons (retinoblastoma) and uveal melanocytes (melanoma).**

MELANOMA

While melanomas, **the most common primary intraocular malignancy,** may arise from melanocytes in any part of the eye, the choroid is the most common site. (Fig. 29-1). Based on the microscopic appearance of uveal melanomas, they have been subdivided into different types (spindle A, spindle B, fascicular, necrotic, mixed, and epithelioid types). Melanomas in the iris present clinically one to two decades earlier than those in the choroid and ciliary body, perhaps because they are more easily seen. Aside from hematogenous spread, uveal melanomas disseminate by traversing the sclera to enter the orbital tissues, usually at sites where blood vessels and nerves pass through the sclera. Unlike melanomas of the skin, those of the uvea do not exhibit lymphatic spread, because the eye lacks lymphatics.

RETINOBLASTOMA

Retinoblastoma, the most common intraocular, potentially fatal, neoplasm of childhood (Fig. 29-2), is estimated to affect one in 20,000 to 34,000 live births. It arises from the retina and most frequently presents within the first two years of life.

Most retinoblastomas (about 95%) occur sporadically, but some (6% to 8%) are inherited. While most retinoblastomas are unilateral, up to 25% of the sporadic cases and most inherited retinoblastomas are bilateral. The retinoblastoma (R*b*) susceptibility gene is located on the long arm of chromosome 13 (13q14). A recent hypothesis suggests that the R*b* gene normally regulates a set of protooncogenes, and that when both alleles of this gene are lost or inactivated, the structural transforming gene is expressed. There is a high inci-

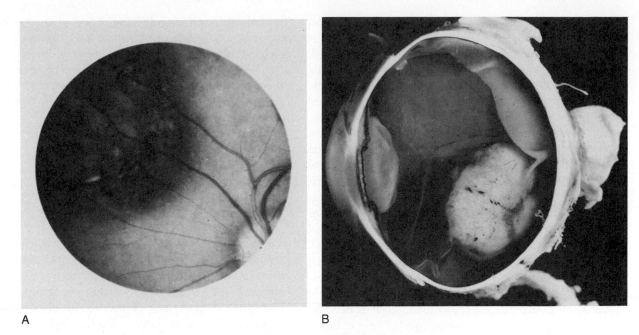

A   B

Figure 29-1. Malignant melanoma. (*A*) A malignant melanoma of the choroid is apparent as a dark mass visible beneath the retinal blood vessels. (*B*) A mushroom-shaped melanoma of the choroid is present in this eye. Choroidal melanomas commonly invade through Bruch's membrane and result in this appearance.

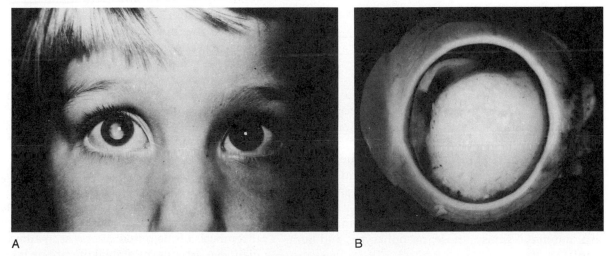

A   B

Figure 29-2. Retinoblastoma. (*A*) The white pupil (leukocoria) in the right eye is the result of an intraocular retinoblastoma. (*B*) This surgically excised eye is almost filled by a cream-colored intraocular retinoblastoma with white calcified flecks.

dence of retinoblastoma in individuals with a deletion of chromosome 13.

This cream-colored tumor usually contains scattered, chalky white, calcified flecks within yellow necrotic zones. Retinoblastomas are intensely cellular and display several morphologic patterns. In some instances, densely packed, round neoplastic cells with hyperchromatic nuclei, scant cytoplasm, and abundant mitoses are randomly distributed. In other tumors the cells are commonly arranged radially around a central cavity (Flexner-Wintersteiner rosettes), as they differentiate towards photoreceptors. In some retinoblastomas the cellular arrangement resembles the fleur-de-lis (fleurette).

Retinoblastomas disseminate by several routes. They commonly extend into the optic nerve, from which they spread intracranially. They also invade blood vessels, especially in the highly vascular choroid, before metastasizing hematogenously throughout the body. The bone marrow is a common site of blood-borne metastases, but surprisingly the lung is rarely involved. Retinoblastomas are almost always fatal if left untreated. However, with early diagnosis and modern therapy, survival is high (about 90%). On rare occasions, spontaneous regression may occur. Individuals with retinoblastomas have an increased susceptibility to other potentially fatal neoplasms, including osteogenic sarcoma, Ewing's sarcoma, and pinealoblastoma.

METASTATIC INTRAOCULAR AND ORBITAL NEOPLASMS

Metastatic neoplasms in the eye are more common than those that arise within the ocular tissues. Most intraocular metastases involve the posterior choroid, and while any malignant tumor may, in theory, metastasize to the ocular tissues, leukemia, carcinoma of the breast, and carcinoma of the lung account for most cases. Neuroblastoma frequently metastasizes to the orbit in infancy and childhood. The orbit may be invaded by malignant neoplasms of the eyelid, conjunctiva, paranasal sinuses, nose, nasopharynx, and intracranial cavity.

VASCULAR DISORDERS

HEMORRHAGE

Retinal hemorrhages are a feature of many disorders, including hypertension, diabetes mellitus, and central retinal vein occlusion. Hemorrhage in the nerve fiber layer spreads between axons and causes a flame-shaped appearance on funduscopy, while deep retinal hemorrhages tend to be round. When located between the retinal pigment and Bruch's membrane, blood appears as a dark mass and clinically resembles a melanoma.

RETINAL OCCLUSIVE VASCULAR DISEASE

Vascular occlusion results from thrombosis, embolism, stenosis (as in atherosclerosis), vascular compression, intravascular sludging or coagulation, and vasoconstriction (for instance, in hypertensive retinopathy and migraine). Thrombosis of the ocular vessels may accompany disease of these vessels, as in giant cell arteritis.

The effect of vascular occlusion depends upon the size of the vessel involved, the degree of resultant ischemia, and the nature of the embolus. Small emboli often do not interfere with retinal function, while septic emboli may cause foci of ocular infection. Certain disorders of the heart and major vessels, such as the carotid arteries, predispose to emboli that lodge in the retina. Ischemia of any cause deprives the retina of oxygen and other essential metabolites and frequently results in the appearance of white fluffy patches that resemble cotton ("cotton-wool patches") on ophthalmoscopic examination. These spots consist of aggregates of varicose swollen axons in the nerve fiber layer of the retina. Cotton-wool spots are reversible if the circulation is restored in time.

CENTRAL RETINAL ARTERY OCCLUSION

The neurons of the retina are extremely susceptible to hypoxia. Central retinal artery occlusions may follow thrombosis of the retinal artery, as in atherosclerosis or giant cell arteritis, or emboli of various types. Intracellular edema, manifested by retinal pallor, is prominent, especially in the macula, where the ganglion cells are most numerous. The vascularized choroid beneath the center of the macula (foveola) stands out in sharp contrast as a prominent "cherry red spot." The lack of retinal circulation reduces the retinal arterioles to delicate threads. Permanent blindness follows central retinal artery obstruction, unless the ischemia is of short duration.

CENTRAL RETINAL VEIN OCCLUSION

Following central retinal vein occlusion, flame-shaped hemorrhages develop in the nerve fiber layer of the retina, especially around the optic disc, as a result of the high intravascular pressure that dilates the veins and collateral vessels. Edema of the optic disc and retina occur because of an impaired absorption of interstitial fluid. Vision is generally poor, but may recover surprisingly well, considering the severity of the funduscopic changes. An intractable closed-angle glaucoma commonly ensues 2 to 3 months after central retinal vein occlusion, owing to neovascularization of the iris and adhesions between the iris and the anterior chamber angle.

Figure 29-3 summarizes differences between retinal artery and vein occlusions.

THE EYE IN SYSTEMIC DISEASE

HYPERTENSIVE VASCULAR DISEASE

Elevated systemic blood pressure commonly affects the retina, causing changes that relate to the severity of the hypertension. Features of hypertensive retinopathy include (1) variable degrees of arteriolar narrowing, (2) hemorrhages in the retinal nerve fiber layer ("flame-shaped hemorrhages"), (3) exudates, including some that fan out around the center of the macula ("macular star"), (4) fluffy white bodies in the superficial retina ("cotton-wool spots"), and (5) microaneurysms. In cases of severe hypertension, the retinal arterioles are much narrower than normal, and edema of the optic nerve head ensues. Arteriolosclerosis accompanies long-standing hypertension and commonly affects the retinal and choroidal vessels. The thickened retinal arterioles become attenuated, increasingly tortuous, and of irregular caliber.

At sites where the arterioles cross veins, the veins may appear kinked (arteriovenous nicking), but the venous diameter is not narrower distal to the compression, an appearance that indicates that the kinked appearance of veins is not due to compression by a taut sclerotic artery. Instead it reflects sclerosis within the venous walls, because retinal arteries and veins share a common adventitia at sites of arteriovenous crossings.

Small superficial or deep retinal hemorrhages often accompany retinal arteriolosclerosis. In malignant hypertension, a necrotizing arteriolitis, with fibrinoid ne-

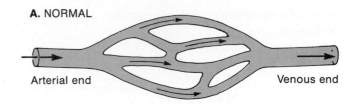

A. NORMAL

Arterial end   Venous end

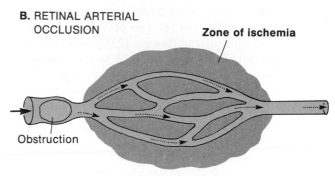

B. RETINAL ARTERIAL OCCLUSION

Zone of ischemia

Obstruction

Neuronal functional impairment → Visual loss

Edema → Pallor

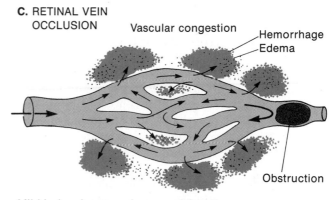

C. RETINAL VEIN OCCLUSION

Vascular congestion

Hemorrhage
Edema

Obstruction

Mild ischemia; normal neuronal function

Figure 29-3. Occlusion of the retinal artery and vein. (*A*) In the retina, as in other parts of the body, blood normally flows through a capillary network. When the retinal arteries become occluded, as with an embolus, a zone of retinal ischemia ensues. This is accompanied by impaired neuronal function and visual loss, and the ischemic retina becomes pale (*B*). Because the intravascular pressure within the ischemic tissue is low, hemorrhage is inconspicuous. On the other hand, with retinal vein occlusion (*C*) vascular congestion, hemorrhage, and edema are prominent, while ischemia is mild and neuronal function remains intact.

crosis and thrombosis of the precapillary retinal arterioles, occurs.

DIABETES MELLITUS

DIABETIC RETINOPATHY

Diabetic retinopathy usually follows 10 to 20 years after the onset of diabetes, and its prevalence increases with the duration of the disease (75% to 90% of patients have retinal changes after 25 years of diabetes (Figs. 29-4 to 29-6). Diabetic retinopathy under the age of 10 is rare, and most cases are over the age of 50 years. Women are not only more prone to diabetes than men, but also develop diabetic retinopathy more frequently. The retinopathy does not seem to be closely related to the severity of the diabetes. Similar to other delayed lesions in diabetes mellitus, the retinopathy is an outcome of vascular disease.

Retinal ischemia accounts for most features of diabetic retinopathy, including cotton-wool spots, capillary closure, microaneurysms, and retinal neovascularization. These result from narrowing or occlusion of retinal arterioles or from atheromatosis of the central retinal or ophthalmic arteries.

The retinopathy of diabetes is characterized by nonproliferative and proliferative stages. Nonproliferative diabetic retinopathy exhibits venous engorgement, small hemorrhages ("dot and blot hemorrhages"), capillary microaneurysms, and exudates. The retinopathy begins at the posterior pole, but eventually may involve the entire retina.

The first discernible clinical abnormality in nonproliferative diabetic retinopathy is engorged retinal veins. This is followed by small hemorrhages in the same area, mostly in the inner nuclear and outer plexiform layers. With time, "waxy" exudates accumulate, chiefly in the vicinity of the microaneurysms. The retinopathy of the elderly diabetic frequently displays numerous exudates, while this is not a feature in juvenile diabetics. Because of the hyperlipoproteinemia of diabetics, the exudates are rich in lipid, and hence appear yellowish ("waxy" exudates). Capillary microaneurysms appear in areas of poor retinal vascular perfusion.

After many years the retinopathy becomes proliferative; delicate new blood vessels, together with fibrous and glial tissue, grow toward the vitreous humor. Neovascularization of the retina is a prominent feature of diabetic retinopathy and of other conditions caused by retinal ischemia. Tortuous new vessels first appear on the surface of the retina and optic nerve head and then grow into the vitreous cavity. The newly formed friable

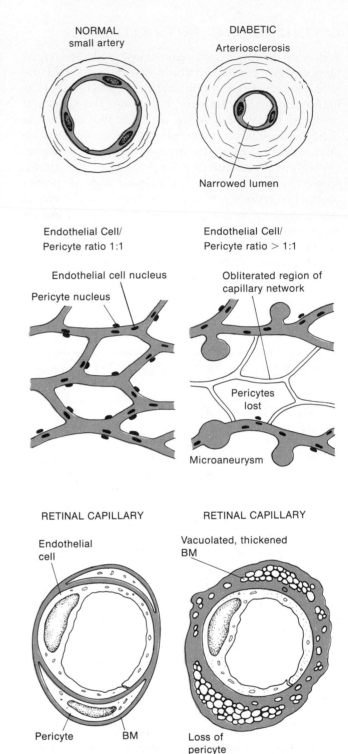

Figure 29-4. Diabetic retinopathy. In diabetic retinopathy the microvasculature is abnormal. Arteriosclerosis narrows the lumen of the small arteries. Pericytes are lost and the endothelial cell:pericyte ratio is greater than 1. Capillary microaneurysms are prominent, and portions of the capillary network become acellular and show no blood flow. The basement membrane of the retinal capillaries is thickened and vacuolated. (BM = basement membranes)

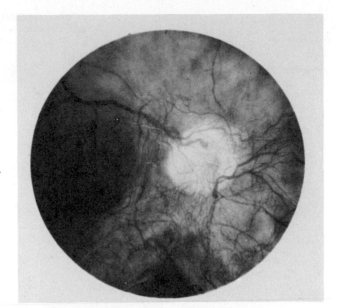

Figure 29-5. Diabetic retinopathy. (*A*) An extensive network of newly formed blood vessels extends into the vitreous cavity from the region of the optic disc in a patient with advanced diabetic retinopathy. (*B*) Numerous microaneurysms are present in this flat preparation of a diabetic retina.

A

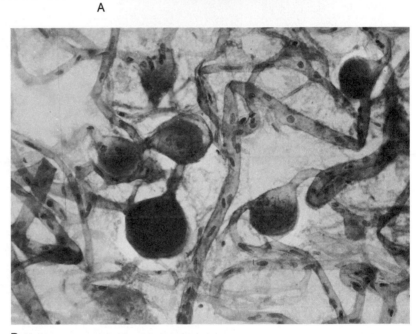

B

vessels bleed easily, and the resultant vitreal hemorrhage obscures vision by impairing the ability of light to reach the retinal photoreceptors. The proliferating, preretinal, fibrovascular, gliotic tissue contracts, often causing retinal detachment and blindness.

In diabetes mellitus blindness results when the macula is involved in the retinopathy, but it also follows vitreous hemorrhage, retinal detachment, and glaucoma. **Diabetic retinopathy now equals glaucoma as a leading cause of irreversible blindness in the United States.** Once blindness ensues it heralds an ominous future for the patient, since the average life expectancy is then less than 6 years, and only one-fifth of blind diabetics survive 10 years.

DIABETIC IRIDOPATHY

In diabetics with severe retinopathy, a fibrovascular layer frequently grows along the anterior surface of the iris and in the anterior chamber angle. The fibrovascular membrane leads to adhesions between the iris and the cornea and between the iris and lens, while traction

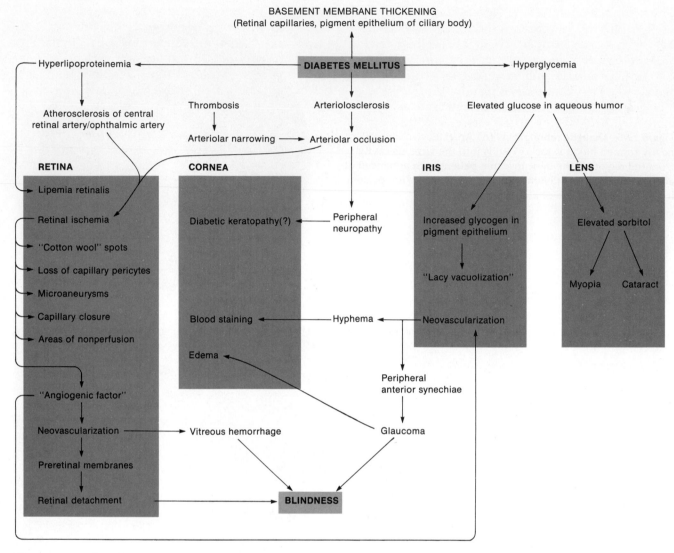

BASEMENT MEMBRANE THICKENING
(Retinal capillaries, pigment epithelium of ciliary body)

Figure 29-6. The effects of diabetes mellitus on the eye.

by the fibrovascular membrane pulls the iris pigment epithelium around the pupillary margin (ectropion uveae). The friable new vessels on the iris bleed easily and cause hyphema. Iris neovascularization frequently culminates in a blind painful eye due to a secondary glaucoma.

DIABETES AND THE LENS

In juvenile diabetics (15 to 25 years old) and, exceptionally, in diabetic infants, a blanket of white needle-shaped opacities may collect in both crystalline lenses immediately beneath the anterior and posterior lens capsule. These opacities, which resemble snowflakes, coalesce within a few weeks in adolescents, and within days in children, until the whole lens becomes opaque. So-called senile cataracts occur in elderly diabetics at an earlier age than in the general population and progress more rapidly to maturity.

RETINOPATHY OF PREMATURITY (RETROLENTAL FIBROPLASIA)

The retinopathy of prematurity remains an important cause of blindness in infants. This bilateral, iatrogenic ocular disorder is almost restricted to premature infants and is caused by the administration of high concentrations of oxygen. When a premature infant is exposed to excessive amounts of oxygen, as in an incubator, the developing retinal blood vessels become obliterated. As a result the peripheral retina, which is normally avascular until the end of fetal life, does not vascularize.

The more mature the retina, the less the vascular obliterative effect of hyperoxia. When the infant eventually returns to ambient air, an intense proliferation of vascular endothelium and glial cells begins at the junction of the avascular and vascularized portions of the retina. In some cases the retinopathy progresses to a cicatricial phase, characterized by retinal detachment and a retrolental, fibrovascular mass.

THYROID DISEASE

Exophthalmos, defined as forward protrusion of the eyeball from the orbit, is most frequently due to Graves' disease. While usually bilateral, one side may be involved earlier or more extensively than the other.

Exophthalmos due to thyroid disease usually occurs in early adult life, especially in women, who are affected more often than men. It may be severe and progressive, particularly in middle life. Dysthyroid exophthalmos may be associated with edema of the eyelid and conjunctiva, and limited ocular motility. Sequelae of severe exophthalmos include corneal exposure with subsequent ulceration, secondary glaucoma, and optic nerve compression. Thyroidectomy enhances the severity and the incidence of dysthyroid exophthalmos.

Dysthyroid exophthalmos results from an increase in the volume of orbital tissue. This is produced largely by an increase in orbital water, imbibed because of the osmotic pressure of glycosaminoglycans, and enlarged extraocular muscles that are infiltrated with lymphocytes and other mononuclear cells.

SARCOIDOSIS

Ocular involvement occurs in one fourth to one third of patients with sarcoidosis. While any of the ocular and orbital tissues may be involved, this granulomatous disease has a predilection for the anterior segment of the eye. Ocular involvement is usually bilateral and most often takes the form of a granulomatous uveitis.

COMMON DISORDERS OF SPECIFIC OCULAR TISSUES

CONJUNCTIVA

DRY EYE SYNDROME

Basal tear production is diminished in certain ocular or systemic diseases. Dry eye syndrome associated with xerostomia and a systemic immune disorder (Sjögren's syndrome) usually affects middle-aged women and is associated with atrophy of the lacrimal and salivary glands and of other mucosal glands. Frequent findings in the blood of patients with Sjögren's syndrome include hypergammaglobulinemia, rheumatoid factor, antinuclear antibodies, and autoantibodies to salivary duct cytoplasm, gastric parietal cells, and thyroglobulin. Affected individuals often develop malignant lymphomas.

PINGUECULA AND PTERYGIUM

The most common conjunctival lump, the pinguecula, is most often located nasal to the corneoscleral limbus. The lesion consists of sun-damaged connective tissue identical to that in similarly injured skin ("actinic elastosis").

Another common conjunctival lesion, the pterygium, consists of a triangular fold of vascularized conjunctival that grows horizontally onto the cornea in the shape of an insect wing.

LENS

CATARACTS

Some ophthalmologists call any opacity in the lens a cataract, while others restrict the term to lens opacities that impair vision (Fig. 29-7). Cataracts can be caused by certain disorders of carbohydrate metabolism or by deficiencies in riboflavin or tryptophan. Numerous cat-

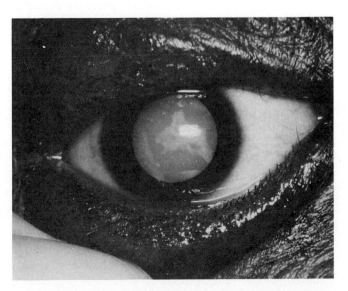

Figure 29-7. Cataract. The white appearance of the pupil in this eye is due to complete opacification of the lens ("mature cataract").

aracts are the result of genetic disorders. Others result from toxins, drugs, or physical agents, such as heat, some categories of electromagnetic radiation (ultraviolet light, microwaves), trauma, intraocular surgery, ultrasound, or electric shock.

The most common cataract in the United States is associated with aging (senile cataract). Degenerated lens material in these cataracts exerts an osmotic pressure, causing the lens to increase in volume by imbibing water. Such a swollen lens may obstruct the pupil and cause glaucoma. After the entire lens degenerates, its volume diminishes because lenticular debris escapes into the aqueous humor through a degenerated lens capsule. After becoming engulfed by macrophages the extruded lenticular material may obstruct the aqueous outflow and produce glaucoma.

Other ocular diseases that may result in cataracts include uveitis, intraocular neoplasms, glaucoma, retinitis pigmentosa, and sensory retinal detachment. Cataracts are also associated with the rubella virus, aging, some skin diseases (atopic dermatitis, scleroderma), and various systemic diseases.

AQUEOUS HUMOR

GLAUCOMA

A delicate balance between the production and drainage of the aqueous humor maintains intraocular pressure within its physiologic range (10 to 20 mm Hg). In certain pathologic states aqueous humor accumulates within the eye, and the intraocular pressure becomes elevated, producing temporary or permanent impairment of vision and damage to the optic nerve. When this occurs the term glaucoma is applied. Vision becomes impaired because of degenerative changes in the retina and optic nerve head (a result of ocular hypertension and resultant ischemia), and because of corneal edema and opacification.

Causes of Glaucoma

Glaucoma almost always follows a lesion of the anterior segment of the eye that mechanically obstructs the aqueous drainage. The obstruction may be located between the iris and lens, in the angle of the anterior chamber, in the trabecular meshwork, in Schlemm's canal, or in the venous drainage of the eye (Fig. 29-8).

Glaucoma may develop in a person with no apparent underlying eye disease (primary glaucoma), or it may follow a known antecedent or concomitant ocular disorder (secondary glaucoma).

Types of Glaucoma

CONGENITAL GLAUCOMA (INFANTILE GLAUCOMA)   The term congenital glaucoma refers to glaucoma caused by an obstruction of the aqueous drainage by developmental anomalies, even though the intraocular pressure may not become elevated until early infancy or childhood. Most cases of congenital glaucoma are in males (60% to 70%), and an X-linked recessive mode of inheritance is common. The developmental anomaly usually involves both eyes and, while often limited to the angle of the anterior chamber, may be accompanied by a variety of other ocular malformations. Congenital glaucoma is often associated with enlarged eyes (buphthalmos).

PRIMARY GLAUCOMA   Primary glaucomas are of two types, namely open-angle glaucoma and closed-angle (narrow-angle) glaucoma.

Primary open-angle glaucoma, the most common type of glaucoma and a major blinding disorder in the United States, is estimated to affect 1% to 3% of the population over the age of 40 years. It occurs principally in the sixth decade. The intraocular pressure becomes elevated insidiously and asymptomatically, and while almost always bilateral, one eye may be affected more severely than the other. With time, damage to the retina and optic nerve causes an irreversible loss of peripheral vision. The angle of the anterior chamber appears normal, but an increased resistance to the outflow of the aqueous humor is present within the vicinity of Schlemm's canal.

Primary narrow-angle glaucoma occurs, especially after the age of 40 years, in individuals who possess an abnormally narrow angle, in which the peripheral iris is displaced anteriorly towards the trabecular meshwork. When the pupil is constricted, the iris remains stretched, so that the chamber angle is not occluded. However, when the pupil dilates, the iris obstructs the anterior chamber angle, thereby impairing aqueous drainage and resulting in sudden episodes of intraocular hypertension. Primary closed-angle glaucoma affects both eyes, but it may become apparent in one eye 2 to 5 years before it becomes apparent in the other. The intraocular pressure is normal between attacks, but after many episodes adhesions form between the iris

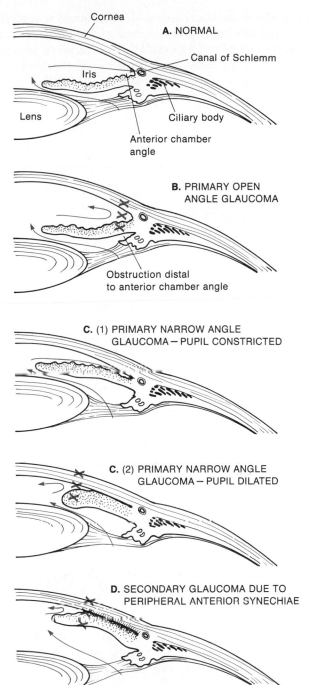

Figure 29-8. Pathogenesis of glaucoma. The anterior segment of the eye is affected differently in various forms of glaucoma. (*A*) The structure of the normal eye. In primary open-angle glaucoma (*B*) the obstruction to the aqueous outflow is distal to the anterior chamber angle, and the anterior segment resembles that of the normal eye. In primary narrow-angle glaucoma (*C*) the anterior chamber angle is open, but narrower than normal when the pupil is constricted (*C1*). When the pupil becomes dilated in such an eye the thickened iris obstructs the anterior chamber angle (*C2*) thereby causing an increase in intraocular pressure. The anterior chamber angle can become obstructed by a variety of pathologic processes, including an adhesion between the iris and the posterior surface of the cornea (peripheral anterior synechia) (*D*).

and the trabecular meshwork and cornea and accentuate the blockage to the outflow of the aqueous humor. **SECONDARY GLAUCOMA**   The causes of secondary glaucoma are many, and the anterior chamber angles may be open or closed. Because the underlying disorder is usually limited to one eye, secondary glaucomas are usually unilateral.

RETINA

RETINAL DETACHMENT

The sensory retina readily separates from the retinal pigment epithelium when fluid (liquid vitreous humor, hemorrhage, or exudate) accumulates within the potential space between these structures. Such a separation is designated a retinal detachment (Fig. 29-9), and three varieties of this common cause of blindness are recognized, namely rhegmatogenous, tractional, and exudative.

Rhegmatogenous retinal detachment, the most common form, is associated with a retinal tear and, often, with degenerative changes in the vitreous or peripheral retina. Retinal detachment follows intraocular hemorrhage (as after trauma) and is a potential complication of cataract extractions and several other ocular operations.

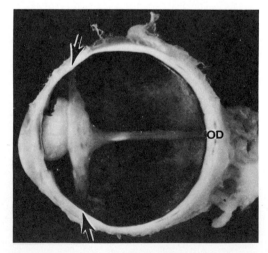

Figure 29-9. Retinal detachment. The sensory retina is completely detached from the retinal pigment epithelium in this eye. It remains attached at the optic disc (OD) and at the boundary of the retina and ciliary body (ora serata, *arrows*).

In tractional retinal detachment, the retina is pulled toward the center of the eye by adherent vitreoretinal adhesions, as occurs in proliferative diabetic retinopathy and the retinopathy of prematurity, and after intraocular infection.

An accumulation of fluid in the potential space between the sensory retina and the retinal pigment epithelium causes an "exudative retinal detachment" in disorders such as choroiditis, choroidal hemangioma, and choroidal melanomas.

RETINITIS PIGMENTOSA

The misnomer "retinitis pigmentosa" is a generic term that comprises a variety of bilateral, progressive, degenerative retinopathies that are characterized by pigment accumulation within the retina and loss of retinal photoreceptors (rods and cones). This noninflammatory reaction presumably results from multiple genetic abnormalities.

The condition ensues when retinal pigment epithelium migrates into the sensory retina, and melanin, which appears within slender processes of spidery cells, accumulates mainly around small branching retinal blood vessels (especially in the equatorial portion of the retina) like spicules of bone. The clinical manifestations often begin with night blindness and end with total blindness.

MACULAR DEGENERATION

With aging, in certain drug toxicities (for example chloroquine), and in several inherited disorders, the macula degenerates, and central vision is impaired. Perhaps the most common cause of reduced vision in the elderly in the United States is senile or involutional macular degeneration, which is sometimes associated with bleeding into the subretinal space (hemorrhagic macular degeneration).

CHERRY RED SPOT AT THE MACULA

In lysosomal storage diseases, including GM_2-gangliosidosis type II (Tay-Sachs disease), a myriad of intracytoplasmic lysosomal inclusions within the multilayered ganglion cell layer of the macula imparts a striking pallor to the affected retina. As a result the central foveola appears bright red ("cherry red spot") because of the underlying choroidal vasculature.

Following a central retinal artery occlusion, a cherry red spot also occurs at the macula, but for a different reason. Edema causes the entire retina to appear pale, a condition which highlights the subfoveolar vascular choroid.

OPTIC NERVE

EDEMA OF OPTIC DISC (PAPILLEDEMA)

Optic disc edema can result from various causes, the most important of which is increased intracranial pressure. Other causes are obstruction to the venous drainage of the eye, such as may occur with compressive lesions of the orbit, an infarct of the optic nerve, inflammation of the optic nerve close to the eyeball, and multiple sclerosis.

OPTIC ATROPHY

The nerve axons within the optic nerve may be lost in many conditions. Longstanding papilledema, optic neuritis, optic nerve compression, glaucoma, and retinal degeneration are all possible causes. Optic atrophy can also be caused by some drugs, examples being ethambutol and isoniazid.

ACKNOWLEDGMENTS

Specific acknowledgment is made for permission to use the following material:

Chapter 4, Figure 10. Photograph from Armed Forces Institute of Pathology.

Chapter 9. All photographs from Armed Forces Institute of Pathology.

Chapter 11, Table 4. Reimer K, Jennings RB: Myocardial ischemia, hypoxia, and infarction. In Fozzard HA, Haber E, Katz AM, et al (eds): The Heart and Cardiovascular System. Raven Press, 1986.

Chapter 11, Figures 9 and 10. Hackel DB: The coronary arteries in acute myocardial infarction. Circulation 68 (suppl 1): 1, 1983

Chapter 11, Figure 23. Hackel DB: Diseases of the pericardium. In Edwards J (ed): Clinical-Pathologic Correlations, I. Cardiovasc Clin 4(2): 147, 1972. By permission FA Davis Company

Chapter 16, Figures 3, 4, 6, 8, 10–15, 17, 19, 22, 26–28, 31, 33, 34, 36. Spargo BH, Seymour AE, Ordonez NG: Renal Biopsy Pathology with Diagnostic and Therapeutic Implications. New York, John Wiley & Sons, 1980

Chapter 16, Figures 30 and 35. Peterson ROP: Urologic Pathology, Philadelphia, JB Lippincott, 1987

Chapter 17, all photographs. Peterson ROP: Urologic Pathology, Philadelphia, JB Lippincott, 1987

Chapter 29, Figures 1B, 2B, 7 and 9. Klintworth GK, Landers MD III: The Eye: Structure and Function in Disease. Baltimore, Williams & Wilkins, 1976

INDEX

Page numbers followed by *f* indicate figures; those followed by *t* indicate tabular material.